K  Y0-BBD-642  eck

S   A   U   N   D   E   R   S

# PHARMACEUTICAL

# WORD
# BOOK

## 1998

Karen Schember

ELLEN DRAKE, CMT
RANDY DRAKE, BS

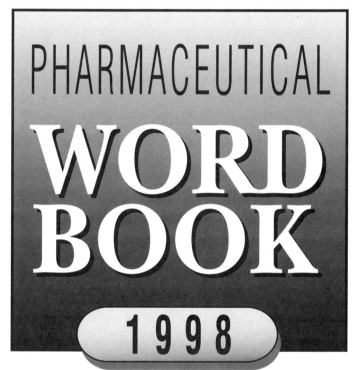

S A U N D E R S

PHARMACEUTICAL
WORD
BOOK
1998

**W.B. SAUNDERS COMPANY**
*A Division of Harcourt Brace & Company*
Philadelphia London Toronto Montreal Sydney Tokyo

**W.B. SAUNDERS COMPANY**
*A Division of*
*Harcourt Brace & Company*

The Curtis Center
Independence Square West
Philadelphia, Pennsylvania 19106

SAUNDERS PHARMACEUTICAL WORD BOOK 1998          ISBN 0-7216-7261-2

Copyright © 1998, 1997, 1996, 1995, 1994, 1992 by W.B. Saunders Company.

All rights reserved. No part of this publication may be reproduced or transmitted in any
form or by any means, electronic or mechanical, including photocopying, recording, or any
information storage and retrieval system, without permission in writing from the publisher.

ISSN 1072-7779

Printed in the United States of America.

Last digit is the print number:     9     8     7     6     5     4     3     2     1

# To the Lord Jesus

"Though the fig tree should not blossom,
And there be no fruit on the vines;
Though the yield of the olive should fail,
And the fields produce no food;
Though the flock should be cut off from the fold,
And there be no cattle in the stalls—
Yet I will exult in the Lord
I will rejoice in the God of my salvation.

"The Lord God is my strength;
And He has made my feet like hind's feet,
And makes me walk on my high places."

— Habakkuk 3:17–19

# Contents

# Preface

The 1998 edition brings with it a milestone in its publication. For the first time, there are over 25,000 entries contained within the main list. The full statistics can be found on the new Contents page.

New to this edition is the inclusion of a comprehensive list of illicit "street drugs" and street drug slang. Notations have also been made in entries for regular, legal medicines that are commonly abused as street drugs, as well as some approved foreign and veterinary products that are abused as street drugs in the United States.

The orphan drugs have been completely reworked this year, with orphan status granted to many new products and withdrawn from others. A description of experimental, investigational, and orphan drugs has been added on page xv, along with a summary of the drug approval process.

We have a new e-mail address listed below that you may use to contact us with your comments, suggestions, or constructive criticisms about the content of the book. We welcome the feedback and use it to improve and expand each edition. (Orders and order fulfillment questions should be directed to the publisher or your local Saunders representative.)

In the main section of the book, drug names, whether trade, generic, or chemical, are in bold print for greater ease of reading. Brand (trade) names appear with appropriate capitalization, with generic and chemical names shown in lower case—the way transcription style guides recommend they be typed.

We think you will find this sixth edition more complete and more valuable than ever; however, no book is ever perfect. We keep our database current by adding and updating entries as the information becomes available. Although we have diligently tried to be as accurate and comprehensive as possible, we certainly welcome your comments regarding additions, inconsistencies, or inaccuracies. Please send them to us via e-mail at the address below, or via regular mail to W.B. Saunders Company, The Curtis Center, Independence Square West, Philadelphia, PA 19106-3399. We welcome your suggestions.

Authors' e-mail address:
PharmaceuticalWordBook@Saunders.net

ELLEN DRAKE, CMT
RANDY DRAKE, BS
Atlanta, Georgia

# Notes on Using the Text

The purpose of the *Saunders Pharmaceutical Word Book* is to provide the medical transcriptionist (as well as medical record administrators and technicians, coders, nurses, ward clerks, court reporters, legal secretaries, medical assistants, allied health students, physicians, and even pharmacists) a quick, easy-to-use reference that gives not only the correct spellings and capitalizations of drugs, but the designated uses of those drugs, the cross-referencing of brand names to generics, and the usual methods of administration (e.g., capsule, IV, cream). The indication of the preferred nonproprietary (generic) names and the agencies adopting these names (e.g., USAN, USP) should be particularly useful to those writing for publication. The reader will also find various trademarked or proprietary names (e.g., Spansule, Dosepak) that are not drugs but are closely associated with the packaging or administration of drugs.

There are four different ways to refer to drugs. One of these ways is not the name of the drug itself but the class to which it belongs—aminoglycosides, for example. Inexperienced transcriptionists sometimes confuse these classes with the names of drugs. We have included some 200 drug classes in the main list, with a brief description of the therapeutic use and/or method of action common to drugs in the class. Beyond a class description, each drug has three names. The first is the *chemical name*, which describes its chemical composition and how the molecules are arranged. It is often long and complex, sometimes containing numbers, Greek letters, italicized letters, and hyphens between elements. This name is rarely used in dictation except in research hospitals and sometimes in the laboratory section when the blood or urine is examined for traces of the drug. The second name for a drug is the *nonproprietary* or *generic name*. This is a name chosen by the discovering manufacturer or agency and submitted to a nomenclature committee (the United States Adopted Names Council, for example). The name is simpler than the chemical name but often reflects the chemical entity. It is arrived at by using guidelines provided by the nomenclature committee—beta-blockers must end in "olol," for example—and must be unique. There is increasing emphasis on the adoption of the same nonproprietary name by various nomenclature committees worldwide (see the list on page xiii). The third name for a drug is the *trade* or *brand name*. There may be several trade names for the same generic drug, each marketed by a different company. These are the ones that are highly advertised, and sometimes have unusual capitalization. An interesting article on the naming of drugs is "Pharmaceutical Nomenclature: The Lawless Language" in *Perspectives on the Medical Transcription Profession*.[1] *Understanding Pharmacology*[2] also discusses the naming of drugs.

We have included many foreign names of drugs for our Canadian friends, and also because we have so many visitors to the United States from other countries (and they get sick, too). The international and British spellings of generic drugs are cross-referenced to the American spellings, and vice versa. Occasionally there will be three different spellings—one American, one international, and another British—which are all cross-referenced to each other. Other special features that may be useful, especially for students, are the commonly used prescribing abbreviations and the sound-alike lists that are found in the appendices. Another appendix gives the investigational codes (assigned to drugs before they are named), cross-referenced to their subsequent generic names. The Most Prescribed Drugs and Therapeutic Drug Levels appendices will be useful as well.

This information was compiled using a variety of sources including direct communication with over 500 drug companies. The orphan entries are taken directly from the latest list issued by the FDA. When sources differed, we ranked our sources as to reliability and went with what we thought was the most reliable source. We recognize that there may be several published ways in which to type a single drug, but we have chosen to use only one of those ways. In the instance of internal capitalization (e.g., pHisoHex), it should be recognized that in most instances it is acceptable to type such words with initial capitalization only (Phisohex).

While we have made every attempt to include as much necessary information as possible, we have by no means tried to provide *prescribing information* as defined by the FDA. The given uses/actions for a particular drug are not all-inclusive, and the indications, contraindications, and side effects are not listed. Physicians should consult the *Physicians' Desk Reference*, package insert, or some other acceptable source for prescribing information.

# How the Book Is Arranged

While other pharmaceutical references have separate listings for brand names and generics, or put entries into separate sections by body system or therapeutic use, we have chosen to list all entries in one comprehensive alphabetical listing. Therefore, it is not necessary to know if the term sought is a brand name, a generic, a drug class, a chemotherapy protocol, approved or investigational, or slang; what it's used for; or which body system it affects. If it's given to a patient, it's in "the list." In addition to strict pharmaceuticals, we have included other "consumable" products, such as *in vitro* testing kits, radiographic contrast and other imaging agents, wound dressings, etc.

All entries are in alphabetical order by word. Initial numbers, chemical prefixes (*N*-, *p*-, L-, *l*-, D-, *d*-, etc.), and punctuation (prime, ampersands, etc.) are ignored. For example, L-dopa would be alphabetized under "dopa," but levodopa under "levo."

We have indicated brand names with initial capital letters unless an unusual combination of capitals and lowercase has been designated by the manufacturer (e.g., pHisoHex, ALternaGEL). Generic names are rendered in lowercase. Where the same name can be either generic or brand, both have been included.

**The general format of a *generic* entry is:**

**entry** council(s) *designated use* [other references] dosages 🕜 sound-alike(s)

| #1 | #2 | #3 | #4 | #5 | #6 |

1. The name of the drug (in bold).
2. The various agencies that have approved the name, shown in small caps, which may be any or all of the following (listed according to appearance in the book):

   USAN   United States Adopted Name Council
   USP    United States Pharmacopeial Convention
   NF     National Formulary
   FDA    U.S. Food and Drug Administration
   INN    International Nonproprietary Name (a project of the World Health Organization)
   BAN    British Approved Name
   JAN    Japanese Accepted Name
   DCF    Dénomination Commune Française (French)

3. The designated use, sometimes referred to as the drug's "therapeutic action." This is provided only for official FDA-approved names or other names for the same substance (e.g., the British name of an official U.S. generic). This entry is always in italic.
4. The entry in brackets is one of four cross-references:

   see:   refers the reader to the "official" name(s).
   now:   for an older generic name no longer used, refers reader to the current official name(s).
   also:  a substance that has two or more different names, each officially recognized by one of the above groups, will cross-reference the other name(s).
   q.v.   Latin for quod vide; which see. Used exclusively for abbreviations, it invites the reader to turn to the reference in parentheses.

   If there is more than one cross-reference, alternate names will follow the order of the above agency list, i.e., U.S. names, then international names, then British, Japanese, and French names. The first cross-reference will always be to the approved U.S. name, unless the entry itself is the U.S. name.

5. Dosage information, including the delivery form(s), is given for medications that may be dispensed generically. No dosage information appears for drugs dispensed only under the brand name, or for those containing multiple ingredients. Some drugs may be available in more than one strength, indicated by a comma in the dosage field:

   **phentermine HCl** USP *anorexiant; CNS stimulant* 8, 15, 18.75, 30, 37.5 mg oral

   A semicolon in the dosage field separates different delivery forms, such as:

   **nitroglycerin** USP *coronary vasodilator; antianginal* [also: glyceryl trinitrate] 2.5, 6.5, 9 mg oral; 5 mg/mL injection; 16–187.5 mg transdermal; 2% topical

   (Note that the oral and transdermal forms come in multiple strengths.)
6. Sound-alike drugs follow the "ear" icon.

**The general format for a *brand name* entry is:**

**Entry** (CAN) form(s) ℞/OTC *designated use* [generics] dosages ② sound-alike(s)

| #1 | #2 | #3 | #4 | #5 | #6 | #7 | #8 |
| --- | --- | --- | --- | --- | --- | --- | --- |

1. The drug name (in bold), which almost always starts with a capital letter.
2. If a brand is not marketed in the United States, an icon designates the country where it is available. Canadian brands are designated by (CAN).
3. The form of administration, e.g., tablets, capsules, syrup. (Sometimes these words are slurred by the dictator causing confusion regarding the name.)
4. The ℞ or OTC status. A few drugs may be either ℞ or OTC depending on strength or various state laws.[3]
5. The designated use in italics as for generics. These are more complete or less complete as supplied by the individual drug companies.
6. The brackets that follow contain the generic names of the active ingredients to which the reader may refer for further information.
7. Dosage information follows the generics. For multi-ingredient drugs, a bullet separates the dosages of each ingredient, listed in the same order as the generics. For example,

    **Ser-Ap-Es** tablets ℞ *antihypertensive* [hydrochlorothiazide; reserpine; hydralazine HCl] 15•0.1•25 mg

    shows a three-ingredient product containing 15 mg hydrochlorothiazide, 0.1 mg reserpine, and 25 mg hydralazine HCl.

    Some drugs may have more than one strength, indicated by a comma in the dosage field:

    **Nitrodisc** transdermal patch ℞ *antianginal* [nitroglycerin] 16, 24, 32 mg

    A semicolon in the dosage field separates either different products listed together, such as:

    **Pred Mild; Pred Forte** eye drop suspension ℞ *ophthalmic topical corticosteroidal anti-inflammatory* [prednisolone acetate] 0.12%; 1%

    Or different delivery forms:

    **Phenergan** tablets, suppositories, injection ℞ *antihistamine; motion sickness; sleep aid; antiemetic; sedative* [promethazine HCl] 12.5, 25 mg; 12.5, 25, 50 mg; 25, 50 mg/mL

    (Note that all three forms of Phenergan come in multiple strengths.)

    Liquid delivery forms show the strength per usual dose where appropriate. Thus injectables and drops are usually shown per milliliter (mL), with oral liquids and syrups shown per 5 mL or 15 mL.

    The ≜ symbol indicates that dosage information has not been supplied by the manufacturer for one or more ingredients.

    The ≜ symbol is used when a value *cannot* be given because the generic entry refers to multiple ingredients.
8. Sound-alike drugs follow the "ear" icon.

# Experimental, Investigational, and Orphan Drugs

Before a drug can be advertised or sold in the United States, it must first be approved for marketing by the U.S. Food and Drug Administration. With a few exceptions, FDA approval is contingent solely upon the manufacturer demonstrating that the proposed drug is both safe and effective.

To provide such proof, the manufacturer undertakes a series of tests. Preclinical (before human) research is done through computer simulation, then *in vitro* (L. "in glass," meaning laboratory) tests, then in animals. In most cases neither the public nor the general medical community hears about "experimental drugs" in this stage of testing. Neither are they listed in this reference.

If safety and efficacy are successfully demonstrated during the preclinical stage, an Investigational New Drug (IND) application is filed with the FDA. There are three phases of clinical trials, designated Phase I, Phase II, and Phase III. After each phase, the FDA will review the findings and approve or deny further testing.

Phase I trials involve 20 to 100 patients, primarily to establish safety. Phase II trials may involve several hundred patients for up to two years. The goal in this phase is to determine the drug's effectiveness for the proposed indication. Phase III trials, which routinely last up to four years and involve several thousand patients, determine the optimum effective, but safe, dosage. The manufacturer will then file a New Drug Application (NDA) with the FDA, requesting final marketing approval. Only 20% of drugs entering Phase I trials will ultimately be approved for marketing, at an average cost of $359 million and 8½ years in testing.[4]

An orphan drug is a drug or biological product for the diagnosis, treatment, or prevention of a rare disease or condition. A rare disease is one that affects less than 200,000 persons or for which there is no reasonable expectation that the cost of development and testing will be recovered through U.S. sales of the product. Federal subsidies are provided to the manufacturer or sponsor for the development of orphan drugs. Applications for orphan status are made through the FDA, and may be made during drug development or after marketing approval.

# A Brief Note on the Transcription of Drugs

Many references are available describing several acceptable ways to transcribe drug information when dictated. We offer the following only as brief guidelines.

Although some institutions favor capitalizing every drug, others promote not capitalizing any drug, and yet others put drugs in all capital letters, the generally accepted style today for the transcription of medical reports for hospital and doctors' office charts (see the American Medical Association *Manual of Style*[5] for publications) is to capitalize the initial letter of brand name drugs and lowercase generic name drugs. The institution may also designate that brand name drugs with unusual capitalization may be typed with initial capital letter only, or typed using the manufacturer's scheme.

In general, commas are omitted between the drug name, the dosage, and the instructions for purposes of simplification. Items in a series may be separated by either commas (if no internal commas are used) or semicolons. A simple series might be typed thus:

Procardia, nitroglycerin sublingual, and Tolinase

or

Procardia 10 mg three times a day, nitroglycerin 1/150 p.r.n., and Tolinase 100 mg twice a day.

or

Procardia 10 mg t.i.d., nitroglycerin 1/150 p.r.n., and Tolinase 100 mg b.i.d.

A more complex or lengthy list of medications, or a list with internal commas, may require the use of semicolons to separate the items in a series. For example,

Procardia 10 mg, one t.i.d.; nitroglycerin 1/150 p.r.n., to take one with onset of pain, a second in five minutes, and a third five minutes later, if no relief to go immediately to the ER; Tolinase 100 mg, one b.i.d.; and Coumadin 2.5 mg on Mondays, Wednesdays, and Fridays, and 5 mg on Tuesdays, Thursdays, and Saturdays...

Note that the "one" following Procardia 10 mg and Tolinase 100 mg is not necessary, but many doctors dictate something like this; when they do, it is acceptable to place a comma after the dosage. In addition, when two numbers are adjacent to each other, write out one number and use a numeral for the other.

The typing of chemicals with superscripts or subscripts, italics, small capitals, and Greek letters often presents a problem to the medical transcriptionist. In general, Greek letters are written out (alpha-, beta-, gamma-, etc.). Italics and small capitals are written as standard letters followed by a hyphen (dl-alpha-tocopherol, L-dopa).

When typing nonproprietary (generic) isotope names, element symbols should be included with the name. It may appear to be redundant, but it is the correct form. Therefore, we would type sodium pertechnetate Tc 99m, iodohippurate sodium I 131, or sodium iodide I 125. Occasionally the physician may simply dictate isotopes such as Tc 99m, iodine 131 or I 131, or sodium iodide I 125, and unless he is indicating a trademarked name, it should be typed with a space, no hyphen, and no superscript. This reference indicates proper capitalization, spacing, and hyphenation of isotope entries.

Other combinations of letters and numbers are usually written without spaces or hyphens (OKT1, OKT3, T101, SC1), but this is a complex subject and is dealt with extensively in the AMA *Manual of Style*.

---

[1] Dirckx, John, M.D.: "Pharmaceutical Nomenclature: The Lawless Language," *Perspectives on the Medical Transcription Profession*, Vol. 1, No. 4. Modesto: Health Professions Institute, 1991, p. 9.

[2] Turley, Susan M., CMT: *Understanding Pharmacology*. Englewood Cliffs: Regents/Prentice Hall, 1991.

[3] Some states are moving toward the creation of a third class of drugs between ℞ and oTc. These medications, while not being readily available on the shelf, could be dispensed by a licensed pharmacist without a doctor's prescription.

[4] *FDA Consumer*, January, 1995. www.fda.gov/fdac/special/newdrug/ndd_toc.html

[5] American Medical Association: *Manual of Style*, 9th ed. Baltimore: Williams & Wilkins, 1997.

**A** *street drug slang* [see: LSD; amphetamines]

**A (vitamin A)** [q.v.]

**A and D** ointment OTC *moisturizer; emollient* [fish liver oil (vitamins A and D); cholecalciferol; lanolin] ≛

**A and D Medicated** ointment OTC *topical diaper rash treatment* [zinc oxide; vitamins A and D] ≛

**A + D (ara-C, daunorubicin)** *chemotherapy protocol*

**A-200** shampoo concentrate (discontinued 1995) OTC *pediculicide* [pyrethrins; piperonyl butoxide] 0.33%•4%

**AA (ara-C, Adriamycin)** *chemotherapy protocol*

**AA-HC Otic** ear drops ℞ *topical corticosteroidal anti-inflammatory; antibacterial/antifungal* [hydrocortisone; acetic acid] 1%•2%

**abacavir succinate** USAN *investigational (Phase I/II) antiviral for HIV*

**abafilcon A** USAN *hydrophilic contact lens material*

**abamectin** USAN, INN *antiparasitic*

**abanoquil** INN, BAN

**Abbokinase** powder for IV or intracoronary artery infusion ℞ *thrombolytic enzymes for pulmonary embolism or coronary artery thrombosis* [urokinase] 250 000 IU/vial

**Abbokinase Open-Cath** powder for catheter clearance ℞ *thrombolytic enzymes* [urokinase] 5000 IU/mL

**Abbo-Pac** (trademarked packaging form) *unit dose package*

**Abbott HIVAB HIV-1 EIA** test kit (name changed to HIVAB HIV-1 EIA in 1995)

**Abbott HIVAG-1** test kit (name changed to HIVAG-1 in 1995)

**Abbott HTLV I EIA** test kit (name changed to Human T-Lymphotropic Virus Type I EIA in 1995)

**Abbott HTLV III Confirmatory EIA** test kit for professional use (discontinued 1995) *in vitro diagnostic aid for HTLV III antibody* [enzyme immunoassay (EIA)]

**Abbott TestPack Plus hCG-Urine Plus** test kit for professional use *in vitro diagnostic aid for urine pregnancy test* [monoclonal antibody-based enzyme immunoassay]

**Abbott TestPack Strep A** kit (name changed to Test Pack in 1995)

**ABC (Adriamycin, BCNU, cyclophosphamide)** *chemotherapy protocol*

**ABC to Z** tablets OTC *vitamin/mineral/iron supplement* [multiple vitamins & minerals; ferrous fumarate; folic acid; biotin] ≛•18 mg•0.4 mg•30 μg

**abciximab** USAN, INN *monoclonal antibody; antiplatelet agent for acute arterial occlusive disorders*

**ABCM (Adriamycin, bleomycin, cyclophosphamide, mitomycin)** *chemotherapy protocol*

**ABD (Adriamycin, bleomycin, DTIC)** *chemotherapy protocol*

**ABDIC (Adriamycin, bleomycin, DIC, [CCNU, prednisone])** *chemotherapy protocol*

**ABDV (Adriamycin, bleomycin, DTIC, vinblastine)** *chemotherapy protocol*

**ABE (antitoxin botulism equine)** [see: botulism equine antitoxin, trivalent]

**abecarnil** INN *investigational anxiolytic*

**Abelcet** suspension for IV infusion ℞ *systemic antifungal for aspergillosis and other resistant fungal infections* [amphotericin B lipid complex (ABLC)] 100 mg/20 mL

**Abenol** ⓒⓐⓝ (U.S. product: Tylenol) suppositories OTC *analgesic; antipyretic* [acetaminophen] 120, 325, 650 mg

**Abitrexate** IV or IM injection ℞ *antineoplastic for leukemia; systemic antipsoriatic; antirheumatic* [methotrexate sodium]

**ABLC** [see: TLC ABLC]

**ABLC (amphotericin B lipid complex)** [q.v.]

**ablukast** USAN, INN *antiasthmatic; leukotriene antagonist*

**ablukast sodium** USAN *antiasthmatic; leukotriene antagonist*

**Abolic** *a veterinary steroid abused as a street drug*

**A-bomb** *street drug slang for marijuana and heroin smoked together in a cigarette* [see: marijuana; heroin]

**abortifacients** *a class of agents that stimulate uterine contractions sufficient to produce uterine evacuation*

**ABP (Adriamycin, bleomycin, prednisone)** *chemotherapy protocol*

**ABPP (aminobromophenylpyrimidinone)** [see: bropirimine]

**absorbable cellulose cotton** [see: cellulose, oxidized]

**absorbable dusting powder** [see: dusting powder, absorbable]

**absorbable gelatin film** [see: gelatin film, absorbable]

**absorbable gelatin powder** [see: gelatin powder, absorbable]

**absorbable gelatin sponge** [see: gelatin sponge, absorbable]

**absorbable surgical suture** [see: suture, absorbable surgical]

**Absorbase** OTC *ointment base* [water-in-oil emulsion of cholesterolized petrolatum and purified water]

**absorbent gauze** [see: gauze, absorbent]

**Absorbine Antifungal** cream, powder OTC *topical antifungal* [tolnaftate] 1%

**Absorbine Antifungal Foot** aerosol powder OTC *topical antifungal* [miconazole nitrate; alcohol 10%] 2%

**Absorbine Arthritic Pain** lotion (discontinued 1994) OTC *counterirritant* [methyl salicylate; camphor; menthol; methyl nicotinate] 10%•3.25%•1.25%•1%

**Absorbine Athlete's Foot Care** liquid OTC *topical antifungal* [tolnaftate] 1%

**Absorbine Jock Itch** powder OTC *topical antifungal* [tolnaftate] 1%

**Absorbine Jr.** liniment OTC *counterirritant* [menthol] 1.27%, 4%

**Absorbine Jr. Antifungal** spray liquid OTC *topical antifungal* [tolnaftate] 1%

**Absorbine Jr. Extra Strength** liquid OTC *counterirritant* [menthol] 4%

**Absorbine Power** gel OTC *counterirritant* [menthol] 4%

**ABT-719** *investigational quinolizidine-type antibiotic*

**abunidazole** INN

**ABV (actimomycin D, bleomycin, vincristine)** *chemotherapy protocol*

**ABV (Adriamycin, bleomycin, vinblastine)** *chemotherapy protocol*

**ABVD (Adriamycin, bleomycin, vinblastine, dacarbazine)** *chemotherapy protocol*

**ABVD/MOPP (alternating cycles of ABVD and MOPP)** *chemotherapy protocol*

**AC (Adriamycin, carmustine)** *chemotherapy protocol*

**AC (Adriamycin, CCNU)** *chemotherapy protocol*

**AC (Adriamycin, cisplatin)** *chemotherapy protocol*

**AC; A-C (Adriamycin, cyclophosphamide)** *chemotherapy protocol*

**AC 137** *investigational antidiabetic*

**AC625** *investigational amylin blocker antihypertensive for overweight patients*

**ACA-147** *investigational AcylCoA cholesterol acyltransferase inhibitor for reducing serum cholesterol*

**acacia** NF, JAN *suspending agent; emollient; demulcent*

**acadesine** USAN, INN, BAN *platelet aggregation inhibitor*

**A-Caine Rectal** ointment (discontinued 1995) OTC *topical anesthetic; vasoconstrictor; astringent* [diperodon HCl; pyrilamine maleate; phenylephrine HCl; bismuth subcarbonate; zinc oxide] 0.25%•0.1%•0.25%•0.2%•5% ᴅ Anocaine

**acamprosate 6473** INN

**acamylophenine** [see: camylofin]

**acaprazine** INN

**Acapulco gold; Acapulco red** *street drug slang for marijuana from southwest Mexico* [see: marijuana]

**acarbose** USAN, INN, BAN *α-glucosidase inhibitor for type 2 diabetes mellitus*

**ACAT (AcylCoA transferase) inhibitor** *investigational agent to lower serum cholesterol levels*

**Accolate** film-coated tablets ℞ *leukotriene receptor antagonist (LTRA) for prevention and chronic treatment of asthma* [zafirlukast] 20 mg

**Accu-Chek Advantage** reagent strips for home use OTC *in vitro diagnostic aid for blood glucose*

**Accu-Pak** (trademarked packaging form) *unit dose blister pack*

**Accupep HPF** powder OTC *enteral nutritional therapy for GI impairment*

**Accupril** film-coated tablets ℞ *antihypertensive; angiotensin-converting enzyme (ACE) inhibitor* [quinapril HCl] 5, 10, 20, 40 mg

**Accurbron** syrup ℞ *antiasthmatic* [theophylline; alcohol 7.5%] 150 mg/15 mL ⊡ Accutane

**Accusens T** multi-sample kit (discontinued 1995) *in vitro diagnostic aid for taste dysfunction*

**AccuSite** injectable gel ℞ *investigational (NDA filed) treatment for genital warts*

**Accutane** capsules ℞ *internal keratolytic for severe recalcitrant cystic acne* [isotretinoin] 10, 20, 40 mg ⊡ Accurbron

**ACD solution (acid citrate dextrose; anticoagulant citrate dextrose)** [see: anticoagulant citrate dextrose solution]

**ACD whole blood** [see: blood, whole]

**ace** *street drug slang* [see: marijuana; PCP]

**ACe (Adriamycin, cyclophosphamide)** *chemotherapy protocol*

**ACE (Adriamycin, cyclophosphamide, etoposide)** *chemotherapy protocol* [also: CAE]

**acebrochol** INN, DCF

**aceburic acid** INN, DCF

**acebutolol** USAN, INN, BAN *antihypertensive; antiarrhythmic; antiadrenergic (β-receptor)* [also: acebutolol HCl]

**acebutolol HCl** JAN *antihypertensive; antiarrhythmic; antiadrenergic (β-receptor)* [also: acebutolol] 200, 400 mg oral

**acecainide** INN *antiarrhythmic* [also: acecainide HCl]

**acecainide HCl** USAN *antiarrhythmic* [also: acecainide]

**acecarbromal** INN *CNS depressant; sedative; hypnotic*

**aceclidine** USAN, INN *cholinergic*

**aceclofenac** INN, BAN

**acedapsone** USAN, INN, BAN *antimalarial; antibacterial; leprostatic*

**acediasulfone sodium** INN, DCF

**acedoben** INN

**acefluranol** INN, BAN

**acefurtiamine** INN

**acefylline clofibrol** INN

**acefylline piperazine** INN, DCF [also: acepifylline]

**aceglaton** JAN [also: aceglatone]

**aceglatone** INN [also: aceglaton]

**aceglutamide** INN *antiulcerative* [also: aceglutamide aluminum]

**aceglutamide aluminum** USAN, JAN *antiulcerative* [also: aceglutamide]

**ACEIs (angiotensin-converting enzyme inhibitors)** [q.v.]

**Acel-Imune** IM injection ℞ *immunization against diphtheria, tetanus and pertussis* [diphtheria & tetanus toxoids & acellular pertussis vaccine (DTaP)] 7.5 LfU•5 LfU•300 HAU per 0.5 mL

**acemannan** USAN, INN *antiviral; immunomodulator; investigational (Phase I) for AIDS*

**acemetacin** INN, BAN, JAN

**acemethadone** [see: methadyl acetate]

**aceneuramic acid** INN

**acenocoumarin** [see: acenocoumarol]

**acenocoumarol** NF, INN [also: nicoumalone]

**Aceon** tablets (discontinued 1994) ℞ *antihypertensive; ACE inhibitor* [perindopril erbumine] 2, 4, 8 mg

**aceperone** INN

**Acephen** suppositories OTC *analgesic; antipyretic* [acetaminophen] 120, 325, 650 mg

**acephenazine dimaleate** [see: acetophenazine maleate]

**acepifylline** BAN [also: acefylline piperazine]

**acepromazine** INN, BAN *veterinary sedative* [also: acepromazine maleate]

**acepromazine maleate** USAN *veterinary sedative* [also: acepromazine]

**aceprometazine** INN, DCF

**acequinoline** INN, DCF

**acesulfame** INN, BAN

**Aceta** tablets, elixir OTC *analgesic; antipyretic* [acetaminophen] 325, 500 mg; 120 mg/5 mL

**Aceta with Codeine** tablets ℞ *narcotic analgesic* [codeine phosphate; acetaminophen] 30•300 mg

**Aceta-Gesic** tablets OTC *antihistamine; analgesic* [phenyltoloxamine citrate; acetaminophen] 30•325 mg

*p*-**acetamidobenzoic acid** [see: acedoben]

**6-acetamidohexanoic acid** [see: acexamic acid]

**4-acetamidophenyl acetate** [see: diacetamate]

**acetaminocaproic acid** [see: acexamic acid]

**acetaminophen** USP *analgesic; antipyretic* [also: paracetamol] 80, 325, 500, 650 mg, 100 mg/mL, 120, 160 mg/5 mL, 500/15 mL oral; 120, 300, 325, 650 mg suppository

**acetaminophen & codeine** *narcotic analgesic* 300•15, 300•30, 300•60 mg oral; 30•12 mg/5 mL oral

**acetaminophenol** [see: acetaminophen]

**acetaminosalol** INN, DCF

**acetanilid (or acetanilide)** NF

**acetannin** [see: acetyltannic acid]

**acetarsol** INN, BAN, DCF [also: acetarsone]

**acetarsone** NF [also: acetarsol]

**acetarsone salt of arecoline** [see: drocarbil]

**Acetasol** ear drops ℞ *antibacterial/antifungal* [acetic acid] 2%

**Acetasol HC** ear drops ℞ *topical corticosteroidal anti-inflammatory; antibacterial/antifungal* [hydrocortisone; acetic acid] 1%•2%

**acetazolamide** USP, INN, BAN, JAN *carbonic anhydrase inhibitor; anticonvulsant* 125, 250 mg oral; 500 mg injection

**acetazolamide sodium** USP, JAN *carbonic anhydrase inhibitor*

**acetcarbromal** [see: acecarbromal]

**acet-dia-mer-sulfonamide (sulfacetamide, sulfadiazine & sulfamerazine)** [q.v.]

**acetergamine** INN

**Acetest** reagent tablets for professional use *in vitro diagnostic aid for acetone (ketones) in the urine or blood*

**acetiamine** INN

**acetic acid** NF, JAN *acidifying agent* 0.25%

**acetic acid, aluminum salt** [see: aluminum acetate]

**acetic acid, calcium salt** [see: calcium acetate]

**acetic acid, diluted** NF *bladder irrigant*

**acetic acid, ethyl ester** [see: ethyl acetate]

**acetic acid, glacial** USP, INN *acidifying agent*

**acetic acid, potassium salt** [see: potassium acetate]

**acetic acid, sodium salt trihydrate** [see: sodium acetate]

**acetic acid, zinc salt dihydrate** [see: zinc acetate]

**acetic acid 5-nitrofurfurylidenehydrazide** [see: nihydrazone]

**aceticyl** [see: aspirin]

**acetilum acidulatum** [see: aspirin]

**acetiromate** INN

**acetohexamide** USAN, USP, INN, BAN, JAN *sulfonylurea-type antidiabetic* 250, 500 mg oral

**acetohydroxamic acid (AHA)** USAN, USP, INN *urease enzyme inhibitor for chronic urea-splitting urinary infections*

**acetol** [see: aspirin]

**acetomenaphthone** BAN

**acetomeroctol**

**acetone** NF *solvent; antiseptic*

**acetophen** [see: aspirin]

**acetophenazine** INN *antipsychotic* [also: acetophenazine maleate]

**acetophenazine maleate** USAN, USP *antipsychotic* [also: acetophenazine]

*p*-**acetophenetidide** (*withdrawn from market*) [see: phenacetin]

**acetophenetidin** (*withdrawn from market*) [now: phenacetin]

**acetorphine** INN, BAN *enkephalinase inhibitor for acute diarrhea; investigational for opioid withdrawal and GERD*

**acetosal** [see: aspirin]

**acetosalic acid** [see: aspirin]

**acetosalin** [see: aspirin]

**acetosulfone sodium** USAN *antibacterial; leprostatic* [also: sulfadiasulfone sodium]

**acetoxyphenylmercury** [see: phenylmercuric acetate]

**acetoxythymoxamine** [see: moxisylyte]

**acetphenarsine** [see: acetarsone]

**acetphenetidin** (*withdrawn from market*) [now: phenacetin]

**acetphenolisatin** [see: oxyphenisatin acetate]

**acetrizoate sodium** USP [also: sodium acetrizoate]

**acetrizoic acid** USP

**acetryptine** INN

**acetsalicylamide** [see: salacetamide]

**acet-theocin sodium** [see: theophylline sodium acetate]

**aceturate** USAN, INN *combining name for radicals or groups*

**acetyl adalin** [see: acetylcarbromal]

**acetyl L-carnitine** [see: levacecarnine]

**acetyl sulfisoxazole** [see: sulfisoxazole acetyl]

*l*-**acetyl-α-methadol (LAAM)** [see: levomethadyl acetate]

*p*-**acetylaminobenzaldehyde thiosemicarbazone** [see: thioacetazone; thiacetazone]

**acetylaminobenzene** [see: acetanilid]

**N-acetyl-*p*-aminophenol (APAP; NAPA)** [see: acetaminophen]

**acetylaniline** [see: acetanilid]

**acetylated polyvinyl alcohol** *viscosity-increasing agent*

**acetyl-bromo-diethylacetylcarbamide** [see: acecarbromal]

**acetylcarbromal** [see: acecarbromal]

**acetylcholine chloride** USP, INN, BAN, JAN *cardiac depressant; cholinergic; miotic; peripheral vasodilator*

**acetylcholinesterase (AChE) inhibitors** *a class of drugs that alter acetylcholine neurotransmitters, used as a cognition adjuvant in Alzheimer's dementia* [also called: cholinesterase inhibitors]

**acetylcysteine (N-acetylcysteine)** USAN, USP, INN, BAN *mucolytic inhaler; investigational immunomodulator for AIDS; investigational (orphan)*

*for severe acetaminophen overdose* [also: N-acetyl-L-cysteine]

**acetylcysteine sodium** *mucolytic* 10%, 20% inhalation

**acetyldigitoxin (α-acetyldigitoxin)** NF, INN

**acetyldihydrocodeinone** [see: thebacon]

**N-acetyl-DL-leucine** [see: acetylleucine]

**acetylin** [see: aspirin]

**acetylkitasamycin** JAN *antibacterial* [also: kitasamycin; kitasamycin tartrate]

**acetyl-L-carnitine (ALCAR)** *investigational cognition enhancer for Alzheimer's disease*

**N-acetyl-L-cysteine** JAN *mucolytic inhaler* [also: acetylcysteine]

**N-acetyl-L-cysteine salicylate** [see: salnacedin]

**acetylleucine (N-acetyl-DL-leucine)** INN

**acetylmethadol** INN, DCF *narcotic analgesic* [also: methadyl acetate]

**acetyloleandomycin** [see: troleandomycin]

**2-acetyloxybenzoic acid** [see: aspirin]

**acetylpheneturide** JAN [also: pheneturide]

**acetylphenylisatin** [see: oxyphenisatin acetate]

**N-acetyl-procainamide (NAPA)** *investigational (orphan) preventative for ventricular arrhythmias in procainamide-induced lupus*

**acetylpropylorvinol** [see: acetorphine]

**acetylresorcinol** [see: resorcinol monoacetate]

**acetylsal** [see: aspirin]

**N-acetylsalicylamide** [see: salacetamide]

**acetylsalicylate aluminum** [see: aspirin aluminum]

**acetylsalicylic acid (ASA)** [now: aspirin]

**acetylsalicylic acid, phenacetin & caffeine** [see: APC]

**acetylspiramycin** JAN *antibacterial* [also: spiramycin]

**acetylsulfamethoxazole** JAN *broad-spectrum sulfonamide bacteriostatic* [also:

sulfamethoxazole; sulphamethoxazole; sulfamethoxazole sodium]

**$N^1$-acetylsulfanilamide** [see: sulfacetamide]

**acetyltannic acid** USP

**acetyltannin** [see: acetyltannic acid]

**acevaltrate** INN

**acexamic acid** INN, DCF

**ACFUCY (actinomycin D, fluorouracil, cyclophosphamide)** *chemotherapy protocol*

**AChE (acetylcholinesterase) inhibitors** [q.v.]

**Aches-N-Pain** tablets (discontinued 1996) OTC *nonsteroidal anti-inflammatory drug (NSAID); antiarthritic; analgesic* [ibuprofen] 200 mg

**Achromycin** eye drop suspension, ophthalmic ointment (discontinued 1995) ℞ *ophthalmic antibiotic* [tetracycline HCl] 10 mg/mL; 10 mg/g ☒ actinomycin; Aureomycin

**Achromycin** topical ointment (discontinued 1995) OTC *broad-spectrum antibacterial* [tetracycline HCl] 3%

**Achromycin V** capsules, oral suspension ℞ *broad-spectrum antibiotic* [tetracycline HCl] 250, 500 mg; 125 mg/5 mL

**aciclovir** INN, JAN *antiviral* [also: acyclovir]

**acid** *street drug slang* [see: LSD]

**acid acriflavine** [see: acriflavine HCl]

**acid alpha-glucosidase, human** [see: human acid alpha-glucosidase]

**acid citrate dextrose (ACD)** [see: anticoagulant citrate dextrose solution]

**acid histamine phosphate** [see: histamine phosphate]

**Acid Mantle** OTC *cream base*

**acid trypaflavine** [see: acriflavine HCl]

**acidogen** [see: glutamic acid HCl]

**acidol HCl** [see: betaine HCl]

**acidophilus** [see: *Lactobacillus acidophilus*]

**acidulated phosphate fluoride (sodium fluoride & hydrofluoric acid)** *dental caries prophylactic*

**acidum acetylsalicylicum** [see: aspirin]

**Acid-X** tablets OTC *analgesic; antipyretic; antacid* [acetaminophen; calcium carbonate] 500•250 mg

**acifran** USAN, INN *antihyperlipoproteinemic*

**aciglumin** [see: glutamic acid HCl]

**Aci-jel** vaginal jelly OTC *acidity modifier* [acetic acid; oxyquinolone sulfate] 0.921%•0.025%

**acinitrazole** BAN *veterinary antibacterial* [also: nithiamide; aminitrozole]

**acipimox** INN, BAN

**acistrate** INN *combining name for radicals or groups*

**acitemate** INN

**acitretin** USAN, INN, BAN *antipsoriatic; synthetic retinoid*

**acivicin** USAN, INN *antineoplastic*

**Aclacin** ℞ *investigational antibiotic antineoplastic for acute nonlymphocytic leukemia* [aclarubicin HCl]

**aclacinomycin A** [now: aclarubicin]

**aclantate** INN

**aclarubicin** USAN, INN, BAN *antibiotic antineoplastic* [also: aclarubicin HCl]

**aclarubicin HCl** JAN *antibiotic antineoplastic* [also: aclarubicin]

**aclatonium napadisilate** INN, BAN, JAN

**Aclophen** long-acting tablets ℞ *decongestant; antihistamine; analgesic* [phenylephrine HCl; chlorpheniramine maleate; acetaminophen] 40•8•500 mg

**Aclovate** ointment, cream ℞ *topical corticosteroidal anti-inflammatory* [alclometasone dipropionate] 0.05%

**ACM (Adriamycin, cyclophosphamide, methotrexate)** *chemotherapy protocol*

**A.C.N.** tablets OTC *vitamin supplement* [vitamins A, $B_3$, and C] 25 000 IU•25 mg•250 mg

**Acne Lotion 10** OTC *antibacterial and exfoliant for acne* [colloidal sulfur] 10%

**Acne-5** lotion, mask OTC *topical keratolytic for acne* [benzoyl peroxide] 5%

**Acne-10** lotion OTC *topical keratolytic for acne* [benzoyl peroxide] 10%

**Acne-Aid** cleansing bar (discontinued 1994) OTC *medicated cleanser for acne* [surfactant blend] 6.3%

**Acne-Aid** cream (discontinued 1994) OTC *keratolytic for acne* [benzoyl peroxide] 10%

**Acnederm** lotion (discontinued 1993) OTC *topical acne treatment* [sulfur; zinc sulfate; zinc oxide; isopropyl alcohol] 5%•1%•10%•21%

**Acno** lotion OTC *topical acne treatment* [sulfur] 3%

**Acno Cleanser** liquid OTC *topical cleanser for acne* [isopropyl alcohol] 60%

**Acnomel** cream OTC *topical acne treatment* [sulfur; resorcinol; alcohol] 8%•2%•11%

**Acnotex** lotion OTC *topical acne treatment* [sulfur; resorcinol; isopropyl alcohol] 8%•2%•20%

**acodazole** INN *antineoplastic* [also: acodazole HCl]

**acodazole HCl** USAN *antineoplastic* [also: acodazole]

**aconiazide** INN *investigational (orphan) for tuberculosis*

**aconitine** USP

**ACOP (Adriamycin, cyclophosphamide, Oncovin, prednisone)** *chemotherapy protocol*

**ACOPP; A-COPP (Adriamycin, cyclophosphamide, Oncovin, procarbazine, prednisone)** *chemotherapy protocol*

**acortan** [see: corticotropin]

**acoxatrine** INN

**9-acridinamine monohydrochloride** [see: aminacrine HCl]

**acridinyl anisidide** [see: amsacrine]

**acridinylamine methanesulfon anisidide (AMSA)** [see: amsacrine]

**acridorex** INN

**acriflavine** NF

**acriflavine HCl** NF [also: acriflavinium chloride]

**acriflavinium chloride** INN [also: acriflavine HCl]

**acrihellin** INN

**acrinol** JAN [also: ethacridine lactate; ethacridine]

**acrisorcin** USAN, USP, INN *antifungal*

**acrivastine** USAN, INN, BAN *antihistamine*

**acrocinonide** INN, DCF

**acronine** USAN, INN *antineoplastic*

**acrosoxacin** BAN *antibacterial* [also: rosoxacin]

**AcryDerm Strands** wound dressing *high-exudate absorbent dressing for cavitated wounds*

**ACT** oral rinse OTC *topical dental caries preventative* [sodium fluoride; alcohol 7%] 0.05%

**actagardin** INN

**Actagen** tablets, syrup OTC *decongestant; antihistamine* [pseudoephedrine HCl; triprolidine HCl] 60•2.5 mg; 30•1.25 mg/5 mL

**Actagen-C Cough** syrup Rx *narcotic antitussive; decongestant; antihistamine* [codeine phosphate; pseudoephedrine HCl; triprolidine HCl] 10•30•2 mg/5 mL

**Actamin; Actamin Extra** tablets OTC *analgesic; antipyretic* [acetaminophen]

**actaplanin** USAN, INN, BAN *veterinary growth stimulant*

**actarit** INN

**ACTH** powder for IM or subcu injection Rx *steroid* [corticotropin] 40 U/vial

**ACTH (adrenocorticotropic hormone)** [see: corticotropin]

**ACTH-40** subcu or IM injection (discontinued 1994) Rx *steroid* [corticotropin repository] 40 U/mL

**ACTH-80** subcu or IM injection Rx *steroid* [corticotropin repository] 80 U/mL

**Acthar** powder for IM or subcu injection Rx *steroid* [corticotropin] 25, 40 U/vial

**Acthar Gel** [see: H.P. Acthar Gel]

**ActHIB** powder for injection Rx *pediatric vaccine for meningitis caused by Haemophilus influenzae type b (HIB) virus* [Hemophilus b conjugate vaccine; tetanus toxoid] 10•24 µg/0.5 mL

**ActHIB/acellular DTP** (formula changed and released as ActHIB/Tripedia in 1996)

**ActHIB/DTacP** (pre-marketing name; released as ActHIB/Tripedia in 1996)

**ActHIB/DTP** IM injection Rx *pediatric vaccine for diphtheria, tetanus, pertussis, and Haemophilus influenzae type b (HIB)* [Hemophilus b conjugate vaccine; diphtheria & tetanus toxoids & pertussis vaccine (DTP)] 20 µg/mL

**ActHIB/Tripedia** injection ℞ *pediatric vaccine for children younger than 5 months old* [Hemophilus b conjugate vaccine; diphtheria & tetanus toxoids & acellular pertussis vaccine] ☲

**Acthrel** ℞ *diagnostic aid for adrenocorticotropic hormone-dependent Cushing syndrome (orphan)* [corticorelin ovine triflutate]

**ActiBath** effervescent tablets OTC *moisturizer; emollient* [colloidal oatmeal] 20%

**Acticel** ℞ *investigational treatment for Parkinson's disease, stroke, burns, and venous ulcers* [fibroblast growth factor]

**Acticort 100** lotion ℞ *topical corticosteroid* [hydrocortisone] 1%

**Actidil** syrup (discontinued 1996) OTC *antihistamine* [triprolidine HCl; alcohol 4%] 1.25 mg/5 mL ☲ Actifed

**Actidil** tablets (discontinued 1993) OTC *antihistamine* [triprolidine HCl] 2.5 mg

**Actidose with Sorbitol** oral suspension OTC *adsorbent antidote for poisoning; reduces intestinal transit time* [activated charcoal; sorbitol] 25• ☲ g/120 mL; 50• ☲ g/240 mL

**Actidose-Aqua** oral suspension OTC *adsorbent antidote for poisoning* [activated charcoal] 25 g/120 mL, 50 g/240 mL

**Actifed** capsules (discontinued 1993) OTC *decongestant; antihistamine* [pseudoephedrine HCl; triprolidine HCl] ☲ Actidil

**Actifed** syrup (discontinued 1995) OTC *decongestant; antihistamine* [pseudoephedrine HCl; triprolidine HCl] 30•1.25 mg/5 mL

**Actifed** tablets OTC *decongestant; antihistamine* [pseudoephedrine HCl; triprolidine HCl] 60•2.5 mg

**Actifed 12-Hour** sustained-release capsules (discontinued 1993) OTC *decongestant; antihistamine* [pseudoephedrine HCl; triprolidine HCl]

**Actifed Allergy** daytime caplets + nighttime caplets OTC *decongestant; (antihistamine/sleep aid added at night)* [pseudoephedrine HCl; (diphenhydramine HCl added at night)] 30 mg; 30•25 mg

**Actifed Plus** caplets, tablets OTC *decongestant; antihistamine; analgesic* [pseudoephedrine HCl; triprolidine HCl; acetaminophen] 30•1.25•500 mg

**Actifed Sinus** daytime caplets + nighttime caplets OTC *decongestant; analgesic; (antihistamine/sleep aid added at night)* [pseudoephedrine HCl; acetaminophen; (diphenhydramine HCl added at night)] 30•325 mg; 30•500•25 mg

**Actifed with Codeine Cough** syrup (discontinued 1997) ℞ *narcotic antitussive; decongestant; antihistamine* [codeine phosphate; pseudoephedrine HCl; triprolidine HCl; alcohol 4.3%] 10•30•1.25 mg/5 mL

**Actigall** capsules ℞ *gallstone dissolving agent; investigational (orphan) for primary biliary cirrhosis* [ursodiol] 300 mg

**Actimmune** subcu injection ℞ *biologic response modifier for chronic granulomatous disease (orphan); investigational (orphan) for renal cell carcinoma and osteopetrosis* [interferon gamma-1b] 100 μg (3 million U)

**Actinex** cream ℞ *antineoplastic for actinic keratoses (AK)* [masoprocol] 10%

**actinium** *element (Ac)*

**actinomycin C** BAN *antibiotic antineoplastic* [also: cactinomycin] ☲ Achromycin; Aureomycin

**actinomycin D** JAN *antibiotic antineoplastic* [also: dactinomycin] ☲ Achromycin; Aureomycin

**actinoquinol** INN *ultraviolet screen* [also: actinoquinol sodium]

**actinoquinol sodium** USAN *ultraviolet screen* [also: actinoquinol]

**actinospectocin** [see: spectinomycin]

**Actiq** oral transmucosal ℞ *investigational (Phase III) opioid delivery system for breakthrough pain in cancer patients* [fentanyl citrate]

**Actisite** periodontal fiber ℞ *oral antibiotic for periodontitis* [tetracycline] 12.7 mg/23 cm

**actisomide** USAN, INN *antiarrhythmic*

**Activase** powder for IV infusion ℞ *tissue plasminogen activator (tPA) for acute myocardial infarction, acute ischemic stroke, or pulmonary embolism* [alteplase] 50, 100 mg/vial (29, 58 million IU/vial)

**activated attapulgite** [see: attapulgite, activated]

**activated carbon**

**activated charcoal** [see: charcoal, activated]

**activated 7-dehydrocholesterol** [see: cholecalciferol]

**activated ergosterol** [see: ergocalciferol]

**activated prothrombin complex** BAN

**actodigin** USAN, INN *cardiotonic*

**Act-O-Vial** (trademarked packaging form) *vial system*

**Actron** tablets OTC *nonsteroidal anti-inflammatory drug (NSAID); analgesic; antiarthritic* [ketoprofen] 12.5 mg

**ACU-dyne** ointment, perineal wash concentrate, prep solution, skin cleanser, prep swabs, swabsticks OTC *broad-spectrum antimicrobial* [povidone-iodine]

**ACU-dyne Douche** concentrate OTC *antiseptic/germicidal; vaginal cleanser and deodorizer* [povidone-iodine]

**Acular** eye drops ℞ *ocular nonsteroidal anti-inflammatory drug (NSAID) for allergic conjunctivitis or following cataract extraction* [ketorolac tromethamine] 0.5%

**Acupaque** ℞ *investigational broad-spectrum contrast agent for x-ray and CT scans (trials discontinued 1996)* [iodixanol]

**AcuTect** ℞ *investigational (NDA filed) radiopharmaceutical diagnostic aid for acute venous thrombosis* [technetium Tc 99m apcitide]

**Acutrim 16 Hour; Acutrim Late Day; Acutrim II** precision-release tablets OTC *diet aid* [phenylpropanolamine HCl] 75 mg

**acycloguanosine** [see: acyclovir]

**acyclovir** USAN, USP, BAN *antiviral* [also: aciclovir] 200, 400, 800 mg oral

**acyclovir redox** [see: redox-acyclovir]

**acyclovir sodium** USAN *antiviral* 200 mg oral; 50 mg/mL injection

**acylpyrin** [see: aspirin]

**AD** *street drug slang* [see: PCP]

**AD-439** *investigational (Phase II) antiviral for HIV and AIDS*

**AD-519** *investigational (Phase II) antiviral for HIV and AIDS*

**ADA (adenosine deaminase)** [see: pegademase bovine; pegademase]

**adafenoxate** INN

**Adagen** IM injection ℞ *adenosine deaminase (ADA) enzyme replacement for severe combined immunodeficiency disease (orphan)* [pegademase bovine] 250 U/mL

**Adalat** capsules ℞ *antianginal* [nifedipine] 10, 20 mg

**Adalat CC; Adalat Oros** sustained-release tablets ℞ *antianginal; antihypertensive* [nifedipine] 30, 60, 90 mg

**Adam** *street drug slang* [see: MDMA]

**Adam and Eve** *street drug slang for the combination of MDMA and MDEA* [see: MDMA; MDEA]

**adamantanamine** [see: amantadine]

**adamantanamine HCl** [see: amantadine HCl]

**adamexine** INN

**adapalene** USAN, INN, BAN *synthetic retinoid for topical treatment of acne*

**Adapettes** solution OTC *rewetting solution for hard contact lenses*

**Adapettes Especially for Sensitive Eyes** solution OTC *rewetting solution for soft contact lenses*

**Adapin** capsules (discontinued 1996) ℞ *tricyclic antidepressant; anxiolytic* [doxepin HCl] 10, 25, 50, 75, 100, 150 mg ② Atabrine; Ativan; Betapen

**adaprolol maleate** USAN *ophthalmic antihypertensive (β-blocker)*

**Adapt** solution (discontinued 1995) OTC *wetting/rewetting solution for hard contact lenses*

**adatanserin** INN *anxiolytic; antidepressant* [also: adatanserin HCl]

**adatanserin HCl** USAN *anxiolytic; antidepressant* [also: adatanserin]

**AdatoSil 5000** intraocular injection ℞ *retinal tamponade for retinal detachment* [polydimethylsiloxane] 10, 15 mL

**Adavite** tablets OTC *vitamin supplement* [multiple vitamins; folic acid; biotin] ±•400•35 µg

**Adavite-M** tablets OTC *vitamin/mineral/iron supplement* [multiple vitamins & minerals; iron; folic acid; biotin] ± •27 mg•0.4 mg•30 μg

**ADBC (Adriamycin, DTIC, bleomycin, CCNU)** *chemotherapy protocol*

**ADC with Fluoride** drops ℞ *pediatric vitamin supplement and dental caries preventative* [vitamins A, C, and D; fluoride] 1500 IU•35 mg•400 IU• 0.5 mg per mL

**Adcon-L** gel ℞ *investigational agent to inhibit excess scar formation following back surgery*

**Adderall** tablets ℞ *CNS stimulant for attention deficit hyperactivity disorder (ADHD), narcolepsy, and obesity* [dextroamphetamine sulfate; dextroamphetamine saccharate; amphetamine aspartate; amphetamine sulfate] 2.5•2.5•2.5•2.5, 5•5•5•5 mg

**ADD-Vantage** (trademarked delivery system) *intravenous drug admixture system*

**ADE (ara-C, daunorubicin, etoposide)** *chemotherapy protocol*

**Adeflor M** tablets ℞ *pediatric vitamin deficiency and dental caries prevention* [multiple vitamins; fluoride; calcium; iron] ± •1•250•30 mg

**adefovir dipivoxil** *investigational (Phase III) oral antiretroviral for HIV and AIDS; investigational (Phase II) treatment for chronic hepatitis B virus (HBV) infection*

**ADEKs** chewable tablets OTC *vitamin/ mineral supplement* [multiple vitamins & minerals; folic acid; biotin] ± •200•50 μg

**ADEKs** pediatric drops OTC *vitamin/ mineral supplement* [multiple vitamins & minerals; biotin] ± •15 μg

**adelmidrol** INN

**ademetionine** INN

**Adenazole** ℞ *investigational antineoplastic* [8-chlorocamp]

**adenine** USP, JAN *amino acid*

**adenine arabinoside (ara-A)** [see: vidarabine]

**adeno-associated viral-based vector cystic fibrosis gene therapy** *investigational (orphan) for cystic fibrosis*

**Adenocard** IV injection ℞ *antiarrhythmic* [adenosine] 3 mg/mL

**Adenoscan** IV infusion ℞ *cardiac diagnostic aid; cardiac stressor; adjunct to thallium 201 myocardial perfusion scintigraphy* [adenosine] 3 mg/mL

**adenosine** USAN, BAN *antiarrhythmic for paroxysmal supraventricular tachycardia; diagnostic aid; orphan status withdrawn 1996*

**adenosine deaminase (ADA)** [see: pegademase bovine; pegademase]

**adenosine monophosphate (AMP)** [see: adenosine phosphate]

**adenosine phosphate** USAN, INN, BAN *nutrient; treatment for varicose veins and herpes infections* 25 mg/mL IM injection

**adenosine triphosphate (ATP) disodium** JAN

**5'-adenylic acid** [see: adenosine phosphate]

**adepsine oil** [see: mineral oil]

**adhesive bandage** [see: bandage, adhesive]

**adhesive tape** [see: tape, adhesive]

**adibendan** INN

**A-DIC (Adriamycin, dacarbazine)** *chemotherapy protocol*

**adicillin** INN, BAN

**adimolol** INN

**adinazolam** USAN, INN, BAN *antidepressant; sedative*

**adinazolam mesylate** USAN *antidepressant*

**Adipex-P** tablets ℞ *anorexiant* [phentermine HCl] 37.5 mg

**adiphenine** INN *smooth muscle relaxant* [also: adiphenine HCl]

**adiphenine HCl** USAN *smooth muscle relaxant* [also: adiphenine]

**adipiodone** INN, JAN [also: iodipamide]

**adipiodone meglumine** JAN *radiopaque medium* [also: iodipamide meglumine]

**Adipost** slow-release capsules ℞ *anorexiant* [phendimetrazine tartrate] 105 mg

**aditeren** INN

**aditoprim** INN

**Adlone** injection ℞ *glucocorticoids* [methylprednisolone acetate] 40, 80 mg/mL

**adnephrine** [see: epinephrine]

**ADOAP (Adriamycin, Oncovin, ara-C, prednisone)** *chemotherapy protocol*

**Adolph's Salt Substitute** OTC *salt substitute* [potassium chloride] 64 mEq/5 g; 35 mEq/5 g

**Adolph's Seasoned Salt Substitute** (discontinued 1997) OTC *salt substitute* [potassium chloride] 35 mEq/5 g

**ADOP (Adriamycin, Oncovin, prednisone)** *chemotherapy protocol*

**Adosar** ℞ *investigational antineoplastic for solid tumors and leukemia* [adozelesin]

**adosopine** INN

**adozelesin** USAN, INN *antineoplastic*

**Adprin-B** coated tablets OTC *analgesic; antipyretic; anti-inflammatory; antirheumatic* [aspirin (buffered with calcium carbonate, magnesium oxide, and magnesium carbonate)] 325, 500 mg

**ADR (Adriamycin)** [see: doxorubicin HCl]

**adrafinil** INN

**adrenal** [see: epinephrine]

**adrenal cortical steroids** *a class of steroid hormones that stimulate the adrenal cortex*

**Adrenalin Chloride** eye drops ℞ *antiglaucoma agent* [epinephrine HCl]

**Adrenalin Chloride** nose drops OTC *nasal decongestant* [epinephrine HCl] 0.1%

**Adrenalin Chloride** solution for inhalation ℞ *bronchodilator for bronchial asthma* [epinephrine HCl] 1:100

**Adrenalin Chloride** subcu, IV, IM or intracardiac injection ℞ *bronchodilator for bronchial asthma, bronchospasm and COPD; vasopressor for shock* [epinephrine HCl] 1:1000 (1 mg/mL)

**adrenaline** BAN *vasoconstrictor; bronchodilator; topical antiglaucoma agent; vasopressor for shock* [also: epinephrine] ☒ adrenalone

**adrenaline bitartrate** [see: epinephrine bitartrate]

**adrenaline HCl** [see: epinephrine HCl]

**adrenalone** USAN, INN *ophthalmic adrenergic* ☒ adrenaline

**adrenamine** [see: epinephrine]

**adrenergic antagonists** *a class of bronchodilators that relax the bronchial muscles, reducing bronchospasm* [also called: sympathomimetics]

**adrenine** [see: epinephrine]

**adrenochromazone** [see: carbazochrome salicylate]

**adrenochrome** [see: carbazochrome salicylate]

**adrenochrome guanylhydrazone mesilate** JAN

**adrenochrome monoaminoguanidine sodium methylsulfonate** [see: adrenochrome guanylhydrazone mesilate]

**adrenochrome monosemicarbazone sodium salicylate** [see: carbazochrome salicylate]

**adrenocorticotrophin** [see: corticotropin]

**adrenocorticotropic hormone (ACTH)** [see: corticotropin]

**adrenone** [see: adrenalone]

**Adria + BCNU (Adriamycin, BCNU)** *chemotherapy protocol*

**Adria-L-PAM (Adriamycin, L-phenylalanine mustard)** *chemotherapy protocol*

**Adriamycin PFS** (preservative-free solution) IV injection ℞ *antibiotic antineoplastic* [doxorubicin HCl] 2 mg/mL

**Adriamycin RDF** (rapid dissolution formula) IV injection ℞ *antibiotic antineoplastic* [doxorubicin HCl] 10, 20, 50, 150 mg/vial

**Adria-Oncoline Chemo-Pin** (trademarked delivery system)

**Adrin** tablets (discontinued 1993) ℞ *peripheral vasodilator* [nylidrin HCl] 6, 12 mg

**Adrucil** IV injection ℞ *antimetabolic antineoplastic; investigational (orphan) adjuvant to colorectal and esophageal cancer* [fluorouracil] 50 mg/mL

**ADS (azodisal sodium)** [now: olsalazine sodium]

**adsorbed diphtheria toxoid** [see: diphtheria toxoid, adsorbed]

**Adsorbocarpine** eye drops ℞ *antiglaucoma agent; direct-acting miotic* [pilocarpine HCl] 1%, 2%, 4%

**Adsorbonac** eye drops OTC *corneal edema-reducing agent* [hypertonic saline solution] 2%, 5%

**Adsorbotear** eye drops OTC *ocular moisturizer/lubricant* [hydroxyethylcellulose] 0.4%

**ADT** (trademarked dosage form) *alternate-day therapy*

**Advance** liquid (discontinued 1993) OTC *total or supplementary infant feeding* 390 mL concentrate, 1 qt. ready-to-use

**Advance** test stick for home use OTC *in vitro diagnostic aid for urine pregnancy test*

**Advanced Care Cholesterol Test** kit for home use OTC *in vitro diagnostic aid for cholesterol in the blood*

**"Advanced Formula"** products [see under product name]

**Advantage 24** vaginal gel OTC *spermicidal contraceptive (for use with a diaphragm)* [nonoxynol 9] 3.5%

**Advera** liquid OTC *enteral nutritional therapy for HIV and AIDS patients* [lactose-free formula] 240 mL

**Advil** tablets, caplets OTC *nonsteroidal anti-inflammatory drug (NSAID); antiarthritic; analgesic* [ibuprofen] 200 mg ⊡ Avail

**Advil, Children's** oral suspension OTC *nonsteroidal anti-inflammatory drug (NSAID); analgesic* [ibuprofen] 100 mg/5 mL

**Advil, Junior Strength** coated tablets OTC *nonsteroidal anti-inflammatory drug (NSAID); analgesic* [ibuprofen] 100 mg

**Advil Cold & Sinus** caplets OTC *decongestant; analgesic* [pseudoephedrine HCl; ibuprofen] 30•200 mg

**AE-0047** *investigational calcium antagonist for hypertension and to improve cerebral blood flow*

**AEDs (anti-epileptic drugs)** [see: anticonvulsants]

**A-E-R** pads OTC *astringent* [hamamelis water] 50%

**Aeroaid** spray OTC *antiseptic; antibacterial; antifungal* [thimerosal; alcohol 72%] 1:1000

**AeroBid; AeroBid-M** oral inhalation aerosol ℞ *corticosteroid for bronchial asthma* [flunisolide] 200 μg/dose

**AeroCaine** aerosol solution OTC *topical local anesthetic* [benzocaine; benzethonium chloride] 13.6%•0.5%

**AeroChamber** (trademarked form) *aerosol holding chamber*

**Aerodine** aerosol OTC *broad-spectrum antimicrobial* [povidone-iodine]

**Aerofreeze** spray OTC *topical vapo-coolant anesthetic* [trichloromonofluoromethane; dichlorodifluoromethane] ≟•≟

**Aerolate** oral solution (discontinued 1993) ℞ *bronchodilator* [theophylline] 150 mg/15 mL

**Aerolate Sr.; Aerolate Jr.; Aerolate III** timed-action capsules ℞ *bronchodilator* [theophylline] 260 mg; 130 mg; 65 mg

**Aeropin** ℞ *investigational (orphan) for cystic fibrosis* [heparin, 2-0-desulfated]

**Aeroseb-Dex** aerosol spray ℞ *topical corticosteroid* [dexamethasone] 0.01%

**Aeroseb-HC** aerosol spray (discontinued 1997) ℞ *topical corticosteroid; antiseborrheic* [hydrocortisone] 0.5%

**aerosol OT** [see: docusate sodium]

**aerosolized pooled immune globulin** [see: globulin, aerosolized pooled immune]

**Aerosporin** powder for IV, IM or intrathecal injection (discontinued 1996) ℞ *bactericidal antibiotic* [polymyxin B sulfate] 500 000 U

**AeroTherm** aerosol solution OTC *topical local anesthetic* [benzocaine; benzethonium chloride] 13.6%•0.5%

**Aerotrol** (trademarked form) *inhalation aerosol*

**AeroZoin** spray OTC *skin protectant* [benzoin; isopropyl alcohol 44.8%] 30%

**AErrane** ℞ *investigational anesthetic* [isoflurane]

**aethylis chloridum** [see: ethyl chloride]

**AF102B** *investigational M-1 agonist for Alzheimer's disease*

**afalanine** INN

**Affirm DP** kit ℞ *investigational microbial identification test system for periodontal disease*

**afloqualone** INN, JAN

**AFM (Adriamycin, fluorouracil, methotrexate [with leucovorin rescue])** *chemotherapy protocol*

**afovirsen** INN

**African black; African bush; African woodbine** *street drug slang* [see: marijuana]

**Afrin** extended-release tablets OTC *nasal decongestant* [pseudoephedrine sulfate] 120 mg ☒ Afrinol; aspirin

**Afrin** nasal spray, nose drops OTC *nasal decongestant* [oxymetazoline HCl] 0.05%

**Afrin Children's Nose Drops** OTC *nasal decongestant* [oxymetazoline HCl] 0.025%

**Afrin Moisturizing Saline Mist** solution OTC *nasal moisturizer* [sodium chloride (saline)] 0.64%

**Afrin Saline Mist** solution (name changed to Afrin Moisturizing Saline Mist in 1996)

**Afrin Sinus** nasal spray OTC *nasal decongestant* [oxymetazoline HCl] 0.05%

**Afrinol** (name changed to Afrin in 1993) ☒ Afrin

**Aftate for Athlete's Foot** gel, powder, spray powder, spray liquid OTC *topical antifungal* [tolnaftate] 1%

**Aftate for Jock Itch** gel, powder, spray powder OTC *topical antifungal* [tolnaftate] 1%

**afurolol** INN

**A/G Pro** tablets OTC *dietary supplement* [protein hydrolysate; multiple vitamins, minerals, and amino acids] 542•± mg

**AG-337** *investigational antineoplastic*

**aganodine** INN

**agar** NF, JAN *suspending agent*

**agar-agar** [see: agar]

**age cross-link breakers** *a class of investigational antiaging compounds that break age-mediated bonds between proteins*

**aggregated albumin** [see: albumin, aggregated]

**aggregated radio-iodinated I 131 serum albumin** [see: albumin, aggregated iodinated I 131 serum]

**aglepristone** INN

**agofollin** [see: estradiol]

**Agoral** emulsion OTC *laxative* [mineral oil; phenolphthalein] 4.2•0.2 g/15 mL ☒ Argyrol

**Agoral Plain** emulsion (discontinued 1997) OTC *emollient laxative* [mineral oil] 1.4 g/5 mL

**Agrylin** capsules ℞ *antithrombotic/ antiplatelet drug for essential thrombocytopenia (orphan); investigational (orphan) for thrombocytosis and polycythemia vera* [anagrelide HCl] 0.5, 1 mg

**agurin** [see: theobromine sodium acetate]

**AHA (acetohydroxamic acid)** [q.v.]

**AHA (alpha hydroxy acids)** [see: glycolic acid]

**AH-chew** chewable tablets ℞ *decongestant; antihistamine; anticholinergic* [phenylephrine HCl; chlorpheniramine maleate; methscopolamine nitrate] 10•2•1.25 mg

**AH-chew D** chewable tablets ℞ *decongestant* [phenylephrine HCl] 10 mg

**AHF (antihemophilic factor)** [q.v.]

**AHG (antihemophilic globulin)** [see: antihemophilic factor]

**ah-pen-yen** *street drug slang* [see: opium]

**A-Hydrocort** IV or IM injection ℞ *glucocorticoids* [hydrocortisone sodium succinate] 100, 250, 500, 1000 mg/vial

**AI204** *investigational T-cell receptor peptide vaccine for rheumatoid arthritis*

**AIDS vaccine** (several different compounds are included in this general category; e.g., gp120, rgp160, rgp160 MN, rp24) *investigational (Phase I to III) antiviral for AIDS/HIV*

**aimies; amys** *street drug slang for amphetamines, amyl nitrite, Amytal (amobarbital; discontinued 1991)* [see: amphetamine; amyl nitrite; Amytal Sodium; amobarbital; amobarbital sodium]

**AIP** *street drug slang for heroin from Afghanistan, Iran, and Pakistan* [see: heroin]

**air, compressed** [see: air, medical]

**air, medical** USP *medicinal gas*

**Airet** solution for inhalation ℞ *bronchodilator* [albuterol sulfate] 0.083%z

**Airomir** metered dose inhaler *investigational CFC-free aerosol propellant to replace CFC-based propellants in other inhalers*

**airplane** *street drug slang* [see: marijuana]

**Al-RSA** *investigational (orphan) for autoimmune uveitis*

**ajmaline** JAN

**Akarpine** eye drops ℞ *antiglaucoma agent; direct-acting miotic* [pilocarpine HCl] 1%, 2%, 4%

**AKBeta** eye drops ℞ *topical antiglaucoma agent (β-blocker)* [levobunolol HCl] 0.25%, 0.5%

**AK-Chlor** eye drops, ophthalmic ointment ℞ *ophthalmic antibiotic* [chloramphenicol] 5 mg/mL; 10 mg/g

**AK-Cide** eye drop suspension, ophthalmic ointment ℞ *ophthalmic topical corticosteroidal anti-inflammatory; bacteriostatic* [prednisolone acetate; sulfacetamide sodium] 0.5%•10%

**AK-Con** eye drops ℞ *topical ocular decongestant/vasoconstrictor* [naphazoline HCl] 0.1%

**AK-Con-A** eye drops (discontinued 1995) ℞ *topical ocular decongestant and antihistamine* [naphazoline HCl; pheniramine maleate] 0.025%•0.3%

**AK-Dex** eye drops, ophthalmic ointment ℞ *ophthalmic topical corticosteroidal anti-inflammatory* [dexamethasone sodium phosphate] 0.1%; 0.05%

**AK-Dilate** eye drops ℞ *ocular decongestant/vasoconstrictor; mydriatic* [phenylephrine HCl] 2.5%, 10%

**AK-Fluor** IV injection ℞ *corneal disclosing agent* [fluorescein] 10%, 25%

**AK-Homatropine** eye drops ℞ *mydriatic; cycloplegic* [homatropine hydrobromide] 5%

**Akineton** IV or IM injection ℞ *anticholinergic; antiparkinsonian agent* [biperiden lactate] 5 mg/mL

**Akineton** tablets ℞ *anticholinergic; antiparkinsonian agent* [biperiden HCl] 2 mg

**aklomide** USAN, INN, BAN *coccidiostat for poultry*

**AK-Mycin** ophthalmic ointment (discontinued 1995) ℞ *ophthalmic antibiotic* [erythromycin] 5 mg/g ⊡ Akne-Mycin

**AK-NaCl** eye drops, ophthalmic ointment OTC *corneal edema-reducing agent* [hypertonic saline solution] 5%

**AK-Nefrin** eye drops OTC *topical ocular decongestant* [phenylephrine HCl] 0.12%

**Akne-mycin** ointment, topical solution ℞ *topical antibiotic for acne* [erythromycin] 2% ⊡ Ak-Mycin

**AK-Neo-Dex** eye drops ℞ *topical ophthalmic corticosteroidal anti-inflammatory; antibiotic* [dexamethasone sodium phosphate; neomycin sulfate] 0.1%•0.35%

**Akoline C.B.** capsules, caplets (discontinued 1995) OTC *dietary lipotropic with vitamin supplementation* [choline; inositol; methionine; multiple B vitamins; vitamin C; lemon bioflavonoids] 111•111•28•±• 100•100 mg

**Akoline CB with Zinc** caplets OTC *dietary lipotropic with vitamin and zinc supplementation* [choline; inositol; methionine; multiple B vitamins; vitamin C; bioflavonoid; zinc amino acid chelate]

**AK-Pentolate** eye drops ℞ *mydriatic; cycloplegic* [cyclopentolate HCl] 1%

**AK-Poly-Bac** ophthalmic ointment ℞ *ophthalmic antibiotic* [polymyxin B sulfate; bacitracin zinc] 10 000•500 U/g

**AK-Pred** eye drops ℞ *ophthalmic topical corticosteroidal anti-inflammatory* [prednisolone sodium phosphate] 0.125%, 1%

**AKPro** eye drops ℞ *antiglaucoma agent* [dipivefrin HCl] 0.1%

**AK-Rinse** ophthalmic solution OTC *extraocular irrigating solution* [sterile isotonic solution]

**AK-Spore** eye drops ℞ *ophthalmic antibiotic* [polymyxin B sulfate; neomycin sulfate; gramicidin] 10 000 U• 1.75 mg•0.025 mg per mL

**AK-Spore** ophthalmic ointment ℞ *ophthalmic antibiotic* [polymyxin B sulfate; neomycin sulfate; bacitracin zinc] 10 000 U•3.5 mg•400 U per g

**AK-Spore H.C.** ear drops, otic suspension ℞ *topical corticosteroidal anti-inflammatory; antibiotic* [hydrocortisone; neomycin sulfate; polymyxin B sulfate] 1%•5 mg•10 000 U per mL

**AK-Spore H.C.** eye drop suspension ℞ *topical ophthalmic corticosteroidal anti-inflammatory; antibiotic* [hydrocortisone; neomycin sulfate; polymyxin B sulfate] 1%•0.35%•10 000 U per mL

**AK-Spore H.C.** ointment ℞ *topical ophthalmic corticosteroidal anti-inflammatory; antibiotic* [hydrocortisone; neomycin sulfate; bacitracin zinc; polymyxin B sulfate] 1%•0.35%• 400 U/g•10 000 U/g

**AK-Sulf** eye drops, ophthalmic ointment ℞ *ophthalmic bacteriostatic* [sulfacetamide sodium] 10%

**AK-Taine** eye drops (discontinued 1995) ℞ *topical ophthalmic anesthetic* [proparacaine HCl] 0.5%

**AKTob** eye drops ℞ *ophthalmic antibiotic* [tobramycin] 0.3%

**AK-Tracin** ophthalmic ointment ℞ *ophthalmic antibiotic* [bacitracin] 500 U/g

**AK-Trol** eye drop suspension, ophthalmic ointment ℞ *topical ophthalmic corticosteroidal anti-inflammatory; antibiotic* [dexamethasone; neomycin sulfate; polymyxin B sulfate] 0.1%• 0.35%•10 000 U/mL; 0.1%• 0.35%•10 000 U/g

**Akwa Tears** eye drops OTC *ocular moisturizer/lubricant* [polyvinyl alcohol] 1.4%

**Akwa Tears** ophthalmic ointment OTC *ocular moisturizer/lubricant* [white petrolatum; mineral oil]

**AK-Zol** tablets (discontinued 1993) ℞ *antiglaucoma; anticonvulsant; diuretic* [acetazolamide] 250 mg

**AL-721** *investigational (Phase I/II) antiviral for HIV and AIDS*

**ALA Photodynamic Therapy** ℞ *investigational (Phase III) treatment for psoriasis and actinic keratoses*

**alacepril** INN, JAN

**Ala-Cort** cream, lotion ℞ *topical corticosteroid* [hydrocortisone] 1%

**alafosfalin** INN, BAN

**Alamag** oral suspension OTC *antacid* [aluminum hydroxide; magnesium hydroxide] 225•200 mg/5 mL ☑ Alma-Mag

**Alamag Plus** oral suspension OTC *antacid; antiflatulent* [aluminum hydroxide; magnesium hydroxide; simethicone] 225•200•25 mg/5 mL

**alamecin** USAN *antibacterial*

**alanine (L-alanine)** USAN, USP, INN *nonessential amino acid; symbols: Ala, A*

**alanine nitrogen mustard** [see: melphalan]

**alanosine** INN

**alaproclate** USAN, INN *antidepressant*

**Ala-Quin** cream ℞ *topical corticosteroid; antifungal; antibacterial* [hydrocortisone; clioquinol] 0.5%•3%

**Ala-Scalp** lotion ℞ *topical corticosteroid* [hydrocortisone] 2%

**AlaSTAT** lab test for professional use ℞ *test for allergic reaction to latex*

**Alasulf** vaginal cream ℞ *bacteriostatic antibiotic; antiseptic; vulnerary* [sulfanilamide; aminacrine HCl; allantoin] 15%•0.2%•2%

**Alatone** tablets (discontinued 1993) ℞ *potassium-sparing diuretic* [spironolactone]

**alatrofloxacin mesylate** USAN *antibacterial*

**alazanine triclofenate** INN

**Alazide** tablets (discontinued 1993) ℞ *diuretic* [spironolactone; hydrochlorothiazide]

**Alazine** tablets (discontinued 1993) ℞ *antihypertensive; vasodilator* [hydralazine HCl]

**Albalon** eye drops ℞ *topical ocular decongestant/vasoconstrictor; ocular lubricant* [naphazoline HCl; polyvinyl alcohol] 0.1%•1.4%

**Albalon-A Liquifilm** eye drops (discontinued 1993) ℞ *topical ocular decongestant and antihistamine* [naphazoline HCl; antazoline phosphate]

**Albamycin** capsules ℞ *bacteriostatic antibiotic* [novobiocin sodium] 250 mg

**Albay** subcu or IM injection ℞ *venom sensitivity testing (subcu); venom*

*desensitization therapy (IM)* [extract of honeybee, yellow jacket, yellow hornet, white-faced hornet, wasp, and mixed vespid]

**albendazole** USAN, INN, BAN *anthelmintic for neurocysticercosis and hydatid cyst disease (orphan); investigational (Phase III) for AIDS-related microsporidiosis*

**albendazole oxide** INN, BAN

**Albenza** Tiltab (film-coated tablets) ℞ *anthelmintic for neurocysticercosis (tapeworm) and cestode-induced hydatid cyst disease (orphan)* [albendazole]

**Albright solution (sodium citrate and citric acid)** *urine alkalizer; compounding agent*

**albucid** [see: sulfacetamide]

**albumin, aggregated** USAN *lung imaging aid (with technetium Tc 99m)*

**albumin, aggregated iodinated I 131 serum** USAN, USP *radioactive agent*

**albumin, chromated Cr 51 serum** USAN *radioactive agent*

**albumin, human** USP *blood volume supporter* 5%, 25% injection

**albumin, human (sonicated)** *ultrasound heart imaging agent; investigational (Phase III) diagnostic aid for infertility due to obstructed fallopian tubes*

**albumin, iodinated ($^{125}$I) human serum** INN *radioactive agent; blood volume test* [also: albumin, iodinated I 125 serum]

**albumin, iodinated ($^{131}$I) human serum** INN, JAN *radioactive agent; intrathecal imaging agent; blood volume test* [also: albumin, iodinated I 131 serum]

**albumin, iodinated I 125** USP *radioactive agent; blood volume test*

**albumin, iodinated I 125 serum** USAN, USP *radioactive agent; blood volume test* [also: iodinated ($^{125}$I) human serum albumin]

**albumin, iodinated I 131** USP *radioactive agent; intrathecal imaging agent; blood volume test*

**albumin, iodinated I 131 serum** USAN, USP *radioactive agent; intrathecal imaging agent; blood volume test*

[also: iodinated ($^{131}$I) human serum albumin]

**albumin, normal human serum** [now: albumin, human]

**Albuminar-5; Albuminar-25** IV infusion ℞ *blood volume expander for shock, burns, and hypoproteinemia* [human albumin] 5%; 25%

**Albunex** injection ℞ *ultrasound heart imaging agent; investigational (Phase III) diagnostic aid for infertility due to obstructed fallopian tubes* [albumin, human (sonicated)] 5%

**Albustix** reagent strips for professional use *in vitro diagnostic aid for albumin (protein) in the urine*

**Albutein 5%; Albutein 25%** IV infusion ℞ *blood volume expander for shock, burns, and hypoproteinemia* [human albumin] 5%; 25%

**albuterol** USAN, USP *bronchodilator* [also: salbutamol]

**albuterol sulfate** USAN, USP *bronchodilator* [also: salbutamol sulfate] 2, 4 mg oral; 2 mg/5 mL oral; 0.083%, 0.5% inhalation; 90 μg aerosol

**albutoin** USAN, INN *anticonvulsant*

**Alcaine** Drop-Tainers (eye drops) ℞ *topical ophthalmic anesthetic* [proparacaine HCl] 0.5%

**Alcar** ℞ *investigational treatment for Alzheimer's disease* [levacecarnine]

**ALCAR (acetyl-L-carnitine)** [q.v.]

**Alcare** foam OTC *topical antiseptic* [ethyl alcohol] 62%

**alclofenac** USAN, INN, BAN, JAN *anti-inflammatory*

**alclometasone** INN, BAN *topical corticosteroidal anti-inflammatory* [also: alclometasone dipropionate]

**alclometasone dipropionate** USAN, USP, JAN *topical corticosteroidal anti-inflammatory* [also: alclometasone]

**alcloxa** USAN, INN *astringent; keratolytic* [also: aluminum chlorohydroxy allantoinate]

**Alco-Gel** OTC *topical antiseptic for instant sanitation of hands* [ethyl alcohol] 60% aloe gel

**alcohol** USP *topical anti-infective/antiseptic; astringent; solvent; a widely* *abused "legal street drug" used to produce euphoria* [also: ethanol]

**alcohol, dehydrated** USP *antidote* [also: ethanol, dehydrated]

**alcohol, diluted** NF *solvent*

**alcohol, rubbing** USP, INN *rubefacient*

**5% Alcohol and 5% Dextrose in Water; 10% Alcohol and 5% Dextrose in Water** IV infusion ℞ *for caloric replacement and rehydration* [alcohol; dextrose] 5%•5%; 10%•5%

**Alcon Saline Especially for Sensitive Eyes** solution OTC *rinsing/storage solution for soft contact lenses* [preserved saline solution]

**Alconefrin** nose drops, nasal spray OTC *nasal decongestant* [phenylephrine HCl] 0.25%, 0.5%

**Alconefrin 12** nose drops OTC *nasal decongestant* [phenylephrine HCl] 0.16%

**alcuronium chloride** USAN, INN, BAN, JAN *skeletal muscle relaxant*

**Aldactazide** tablets ℞ *diuretic; antihypertensive* [spironolactone; hydrochlorothiazide] 25•25, 50•50 mg ▣ Aldactone

**Aldactone** tablets ℞ *potassium-sparing diuretic* [spironolactone] 25, 50, 100 mg ▣ Aldactazide

**Aldara** cream (250 mg single-use packets) ℞ *immunomodulator for external genital and perianal warts* [imiquimod] 5%

**alderlin** [see: pronethalol]

**aldesleukin** USAN, INN, BAN *antineoplastic; biologic response modifier; immunostimulant; investigational (orphan) for immunodeficiency diseases*

**aldesulfone sodium** INN, DCF *antibacterial; leprostatic* [also: sulfoxone sodium]

**aldioxa** USAN, INN, JAN *astringent; keratolytic*

**Aldoclor-150; Aldoclor-250** film-coated tablets ℞ *antihypertensive* [chlorothiazide; methyldopa] 150•250 mg; 250•250 mg

**aldocorten** [see: aldosterone]

**Aldomet** film-coated tablets, oral suspension ℞ *antihypertensive* [methyldopa] 125, 250, 500 mg; 250 mg/5 mL

**Aldomet** IV injection ℞ *antihypertensive* [methyldopate HCl] 50 mg/mL ▣ Aldoril

**Aldoril 15; Aldoril 25; Aldoril D30; Aldoril D50** film-coated tablets ℞ *antihypertensive* [hydrochlorothiazide; methyldopa] 15•250 mg; 25•250 mg; 30•500 mg; 50•500 mg ▣ Aldomet; Elavil

**aldosterone** INN, BAN, DCF

**Alec** ℞ *investigational (orphan) for neonatal respiratory distress syndrome* [colfosceril palmitate; phosphatidylglycerol]

**alendronate sodium** USAN *bisphosphonate bone resorption inhibitor for postmenopausal osteoporosis and Paget's disease*

**alendronic acid** INN, BAN

**Alenic Alka** chewable tablets OTC *antacid* [aluminum hydroxide; magnesium trisilicate] 80•20 mg

**Alenic Alka** liquid OTC *antacid* [aluminum hydroxide; magnesium carbonate] 31.7•137.3 mg/5 mL

**Alenic Alka, Extra Strength** chewable tablets OTC *antacid* [aluminum hydroxide; magnesium carbonate] 160•105 mg

**alentemol** INN *antipsychotic; dopamine agonist* [also: alentemol hydrobromide]

**alentemol hydrobromide** USAN *antipsychotic; dopamine agonist* [also: alentemol]

**alepride** INN

**Alersule** sustained-release capsules (discontinued 1995) ℞ *decongestant; antihistamine* [phenylephrine HCl; chlorpheniramine maleate] 20•8 mg

**Alesse** tablets (21 or 28 per pack) ℞ *monophasic oral contraceptive* [levonorgestrel; ethinyl estradiol] 100•20 μg

**alestramustine** INN

**aletamine HCl** USAN *antidepressant* [also: alfetamine]

**Aleve** tablets OTC *nonsteroidal anti-inflammatory drug (NSAID); antiarthritic; analgesic* [naproxen (from naproxen sodium)] 200 (220) mg

**alexidine** USAN, INN *antibacterial*

**alexitol sodium** INN, BAN

**alexomycin** USAN *veterinary growth promoter for poultry and swine*

**alfacalcidol** INN, BAN, JAN
**alfadex** INN
**alfadolone** INN, DCF [also: alphadolone]
**alfaprostol** USAN, INN, BAN *veterinary prostaglandin*
**alfaxalone** INN, JAN, DCF [also: alphaxalone]
**Alfenta** IV or IM injection ℞ *narcotic agonist analgesic; anesthetic* [alfentanil HCl] 500 μg/mL
**alfentanil** INN, BAN *narcotic agonist analgesic* [also: alfentanil HCl]
**alfentanil HCl** USAN *narcotic agonist analgesic* [also: alfentanil]
**Alferon LDO** (low dose oral) ℞ *investigational (Phase I/II) cytokine for AIDS and ARC* [interferon alfa-n3]
**Alferon N** intralesional injection ℞ *antineoplastic for condylomata acuminata; investigational (Phase III) cytokine for HIV, AIDS, ARC, and hepatitis C* [interferon alfa-n3] 5 mIU
**alfetamine** INN *antidepressant* [also: aletamine HCl]
**alfetamine HCl** [see: aletamine HCl]
**alfuzosin** INN, BAN *antihypertensive (α-blocker); investigational treatment for urinary incontinence* [also: alfuzosin HCl]
**alfuzosin HCl** USAN *antihypertensive (α-blocker); investigational treatment for urinary incontinence* [also: alfuzosin]
**algeldrate** USAN, INN *antacid*
**Algenic Alka** liquid OTC *antacid* [aluminum hydroxide; magnesium carbonate; EDTA]
**Algenic Alka Improved** chewable tablets OTC *antacid* [aluminum hydroxide; sodium bicarbonate; magnesium trisilicate]
**algestone** INN *anti-inflammatory* [also: algestone acetonide]
**algestone acetonide** USAN, BAN *anti-inflammatory* [also: algestone]
**algestone acetophenide** USAN *progestin*
**algin** [see: sodium alginate]
**alginic acid** NF, BAN *tablet binder and emulsifying agent*
**alginic acid, sodium salt** [see: sodium alginate]

**alglucerase** USAN, INN, BAN *glucocerebrosidase enzyme replacement for Gaucher's disease type I (orphan); investigational (orphan) for type II and III*
**alibendol** INN, DCF
**Alice B. Toklas** *street drug slang for marijuana brownies* [see: marijuana]
**aliconazole** INN
**alidine dihydrochloride** [see: anileridine]
**alidine phosphate** [see: anileridine]
**alifedrine** INN
**aliflurane** USAN, INN *inhalation anesthetic*
**alimadol** INN
**alimemazine** INN *antipruritic; antihistamine* [also: trimeprazine tartrate; trimeprazine; alimemazine tartrate]
**alimemazine tartrate** JAN *antipruritic; antihistamine* [also: trimeprazine tartrate; alimemazine; trimeprazine]
**Alimentum** ready-to-use liquid OTC *hypoallergenic infant food* [casein protein formula]
**alinidine** INN, BAN
**alipamide** USAN, INN, BAN *diuretic; antihypertensive*
**aliphatic alcohol compound** *investigational (Phase III) topical antiviral treatment for herpes simplex*
**alisactide** [see: alsactide]
**alisobumal** [see: butalbital]
**alitame** USAN *sweetener*
**alizapride** INN
**Alkaban-AQ** IV injection (discontinued 1995) ℞ *antineoplastic* [vinblastine sulfate] 1 mg/mL
**Alka-Mints** chewable tablets OTC *antacid* [calcium carbonate] 850 mg
**Alka-Seltzer** effervescent tablets OTC *antacid; analgesic* [sodium bicarbonate; citric acid; aspirin; phenylalanine] 1700•1000•325•9 mg
**Alka-Seltzer, Extra Strength** effervescent tablets OTC *antacid; analgesic* [sodium bicarbonate; citric acid; aspirin] 1985•1000•500 mg
**Alka-Seltzer, Gold** effervescent tablets OTC *antacid* [sodium bicarbonate; citric acid; potassium bicarbonate] 958•832•312 mg
**Alka-Seltzer, Original** effervescent tablets OTC *antacid; analgesic* [sodium

bicarbonate; citric acid; aspirin]
1916•1000•325 mg

**Alka-Seltzer Advanced Formula**
effervescent tablets (discontinued
1994) OTC *antacid; analgesic* [sodium
bicarbonate; calcium carbonate;
acetaminophen; citric acid; potassium bicarbonate] 465•280•325•
900•300 mg

**Alka-Seltzer Plus Allergy Liqui-Gels;
Alka-Seltzer Plus Cold Liqui-Gels**
(capsules) OTC *decongestant; antihistamine; analgesic* [pseudoephedrine HCl;
chlorpheniramine maleate; acetamin-
ophen] 30•2•250 mg

**Alka-Seltzer Plus Cold & Cough**
tablets OTC *antitussive; decongestant;
antihistamine; analgesic; antipyretic*
[dextromethorphan hydrobromide;
phenylpropanolamine bitartrate;
chlorpheniramine maleate; aspirin]
10•20•2•325 mg

**Alka-Seltzer Plus Cold & Cough
Liqui-Gels** (capsules) OTC *antitussive; decongestant; antihistamine; analgesic* [dextromethorphan hydrobromide; pseudoephedrine HCl;
chlorpheniramine maleate; aceta-
minophen] 10•30•2•250 mg

**Alka-Seltzer Plus Cold Medicine;
Alka-Seltzer Plus Cold Tablets**
for oral solution OTC *decongestant;
antihistamine; analgesic; antipyretic*
[phenylpropanolamine bitartrate;
brompheniramine maleate; aspirin]
20•2•325 mg; 24.08•2•325 mg

**Alka-Seltzer Plus Flu & Body
Aches Non-Drowsy Liqui-Gels**
(capsules) OTC *antitussive; decongestant; analgesic* [dextromethorphan
hydrobromide; pseudoephedrine HCl;
acetaminophen] 10•30•250 mg

**Alka-Seltzer Plus Night-Time Cold**
tablets OTC *antitussive; decongestant;
antihistamine; analgesic; antipyretic*
[dextromethorphan hydrobromide;
phenylpropanolamine bitartrate;
doxylamine succinate; aspirin] 10•
20•6.25•500 mg

**Alka-Seltzer Plus Night-Time Cold
Liqui-Gels** (capsules) OTC *antitussive; decongestant; antihistamine; analgesic* [dextromethorphan hydrobromide; pseudoephedrine HCl; doxylamine succinate; acetaminophen]
10•30•6.25•250 mg

**Alka-Seltzer Plus Sinus** tablets OTC
*decongestant; analgesic; antipyretic*
[phenylpropanolamine bitartrate;
aspirin] 20•325 mg

**Alka-Seltzer Plus Sinus Allergy** tablets (discontinued 1995) OTC *decongestant; antihistamine; analgesic; antipyretic* [phenylpropanolamine
bitartrate; brompheniramine maleate; aspirin] 24.08•2•500 mg

**Alka-Seltzer with Aspirin** effervescent tablets OTC *antacid; analgesic*
[sodium bicarbonate; citric acid;
aspirin] 1900•1000•325, 1900•
1000•500 mg

**alkavervir (Veratrum viride alka-
loids)**

**Alkeran** tablets, powder for IV infusion ℞ *nitrogen mustard-type alkylating antineoplastic for multiple myeloma
and ovarian cancer; investigational
(orphan) for metastatic melanoma*
[melphalan] 2 mg; 50 mg

**Alkets** chewable tablets OTC *antacid*
[calcium carbonate] 500, 750 mg

**alkyl aryl sulfonate** *surfactant/wet-
ting agent*

**alkylamines** *a class of antihistamines*

**alkylbenzyldimethylammonium
chloride** [see: benzalkonium chloride]

**alkyldimethylbenzylammonium
chloride** [see: benzalkonium chloride]

**alkylpolyaminoethylglycine** JAN

**alkylpolyaminoethylglycine HCl** JAN

**all-American drug** *street drug slang*
[see: cocaine]

**allantoin** USAN, BAN *topical vulnerary*

**Allbee C-800** film-coated tablets OTC
*vitamin supplement* [multiple B vitamins; vitamins C and E] ≛•800•45
mg

**Allbee C-800 plus Iron** film-coated
tablets OTC *vitamin/iron supplement*
[ferrous fumarate; multiple B vitamins; vitamins C and E; folic acid]
27 mg•≛•800 mg•45 IU•0.4 mg

**Allbee with C** caplets OTC *vitamin supplement* [multiple B vitamins; vitamin C] ≜ •300 mg

**Allbee-T** tablets OTC *vitamin supplement* [multiple B vitamins; vitamin C] ≜ •500 mg

**Allegra** capsules ℞ *nonsedating antihistamine* [fexofenadine HCl] 60 mg

**allegron** [see: nortriptyline]

**Allent** sustained-release capsules ℞ *decongestant; antihistamine* [pseudoephedrine HCl; brompheniramine maleate] 120•12 mg

**Aller-Chlor** tablets, syrup OTC *antihistamine* [chlorpheniramine maleate] 4 mg; 2 mg/5 mL

**Allercon** tablets OTC *decongestant; antihistamine* [pseudoephedrine HCl; triprolidine HCl] 60•2.5 mg

**Allercreme Skin** lotion OTC *moisturizer; emollient*

**Allercreme Ultra Emollient** cream OTC *moisturizer; emollient*

**Allerest** eye drops OTC *topical ocular decongestant/vasoconstrictor* [naphazoline HCl] 0.012%

**Allerest** tablets OTC *decongestant; antihistamine* [pseudoephedrine HCl; chlorpheniramine maleate] 30•2 mg

**Allerest, Children's** chewable tablets OTC *pediatric decongestant and antihistamine* [phenylpropanolamine HCl; chlorpheniramine maleate] 9.4•1 mg

**Allerest 12 Hour** nasal spray OTC *nasal decongestant* [oxymetazoline HCl] 0.05%

**Allerest 12 Hour** sustained-release caplets OTC *decongestant; antihistamine* [phenylpropanolamine HCl; chlorpheniramine maleate] 75•12 mg

**Allerest Headache; Allerest Sinus Pain Formula** tablets OTC *decongestant; antihistamine; analgesic* [pseudoephedrine HCl; chlorpheniramine maleate; acetaminophen] 30•2•325 mg; 30•2•500 mg

**Allerest No Drowsiness** tablets OTC *decongestant; analgesic* [pseudoephedrine HCl; acetaminophen] 30•325 mg

**Allerfrim** tablets, syrup OTC *decongestant; antihistamine* [pseudoephedrine HCl; triprolidine HCl] 60•2.5 mg; 30•1.25 mg/5 mL

**Allerfrin with Codeine** syrup ℞ *narcotic antitussive; decongestant; antihistamine* [codeine phosphate; pseudoephedrine HCl; triprolidine HCl] 10•30•1.25 mg/5 mL

**Allergan Enzymatic** tablets OTC *enzymatic cleaner for soft contact lenses* [papain] ⑫ allergen; Auralgan

**Allergan Hydrocare** [see: Hydrocare]

**Allergen Ear Drops** ℞ *topical local anesthetic; analgesic* [benzocaine; antipyrine] 1.4%•5.4%

**allergenic extracts** *a class of agents derived from various biological sources containing antigens which possess immunologic activity*

**allergenic extracts (aqueous, glycerinated, or alum-precipitated)** *over 900 allergens available for diagnosis of and desensitization to specific allergies*

**Allergy** tablets OTC *antihistamine* [chlorpheniramine maleate] 4 mg

**Allergy Cold** tablets (discontinued 1995) OTC *decongestant; antihistamine* [pseudoephedrine HCl; triprolidine HCl] 60•2.5 mg

**Allergy Drops** eye drops OTC *topical ocular decongestant/vasoconstrictor* [naphazoline HCl] 0.012%; 0.03%

**Allergy Relief Medicine** tablets (discontinued 1995) OTC *decongestant; antihistamine* [phenylpropanolamine HCl; chlorpheniramine maleate] 25•4 mg

**AlleRid** capsules OTC *decongestant* [pseudoephedrine HCl]

**AllerMax** caplets, oral liquid OTC *antihistamine* [diphenhydramine HCl] 25, 50 mg; 12.5 mg/5 mL

**Allermed** capsules OTC *nasal decongestant* [pseudoephedrine HCl] 60 mg

**Allerphed** syrup OTC *decongestant; antihistamine* [pseudoephedrine HCl; triprolidine HCl] 30•1.25 mg/5 mL

**Allervax** ℞ *investigational antiallergic*

**alletorphine** BAN, INN

**All-Nite Cold Formula** liquid OTC *antitussive; decongestant; antihistamine; analgesic* [dextromethorphan hydrobromide; pseudoephedrine HCl; doxylamine succinate; acetaminophen; alcohol 25%] 5•10•1.25•167 mg/5 mL

**allobarbital** USAN, INN *hypnotic*

**allobarbitone** [see: allobarbital]

**alloclamide** INN, DCF

**allocupreide sodium** INN, DCF

**Alloderm** *investigational skin graft for third-degree burns and plastic surgery* [processed human donor skin]

**allomethadione** INN, DCF [also: aloxidone]

**allopurinol** USAN, USP, INN, BAN, JAN *xanthine oxidase inhibitor for gout and hyperuricemia; orphan status withdrawn 1994* 100, 300 mg oral

**allopurinol riboside** *orphan status withdrawn 1996*

**allopurinol sodium** *antineoplastic for leukemia, lymphoma, and solid tumor malignancies (orphan)*

**Allpyral** subcu or IM injection ℞ *allergenic sensitivity testing (subcu); allergenic desensitization therapy (IM)* [allergenic extracts, alum-precipitated]

**all-*trans*-retinoic acid** [see: tretinoin]

**allyl isothiocyanate** USAN, USP

**allylamines** *a class of antifungals*

**allylbarbituric acid** [now: butalbital]

**allylestrenol** INN, JAN [also: allyloestrenol]

**allyl-isobutylbarbituric acid** [see: butalbital]

**allylisopropylmalonylurea** [see: aprobarbital]

**4-allyl-2-methoxyphenol** [see: eugenol]

**N-allylnoretorphine** [see: alletorphine]

**N-allylnoroxymorphone HCl** [see: naloxone HCl]

**allyloestrenol** BAN [also: allylestrenol]

**allylprodine** INN, BAN, DCF

**5-allyl-5-*sec*-butylbarbituric acid** [see: talbutal]

**allylthiourea** INN

**allypropymal** [see: aprobarbital]

**Almacone** chewable tablets, liquid OTC *antacid; antiflatulent* [aluminum hydroxide; magnesium hydroxide; simethicone] 200•200•20 mg; 200•200•20 mg/5 mL

**Almacone II** liquid OTC *antacid; antiflatulent* [aluminum hydroxide; magnesium hydroxide; simethicone] 400•400•40 mg/5 mL

**almadrate sulfate** USAN, INN *antacid*

**almagate** USAN, INN *antacid*

**almagodrate** INN

**Alma-Mag** oral suspension (discontinued 1994) OTC *antacid* [aluminum hydroxide; magnesium hydroxide] ℞ Alamag

**Alma-Mag, Improved** liquid (discontinued 1994) OTC *antacid; antiflatulent* [aluminum hydroxide; magnesium hydroxide; simethicone] 40•40•5 mg/mL

**Alma-Mag #4 Improved** chewable tablets (discontinued 1994) OTC *antacid; antiflatulent* [aluminum hydroxide; magnesium hydroxide; simethicone] 200•200•25 mg

**almasilate** INN, BAN

**Almebex Plus B₁₂** liquid OTC *vitamin supplement* [multiple B vitamins] ≐

**almecillin** INN

**almestrone** INN

**alminoprofen** INN, JAN

**almitrine** INN, BAN

**almokalant** INN *investigational antiarrhythmic*

**almond oil** NF *emollient and perfume; oleaginous vehicle*

**Almora** tablets OTC *magnesium supplement* [magnesium gluconate] 500 mg

**almoxatone** INN

**alnespirone** INN

**alniditan dihydrochloride** USAN *serotonin 5-HT₁D agonist for migraine*

**Alodopa-15; Alodopa-25** tablets ℞ *antihypertensive* [hydrochlorothiazide; methyldopa]

**aloe** USP ℞ Alco-Gel

**Aloe Grande** lotion OTC *moisturizer; emollient; skin protectant* [vitamins A and E; aloe] 3333.3•50•≐ U/g

**Aloe Vesta Perineal** solution OTC *emollient/protectant* [propylene glycol; aloe vera gel]

**alofilcon A** USAN *hydrophilic contact lens material*

**aloin** BAN

**ALOMAD (Adriamycin, Leukeran, Oncovin, methotrexate, actino-mycin D, dacarbazine)** *chemother-apy protocol* ⑨ Alomide

**Alomide** Drop-Tainers (eye drops) ℞ *antiallergic agent for vernal keratocon-junctivitis (orphan)* [lodoxamide tro-methamine] 0.1% ⑨ ALOMAD

**alonacic** INN

**alonimid** USAN, INN *sedative; hypnotic*

**Alophen Pills** tablets OTC *laxative* [phenolphthalein] 60 mg

**Alophen Pills No. 973** tablets (name changed to Alophen Pills in 1995)

**Alor 5/500** tablets ℞ *narcotic analge-sic* [hydrocodone bitartrate; aspirin] 5•500 mg

**Alora** transdermal patch ℞ *estrogen replacement therapy for postmenopausal disorders* [estradiol] 50, 75, 100 μg/day

**aloracetam** INN

**alosetron** INN, BAN *antiemetic* [also: alosetron HCl]

**alosetron HCl** USAN *antiemetic; inves-tigational antipsychotic for schizophre-nia (clinical trials discontinued 1994)* [also: alosetron]

**alovudine** USAN, INN *antiviral*

**aloxidone** BAN [also: allomethadione]

**aloxiprin** INN, BAN, DCF

**aloxistatin** INN

**alozafone** INN

**alpertine** USAN, INN *antipsychotic*

**alpha amylase (α-amylase)** USAN *anti-inflammatory*

**alpha hydroxy acids (AHA)** [see: glycolic acid]

**alpha interferon-2A** [see: interferon alfa-2A]

**alpha interferon-2B** [see: interferon alfa-2B]

**alpha interferon-N1** [see: interferon alfa-N1]

**alpha interferon-N3** [see: interferon alfa-N3]

**Alpha Keri Moisturizing Soap** bar OTC *therapeutic skin cleanser*

**Alpha Keri Spray; Alpha Keri Therapeutic Bath Oil** OTC *bath emollient*

**d-alpha tocopherol** [see: vitamin E]

**dl-alpha tocopherol** [see: vitamin E]

**d-alpha tocopheryl acetate** [see: vit-amin E]

**dl-alpha tocopheryl acetate** [see: vitamin E]

**d-alpha tocopheryl acid succinate** [see: vitamin E]

**dl-alpha tocopheryl acid succinate** [see: vitamin E]

**Alpha Zeta** tablets (discontinued 1994) OTC *vitamin/mineral/iron sup-plement* [ferrous fumarate; multiple vitamins & minerals; folic acid; bio-tin] 27 mg• ± •0.4 mg•45 μg

**alpha$_1$ PI (alpha$_1$-proteinase inhibi-tor)** [q.v.]

**alpha$_1$-antitrypsin, recombinant** *investigational (orphan) for alpha$_1$-antitrypsin deficiency in the ZZ pheno-type population*

**alpha$_1$-proteinase inhibitor (alpha$_1$ PI)** *investigational (Phase II) antiviral for HIV; replacement therapy for con-genital alpha$_1$ PI deficiency (orphan)*

**l-alpha-acetyl-methadol (LAAM)** *orphan status withdrawn 1996*

**alphacemethadone** [see: alphacetyl-methadol]

**alphacetylmethadol** BAN, INN, DCF

**alpha-chymotrypsin** [see: chymotryp-sin]

**alpha-cypermethrin** BAN

**alpha-D-galactosidase** *digestive enzyme*

**alphadolone** BAN [also: alfadolone]

**alpha-estradiol** [see: estradiol]

**alpha-estradiol benzoate** [see: estra-diol benzoate]

**alpha-ET** *street drug slang* [see: alpha-ethyltryptamine]

**alpha-ethyltryptamine (alpha-EtT)** *a hallucinogenic street drug chemically related to MDMA* [see also: MDMA; alpha-methyltryptamine]

**alphafilcon A** USAN *hydrophilic contact lens material*

**alpha-galactosidase A** *investigational (orphan) for Fabry's disease*

**alpha-galactosidase A & ceramide trihexosidase (CTH)** *investigational (orphan) for Fabry's disease*

**Alphagan** eye drops ℞ *selective α$_2$ ago-nist for open-angle glaucoma and ocu-*

*lar hypertension* [brimonidine tartrate] 0.2%

**alpha-glucosidase, human acid** [see: human acid alpha-glucosidase]

**1-alpha-hydroxy vitamin D$_2$** *investigational osteoporosis treatment*

**alpha-hypophamine** [see: oxytocin]

**alphameprodine** INN, BAN, DCF

**alphamethadol** INN, BAN, DCF

**alpha-methyldopa** [now: methyldopa]

**alpha-methyltryptamine (alpha-MeT)** *a hallucinogenic street drug chemically related to MDMA* [see also: MDMA; alpha-ethyltryptamine]

**Alphamin** IM injection (discontinued 1994) ℞ *antianemic; vitamin B$_{12}$ supplement* [hydroxocobalamin] 1000 µg/mL

**Alphamul** emulsion (discontinued 1994) OTC *stimulant laxative* [castor oil] 60%

**Alphanate** powder for IV injection ℞ *antihemophilic; investigational (orphan) for von Willebrand's disease* [antihemophilic factor VIII:C, solvent/detergent treated] ²

**AlphaNine** IV injection (discontinued 1997; replaced by AlphaNine SD) ℞ *antihemophilic for factor IX deficiency (hemophilia B; Christmas disease) (orphan)* [coagulation factor IX (human)]

**AlphaNine SD** IV injection ℞ *antihemophilic for factor IX deficiency (hemophilia B; Christmas disease) (orphan)* [coagulation factors II, VII, IX, and X, solvent/detergent treated]

**alpha-phenoxyethyl penicillin, potassium** [see: phenethicillin potassium]

**alphaprodine** INN, BAN [also: alphaprodine HCl]

**alphaprodine HCl** USP [also: alphaprodine]

**alphasone acetophenide** [now: algestone acetonide]

**Alphatrex** cream, ointment, lotion ℞ *topical corticosteroid* [betamethasone dipropionate] 0.05%

**alphaxalone** BAN [also: alfaxalone]

**Alphosyl** lotion OTC *topical antipsoriatic; antiseborrheic; vulnerary* [coal tar extract; allantoin]

**alpidem** USAN, INN, BAN *anxiolytic*

**alpiropride** INN

**alprafenone** INN

**alprazolam** USAN, USP, INN, BAN, JAN *anxiolytic; sedative; treatment of panic disorders and agoraphobia* 0.25, 0.5, 1, 2 mg, 0.5 mg/5 mL, 1 mg/mL oral

**alprenolol** INN, BAN *antiadrenergic (β-receptor)* [also: alprenolol HCl]

**alprenolol HCl** USAN, JAN *antiadrenergic (β-receptor)* [also: alprenolol]

**alprenoxime HCl** USAN *antiglaucoma agent*

**alprostadil** USAN, USP, INN, BAN, JAN *vasodilator for erectile dysfunction; platelet aggregation inhibitor; investigational (orphan) for peripheral arterial occlusive disease*

**alprostadil, liposomal** *investigational (Phase III) for erectile dysfunction; investigational (orphan) for ischemic ulcerations of peripheral artery disease and acute respiratory distress*

**alprostadil alfadex** BAN

**Alramucil** effervescent powder OTC *bulk laxative* [psyllium hydrophilic mucilloid] 3.6 g/packet

**Alredase** ℞ *investigational aldose reductase inhibitor for diabetic neuropathy* [tolrestat]

**alrestatin** INN *aldose reductase enzyme inhibitor* [also: alrestatin sodium]

**alrestatin sodium** USAN *aldose reductase enzyme inhibitor* [also: alrestatin]

**alsactide** INN

**alseroxylon** JAN *antihypertensive; rauwolfia derivative*

**ALT (autolymphocyte therapy)** [q.v.]

**Altace** capsules ℞ *antihypertensive; angiotensin-converting enzyme (ACE) inhibitor* [ramipril] 1.25, 2.5, 5, 10 mg

**altanserin** INN *serotonin antagonist* [also: altanserin tartrate]

**altanserin tartrate** USAN *serotonin antagonist* [also: altanserin]

**altapizone** INN

**alteconazole** INN

**alteplase** USAN, INN, BAN, JAN *tissue plasminogen activator (tPA) for acute* *myocardial infarction, acute ischemic stroke, or pulmonary embolism*

**ALternaGEL** liquid OTC *antacid* [aluminum hydroxide gel] 600 mg/5 mL

**althiazide** USAN *antihypertensive* [also: altizide]

**altiprimod dihydrochloride** USAN *immunomodulator; anti-inflammatory; antiarthritic*

**altizide** INN, DCF *antihypertensive* [also: althiazide]

**altoqualine** INN

**Altracin** *investigational (orphan) for pseudomembranous enterocolitis* [bacitracin]

**altrenogest** USAN, INN, BAN *veterinary progestin*

**altretamine** USAN, INN, BAN *antineoplastic for advanced ovarian adenocarcinoma (orphan)*

**altumomab** USAN, INN *radiodiagnostic monoclonal antibody for colorectal carcinoma; anticarcinoembryonic antigen (anti-CEA)* [also: indium In 111 altumomab pentetate]

**altumomab pentetate** USAN *monoclonal antibody conjugate* [also: indium In 111 altumomab pentetate]

**Alu-Cap** capsules OTC *antacid* [aluminum hydroxide gel] 400 mg

**Aludrox** oral suspension OTC *antacid; antiflatulent* [aluminum hydroxide; magnesium hydroxide; simethicone] 307•103• $\frac{?}{}$ mg/5 mL

**alukalin** [see: kaolin]

**alum, ammonium** USP *topical astringent*

**alum, potassium** USP *topical astringent* [also: aluminum potassium sulfate]

**Alumadrine** tablets ℞ *decongestant; antihistamine; analgesic* [phenylpropanolamine HCl; chlorpheniramine maleate; acetaminophen] 25•4•500 mg

**alumina & magnesia** USP *antacid*

**aluminopara-aminosalicylate calcium (alumino *p*-aminosalicylate calcium)** JAN

**aluminosilicic acid, magnesium salt hydrate** [see: silodrate]

**aluminum** *element (Al)*

**aluminum, micronized** *astringent*

**aluminum acetate** USP *topical astringent; Burow solution*

**aluminum aminoacetate** [see: dihydroxyaluminum aminoacetate]

**aluminum ammonium sulfate dodecahydrate** [see: alum, ammonium]

**aluminum bismuth oxide** [see: bismuth aluminate]

**aluminum carbonate, basic** USAN, USP *antacid*

**aluminum chlorhydroxide** [now: aluminum chlorhydrate]

**aluminum chlorhydroxide alcohol soluble complex** [now: aluminum chlorhydrex]

**aluminum chloride** USP *topical astringent for hyperhidrosis*

**aluminum chloride, basic** [see: aluminum sesquichlorohydrate]

**aluminum chloride hexahydrate** [see: aluminum chloride]

**aluminum chloride hydroxide hydrate** [see: aluminum chlorohydrate]

**aluminum chlorohydrate** USAN *anhidrotic*

**aluminum chlorohydrex** USAN *topical astringent*

**aluminum chlorohydrol propylene glycol complex** [now: aluminum chlorohydrex]

**aluminum chlorohydroxy allantoinate** JAN *astringent; keratolytic* [also: alcloxa]

**aluminum clofibrate** INN, BAN, JAN

**aluminum dihydroxyaminoacetate** [see: dihydroxyaluminum aminoacetate]

**aluminum flufenamate** JAN

**aluminum glycinate, basic** [see: dihydroxyaluminum aminoacetate]

**aluminum hydroxide gel** USP *antacid* 320, 450, 600 mg/5 mL oral

**aluminum hydroxide gel, dried** USP, JAN *antacid*

**aluminum hydroxide glycine** [see: dihydroxyaluminum aminoacetate]

**aluminum hydroxide hydrate** [see: algeldrate]

**aluminum hydroxychloride** [now: aluminum chlorohydrate]

**aluminum magnesium carbonate hydroxide dihydrate** [see: almagate] aluminum magnesium hydroxide carbonate hydrate [see: hydrotalcite]

aluminum magnesium hydroxide oxide sulfate [see: almadrate sulfate]

aluminum magnesium hydroxide oxide sulfate hydrate [see: almadrate sulfate]

aluminum magnesium hydroxide sulfate [see: magaldrate]

aluminum magnesium hydroxide sulfate hydrate [see: magaldrate]

aluminum monostearate NF, JAN

aluminum oxide

Aluminum Paste ointment OTC *occlusive skin protectant* [metallic aluminum] 10%

aluminum phosphate gel USP *antacid (disapproved for use as an antacid in 1989)*

aluminum potassium sulfate JAN *topical astringent* [also: alum, potassium]

aluminum potassium sulfate dodecahydrate [see: alum, potassium]

aluminum sesquichlorohydrate USAN *anhidrotic*

aluminum silicate, natural JAN

aluminum silicate, synthetic JAN

aluminum sodium carbonate hydroxide [see: dihydroxyaluminum sodium carbonate]

aluminum subacetate USP *topical astringent*

aluminum sulfate USP

aluminum sulfate hydrate [see: aluminum sulfate]

aluminum zirconium glycine tetrachloro hydrate complex [see: aluminum zirconium tetrachlorohydrex gly]

aluminum zirconium glycine trichloro hydrate complex [see: aluminum zirconium trichlorohydrex gly]

aluminum zirconium octachlorohydrate USP *anhidrotic*

aluminum zirconium octachlorohydrex gly USP *anhidrotic*

aluminum zirconium pentachlorohydrate USP *anhidrotic*

aluminum zirconium pentachlorohydrex gly USP *anhidrotic*

aluminum zirconium tetrachlorohydrate USP *anhidrotic*

aluminum zirconium tetrachlorohydrex gly USAN, USP *anhidrotic*

aluminum zirconium trichlorohydrate USP *anhidrotic*

aluminum zirconium trichlorohydrex gly USAN, USP *anhidrotic*

Alupent tablets, syrup, inhalation aerosol powder, solution for inhalation ℞ *bronchodilator* [metaproterenol sulfate] 10, 20 mg; 10 mg/5 mL; 0.65 mg/dose; 0.4%, 0.6%, 5%

Alurate elixir ℞ *sedative; hypnotic* [aprobarbital] 40 mg/5 mL

alusulf INN

Alu-Tab film-coated tablets OTC *antacid* [aluminum hydroxide gel] 500 mg

ALVAC-120TMG *investigational (Phase I) vaccine for HIV*

ALVAC-HIV 1 *investigational (Phase I) vaccine for HIV*

alverine INN, BAN *anticholinergic* [also: alverine citrate]

alverine citrate USAN, NF *anticholinergic* [also: alverine]

alvircept sudotox USAN, INN *antiviral; investigational (Phase II) for AIDS*

Al-Vite tablets (discontinued 1993) ℞ *vitamin supplement* [multiple vitamins]

Alzene ℞ *investigational treatment for Alzheimer's disease and epilepsy*

amabevan [see: carbarsone]

amacetam HCl [now: pramiracetam HCl]

amacetam sulfate [now: pramiracetam sulfate]

Amacodone tablets (discontinued 1995) ℞ *narcotic analgesic* [hydrocodone bitartrate; acetaminophen] 5 • 500 mg

amadinone INN *progestin* [also: amadinone acetate]

amadinone acetate USAN *progestin* [also: amadinone]

amafolone INN, BAN

amalgucin

*Amanita muscaria* mushrooms *a species that produces muscarine and ibotenic acid, a psychotropic substance ingested as a street drug*

amanozine INN

**amantadine** INN, BAN *antiviral for influenza A virus; antiparkinsonian* [also: amantadine HCl]

**amantadine HCl** USAN, USP, JAN *antiviral for influenza A virus; antiparkinsonian* [also: amantadine] 100 mg oral; 50 mg/5 mL oral

**amantanium bromide** INN

**amantocillin** INN

**Amaphen** capsules ℞ *analgesic; antipyretic; sedative* [acetaminophen; caffeine; butalbital] 325•40•50 mg

**Amaphen with Codeine #3** capsules (discontinued 1995) ℞ *narcotic analgesic; sedative* [codeine phosphate; acetaminophen; caffeine; butalbital] 30•325•40•50 mg

**amaranth (FD&C Red No. 2)** USP

**amarsan** [see: acetarsone]

**Amaryl** tablets ℞ *once-daily sulfonylurea-type antidiabetic* [glimepiride] 1, 2, 4 mg

**Amatine** (name changed to ProAmatine upon release in 1996)

**ambamustine** INN

**ambasilide** INN *investigational antiarrhythmic*

**ambazone** INN, BAN, DCF

**ambenonium chloride** USP, INN, BAN, JAN *anticholinesterase muscle stimulant*

**ambenoxan** INN, BAN

**Ambenyl Cough** syrup ℞ *narcotic antitussive; antihistamine* [codeine phosphate; bromodiphenhydramine HCl; alcohol 5%] 10•12.5 mg/5 mL ⓓ Aventyl

**Ambenyl-D** liquid OTC *antitussive; decongestant; expectorant* [dextromethorphan hydrobromide; pseudoephedrine HCl; guaifenesin; alcohol 9.5%] 10•30•100 mg/5 mL

**Ambi 10** bar OTC *therapeutic skin cleanser*

**Ambi 10** cream OTC *topical keratolytic for acne* [benzoyl peroxide] 10%

**Ambi Skin Tone** cream OTC *hyperpigmentation bleaching agent; sunscreen* [hydroquinone; padimate O]

**ambicromil** INN, BAN *prophylactic antiallergic* [also: probicromil calcium]

**ambicromil calcium** [see: probicromil calcium]

**Ambien** film-coated tablets ℞ *imidazopyridine-type sedative/hypnotic* [zolpidem tartrate] 5, 10 mg

**AmBisome** ℞ *investigational (orphan) antifungal for cryptococcal meningitis, visceral leishmaniasis, and histoplasmosis* [amphotericin B lipid complex (ABLC)]

**ambomycin** USAN, INN *antineoplastic*

**ambroxol** INN [also: ambroxol HCl]

**ambroxol HCl** JAN [also: ambroxol]

**ambruticin** USAN, INN *antifungal*

**ambucaine** INN, DCF

**ambucetamide** INN, BAN

**ambuphylline** USAN *diuretic; smooth muscle relaxant* [also: bufylline]

**ambuside** USAN, INN, BAN *diuretic*

**ambuterol** [see: mabuterol]

**ambutonium bromide** BAN

**ambutoxate** [see: ambucaine]

**amcinafal** USAN, INN *anti-inflammatory*

**amcinafide** USAN, INN *anti-inflammatory*

**amcinonide** USAN, USP, INN, BAN, JAN *topical corticosteroid*

**Amcort** IM injection ℞ *glucocorticoid* [triamcinolone diacetate] 40 mg/mL

**amdinocillin** USAN, USP *antibacterial* [also: mecillinam]

**amdinocillin pivoxil** USAN *antibacterial* [also: pivmecillinam; pivmecillinam HCl]

**ameban** [see: carbarsone]

**amebarsone** [see: carbarsone]

**amebicides** *a class of drugs that kill amoebae*

**amebucort** INN

**amechol** [see: methacholine chloride]

**amedalin** INN *antidepressant* [also: amedalin HCl]

**amedalin HCl** USAN *antidepressant* [also: amedalin]

**ameltolide** USAN, INN, BAN *anticonvulsant*

**Amen** tablets ℞ *progestin for secondary amenorrhea or abnormal uterine bleeding* [medroxyprogesterone acetate] 10 mg

**amenozine** [see: amanozine]

**Amerge** tablets ℞ *investigational (Phase III) migraine therapy* [naratriptan]

**Americaine** ointment, anorectal ointment, aerosol spray OTC *topical local anesthetic* [benzocaine] 20%

**Americaine Anesthetic Lubricant** gel Ŗ *anesthetic lubricant for upper GI procedures* [benzocaine] 20%

**Americaine First Aid** ointment OTC *topical local anesthetic* [benzocaine] 20%

**Americaine Otic** ear drops Ŗ *topical local anesthetic* [benzocaine] 20%

**americium** *element (Am)*

**Amesec** capsules (discontinued 1993) OTC *antiasthmatic; bronchodilator; decongestant* [aminophylline; ephedrine HCl]

**amesergide** USAN, INN *serotonin antagonist; investigational antidepressant*

**ametantrone** INN *antineoplastic* [also: ametantrone acetate]

**ametantrone acetate** USAN *antineoplastic* [also: ametantrone]

**ametazole** BAN [also: betazole HCl; betazole]

**A-Methapred** powder for injection Ŗ *glucocorticoid; anti-inflammatory; immunosuppressant* [methylprednisolone sodium succinate] 40, 125, 500, 1000 mg/vial

**amethocaine** BAN *topical anesthetic* [also: tetracaine]

**amethocaine HCl** BAN *local anesthetic* [also: tetracaine HCl]

**amethopterin** [now: methotrexate]

**amezepine** INN

**amezinium metilsulfate** INN, JAN

**amfebutamone** INN *aminoketone antidepressant; non-nicotine aid to smoking cessation* [also: bupropion HCl; bupropion]

**amfebutamone HCl** [see: bupropion HCl]

**amfecloral** INN, BAN *anorectic* [also: amphecloral]

**amfenac** INN, BAN *anti-inflammatory* [also: amfenac sodium]

**amfenac sodium** USAN, JAN *anti-inflammatory* [also: amfenac]

**amfepentorex** INN, DCF

**amfepramone** INN, DCF *anorexiant* [also: diethylpropion HCl; diethylpropion]

**amfepramone HCl** *anorexiant* [see: diethylpropion HCl]

**amfetamine** INN *CNS stimulant* [also: amphetamine sulfate; amphetamine]

**amfetaminil** INN

**amfilcon A** USAN *hydrophilic contact lens material*

**amflutizole** USAN, INN *gout suppressant*

**amfodyne** [see: imidecyl iodine]

**amfomycin** INN, DCF *antibacterial* [also: amphomycin]

**amfonelic acid** USAN, INN, BAN *CNS stimulant*

**Amgenal Cough** syrup Ŗ *narcotic antitussive; antihistamine* [codeine phosphate; bromodiphenhydramine HCl] 10•12.5 mg/5 mL

**AMI-227** *investigational contrast agent for magnetic imaging of the heart, brain, and lymphatic system*

**amibiarson** [see: carbarsone]

**Amicar** tablets, syrup, IV infusion Ŗ *systemic hemostatic to control excessive bleeding* [aminocaproic acid] 500 mg; 250 mg/mL; 250 mg/mL ⟲ Amikin

**amicarbalide** INN, BAN

**amicibone** INN

**amicloral** USAN *veterinary food additive*

**amicycline** USAN, INN *antibacterial*

**amidantel** INN, BAN

**amidapsone** USAN, INN *antiviral for poultry*

**Amidate** IV injection Ŗ *rapid-acting nonbarbiturate general anesthetic* [etomidate] 2 mg/mL

**amidefrine mesilate** INN *adrenergic* [also: amidephrine mesylate; amidephrine]

**amidephrine** BAN *adrenergic* [also: amidephrine mesylate; amidefrine mesilate]

**amidephrine mesylate** USAN *adrenergic* [also: amidefrine mesilate; amidephrine]

**amidofebrin** [see: aminopyrine]

**amidol** [see: dimepheptanol]

**amidone HCl** [see: methadone HCl]

**amidopyrazoline** [see: aminopyrine]

**amidopyrine** [now: aminopyrine]

**amidotrizoate sodium** [see: diatrizoate sodium]

**amidotrizoic acid** JAN *radiopaque medium* [also: diatrizoic acid]

**Ami-Drix** sustained-release tablets (discontinued 1995) Ŗ *decongestant; antihistamine* [pseudoephedrine sulfate; dexbrompheniramine maleate] 120•6 mg

**amiflamine** INN

**amifloverine** INN, DCF

**amifloxacin** USAN, INN, BAN *broad-spectrum fluoroquinolone-type antibiotic*

**amifloxacin mesylate** USAN *antibacterial*

**amifostine** USAN, INN, BAN *topical radioprotectant; chemoprotective agent for cisplatin and paclitaxel (orphan); investigational (orphan) for cyclophosphamide rescue* [USAN *previously used:* ethiofos]

**Amigesic** film-coated tablets, film-coated caplets, capsules ℞ *analgesic; antipyretic; anti-inflammatory; antirheumatic* [salsalate] 500 mg; 750 mg; 500 mg

**AMI-HS** *investigational contrast agent for magnetic imaging of the liver*

**amikacin** USP, INN, BAN *antibacterial*

**amikacin sulfate** USAN, USP, JAN *aminoglycoside bactericidal antibiotic* 50, 250 mg/mL injection

**amikhelline** INN

**Amikin** IV or IM injection, pediatric injection ℞ *aminoglycoside-type antibiotic* [amikacin sulfate] 250 mg/mL; 50 mg/mL ☑ Amicar

**amilomer** INN

**amiloride** INN, BAN *potassium-sparing diuretic* [also: amiloride HCl]

**amiloride HCl** USAN, USP *potassium-sparing diuretic; investigational (orphan) for cystic fibrosis* [also: amiloride]

**aminacrine** BAN *topical anti-infective/antiseptic* [also: aminacrine HCl; aminoacridine]

**aminacrine HCl** USAN *topical anti-infective/antiseptic* [also: aminoacridine; aminacrine]

**Amin-Aid Instant Drink** powder (discontinued 1997) OTC *enteral nutritional therapy for acute or chronic renal failure* [essential amino acids]

**aminarsone** [see: carbarsone]

**amindocate** INN

**amine resin** [see: polyamine-methylene resin]

**amineptine** INN

**Aminess 5.2%** IV infusion ℞ *nutritional therapy for renal failure* [multiple essential amino acids]

**aminicotin** [see: niacinamide]

**aminitrozole** INN *veterinary antibacterial* [also: nithiamide; acinitrazole]

**aminoacetic acid** JAN *nonessential amino acid; urologic irrigant; symbols:* Gly, G [also: glycine]

**aminoacridine** INN *topical anti-infective/antiseptic* [also: aminacrine HCl; aminacrine]

**aminoacridine HCl** [see: aminacrine HCl]

**9-aminoacridine monohydrochloride** [see: aminacrine HCl]

*p*-**aminobenzenearsonic acid** [see: arsanilic acid]

*p*-**aminobenzenesulfonamide** [see: sulfanilamide]

*p*-**aminobenzene-sulfonylacetylimide** [see: sulfacetamide]

**aminobenzoate potassium** USP *analgesic; "possibly effective" for scleroderma and other skin diseases*

**aminobenzoate sodium** USP *analgesic*

*p*-**aminobenzoic acid** [see: aminobenzoic acid]

**aminobenzoic acid (4-aminobenzoic acid)** USP *ultraviolet screen*

**aminobenzylpenicillin** [see: ampicillin]

γ-**amino-β-hydroxybutyric acid** JAN

**aminobromophenylpyrimidinone (ABPP)** [see: bropirimine]

γ-**aminobutyric acid** JAN

**aminocaproic acid** USAN, USP, INN, BAN *systemic hemostatic; investigational (orphan) for traumatic hyphema of the eye* [also: ∈-aminocaproic acid] 250 mg/mL injection

JAN *systemic hemostatic* [also: aminocaproic acid]

**aminocardol** [see: aminophylline]

**Amino-Cerv pH 5.5** vaginal cream ℞ *emollient; antifungal; anti-inflammatory* [urea; sodium propionate; methionine; cystine; inositol] 8.34%•0.5%•0.83%•0.35%•0.83%

**aminodeoxykanamycin** [see: bekanamycin]

**2-aminoethanethiol** [see: cysteamine]

**2-aminoethanethiol HCl** [see: cysteamine HCl]

**2-aminoethanol** [see: monoethanolamine]

**aminoethyl nitrate (2-aminoethyl nitrate)** INN, DCF

**amino-ethyl-propanol** [see: ambuphylline]

**aminoethylsulfonic acid** JAN [also: taurine]

**aminoform** [see: methenamine]

**aminoglutethimide** USP, INN, BAN *adrenocortical suppressant; antineoplastic*

**aminoglycosides** *a class of bactericidal antibiotics effective against gram-negative organisms*

**aminoguanidine monohydrochloride** [see: pimagedine HCl]

**6-aminohexanoic acid** [see: aminocaproic acid]

**aminohippurate sodium** USP *renal function test* [also: *p*-aminohippurate sodium] 20% injection

***p*-aminohippurate sodium** JAN *renal function test* [also: aminohippurate sodium]

**aminohippuric acid (*p*-aminohippuric acid)** USP

**aminohydroxypropylidene diphosphonate (APD)** [see: pamidronate disodium]

**aminoisobutanol** [see: ambuphylline]

**aminoisometradine** [see: methionine]

**5-aminolevulinic acid** *investigational (Phase III) photodynamic therapy for precancerous actinic keratoses of the skin*

**aminometradine** INN, BAN

**Amino-Min-D** capsules OTC *dietary supplement* [calcium carbonate; multiple minerals; vitamin D] 250 mg• ± •100 IU

**aminonat** [see: protein hydrolysate]

**Amino-Opti-C** sustained-release tablets OTC *dietary supplement* [vitamin C; lemon & rose hips bioflavonoids; rutin; hesperidin] 1000• 250•±•± mg

**Amino-Opti-E** capsules OTC *dietary supplement* [vitamin E] 165 mg

**aminopenicillins** *a class of bactericidal antibiotics*

**aminopentamide sulfate** [see: dimevamide]

**aminophenazone** INN [also: aminopyrine]

**aminophenazone cyclamate** INN

***p*-aminophenylarsonic acid** [see: arsanilic acid]

**aminophylline** USP, INN, BAN, JAN *smooth muscle relaxant; bronchodilator* 100, 200 mg oral; 105 mg/5 mL oral; 250 mg/10 mL injection; 250, 500 suppositories

**aminopromazine** INN, DCF [also: proquamezine]

**aminopterin sodium** INN, BAN, DCF *investigational antineoplastic for breast and ovarian cancer*

**4-aminopyridine** [see: fampridine]

**aminopyrine** NF, JAN [also: aminophenazone]

**aminoquin naphthoate** [see: pamaquine naphthoate]

**aminoquinol** INN

**aminoquinoline** [see: aminoquinol]

**4-aminoquinoline** [see: chloroquine phosphate]

**8-aminoquinoline** [see: primaquine phosphate]

**aminoquinuride** INN

**aminorex** USAN, INN, BAN *anorectic*

**aminosalicylate calcium** USP [also: calcium para-aminosalicylate]

**aminosalicylate potassium** USP

**aminosalicylate sodium (*p*-aminosalicylate sodium)** USP *bacteriostatic; tuberculosis retreatment agent; investigational (orphan) for Crohn's disease*

**aminosalicylic acid (4-aminosalicylic acid)** USP *antibacterial; tuberculostatic (orphan); investigational (orphan) for ulcerative colitis*

**5-aminosalicylic acid (5-ASA)** [see: mesalamine]

**aminosalyle sodium** [see: aminosalicylate sodium]

**aminosidine** *investigational (orphan) for tuberculosis, Mycobacterium avium complex, and visceral leishmaniasis*

**aminosidine sulfate** [see: paromomycin sulfate]

**aminosuccinic acid** [see: aspartic acid]

**Aminosyn 3.5% (5%, 7%, 8.5%, 10%); Aminosyn (pH6) 10%; Aminosyn II 3.5% (5%, 7%, 8.5%, 10%, 15%); Aminosyn-PF 7% (10%)** IV infusion ℞ *total parenteral nutrition (except 3.5%); peripheral parenteral nutrition (all)* [multiple essential and nonessential amino acids]

**Aminosyn 3.5% M; Aminosyn II 3.5% M** IV infusion ℞ *peripheral parenteral nutrition* [multiple essential and nonessential amino acids; electrolytes]

**Aminosyn 7% (8.5%) with Electrolytes; Aminosyn II 7% (8.5%, 10%) with Electrolytes** IV infusion ℞ *total parenteral nutrition; peripheral parenteral nutrition* [multiple essential and nonessential amino acids; electrolytes]

**Aminosyn II 3.5% in 5% (25%) Dextrose; Aminosyn II 4.25% in 10% (20%, 25%) Dextrose; Aminosyn II 5% in 25% Dextrose** IV infusion ℞ *total parenteral nutrition (except 3.5% in 5%); peripheral parenteral nutrition (not 20% and 25%)* [multiple essential and nonessential amino acids; dextrose]

**Aminosyn II 3.5% M in 5% Dextrose; Aminosyn II 4.25% M in 10% Dextrose** IV infusion ℞ *total parenteral nutrition (4.25% in 10% only); peripheral parenteral nutrition (both)* [multiple essential and nonessential amino acids & electrolytes; dextrose]

**Aminosyn-HBC 7%** IV infusion ℞ *nutritional therapy for high metabolic stress* [multiple branched-chain essential and nonessential amino acids; electrolytes]

**Aminosyn-RF 5.2%** IV infusion ℞ *nutritional therapy for renal failure* [multiple essential amino acids]

**aminothiazole** INN

**aminotrate phosphate** [see: trolnitrate phosphate]

**aminoxaphen** [see: aminorex]

**aminoxytriphene** INN

**aminoxytropine tropate HCl** [see: atropine oxide HCl]

**Amio-Aqueous** ℞ *antiarrhythmic for acute ventricular tachycardia and fibrillation (orphan)* [amiodarone HCl]

**amiodarone** USAN, INN, BAN *ventricular antiarrhythmic*

**amiodarone HCl** *ventricular antiarrhythmic for acute ventricular tachycardia and fibrillation (orphan)*

**Amipaque** powder for injection ℞ *parenteral radiopaque agent* [metrizamide] 13.5%, 18.75%

**amiperone** INN

**amiphenazole** INN, BAN

**amipizone** INN

**amipramidine** [see: amiloride HCl]

**amiprilose** INN *anti-inflammatory* [also: amiprilose HCl]

**amiprilose HCl** USAN *investigational (Phase III) anti-inflammatory for rheumatoid arthritis* [also: amiprilose]

**amiquinsin** INN *antihypertensive* [also: amiquinsin HCl]

**amiquinsin HCl** USAN *antihypertensive* [also: amiquinsin]

**amisometradine** NF, INN, BAN

**amisulpride** INN

**amiterol** INN

**Ami-Tex LA** long-acting tablets ℞ *decongestant; expectorant* [phenylpropanolamine HCl; guaifenesin] 75•400 mg

**amithiozone** [see: thioacetazone; thiacetazone]

**amitivir** INN *investigational influenza vaccine*

**Amitone** chewable tablets OTC *antacid* [calcium carbonate] 350 mg

**amitraz** USAN, INN, BAN *scabicide*

**amitriptyline** INN, BAN *tricyclic antidepressant* [also: amitriptyline HCl] ⊠ nortriptyline

**amitriptyline HCl (AMT)** USP, JAN *tricyclic antidepressant* [also: amitriptyline] 10, 25, 50, 75, 100, 150 mg oral

**amitriptylinoxide** INN

**amixetrine** INN, DCF

**amlexanox** USAN, INN, JAN *antiallergic; anti-inflammatory; aphthous ulcer treatment*

**amlintide** USAN *antidiabetic for type 1 diabetes mellitus*

**amlodipine** INN, BAN *antianginal; antihypertensive; calcium channel blocker* [also: amlodipine besylate]

**amlodipine besylate** USAN *antianginal; antihypertensive; calcium channel blocker* [also: amlodipine]

**amlodipine maleate** USAN *antianginal; antihypertensive*

**ammoidin** [see: methoxsalen]

**[$^{13}$N]ammonia** [see: ammonia N 13]

**ammonia** [see: ammonia spirit, aromatic]

**ammonia N 13** USAN, USP *radioactive diagnostic aid for cardiac and liver imaging*

**ammonia solution, strong** NF *solvent; source of ammonia* [also: ammonia water]

**ammonia spirit, aromatic** USP *respiratory stimulant*

**ammonia water** JAN *solvent; source of ammonia* [also: ammonia solution, strong]

**ammoniated mercury** [see: mercury, ammoniated]

**ammonio methacrylate copolymer** NF *coating agent*

**ammonium alum** [see: alum, ammonium]

**ammonium benzoate** USP

**ammonium biphosphate** *urinary acidifier*

**ammonium carbonate** NF *source of ammonia*

**ammonium chloride** USP, JAN *urinary acidifier; nonprescription diuretic* 486, 500 mg oral; 5 mEq/mL (26.75%) injection

**ammonium 2-hydroxypropanoate** [see: ammonium lactate]

**ammonium ichthosulfonate** [see: ichthammol]

**ammonium lactate (lactic acid neutralized with ammonium hydroxide)** USAN *antipruritic; emollient for xerosis*

**ammonium mandelate** USP

**ammonium molybdate** USP *dietary molybdenum supplement* 25 µg/mL injection

**ammonium molybdate tetrahydrate** [see: ammonium molybdate]

**ammonium phosphate** NF *pharmaceutic aid*

**ammonium salicylate** NF

**ammonium tetrathiomolybdate** *investigational (orphan) for Wilson's disease*

**ammonium valerate** NF

**ammophylline** [see: aminophylline]

**AMO Endosol; AMO Endosol Extra** ophthalmic solution ℞ *intraocular irrigating solution* [balanced saline solution]

**AMO Vitrax** intraocular injection ℞ *viscoelastic agent for ophthalmic surgery* [hyaluronate sodium] 30 mg/mL

**amobarbital** USP, INN, JAN *sedative; hypnotic; anticonvulsant; also abused as a street drug* [also: amylobarbitone]

**amobarbital sodium** USP, JAN *hypnotic; sedative; anticonvulsant; also abused as a street drug*

**amocaine chloride** [see: amolanone HCl]

**amocarzine** INN

**amodiaquine** USP, INN, BAN *antiprotozoal*

**amodiaquine HCl** USP *antimalarial*

**Amodopa** tablets (discontinued 1998) ℞ *antihypertensive* [methyldopa] 125, 250, 500 mg

**amoeba** *street drug slang* [see: PCP]

**amogastrin** INN, JAN

**amolanone** INN

**amolanone HCl** [see: amolanone]

**amonafide** INN *investigational antineoplastic*

**Amonidrin** tablets (discontinued 1994) OTC *expectorant* [guaifenesin] 200 mg

**Amoni-Opti-E** capsules OTC *vitamin supplement* [vitamin E]

**amoproxan** INN, DCF

**amopyroquine** INN

**amorolfine** USAN, INN, BAN *antimycotic*

**Amosan** powder OTC *oral antibacterial* [sodium peroxyborate monohydrate]

**amoscanate** INN

**amosulalol** INN [also: amosulalol HCl]

**amosulalol HCl** JAN [also: amosulalol]

**amotriphene** [see: aminoxytriphene]

**amoxapine** USAN, USP, INN, BAN, JAN *tricyclic antidepressant* 25, 50, 100, 150 mg oral ☒ amoxicillin; Amoxil

**amoxecaine** INN

**amoxicillin** USAN, USP, JAN *bactericidal antibiotic* [also: amoxicilline; amoxycillin] 250 mg oral ☒ amoxapine

**amoxicillin trihydrate** *bactericidal antibiotic* 250, 500 mg oral; 125, 250 mg/5 mL oral; 50 mg/mL oral

**amoxicilline** INN *bactericidal antibiotic* [also: amoxicillin; amoxycillin]

**Amoxil** capsules, powder for oral suspension, chewable tablets, pediatric drops ℞ *penicillin-type antibiotic* [amoxicillin trihydrate] 250, 500 mg; 125, 250 mg/5 mL; 125, 250 mg; 50 mg/mL ☒ amoxapine

**amoxycillin** BAN *bactericidal antibiotic* [also: amoxicillin; amoxicilline]

**amoxydramine camsilate** INN [also: amoxydramine camsylate]

**amoxydramine camsylate** DCF [also: amoxydramine camsilate]

**amp** *street drug slang* [see: amphetamines]

**AMP; A₅MP (adenosine monophosphate)** [see: adenosine phosphate]

**amp joint** *street drug slang for a marijuana cigarette laced with a narcotic* [see: marijuana]

**amperozide** INN, BAN *investigational antipsychotic for schizophrenia*

**amphecloral** USAN *anorectic* [also: amfecloral]

**amphenidone** INN

**amphetamine** BAN *CNS stimulant; widely abused as a street drug, which causes strong psychic dependence* [also: amphetamine sulfate; amfetamine]

*d*-**amphetamine** [see: dextroamphetamine]

**(+)-amphetamine** [see: dextroamphetamine]

*l*-**amphetamine** [see: levamphetamine]

**(−)-amphetamine** [see: levamphetamine]

**amphetamine aspartate** *CNS stimulant*

**amphetamine complex (resin complex of amphetamine & dextroamphetamine)** [q.v.]

**amphetamine phosphate, dextro** [see: dextroamphetamine phosphate]

**amphetamine succinate, levo** [see: levamphetamine succinate]

**amphetamine sulfate** USP *CNS stimulant; widely abused as a street drug, which causes strong psychic dependence* [also: amfetamine; amphetamine] 5, 10 mg oral

**amphetamine sulfate, dextro** [see: dextroamphetamine sulfate]

**amphetamines** *a class of CNS stimulants that includes amphetamine, dextroamphetamine, levamphetamine, methamphetamine, and their salts*

**Amphocil** ℞ *investigational antifungal for immunocompromised patients* [lipid-complex formulation of amphotericin B]

**amphocortrin** [see: amphomycin]

**Amphojel** tablets, oral suspension OTC *antacid* [aluminum hydroxide gel] 300, 600 mg; 320 mg/5 mL

**amphomycin** USAN, BAN *antibacterial* [also: amfomycin]

**amphotalide** INN, DCF

**Amphotec** powder for IV infusion ℞ *systemic antifungal for invasive aspergillosis* [amphotericin B cholesteryl sulfate] 50, 100 mg

**amphotericin B** USP, INN, BAN, JAN *polyene antifungal*

**amphotericin B cholesteryl sulfate** *systemic polyene antifungal for invasive aspergillosis*

**amphotericin B deoxycholate** *polyene antifungal* 50 mg injection

**amphotericin B lipid complex (ABLC)** *systemic polyene antifungal for invasive infections (orphan); investigational (orphan) for meningitis, leishmaniasis, and histoplasmosis*

**ampicillin** USAN, USP, INN, BAN, JAN *bactericidal antibiotic*

**ampicillin sodium** USAN, USP, JAN *bactericidal antibiotic* 125, 250, 500, 1000, 2000, 10 000 g/vial injection

**ampicillin trihydrate** *bactericidal antibiotic* 250, 500 mg oral; 125, 250, 500 mg/5 mL oral; 100 mg/mL oral

**ampiroxicam** INN, BAN

**Amplicor Chlamydia** test kit for professional use *in vitro diagnostic aid for Chlamydia trachomatis* [DNA amplification test]

**Amplicor HIV-1 Monitor** test kit for professional use *in vitro diagnostic aid for HIV-1 in blood* [polymerase chain reaction (PCR) test]

**Amplicor MTB** test kit for professional use *in vitro diagnostic aid for Mycobacterium tuberculosis* [polymerase chain reaction (PCR) test]

**Ampligen** ℞ *investigational (Phase III, orphan) antiviral/immunomodulator for AIDS, renal cell carcinoma, metastatic melanoma, and chronic fatigue syndrome* [poly I: poly C12U]

**amprocidum** [see: amprolium]

**amprolium** USP, INN, BAN *coccidiostat for poultry*

**amprotropine phosphate**

**ampyrimine** INN

**ampyzine** INN *CNS stimulant* [also: ampyzine sulfate]

**ampyzine sulfate** USAN *CNS stimulant* [also: ampyzine]

**amquinate** USAN, INN *antimalarial*

**amrinone** USAN, INN, BAN *cardiotonic*

**amrinone lactate** *vasodilator for congestive heart failure*

**amrubicin** INN

**AMSA; *m*-AMSA (acridinylamine methanesulfon anisidide)** [see: amsacrine]

**amsacrine** USAN, INN, BAN *investigational (NDA filed) antineoplastic for acute adult leukemias (AML, APL, and ALL) and lymphomas*

**Amsidyl** ℞ *investigational (NDA filed) antineoplastic for acute adult leukemias (AML, APL, and ALL) and lymphomas* [amsacrine]

**amsonate** INN, BAN *combining name for radicals or groups*

**AMT (amitriptyline HCl)** [q.v.]

**amtolmetin guacil** INN

**Amvisc; Amvisc Plus** intraocular injection ℞ *viscoelastic agent for ophthalmic surgery* [hyaluronate sodium] 12 mg/mL; 16 mg/mL

**amyl alcohol, tertiary** [see: amylene hydrate]

**amyl nitrite** USP, JAN *vasodilator; antianginal; also abused as a euphoric street drug and sexual stimulant* 0.3 mL inhalant

**amylase** [see: alpha amylase]

**amylene hydrate** NF *solvent*

**amylin** [see: amlintide]

**amylmetacresol** INN, BAN

**amylobarbitone** BAN *sedative; hypnotic; anticonvulsant* [also: amobarbital]

**amylocaine** BAN

**amylopectin sulfate, sodium salt** [see: sodium amylosulfate]

**amylosulfate sodium** [see: sodium amylosulfate]

**amys; aimies** *street drug slang for amphetamines, amyl nitrite, or Amytal (amobarbital; discontinued 1991)* [see: amphetamines; amyl nitrite; Amytal Sodium; amobarbital; amobarbital sodium]

**Amytal Sodium** powder for injection ℞ *sedative; hypnotic; anxiolytic; anticonvulsant; also abused as a street drug* [amobarbital sodium]

**ANA-756** *investigational once-daily vasodilator for hypertension*

**anabolic steroids** *a class of hormones that increase anabolic (tissue-building) and decrease catabolic (tissue-depleting) processes*

**Anacin** caplets, tablets OTC *analgesic; antipyretic; anti-inflammatory* [aspirin; caffeine] 400•32 mg; 400•32, 500•32 mg

**Anacin, Aspirin Free** tablets, caplets, gelcaps OTC *analgesic; antipyretic* [acetaminophen] 500 mg

**Anacin P.M., Aspirin Free** film-coated caplets OTC *antihistaminic sleep aid; analgesic* [diphenhydramine HCl; acetaminophen] 25•500 mg

**Anacin-3, Children's** chewable tablets, liquid (discontinued 1993) OTC *analgesic; antipyretic* [acetaminophen] 80 mg; 160 mg/5 mL

**Anacin-3, Infants'** drops (discontinued 1993) OTC *analgesic; antipyretic* [acetaminophen] 100 mg/mL

**Anadrol-50** tablets ℞ *anabolic steroid for anemias; also abused as a street drug* [oxymetholone] 50 mg

**anafebrina** [see: aminopyrine]

**Anafranil** capsules ℞ *tricyclic antidepressant for obsessive-compulsive disor-*

*ders* [clomipramine HCl] 25, 50, 75 mg ② enalapril

**anagestone** INN *progestin* [also: anagestone acetate]

**anagestone acetate** USAN *progestin* [also: anagestone]

**anagrelide** INN *antithrombotic/ antiplatelet drug for essential thrombocythemia (orphan); investigational (orphan) for thrombocytosis and polycythemia vera* [also: anagrelide HCl]

**anagrelide HCl** USAN *antithrombotic/ antiplatelet drug for essential thrombocythemia (orphan); investigational (orphan) for thrombocytosis and polycythemia vera* [also: anagrelide]

**Ana-Guard Epinephrine** injection ℞ *emergency treatment of anaphylaxis* [epinephrine] 1:1000

**Anaids** tablets (discontinued 1994) ℞ *antacid; sedative* [calcium carbonate; phenobarbital sodium]

**anakinra** USAN, INN *nonsteroidal antiinflammatory for inflammatory bowel disease; investigational (orphan) for juvenile rheumatoid arthritis and GVH disease*

**Ana-Kit** ℞ *emergency treatment of anaphylaxis* [epinephrine; chlorpheniramine maleate; alcohol pads; tourniquet] 1:100 000•2 mg

**Analbalm** emulsion (discontinued 1994) OTC *counterirritant* [methyl salicylate; camphor; menthol] 10%• 3%•1.25% ② Analpram

**analeptics** *a class of central nervous system stimulants used to maintain or improve alertness*

**Analgesia Creme** OTC *topical analgesic* [trolamine salicylate] 10%

**Analgesic Balm** OTC *counterirritant* [methyl salicylate; menthol]

**analgesics** *a class of drugs that relieve pain or reduce sensitivity to pain without causing loss of consciousness*

**analgesine** [see: antipyrine]

**Analpram-HC** anorectal cream ℞ *topical corticosteroidal anti-inflammatory; local anesthetic* [hydrocortisone acetate; pramoxine] 1%•1%, 2.5%• 1% ② Analbalm

**Anamine** syrup ℞ *decongestant; antihistamine* [pseudoephedrine HCl; chlorpheniramine maleate] 30•2 mg/5 mL

**Anamine T.D.** sustained-release capsules ℞ *decongestant; antihistamine* [pseudoephedrine HCl; chlorpheniramine maleate] 120•8 mg

**ananain** *investigational (orphan) for enzymatic debridement of severe burns*

**Anandron** ⊛ (U.S. product: Nilandron) tablets (also available in Europe and Latin America) ℞ *antiandrogen antineoplastic adjunct to surgical or chemical castration for metastatic prostate cancer* [nilutamide] 50, 100 mg

**Anaplex** liquid ℞ *decongestant; antihistamine* [pseudoephedrine HCl; chlorpheniramine maleate] 30•2 mg/5 mL

**Anaplex HD** syrup ℞ *narcotic antitussive; decongestant; antihistamine* [hydrocodone bitartrate; phenylephrine HCl; chlorpheniramine maleate] 1.7•5•2 mg/5 mL

**Anaplex SR** sustained-release capsules (discontinued 1995) ℞ *decongestant; antihistamine* [pseudoephedrine HCl; chlorpheniramine maleate] 120•8 mg

**Anaprox; Anaprox DS** film-coated tablets ℞ *nonsteroidal anti-inflammatory drug (NSAID); antiarthritic; analgesic* [naproxen (from naproxen sodium)] 250 (275) mg; 500 (550) mg

**anarel** [see: guanadrel sulfate]

**anaritide** INN, BAN *antihypertensive; diuretic* [also: anaritide acetate]

**anaritide acetate** USAN *antihypertensive; diuretic; investigational (orphan) for acute renal failure and renal transplants; clinical trials discontinued 1997*

**Anaspaz** tablets ℞ *anticholinergic; antispasmodic* [hyoscyamine sulfate] 0.125 mg

**anastrozole** USAN, INN, BAN *hormonal antineoplastic for advanced breast cancer; aromatase inhibitor*

**Anatrast** paste ℞ *GI contrast radiopaque agent* [barium sulfate] 100%

**Anatrofin** brand name for stenbolone acetate, an anabolic steroid abused as a street drug

**Anatuss** film-coated tablets ℞ *antitus-sive; decongestant; expectorant; anal-gesic* [dextromethorphan hydrobro-mide; phenylpropanolamine HCl; guaifenesin; acetaminophen] 15•25•100•325 mg

**Anatuss** syrup OTC *antitussive; decon-gestant; expectorant* [dextromethor-phan hydrobromide; phenylpropa-nolamine HCl; guaifenesin] 15•25•100 mg/5 mL

**Anatuss DM** tablets, syrup OTC *anti-tussive; decongestant; expectorant* [dex-tromethorphan hydrobromide; pseu-doephedrine HCl; guaifenesin] 20•60•400 mg; 10•30•100 mg/5 mL

**Anatuss LA** long-acting tablets ℞ *decongestant; expectorant* [pseudo-ephedrine HCl; guaifenesin] 120•400 mg

**Anavar** *brand name for oxandrolone, an anabolic steroid abused as a street drug*

**anaxirone** INN

**anayodin** [see: chiniofon]

**anazocine** INN

**anazolene sodium** USAN, INN *blood volume and cardiac output test* [also: sodium anoxynaphthonate]

**Anbesol** liquid, gel OTC *topical oral anesthetic; antipruritic/counterirritant; antiseptic* [benzocaine; phenol; alco-hol 70%] 6.3%•0.5%

**Anbesol, Baby** gel OTC *topical oral anesthetic* [benzocaine] 7.5%

**Anbesol, Maximum Strength** liquid, gel OTC *mucous membrane anesthetic* [benzocaine; alcohol 60%] 20%

**ancarolol** INN

**Ancef** powder for IV or IM injection ℞ *cephalosporin-type antibiotic* [cefaz-olin sodium] 0.25, 0.5, 1, 5, 10 g

**Ancet** liquid OTC *soap-free therapeutic skin cleanser*

**ancitabine** INN [also: ancitabine HCl]

**ancitabine HCl** JAN [also: ancitabine]

**Ancobon** capsules ℞ *antifungal* [flucy-tosine] 250, 500 mg ☒ Oncovin

**ancrod** USAN, INN, BAN *anticoagulant; investigational (orphan) antithrombotic for heparin-induced thrombocytopenia or thrombosis*

**andolast** INN

**Andozac** ℞ *investigational treatment for benign prostatic hyperplasia*

**Andro 100** IM injection (discontin-ued 1994) ℞ *androgen replacement for delayed puberty or breast cancer* [testosterone] 100 mg/mL

**Andro 100; Andro 200** [see: depAn-dro 100; depAndro 200]

**Andro L.A. 200** IM injection ℞ *androgen replacement for delayed puberty or breast cancer* [testosterone enanthate] 200 mg/mL

**Androcur** *orphan status withdrawn 1996* [cyproterone acetate]

**Andro-Cyp 100; Andro-Cyp 200** IM injection (discontinued 1994) ℞ *androgen replacement for delayed puberty or breast cancer* [testosterone cypionate] 100 mg/mL; 200 mg/mL

**Androderm** transdermal patch (for nonscrotal area) ℞ *hormone replace-ment therapy for hypogonadism* [testos-terone] 2.5, 5 mg/day

**Andro/Fem** IM injection (discontin-ued 1995) ℞ *estrogen/androgen for menopausal vasomotor symptoms* [estradiol cypionate; testosterone cypionate] 2•50 mg/mL

**Androgel** *investigational (orphan) for AIDS-wasting syndrome; investiga-tional (Phase III) for testosterone defi-ciency in men* [testosterone]

**Androgel-DHT** *investigational (orphan) for AIDS-wasting syndrome* [dihydrotestosterone]

**androgens** *a class of sex hormones responsible for the development of the male sex organs and secondary sex characteristics*

**Androgyn** [see: depAndrogyn]

**Androgyn L.A.** IM injection (discon-tinued 1994) ℞ *estrogen/androgen for menopausal vasomotor symptoms* [estradiol valerate; testosterone enanthate] 4•90 mg/mL

**Android-10; Android-25** tablets ℞ *androgen for male hypogonadism, cryp-torchidism, impotence, and female breast cancer* [methyltestosterone] 10 mg; 25 mg

**Androlone-D 200** IM injection ℞ *anabolic steroid for anemia of renal*

*insufficiency* [nandrolone decanoate] 200 mg/mL

**Andronate 100; Andronate 200** IM injection (discontinued 1994) ℞ *androgen replacement for delayed puberty or breast cancer* [testosterone cypionate] 100 mg/mL; 200 mg/mL

**Andropository-200** IM injection ℞ *androgen replacement for delayed puberty or breast cancer* [testosterone enanthate] 200 mg/mL

**androstanazole** [now: stanozolol]

**androstane** [see: androstanolone; stanolone]

**androstanolone** INN *investigational (orphan) for AIDS-wasting syndrome* [also: stanolone]

**androtest P** [see: testosterone propionate]

**Androtest-SL** sublingual tablets ℞ *investigational (NDA filed) treatment for hypogonadism* [testosterone]

**Androvite** tablets OTC *vitamin/mineral/iron supplement* [multiple vitamins & minerals; iron; folic acid; biotin] ±•3•0.06•² mg

**Anectine** IV or IM injection, Flo-Pack (powder for injection) ℞ *muscle relaxant; anesthesia adjunct* [succinylcholine chloride] 20 mg/mL; 500, 1000 mg

**Anergan 25** injection (discontinued 1995) ℞ *antihistamine; motion sickness; sleep aid; antiemetic; sedative* [promethazine HCl] 25 mg/mL

**Anergan 50** injection ℞ *antihistamine; motion sickness; sleep aid; antiemetic; sedative* [promethazine HCl] 50 mg/mL

**anertan** [see: testosterone propionate]

**Anestacon** jelly ℞ *mucous membrane anesthetic* [lidocaine HCl] 2%

**anesthesin** [see: benzocaine]

**anesthrone** [see: benzocaine]

**anethaine** [see: tetracaine HCl]

**anethole** NF *flavoring agent*

**anetholtrithion** JAN

**aneurine HCl** [see: thiamine HCl]

**Anexsia 5/500; Anexsia 7.5/650; Anexsia 10/660** tablets ℞ *narcotic analgesic* [hydrocodone bitartrate;

acetaminophen] 5•500 mg; 7.5•650 mg; 10•660 mg

**angel; angel dust; angel hair; angel mist; angel poke** *street drug slang* [see: PCP]

**angie** *street drug slang* [see: cocaine]

**Angio-Conray** injection ℞ *parenteral angiography radiopaque agent* [iothalamate sodium] 80%

**angiotensin II** INN

**angiotensin II receptor antagonists** *a class of antihypertensives*

**angiotensin amide** USAN, NF, BAN *vasoconstrictor* [also: angiotensinamide]

**angiotensin converting enzyme inhibitors (ACEI)** *a class of antihypertensive agents*

**angiotensinamide** INN *vasoconstrictor* [also: angiotensin amide]

**Angiovist 282** injection ℞ *parenteral radiopaque agent* [diatrizoate meglumine] 60%

**Angiovist 292; Angiovist 370** injection ℞ *parenteral radiopaque agent* [diatrizoate meglumine; diatrizoate sodium] 52%•8%; 66%•10%

**Angola** *street drug slang* [see: marijuana]

**anhydrohydroxyprogesterone** [now: ethisterone]

**anhydrous lanolin** [see: lanolin, anhydrous]

**anidoxime** USAN, INN, BAN *analgesic*

**anilamate** INN

**anileridine** USP, INN, BAN *narcotic analgesic*

**anileridine HCl** USP *narcotic analgesic*

**anilopam** INN *analgesic* [also: anilopam HCl]

**anilopam HCl** USAN *analgesic* [also: anilopam]

**animal** *street drug slang* [see: LSD]

**Animal Shapes** chewable tablets OTC *vitamin supplement* [multiple vitamins; folic acid] ±•0.3 mg

**Animal Shapes + Iron** chewable tablets OTC *vitamin/iron supplement* [multiple vitamins; iron; folic acid] ±•15•0.3 mg

**animal trank; animal tranquilizer** *street drug slang* [see: PCP]

**anion exchange resin** [see: polyamine-methylene resin]

**anipamil** INN

**aniracetam** USAN, INN *mental performance enhancer*

**anirolac** USAN, INN *anti-inflammatory; analgesic*

**anisacril** INN

**anisatil** USAN *combining name for radicals or groups*

**anise oil** NF

**anisindione** NF, INN, BAN *indandione-derivative anticoagulant*

**anisopirol** INN

**anisopyradamine** [see: pyrilamine maleate]

**anisotropine methylbromide** USAN, JAN *anticholinergic; peptic ulcer adjunct* [also: octatropine methylbromide] 50 mg oral

**anisoylated plasminogen streptokinase activator complex (APSAC)** [see: anistreplase]

**anistreplase** USAN, INN, BAN *fibrinolytic; thrombolytic enzyme for acute myocardial infarction*

**anitrazafen** USAN, INN *topical anti-inflammatory*

**anodynine** [see: antipyrine]

**anodynon** [see: ethyl chloride]

**Anodynos** tablets (discontinued 1995) OTC *analgesic; antipyretic; anti-inflammatory* [aspirin; salicylamide; caffeine] 420.6•34.4•34.4 mg

**Anodynos DHC** tablets (discontinued 1994) Ŗ *narcotic analgesic* [hydrocodone bitartrate; acetaminophen]

**Anoquan** capsules Ŗ *analgesic; antipyretic; sedative* [acetaminophen; caffeine; butalbital] 325•40•50 mg

**anorectics** *a class of central nervous system stimulants that suppress the appetite* [also called: anorexiants; anorexigenics]

**Anorex** capsules (discontinued 1996) Ŗ *anorexiant* [phendimetrazine tartrate] 35 mg

**anorexiants** *a class of central nervous system stimulants that suppress the appetite* [also called: anorectics; anorexigenics]

**anorexigenics** *a class of central nervous system stimulants that suppress the*

*appetite* [also called: anorexiants; anorectics]

**anovlar** [see: norethindrone & ethinyl estradiol]

**anoxomer** USAN *antioxidant; food additive*

**anoxynaphthonate sodium** [see: anazolene sodium]

**anpirtoline** INN

**Ansaid** tablets Ŗ *nonsteroidal anti-inflammatory drug (NSAID); antiarthritic* [flurbiprofen] 50, 100 mg

**ansamycin** [see: rifabutin]

**ansoxetine** INN

**Answer; Answer 2; Answer Plus 2** test kit for home use (discontinued 1995) OTC *in vitro diagnostic aid for urine pregnancy test*

**Answer Ovulation** test kit for home use OTC *in vitro diagnostic aid to predict ovulation time*

**Answer Plus; Answer Quick & Simple** test kit for home use OTC *in vitro diagnostic aid for urine pregnancy test*

**Antabuse** tablets Ŗ *deterrent to alcohol consumption* [disulfiram] 250, 500 mg

**Antacid** chewable tablets OTC *antacid* [calcium carbonate] 500, 750 mg

**Antacid** oral suspension OTC *antacid* [aluminum hydroxide; magnesium hydroxide] 225•200 mg/5 mL

**antacids** *a class of drugs that neutralize gastric acid*

**antafenite** INN

**Anta-Gel; Anta-Gel II** oral suspension (discontinued 1994) OTC *antacid; antiflatulent* [aluminum hydroxide; magnesium hydroxide; simethicone] 40•40•4 mg/mL; 80•80•6 mg/mL

**antastan** [see: antazoline HCl]

**antazoline** INN, BAN [also: antazoline HCl]

**antazoline HCl** USP [also: antazoline]

**antazoline phosphate** USP *antihistamine*

**antazoline phosphate & naphazoline HCl** *topical ocular antihistamine and decongestant* 0.5%•0.05%

**Antazoline-V** eye drops (discontinued 1995) Ŗ *topical ocular decongestant and antihistamine* [naphazoline HCl; antazoline phosphate] 0.05%•0.5%

**antazonite** INN

**antelmycin** INN *anthelmintic* [also: anthelmycin]

**anterior pituitary**

**anthelmintics** *a class of drugs effective against parasitic infections*

**anthelmycin** USAN *anthelmintic* [also: antelmycin]

**anthiolimine** INN

**anthracyclines** *a class of antibiotic antineoplastics*

**Anthra-Derm** ointment ℞ *topical antipsoriatic* [anthralin] 0.1%, 0.25%, 0.5%, 1%

**anthralin** USP *antipsoriatic* [also: dithranol]

**anthramycin** USAN *antineoplastic* [also: antramycin]

**anthraquinone of cascara** [see: cascara sagrada]

**anti pan T lymphocyte MAb** *orphan status withdrawn 1996* [also: anti-T lymphocyte immunotoxin XMMLY-H65-RTA]

**anti-A blood grouping serum** USP *in vitro blood testing*

**antiadrenergics** *a class of cardiovascular drugs that block the passage of impulses through the sympathetic nervous system* [also called: sympatholytics]

**antiandrogens** *a class of hormonal antineoplastics*

**antib** [see: thioacetazone; thiacetazone]

**anti-B blood grouping serum** USP *in vitro blood testing*

**anti-B4-blocked ricin** [see: ricin (blocked) ...]

**antibason** [see: methylthiouracil]

**AntibiŌtic** ear drops, otic suspension ℞ *topical corticosteroidal anti-inflammatory; antibiotic* [hydrocortisone; neomycin sulfate; polymyxin B sulfate] 1%•5 mg•10 000 U per mL

**Antibiotic Ear Solution** ℞ *topical corticosteroidal anti-inflammatory; antibiotic* [hydrocortisone; neomycin sulfate; polymyxin B sulfate] 1%•5 mg•10 000 U per mL

**Antibiotic Ear Suspension** ℞ *topical corticosteroidal anti-inflammatory; antibiotic* [hydrocortisone; neomycin

sulfate; polymyxin B sulfate] 1%•5 mg•10 000 U per mL

**anti-C blood grouping serum** [see: blood grouping serum, anti-C]

**anti-c blood grouping serum** [see: blood grouping serum, anti-c]

**anti-CD3** [see: muromonab-CD3]

**anti-CD5 monoclonal antibodies** *investigational treatment for graft vs. host disease, rheumatoid arthritis, and type 1 diabetes*

**anticholinergics** *a class of agents that block parasympathetic nerve impulses, producing antiemetic, antinausea, and antispasmodic effects*

**anticoagulant citrate dextrose (ACD) solution** USP *anticoagulant for storage of whole blood and during cardiac surgery*

**anticoagulant citrate phosphate dextrose adenine solution** USP *anticoagulant for storage of whole blood*

**anticoagulant citrate phosphate dextrose solution** USP *anticoagulant for storage of whole blood*

**anticoagulant heparin solution** USP *anticoagulant for storage of whole blood*

**anticoagulant sodium citrate solution** USP *anticoagulant for plasma and for blood for fractionation*

**anticoagulants** *a class of therapeutic agents that inhibit or inactivate blood clotting factors*

**anticonvulsants** *a class of agents that prevent seizures by suppressing abnormal neuronal discharges in the central nervous system* [also called: antiepileptic drugs (AEDs)]

**anticytomegalovirus monoclonal antibodies** *orphan status withdrawn 1994*

**anti-D antibodies** [see: $Rh_0(D)$ immune globulin]

**Antide** ℞ *investigational LHRH antagonist for hormone-dependent cancers and gynecologic disorders*

**antidopaminergics** *a class of antiemetic drugs*

**antidotes** *a class of drugs that counteract the effects of toxic doses of other drugs or toxic substances*

**anti-E blood grouping serum** [see: blood grouping serum, anti-E]

**anti-e blood grouping serum** [see: blood grouping serum, anti-e]

**antiendotoxin MAb E5** [now: edobacomab]

**antienite** INN

**antiepilepsirine** [now: ilepcimide]

**anti-epileptic drugs (AEDs)** *a class of agents that prevent seizures by suppressing abnormal neuronal discharges in the central nervous system* [also called: anticonvulsants]

**antiestrogen** [see: tamoxifen citrate]

**antiestrogens** *a class of hormonal antineoplastics*

**antifebrin** [see: acetanilide]

**antifolic acid** [see: methotrexate]

**antiformin, dental** JAN [also: sodium hypochlorite, diluted]

**antifreeze** *street drug slang* [see: heroin]

**antihemophilic factor (AHF)** USP *antihemophilic; investigational (orphan) for von Willebrand's disease*

**Antihemophilic Factor (Porcine) Hyate:C** *powder for IV injection* ℞ *antihemophilic to correct coagulation deficiency* [antihemophilic factor VIII:C] 400–700 porcine units/vial

**antihemophilic factor, human** [now: antihemophilic factor]

**antihemophilic factor, recombinant (rFVIII)** *antihemophilic for treatment of hemophilia A and presurgical prophylaxis for hemophiliacs (orphan)*

**antihemophilic factor A** [see: antihemophilic factor]

**antihemophilic factor B** [see: factor IX complex]

**antihemophilic globulin (AHG)** [see: antihemophilic factor]

**antihemophilic human plasma** [now: plasma, antihemophilic human]

**antihemophilic plasma, human** [now: plasma, antihemophilic human]

**antiheparin** [see: protamine sulfate]

**Antihist-1** *tablets* OTC *antihistamine* [clemastine fumarate] 1.34 mg

**antihistamines** *a class of drugs that counteract the effect of histamine*

**Antihist-D** *tablets* OTC *decongestant; antihistamine* [phenylpropanolamine HCl (extended release); clemastine fumarate (immediate release)] 75• 1.34 mg

**anti-HIV T-cell** *investigational (Phase I/II) gene therapy for HIV*

**anti-human thymocyte immunoglobulin, rabbit** *investigational (Phase III) immunosuppressant for kidney transplants*

**antihyperlipidemic agents** *a class of drugs that lower serum lipid levels* [also called: antilipemics]

**anti-idiotypic antibody vaccine** *investigational treatment for small cell lung cancer*

**anti-IgE humanized MAb** *investigational treatment for allergic rhinitis and asthma*

**anti-inhibitor coagulant complex** *antihemophilic*

**anti-J5MAB** *orphan status withdrawn 1993*

**antilipemics** *a class of drugs that lower serum lipid levels* [also called: antihyperlipidemics]

**Antilirium** *IV or IM injection* ℞ *cholinergic to reverse anticholinergic overdose; investigational (orphan) for Friedreich's and other inherited ataxias* [physostigmine salicylate] 1 mg/mL

**antilymphocyte immunoglobulin** BAN

**antimelanoma antibody XMMME-001-DTPA 111 indium** *orphan status withdrawn 1996*

**antimelanoma antibody XMMME-001-RTA** *orphan status withdrawn 1996*

**Antiminth** *oral suspension* OTC *anthelmintic for ascariasis (roundworm) and enterobiasis (pinworm)* [pyrantel pamoate] 50 mg/mL

**antimony** *element (Sb)*

**antimony potassium tartrate** USP *antischistosomal*

**antimony sodium tartrate** USP, JAN *antischistosomal*

**antimony sodium thioglycollate** USP

**antimony sulfide** [see: antimony trisulfide colloid]

**antimony trisulfide colloid** USAN *pharmaceutic aid*

**antimonyl potassium tartrate** [see: antimony potassium tartrate]

**antimuscarinics** *a class of anticholinergic agents*

**anti-MY9-blocked ricin** [see: ricin (blocked) ...]

**antineoplastics** *a class of chemotherapeutic agents capable of selective action on neoplastic (abnormally proliferating) tissues*

**antineoplastons** *a class of naturally occurring peptides that suppress cancer oncogenes and stimulate the body's cancer suppressor genes*

**Antiox** capsules OTC *vitamin supplement* [vitamins C and E; beta carotene] 120 mg•100 IU•25 mg

**anti-pellagra vitamin** [see: niacin]

**anti-pernicious anemia principle** [see: cyanocobalamin]

**antipyrine** USP, JAN *analgesic; orphan status withdrawn 1996* [also: phenazone]

**N-antipyrinylnicotinamide** [see: nifenazone]

**antirabies serum (ARS)** USP *passive immunizing agent*

**anti-Rh antibodies** [see: $Rh_0$(D) immune globulin]

**anti-Rh typing serums** [now: blood grouping serums]

**antiscorbutic vitamin** [see: ascorbic acid]

**antisense drugs** *a class of antiviral drugs that interfere with the replication of viral protein*

**antiseptics** *a class of agents that inhibit the growth and development of microorganisms without necessarily killing them* [compare to: germicides]

**Antispas** IM injection ℞ *gastrointestinal antispasmodic* [dicyclomine HCl] 10 mg/mL

**Antispasmodic** elixir ℞ *GI anticholinergic; sedative* [atropine sulfate; scopolamine hydrobromide; hyoscyamine sulfate; phenobarbital] 0.0194•0.0065•0.1037•16.2 mg/5 mL

**antisterility vitamin** [see: vitamin E]

**anti-T lymphocyte immunotoxin XMMLY-H65-RTA** *orphan status withdrawn 1996* [also: anti pan T lymphocyte monoclonal antibody]

**anti-tac, humanized; SMART anti-tac** [now: dacliximab]

**anti-TAP-72 immunotoxin** *orphan status withdrawn 1996*

**antithrombin III (AT-III)** INN, BAN *for thrombosis and pulmonary emboli of congenital AT-III deficiency (orphan); investigational (Phase II) for coronary artery bypass grafts*

**antithrombin III, human** [see: antithrombin III]

**antithrombin III concentrate IV** [see: antithrombin III]

**antithymocyte globulin** [see: lymphocyte immune globulin, antithymocyte]

**antithymocyte serum** [see: lymphocyte immune globulin, antithymocyte]

**anti-TNF (tumor necrosis factor) MAb** [now: nerelimomab]

**antitoxin botulism equine (ABE)** [see: botulism equine antitoxin, trivalent]

**antitoxins** *a class of drugs used for passive immunization that consist of antibodies which combine with toxins to neutralize them*

**$\alpha_1$-antitrypsin** [see: alpha$_1$-antitrypsin]

**antituberculous agents** *a class of antibiotics, divided into primary and retreatment agents*

**Anti-Tuss** syrup OTC *expectorant* [guaifenesin; alcohol 3.5%] 100 mg/5 mL

**antitussives** *a class of drugs that prevent or relieve cough*

**antivenin (Crotalidae) polyvalent** USP *passive immunizing agent for pit viper (rattlesnake, copperhead, and cottonmouth moccasin) bites*

**antivenin (Crotalidae) polyvalent (ovine) Fab** *investigational (orphan) treatment of Crotalidae snake bites*

**antivenin (Crotalidae) purified (avian)** *investigational (orphan) treatment of Crotalidae snake bites*

**antivenin (Latrodectus mactans)** USP *passive immunizing agent for black widow spider bites* 6000 U/vial

**antivenin (Micrurus fulvius)** USP *passive immunizing agent for coral snake bites*

**antivenins** *a class of drugs used for passive immunization against venomous bites and stings*

**Antivert; Antivert/25; Antivert/50** tablets ℞ *anticholinergic; antihistamine; antivertigo agent; motion sickness preventative* [meclizine HCl] 12.5 mg; 25 mg; 50 mg

**Antivert/25** chewable tablets (discontinued 1995) ℞ *anticholinergic; antihistamine; antivertigo agent; motion sickness preventative* [meclizine HCl] 25 mg

**antivirals** *a class of drugs effective against viral infections*

**antixerophthalmic vitamin** [see: vitamin A]

**Antizol** *investigational (orphan) alcohol dehydrogenase inhibitor for methanol or ethylene glycol poisoning* [fomepizole]

**antrafenine** INN

**antramycin** INN *antineoplastic* [also: anthramycin]

**Antril** ℞ *nonsteroidal anti-inflammatory drug (NSAID); investigational (orphan) for juvenile rheumatoid arthritis and graft vs. host disease* [anakinra]

**Antrizine** tablets ℞ *anticholinergic; antihistamine; antivertigo agent; motion sickness preventative* [meclizine HCl] 12.5, 25, 50 mg

**Antrocol** capsules, tablets (discontinued 1995) ℞ *GI anticholinergic; sedative* [atropine sulfate; phenobarbital] 0.195•16 mg

**Antrocol** elixir ℞ *GI anticholinergic; sedative* [atropine sulfate; phenobarbital] 0.195•16 mg/5 mL

**Antrypol** (available only from the Centers for Disease Control) ℞ *investigational anti-infective for trypanosomiasis and onchocerciasis* [suramin sodium]

**antrypol** [see: suramin sodium]

**Anturane** tablets, capsules ℞ *uricosuric for gout* [sulfinpyrazone] 100 mg; 200 mg ☑ Artane

**Anucort HC** rectal suppositories ℞ *topical corticosteroidal anti-inflammatory* [hydrocortisone acetate] 25 mg

**Anumed** rectal suppositories OTC *temporary relief of hemorrhoidal symptoms* [bismuth subgallate; bismuth resorcin compound; benzyl benzoate; zinc oxide; peruvian balsam] 2.25%•1.75%•1.2%•11%•1.8%

**Anumed HC** rectal suppositories ℞ *topical corticosteroidal anti-inflammatory* [hydrocortisone acetate] 10 mg

**Anuprep HC** rectal suppositories (discontinued 1995) ℞ *topical corticosteroidal anti-inflammatory; antipruritic* [hydrocortisone acetate] 25 mg

**Anuprep Hemorrhoidal** rectal suppositories (discontinued 1995) OTC *temporary relief of hemorrhoidal symptoms* [bismuth subgallate; bismuth resorcin compound; benzyl benzoate; peruvian balsam; zinc oxide] 2.25%•1.75%•1.2%•1.8%•11%

**Anusol** anorectal ointment OTC *topical local anesthetic; astringent* [pramoxine HCl; zinc oxide] 1%•12.5% ☑ Aplisol

**Anusol** rectal suppositories OTC *emollient* [topical starch] 51%

**Anusol-HC** anorectal cream ℞ *topical corticosteroidal anti-inflammatory* [hydrocortisone] 2.5%

**Anusol-HC** rectal suppositories ℞ *topical corticosteroidal anti-inflammatory* [hydrocortisone acetate] 25 mg

**Anusol-HC 1** ointment ℞ *topical corticosteroid* [hydrocortisone acetate] 1%

**Anxanil** film-coated tablets ℞ *anxiolytic* [hydroxyzine HCl] 25 mg

**Anzemet** injection ℞ *investigational antiemetic for nausea following chemotherapy, radiation therapy, or operations* [dolasetron mesylate]

**AOPA (ara-C, Oncovin, prednisone, asparaginase)** *chemotherapy protocol*

**AOPE (Adriamycin, Oncovin, prednisone, etoposide)** *chemotherapy protocol*

**Aosept** solution + Aodisc (tablet) OTC *two-step chemical disinfecting system for soft contact lenses* [hydrogen peroxide based] 3%

**AP (Adriamycin, Platinol)** *chemotherapy protocol*

**Apacet** chewable tablets, drops OTC *analgesic; antipyretic* [acetaminophen] 80 mg; 100 mg/mL

**Apache** *street drug slang* [see: fentanyl (citrate)]

**apafant** INN

**apalcillin sodium** USAN, INN *antibacterial*

**APAP (N-acetyl-*p*-aminophenol)** [see: acetaminophen]

**Apatate** chewable tablets, liquid OTC *vitamin supplement* [vitamins $B_1$, $B_6$, and $B_{12}$] 15•0.5•0.025 mg; 15•0.5•0.025 mg/5 mL

**Apatate with Fluoride** liquid ℞ *pediatric vitamin supplement and dental caries preventative* [vitamins $B_1$, $B_6$, and $B_{12}$; fluoride] 15•0.5•0.025•0.5 mg/5 mL

**apaxifylline** USAN, INN *selective adenosine $A_1$ antagonist for cognitive deficits*

**apazone** USAN *anti-inflammatory* [also: azapropazone]

**APC (AMSA, prednisone, chlorambucil)** *chemotherapy protocol*

**APC (aspirin, phenacetin & caffeine)** [q.v.]

**APD (aminohydroxypropylidene diphosphonate)** [see: pamidronate disodium]

**APE (Adriamycin, Platinol, etoposide)** *chemotherapy protocol*

**APE (ara-C, Platinol, etoposide)** *chemotherapy protocol*

**Apetil** liquid OTC *vitamin/mineral supplement* [multiple B vitamins; multiple minerals] ±•±

**Aphrodyne** tablets ℞ *no approved uses; sympatholytic; mydriatic; aphrodisiac* [yohimbine HCl] 5.4 mg

**Aphthasol** oral paste ℞ *anti-inflammatory for aphthous ulcers* [amlexanox] 5%

**apicillin** [see: ampicillin]

**apicycline** INN

**apiquel fumarate** [see: aminorex]

**A.P.L.** powder for IM injection ℞ *hormone for prepubertal cryptorchidism and hypogonadism; ovulation stimulant* [chorionic gonadotropin] 500, 1000, 2000 U/mL

**APL 400-020** *investigational (orphan) for cutaneous T-cell lymphoma*

**Aplisol** intradermal injection ℞ *tuberculosis skin test* [tuberculin purified protein derivative] 5 U/0.1 mL ☑ Anusol; Apresoline

**Aplitest** single-use intradermal puncture test device ℞ *tuberculosis skin test* [tuberculin purified protein derivative] 5 U

**aplonidine HCl** [see: apraclonidine HCl]

**APO (Adriamycin, prednisone, Oncovin)** *chemotherapy protocol*

**apodol** [see: anileridine HCl]

**Apo-Gemfibrozil** ⒸⒶⓃ (U.S. product: Lopid) capsules, tablets ℞ *antihyperlipidemic for hypertriglyceridemia and coronary heart disease* [gemfibrozil] 300 mg; 600 mg

**Apo-Ipravent** ⒸⒶⓃ (U.S. product: Atrovent) solution for inhalation ℞ *bronchodilator* [ipratropium bromide] 250 μg/mL

**apomorphine** BAN *emetic* [also: apomorphine HCl]

**apomorphine HCl** USP *emetic; investigational (orphan) for late-stage Parkinson's disease* [also: apomorphine]

**apovincamine** INN

**Appedrine** tablets OTC *nonprescription diet aid; vitamin/mineral supplement* [phenylpropanolamine HCl; multiple vitamins and minerals; folic acid] 25•±•0.4 mg ☑ aprindine; ephedrine

**APPG (aqueous penicillin G procaine)** [see: penicillin G procaine]

**apple jacks** *street drug slang* [see: cocaine, crack]

**Appli-Kit** (trademarked form) *ointment and adhesive dosage covers*

**Appli-Ruler** (trademarked name) OTC *dose-determining pads*

**Appli-Tape** (trademarked name) OTC *dosage covers*

**apraclonidine** INN, BAN *topical adrenergic for glaucoma* [also: apraclonidine HCl]

**apraclonidine HCl** USAN *topical adrenergic for glaucoma* [also: apraclonidine]

**apramycin** USAN, INN, BAN *antibacterial*

**Aprazone** capsules ℞ *uricosuric for gout* [sulfinpyrazone]

**Apresazide 25/25; Apresazide 50/
50; Apresazide 100/50** capsules ℞
*antihypertensive* [hydralazine HCl;
hydrochlorothiazide] 25•25 mg; 50•
50 mg; 100•50 mg

**Apresoline** IV or IM injection (discontinued 1993) ℞ *antihypertensive;
vasodilator* [hydralazine HCl] 20
mg/mL 🔲 Aplisol; Priscoline

**Apresoline** tablets ℞ *antihypertensive;
vasodilator* [hydralazine HCl] 10, 25,
50, 100 mg

**apricot kernel water** JAN

**aprikalim** INN *investigational antianginal*

**Aprim** ℞ *investigational potassium channel opener for angina* [aprikalim]

**aprindine** USAN, INN, BAN *antiarrhythmic* 🔲 Appedrine; ephedrine

**aprindine HCl** USAN, JAN *antiarrhythmic*

**aprobarbital** NF, INN, DCF *sedative*

**Aprodine** tablets, syrup OTC *decongestant; antihistamine* [pseudoephedrine
HCl; triprolidine HCl] 60•2.5 mg;
30•1.25 mg/5 mL

**Aprodine with Codeine** syrup ℞ *narcotic antitussive; decongestant; antihistamine* [codeine phosphate; pseudoephedrine HCl; triprolidine HCl]
10•30•1.25 mg/5 mL

**aprofene** INN

**aprosulate sodium** INN

**aprotinin** USAN, INN, BAN, JAN *systemic hemostatic to reduce blood loss in
coronary surgery (orphan); protease
inhibitor*

**Aprozide 25/25; Aprozide 50/50;
Aprozide 100/50** capsules ℞ *antihypertensive* [hydrochlorothiazide;
hydralazine HCl]

**A.P.S. (aspirin, phenacetin & sali-
cylamide)** [q.v.]

**APSAC (anisoylated plasminogen
streptokinase activator complex)**
[see: anistreplase]

**aptazapine** INN *antidepressant* [also:
aptazapine maleate]

**aptazapine maleate** USAN *antidepressant* [also: aptazapine]

**aptiganel HCl** USAN *investigational
(Phase III) NMDA ion channel blocker
for stroke and traumatic brain injury*

**aptocaine** INN, BAN, DCF

**apyron** [see: magnesium salicylate]

**Aqua-Ban** enteric-coated tablets OTC
*diuretic* [ammonium chloride; caf-
feine] 325•100 mg

**Aqua-Ban, Maximum Strength** tablets OTC *diuretic* [pamabrom] 50 mg

**Aqua-Ban Plus** enteric-coated tablets
OTC *diuretic* [ammonium chloride; caffeine; ferrous sulfate] 650•200•6 mg

**Aquabase** OTC *ointment base*

**Aquacare** cream, lotion OTC *moisturizer; emollient; keratolytic* [urea] 10%

**Aquachloral** Supprettes (suppositories) ℞ *sedative; hypnotic* [chloral
hydrate] 324, 648 mg

**aquaday** [see: menadione]

**aquakay** [see: menadione]

**AquaMEPHYTON** IM or subcu
injection ℞ *coagulant; correct anticoagulant-induced prothrombin deficiency; vitamin K supplement* [phyto-
nadione] 2, 10 mg/mL

**Aquanil** lotion OTC *moisturizer; emollient*

**Aquanil Cleanser** lotion OTC *soap-
free therapeutic skin cleanser*

**Aquaphilic** OTC *ointment base*

**Aquaphilic with Carbamide** OTC
*ointment base* [urea] 10%, 20%

**Aquaphor** OTC *ointment base*

**Aquaphor Antibiotic** ointment (discontinued 1994) OTC *topical antibiotic* [polymyxin B sulfate; bacitracin
zinc] 10 000•500 U/g

**Aquaphyllin** syrup ℞ *bronchodilator*
[theophylline] 80 mg/15 mL

**AquaSite** eye drops OTC *ocular mois-
turizer/lubricant* [polyethylene glycol
400] 0.2%

**Aquasol A** capsules, IM injection ℞
*vitamin deficiency therapy* [vitamin A]
25 000, 50 000 IU; 50 000 IU/mL

**Aquasol A** drops OTC *vitamin supplement* [vitamin A] 5000 IU/0.1 mL

**Aquasol E** capsules, drops OTC *vitamin
supplement* [vitamin E] 73.5 mg, 400
IU; 50 mg/mL

**AquaTar** gel OTC *topical antipsoriatic;
antiseborrheic* [coal tar extract] 2.5%

**Aquatensen** tablets ℞ *diuretic; antihypertensive* [methyclothiazide] 5 mg

**aqueous penicillin G procaine
(APPG)** [see: penicillin G procaine]

**Aquest** IM injection ℞ *estrogen replacement therapy; antineoplastic for prostatic and breast cancer* [estrone] 2 mg/mL

**aquinone** [see: menadione]

**AR-177** *investigational (Phase I) antiviral/ oligonucleotide/integrase inhibitor for HIV*

**AR-623** *investigational antineoplastic for leukemia and Kaposi sarcoma; orphan status withdrawn 1994*

**ara-A (adenine arabinoside)** [see: vidarabine]

**ara-AC (azacytosine arabinoside)** [see: fazarabine]

**arabinofuranosylcytosine** [see: cytarabine]

**arabinoluranosylcytosine HCl** [see: cytarabine HCl]

**arabinosyl cytosine** [see: cytarabine]

**ara-C (cytosine arabinoside)** [see: cytarabine] ② ERYC

**ara-C, DepoFoam encapsulated** *investigational (Phase II) antineoplastic for leptomeningeal leukemia, lymphoma, and solid tumors*

**ara-C + 6-TG (ara-C, thioguanine)** *chemotherapy protocol*

**ara-C + ADR (ara-C, Adriamycin)** *chemotherapy protocol*

**ara-C + DNR + PRED + MP (ara-C, daunorubicin, prednisolone, mercaptopurine)** *chemotherapy protocol*

**arachis oil** [see: peanut oil]

**ara-C-HU (ara-C, hydroxyurea)** *chemotherapy protocol*

**ara-cytidine** [see: cytarabine]

**Aralen HCl** IM injection ℞ *antimalarial; amebicide* [chloroquine HCl] 50 mg/mL ② Arlidin

**Aralen Phosphate** film-coated tablets ℞ *antimalarial; amebicide* [chloroquine phosphate] 500 mg

**Aralen Phosphate** injection (discontinued 1996) ℞ *antimalarial; amebicide* [chloroquine phosphate] 5 mg

**Aralen Phosphate with Primaquine Phosphate** tablets (discontinued 1996) ℞ *malaria prophylaxis* [chloroquine phosphate; primaquine phosphate] 500•79 mg

**Aramine** IV, subcu or IM injection ℞ *vasopressor for acute hypotensive*

shock, anaphylaxis, or traumatic shock [metaraminol bitartrate] 10 mg/mL

**aranidipine** INN

**aranotin** USAN, INN *antiviral*

**araprofen** INN

**arbaprostil** USAN, INN *gastric antisecretory*

**arbekacin** INN

**Arbon** tablets (discontinued 1994) OTC *vitamin/mineral/iron supplement* [multiple vitamins & minerals; ferrous fumarate; folic acid] ≐•18•0.4 mg

**Arbon Plus** tablets (discontinued 1994) OTC *vitamin/mineral/iron supplement* [multiple vitamins & minerals; ferrous fumarate; folic acid; biotin] ≐•27 mg•0.4 mg•150 μg

**arbutamine** INN, BAN *cardiac stimulant* [also: arbutamine HCl]

**arbutamine HCl** USAN *cardiac stimulant* [also: arbutamine]

**Arcet** tablets (discontinued 1995) ℞ *sedative; analgesic; antipyretic* [butalbital; acetaminophen; caffeine] 50•325•40 mg

**arcitumomab** USAN *investigational (orphan) imaging agent for detection of recurrent or metastatic thyroid and colorectal cancers*

**arclofenin** USAN, INN *hepatic function test*

**Arcobee with C** caplets OTC *vitamin supplement* [multiple B vitamins; vitamin C] ≐•300 mg

**Arco-Lase** chewable tablets OTC *digestive enzymes* [amylase; protease; lipase; cellulase] 30•6•25•2 mg

**Arco-Lase Plus** tablets ℞ *digestive enzymes; antispasmodic; sedative* [amylase; protease; lipase; cellulase; hyoscyamine sulfate; atropine sulfate; phenobarbital] 30•6•25•2•0.1•0.02•7.5 mg

**Arcotinic** tablets (discontinued 1995) OTC *hematinic* [ferrous fumarate & ferrous sulfate; desiccated liver; ascorbic acid] 102.5•200•250 mg

**ardacin** INN

**ardeparin sodium** USAN, INN *low molecular weight heparin-type anticoagulant and antithrombotic for prevention of deep vein thrombosis (DVT)*

**Arduan** powder for IV injection ℞ *nondepolarizing neuromuscular blocker; adjunct to anesthesia* [pipecuronium bromide] 10 mg/vial

**arecoline acetarsone salt** [see: dro-carbil]

**arecoline hydrobromide** NF

**Aredia** powder for IV infusion ℞ *bis-phosphonate bone resorption suppressant for Paget's disease, hypercalcemia of malignancy, and multiple myeloma* [pamidronate disodium] 30, 60, 90 mg

**arfalasin** INN

**arfendazam** INN

**Arfonad** IV infusion (discontinued 1995) ℞ *antihypertensive for hyperten-sive emergencies* [trimethaphan cam-sylate] 50 mg/mL

**argatroban** INN, JAN *investigational (Phase III) thrombin inhibitor for hepa-rin-induced thrombocytopenia (HIT) and thrombosis; investigational (Phase II) for myocardial infarction*

**Argesic** cream OTC *topical analgesic; counterirritant* [methyl salicylate; tro-lamine]

**Argesic-SA** tablets ℞ *analgesic; anti-inflammatory* [salsalate] 500 mg

**argimesna** INN

**arginine (L-arginine)** USP, INN *nones-sential amino acid; ammonia detoxi-cant; pituitary function diagnostic aid; symbols: Arg, R*

**arginine butanoate** [see: arginine butyrate]

**arginine butyrate (L-arginine butyrate)** USAN *investigational (orphan) for beta-hemoglobinopathies, beta-thalassemia, and sickle cell disease*

**arginine glutamate (L-arginine L-glutamate)** USAN, BAN, JAN *ammo-nia detoxicant*

**arginine HCl** USAN, USP, JAN *ammonia detoxicant; pituitary (growth hormone) function diagnostic aid*

**L-arginine monohydrochloride** [see: arginine HCl]

**8-L-arginine vasopressin** [see: vaso-pressin]

**8-arginineoxytocin** [see: argiprestocin]

**8-L-argininevasopressin tannate** [see: argipressin tannate]

**argipressin** INN, BAN *antidiuretic* [also: argipressin tannate]

**argipressin tannate** USAN *antidiuretic* [also: argipressin]

**argiprestocin** INN

**argon** *element (Ar)*

**argyn** [see: silver protein, mild]

**Argyrol S.S. 10%** eye drops (discon-tinued 1994) OTC *ophthalmic antiseptic* [silver protein, mild] 10% ⌦ Agoral

**Argyrol S.S. 20%** eye drops (discon-tinued 1995) ℞ *ophthalmic mucus staining and coagulating agent; topical antiseptic* [silver protein, mild] 20%

**ARI-509** *investigational aldose reductase inhibitor for the secondary complica-tions of long-term diabetes*

**Aricept** tablets ℞ *reversible acetyl-cholinesterase (AChE) inhibitor; cogni-tion adjuvant for Alzheimer's dementia* [donepezil HCl] 5, 10 mg ⌦ Erycette

**Aries** *street drug slang* [see: heroin]

**arildone** USAN, INN *antiviral*

**Arimidex** film-coated tablets ℞ *hor-monal antineoplastic and aromatase inhibitor for advanced breast cancer* [anastrozole] 1 mg

**aripiprazole** USAN *antischizophrenic*

**Aristocort** ointment, cream ℞ *topical corticosteroid* [triamcinolone acetonide] 0.1%, 0.5%; 0.025%, 0.1%, 0.5%

**Aristocort** tablets ℞ *glucocorticoid* [tri-amcinolone] 1, 2, 4, 8 mg

**Aristocort A** ointment, cream ℞ *topi-cal corticosteroid* [triamcinolone ace-tonide in a water-washable base] 0.1%; 0.025%, 0.1%, 0.5%

**Aristocort Forte** IM injection ℞ *glu-cocorticoid* [triamcinolone diacetate] 40 mg/mL

**Aristocort Intralesional** injection ℞ *glucocorticoid* [triamcinolone diace-tate] 25 mg/mL

**Aristospan Intra-articular** injection ℞ *glucocorticoid* [triamcinolone hexacetonide] 20 mg/mL

**Aristospan Intralesional** injection ℞ *glucocorticoid* [triamcinolone hexace-tonide] 5 mg/mL

**Arkin Z** (commercially available in Japan) ℞ *investigational treatment for congestive heart failure* [vesnarinone]

**Arlidin** tablets (discontinued 1993) ℞ *peripheral vasodilator* [nylidrin HCl] 6, 12 mg ⊡ Aralen

**A.R.M. (Allergy Relief Medicine)** caplets OTC *decongestant; antihistamine* [phenylpropanolamine HCl; chlorpheniramine maleate] 25•4 mg

**Arm-A-Med** (trademarked packaging form) *single-dose plastic vial*

**Arm-A-Vial** (trademarked packaging form) *single-dose plastic vial*

**Armour Thyroid** tablets ℞ *hypothyroidism; thyroid cancer* [thyroid, desiccated] 15, 30, 60, 90, 120, 180, 240, 300 mg

**arnica** *claimed to relieve sprains and bruises (of dubious value)*

**arnolol** INN

**aroma of men** *street drug slang* [see: isobutyl nitrite]

**aromatase inhibitors** *a class of hormonal antineoplastics*

**aromatic ammonia spirit** [see: ammonia spirit, aromatic]

**aromatic cascara fluidextract** [see: cascara fluidextract, aromatic]

**aromatic cascara sagrada** [see: cascara fluidextract, aromatic]

**aromatic elixir** NF *flavored and sweetened vehicle*

**aronixil** INN

**arotinolol** INN [also: arotinolol HCl]

**arotinolol HCl** JAN [also: arotinolol]

**arprinocid** USAN, INN, BAN *coccidiostat*

**arpromidine** INN

**Arrestin** IM injection ℞ *anticholinergic; antiemetic* [trimethobenzamide HCl] 100 mg/mL

**ARS (antirabies serum)** [q.v.]

**arsambide** [see: carbarsone]

**arsanilic acid** INN, BAN *investigational (Phase I/II) immunomodulator for AIDS; orphan status withdrawn 1996*

**arseclor** [see: dichlorophenarsine HCl]

**arsenic** *element (As)*

**arsenic acid, sodium salt** [see: sodium arsenate]

**arsenic trioxide** JAN

**arsenobenzene** [see: arsphenamine]

**arsenobenzol** [see: arsphenamine]

**arsenphenolamine** [see: arsphenamine]

**Arsobal** (available only from the Centers for Disease Control) ℞ *investigational anti-infective for trypanosomiasis* [melarsoprol]

**arsphenamine** USP

**arsthinenol** DCF [also: arsthinol]

**arsthinol** INN [also: arsthinenol]

**Artane** tablets, elixir, Sequels (sustained-release capsules) ℞ *anticholinergic; antiparkinsonian agent* [trihexyphenidyl HCl] 2, 5 mg; 2 mg/5 mL; 5 mg ⊡ Anturane

**arteflene** USAN, INN *antimalarial*

**artegraft** USAN *arterial prosthetic aid*

**artemether** INN

**artemisinin** INN

**arterenol** [see: norepinephrine bitartrate]

**artesunate** INN

**Artha-G** tablets OTC *analgesic; anti-inflammatory* [salsalate] 750 mg

**ArthriCare, Double Ice** gel OTC *counterirritant* [menthol; camphor] 4%•3.1%

**ArthriCare, Odor Free** rub OTC *counterirritant* [menthol; methyl nicotinate; capsaicin] 1.25%•0.25%•0.025%

**ArthriCare Triple Medicated** gel OTC *counterirritant* [methyl salicylate; menthol; methyl nicotinate] 30%•1.5%•0.7%

**Arthriten** tablets OTC *analgesic; antipyretic* [acetaminophen; magnesium salicylate; caffeine (buffered with magnesium carbonate, magnesium oxide, and calcium carbonate)] 250•250•32.5 mg

**Arthritis Foundation Ibuprofen** tablets (discontinued 1997) OTC *nonsteroidal anti-inflammatory drug (NSAID); antiarthritic; analgesic* [ibuprofen] 200 mg

**Arthritis Foundation Nighttime** caplets (discontinued 1997) OTC *antihistaminic sleep aid; analgesic* [diphenhydramine HCl; acetaminophen] 25•500 mg

**Arthritis Foundation Pain Reliever** tablets OTC *analgesic; antipyretic; anti-inflammatory; antirheumatic* [aspirin] 500 mg

**Arthritis Foundation Pain Reliever, Aspirin Free** caplets (discontinued 1997) OTC *analgesic; antipyretic* [acetaminophen] 500 mg

**Arthritis Hot Creme** OTC *counterirritant* [methyl salicylate; menthol] 15%•10%

**Arthritis Pain Formula** caplets OTC *analgesic; antipyretic; anti-inflammatory; antirheumatic* [aspirin (buffered with magnesium hydroxide and aluminum hydroxide)] 500 mg

**Arthritis Pain Formula Aspirin-Free** tablets (discontinued 1997) OTC *analgesic; antipyretic* [acetaminophen] 500 mg

**"Arthritis Strength"** products [see: under product name]

**Arthropan** IM injection ℞ *analgesic; antipyretic; anti-inflammatory; antirheumatic* [choline salicylate] 870 mg/5 mL

**Arthrotec** ℞ *investigational antiarthritic* [diclofenac sodium; misoprostol]

**articaine** INN [also: carticaine]

**Articulose L.A.** IM injection ℞ *glucocorticoids* [triamcinolone diacetate] 40 mg/mL

**Articulose-50** IM injection ℞ *glucocorticoids* [prednisolone acetate] 50 mg/mL

**Artificial Tears** eye drops OTC *ocular moisturizer/lubricant*

**Artificial Tears** ophthalmic ointment OTC *ocular moisturizer/lubricant* [white petrolatum; mineral oil; lanolin]

**Artificial Tears Plus** eye drops OTC *ocular moisturizer/lubricant* [polyvinyl alcohol] 1.4%

**artilide** INN *antiarrhythmic* [also: artilide fumarate]

**artilide fumarate** USAN *antiarrhythmic* [also: artilide]

**Arvin** orphan status withdrawn 1997 [ancrod]

**AS-013** *investigational prostaglandin for peripheral arterial occlusive disease*

**⁷⁴As** [see: sodium arsenate As 74]

**A.S.A.** Enseals (enteric-release tablets), suppositories OTC *analgesic; antipyretic; anti-inflammatory* [aspirin]

**5-ASA (5-aminosalicylic acid)** [see: mesalamine]

**ASA (acetylsalicylic acid)** [see: aspirin]

**Asacol** delayed-release tablets ℞ *treatment of active ulcerative colitis, proctosigmoiditis and proctitis* [mesalamine] 400 mg

**Asbron-G** Inlay-Tabs (tablets), elixir (discontinued 1996) ℞ *antiasthmatic; bronchodilator; expectorant* [theophylline; guaifenesin] 150•100 mg; 150•100 mg/15 mL

**ascorbic acid (L-ascorbic acid)** USP, INN, BAN, JAN *vitamin C; antiscorbutic; urinary acidifier* 25, 50, 100, 250, 500, 1000, 1500 oral; 500 mg/5 mL oral; 250, 500 mg/mL injection

**L-ascorbic acid, monosodium salt** [see: sodium ascorbate]

**L-ascorbic acid 6-palmitate** [see: ascorbyl palmitate]

**Ascorbicap** timed-release capsules OTC *vitamin supplement* [ascorbic acid] 500 mg

**ascorbyl palmitate** NF *antioxidant*

**Ascriptin; Ascriptin A/D** coated tablets OTC *analgesic; antipyretic; anti-inflammatory; antirheumatic* [aspirin (buffered with magnesium hydroxide, aluminum hydroxide, and calcium carbonate)] 325, 500 mg; 325 mg

**Asendin** tablets ℞ *tricyclic antidepressant* [amoxapine] 25, 50, 100, 150 mg

**aseptichrome** [see: merbromin]

**ASHAP; A-SHAP (Adriamycin, Solu-Medrol, high-dose ara-C, Platinol)** *chemotherapy protocol*

**ashes** *street drug slang* [see: marijuana]

**Asmalix** elixir ℞ *bronchodilator* [theophylline] 80 mg/15 mL

**asobamast** INN, BAN

**asocainol** INN

**asparaginase (L-asparaginase)** USAN, JAN *antineoplastic for acute lymphocytic leukemia* [also: colaspase]

**asparagine (L-asparagine)** *nonessential amino acid; symbols: Asn, N*

**L-asparagine amidohydrolase** [see: asparaginase]

**aspartame** USAN, NF, INN, BAN *sweetener*

**L-aspartate potassium** JAN

**aspartic acid (L-aspartic acid)** USAN, INN *nonessential amino acid; symbols: Asp, D*

**aspartocin** USAN, INN *antibacterial*

**A-Spas S/L** sublingual tablets ℞ *anticholinergic; antispasmodic* [hyoscyamine sulfate] 0.125 mg

**Aspegic** ℞ *orphan status withdrawn 1993* [lysine acetylsalicylate]

**Aspercreme** cream OTC *topical analgesic* [trolamine salicylate] 10%

**Aspercreme Rub** lotion OTC *topical analgesic* [trolamine salicylate] 10%

*Aspergillus oryase* **proteinase** [see: asperkinase]

**Aspergum** chewing gum tablets OTC *analgesic; antipyretic; anti-inflammatory; antirheumatic* [aspirin] 227.5 mg

**asperkinase**

**asperlin** USAN *antibacterial; antineoplastic*

**aspidosperma** USP

**aspirin** USP, BAN, JAN *analgesic; antipyretic; anti-inflammatory; antirheumatic* 325, 500, 650, 975 mg oral; 120, 200, 300, 600 mg suppositories ☑ Afrin

**aspirin, buffered** USP *analgesic; antipyretic; anti-inflammatory; antirheumatic* 325 mg oral

**aspirin aluminum** NF, JAN

**aspirin DL-lysine** JAN

**Aspirin with Codeine No. 2, No. 3, and No. 4** tablets ℞ *narcotic analgesic* [codeine phosphate; aspirin] 15•325 mg; 30•325 mg; 60•325 mg

**Aspirin-Free Pain Relief** tablets, caplets OTC *analgesic; antipyretic* [acetaminophen] 325, 500 mg; 500 mg

**Aspirol** (trademarked delivery form) *crushable ampule for inhalation*

**aspogen** [see: dihydroxyaluminum aminoacetate]

**aspoxicillin** INN, JAN

**Asprimox; Asprimox Extra Protection for Arthritis Pain** tablets, caplets OTC *analgesic; antipyretic; anti-inflammatory; antirheumatic* [aspirin (buffered with aluminum hydroxide, magnesium hydroxide, and calcium carbonate)] 325 mg

**aspro** [see: aspirin]

**Assassin of Youth** *street drug slang, from a 1930s film of the same name* [see: marijuana]

**astatine** *element (At)*

**Astelin** nasal spray ℞ *antihistamine for seasonal allergic rhinitis; H₁ receptor antagonist* [azelastine HCl] 137 μg/spray

**astemizole** USAN, INN, BAN *antiallergic; antihistamine*

**Astenose** ℞ *investigational anticoagulant to block vascular restenosis following cardiac surgery*

**AsthmaHaler** inhalation aerosol OTC *bronchodilator for bronchial asthma* [epinephrine bitartrate] 0.3 mg/dose

**AsthmaNefrin** solution for inhalation OTC *bronchodilator for bronchial asthma* [racepinephrine] 2.25%

**astifilcon A** USAN *hydrophilic contact lens material*

**Astramorph PF** IV, subcu or IM injection ℞ *narcotic analgesic; preoperative sedative and anxiolytic* [morphine sulfate] 0.5, 1 mg/mL

**Astroglide** vaginal gel OTC *lubricant* [glycerin; propylene glycol]

**astromicin** INN *antibacterial* [also: astromicin sulfate]

**astromicin sulfate** USAN, JAN *antibacterial* [also: astromicin]

**AT-III (antithrombin III)** [q.v.]

**Atabrine HCl** tablets (discontinued 1993) ℞ *antimalarial; anthelmintic for giardiasis and cestodiasis (tapeworm)* [quinacrine HCl] 100 mg ☑ Adapin

**atamestane** INN *investigational aromatase inhibitor for cancer*

**ataprost** INN

**Atarax** tablets, syrup ℞ *anxiolytic* [hydroxyzine HCl] 10, 25, 50 mg; 10 mg/5 mL ☑ Marax

**Atarax 100** tablets ℞ *anxiolytic* [hydroxyzine HCl] 100 mg

**atarvet** [see: acepromazine]

**atenolol** USAN, INN, BAN, JAN *antiadrenergic (β-receptor)* 25, 50, 100 mg oral ☑ timolol

**atevirdine** INN *antiviral* [also: atevirdine mesylate]

**atevirdine mesylate** USAN *antiviral; investigational (Phase II) for HIV and AIDS* [also: atevirdine]

**Atgam** IV infusion ℞ *immunizing agent for allograft rejection* [lymphocyte immune globulin, antithymocyte globulin (equine)] 50 mg/mL

**athyromazole** [see: carbimazole]

**atipamezole** USAN, INN, BAN $\alpha_2$-*receptor antagonist*

**atiprosin** INN *antihypertensive* [also: atiprosin maleate]

**atiprosin maleate** USAN *antihypertensive* [also: atiprosin]

**Ativan** tablets, IV or IM injection ℞ *anxiolytic* [lorazepam] 0.5, 1, 2 mg; 2, 4 mg/mL ⊘ Adapin; Avitene

**atlafilcon A** USAN *hydrophilic contact lens material*

**ATnativ** powder for IV infusion ℞ *for thrombosis and pulmonary emboli of congenital AT-III deficiency (orphan)* [antithrombin III, human] 500 IU

**atolide** USAN, INN *anticonvulsant*

**Atolone** tablets ℞ *glucocorticoid* [triamcinolone] 4 mg

**atom bomb** *street drug slang for a combination of marijuana and heroin* [see: marijuana; heroin]

**atorvastatin calcium** USAN *antihyperlipidemic; HMG-CoA reductase inhibitor*

**atosiban** USAN, INN *oxytocin antagonist*

**atovaquone** USAN, INN, BAN *antipneumocystic for Pneumocystis carinii pneumonia (orphan); investigational (orphan) antiprotozoal for Toxoplasma gondii encephalitis*

**ATP (adenosine triphosphate)** [see: adenosine triphosphate disodium]

**ATPase (adenosine triphosphatase) inhibitors** *a class of gastric antisecretory agents that inhibit the ATPase "proton pump" within the cell* [also called: proton pump inhibitors; substituted benzimidazoles]

**atracurium besilate** INN *skeletal muscle relaxant; nondepolarizing neuromuscular blocker; adjunct to anesthesia* [also: atracurium besylate]

**atracurium besylate** USAN, BAN *skeletal muscle relaxant; nondepolarizing neuromuscular blocker; adjunct to anesthesia* [also: atracurium besilate]

**Atragen** *antineoplastic for acute promyelocytic leukemia (orphan); investigational (orphan) for other leukemias and ophthalmic squamous metaplasia* [tretinoin]

**Atretol** tablets ℞ *anticonvulsant; analgesic for trigeminal neuralgia* [carbamazepine] 200 mg

**Atridox** ℞ *investigational (Phase III) treatment for periodontal disease*

**Atrigel** (trademarked delivery system) *sustained-release delivery*

**atrimustine** INN

**atrinositol** INN

**Atrofed** tablets (discontinued 1993) OTC *decongestant; antihistamine* [pseudoephedrine HCl; triprolidine HCl]

**Atrohist L.A.** sustained-release tablets (discontinued 1993) ℞ *antihistamine; decongestant; anticholinergic* [brompheniramine maleate; phenyltoloxamine citrate; pseudoephedrine HCl; atropine sulfate]

**Atrohist Pediatric** oral suspension ℞ *pediatric decongestant and antihistamine* [phenylephrine tannate; chlorpheniramine tannate; pyrilamine tannate] 5•2•12.5 mg/5 mL

**Atrohist Pediatric** sustained-release capsules ℞ *pediatric decongestant and antihistamine* [pseudoephedrine HCl; chlorpheniramine maleate] 60•4 mg

**Atrohist Plus** sustained-release tablets ℞ *decongestant; antihistamine; anticholinergic* [phenylpropanolamine HCl; phenylephrine HCl; chlorpheniramine maleate; hyoscyamine sulfate; atropine sulfate; scopolamine hydrobromide] 50•25•8•0.19• 0.04•0.01 mg

**Atrohist Sprinkle** sustained-release capsules (name changed to Atrohist Pediatric in 1995)

**atromepine** INN, DCF

**Atromid-S** capsules ℞ *cholesterol-lowering antihyperlipidemic; also for primary dysbetalipoproteinemia* [clofibrate] 500 mg (1 g available in Canada)

**AtroPen** auto-injector (automatic IM injection device) ℞ *antidote for* *organophosphorous or carbamate insecticides* [atropine sulfate] ≟

**atropine** USP, BAN *anticholinergic*

**Atropine Care** eye drops ℞ *mydriatic; cycloplegic* [atropine sulfate] 1%

**Atropine Care** ophthalmic ointment (discontinued 1993) ℞ *mydriatic; cycloplegic* [atropine sulfate]

**atropine methonitrate** INN, BAN *anticholinergic* [also: methylatropine nitrate]

**atropine methylnitrate** [see: methylatropine nitrate]

**atropine oxide** INN *anticholinergic* [also: atropine oxide HCl]

**atropine oxide HCl** USAN *anticholinergic* [also: atropine oxide]

**atropine propionate** [see: prampine]

**atropine sulfate** USP, JAN *GI antispasmodic; bronchodilator; cycloplegic; mydriatic* [also: atropine sulphate] 0.4, 0.6 mg oral; 1%, 2% eye drops; 0.05, 0.1, 0.3, 0.4, 0.5, 0.8, 1 mg/mL injection

**atropine sulphate** BAN *GI antispasmodic; bronchodilator; cycloplegic; mydriatic* [also: atropine sulfate]

**Atropine-1** eye drops ℞ *mydriatic; cycloplegic* [atropine sulfate] 1%

**Atropisol** Dropperettes (eye drops) ℞ *cycloplegic; mydriatic* [atropine sulfate] 1%

**Atrosept** sugar-coated tablets ℞ *urinary anti-infective; analgesic; antispasmodic; acidifier* [methenamine; phenyl salicylate; atropine sulfate; methylene blue; hyoscyamine sulfate; benzoic acid] 40.8•18.1•0.03•5.4•0.03•4.5 mg

**Atrovent** nasal spray, solution for inhalation, inhalation aerosol ℞ *bronchodilator* [ipratropium bromide] 0.03%, 0.06%; 0.02%; 18 μg/dose

**A/T/S** topical solution, gel ℞ *topical antibiotic for acne* [erythromycin] 2%

**atshitshi** *street drug slang* [see: marijuana]

**Attain** liquid OTC *enteral nutritional therapy* [lactose-free formula]

**attapulgite, activated** USP *suspending agent; GI adsorbent*

**Attenuvax** powder for subcu injection ℞ *measles vaccine* [measles virus vaccine, live attenuated] 0.5 mL

**Atuss DM** syrup ℞ *antitussive; decongestant; antihistamine* [dextromethorphan hydrobromide; phenylephrine HCl; chlorpheniramine maleate] 15•5•2 mg/5 mL

**Atuss EX** syrup ℞ *narcotic antitussive; expectorant* [hydrocodone bitartrate; guaifenesin] 5•100 mg/5 mL

**Atuss G** syrup ℞ *narcotic antitussive; decongestant; expectorant* [hydrocodone bitartrate; phenylephrine HCl; guaifenesin] 2•10•100 mg/5 mL

**Atuss HD** liquid ℞ *narcotic antitussive; decongestant; antihistamine* [hydrocodone bitartrate; phenylephrine HCl; chlorpheniramine maleate] 2.5•5•2 mg/5 mL

**$^{198}$Au** [see: gold Au 198]

**augmented betamethasone dipropionate** *topical corticosteroid*

**Augmentin** tablets, chewable tablets ℞ *penicillin-type antibiotic* [amoxicillin trihydrate; clavulanate potassium] 250•125, 500•125, 875•125 mg; 125•31.25, 200•28.5, 250•62.5 400•57 mg

**Augmentin** powder for oral suspension ℞ *penicillin-type antibiotic* [amoxicillin trihydrate; clavulanate potassium] 125•31.25, 200•28.5, 250•62.5, 400•57 mg/5 mL

**aunt Hazel** *street drug slang* [see: heroin]

**aunt Mary** *street drug slang* [see: marijuana]

**aunt Nora** *street drug slang* [see: cocaine]

**auntie; auntie Emma** *street drug slang* [see: opium]

**Auralgan Otic** ear drops ℞ *topical local anesthetic; analgesic* [benzocaine; antipyrine] 1.4%•5.4% ② Allergan; allergen

**auranofin** USAN, INN, BAN, JAN *antirheumatic (29% gold)*

**Aureomycin** ointment (discontinued 1996) OTC *topical antibiotic* [chlortetracycline HCl] 3% ② Achromycin; actinomycin

**Aureomycin** ophthalmic ointment (discontinued 1995) ℞ *ophthalmic antibiotic and antiprotozoal* [chlortetracycline HCl] 10 mg/g

**aureoquin** [now: quinetolate]

**Auriculin** *investigational (orphan) for acute renal failure and renal transplants; clinical trials discontinued 1997* [anaritide acetate]

**Auro Ear Drops** OTC *agent to emulsify and disperse ear wax* [carbamide peroxide] 6.5%

**Auro-Dri** ear drops OTC *antibacterial/ antifungal* [boric acid] 2.75%

**Aurolate** IM injection ℞ *antirheumatic* [gold sodium thiomalate] 50 mg/mL

**aurolin** [see: gold sodium thiosulfate]

**auropin** [see: gold sodium thiosulfate]

**aurora borealis** *street drug slang* [see: PCP]

**Aurorix** (available in Canada as Manerex) ℞ *investigational antidepressant* [moclobemide]

**aurosan** [see: gold sodium thiosulfate]

**aurothioglucose** USP *antirheumatic (50% gold)*

**aurothioglycanide** INN, DCF

**aurothiomalate disodium** [see: gold sodium thiomalate]

**aurothiomalate sodium** [see: gold sodium thiomalate]

**Auroto Otic** ear drops ℞ *topical local anesthetic; analgesic* [antipyrine; benzocaine] 1.4%•5.4%

**Autohaler** (delivery form) *breath-activated metered-dose inhaler*

**auto-injector** (delivery device) *automatic IM injection device*

**autolymphocyte therapy (ALT)** *investigational (orphan) for renal cell carcinoma*

**Autoplex T** IV injection or drip ℞ *antihemophilic to correct factor VIII deficiency and coagulation deficiency* [anti-inhibitor coagulant complex, heat treated] (each bottle is labeled with dosage)

**autoprothrombin I** [see: factor VII]

**autoprothrombin II** [see: factor IX]

**AV (Adriamycin, vincristine)** *chemotherapy protocol*

**Avail** tablets OTC *vitamin/mineral/iron supplement* [multiple vitamins & minerals; iron; folic acid] ±•18•0.4 mg ⦸ Advil

**Avalgesic** lotion (discontinued 1994) OTC *counterirritant* [methyl salicylate; menthol; camphor; methyl nicotinate; capsicum oleoresin]

**Avan** ℞ *investigational treatment for Alzheimer's disease* [idebenone]

**AVC** vaginal cream, vaginal suppositories ℞ *broad-spectrum bacteriostatic* [sulfanilamide] 15%; 1.05 g

**Aveeno** lotion OTC *moisturizer; emollient* [colloidal oatmeal] 1%

**Aveeno Anti-Itch** cream, lotion OTC *topical poison ivy treatment* [calamine; pramoxine HCl; camphor] 3%• 1%•0.3%

**Aveeno Cleansing** bar OTC *soap-free therapeutic skin cleanser* [colloidal oatmeal] 51%

**Aveeno Cleansing for Acne-Prone Skin** bar OTC *medicated cleanser for acne* [salicylic acid; colloidal oatmeal]

**Aveeno Moisturizing** cream OTC *moisturizer; emollient* [colloidal oatmeal] 1%

**Aveeno Oilated Bath** packets OTC *bath emollient* [colloidal oatmeal; mineral oil] 43%• ≜

**Aveeno Regular Bath** packets OTC *bath emollient* [colloidal oatmeal] 100%

**Aveeno Shave** gel OTC *moisturizer; emollient* [oatmeal flour] ≜

**Aveeno Shower & Bath** oil OTC *bath emollient* [colloidal oatmeal] 5%

**Aventyl** Pulvules (capsules), solution ℞ *tricyclic antidepressant* [nortriptyline HCl] 10, 25 mg; 10 mg/5 mL ⦸ Ambenyl; Bentyl

**avertin** [see: tribromoethanol]

**avicatonin** INN

**avilamycin** USAN, INN, BAN *antibacterial*

**avinar** [see: uredepa]

**Avita** cream ℞ *topical keratolytic for acne* [tretinoin] 0.025%

**Avitene Hemostat** fiber (discontinued 1996) ℞ *topical hemostatic aid for surgery* [microfibrillar collagen hemostat] ⦸ Ativan

**Avitene Hemostat** nonwoven web ℞ *topical hemostatic aid in surgery* [microfibrillar collagen hemostat] ② Ativan

**avitriptan fumarate** USAN *serotonin 5-HT₁ agonist for migraine*

**Aviva** ℞ *investigational treatment for Alzheimer's disease (clinical trials discontinued 1994)* [linopirdine]

**avizafone** INN, BAN

**avobenzone** USAN, INN *sunscreen*

**Avonex** powder for IM injection ℞ *immunomodulator for relapsing multiple sclerosis (orphan); investigational (orphan) for non-A, non-B hepatitis and brain tumors* [interferon beta-1a] 33 μg (6.6 million IU)/vial

**avoparcin** USAN, INN, BAN *glycopeptide antibiotic*

**AVP (actinomycin D, vincristine, Platinol)** *chemotherapy protocol*

**avridine** USAN, INN *antiviral*

**axamozide** INN

**axerophthol** [see: vitamin A]

**axetil** USAN, INN *combining name for radicals or groups*

**Axid** Pulvules (capsules) ℞ *histamine H₂ antagonist for treatment of gastric and duodenal ulcers* [nizatidine] 150, 300 mg

**Axid AR** tablets OTC *histamine H₂ antagonist for gastric and duodenal ulcers* [nizatidine] 75 mg

**Axocet** capsules ℞ *analgesic; antipyretic; sedative* [acetaminophen; butalbital] 650•50 mg

**Axotal** tablets (discontinued 1997) ℞ *analgesic; antipyretic; anti-inflammatory; sedative* [aspirin; butalbital] 650•50 mg

**Aygestin** tablets ℞ *progestin for amenorrhea, abnormal uterine bleeding, or endometriosis* [norethindrone acetate] 5 mg

**Ayr Saline** nasal mist, nose drops, nasal gel OTC *nasal moisturizer* [sodium chloride (saline)] 0.65%

**5-AZA (5-azacitidine)** [see: azacitidine]

**azabon** USAN, INN *CNS stimulant*

**azabuperone** INN

**azacitidine (5-AZA; 5-AZC)** USAN, INN *antineoplastic*

**azaclorzine** INN *coronary vasodilator* [also: azaclorzine HCl]

**azaclorzine HCl** USAN *coronary vasodilator* [also: azaclorzine]

**azaconazole** USAN, INN *antifungal*

**azacosterol** INN *avian chemosterilant* [also: azacosterol HCl]

**azacosterol HCl** USAN *avian chemosterilant* [also: azacosterol]

**AZA-CR** [see: azacitidine]

**Azactam** powder for IV or IM injection ℞ *monobactam-type bactericidal antibiotic* [aztreonam] 0.5, 1, 2 g

**azacyclonol** INN, BAN [also: azacyclonol HCl]

**azacyclonol HCl** NF [also: azacyclonol]

**5-azacytosine arabinoside (ara-AC)** [see: fazarabine]

**5-AZA-2'-deoxycytidine** *investigational (orphan) for acute leukemia*

**azaftozine** INN

**azalanstat dihydrochloride** USAN *hypolipidemic*

**azalomycin** INN, BAN

**azaloxan** INN *antidepressant* [also: azaloxan fumarate]

**azaloxan fumarate** USAN *antidepressant* [also: azaloxan]

**azamethiphos** BAN

**azamethonium bromide** INN, BAN

**azamulin** INN

**azanator** INN *bronchodilator* [also: azanator maleate]

**azanator maleate** USAN *bronchodilator* [also: azanator]

**azanidazole** USAN, INN, BAN *antiprotozoal*

**azaperone** USAN, INN, BAN *antipsychotic*

**azapetine** BAN

**azapetine phosphate** [see: azapetine]

**azapirones** *a class of anxiolytics*

**azaprocin** INN

**azapropazone** INN, BAN, DCF *anti-inflammatory* [also: apazone]

**azaquinzole** INN

**azaribine** USAN, INN, BAN *antipsoriatic*

**azarole** USAN *immunoregulator*

**azaserine** USAN, INN *antifungal*

**azasetron** INN

**azaspirium chloride** INN

**azastene**

**azatadine** INN, BAN *antihistamine* [also: azatadine maleate]

**azatadine maleate** USAN, USP *antihistamine* [also: azatadine]

**azatepa** INN *antineoplastic* [also: azetepa]

**azathioprine** USAN, USP, INN, BAN, JAN *immunosuppressant*

**azathioprine sodium** USP *immunosuppressant* 100 mg injection

**5-AZC (5-azacitidine)** [see: azacitidine]

**Azdone** tablets ℞ *narcotic analgesic* [hydrocodone bitartrate; aspirin] 5•500 mg

**azdU (azidouridine)** [q.v.]

**azelaic acid** USAN, INN *topical antimicrobial and keratolytic*

**azelastine** INN, BAN *antihistamine; antiallergic; antiasthmatic* [also: azelastine HCl]

**azelastine HCl** USAN, JAN *antihistamine; antiallergic; antiasthmatic* [also: azelastine]

**Azelex** cream ℞ *antimicrobial and keratolytic for inflammatory acne vulgaris* [azelaic acid] 20%

**azelnidipine** INN

**azepexole** INN, BAN

**azephine** [see: azapetine phosphate]

**azepinamide** [see: glypinamide]

**azepindole** USAN, INN *antidepressant*

**azetepa** USAN, BAN *antineoplastic* [also: azatepa]

**azetirelin** INN

**azidamfenicol** INN, BAN, DCF

**3'-azido-2',3'dideoxyuridine** *orphan status withdrawn 1994*

**azidoamphenicol** [see: azidamfenicol]

**azidocillin** INN, BAN

**azidothymidine (AZT)** [now: zidovudine]

**azidouridine (azdU)** *investigational (Phase I) antiviral for HIV and AIDS*

**azimexon** INN

**azimilide dihydrochloride** USAN *antiarrhythmic; antifibrillatory*

**azintamide** INN

**azinthiamide** [see: azintamide]

**azipramine** INN *antidepressant* [also: azipramine HCl]

**azipramine HCl** USAN *antidepressant* [also: azipramine]

**aziridinyl benzoquinone** [see: diaziquone]

**azithromycin** USAN, USP, INN, BAN *macrolide antibacterial antibiotic*

**azlocillin** USAN, INN, BAN *antibacterial*

**azlocillin sodium** USP *antibacterial*

**Azmacort** oral inhalation aerosol ℞ *corticosteroid for prevention or treatment of bronchial asthma episodes* [triamcinolone acetonide] 100 μg/dose

**Azo Gantanol** film-coated tablets (discontinued 1995) ℞ *urinary anti-infective; urinary analgesic* [sulfamethoxazole; phenazopyridine HCl] 500•100 mg

**Azo Gantrisin** film-coated tablets (discontinued 1995) ℞ *urinary anti-infective; urinary analgesic* [sulfisoxazole; phenazopyridine HCl] 500•50 mg

**azoconazole** [now: azaconazole]

**azodisal sodium (ADS)** [now: olsalazine sodium]

**azolimine** USAN, INN *diuretic* ② Azulfidine

**azosemide** USAN, INN, JAN *diuretic*

**Azo-Standard** tablets OTC *urinary analgesic* [phenazopyridine HCl] 95 mg

**Azostix** reagent strips for professional use *in vitro diagnostic aid to estimate the amount of BUN in whole blood*

**Azo-Sulfisoxazole** tablets ℞ *urinary anti-infective; urinary analgesic* [sulfisoxazole; phenazopyridine HCl] 500•50 mg

**azotomycin** USAN, INN *antibiotic antineoplastic*

**azovan blue** BAN *blood volume test* [also: Evans blue]

**azovan sodium** [see: Evans blue]

**AZT (azidothymidine)** [now: zidovudine]

**Aztec** ℞ *investigational (Phase III) controlled-release formulation for early HIV and AIDS* [zidovudine]

**AZT-P-ddI** *investigational (Phase I) antiviral for AIDS*

**aztreonam** USAN, USP, INN, BAN, JAN *monobactam-type bactericidal antibiotic*

**azulene sulfonate sodium** JAN [also: sodium gualenate]

**Azulfidine** oral suspension (discontinued 1995) ℞ *broad-spectrum bacteriostatic; anti-inflammatory for ulcerative colitis* [sulfasalazine] 250 mg/5 mL ⚕ azolimine

**Azulfidine** tablets ℞ *broad-spectrum bacteriostatic; anti-inflammatory for ulcerative colitis* [sulfasalazine] 500 mg

**Azulfidine EN-tabs** enteric-coated tablets ℞ *broad-spectrum bacteriosta-tic; anti-inflammatory for ulcerative colitis and rheumatoid arthritis* [sulfasalazine] 500 mg

**azumolene** INN *skeletal muscle relaxant* [also: azumolene sodium]

**azumolene sodium** USAN *skeletal muscle relaxant* [also: azumolene]

**azure A carbacrylic resin** [see: azuresin]

**azuresin** NF, BAN

# B

**B Complex + C** timed-release tablets OTC *vitamin supplement* [multiple B vitamins; vitamin C] ± • 500 mg

**B Complex with C and B-12** injection ℞ *parenteral vitamin supplement* [multiple vitamins] ±

**B Complex-50** sustained-release tablets OTC *vitamin supplement* [multiple B vitamins; folic acid; biotin] ± • 400 • 50 μg

**B Complex-150** sustained-release tablets OTC *vitamin supplement* [multiple B vitamins; folic acid; biotin] ± • 400 • 150 μg

**B & O Supprettes No. 15A; B & O Supprettes No. 16A** suppositories ℞ *narcotic analgesic* [belladonna extract; opium] 16.2 • 30 mg; 16.2 • 60 mg

**B vitamins** [see: vitamin B]

**$B_1$ (vitamin $B_1$)** [see: thiamine HCl]

**$B_2$ (vitamin $B_2$)** [see: riboflavin]

**$B_3$ (vitamin $B_3$)** [see: niacin; niacinamide]

**$B_5$ (vitamin $B_5$)** [see: calcium pantothenate]

**$B_6$ (vitamin $B_6$)** [see: pyridoxine HCl]

**$B_8$ (vitamin $B_8$)** [see: adenosine phosphate]

**$B_{12}$ (vitamin $B_{12}$)** [see: cyanocobalamin]

**$B_{12a}$ (vitamin $B_{12a}$)** [see: hydroxocobalamin]

**$B_{12b}$ (vitamin $B_{12b}$)** [see: hydroxocobalamin]

**B-50** tablets OTC *vitamin supplement* [multiple B vitamins; folic acid; biotin] ± • 100 • 50 μg

**B-50** timed-release tablets (discontinued 1995) OTC *vitamin supplement* [multiple B vitamins; folic acid; biotin] ± • 100 • 50 μg

**B-100** tablets, timed-release tablets OTC *vitamin supplement* [multiple B vitamins; folic acid; biotin] ± • 100 • 100 μg; ± • 400 • 50 μg

**$B_c$ (vitamin $B_c$)** [see: folic acid]

**$B_t$ (vitamin $B_t$)** [see: carnitine]

**Babee Teething** lotion OTC *topical oral anesthetic; antiseptic* [benzocaine; cetalkonium chloride] 2.5% • 0.02%

**baby; baby bhang** *street drug slang* [see: marijuana]

**baby T** *street drug slang* [see: cocaine, crack]

**Baby Vitamin** drops OTC *vitamin supplement* [multiple vitamins] ±

**Baby Vitamin with Iron** drops OTC *vitamin/iron supplement* [multiple vitamins; iron] ± • 10 mg/mL

**Babylax** [see: Fleet Babylax]

**BAC (BCNU, ara-C, cyclophosphamide)** *chemotherapy protocol*

**BAC (benzalkonium chloride)** [q.v.]

**bacampicillin** INN, BAN *bactericidal antibiotic* [also: bacampicillin HCl]

**bacampicillin HCl** USAN, USP, JAN *bactericidal antibiotic* [also: bacampicillin]

**BACI** ℞ *investigational anti-infective for AIDS-related cryptosporidiosis* [cryptosporidium hyperimmune bovine colostrum IgG concentrate]

**Bacid** capsules OTC *dietary supplement; fever blister treatment; not generally regarded as safe and effective as an antidiarrheal* [*Lactobacillus acidophilus*] 500 million cultures ⊡ Banacid

**Baciguent** ointment OTC *topical antibiotic* [bacitracin] 500 U/g

**Baci-IM** powder for IM injection ℞ *bactericidal antibiotic* [bacitracin] 50 000 U

**bacillus Calmette-Guérin (BCG) vaccine** [see: BCG vaccine]

**bacitracin** USP, INN, BAN, JAN *bactericidal antibiotic; investigational (orphan) for pseudomembranous enterocolitis* 500 U/g topical; 50 000 U/ vial injection ⊡ Bacitrin; Bactrim

**bacitracin zinc** USP, BAN *bactericidal antibiotic*

**bacitracins zinc complex** [see: bacitracin zinc]

**Backache Maximum Strength Relief** film-coated caplets OTC *analgesic; antirheumatic* [magnesium salicylate] 467 mg

**backbreakers** *street drug slang for a combination of LSD and strychnine* [see: LSD; strychnine]

**Back-Pack** (trademarked packaging form) *unit-of-use package*

**back-to-back** *street drug slang for smoking crack after injecting heroin or vice versa* [see: heroin; cocaine, crack]

**backwards** *street drug slang for various CNS depressants*

**baclofen** (L-baclofen) USAN, USP, INN, BAN, JAN *skeletal muscle relaxant for intractable spasticity due to spinal cord injury or disease* (orphan) 10, 20 mg oral

**bacmecillinam** INN

**Bacmin** tablets ℞ *vitamin/mineral/iron supplement* [multiple vitamins & minerals; iron; folic acid; biotin] ≜ • 27•0.8•0.15 mg

**BACOD (bleomycin, Adriamycin, CCNU, Oncovin, dexamethasone)** *chemotherapy protocol*

**BACON (bleomycin, Adriamycin, CCNU, Oncovin, nitrogen mustard)** *chemotherapy protocol*

**BACOP (bleomycin, Adriamycin, cyclophosphamide, Oncovin, prednisone)** *chemotherapy protocol*

**BACT (BCNU, ara-C, cyclophosphamide, thioguanine)** *chemotherapy protocol*

**bactericidal and permeability-increasing (BPI) protein** *investigational (Phase III) treatment for gram-negative sepsis*

**bactericidal/permeability-increasing protein** [see: rBPI-21]

**bacteriostatic sodium chloride** [see: sodium chloride]

**Bacteriostatic Sodium Chloride Injection** ℞ *IV diluent* [sodium chloride (saline)] 0.9% (normal)

**Bacti-Cleanse** liquid OTC *soap-free therapeutic skin cleanser* [benzalkonium chloride] ≜

**Bacticort** eye drop suspension (discontinued 1995) ℞ *topical ophthalmic corticosteroidal anti-inflammatory; antibiotic* [hydrocortisone; neomycin sulfate; polymyxin B sulfate] 1%• 0.35%•10 000 U/mL

**Bactigen B Streptococcus-CS** slide test for professional use *in vitro diagnostic aid for Group B streptococcal antigens in vaginal and cervical swabs*

**Bactigen Meningitis Panel** slide test for professional use *in vitro diagnostic aid for H influenzae, N meningitidis, and S pneumoniae in various fluids* [latex agglutination test]

**Bactigen N meningitidis** slide test for professional use ℞ *in vitro diagnostic aid for Neisseria meningitidis* [latex agglutination test]

**Bactigen S Pneumonia** test kit for professional use (discontinued 1996) *in vitro diagnostic aid for Streptococcus pneumoniae antigens in various fluids*

**Bactigen Salmonella-Shigella** slide test for professional use *in vitro diagnostic aid for salmonella and shigella* [latex agglutination test]

**Bactigen Strep B** slide test for professional use (discontinued 1996) *in*

*vitro diagnostic aid for Group B strep-
tococcal antigens in various fluids*

**Bactine Antiseptic Anesthetic** aerosol
(discontinued 1995) OTC *topical local
anesthetic; antiseptic* [lidocaine HCl;
benzalkonium chloride] 2.5%•0.13%

**Bactine Antiseptic Anesthetic** liquid, spray OTC *topical local anesthetic;
antiseptic* [lidocaine HCl; benzalkonium chloride] 2.5%•0.13%

**Bactine First Aid Antibiotic** ointment OTC *topical antibiotic* [poly-
myxin B sulfate; neomycin sulfate;
bacitracin]

**Bactine First Aid Antibiotic Plus
Anesthetic** ointment OTC *topical
antibiotic; topical local anesthetic*
[polymyxin B sulfate; neomycin sulfate; bacitracin; diperodon HCl]
5000 U•3.5 mg•400 U•10 mg per g

**Bactine Hydrocortisone; Maxi-
mum Strength Bactine** cream OTC
*topical corticosteroid* [hydrocortisone]
0.5%; 1%

**Bactocill** capsules, powder for IV or
IM injection ℞ *bactericidal antibiotic
(penicillinase-resistant penicillin)*
[oxacillin sodium] 250, 500 mg;
0.25, 0.5, 1, 2, 4, 10 g ⑨ Pathocil

**BactoShield** aerosol foam, solution
OTC *broad-spectrum antimicrobial; germicidal* [chlorhexidine gluconate;
alcohol 4%] 4%

**BactoShield 2** solution OTC *broad-spectrum antimicrobial; germicidal* [chlor-
hexidine gluconate; alcohol 4%] 2%

**Bactrim; Bactrim DS** tablets ℞ *anti-
infective; antibacterial* [trimethoprim;
sulfamethoxazole] 80•400 mg; 160•
800 mg ⑨ bacitracin

**Bactrim IV** infusion ℞ *anti-infective;
antibacterial* [trimethoprim; sulfa-
methoxazole] 80•400 mg/5 mL

**Bactrim Pediatric** oral suspension ℞
*anti-infective; antibacterial* [trimetho-
prim; sulfamethoxazole] 40•200
mg/5 mL

**Bactroban** ointment ℞ *topical antibiotic for impetigo* [mupirocin] 2%

**Bactroban Nasal** ointment in single-
use tubes ℞ *antibiotic for iatrogenic
methicillin-resistant Staphylococcus*

*aureus (MRSA) infections* [mupirocin
calcium] 2%

**bad** *street drug slang* [see: cocaine, crack]

**bad pizza** *street drug slang* [see: PCP]

**bad seed** *street drug slang* [see: mescaline; heroin; marijuana]

**bag** *street drug slang for 1 to 15 g of heroin; also known as a "deck"* [see: her-
oin]

**bah-say** *street drug slang* [see: cocaine,
crack; coca paste]

**bakeprofen** INN

**baker's yeast** *natural source of protein
and B-complex vitamins*

**BAL (British antilewisite)** [now:
dimercaprol]

**BAL in Oil** deep IM injection ℞ *antidote for arsenic, gold, and mercury poisoning; lead poisoning adjunct* [dimer-
caprol in peanut oil] 100 mg/mL

**balafilcon A** USAN *hydrophilic contact
lens material*

**Baldex** eye drops, ophthalmic ointment (discontinued 1993) ℞ *ophthalmic topical corticosteroidal anti-
inflammatory* [dexamethasone
sodium phosphate]

**bale** *street drug slang for 1 pound of
marijuana* [see: marijuana]

**balipramine** BAN [also: depramine]

**ball** *street drug slang* [see: cocaine, crack]

**ballot** *street drug slang* [see: heroin]

**Balmex** ointment OTC *moisturizer;
emollient; astringent; antiseptic* [peru-
vian balsam; zinc oxide; bismuth
subnitrate]

**Balmex Baby** powder OTC *topical diaper rash treatment* [zinc oxide; balsam
Peru; corn starch]

**Balmex Emollient** lotion OTC *moisturizer; emollient*

**Balneol Perianal Cleansing** lotion
OTC *emollient/protectant* [mineral oil;
lanolin]

**Balnetar** bath oil OTC *antipsoriatic;
antiseborrheic; antipruritic; emollient*
[coal tar] 2.5%

**balsalazide** INN, BAN *investigational
(Phase III) gastrointestinal anti-inflammatory for ulcerative colitis* [also: balsalazide disodium]

**balsalazide disodium** USAN *investigational (Phase III) gastrointestinal anti-inflammatory for ulcerative colitis* [also: balsalazide]

**balsalazide sodium** [see: balsalazide disodium]

**balsalazine** [see: balsalazide disodium; balsalazide]

**balsam Peru** [see: peruvian balsam; balsam tree]

**balsan** [see: peruvian balsam]

**bam** *street drug slang for various CNS depressants or amphetamines* [see: amphetamines]

**bamaluzole** INN

**bambalacha** *street drug slang* [see: marijuana]

**bambermycin** INN, BAN *antibacterial antibiotic* [also: bambermycins]

**bambermycins** USAN *antibacterial antibiotic* [also: bambermycin]

**bambs** *street drug slang for various CNS depressants*

**bambuterol** INN, BAN

**bamethan** INN, BAN *vasodilator* [also: bamethan sulfate]

**bamethan sulfate** USAN, JAN *vasodilator* [also: bamethan]

**bamifylline** INN, BAN *bronchodilator* [also: bamifylline HCl]

**bamifylline HCl** USAN *bronchodilator* [also: bamifylline]

**bamipine** INN, BAN, DCF

**bammy** *street drug slang* [see: marijuana]

**bamnidazole** USAN, INN *antiprotozoal (Trichomonas)*

**BAMON (bleomycin, Adriamycin, methotrexate, Oncovin, nitrogen mustard)** *chemotherapy protocol*

**Banacid** tablets OTC *antacid* [magnesium hydroxide; aluminum hydroxide; magnesium trisilicate] ☒ Bacid

**Banadyne-3** solution OTC *topical oral anesthetic; antipruritic/counterirritant; antiseptic* [lidocaine; menthol; alcohol 45%] 4%•1%

**Banalg** lotion OTC *counterirritant* [methyl salicylate; camphor; menthol] 4.9%•2%•1%

**Banalg Hospital Strength** lotion OTC *counterirritant* [methyl salicylate; menthol] 14%•3%

**banano** (Spanish for "banana tree") *street drug slang for a marijuana or tobacco cigarette laced with cocaine* [see: marijuana; tobacco; cocaine]

**Bancap** capsules (discontinued 1994) ℞ *analgesic; antipyretic; sedative* [acetaminophen; butalbital] 325•50 mg

**Bancap HC** capsules ℞ *narcotic analgesic* [hydrocodone bitartrate; acetaminophen] 5•500 mg

**bandage, adhesive** USP *surgical aid*

**bandage, gauze** USP *surgical aid*

**Banesin** tablets (discontinued 1994) OTC *analgesic; antipyretic* [acetaminophen] 500 mg

**Banex** liquid ℞ *decongestant; antihistamine; expectorant* [phenylpropanolamine HCl; phenylephrine HCl; guaifenesin]

**Banflex** IV or IM injection ℞ *skeletal muscle relaxant* [orphenadrine citrate] 30 mg/mL

**Bangesic** liniment (discontinued 1994) OTC *counterirritant* [menthol; camphor; methyl salicylate; eucalyptus oil]

**bank bandit pills** *street drug slang for various CNS depressants*

**banocide** [see: diethylcarbamazine citrate]

**Banophen** elixir OTC *antihistamine* [diphenhydramine HCl] 12.5 mg/5 mL

**Banophen Decongestant** capsules OTC *decongestant; antihistamine* [pseudoephedrine HCl; diphenhydramine HCl] 60•25 mg ☒ Barophen

**BanSmoke** gum (discontinued 1995) OTC *smoking deterrent* [benzocaine] 6 mg

**Banthīne** tablets ℞ *anticholinergic; peptic ulcer treatment adjunct* [methantheline bromide] 50 mg ☒ Brethine

**Bantron** tablets OTC *smoking deterrent* [lobeline sulfate alkaloids; tribasic calcium phosphate; magnesium carbonate] 2•130•130 mg

**baquiloprim** INN, BAN

**bar** *street drug slang* [see: marijuana]

**barb; barbie doll; barbies; barbs**
*street drug slang for various CNS
depressants, primarily barbiturates*

**barbenyl** [see: phenobarbital]

**barbexaclone** INN

**Barbidonna** elixir (discontinued
1995) ℞ *anticholinergic; sedative*
[atropine sulfate; scopolamine
hydrobromide; hyoscyamine hydrobromide; phenobarbital] 0.034•
0.01•0.174•21.6 mg/5 mL

**Barbidonna; Barbidonna No. 2** tablets ℞ *GI anticholinergic; sedative*
[atropine sulfate; scopolamine
hydrobromide; hyoscyamine hydrobromide; phenobarbital] 0.025•
0.0074•0.1286•16 mg; 0.025•
0.0074•0.1286•32 mg

**barbiphenyl** [see: phenobarbital]

**Barbita** sugar-coated tablets (discontinued 1993) ℞ *long-acting barbiturate sedative, hypnotic and anticonvulsant* [phenobarbital]

**barbital** NF, INN, JAN [also: barbitone]

**barbital, soluble** [now: barbital sodium]

**barbital sodium** NF, INN [also: barbitone sodium]

**barbitone** BAN [also: barbital]

**barbitone sodium** BAN [also: barbital
sodium]

**barbiturates** *a class of sedative/hyp-
notics that produce a wide range of
mood alteration; also widely abused as
addictive street drugs*

**barbs** *street drug slang* [see: cocaine]

**Barc** liquid OTC *pediculicide* [pyre-
thrins; piperonyl butoxide; petroleum distillate] 0.18%•2.2%•5.52%

**Baricon** powder for suspension ℞ *GI
contrast radiopaque agent* [barium sul-
fate] 98%

**Baridium** tablets ℞ *urinary analgesic*
[phenazopyridine HCl] 100 mg

**barium** *element (Ba)*

**barium hydroxide lime** USP *carbon
dioxide absorbent*

**barium sulfate** USP, JAN *GI radiopaque medium*

**barmastine** USAN, INN *antihistamine*

**BarnesHind Saline for Sensitive
Eyes** solution OTC *rinsing/storage

solution for soft contact lenses* [pre-
served saline solution]

**barnidipine** INN

**Barobag** suspension (discontinued
1993) ℞ *GI contrast radiopaque agent*
[barium sulfate] 97%

**Baro-cat** suspension ℞ *GI contrast radiopaque agent* [barium sulfate] 1.5%

**Baroflave** powder ℞ *GI contrast radiopaque agent* [barium sulfate]

**Barophen** elixir (discontinued 1995)
℞ *GI anticholinergic; sedative* [atro-
pine sulfate; scopolamine hydrobromide; hyoscyamine sulfate; pheno-
barbital] 0.0194•0.0065•0.1037•
16.2 mg/5 mL ② Banophen

**Baros** effervescent granules ℞ *GI contrast radiopaque agent* [sodium bicarbonate; tartaric acid; simethicone]
460•420• ² mg/g

**barosmin** [see: diosmin]

**Barosperse** powder for suspension ℞
*GI contrast radiopaque agent* [barium
sulfate] 95%

**Barosperse, Liquid** suspension ℞ *GI
contrast radiopaque agent* [barium sul-
fate] 60%

**barrels** *street drug slang* [see: LSD]

**Barriere** cream *investigational protective
hand cream*

**barucainide** INN

**BAS (benzyl analogue of sero-
tonin)** [see: benanserin HCl]

**Basaljel** tablets, capsules, suspension
OTC *antacid* [aluminum carbonate gel,
basic] 500 mg; 500 mg; 400 mg/5 mL

**base; baseball** *street drug slang, from
"freebase"* [see: cocaine, crack]

**bash** *street drug slang* [see: marijuana]

**basic aluminum acetate** [see: aluminum subacetate]

**basic aluminum aminoacetate** [see:
dihydroxyaluminum aminoacetate]

**basic aluminum carbonate** [see: aluminum carbonate, basic]

**basic aluminum chloride** [see: aluminum sesquichlorohydrate]

**basic aluminum glycinate** [see: dihydroxyaluminum aminoacetate]

**basic bismuth carbonate** [see: bismuth subcarbonate]

**basic bismuth gallate** [see: bismuth subgallate]

**basic bismuth nitrate** [see: bismuth subnitrate]

**basic bismuth potassium bismuthotartrate** [see: bismuth potassium tartrate]

**basic bismuth salicylate** [see: bismuth subsalicylate]

**basic fibroblast growth factor (bFGF)** [see: ersofermin]

**basic fuchsin** [see: fuchsin, basic]

**basic zinc acetate** [see: zinc acetate, basic]

**basifungin** USAN, INN *antifungal*

**basuco** *street drug slang for coca paste or coca paste residue sprinkled on a marijuana or tobacco cigarette* [see: coca paste; marijuana; tobacco]

**batanopride** INN *antiemetic* [also: batanopride HCl]

**batanopride HCl** USAN *antiemetic* [also: batanopride]

**batebulast** INN

**batelapine** INN *antipsychotic* [also: batelapine HCl]

**batelapine maleate** USAN *antipsychotic* [also: batelapine]

**bathtub speed** *street drug slang* [see: methcathinone]

**batilol** INN

**batimastat** USAN, INN *investigational (Phase III) antineoplastic; matrix metalloproteinase (MMP) inhibitor*

**batoprazine** INN

**batroxobin** INN, JAN

**battery acid** *street drug slang* [see: LSD]

**batu** *street drug slang for smokable methamphetamine* [see: methamphetamine HCl]

**batyl alcohol** [see: batilol]

**batylol** [see: batilol]

**BAVIP (bleomycin, Adriamycin, vinblastine, imidazole carboxamide, prednisone)** *chemotherapy protocol*

**baxitozine** INN

**Baycol** tablets R̥ *cholesterol-lowering antihyperlipidemic; HMG-CoA reductase inhibitor* [cerivastatin sodium] 0.2, 0.3 mg

**Bayer, Therapy** caplets (name changed to Bayer Enteric Coated in 1994)

**Bayer Arthritis Regimen** delayed-release enteric-coated tablets OTC *analgesic; antipyretic; anti-inflammatory; antirheumatic* [aspirin] 500 mg

**Bayer Aspirin, Genuine; Maximum Bayer Aspirin** film-coated tablets, film-coated caplets OTC *analgesic; antipyretic; anti-inflammatory; antirheumatic* [aspirin] 325 mg; 500 mg

**Bayer Aspirin Regimen** delayed-release enteric-coated tablets and caplets OTC *analgesic; antipyretic; anti-inflammatory; antirheumatic* [aspirin] 81, 325 mg

**Bayer Buffered Aspirin** tablets OTC *analgesic; antipyretic; anti-inflammatory; antirheumatic* [aspirin, buffered] 325 mg

**Bayer Children's Aspirin** chewable tablets OTC *analgesic; antipyretic; anti-inflammatory; antirheumatic* [aspirin] 81 mg

**Bayer Enteric 500** delayed-release enteric-coated caplets (name changed to Bayer Arthritis Regimen in 1995)

**Bayer Enteric Coated** delayed-release enteric-coated caplets (name changed to Bayer Aspirin Regimen in 1995)

**Bayer Low Adult Strength** delayed-release enteric-coated tablets (name changed to Bayer Aspirin Regimen in 1995)

**Bayer Plus** caplets OTC *analgesic; antipyretic; anti-inflammatory; antirheumatic* [aspirin (buffered with calcium carbonate, magnesium carbonate and magnesium oxide)] 500 mg

**Bayer Select Allergy Sinus, Aspirin-Free** caplets OTC *decongestant; antihistamine; analgesic* [pseudoephedrine HCl; chlorpheniramine maleate; acetaminophen] 30•2•500 mg

**Bayer Select Backache** caplets OTC *analgesic; antipyretic; anti-inflammatory; antirheumatic* [magnesium salicylate] 580 mg

**Bayer Select Chest Cold** caplets OTC *antitussive; analgesic* [dextromethor-

phan hydrobromide; acetamino-
phen] 15•500 mg

**Bayer Select Flu Relief** caplets OTC
*antitussive; decongestant; antihista-
mine; analgesic* [dextromethorphan
hydrobromide; pseudoephedrine
HCl; chlorpheniramine maleate;
acetaminophen] 15•30•2•500 mg

**Bayer Select Head & Chest Cold,
Aspirin-Free** caplets OTC *antitussive;
decongestant; expectorant; analgesic*
[dextromethorphan hydrobromide;
pseudoephedrine HCl; guaifenesin;
acetaminophen] 10•30•100•325 mg

**Bayer Select Head Cold; Bayer
Select Sinus Pain Relief** caplets
OTC *decongestant; analgesic; antipyretic* [pseudoephedrine HCl; aceta-
minophen] 30•500 mg

**Bayer Select Headache** caplets OTC
*analgesic; antipyretic* [acetaminophen;
caffeine] 500•65 mg

**Bayer Select Menstrual** caplets OTC
*analgesic; antipyretic; diuretic* [aceta-
minophen; pamabrom] 500•25 mg

**Bayer Select Night Time Cold** caplets OTC *antitussive; decongestant;
antihistamine; analgesic* [dextometh-
orphan hydrobromide; pseudoephedrine HCl; triprolidine HCl; aceta-
minophen] 15•30•1.25•500 mg

**Bayer Select Night Time Pain
Relief** caplets OTC *antihistaminic
sleep aid; analgesic* [diphenhydramine
HCl; acetaminophen] 25•500 mg

**Bayer Select Pain Relief Formula**
caplets OTC *nonsteroidal anti-inflammatory drug (NSAID); analgesic* [ibu-
profen] 200 mg

**Bayer Timed Release, 8-Hour** caplets
OTC *analgesic; antipyretic; anti-inflammatory; antirheumatic* [aspirin] 650 mg

**Baylocaine 2% Viscous; Baylo-
caine 4%** solution R̲ *topical anesthetic for mouth and pharynx* [lido-
caine HCl]

**Baypress** R̲ *investigational antihypertensive; calcium channel blocker* [nitren-
dipine]

**bazinaprine** INN

**bazooka** *street drug slang for crack or a
combination of coca paste and mari-*
*juana* [see: cocaine, crack; coca
paste; marijuana]

**bazulco** *street drug slang* [see: cocaine]

**B-bomb** *1940s street drug slang for a
Benzedrine inhaler (amphetamine sulfate; discontinued)*

**BBVP-M (BCNU, bleomycin,
VePesid, prednisone, methotrexate)** *chemotherapy protocol*

**BC** tablets, powder OTC *analgesic; antipyretic; anti-inflammatory* [aspirin;
salicylamide; caffeine] 325•95•16
mg; 650•145•32 mg/packet

**B$_c$ (vitamin B$_c$)** [see: folic acid]

**BC Arthritis Strength** powder OTC
*analgesic; antipyretic; anti-inflamma-
tory* [aspirin; salicylamide; caffeine]
742•222•36 mg

**BC Cold Powder Non-Drowsy For-
mula** packets (name changed to BC
Cold-Sinus Powder in 1995)

**BC Cold-Sinus Powder** packets OTC
*decongestant; analgesic; antipyretic*
[phenylpropanolamine HCl; aspirin]
25•650 mg

**BC Cold-Sinus-Allergy Powder**
packets OTC *decongestant; antihistamine; analgesic; antipyretic* [phenylpro-
panolamine HCl; chlorpheniramine
maleate; aspirin] 25•4•650 mg

**BC Multi Symptom Cold Powder**
packets (name changed to BC Cold-
Sinus-Allergy Powder in 1995)

**B-C with Folic Acid** tablets R̲ *vitamin
supplement* [multiple B vitamins; vitamin C; folic acid] ±•500•0.5 mg

**B-C with Folic Acid Plus** tablets R̲
*vitamin/mineral/iron supplement* [mul-
tiple vitamins & minerals; ferrous
fumarate; folic acid; biotin] ±•27•
0.8•0.15 mg

**BCAA (branched-chain amino
acids)** [see: isoleucine; leucine; valine]

**BCAP (BCNU, cyclophosphamide,
Adriamycin, prednisone)** *chemotherapy protocol*

**BCAVe; B-CAVe (bleomycin,
CCNU, Adriamycin, Velban)** *chemotherapy protocol*

**B-C-Bid** caplets OTC *vitamin supplement* [multiple B vitamins; vitamin
C] ±•300 mg

**BCD (bleomycin, cyclophospha-
mide, dactinomycin)** *chemotherapy
protocol*
**B-C-E & Zinc** tablets (discontinued
1993) OTC *vitamin/zinc supplement*
[vitamin E; vitamin C; multiple B
vitamins; zinc]
**BCG vaccine (bacillus Calmette-
Guérin)** USP *active bacterin for tuberculosis*
**B-CHOP (bleomycin, Cytoxin,
hydroxydaunomycin, Oncovin,
prednisone)** *chemotherapy protocol*
**BCMF (bleomycin, cyclophospha-
mide, methotrexate, fluorouracil)** *chemotherapy protocol*
**BCNU (bis-chloroethyl-nitroso-
urea)** [see: carmustine]
**B-Complex** elixir OTC *vitamin supplement* [multiple B vitamins] ±
**B-Complex and B-12** tablets OTC *vitamin supplement* [multiple B vitamins; protease] ± • 10 mg
**B-Complex with B-12** tablets OTC
*vitamin supplement* [multiple B vita-
mins] ±
**B-Complex/Vitamin C** caplets OTC
*vitamin supplement* [multiple B vitamins; vitamin C] ± • 300 mg
**BCOP (BCNU, cyclophosphamide,
Oncovin, prednisone)** *chemotherapy protocol*
**BCP (BCNU, cyclophosphamide,
prednisone)** *chemotherapy protocol*
**BC-Vite** tablets OTC *vitamin supplement*
[multiple B vitamins; vitamin C]
**BCVP (BCNU, cyclophosphamide,
vincristine, prednisone)** *chemotherapy protocol*
**BCVPP (BCNU, cyclophospha-
mide, vinblastine, procarbazine,
prednisone)** *chemotherapy protocol*
**B-D glucose** chewable tablets OTC
*glucose elevating agent* [glucose] 5 g
**bDNA (branched DNA) assay**
*investigational in vitro diagnostic aid for
HIV in the blood*
**BDNF (brain-derived neurotrophic
factor)** [q.v.]
**B-DOPA (bleomycin, DTIC,
Oncovin, prednisone, Adriamycin)** *chemotherapy protocol*

**BEAC (BCNU, etoposide, ara-C,
cyclophosphamide)** *chemotherapy
protocol*
**BEAM (BCNU, etoposide, ara-C,
melphalan)** *chemotherapy protocol*
**beam me up Scottie** *street drug slang
for crack dipped in PCP* [see: cocaine,
crack; PCP]
**Beano** liquid, tablets OTC *digestive aid*
[alpha-D-galactosidase enzyme]
**beans** *street drug slang for amphetamines,
various CNS depressants, or mescaline*
[see: amphetamines; mescaline]
**beast** *street drug slang* [see: LSD]
**beautiful boulders** *street drug slang*
[see: cocaine, crack]
**bebe** *street drug slang* [see: cocaine,
crack]
**Bebulin VH** Ŗ *investigational coagulant
for hemophilia B* [factor IX complex]
**BEC-2** *investigational (Phase III) cancer vaccine*
**becanthone HCl** USAN *antischistosomal* [also: becantone]
**becantone** INN *antischistosomal* [also:
becanthone HCl]
**becantone HCl** [see: becanthone HCl]
**becaplermin** USAN *recombinant
platelet-derived growth factor B for
chronic dermal ulcers*
**Because** vaginal foam OTC *spermicidal
contraceptive* [nonoxynol 9] 8%
**beciparcil** INN
**beclamide** INN, BAN, DCF
**becliconazole** INN
**beclobrate** INN, BAN
**beclometasone** INN *corticosteroidal
inhalant for asthma; intranasal steroid*
[also: beclomethasone dipropionate;
beclomethasone; beclometasone
dipropionate]
**beclometasone dipropionate** JAN
*corticosteroidal inhalant for asthma;
intranasal steroid* [also: beclomethasone dipropionate; beclomethasone;
beclometasone]
**beclomethasone** BAN *corticosteroidal
inhalant for asthma; intranasal steroid*
[also: beclomethasone dipropionate;
beclomethasone; beclometasone
dipropionate]

**beclomethasone dipropionate** USAN, USP *corticosteroidal inhalant for asthma; intranasal steroid* [also: beclometasone; beclomethasone; beclomethasone dipropionate]

**beclotiamine** INN

**Beclovent** oral inhalation aerosol ℞ *corticosteroid for bronchial asthma* [beclomethasone dipropionate] 42 μg/dose

**Becomject-100** injection (discontinued 1996) ℞ *parenteral vitamin therapy* [multiple B vitamins] ±

**Beconase** nasal inhalation aerosol ℞ *intranasal steroidal anti-inflammatory* [beclomethasone dipropionate] 42 μg/dose

**Beconase AQ** nasal spray ℞ *intranasal steroidal anti-inflammatory* [beclomethasone dipropionate] 0.042%

**bectumomab** USAN *monoclonal antibody; investigational (Phase III, orphan) diagnostic aid for non-Hodgkin's lymphoma and AIDS-related lymphoma* [also: technetium Tc 99m bectumomab]

**beechwood creosote** [see: creosote carbonate]

**beef tallow** JAN

**Beelith** tablets OTC *dietary supplement* [vitamin B$_6$; magnesium oxide] 20•362 mg

**beemers** *street drug slang* [see: cocaine, crack]

**Beepen-VK** tablets, powder for oral solution ℞ *bactericidal antibiotic* [penicillin V potassium] 250, 500 mg; 125, 250 mg/5 mL

**Beesix** IM or IV injection (discontinued 1994) ℞ *vitamin deficiency therapy; antidote to isoniazid poisoning* [pyridoxine HCl] 100 mg/mL

**beeswax, white** JAN [also: wax, white]

**beeswax, yellow** JAN [also: wax, yellow]

**Bee-T-Vites** film-coated tablets (discontinued 1995) OTC *vitamin supplement* [multiple B vitamins; vitamin C] ±•300 mg

**Bee-Zee** tablets OTC *vitamin/zinc supplement* [multiple vitamins; zinc] ±•22.5 mg

**befiperide** INN

**befloxatone** INN

**befunolol** INN [also: befunolol HCl]

**befunolol HCl** JAN [also: befunolol]

**befuraline** INN

**behepan** [see: cyanocobalamin]

**bekanamycin** INN *antibiotic* [also: bekanamycin sulfate]

**bekanamycin sulfate** JAN *antibiotic* [also: bekanamycin]

**belarizine** INN

**belfosdil** USAN, INN *antihypertensive; calcium channel blocker*

**Belganyl** (available only from the Centers for Disease Control) ℞ *investigational anti-infective for trypanosomiasis and onchocerciasis* [suramin sodium]

**Belix** elixir OTC *antihistamine* [diphenhydramine HCl] 12.5 mg/5 mL

**Bellacane** elixir ℞ *GI anticholinergic; sedative* [atropine sulfate; scopolamine hydrobromide; hyoscyamine sulfate; phenobarbital] 0.0194•0.0065•0.1037•16.2 mg/5 mL

**Bellacane** tablets ℞ *GI anticholinergic; sedative* [hyoscyamine sulfate; phenobarbital] 0.125•15 mg

**Bellacane SR** sustained-release tablets ℞ *GI anticholinergic; sedative; analgesic* [belladonna alkaloids; phenobarbital; ergotamine tartrate] 0.2•40•0.6 mg

**belladonna extract** USP *GI/GU anticholinergic/antispasmodic; antiparkinsonian* 27–33 mg/100 mL oral

**Bellafoline** tablets ℞ *GI anticholinergic; antispasmodic; antiparkinsonian agent* [belladonna extract] 0.25 mg

**Bell/ans** tablets OTC *antacid* [sodium bicarbonate] 520 mg

**Bellatal** tablets ℞ *long-acting barbiturate sedative, hypnotic, and anticonvulsant* [phenobarbital] 16.2 mg

**Bellergal-S** tablets ℞ *GI anticholinergic; sedative; analgesic* [belladonna extract; phenobarbital; ergotamine tartrate] 0.2•40•0.6 mg

**beloxamide** USAN, INN *antihyperlipoproteinemic*

**Bel-Phen-Ergot SR** sustained-release tablets ℞ *GI anticholinergic; sedative; analgesic* [belladonna alkaloids; phenobarbital; ergotamine tartrate] 0.2•40•0.6 mg

**Belushi** *street drug slang for a combination of cocaine and heroin (from the actor John Belushi, who died of an overdose)* [see: cocaine; heroin]

**belyando spruce** *street drug slang* [see: marijuana]

**bemarinone** INN *cardiotonic; positive inotropic; vasodilator* [also: bemarinone HCl]

**bemarinone HCl** USAN *cardiotonic; positive inotropic; vasodilator* [also: bemarinone]

**bemegride** USP, INN, BAN, JAN

**bemesetron** USAN, INN *antiemetic*

**bemetizide** INN, BAN

**Beminal 500** tablets OTC *vitamin supplement* [multiple B vitamins; vitamin C] $\pm$•500 mg ℞ Benemid

**bemitradine** USAN, INN *antihypertensive; diuretic*

**bemoradan** USAN, INN *cardiotonic*

**BEMP (bleomycin, Eldisine, mitomycin, Platinol)** *chemotherapy protocol*

**benactyzine** INN, BAN

**benactyzine HCl** *mild antidepressant; anticholinergic*

**Bena-D 10; Bena-D 50** injection (discontinued 1996) ℞ *antihistamine; motion sickness preventative; sleep aid; antiparkinsonian* [diphenhydramine HCl] 10 mg/mL; 50 mg/mL

**Benadryl** elixir (name changed to Benadryl Allergy in 1995) ℞ Bentyl; Benylin; Caladryl

**Benadryl** tablets, capsules, Kapseals (capsules), injection OTC *antihistamine; motion sickness preventative; sleep aid; antiparkinsonian* [diphenhydramine HCl] 25 mg; 25 mg; 50 mg; 10, 50 mg/mL ℞ Bentyl; Benylin; Caladryl

**Benadryl; Benadryl 2%** cream, spray OTC *topical antihistamine* [diphenhydramine HCl] 1%; 2% ℞ Bentyl; Benylin; Caladryl

**Benadryl Allergy** Kapseals (sealed capsules), tablets, chewable tablets, liquid OTC *antihistamine; motion sickness preventative; sleep aid; antiparkinsonian* [diphenhydramine HCl] 25 mg; 25 mg; 12.5 mg; 12.5 mg/5 mL ℞ Bentyl; Benylin; Caladryl

**Benadryl Allergy Decongestant** liquid OTC *pediatric decongestant and antihistamine* [pseudoephedrine HCl; diphenhydramine HCl] 30•12.5 mg/5 mL ℞ Bentyl; Benylin; Caladryl

**Benadryl Allergy/Sinus Headache** caplets OTC *decongestant; antihistamine; analgesic* [pseudoephedrine HCl; diphenhydramine HCl; acetaminophen] 30•12.5•500 mg ℞ Bentyl; Benylin; Caladryl

**Benadryl Cold Nighttime Formula** liquid (discontinued 1995) OTC *decongestant; antihistamine; analgesic* [pseudoephedrine HCl; diphenhydramine HCl; acetaminophen; alcohol 10%] 10•8.3•167 mg/5 mL ℞ Bentyl; Benylin; Caladryl

**Benadryl Cold/Flu** tablets (discontinued 1996) OTC *decongestant; antihistamine; analgesic* [pseudoephedrine HCl; diphenhydramine HCl; acetaminophen] 30•12.5•500 mg ℞ Bentyl; Benylin; Caladryl

**Benadryl Decongestant** elixir (name changed to Benadryl Allergy Decongestant in 1995) ℞ Bentyl; Benylin; Caladryl

**Benadryl Decongestant** Kapseals (capsules) (discontinued 1993) OTC *decongestant; antihistamine* [pseudoephedrine HCl; diphenhydramine HCl] ℞ Bentyl; Benylin; Caladryl

**Benadryl Decongestant Allergy** film-coated tablets OTC *decongestant; antihistamine* [pseudoephedrine HCl; diphenhydramine HCl] 60•25 mg ℞ Bentyl; Benylin; Caladryl

**Benadryl Dye-Free Allergy** liquid, Liqui Gels (soft capsules) OTC *antihistamine* [diphenhydramine HCl] 12.5 mg/5 mL; 25 mg ℞ Bentyl; Benylin; Caladryl

**Benadryl Itch Relief** spray, cream, stick OTC *topical antihistamine; astringent* [diphenhydramine HCl; zinc acetate] 2%•0.1% ℞ Bentyl; Benylin; Caladryl

**Benadryl Itch Relief, Children's** spray, cream OTC *topical antihista-*

*mine; astringent* [diphenhydramine HCl; zinc acetate] 1%•0.1% ⓘ Bentyl; Benylin; Caladryl

**Benadryl Itch Stopping Gel; Benadryl Itch Stopping Gel Children's Formula** OTC *topical antihistamine; astringent* [diphenhydramine HCl; zinc acetate] 2%•1%; 1%•1% ⓘ Bentyl; Benylin; Caladryl

**benafentrine** INN

**Benahist 10; Benahist 50** injection (discontinued 1996) ℞ *antihistamine; motion sickness preventative; sleep aid; antiparkinsonian* [diphenhydramine HCl] 10 mg/mL; 50 mg/mL

**Ben-Allergin-50** injection ℞ *antihistamine; motion sickness preventative; sleep aid; antiparkinsonian* [diphenhydramine HCl] 50 mg/mL

**benanserin HCl**

**benapen** [see: benethamine penicillin]

**benaprizine** INN *anticholinergic* [also: benapryzine HCl; benapryzine]

**benapryzine** BAN *anticholinergic* [also: benapryzine HCl; benaprizine]

**benapryzine HCl** USAN *anticholinergic* [also: benaprizine; benapryzine]

**Ben-Aqua 5; Ben-Aqua 10** gel OTC *topical keratolytic for acne* [benzoyl peroxide] 5%; 10%

**Ben-Aqua 5; Ben-Aqua 10** lotion (discontinued 1994) OTC *topical keratolytic for acne* [benzoyl peroxide]

**Benatol** ℞ *investigational beta blocker for hypertension* [bevantolol]

**benaxibine** INN

**benazepril** INN, BAN *antihypertensive; angiotensin-converting enzyme (ACE) inhibitor* [also: benazepril HCl]

**benazepril HCl** USAN *antihypertensive; angiotensin-converting enzyme (ACE) inhibitor* [also: benazepril]

**benazeprilat** USAN, INN *angiotensin-converting enzyme inhibitor*

**bencianol** INN

**bencisteine** INN, DCF

**benclonidine** INN

**bencyclane** INN [also: bencyclane fumarate]

**bencyclane fumarate** JAN [also: bencyclane]

**bendacalol mesylate** USAN *antihypertensive*

**bendamustine** INN

**bendazac** USAN, INN, BAN, JAN *antiinflammatory*

**bendazol** INN, DCF

**benderizine** INN

**bendrofluazide** BAN *diuretic; antihypertensive* [also: bendroflumethiazide]

**bendroflumethiazide** USP, INN *diuretic; antihypertensive* [also: bendrofluazide]

**Benefix** powder for IV injection ℞ *antihemophilic for factor IX deficiency (hemophilia B; Christmas disease) (orphan)* [coagulation factor IX (recombinant)] 250, 500, 1000 IU

**Benegyn** vaginal cream (discontinued 1993) ℞ *bacteriostatic antibiotic; antiseptic; vulnerary* [sulfanilamide; aminacrine HCl; allantoin] 15%•0.2%•2%

**Benemid** ⓐ tablets (discontinued in U.S. 1996) ℞ *uricosuric for gout* [probenecid] 500 mg ⓘ Beminal

**benethamine penicillin** INN, BAN

**benexate** INN

**benexate HCl** JAN

**benfluorex** INN, DCF

**benfosformin** INN, DCF

**benfotiamine** INN, JAN, DCF

**benfurodil hemisuccinate** INN, DCF

**bengal gelatin** [see: agar]

**Ben-Gay Original** ointment OTC *counterirritant* [methyl salicylate; menthol] 18.3%•16%

**Ben-Gay Regular Strength; Ben-Gay Extra Strength** cream OTC *counterirritant* [methyl salicylate; menthol] 15%•10%; 30%•8%

**Ben-Gay Ultra Strength** cream OTC *counterirritant* [methyl salicylate; menthol; camphor] 30%•10%•4%

**Ben-Gay Vanishing Scent** gel OTC *counterirritant* [menthol; camphor] 3%• ?

**benhepazone** INN

**benidipine** INN

**benmoxin** INN, DCF

**bennie; bennies; Benny and the Jets** *street drug slang for Benzedrine (amphetamine sulfate; discontinued*

*1982) or any of the amphetamines* [see: amphetamine sulfate; amphetamines]

**Benoject-10; Benoject-50** injection (discontinued 1996) ℞ *antihistamine; motion sickness preventative; sleep aid; antiparkinsonian* [diphenhydramine HCl] 10 mg/mL; 50 mg/mL

**benolizime** INN

**Benoquin** cream ℞ *depigmenting agent for vitiligo* [monobenzone] 20%

**benorilate** INN, DCF [also: benorylate]

**benorterone** USAN, INN *antiandrogen*

**benorylate** BAN [also: benorilate]

**benoxafos** INN

**benoxaprofen** USAN, INN, BAN *antiinflammatory; analgesic*

**benoxinate HCl** USP *topical anesthetic* [also: oxybuprocaine; oxybuprocaine HCl]

**Benoxyl #5** lotion, mask OTC *topical keratolytic for acne* [benzoyl peroxide] 5% ⊡ PanOxyl

**Benoxyl 10** lotion OTC *topical keratolytic for acne* [benzoyl peroxide] 10%

**benpenolisin** INN

**benperidol** USAN, INN, BAN *antipsychotic*

**benproperine** INN [also: benproperine phosphate]

**benproperine phosphate** JAN [also: benproperine]

**benrixate** INN, DCF

**bensalan** USAN, INN *disinfectant*

**benserazide** USAN, INN, BAN *decarboxylase inhibitor* [also: benserazide HCl]

**benserazide HCl** JAN *decarboxylase inhibitor* [also: benserazide]

**bensuldazic acid** INN, BAN

**Bensulfoid** cream OTC *topical acne treatment* [colloidal sulfur; resorcinol; alcohol] 8%•2%•12%

**Bensulfoid** tablets (discontinued 1994) ℞ *antibacterial and exfoliant for acne* [sulfur] 130 mg

**bensylyte HCl** [see: phenoxybenzamine HCl]

**bentazepam** USAN, INN *sedative*

**bentemazole** INN

**bentiamine** INN

**bentipimine** INN

**bentiromide** USAN, INN, BAN, JAN *pancreas function test*

**bentonite** NF, JAN *suspending agent*

**bentoquatam** USAN *topical skin protectant for allergic contact dermatitis*

**Bentyl** capsules, tablets, IM injection, syrup ℞ *gastrointestinal antispasmodic* [dicyclomine HCl] 10 mg; 20 mg; 10 mg/mL; 10 mg/5 mL ⊡ Aventyl; Benadryl; Bontril

**benurestat** USAN, INN *urease enzyme inhibitor*

**Benuryl** ⊛ tablets ℞ *uricosuric for gout* [probenecid] 500 mg

**Benylin Adult** oral liquid OTC *antitussive* [dextromethorphan hydrobromide; alcohol 5%] 15 mg/5 mL ⊡ Benadryl

**Benylin Cough** syrup (name changed to Benylin Adult in 1995) ⊡ Benadryl

**Benylin Decongestant** liquid (discontinued 1995) OTC *decongestant; antihistamine* [pseudoephedrine HCl; diphenhydramine HCl; alcohol 5%] 30•12.5 mg/5 mL ⊡ Benadryl

**Benylin DM** syrup OTC *antitussive* [dextromethorphan hydrobromide] 10 mg/5 mL ⊡ Benadryl

**Benylin DM-D; Children's Benylin DM-D** ⊛ syrup OTC *antitussive; decongestant* [dextromethorphan hydrobromide; pseudoephedrine HCl] 15•30 mg/5 mL; 7.5•15 mg/5 mL ⊡ Benadryl

**Benylin DM-D-E** ⊛ syrup OTC *antitussive; decongestant; expectorant* [dextromethorphan hydrobromide; pseudoephedrine HCl; guaifenesin; alcohol 5%] 15•30•100, 15•30•200 mg/5 mL ⊡ Benadryl

**Benylin DM-E** ⊛ syrup OTC *antitussive; expectorant* [dextromethorphan hydrobromide; guaifenesin; alcohol 5%] 15•100 mg/5 mL ⊡ Benadryl

**Benylin Expectorant** liquid OTC *antitussive; expectorant* [dextromethorphan hydrobromide; guaifenesin] 5•100 mg/5 mL ⊡ Benadryl

**Benylin Multi-Symptom** liquid OTC *antitussive; decongestant; expectorant* [dextromethorphan hydrobromide; pseudoephedrine HCl; guaifenesin] 5•15•100 mg/5 mL ⊡ Benadryl

**Benylin Pediatric** oral liquid OTC *antitussive* [dextromethorphan hydrobromide] 7.5 mg/5 mL ☑ Benadryl

**benz** *street drug slang for Benzedrine (amphetamine sulfate; discontinued 1982) or any of the amphetamines* [see: amphetamine sulfate; amphetamines]

**Benza** solution OTC *topical antiseptic* [benzalkonium chloride] 1:750

**Benzac AC 2½; Benzac W 2½; Benzac 5; Benzac AC 5; Benzac W 5; Benzac 10; Benzac AC 10; Benzac W 10** gel ℞ *topical keratolytic for acne* [benzoyl peroxide] 2.5%; 2.5%; 5%; 5%; 5%; 10%; 10%; 10%

**Benzac AC Wash 2½; Benzac AC Wash 5; Benzac W Wash 5; Benzac AC Wash 10; Benzac W Wash 10** liquid ℞ *topical keratolytic for acne* [benzoyl peroxide] 2.5%; 5%; 5%; 10%; 10%

**5 Benzagel; 10 Benzagel** gel ℞ *topical keratolytic for acne* [benzoyl peroxide] 5%; 10%

**benzaldehyde** NF *flavoring agent*

**benzalkonium chloride (BAC)** NF, INN, BAN, JAN *preservative; bacteriostatic antiseptic; surfactant/wetting agent* 17% topical

**Benzamycin** gel ℞ *topical antibiotic and keratolytic for acne* [erythromycin; benzoyl peroxide] 30•50 mg/mL

**benzaprinoxide** INN

**benzarone** INN, DCF

**Benzashave** shaving cream ℞ *topical keratolytic for acne* [benzoyl peroxide] 5%, 10%

**benzathine benzylpenicillin** INN *bactericidal antibiotic* [also: penicillin G benzathine; benzathine penicillin; benzylpenicillin benzathine]

**benzathine penicillin** BAN *bactericidal antibiotic* [also: penicillin G benzathine; benzathine benzylpenicillin; benzylpenicillin benzathine]

**benzathine penicillin G** [see: penicillin G benzathine]

**benzatropine** INN *antiparkinsonian; anticholinergic* [also: benztropine mesylate; benztropine]

**benzazoline HCl** [see: tolazoline HCl]

**benzbromaron** JAN *uricosuric* [also: benzbromarone]

**benzbromarone** USAN, INN, BAN *uricosuric* [also: benzbromaron]

**benzchinamide** [see: benzquinamide]

**benzchlorpropamide** [see: beclamide]

**Benzedrex** inhaler ℞ *nasal decongestant* [propylhexedrine] 250 mg

**benzene ethanol** [see: phenylethyl alcohol]

**benzene hexachloride, gamma** [now: lindane]

**benzeneacetic acid, sodium salt** [see: sodium phenylacetate]

**benzenebutanoic acid, sodium salt** [see: sodium phenylbutyrate]

**1,3-benzenediol** [see: resorcinol]

**benzenemethanol** [see: benzyl alcohol]

**benzestrofol** [see: estradiol benzoate]

**benzestrol** USP, INN, BAN

**benzethacil** [see: penicillin G benzathine]

**benzethidine** INN, BAN, DCF

**benzethonium chloride** USP, INN, BAN, JAN *topical anti-infective; preservative*

**benzetimide** INN *anticholinergic* [also: benzetimide HCl]

**benzetimide HCl** USAN *anticholinergic* [also: benzetimide]

**benzfetamine** INN *anorexiant; CNS stimulant* [also: benzphetamine HCl; benzphetamine]

**benzhexol** BAN *anticholinergic; antiparkinsonian* [also: trihexyphenidyl HCl; trihexyphenidyl]

**N-benzhydryl-N-methylpiperazine** [see: cyclizine HCl]

**benzilone bromide** [see: benzilonium bromide]

**benzilonium bromide** USAN, INN, BAN *anticholinergic*

**2-benzimidazolepropionic acid** [see: procodazole]

**benzimidazoles, substituted** *a class of gastric antisecretory agents that inhibit the ATPase "proton pump" within the cell* [also called: proton pump inhibitors; ATPase inhibitors]

**benzin, petroleum** JAN

**benzindamine HCl** [see: benzydamine HCl]

**benzindopyrine** INN *antipsychotic* [also: benzindopyrine HCl]

**benzindopyrine HCl** USAN *antipsychotic* [also: benzindopyrine]

**benzinoform** [see: carbon tetrachloride]

**benziodarone** INN, BAN, DCF

**benzisoxazoles** *a class of antipsychotic agents*

**benzmalecene** INN

**benzmethoxazone** [see: chlorthenoxazine]

**benznidazole** INN

**benzoaric acid** [see: ellagic acid]

**benzoate & phenylacetate** [see: sodium benzoate & sodium phenylacetate]

**benzobarbital** INN

**benzocaine** USP, INN, BAN *topical anesthetic; nonprescription diet aid* [also: ethyl aminobenzoate] 5% topical

**benzoclidine** INN

**Benzocol** cream (discontinued 1995) OTC *topical local anesthetic* [benzocaine] 5%

**benzoctamine** INN, BAN *sedative; muscle relaxant* [also: benzoctamine HCl]

**benzoctamine HCl** USAN, INN *sedative; muscle relaxant* [also: benzoctamine]

**Benzodent** ointment OTC *topical oral anesthetic* [benzocaine] 20%

**benzodepa** USAN, INN *antineoplastic*

**benzodiazepine HCl** [see: medazepam HCl]

**benzodiazepines** *a class of nonbarbiturate sedative/hypnotics and anticonvulsants*

**benzododecinium chloride** INN

**benzogynestryl** [see: estradiol benzoate]

**benzoic acid** USP, JAN *antifungal; urinary acidifier*

**benzoic acid, phenylmethyl ester** [see: benzyl benzoate]

**benzoic acid, potassium salt** [see: potassium benzoate]

**benzoic acid, sodium salt** [see: sodium benzoate]

**benzoin** USP, JAN *topical protectant*

**Benzoin Compound** tincture OTC *skin protectant* [benzoin; aloe; alcohol 74–80%]

**benzol** [see: benzene ...]

**benzonatate** USP, INN, BAN *antitussive* 100 mg oral

**benzophenone**

**benzopyrrolate** [see: benzopyrronium]

**benzopyrronium bromide** INN

**benzoquinone amidoinohydrazone thiosemicarbazone hydrate** [see: ambazone]

**benzoquinonium chloride**

**benzorphanol** [see: levophenacylmorphan]

**benzosulfinide** [see: saccharin]

**benzosulphinide sodium** [see: saccharin sodium]

**benzothiazepines** *a class of calcium channel blockers*

**benzothiozon** [see: thioacetazone; thiacetazone]

**benzotript** INN

**Benzox-10** gel ℞ *topical keratolytic for acne* [benzoyl peroxide] 10%

**benzoxiquine** USAN, INN *antiseptic/disinfectant*

**benzoxonium chloride** INN

**benzoyl p-aminosalicylate (B-PAS)** [see: benzoylpas calcium]

**benzoyl peroxide** USAN, USP *keratolytic* 5%, 10% topical

**m-benzoylhydratropic acid** [see: ketoprofen]

**benzoylmethylecgonine** [see: cocaine]

**benzoylpas calcium** USAN, USP *antibacterial; tuberculostatic* [also: calcium benzamidosalicylate]

**benzoylsulfanilamide** [see: sulfabenzamide]

**benzoylthiamindisulfide** [see: bisbentiamine]

**benzoylthiaminmonophosphate** [see: benfotiamine]

**benzphetamine** BAN *anorexiant; CNS stimulant* [also: benzphetamine HCl; benzfetamine]

**benzphetamine chloride** [see: benzphetamine HCl]

**benzphetamine HCl** NF *anorexiant; CNS stimulant* [also: benzfetamine; benzphetamine]

**benzpiperylon** [see: benzpiperylone]

**benzpiperylone** INN

**benzpyrinium bromide** NF, INN

**benzquercin** INN

**benzquinamide** USAN, INN, BAN *postanesthesia antinauseant and antiemetic*

**benzthiazide** USP, INN, BAN *diuretic; antihypertensive*

**benztropine** BAN *antiparkinsonian; anticholinergic* [also: benztropine mesylate; benzatropine]

**benztropine mesylate** USP *antiparkinsonian; anticholinergic* [also: benzatropine; benztropine] 0.5, 1, 2 mg oral

**benztropine methanesulfonate** [see: benztropine mesylate]

**benzydamine** INN, BAN *analgesic; antipyretic; anti-inflammatory* [also: benzydamine HCl]

**benzydamine HCl** USAN, JAN *analgesic; antipyretic; anti-inflammatory* [also: benzydamine]

**benzydroflumethiazide** [see: bendroflumethiazide]

**benzyl alcohol** NF, INN, JAN *antimicrobial agent; antiseptic; local anesthetic*

**benzyl analogue of serotonin (BAS)** [see: benanserin HCl]

**benzyl antiserotonin** [see: benanserin HCl]

**benzyl benzoate** USP, JAN

**benzyl carbinol** [see: phenylethyl alcohol]

*S*-**benzyl thiobenzoate** [see: tibenzate]

**benzylamide** [see: beclamide]

**benzylamines** *a class of antifungals structurally related to the allylamines*

*N*-**benzylanilinoacetamidoxime** [see: cetoxime]

**2-benzylbenzimidazole** [see: bendazol]

**benzyldimethyltetradecylammonium chloride** [see: miristalkonium chloride]

**benzyldodecyldimethylammonium chloride** [see: benzododecinium chloride]

**benzylhexadecyldimethylammonium** [see: cetalkonium]

**benzylhexadecyldimethylammonium chloride** [see: cetalkonium chloride]

**benzylhydrochlorothiazide** JAN

*p*-**benzyloxyphenol** [see: monobenzone]

**benzylpenicillin** INN, BAN *investigational (orphan) for penicillin hypersensitivity assessment*

**benzylpenicillin benzathine** JAN *bactericidal antibiotic* [also: penicillin G benzathine; benzathine benzylpenicillin; benzathine penicillin]

**benzylpenicillin potassium** BAN, JAN *antibacterial* [also: penicillin G potassium]

**benzylpenicillin procaine** [see: penicillin G procaine]

**benzylpenicillin sodium** BAN *antibacterial* [also: penicillin G sodium]

**benzylpenicilloic acid** [see: benzylpenicillin]

**benzylpenicilloyl polylysine** USP *penicillin sensitivity test*

**benzylpenilloic acid** [see: benzylpenicillin]

**benzylsulfamide** INN, DCF

**benzylsulfanilamide** [see: benzylsulfamide]

**BEP (bleomycin, etoposide, Platinol)** *chemotherapy protocol*

**bepafant** INN

**bepanthen** [see: panthenol]

**beperidium iodide** INN

**bephene oxinaphthoate** [see: bephenium hydroxynaphthoate]

**bephenium embonate** [see: bephenium hydroxynaphthoate]

**bephenium hydroxynaphthoate** USP, INN, BAN

**bepiastine** INN, DCF

**bepridil** INN, BAN *vasodilator; antianginal; calcium channel blocker* [also: bepridil HCl]

**bepridil HCl** USAN *vasodilator; antianginal; calcium channel blocker* [also: bepridil]

**beractant** USAN *pulmonary surfactant for neonatal respiratory distress syndrome or respiratory failure (orphan)*

**beraprost** USAN, INN *platelet aggregation inhibitor*

**beraprost sodium** USAN *platelet aggregation inhibitor*

**berberine chloride** JAN

**berberine sulfate** JAN

**berberine tannate** JAN

**berculon A** [see: thioacetazone; thia-
cetazone]

**berefrine** USAN, INN *mydriatic*

**bergenin** JAN

**Berinert-P** *investigational (orphan) for
acute angioedema* [C1-esterase-inhibi-
tor, human]

**berkelium** *element (Bk)*

**berlafenone** INN

**bermastine** [see: barmastine]

**bermoprofen** INN

**Bernice; Bernie; Bernie's flakes;
Bernie's gold dust** *street drug slang*
[see: cocaine]

**Berocca** tablets ℞ *vitamin supplement*
[multiple B vitamins; vitamin C;
folic acid] ≛•500•0.5 mg

**Berocca Parenteral Nutrition** injection (discontinued 1997) ℞ *parenteral vitamin supplement* [multiple
vitamins; folic acid; biotin] ≛•400•
60 μg/mL

**Berocca Plus** tablets ℞ *vitamin/min-
eral/iron supplement* [multiple vitamins
& minerals; ferrous fumarate; folic
acid; biotin] ≛•27•0.8•0.15 mg

**Berotec** ℞ *investigational bronchodilator;
antiasthmatic* [fenoterol hydrobromide]

**Berplex Plus** tablets ℞ *vitamin/mineral/
iron supplement* [multiple vitamins &
minerals; ferrous fumarate; folic acid;
biotin] ≛•27•0.8•0.15 mg

**bertosamil** INN

**beryllium** *element (Be)*

**berythromycin** USAN, INN *antiamebic;
antibacterial*

**besigomsin** INN

**besilate** INN *combining name for radicals
or groups* [also: besylate]

**besipirdine** INN *investigational cognition
enhancer for Alzheimer's disease*

**besipirdine HCl** USAN *investigational
cognition enhancer for Alzheimer's disease*

**Besta** capsules (discontinued 1993)
OTC *vitamin/mineral supplement* [mul-
tiple vitamins & minerals]

**besulpamide** INN

**besunide** INN

**besylate** USAN *combining name for radicals or groups* [also: besilate]

**beta alethine** *investigational (orphan)
for multiple myeloma and metastatic
melanoma*

**beta blockers** (β-blockers) *a class of
cardiac agents characterized by their
antihypertensive, antiarrhythmic, and
antianginal actions* [also called: beta-
adrenergic antagonists]

**beta carotene** USAN, USP *ultraviolet
screen; vitamin A precursor* [also:
betacarotene]

**beta cyclodextrin** NF *sequestering
agent* [also: betadex]

**Beta-2** solution for inhalation ℞ *bronchodilator* [isoetharine HCl] 1%

**betacarotene** INN *ultraviolet screen; vitamin A precursor* [also: beta carotene]

**betacetylmethadol** INN, BAN

**Betachron E-R** extended-release capsules ℞ *antianginal; antihypertensive;
migraine preventative* [propranolol
HCl] 60, 80, 120, 160 mg

**betadex** INN *sequestering agent* [also:
beta cyclodextrin]

**beta-D-galactosidase** *digestive enzyme*
[see: tilactase]

**Betadine** aerosol, gauze pads, lubricating gel, cream, mouthwash, ointment, perineal wash, skin cleanser,
foam, solution, swab, swabsticks, surgical scrub OTC *broad-spectrum antimicrobial* [povidone-iodine] 5%;
10%; 5%; 5%; 0.5%; 10%; 10%;
7.5%; 7.5%; 10%; 10%; 10%; 7.5%

**Betadine** shampoo OTC *broad-spectrum
antimicrobial for dandruff* [povidone-
iodine] 7.5%

**Betadine 5% Sterile Ophthalmic
Prep** solution ℞ *broad-spectrum antimicrobial for eye surgery* [povidone-
iodine] 5%

**Betadine First Aid Antibiotics +
Moisturizer** ointment OTC *topical
antibiotic* [polymyxin B sulfate; bacitracin zinc] 10 000•500 IU/g

**Betadine Medicated** vaginal suppositories, vaginal gel OTC *broad-spectrum
antimicrobial* [povidone-iodine] 10%

**Betadine Medicated Douche; Beta-
dine Medicated Disposable
Douche; Betadine Premixed
Medicated Disposable Douche**

solution OTC *broad-spectrum antimicrobial* [povidone-iodine] 10%

**beta-estradiol** [see: estradiol]

**beta-estradiol benzoate** [see: estradiol benzoate]

**betaeucaine HCl** [now: eucaine HCl]

**Betafectin** ℞ *investigational (Phase III) immunotherapeutic to prevent postsurgical infections* [PGG glucan]

**Betagan Liquifilm** eye drops ℞ *topical antiglaucoma agent (β-blocker)* [levobunolol HCl] 0.25%, 0.5% ⊡ Betagen

**Betagen** ointment, solution, surgical scrub OTC *broad-spectrum antimicrobial* [povidone-iodine] 1%; 10%; 7.5% ⊡ Betagan

**beta-glucocerebrosidase** [see: alglucerase]

**betahistine** INN, BAN *vasodilator* [also: betahistine HCl; betahistine mesilate]

**betahistine HCl** USAN *vasodilator* [also: betahistine; betahistine mesilate]

**betahistine mesilate** JAN *vasodilator* [also: betahistine HCl; betahistine]

**beta-hypophamine** [see: vasopressin]

**betaine HCl** USP *electrolyte replenisher for homocystinuria (orphan)*

**BetaKine** ℞ *investigational connective tissue growth stimulator for chronic ulcers and macular holes* [transforming growth factor beta]

**beta-lactams** *a class of antibiotics*

**beta-lactone** [see: propiolactone]

**betameprodine** INN, BAN, DCF

**betamethadol** INN, BAN, DCF

**betamethasone** USAN, USP, INN, BAN, JAN *corticosteroid*

**betamethasone acetate** USP, JAN *corticosteroid*

**betamethasone acibutate** INN, BAN *corticosteroid*

**betamethasone benzoate** USAN, USP, BAN *corticosteroid*

**betamethasone dipropionate** USAN, USP, BAN, JAN *corticosteroid* 0.05% topical

**betamethasone dipropionate, augmented** *corticosteroid*

**betamethasone sodium phosphate** USP, BAN, JAN *corticosteroid* 4 mg/mL injection

**betamethasone valerate** USAN, USP, BAN, JAN *corticosteroid; investigational (Phase III) mousse for scalp psoriasis* 0.1% topical

**betamicin** INN *antibacterial* [also: betamicin sulfate]

**betamicin sulfate** USAN *antibacterial* [also: betamicin]

**betamipron** INN

**betanaphthol** NF

**betanidine** INN *antihypertensive* [also: bethanidine sulfate; bethanidine; betanidine sulfate]

**betanidine sulfate** JAN *antihypertensive* [also: bethanidine sulfate; betanidine; bethanidine]

**Betapace** tablets ℞ *antiarrhythmic (β-blocker) for life-threatening ventricular arrhythmias (orphan)* [sotalol HCl] 80, 120, 160, 240 mg

**Betapen-VK** film-coated tablets, powder for oral solution ℞ *bactericidal antibiotic* [penicillin V potassium] 250, 500 mg; 125, 250 mg/5 mL ⊡ Adapin; Phenaphen

**betaprodine** INN, BAN, DCF

**beta-propiolactone** [see: propiolactone]

**beta-pyridylcarbinol** [see: nicotinyl alcohol]

**BetaRx** *investigational (orphan) antidiabetic for type 1 patients on immunosuppression* [encapsulated porcine islet preparation]

**Betasept** liquid OTC *broad-spectrum antimicrobial; germicidal* [chlorhexidine gluconate; alcohol 4%] 4%

**Betaseron** powder for subcu injection ℞ *immunomodulator for relapsing-remitting multiple sclerosis (orphan)* [interferon beta-1b] 0.3 mg (9.6 mIU)/vial

**Betathine** *investigational (orphan) for multiple myeloma and metastatic melanoma* [beta alethine]

**Beta-Tim** ⒸⒶⓃ (U.S. product: Timoptic) eye drops ℞ *antiglaucoma agent (β-blocker)* [timolol maleate] 0.25%, 0.5%

**Betatrex** cream, ointment, lotion ℞ *topical corticosteroid* [betamethasone valerate] 0.1%

**Beta-Val** cream, lotion ℞ *topical corticosteroid* [betamethasone valerate] 0.1%

**Beta-Val** ointment (discontinued 1994) ℞ *topical corticosteroid* [betamethasone valerate] 0.1%

**betaxolol** INN, BAN *antianginal; antihypertensive; topical antiglaucoma agent (β-blocker)* [also: betaxolol HCl]

**betaxolol HCl** USAN, USP *antianginal; antihypertensive; topical antiglaucoma agent (β-blocker)* [also: betaxolol]

**betazole** INN [also: betazole HCl; ametazole]

**betazole HCl** USP [also: betazole; ametazole]

**betazolium chloride** [see: betazole HCl]

**bethanechol chloride** USP, BAN, JAN *cholinergic urinary stimulant for postsurgical and postpartum urinary retention* 5, 10, 25, 50 mg oral

**bethanidine** BAN *antihypertensive* [also: bethanidine sulfate; betanidine; betanidine sulfate]

**bethanidine sulfate** USAN *antihypertensive; orphan status withdrawn 1996* [also: betanidine; bethanidine; betanidine sulfate]

**betiatide** USAN, INN, BAN *pharmaceutic aid*

**Betimol** eye drops ℞ *ocular antihypertensive; antiglaucoma agent (β-blocker)* [timolol hemihydrate] 0.25%, 0.5%

**Betnesol** ℞ *investigational topical steroidal anti-inflammatory*

**Betoptic; Betoptic S** Drop-Tainer (eye drops) ℞ *topical antiglaucoma agent (β-blocker)* [betaxolol HCl] 0.5% (5.6 mg/mL); 0.25% (2.8 mg/mL)

**betoxycaine** INN

**betoxycaine HCl** [see: betoxycaine]

**betula oil** [see: methyl salicylate]

**Betuline** lotion OTC *counterirritant* [methyl salicylate; camphor; menthol; peppermint oil]

**bevantolol** INN, BAN *antianginal; antihypertensive; antiarrhythmic* [also: bevantolol HCl]

**bevantolol HCl** USAN *antianginal; antihypertensive; antiarrhythmic* [also: bevantolol]

**bevonium methylsulphate** BAN [also: bevonium metilsulfate]

**bevonium metilsulfate** INN [also: bevonium methylsulphate]

**bezafibrate** USAN, INN, BAN, JAN *antihyperlipoproteinemic*

**bezitramide** INN, BAN, DCF

**bezomil** INN *combining name for radicals or groups*

**bFGF (basic fibroblast growth factor)** [see: ersofermin]

**B.F.I. Antiseptic** powder OTC *topical antiseptic* [bismuth-formic-iodide] 16%

**BHA (butylated hydroxyanisole)** [q.v.]

**bhang** *street drug slang (an Indian term)* [see: marijuana]

**BHAPs (bisheteroarylpiperazines)** *a class of antiviral drugs*

**BHD (BCNU, hydroxyurea, dacarbazine)** *chemotherapy protocol*

**BHDV; BHD-V (BCNU, hydroxyurea, dacarbazine, vincristine)** *chemotherapy protocol*

**BHT (butylated hydroxytoluene)** [q.v.]

**bialamicol** INN, BAN *antiamebic* [also: bialamicol HCl]

**bialamicol HCl** USAN *antiamebic* [also: bialamicol]

**biallylamicol** [see: bialamicol]

**biantrazole** [now: losoxantrone HCl]

**biapenem** USAN, INN *antibacterial*

**Biavax II** powder for subcu injection ℞ *rubella and mumps vaccine* [rubella & mumps virus vaccine, live] 1000• 20 000 U/0.5 mL

**Biaxin** Filmtabs (film-coated tablets), granules for oral suspension ℞ *macrolide antibacterial antibiotic* [clarithromycin] 250, 500 mg; 125, 250 mg/5 mL

**bibenzonium bromide** INN, BAN

**bibrocathin** [see: bibrocathol]

**bibrocathol** INN, DCF

**Bicalma** chewable tablets (discontinued 1994) OTC *antacid* [calcium carbonate; magnesium trisilicate]

**bicalutamide** USAN, INN, BAN *antiandrogen for prostatic cancer*

**Bichloracetic Acid** liquid ℞ *cauterant; keratolytic* [dichloroacetic acid] 10 mL ② dichloroacetic acid

**bicifadine** INN *analgesic* [also: bicifadine HCl]

**bicifadine HCl** USAN *analgesic* [also: bicifadine]

**Bicillin C-R; Bicillin C-R 900/300** IM injection, Tubex (cartridge-needle unit) ℞ *bactericidal antibiotic* [penicillin G benzathine; penicillin G procaine] 150 000•150 000 U/mL; 900 000•300 000 U ⌷ V-Cillin; Wycillin

**Bicillin L-A** IM injection, Tubex (cartridge-needle units) ℞ *bactericidal antibiotic* [penicillin G benzathine] 300 000 U/mL; 600 000 U/mL

**biciromab** USAN, INN, BAN *antifibrin monoclonal antibody*

**Bicitra** oral solution ℞ *urinary alkalinizing agent* [sodium citrate; citric acid] 500•334 mg/5 mL

**biclodil** *antihypertensive; vasodilator* [also: biclodil HCl]

**biclodil HCl** USAN *antihypertensive; vasodilator* [also: biclodil]

**biclofibrate** INN, DCF

**biclotymol** INN, DCF

**BiCNU** powder for IV injection ℞ *nitrosourea-type alkylating antineoplastic* [carmustine] 100 mg

**bicozamycin** INN

**Bicozene** cream OTC *topical local anesthetic; antifungal* [benzocaine; resorcinol] 6%•1.67%

**bicyclomycin** [see: bicozamycin]

**bidCAP** (trademarked dosage form) *twice-daily capsule*

**Bidil** ℞ *investigational vasodilator for congestive heart failure* [hydralazine; isosorbide]

**bidimazium iodide** INN, BAN

**bidisomide** USAN, INN *antiarrhythmic*

**Biebrich scarlet red** [see: scarlet red]

**Biebrich scarlet-picroaniline blue**

**bietamiverine** INN

**bietamiverine HCl** [see: bietamiverine]

**bietaserpine** INN, DCF

**bifemelane** INN [also: bifemelane HCl]

**bifemelane HCl** JAN [also: bifemelane]

**bifepramide** INN

**bifeprofen** INN

**bifluranol** INN, BAN

**bifonazole** USAN, INN, BAN, JAN *antifungal*

**big 8** *street drug slang for 1/8 kg of crack (about 4½ ounces)* [see: cocaine, crack]

**big bag** *street drug slang* [see: heroin]

**big C** *street drug slang* [see: cocaine]

**big chief** *street drug slang* [see: mescaline]

**big D** *street drug slang* [see: LSD]

**big flake** *street drug slang* [see: cocaine]

**big H; big Harry** *street drug slang* [see: heroin]

**big O** *street drug slang* [see: opium]

**big rush** *street drug slang* [see: cocaine]

**bile acid sequestrants** *a class of antihyperlipidemic agents*

**bile acids, oxidized** [see: dehydrocholic acid]

**bile salts** BAN *laxative*

**Bilezyme** tablets (discontinued 1995) ℞ *digestive enzymes* [amylase; protease; dehydrocholic acid; desoxycholic acid] 30•6•200•50 mg

**Bili-Labstix** reagent strips *in vitro diagnostic aid for multiple urine products*

**Bilivist** capsules ℞ *oral cholecystographic radiopaque agent* [ipodate sodium] 500 mg

**Bill Blass** *street drug slang* [see: cocaine, crack]

**Billie hoke** *street drug slang* [see: cocaine]

**Bilopaque** capsules ℞ *oral cholecystographic radiopaque agent* [tyropanoate sodium] 750 mg

**Biltricide** film-coated tablets ℞ *anthelmintic for schistosomiasis (flukes)* [praziquantel] 600 mg

**bimakalim** INN

**bimazol** [see: carbimazole]

**bimethadol** [see: dimepheptanol]

**bimethoxycaine lactate**

**bindarit** USAN, INN *antirheumatic*

**bindazac** [see: bendazac]

**binedaline** INN

**binfloxacin** USAN, INN *veterinary antibacterial*

**bings** *street drug slang* [see: cocaine, crack]

**binifibrate** INN

**biniramycin** USAN, INN *antibacterial antibiotic*

**binizolast** INN

**binodaline** [see: binedaline]

**binospirone** INN *anxiolytic* [also: binospirone mesylate]

**binospirone mesylate** USAN *anxiolytic* [also: binospirone]

**Bio-Acerola C Complex** wafers OTC *dietary supplement* [vitamin C; citrus bioflavonoids; rutin] 500•10•5 mg

**bioallethrin** BAN

**Biocef** capsules, powder for oral suspension R *cephalosporin-type antibiotic* [cephalexin monohydrate] 500 mg; 125, 250 mg/5 mL

**Bioclate** powder for IV injection R *antihemophilic to correct coagulation deficiency* [antihemophilic factor VIII, recombinant] 250, 500, 1000 IU

**BioCox** intradermal injection R *diagnostic aid for coccidioidomycosis* [coccidioidin] 1:100, 1:10

**Biocult-GC** culture paddles for professional use *in vitro diagnostic aid for Neisseria gonorrhoeae*

**Bioday with Iron** tablets OTC *vitamin/ iron supplement* [multiple vitamins; iron; folic acid]

**Biodel Implant/BCNU** (name changed to Gliadel upon marketing release in 1998)

**Biodine Topical** solution OTC *broad- spectrum antimicrobial* [povidone- iodine] 1%

**Bioferon** (working name during investigational testing; name changed to Avonex upon product launch in 1996)

**bioflavonoids** *vitamin P*

**biogastrone** [see: carbenoxolone]

**Biohist-LA** timed-release tablets R *decongestant; antihistamine* [pseudo- ephedrine HCl; carbinoxamine maleate] 120•8 mg

**biological indicator for dry-heat sterilization** USP *sterilization indicator*

**biological indicator for ethylene oxide sterilization** USP *sterilization indicator*

**biological indicator for steam sterilization** USP *sterilization indicator*

**Biomox** capsules, powder for oral suspension R *penicillin-type antibiotic* [amoxicillin trihydrate] 250, 500 mg; 250 mg/5 mL

**Bion Tears** eye drops OTC *ocular mois- turizer/lubricant* [hydroxypropyl methylcellulose] 0.3%

**bioral** [see: carbenoxolone]

**Bio-Rescue** R *investigational (orphan) for acute iron poisoning* [dextran; deferoxamine]

**bioresmethrin** INN

**bios I** [see: inositol]

**bios II** [see: biotin]

**Biosynject** R *investigational (orphan) for newborn hemolytic disease and ABO blood incompatibility of organ or bone marrow transplants* [trisaccha- rides A and B]

**biosynthetic human parathyroid hormone (1-34)** [see: teriparatide]

**Bio-Tab** film-coated tablets R *tetracy- cline-type antibiotic* [doxycycline hyclate] 100 mg

**Biotab** tablets OTC *decongestant; anti- histamine; analgesic* [phenylpropanol- amine HCl; phenyltoloxamine cit- rate; acetaminophen]

**Biotel diabetes** test kit (discontinued 1995) *in vitro diagnostic aid for urine glucose*

**Biotel kidney** reagent strips *in vitro diagnostic aid for urine hemoglobin, RBCs, and albumin (predictor of kid- ney diseases)*

**Biotel u.t.i.** test kit for home use (dis- continued 1995) *in vitro diagnostic aid for urine nitrite (predictor of uri- nary tract infections)*

**biotexin** [see: novobiocin]

**biotin** USP, INN, JAN *B complex vitamin; vitamin H*

**Biotin Forte** tablets (discontinued 1997) OTC *vitamin supplement* [multi- ple B vitamins; vitamin C; folic acid; biotin] ±•200 mg•800 μg•3 mg, ±•100 mg•800 μg•5 mg

**BioTropin** R *orphan status withdrawn 1997* [somatropin]

**BIP (bleomycin, ifosfamide [with mesna rescue], Platinol)** *chemo- therapy protocol*

**bipenamol** INN *antidepressant* [also: bipenamol HCl]

**bipenamol HCl** USAN *antidepressant* [also: bipenamol]

**biperiden** USP, INN, BAN, JAN *anticholinergic; antiparkinsonian*

**biperiden HCl** USP, BAN, JAN *anticholinergic; antiparkinsonian*

**biperiden lactate** USP, BAN, JAN *anticholinergic; antiparkinsonian*

**biphasic insulin** [see: insulin, biphasic]

**biphenamine HCl** USAN *topical anesthetic; antibacterial; antifungal* [also: xenysalate]

**Biphetamine 12½; Biphetamine 20** capsules (discontinued 1993) ℞ *CNS stimulant; amphetamine* [dextroamphetamine; amphetamine] 6.25•6.25 mg; 10•10 mg

**biprofenide** [see: bifepramide]

**birch oil, sweet** [see: methyl salicylate]

**birdie powder** *street drug slang* [see: heroin; cocaine]

**biriperone** INN

**bisacodyl** USP, INN, BAN, JAN *stimulant laxative* 5 mg oral; 10 mg suppositories

**bisacodyl tannex** USAN *laxative*

**bisantrene** INN *antineoplastic* [also: bisantrene HCl]

**bisantrene HCl** USAN *antineoplastic* [also: bisantrene]

**bisaramil** INN

**bisatin** [see: oxyphenisatin acetate]

**bisbendazole** INN

**bisbentiamine** INN, JAN

**bisbutiamine** [see: bisbutitiamine]

**bisbutitiamine** JAN

**bis-chloroethyl-nitrosourea (BCNU)** [see: carmustine]

**Bisco-Lax** suppositories OTC *stimulant laxative* [bisacodyl] 10 mg

**biscuit** *street drug slang for 50 rocks of crack* [see: cocaine, crack]

**bisdequalinium diacetate** JAN

**bisfenazone** INN, DCF

**bisfentidine** INN

**bisheteroarylpiperazines (BHAPs)** *a class of antiviral drugs*

**bishydroxycoumarin** [now: dicumarol]

**bisibutiamine** JAN [also: sulbutiamine]

**Bismatrol** chewable tablets, liquid OTC *antidiarrheal; antinauseant* [bismuth subsalicylate] 262 mg; 524 mg/5 mL

**bismucatebrol** [see: bibrocathol]

**bismuth** *element (Bi)*

**bismuth, milk of** USP *antacid; astringent*

**bismuth aluminate** USAN

**bismuth betanaphthol** USP

**bismuth carbonate** USAN

**bismuth carbonate, basic** [see: bismuth subcarbonate]

**bismuth citrate** USP

**bismuth cream** [see: bismuth, milk of]

**bismuth gallate, basic** [see: bismuth subgallate]

**bismuth glycollylarsanilate** BAN [also: glycobiarsol]

**bismuth hydroxide** [see: bismuth, milk of]

**bismuth hydroxide nitrate oxide** [see: bismuth subnitrate]

**bismuth magma** [now: bismuth, milk of]

**bismuth magnesium aluminosilicate** JAN

**bismuth oxycarbonate** [see: bismuth subcarbonate]

**bismuth potassium tartrate** NF

**bismuth sodium triglycollamate** USP

**bismuth subcarbonate** USAN, JAN *antacid; GI adsorbent*

**bismuth subgallate** USAN, USP *antacid; GI adsorbent*

**bismuth subnitrate** USP, JAN *skin protectant*

**bismuth subsalicylate (BSS)** USAN, JAN *antiperistaltic; antacid; GI adsorbent*

**bisnafide dimesylate** USAN *antineoplastic; DNA and RNA synthesis inhibitor*

**bisobrin** INN *fibrinolytic* [also: bisobrin lactate]

**bisobrin lactate** USAN *fibrinolytic* [also: bisobrin]

**Bisodol** chewable tablets (discontinued 1994) OTC *antacid* [magnesium hydroxide; calcium carbonate]

**Bisodol** powder (discontinued 1994) OTC *antacid* [sodium bicarbonate; magnesium carbonate]

**bisoprolol** USAN, INN, BAN *antihypertensive (β-blocker)*

**bisoprolol fumarate** USAN, JAN *antihypertensive (β-blocker)*

**bisorcic** INN

**bisoxatin** INN, BAN *laxative* [also: bisoxatin acetate]

**bisoxatin acetate** USAN *laxative* [also: bisoxatin]

**bispecific antibody 520C9x22** *investigational (orphan) for ovarian cancer*

**bisphosphonates** *a class of calcium-regulating agents that act primarily on bone density and resorption*

**bispyrithione magsulfex** USAN *antibacterial; antidandruff; antifungal*

**bis-tropamide** [now: tropicamide]

**bithionol** NF, INN, BAN, JAN *investigational anti-infective for paragonimiasis and fascioliasis*

**bithionolate sodium** USAN *topical anti-infective* [also: sodium bitionolate]

**bithionoloxide** INN

**Bitin** (available only from the Centers for Disease Control) ℞ *investigational anti-infective for paragonimiasis and fascioliasis* [bithionol]

**bitipazone** INN

**bitolterol** INN, BAN *bronchodilator* [also: bitolterol mesylate; bitolterol mesilate]

**bitolterol mesilate** JAN *bronchodilator* [also: bitolterol mesylate; bitolterol]

**bitolterol mesylate** USAN *bronchodilator* [also: bitolterol; bitolterol mesilate]

**bitoscanate** INN

**bivalirudin** USAN *antithrombotic; anticoagulant*

**bizelesin** USAN, INN *antineoplastic*

**B-Ject-100** injection ℞ *parenteral vitamin therapy* [multiple B vitamins] ≛

**black** *street drug slang* [see: opium; marijuana]

**black acid** *street drug slang for LSD or a combination of LSD and PCP* [see: LSD; PCP]

**black and white** *street drug slang* [see: amphetamines]

**black Bart** *street drug slang* [see: marijuana]

**black beauties** *street drug slang for amphetamines or various CNS depressants* [see: amphetamines]

**black beauties** *street drug slang for Biphetamine (amphetamine + dextroamphetamine; discontinued 1993)* [see: amphetamines; amphetamine sulfate; dextroamphetamine]

**black birds; black bombers** *street drug slang* [see: amphetamines]

**black ganga** *street drug slang for marijuana resin* [see: marijuana]

**black gold** *street drug slang for a high-potency marijuana* [see: marijuana]

**black gungi** *street drug slang for marijuana from India* [see: marijuana]

**black gunion** *street drug slang* [see: marijuana]

**black hash** *street drug slang for a combination of opium and hashish* [see: opium; hashish]

**black mo; black moat** *street drug slang for highly potent marijuana* [see: marijuana]

**black mollies** *street drug slang* [see: amphetamines]

**black mote** *street drug slang for marijuana mixed with honey* [see: marijuana]

**black pearl** *street drug slang* [see: heroin]

**black pill** *street drug slang for an opium pill* [see: opium]

**black rock** *street drug slang* [see: cocaine, crack]

**black Russian** *street drug slang for very potent hashish or a combination of hashish and opium* [see: hashish; opium]

**black star** *street drug slang* [see: LSD]

**black stuff** *street drug slang* [see: heroin]

**black stuff; black tar opium** *street drug slang for a tar-like opium for smoking* [see: opium]

**black sunshine** *street drug slang* [see: LSD]

**black tabs** *street drug slang* [see: LSD]

**black tar** *street drug slang* [see: heroin; opium]

**black tar heroin; black Tootsie Roll** *street drug slang for a potent form of heroin from Mexico* [see: heroin]

**black whack** *street drug slang* [see: PCP]

**black widow spider antivenin** [see: antivenin (Latrodectus mactans)]

**Black-Draught** syrup OTC *laxative* [casanthranol; senna extract] 90• ≛ mg/15 mL

**Black-Draught** tablets, granules OTC *laxative* [senna concentrate] 600 mg; 1.65 g per ½ tsp.

**blacks** *street drug slang* [see: amphetamines]

**Blairex Hard Contact Lens Cleaner** solution (discontinued 1993) OTC *cleaning solution for hard contact lenses*

**Blairex Lens Lubricant** solution OTC *rewetting solution for soft contact lenses*

**Blairex Sterile Saline** aerosol solution OTC *rinsing/storage solution for soft contact lenses* [preservative-free saline solution]

**blanco** (Spanish for "white") *street drug slang* [see: heroin]

**blanket** *street drug slang for a marijuana cigarette* [see: marijuana]

**blastomycin** NF

**BlemErase** lotion OTC *topical keratolytic for acne* [benzoyl peroxide] 10%

**Blenoxane** powder for IM, IV, subcu, or intrapleural injection ℞ *antibiotic antineoplastic for lymphomas, testicular and squamous cell carcinomas and malignant pleural effusion (orphan)* [bleomycin sulfate] 15 U

**BLEO-COMF (bleomycin, cyclophosphamide, Oncovin, methotrexate, fluorouracil)** *chemotherapy protocol*

**bleomycin (BLM)** INN, BAN *glycopeptide antibiotic antineoplastic* [also: bleomycin sulfate; bleomycin HCl] ② Cleocin

**bleomycin HCl** JAN *glycopeptide antibiotic antineoplastic* [also: bleomycin sulfate; bleomycin]

**bleomycin sulfate** USAN, USP, JAN *glycopeptide antibiotic antineoplastic for multiple carcinomas and malignant pleural effusion (orphan)* [also: bleomycin; bleomycin HCl]

**Bleph-10** eye drops, ophthalmic ointment ℞ *ophthalmic bacteriostatic* [sulfacetamide sodium] 10%

**Blephamide** eye drop suspension, ophthalmic ointment ℞ *ophthalmic topical corticosteroidal anti-inflammatory; bacteriostatic* [prednisolone acetate; sulfacetamide sodium] 0.2%•10%

**Blinx** ophthalmic solution OTC *extraocular irrigating solution* [sterile isotonic solution]

**BlisterGard** liquid OTC *skin protectant*

**Blistex** ointment OTC *topical antipruritic/counterirritant; mild local anesthetic; vulnerary* [camphor; phenol; allantoin] 0.5%•0.5%•1%

**Blistik** lip balm OTC *antipruritic/counterirritant; mild local anesthetic; skin protectant; sunscreen (SPF 10)* [camphor; phenol; allantoin; dimethicone; padimate O; oxybenzone] 0.5%•0.5%•1%•2%•6.6%•2.5%

**Blis-To-Sol** liquid OTC *topical antifungal; keratolytic* [tolnaftate] 1%

**Blis-To-Sol** powder OTC *topical antifungal* [zinc undecylenate] 12%

**BLM (bleomycin)** [q.v.]

**Blocadren** tablets ℞ *antihypertensive; migraine preventative; β-blocker* [timolol maleate] 5, 10, 20 mg

**block** *street drug slang for marijuana or crude opium or a cube of morphine* [see: marijuana; opium; morphine]

**blockbusters** *street drug slang for Nembutal (pentobarbital; discontinued 1979) or various CNS depressants*

**blocked ricin conjugated murine MAb** [see: ricin (blocked) conjugated murine MAb]

**blonde** *street drug slang* [see: marijuana]

**blood, whole** USP *blood replenisher*

**blood, whole human** [now: blood, whole]

**blood cell growth factor** *investigational antineoplastic*

**blood cells, human red** [now: blood cells, red]

**blood cells, red** USP *blood replenisher*

**blood group specific substances A, B & AB** USP *blood neutralizer*

**blood grouping serum, anti-A** [see: anti-A blood grouping serum]

**blood grouping serum, anti-B** [see: anti-B blood grouping serum]

**blood grouping serum, anti-C** USP *for in vitro blood testing*

**blood grouping serum, anti-c** USP *for in vitro blood testing*

**blood grouping serum, anti-D** USP *for in vitro blood testing*

**blood grouping serum, anti-E** USP *for in vitro blood testing*

**blood grouping serum, anti-e** USP *for in vitro blood testing*

**blood madman** *street drug slang* [see: PCP]

**blotter** *street drug slang* [see: LSD; cocaine]

**blotter acid; blotter cube** *street drug slang* [see: LSD]

**blow up** *street drug slang for crack cut (diluted) with lidocaine to increase size and weight* [see: cocaine, crack]

**blowcaine** *street drug slang for crack cut (diluted) with cocaine* [see: cocaine, crack; cocaine]

**blowing smoke** *street drug slang* [see: marijuana]

**blowout** *street drug slang* [see: cocaine, crack]

**Bluboro** powder packets OTC *astringent wet dressing (modified Burow solution)* [aluminum sulfate; calcium acetate]

**blue** *street drug slang for crack or various CNS depressants* [see: cocaine, crack]

**blue acid** *street drug slang* [see: LSD]

**blue and clears** *street drug slang for Fastin (phentermine HCl), which is a blue and clear capsule filled with blue and white balls* [see: Fastin; phentermine]

**blue angels** *street drug slang for various CND depressants*

**blue barrels** *street drug slang* [see: LSD]

**blue boy** *street drug slang* [see: amphetamines]

**blue bullets** *street drug slang for various CNS depressants*

**blue caps** *street drug slang* [see: mescaline]

**blue chairs; blue cheers** *street drug slang* [see: LSD]

**blue de hue** *street drug slang for marijuana from Vietnam* [see: marijuana]

**blue devil** *street drug slang for various CNS depressants*

**blue dolls** *street drug slang for various CNS depressants*

**Blue Gel** OTC *pediculicide* [pyrethrins; piperonyl butoxide; petroleum distillate] 0.3%•3%•1.2%

**Blue Gel Muscular Pain Reliever** gel OTC *counterirritant* [menthol] ≟

**blue heaven** *street drug slang* [see: LSD]

**blue heavens; bluebirds** *street drug slang for Amytal (amobarbital; discontinued 1991), Amytal Sodium (amobarbital sodium), or other depressants*

[see: Amytal Sodium; amobarbital; amobarbital sodium]

**blue microdot; blue mist; blue moons** *street drug slang* [see: LSD]

**blue sage** *street drug slang* [see: marijuana]

**blue sky bond** *street drug slang for high-potency marijuana from Colombia* [see: marijuana]

**blue star** *street drug slang for a type of blotter LSD* [see: LSD]

**blue tabs** *street drug slang* [see: LSD]

**blue tips** *street drug slang for various CNS depressants*

**blue velvet** *street drug slang for a combination of paregoric and tripelennamine, used as a weak heroin substitute*

**blue velvet** *street drug slang for a combination of terpin hydrate, codeine, and tripelennamine, used as a weak heroin substitute*

**blue vials** *street drug slang* [see: LSD]

**bluebirds; blue heavens** *street drug slang for Amytal (amobarbital; discontinued 1991), Amytal Sodium (amobarbital sodium), or other depressants* [see: Amytal Sodium; amobarbital; amobarbital sodium]

**bluensomycin** INN *antibiotic*

**blues** *street drug slang for Amytal (amobarbital; discontinued 1991), named for the blue-colored capsules* [see: Amytal Sodium; amobarbital; amobarbital sodium]

**blues and reds** *street drug slang for Amytal (amobarbital; discontinued 1991) and Seconal (secobarbital; discontinued 1990)* [see: Amytal Sodium; amobarbital; Seconal Sodium; secobarbital]

**blunt** *street drug slang for marijuana or a combination of marijuana and cocaine in a cigar* [see: marijuana; cocaine]

**BM 14802** *investigational antipsychotic for schizophrenia (clinical trials discontinued 1994)*

**B-MOPP (bleomycin, nitrogen mustard, Oncovin, procarbazine, prednisone)** *chemotherapy protocol*

**BMP (BCNU, methotrexate, procarbazine)** *chemotherapy protocol*

**BMP-1 to BMP-8 (bone morpho-genetic proteins)** [q.v.]

**BMS 181101** *investigational antidepressant*

**BMY 14802** *investigational antipsychotic for schizophrenia*

**BMY-45622** *orphan status withdrawn 1994*

**BOAP (bleomycin, Oncovin, Adriamycin, prednisone)** *chemotherapy protocol*

**boat** *street drug slang* [see: PCP]

**bobo; boubou; bobo bush** (Spanish for "fool" or 'idiot") *street drug slang* [see: marijuana; cocaine, crack]

**Bo-Cal** *tablets* OTC *dietary supplement* [calcium; vitamin D; magnesium] 250 mg•100 IU•125 mg

**boforsin** [see: colforsin]

**bofumustine** INN

**bohd** *street drug slang* [see: marijuana; PCP]

**Boil-Ease** *ointment* OTC *topical local anesthetic* [benzocaine] 20%

**bolandiol** INN *anabolic* [also: bolandiol dipropionate]

**bolandiol dipropionate** USAN, JAN *anabolic* [also: bolandiol]

**bolasterone** USAN, INN *anabolic steroid; also abused as a street drug*

**bolazine** INN

**BOLD (bleomycin, Oncovin, lomustine, dacarbazine)** *chemotherapy protocol*

**boldenone** INN, BAN *veterinary anabolic steroid; also abused as a street drug* [also: boldenone undecylenate]

**boldenone undecylenate** USAN *veterinary anabolic steroid; also abused as a street drug* [also: boldenone]

**bolenol** USAN, INN *anabolic*

**Bolivian marching powder** *street drug slang* [see: cocaine]

**bolmantalate** USAN, INN, BAN *anabolic*

**bolo** (Spanish and Italian for "bolus") *street drug slang* [see: cocaine, crack]

**bolt** *street drug slang* [see: butyl nitrite; isobutyl nitrite]

**bolus alba** [see: kaolin]

**Bolvidon** ℞ *investigational antidepressant* [mianserin]

**bomb** *street drug slang* [see: cocaine, crack; heroin; marijuana]

**bomber** *street drug slang for a marijuana cigarette* [see: marijuana]

**bombido; bombita** *street drug slang for injectable amphetamines, heroin, or various CNS depressants* [see: amphetamines; heroin]

**bombita** (Spanish for "little bomb") *street drug slang for injectable Desoxyn* (*methamphetamine HCl; discontinued 1980*) [see: methamphetamine HCl; amphetamines]

**bombs away** *street drug slang* [see: heroin]

**bometolol** INN

**BOMP (bleomycin, Oncovin, Matulane, prednisone)** *chemotherapy protocol*

**BOMP (bleomycin, Oncovin, mitomycin, Platinol)** *chemotherapy protocol*

**Bonamil Infant Formula with Iron** *powder, oral liquid* OTC *total or supplementary infant feeding* 453 g; 384, 946 mL

**bone** *street drug slang for marijuana or a $50 piece of crack* [see: marijuana; cocaine, crack]

**bone ash** [see: calcium phosphate, tribasic]

**Bone Meal** *tablets* OTC *dietary supplement* [calcium; phosphorus] 236•118 mg

**bone morphogenetic protein-2 (BMP-2)** *investigational bone growth stimulant*

**bone morphogenetic proteins (BMPs)** *a class of factors that regulate bone formation, growth, and development (investigational)*

**bone powder, purified** [see: calcium phosphate, tribasic]

**bonecrusher; bones** *street drug slang* [see: cocaine, crack]

**Bonefos** ℞ *investigational (orphan) for increased bone resorption due to malignancy* [disodium clodronate tetrahydrate]

**Bonine** *chewable tablets* OTC *anticholinergic; antihistamine; antivertigo* agent; motion sickness preventative [meclizine HCl] 25 mg

**bonita** (Spanish for "beautiful") *street drug slang* [see: heroin]

**Bontril** slow-release capsules R̥ *anorexiant* [phendimetrazine tartrate] 105 mg ② Bentyl; Vontrol

**Bontril PDM** tablets R̥ *anorexiant* [phendimetrazine tartrate] 35 mg

**boo** *street drug slang* [see: marijuana]

**boom** *street drug slang* [see: marijuana]

**boomers** *street drug slang* [see: psilocybin; psilocin]

**Boost** liquid OTC *enteral nutritional therapy* [milk-based formula] 237 mL

**booster** *street drug slang for inhaled (snorted) cocaine* [see: cocaine]

**BOP (BCNU, Oncovin, prednisone)** *chemotherapy protocol*

**BOPAM (bleomycin, Oncovin, prednisone, Adriamycin, mechlorethamine, methotrexate)** *chemotherapy protocol*

**bopindolol** INN

**BOPP (BCNU, Oncovin, procarbazine, prednisone)** *chemotherapy protocol*

**boppers** *street drug slang* [see: amyl nitrite]

**boracic acid** [see: boric acid]

**borax** [see: sodium borate]

**boric acid** NF, JAN *acidifying agent; ocular emollient; antiseptic; astringent* 10% topical

**2-bornanone** [see: camphor]

**bornaprine** INN, BAN

**bornaprolol** INN

**bornelone** USAN, INN *ultraviolet screen*

**bornyl acetate** USAN

**borocaptate sodium B 10** USAN *antineoplastic; radioactive agent* [also: sodium borocaptate ($^{10}$B)]

**Borocell** R̥ *investigational (orphan) for boron neutron capture therapy (BNCT) for glioblastoma multiforme* [sodium monomercaptoundecahydro-closo-dodecaborate]

**Borofair Otic** ear drops R̥ *antibacterial/antifungal; astringent* [acetic acid; aluminum acetate] 2%•≟

**Borofax Skin Protectant** ointment OTC *astringent* [zinc oxide] 15%

**boroglycerin** NF

**boron** *element (B)*

**Boropak** powder packets OTC *astringent wet dressing (modified Burrow solution)* [aluminum sulfate; calcium acetate]

**bosentan** USAN, INN *endothelin receptor antagonist for vasospastic diseases*

**Boston Advance Cleaner; Boston Cleaner** solution OTC *cleaning solution for rigid gas permeable contact lenses*

**Boston Advance Comfort Formula** solution OTC *disinfecting/wetting/soaking solution for rigid gas permeable contact lenses*

**Boston Advance Conditioning Solution** (name changed to Boston Advance Comfort Formula in 1995)

**Boston Advance Rewetting Drops** (name changed to Boston Rewetting Drops in 1995)

**Boston Conditioning Solution** OTC *disinfecting/wetting/soaking solution for rigid gas permeable contact lenses*

**Boston Reconditioning Drops** (discontinued 1993) OTC *cleaning/soaking solution for hard contact lenses*

**Boston Rewetting Drops** OTC *rewetting solution for rigid gas permeable contact lenses*

**botiacrine** INN

**Botox** powder for extraocular muscle injection R̥ *blepharospasm and strabismus of dystonia (orphan); investigational (orphan) for pediatric cerebral palsy and cervical dystonia* [botulinum toxin, type A] 100 U

**botray** *street drug slang* [see: cocaine, crack]

**bottles** *street drug slang* [see: amphetamines]

**BottomBetter** ointment OTC *topical diaper rash treatment*

**botulinum toxin, type A** *blepharospasm and strabismus of dystonia (orphan); investigational (orphan) for pediatric cerebral palsy and cervical dystonia*

**botulinum toxin, type B** *investigational (orphan) for cervical dystonia*

**botulinum toxin, type F** *investigational (orphan) for spasmodic torticollis (cervical dystonia) and essential blepharospasm*

**botulinum toxoid, pentavalent (ABCDE)** *investigational vaccine (available only from the Centers for Disease Control and Prevention)*

**botulism antitoxin** USP *passive immunizing agent*

**botulism equine antitoxin, trivalent** *passive immunizing agent*

**botulism immune globulin** *investigational (orphan) for infant botulism*

**boubou; bobo** *street drug slang* [see: cocaine, crack]

**boulder** *street drug slang for a $20 piece of crack, or for crack in general* [see: cocaine, crack]

**boulya** *street drug slang* [see: cocaine, crack]

**Bounty Bears** chewable tablets OTC *vitamin supplement* [multiple vitamins; folic acid] ±•0.3 mg

**Bounty Bears Plus Iron** chewable tablets OTC *vitamin/iron supplement* [multiple vitamins; iron; folic acid] ±•15•0.3 mg

**bourbonal** [see: ethyl vanillin]

**bovactant** BAN

**bovine colostrum** *investigational (orphan) for AIDS-related diarrhea*

**bovine fibrin** BAN

**bovine immunoglobulin concentrate, Cryptosporidium parvum** *investigational (orphan) for treatment of cryptosporidiosis in immunocompromised patients*

**bovine myelin** *investigational (Phase III) oral treatment for multiple sclerosis*

**bovine superoxide dismutase (bSOD)** [see: orgotein]

**bovine whey protein concentrate** *investigational (orphan) for treatment of cryptosporidiosis in immunocompromised patients*

**boxidine** USAN, INN *antihyperlipoproteinemic*

**boy** *street drug slang* [see: heroin]

**Boyol** salve OTC *topical anti-infective; anesthetic* [ichthammol; benzocaine] 10%•± ⑨ boil

**bozo** *street drug slang* [see: heroin]

**B-PAS (benzoyl para-aminosalicylate)** [see: benzoylpas calcium]

**BPD-MA (benzoporphyrin derivative)** [see: verteporfin]

**BPI (bactericidal and permeability-increasing) protein** [q.v.]

**B-Plex** tablets ℞ *vitamin supplement* [multiple B vitamins; vitamin C; folic acid] ±•500•0.5 mg

**BQ** tablets (discontinued 1993) OTC *decongestant; antihistamine; analgesic* [phenylpropanolamine HCl; chlorpheniramine maleate; acetaminophen]

**BR-96** *investigational antineoplastic* [doxorubicin monoclonal antibody immunoconjugate]

**Bradycor** ℞ *investigational analgesic for systemic inflammatory response syndrome and sepsis*

**brain ticklers** *street drug slang* [see: amphetamines]

**brain-derived neurotrophic factor (BDNF)** *investigational (Phase III) treatment for brain and nerve degenerative diseases; clinical trials for ALS discontinued 1997*

**brallobarbital** INN

**BranchAmin 4%** IV infusion ℞ *nutritional therapy for high metabolic stress* [multiple branched-chain essential amino acids]

**branched DNA (bDNA) assay** *investigational in vitro diagnostic aid for HIV in the blood*

**branched-chain amino acids (BCAA)** *investigational (orphan) for amyotrophic lateral sclerosis* [see: isoleucine; leucine; valine]

**Brasivol** cream OTC *abrasive cleanser for acne* [aluminum oxide]

**Brasivol Base** (discontinued 1994) OTC *topical acne cleanser* [surfactant cleansing base with neutral soaps]

**Bravavir** ℞ *investigational (NDA filed) antiviral for varicella zoster and herpes zoster in AIDS; orphan status withdrawn 1997* [sorivudine]

**brazergoline** INN

**breakdowns** *street drug slang for a $40 piece of crack sold for $20* [see: cocaine, crack]

**Breathe Free** nasal spray OTC *nasal moisturizer* [sodium chloride (saline)] 0.65%

**Breezee Mist Aerosol** powder OTC *topical antifungal; anhidrotic* [undecylenic acid; menthol; aluminum chlorhydrate]

**Breezee Mist Antifungal** powder OTC *topical antifungal* [tolnaftate] 1%

**brefonalol** INN

**bremazocine** INN

**Breonesin** capsules OTC *expectorant* [guaifenesin] 200 mg

**brequinar** INN *antineoplastic* [also: brequinar sodium]

**brequinar sodium** USAN *antineoplastic* [also: brequinar]

**bretazenil** USAN, INN *anxiolytic*

**Brethaire** oral inhalation aerosol R̶ *bronchodilator* [terbutaline sulfate] 0.2 mg/dose

**Brethine** tablets, IV or subcu injection R̶ *bronchodilator* [terbutaline sulfate] 2.5, 5 mg; 1 mg/mL ⧉ Banthine

**bretylium tosilate** INN *antiadrenergic; antiarrhythmic* [also: bretylium tosylate]

**bretylium tosylate** USAN, BAN *antiadrenergic; antiarrhythmic* [also: bretylium tosilate] 500, 1000 mg/vial injection

**Bretylol** IV or IM injection R̶ *antiarrhythmic* [bretylium tosylate] 50 mg/mL ⧉ Brevital

**Brevibloc** IV infusion R̶ *β-blocker for supraventricular tachycardia* [esmolol HCl] 10, 250 mg/mL

**Brevicon** tablets R̶ *monophasic oral contraceptive* [norethindrone; ethinyl estradiol] 0.5 mg•35 μg

**Brevital Sodium** powder for IV injection R̶ *barbiturate general anesthetic* [methohexital sodium] 0.5, 2.5, 5 g ⧉ Bretylol

**Brevoxyl** gel R̶ *keratolytic for acne* [benzoyl peroxide] 4%

**brewer's yeast** *natural source of protein and B-complex vitamins*

**Brexidol** *investigational analgesic, antiinflammatory, and antirheumatic* [piroxicam betadex]

**Brexin-L.A.** sustained-release capsules R̶ *decongestant; antihistamine* [pseudoephedrine HCl; chlorpheniramine maleate] 120•8 mg

**Bricanyl** tablets, IV or subcu injection R̶ *bronchodilator* [terbutaline sulfate] 2.5, 5 mg; 1 mg/mL

**brick** *street drug slang for 1 kilo (kg) of marijuana, or for crack in general* [see: marijuana; cocaine, crack]

**brick gum** *street drug slang* [see: heroin]

**Brietal Sodium** ⒸⒶⓃ (U.S. product: Brevital Sodium) powder for IV injection R̶ *barbiturate general anesthetic* [methohexital sodium] 10 mg/mL

**brifentanil** INN *narcotic analgesic* [also: brifentanil HCl]

**brifentanil HCl** USAN *narcotic analgesic* [also: brifentanil]

**Brik-Paks** (trademarked delivery form) *ready-to-use liquid containers*

**brimonidine** INN *ophthalmic $\alpha_2$-adrenergic agonist for open-angle glaucoma and ocular hypertension* [also: brimonidine tartrate]

**brimonidine tartrate** USAN *ophthalmic $\alpha_2$-adrenergic agonist for open-angle glaucoma and ocular hypertension* [also: brimonidine]

**brinaldix** [see: clopamide]

**brinase** INN [also: brinolase]

**brinazarone** INN

**brindoxime** INN

**brinolase** USAN *fibrinolytic enzyme* [also: brinase]

**brinzolamide** USAN *carbonic anhydrase inhibitor for glaucoma*

**Bristoject** (trademarked delivery form) *prefilled disposable syringe*

**British antilewisite (BAL)** [now: dimercaprol]

**Britton** *street drug slang* [see: mescaline]

**brivudine** INN

**BRL 46470** *investigational antipsychotic for schizophrenia (clinical trials discontinued 1994)*

**BRL 55834** *investigational antiasthmatic*

**brobactam** INN

**brobenzoxaldine** [see: broxaldine]

**broccoli** *street drug slang* [see: marijuana]

**broclepride** INN

**brocresine** USAN, INN, BAN *histidine decarboxylase inhibitor*

**brocrinat** USAN, INN *diuretic*

**brodimoprim** INN

**brofaromine** INN *investigational reversible/selective MAO inhibitor*

**Brofed** elixir R *decongestant; antihistamine* [pseudoephedrine HCl; brompheniramine maleate] 30•4 mg/5 mL

**brofezil** INN, BAN

**brofoxine** USAN, INN *antipsychotic*

**brolaconazole** INN

**brolamfetamine** INN

**Brolene** *orphan status withdrawn 1996* [propamidine isethionate] 0.1%

**bromacrylide** INN

**bromadel** [see: carbromal]

**Bromadine-DX** syrup R *antitussive; decongestant; antihistamine* [dextromethorphan hydrobromide; pseudoephedrine HCl; brompheniramine maleate] 10•30•2 mg/5 mL

**bromadoline** INN *analgesic* [also: bromadoline maleate]

**bromadoline maleate** USAN *analgesic* [also: bromadoline]

**Bromaline** elixir OTC *decongestant; antihistamine* [phenylpropanolamine HCl; brompheniramine maleate] 12.5•2 mg/5 mL

**Bromaline Plus** captabs (discontinued 1995) OTC *decongestant; antihistamine; analgesic* [phenylpropanolamine HCl; brompheniramine maleate; acetaminophen] 12.5•2•500 mg

**bromamid** INN

**Bromanate** elixir OTC *decongestant; antihistamine* [phenylpropanolamine HCl; brompheniramine maleate] 12.5•2 mg/5 mL

**Bromanate DC Cough** syrup R *narcotic antitussive; decongestant; antihistamine* [codeine phosphate; phenylpropanolamine HCl; brompheniramine maleate; alcohol] 10•12.5•2 mg/5 mL

**Bromanyl** syrup R *narcotic antitussive; antihistamine* [codeine phosphate; bromodiphenhydramine HCl] 10•12.5 mg/5 mL

**bromanylpromide** [see: bromamid]

**Bromarest DX Cough** syrup R *antitussive; decongestant; antihistamine* [dextromethorphan hydrobromide; pseudoephedrine HCl; brompheniramine maleate; alcohol 0.95%] 10•30•2 mg/5 mL

**Bromatane DX Cough** syrup R *antitussive; decongestant; antihistamine* [dextromethorphan hydrobromide; pseudoephedrine HCl; brompheniramine maleate] 10•30•2 mg/5 mL

**Bromatapp** elixir (name changed to Cold & Allergy in 1995)

**Bromatapp** extended-release tablets OTC *decongestant; antihistamine* [phenylpropanolamine HCl; brompheniramine maleate] 75•12 mg

**Bromatapp Extended** timed-release tablets (discontinued 1993) R *decongestant; antihistamine* [phenylpropanolamine HCl; phenylephrine HCl; brompheniramine maleate]

**bromauric acid** NF

**bromazepam** USAN, INN, BAN, JAN *minor tranquilizer*

**bromazine** INN, DCF *antihistamine* [also: bromodiphenhydramine HCl; bromodiphenhydramine]

**bromazine HCl** [see: bromodiphenhydramine HCl]

**brombenzonium** [see: bromhexine HCl]

**bromchlorenone** USAN, INN *topical anti-infective*

**bromebric acid** INN, BAN

**bromelain** JAN *anti-inflammatory; proteolytic enzymes* [also: bromelains]

**bromelains** USAN, INN, BAN *anti-inflammatory; proteolytic enzymes* [also: bromelain]

**bromelin** [see: bromelains]

**bromerguride** INN

**brometenamine** INN, DCF

**bromethol** [see: tribromoethanol]

**Bromfed** syrup OTC *decongestant; antihistamine* [pseudoephedrine HCl; brompheniramine maleate] 30•2 mg/5 mL ☑ Bromphen

**Bromfed** tablets, timed-release capsules R *decongestant; antihistamine* [pseudoephedrine HCl; brompheniramine maleate] 60•4 mg; 120•12 mg

**Bromfed-DM Cough** syrup ℞ *antitussive; decongestant; antihistamine* [dextromethorphan hydrobromide; pseudoephedrine HCl; brompheniramine maleate] 10•30•2 mg/5 mL

**Bromfed-PD** timed-release capsules ℞ *pediatric decongestant and antihistamine* [pseudoephedrine HCl; brompheniramine maleate] 60•6 mg

**bromfenac** INN *long-acting nonsteroidal anti-inflammatory drug (NSAID); analgesic; antipyretic* [also: bromfenac sodium]

**bromfenac sodium** USAN *long-acting nonsteroidal anti-inflammatory drug (NSAID); analgesic; antipyretic* [also: bromfenac]

**Bromfenex** extended-release capsules ℞ *decongestant; antihistamine* [pseudoephedrine HCl; brompheniramine maleate] 120•12 mg

**Bromfenex PD** extended-release capsules ℞ *pediatric decongestant and antihistamine* [pseudoephedrine HCl; brompheniramine maleate] 60•6 mg

**bromhexine** INN, BAN *expectorant; mucolytic; investigational (orphan) for keratoconjunctivitis sicca of Sjögren syndrome* [also: bromhexine HCl]

**bromhexine HCl** USAN, JAN *expectorant; mucolytic* [also: bromhexine]

**bromindione** USAN, INN, BAN *anticoagulant*

**bromine** *element (Br)*

**bromisoval** INN [also: bromisovalum; bromvalerylurea; bromovaluree]

**bromisovalum** NF [also: bromisoval; bromvalerylurea; bromovaluree]

**2-bromo-α-ergocryptine** [see: bromocriptine]

**bromocamphor** [see: camphor, monobromated]

**bromociclen** INN [also: bromocyclen]

**bromocriptine** USAN, INN, BAN *prolactin enzyme inhibitor; antiparkinsonian; investigational (Phase III) for diabetic control of hypoglycemia; investigational (Phase II/III) treatment for obesity*

**bromocriptine mesilate** JAN *prolactin enzyme inhibitor; antiparkinsonian* [also: bromocriptine mesylate]

**bromocriptine mesylate** USAN, USP *prolactin enzyme inhibitor; antiparkinsonian* [also: bromocriptine mesilate]

**bromocyclen** BAN [also: bromociclen]

**bromodeoxyuridine** *investigational (orphan) radiation sensitizer for primary brain tumors*

**bromodiethylacetylurea** [see: carbromal]

**bromodiphenhydramine** BAN *antihistamine* [also: bromodiphenhydramine HCl; bromazine]

**bromodiphenhydramine HCl** USP *antihistamine* [also: bromazine; bromodiphenhydramine]

**bromofenofos** INN

**bromoform** USP

**bromofos** INN

**1-bromoheptadecafluorooctane** [see: perflubron]

**bromoisovaleryl urea (BVU)** [see: bromisovalum]

**Bromophen T.D.** sustained-release tablets ℞ *decongestant; antihistamine* [phenylpropanolamine HCl; phenylephrine HCl; brompheniramine maleate] 15•15•12 mg ▣ Bromphen

**bromophenol blue**

**bromophin** [see: apomorphine HCl]

**bromophos** [see: bromofos]

**bromopride** INN, DCF

**Bromo-Seltzer** effervescent granules OTC *antacid; analgesic; antipyretic* [sodium bicarbonate; citric acid; acetaminophen] 2781•2224•325 mg/dose

**bromotheophyllinate aminoisobutanol** [see: pamabrom]

**bromotheophyllinate pyranisamine** [see: pyrabrom]

**bromotheophyllinate pyrilamine** [see: pyrabrom]

**8-bromotheophylline** [see: pamabrom]

**Bromotuss with Codeine** syrup ℞ *narcotic antitussive; antihistamine* [codeine phosphate; bromodiphenhydramine HCl] 10•12.5 mg/5 mL

**bromovaluree** DCF [also: bromisovalum; bromisoval; bromvalerylurea]

**11-bromovincamine** [see: brovincamine]

**bromovinyl arabinosyluracil (BV-araU)** [see: sorivudine]

**bromoxanide** USAN, INN *anthelmintic*

**bromperidol** USAN, INN, BAN, JAN *antipsychotic*

**bromperidol decanoate** USAN, BAN *antipsychotic*

**Bromphen** elixir OTC *antihistamine* [brompheniramine maleate] 2 mg/5 mL ⊡ Bromfed; Bromophen

**Bromphen** sustained-release tablets, elixir (discontinued 1995) OTC *decongestant; antihistamine* [phenylpropanolamine HCl; brompheniramine maleate] 75•12 mg; 12.5•2 mg/5 mL ⊡ Bromfed; Bromophen

**Bromphen DC with Codeine Cough** syrup ℞ *narcotic antitussive; decongestant; antihistamine* [codeine phosphate; phenylpropanolamine HCl; brompheniramine maleate] 10•12.5•2 mg/5 mL

**Bromphen DX Cough** syrup ℞ *antitussive; decongestant; antihistamine* [dextromethorphan hydrobromide; pseudoephedrine HCl; brompheniramine maleate; alcohol 0.95%] 10•30•2 mg/5 mL

**brompheniramine** INN, BAN *antihistamine* [also: brompheniramine maleate]

**Brompheniramine Cough** syrup OTC *antitussive; decongestant; antihistamine* [dextromethorphan hydrobromide; pseudoephedrine HCl; brompheniramine maleate; alcohol 0.95%] 10•30•2 mg/5 mL

**Brompheniramine DC Cough** syrup ℞ *narcotic antitussive; decongestant; antihistamine* [codeine phosphate; phenylpropanolamine HCl; brompheniramine maleate; alcohol 1.15%] 10•12.5•2 mg/5 mL

**brompheniramine maleate** USP *antihistamine* [also: brompheniramine] 4, 8, 12 mg oral; 2 mg/5 mL oral

**Brompton's Cocktail; Brompton's Mixture** (refers to any oral narcotic/alcoholic solution containing morphine and either cocaine or a phenothiazine derivative) *prophylaxis for chronic, severe pain*

**bromvalerylurea** JAN [also: bromisovalum; bromisoval; bromovaluree]

**Bronchial** capsules ℞ *antiasthmatic; bronchodilator; expectorant* [theophylline; guaifenesin] 150•90 mg

**Broncho Saline** solution OTC *diluent for inhalation bronchodilators; solution for tracheal lavage* [saline solution] 0.9%

**Broncholate** softgels, syrup ℞ *decongestant; expectorant* [ephedrine HCl; guaifenesin] 12.5•200 mg; 6.25•100 mg/5 mL ⊡ Brondelate

**Broncholate CS** liquid (discontinued 1994) ℞ *narcotic antitussive; decongestant; expectorant* [codeine phosphate; ephedrine HCl; guaifenesin]

**Brondecon** tablets, elixir (discontinued 1993) ℞ *antiasthmatic; bronchodilator; expectorant* [oxtriphylline; guaifenesin] ⊡ Bronitin

**Brondelate** elixir ℞ *antiasthmatic; bronchodilator; expectorant* [theophylline; guaifenesin] 192•150 mg/15 mL ⊡ Broncholate

**Bronitin** tablets (discontinued 1993) OTC *antiasthmatic; bronchodilator; decongestant; expectorant; antihistamine* [theophylline; ephedrine HCl; guaifenesin; pyrilamine maleate] ⊡ Brondecon

**Bronitin Mist** inhalation aerosol OTC *bronchodilator for bronchial asthma* [epinephrine bitartrate] 0.3 mg/dose

**Bronkaid** tablets (discontinued 1995) OTC *antiasthmatic; bronchodilator; decongestant; expectorant* [theophylline; ephedrine sulfate; guaifenesin] 100•24•100 mg

**Bronkaid Dual Action** caplets OTC *decongestant; expectorant* [ephedrine sulfate; guaifenesin] 25•400 mg

**Bronkaid Mist** inhalation aerosol OTC *bronchodilator for bronchial asthma* [epinephrine nitrate & epinephrine HCl] 0.5%

**Bronkephrine** subcu or IM injection (discontinued 1996) ℞ *bronchodilator* [ethylnorepinephrine HCl] 2 mg/mL

**Bronkodyl** capsules ℞ *bronchodilator* [theophylline] 100, 200 mg

**Bronkolixir** elixir (discontinued 1995) OTC *antiasthmatic; bronchodilator; decongestant; expectorant; sedative* [theophylline; ephedrine sulfate;

guaifenesin; phenobarbital] 3•2.4•10•0.8 mg/mL

**Bronkometer** inhalation aerosol ℞ *bronchodilator* [isoetharine mesylate] 0.61% (340 μg/dose)

**Bronkosol** solution for inhalation ℞ *bronchodilator* [isoetharine HCl] 1%

**Bronkotabs** tablets (discontinued 1995) OTC *antiasthmatic; bronchodilator; decongestant; expectorant; sedative* [theophylline; ephedrine sulfate; guaifenesin; phenobarbital] 100•24•100•8 mg

**Bronkotuss Expectorant** liquid ℞ *decongestant; antihistamine; expectorant* [ephedrine sulfate; chlorpheniramine maleate; guaifenesin; hydriodic acid; alcohol 5%] 8.2•4•100•1.67 mg/5 mL

**bronopol** INN, BAN, JAN

**Brontex** tablets, liquid ℞ *narcotic antitussive; expectorant* [codeine phosphate; guaifenesin] 10•300 mg; 2.5•75 mg/5 mL

**broparestrol** INN, DCF

**broperamole** USAN, INN *anti-inflammatory*

**bropirimine** USAN, INN *antineoplastic; antiviral*

**broquinaldol** INN

**brosotamide** INN, DCF

**brosuximide** INN

**Brotane DX Cough** syrup ℞ *antihistamine; antitussive* [pseudoephedrine HCl; brompheniramine maleate; dextromethorphan hydrobromide]

**brother** *street drug slang* [see: heroin]

**brotianide** INN, BAN

**brotizolam** USAN, INN, BAN, JAN *hypnotic*

**brovanexine** INN

**brovavir** [see: sorivudine]

**brovincamine** INN [also: brovincamine fumarate]

**brovincamine fumarate** JAN [also: brovinacamine]

**brown** *street drug slang* [see: heroin; marijuana]

**brown and clears** *street drug slang for Dexedrine (dextroamphetamine sulfate) Spansules (brown and clear capsules)*

[see: Dexedrine; dextroamphetamine sulfate; amphetamines]

**brown bombers** *street drug slang* [see: LSD]

**brown crystal** *street drug slang* [see: heroin]

**brown dots** *street drug slang* [see: LSD]

**brown rhine; brown sugar** *street drug slang* [see: heroin]

**brownies; browns** *street drug slang for amphetamines, especially Dexedrine Spansules (dextroamphetamine sulfate in brown capsules)* [see: Dexedrine; dextroamphetamine sulfate; amphetamines]

**broxaldine** INN, DCF

**broxaterol** INN

**broxitalamic acid** INN

**broxuridine** INN *investigational (NDA filed) radiosensitizer for breast and brain tumors*

**broxyquinoline** INN, DCF

**brucine sulfate** NF

**B-Salt Forte** ophthalmic solution ℞ *intraocular irrigating solution* [balanced saline solution]

**bSOD (bovine superoxide dismutase)** [see: orgotein]

**BSS (bismuth subsalicylate)** [q.v.]

**BSS; BSS Plus** ophthalmic solution ℞ *intraocular irrigating solution* [balanced saline solution]

**BTA Rapid Urine Test** test kit for professional use ℞ *in vitro diagnostic aid for bladder tumor analytes in the urine*

**BTS67,583** *investigational antidiabetic*

**bubble gum** *street drug slang* [see: cocaine; cocaine, crack]

**bucainide** INN *antiarrhythmic* [also: bucainide maleate]

**bucainide maleate** USAN *antiarrhythmic* [also: bucainide]

**Bucast** ℞ *investigational (Phase II) antiviral glucosidase inhibitor for HIV* [MDL 28,574 (code name—generic name not yet approved)]

**Bucet** capsules ℞ *sedative; analgesic* [butalbital; acetaminophen] 50•650 mg

**bucetin** INN, BAN, JAN

**buciclovir** INN

**bucillamine** INN, JAN

**bucindolol** INN, BAN *antihypertensive; investigational treatment for congestive heart failure* [also: bucindolol HCl]

**bucindolol HCl** USAN *antihypertensive; investigational treatment for congestive heart failure* [also: bucindolol]

**bucladesine** INN [also: bucladesine sodium]

**bucladesine sodium** JAN [also: bucladesine]

**Bucladin-S** Softabs (discontinued 1994) ℞ *anticholinergic; antiemetic; motion sickness preventative* [buclizine HCl] 50 mg

**buclizine** INN, BAN *antinauseant; antiemetic; anticholinergic; motion sickness relief* [also: buclizine HCl]

**buclizine HCl** USAN *antinauseant; antiemetic; anticholinergic; motion sickness relief* [also: buclizine]

**buclosamide** INN, BAN, DCF

**bucloxic acid** INN, DCF

**bucolome** INN, JAN

**bucricaine** INN

**bucrilate** INN *tissue adhesive* [also: bucrylate]

**bucromarone** USAN, INN *antiarrhythmic*

**bucrylate** USAN *tissue adhesive* [also: bucrilate]

**bucumolol** INN [also: bucumolol HCl]

**bucumolol HCl** JAN [also: bucumolol]

**bud** *street drug slang* [see: marijuana]

**buda; budda; buddha** *street drug slang for potent, high-grade marijuana mixed with opium or crack* [see: marijuana; opium; cocaine, crack]

**budesonide** USAN, INN, BAN, JAN *anti-inflammatory*

**budipine** INN

**budotitane** INN

**budralazine** INN, JAN

**Buf-Bar** (discontinued 1994) OTC *medicated cleanser for acne* [sulfur] 3%

**bufenadine** [see: bufenadrine]

**bufenadrine** INN

**bufeniode** INN, DCF

**bufetolol** INN [also: bufetolol HCl]

**bufetolol HCl** JAN [also: bufetolol]

**bufexamac** INN, BAN, JAN, DCF

**bufezolac** INN

**buffered aspirin** [see: aspirin, buffered]

**Bufferin** coated tablets, coated caplets OTC *analgesic; antipyretic; anti-inflammatory; antirheumatic* [aspirin (buffered with calcium carbonate, magnesium oxide, and magnesium carbonate)] 325, 500 mg

**Bufferin, Arthritis Strength; Bufferin Extra Strength** tablets (discontinued 1993) OTC *analgesic; antipyretic; anti-inflammatory; antirheumatic* [aspirin (buffered with magnesium carbonate and aluminum glycinate)]

**Bufferin, Tri-Buffered** caplets (discontinued 1993) OTC *analgesic; antipyretic; anti-inflammatory; antirheumatic* [aspirin (buffered with calcium carbonate, magnesium oxide, and magnesium carbonate)]

**Bufferin, Tri-Buffered** tablets (discontinued 1993) OTC *analgesic; antipyretic; anti-inflammatory; antirheumatic* [aspirin (buffered with calcium carbonate, magnesium oxide, and magnesium carbonate)] 325 mg

**Bufferin AF Nite Time** tablets OTC *antihistaminic sleep aid; analgesic* [diphenhydramine HCl; acetaminophen] 30•500 mg

**Buffets II** tablets OTC *analgesic; antipyretic; anti-inflammatory; antacid* [acetaminophen; aspirin; caffeine; aluminum hydroxide] 162•227•32.4•50 mg

**Buffex** tablets OTC *analgesic; antipyretic; anti-inflammatory; antirheumatic* [aspirin (buffered with aluminum glycinate and magnesium carbonate)] 325 mg

**bufilcon A** USAN *hydrophilic contact lens material*

**buflomedil** INN, BAN, DCF

**bufogenin** INN

**buformin** USAN, INN *antidiabetic*

**Buf-Puf Acne Cleansing** bar (discontinued 1997) OTC *medicated cleanser for acne* [salicylic acid; vitamin E] 2%• ²⁄

**Buf-Puf Medicated** pads OTC *medicated cleansing pad for acne* [salicylic acid; alcohol]

**bufrolin** INN, BAN

**bufuralol** INN, BAN
**bufylline** BAN *diuretic; smooth muscle relaxant* [also: ambuphylline]
**Bugs Bunny Children's** chewable tablets (discontinued 1994) OTC *vitamin supplement* [multiple vitamins; folic acid] ≛•0.3 mg
**Bugs Bunny Complete** chewable tablets OTC *vitamin/mineral/calcium/ iron supplement* [multiple vitamins & minerals; calcium; iron; folic acid; biotin] ≛•100•18•0.4•0.04 mg
**Bugs Bunny Plus Iron** chewable tablets OTC *vitamin/iron supplement* [multiple vitamins; iron; folic acid] ≛•15•0.3 mg
**Bugs Bunny Vitamins and Minerals** (name changed to Bugs Bunny Complete in 1993)
**Bugs Bunny with Extra C Children's** chewable tablets OTC *vitamin supplement* [multiple vitamins; folic acid] ≛•0.3 mg
**bullet** *street drug slang* [see: isobutyl nitrite]
**bullet bolt** *street drug slang for various inhalants*
**bullia capital** *street drug slang* [see: cocaine, crack]
**bullion; bullyon** *street drug slang* [see: cocaine, crack; marijuana]
**bumadizone** INN, DCF
**bumblebees** *street drug slang* [see: amphetamines]
**bumecaine** INN
**bumepidil** INN
**bumetanide** USAN, USP, INN, BAN, JAN *loop diuretic* 0.25 mg/mL injection
**bumetrizole** USAN, INN *ultraviolet screen*
**Bumex** tablets, IV or IM injection ℞ *loop diuretic* [bumetanide] 0.5, 1, 2 mg; 0.25 mg/mL
**Buminate 5%; Buminate 25%** IV infusion ℞ *blood volume expander for shock, burns, and hypoproteinemia* [human albumin] 5%; 25%
**bump** *street drug slang for crack, fake crack, or a $20 hit of ketamine* [see: cocaine, crack; ketamine HCl]
**bunaftine** INN
**bunamidine** INN, BAN *anthelmintic* [also: bunamidine HCl]

**bunamidine HCl** USAN *anthelmintic* [also: bunamidine]
**bunamiodyl** INN [also: buniodyl]
**bunamiodyl sodium** [see: bunamiodyl; buniodyl]
**bunaprolast** USAN, INN *antiasthmatic; 5-lipoxygenase inhibitor*
**bunapsilate** INN *combining name for radicals or groups*
**bunazosin** INN [also: bunazosin HCl]
**bunazosin HCl** JAN [also: bunazosin]
**bundle** *street drug slang* [see: heroin]
**bundlin** [now: sedecamycin]
**buniodyl** BAN [also: bunamiodyl]
**bunitrolol** INN [also: bunitrolol HCl]
**bunitrolol HCl** JAN [also: bunitrolol]
**bunk** *street drug slang for fake cocaine* [see: cocaine]
**bunolol** INN *antiadrenergic (β-receptor)* [also: bunolol HCl]
**bunolol HCl** USAN *antiadrenergic (β-receptor)* [also: bunolol]
**buparvaquone** INN, BAN
**buphenine** INN, BAN *peripheral vasodilator* [also: nylidrin HCl]
**Buphenyl** tablets, powder for oral solution ℞ *antihyperammonemic for urea cycle disorders (orphan); investigational (orphan) for various sickling disorders* [sodium phenylbutyrate] 500 mg; 3 g/tsp, 8.6 g/tbsp
**bupicomide** USAN, INN *antihypertensive*
**bupivacaine** INN, BAN *injectable local anesthetic* [also: bupivacaine HCl]
**bupivacaine HCl** USAN, USP, JAN *injectable local anesthetic* [also: bupivacaine] 0.25%, 0.5%, 0.75%
**bupranol** [see: bupranolol]
**bupranolol** INN, DCF [also: bupranolol HCl]
**bupranolol HCl** JAN [also: bupranolol]
**Buprenex** IV or IM injection ℞ *narcotic agonist-antagonist analgesic* [buprenorphine HCl] 0.324 mg/mL
**buprenorphine** INN, BAN *narcotic agonist-antagonist analgesic* [also: buprenorphine HCl]
**buprenorphine HCl** USAN, JAN *narcotic agonist-antagonist analgesic; investigational (orphan) for opiate addictions* [also: buprenorphine]

**buprenorphine & naloxone** *orphan status withdrawn 1996*

**bupropion** BAN *aminoketone antidepressant; non-nicotine aid to smoking cessation* [also: bupropion HCl; amfebutamone]

**bupropion HCl** USAN *aminoketone antidepressant; non-nicotine aid to smoking cessation* [also: amfebutamone; bupropion]

**buquineran** INN, BAN

**buquinolate** USAN, INN *coccidiostat for poultry*

**buquiterine** INN

**buramate** USAN, INN *anticonvulsant; antipsychotic*

**burefrine** [now: berefrine]

**Burese** *street drug slang* [see: cocaine]

**burnie** *street drug slang* [see: marijuana]

**burodiline** INN

**Buro-Sol** solution OTC *astringent wet dressing (Burow solution)* [aluminum sulfate] 0.23%

**Burow solution** [see: aluminum acetate]

**burrito** *street drug slang* [see: marijuana]

**buserelin** INN, BAN *gonad-stimulating principle; antineoplastic* [also: buserelin acetate]

**buserelin acetate** USAN, JAN *gonad-stimulating principle; antineoplastic* [also: buserelin]

**bush** *street drug slang* [see: cocaine; marijuana]

**businessman's LSD; businessman's special; businessman's trip** *street drug slang* [see: dimethyltryptamine]

**BuSpar** tablets ℞ *azapirone anxiolytic* [buspirone HCl] 5, 10, 15 mg

**BuSpar** transdermal patch ℞ *investigational (Phase III) delivery form for anxiety and ADHD* [buspirone HCl]

**BuSpar ER** ℞ *investigational once-daily anxiolytic* [buspirone HCl]

**buspirone** INN, BAN *azaspirone anxiolytic; minor tranquilizer* [also: buspirone HCl]

**buspirone HCl** USAN *azapirone anxiolytic; minor tranquilizer; investigational (Phase III) transdermal delivery form for anxiety and ADHD* [also: buspirone]

**busters** *street drug slang for various CNS depressants*

**busulfan** USP, INN, JAN *alkylating antineoplastic for chronic myelogenous leukemia investigational (orphan) for bone marrow transplants* [also: busulphan]

**Busulfanex** *investigational (orphan) for bone marrow transplants* [busulfan]

**busulphan** BAN *alkylating antineoplastic* [also: busulfan]

**busy bee** *street drug slang* [see: PCP]

**butabarbital** USP *sedative; hypnotic* [also: secbutobarbitone] 🔁 butalbital

**butabarbital sodium** USP *sedative; hypnotic* [also: secbutabarbital sodium] 15, 30 mg oral; 30 mg/5 mL oral

**butacaine** INN, BAN [also: butacaine sulfate]

**butacaine sulfate** USP [also: butacaine]

**Butace** capsules (discontinued 1994) ℞ *analgesic; antipyretic; sedative* [acetaminophen; caffeine; butalbital] 325•40•50 mg

**butacetin** USAN *analgesic; antidepressant*

**butacetoluide** [see: butanilicaine]

**butaclamol** INN *antipsychotic* [also: butaclamol HCl]

**butaclamol HCl** USAN *antipsychotic* [also: butaclamol]

**butadiazamide** INN

**butafosfan** INN, BAN

**butalamine** INN, BAN

**Butalan** elixir (discontinued 1993) ℞ *sedative; hypnotic* [butabarbital sodium]

**butalbital** USAN, USP, INN *sedative* 🔁 butabarbital; Butibel

**Butalbital Compound** tablets, capsules ℞ *analgesic; antipyretic; anti-inflammatory; sedative* [aspirin; caffeine; butalbital] 325•40•50 mg

**butalgin** [see: methadone HCl]

**butallylonal** NF

**butamben** USAN, USP *topical anesthetic*

**butamben picrate** USAN *topical local anesthetic* 1% topical

**butamirate** INN *antitussive* [also: butamirate citrate; butamyrate]

**butamirate citrate** USAN *antitussive* [also: butamirate; butamyrate]

**butamisole** INN *veterinary anthelmintic* [also: butamisole HCl]

**butamisole HCl** USAN *veterinary anthelmintic* [also: butamisole]

**butamiverine** [see: butaverine]

**butamoxane** INN

**butamyrate** BAN *antitussive* [also: butamirate citrate; butamirate]

**butane (n-butane)** NF *aerosol propellant*

**butanilicaine** INN, BAN

**butanixin** INN

**butanserin** INN

**butantrone** INN

**butaperazine** USAN, INN *antipsychotic*

**butaperazine maleate** USAN *antipsychotic*

**butaprost** USAN, INN, BAN *bronchodilator*

**butaverine** INN, DCF

**butaxamine** INN *antidiabetic; antihyperlipoproteinemic* [also: butoxamine HCl; butoxamine]

**butedronate tetrasodium** USAN *bone imaging aid*

**butedronic acid** INN

**butelline** [see: butacaine sulfate]

**butenafine** INN *antifungal*

**butenafine HCl** USAN *topical benzylamine antifungal*

**butenemal** [see: vinbarbital]

**buteprate** USAN, INN *combining name for radicals or groups*

**buterizine** USAN, INN *peripheral vasodilator*

**Butesin Picrate** ointment OTC *topical local anesthetic* [butamben picrate] 1%

**butetamate** INN [also: butethamate]

**butethal** NF [also: butobarbitone]

**butethamate** BAN [also: butetamate]

**butethamine HCl** NF

**butethanol** [see: tetracaine]

**buthalital sodium** INN [also: buthalitone sodium]

**buthalitone sodium** BAN [also: buthalital sodium]

**buthiazide** USAN *diuretic; antihypertensive* [also: butizide]

**Butibel** tablets, elixir ℞ *GI anticholinergic; sedative* [belladonna extract; butabarbital sodium] 15•15 mg; 15•15 mg/5 mL ☒ butalbital

**butibufen** INN

**butidrine** INN, DCF

**butikacin** USAN, INN, BAN *antibacterial*

**butilfenin** USAN, INN *hepatic function test*

**butinazocine** INN

**butinoline** INN

**butirosin** INN *antibacterial antibiotic* [also: butirosin sulfate; butirosin sulphate]

**butirosin sulfate** USAN *antibacterial antibiotic* [also: butirosin; butirosin sulphate]

**butirosin sulphate** BAN *antibacterial antibiotic* [also: butirosin sulfate; butirosin]

**Butisol Sodium** tablets, elixir ℞ *sedative; hypnotic* [butabarbital sodium] 15, 30, 50, 100 mg; 30 mg/5 mL ☒ Butazolidin

**butixirate** USAN, INN *analgesic; antirheumatic*

**butixocort** INN

**butizide** INN *diuretic; antihypertensive* [also: buthiazide]

**butobarbitone** BAN [also: butethal]

**butobendine** INN

**butoconazole** INN, BAN *antifungal* [also: butoconazole nitrate]

**butoconazole nitrate** USAN, USP *antifungal* [also: butoconazole]

**butocrolol** INN

**butoctamide** INN [also: butoctamide semisuccinate]

**butoctamide semisuccinate** JAN [also: butoctamide]

**butofilolol** INN

**butonate** USAN, INN *anthelmintic*

**butopamine** USAN, INN *cardiotonic*

**butopiprine** INN, DCF

**butoprozine** INN *antiarrhythmic; antianginal* [also: butoprozine HCl]

**butoprozine HCl** USAN *antiarrhythmic; antianginal* [also: butoprozine]

**butopyrammonium iodide** INN

**butopyronoxyl** USP

**butorphanol** USAN, INN, BAN *analgesic; antitussive*

**butorphanol tartrate** USAN, USP, BAN, JAN *narcotic agonist-antagonist analgesic; antitussive*

**butoxamine** BAN *antidiabetic; antihyperlipoproteinemic* [also: butoxamine HCl; butaxamine]

**butoxamine HCl** USAN *antidiabetic; antihyperlipoproteinemic* [also: butaxamine; butoxamine]

**2-butoxyethyl nicotinate** [see: nicoboxil]

**butoxylate** INN

**butoxyphenylacethydroxamic acid** [see: bufexamac]

**butriptyline** INN, BAN *antidepressant* [also: butriptyline HCl]

**butriptyline HCl** USAN *antidepressant* [also: butriptyline]

**butropium bromide** INN, JAN

**butt naked** *street drug slang* [see: PCP]

**butter** *street drug slang* [see: marijuana; cocaine, crack]

**butter flower** *street drug slang* [see: marijuana]

**buttons** *street drug slang* [see: mescaline]

**butu** *street drug slang* [see: heroin]

**butydrine** [see: butidrine]

**butyl alcohol** NF *solvent*

**butyl aminobenzoate (butyl *p*-aminobenzoate)** [now: butamben]

**butyl *p*-aminobenzoate picrate** [see: butamben picrate]

**butyl chloride** NF

**butyl 2-cyanoacrylate** [see: enbucrilate]

**butyl DNJ (deoxynojirimycin)** [see: deoxynojirimycin]

**butyl *p*-hydroxybenzoate** [see: butylparaben]

**butyl methoxydibenzoylmethane** [see: avobenzone]

**butyl nitrite; isobutyl nitrite** *amyl nitrite substitutes, sold as euphoric street drugs, which produce a quick but short-lived "rush"* [see also: amyl nitrite; volatile nitrites]

**butyl parahydroxybenzoate** JAN *antifungal agent* [also: butylparaben]

**butyl parahydroxybenzoate** JAN *antifungal agent* [also: butylparaben]

***p*-butylaminobenzoyldiethylaminoethyl HCl** JAN

**butylated hydroxyanisole (BHA)** NF, BAN *antioxidant*

**butylated hydroxytoluene (BHT)** NF, BAN *antioxidant*

**α-butylbenzyl alcohol** [see: fenipentol]

**1-butylbiguanide** [see: buformin]

**N-butyl-deoxynojirimycin** [see: deoxynojirimycin]

**butylmesityl oxide** [see: butopyronoxyl]

**butylparaben** NF *antifungal agent* [also: butyl parahydroxybenzoate]

**butylphenamide**

**butylphenylsalicylamide** [see: butylphenamide]

**butylscopolamine bromide** JAN

**butynamine** INN

**butyrophenones** *a class of antipsychotic agents*

**butyrylcholesterinase** *investigational (orphan) for reduction and clearance of serum cocaine levels and postsurgical apnea*

**butyrylperazine** [see: butaperazine]

**O-butyrylthiamine disulfide** [see: bisbutitiamine]

**butyvinyl** [see: vinylbital]

**buzepide metiodide** INN, DCF

**buzz bomb** *street drug slang for nitrous oxide or a device for inhaling nitrous oxide from small canisters* [see: nitrous oxide]

**BVAP (BCNU, vincristine, Adriamycin, prednisone)** *chemotherapy protocol*

**BV-araU (bromovinyl arabinosyluracil)** [see: sorivudine]

**BVCPP (BCNU, vinblastine, cyclophosphamide, procarbazine, prednisone)** *chemotherapy protocol*

**BVDS (bleomycin, Velban, doxorubicin, streptozocin)** *chemotherapy protocol*

**BVPP (BCNU, vincristine, procarbazine, prednisone)** *chemotherapy protocol*

**BVU (bromoisovaleryl urea)** [see: bromisovalum]

**BW 12C** *orphan status discontinued 1996*

**Byclomine** *capsules, tablets* ℞ *gastrointestinal antispasmodic* [dicyclomine HCl] 10 mg; 20 mg ⊡ Hycomine

**Bydramine Cough Syrup** OTC *antihistamine; antitussive* [diphenhydramine HCl; alcohol 5%] 12.5 mg/5 mL ⊡ Hydramine

C (vitamin C) [see: ascorbic acid]

C & E softgels OTC *vitamin supplement* [vitamins C and E] 500•400 mg

C Factors "1000" Plus tablets OTC *dietary supplement* [vitamin C; citrus & rose hips bioflavonoids; rutin; hesperidin complex] 1000•250•50•25 mg

C Speridin sustained-release tablets OTC *dietary supplement* [ascorbic acid; hesperidin; lemon bioflavonoids] 500•100•100

C vitamin [see: ascorbic acid]

C1-esterase-inhibitor, human *investigational (orphan) for acute angioedema*

CA (cyclophosphamide, Adriamycin) *chemotherapy protocol*

cA2 MAb (chimeric A2 MAb) [q.v.]

⁴⁵Ca [see: calcium chloride Ca 45]

⁴⁷Ca [see: calcium chloride Ca 47]

caballo (Spanish for "horse") *street drug slang* [see: heroin]

cabastine INN

cabello (Spanish for "hair") *street drug slang* [see: cocaine]

cabergoline USAN, INN *dopamine agonist for hyperprolactinemia; investigational treatment for Parkinson's disease and gynecologic disorders*

cabis bromatum [see: bibrocathol]

CABOP; CA-BOP (Cytoxin, Adriamycin, bleomycin, Oncovin, prednisone) *chemotherapy protocol*

CABS (CCNU, Adriamycin bleomycin, streptozocin) *chemotherapy protocol*

cabufocon A USAN *hydrophobic contact lens material*

cabufocon B USAN *hydrophobic contact lens material*

CAC (cisplatin, ara-C, caffeine) *chemotherapy protocol*

cacao butter JAN

Cachexon B *investigational (orphan) for AIDS-related cachexia* [L-glutathione, reduced]

cactinomycin USAN, INN *antibiotic antineoplastic* [also: actinomycin C]

cactus; cactus buttons; cactus head *street drug slang* [see: mescaline]

CAD (cyclophosphamide, Adriamycin, dacarbazine) *chemotherapy protocol*

CAD (cytarabine [and] daunorubicin) *chemotherapy protocol*

cade oil [see: juniper tar]

cadexomer INN

cadexomer iodine USAN, INN, BAN *antiseptic; antiulcerative*

Cadillac *street drug slang* [see: PCP]

Cadillac express *street drug slang* [see: methcathinone]

cadmium *element (Cd)*

cadralazine INN, BAN, JAN

CAE (cyclophosphamide, Adriamycin, etoposide) *chemotherapy protocol* also: ACE

CAF (cyclophosphamide, Adriamycin, fluorouracil) *chemotherapy protocol*

cafaminol INN

Cafatine suppositories R *migraine-specific vasoconstrictor* [ergotamine tartrate; caffeine] 2•200 mg

Cafatine-PB tablets R *migraine treatment; vasoconstrictor; anticholinergic; sedative* [ergotamine tartrate; caffeine; sodium pentobarbital; belladonna extract] 1•100•30•0.125 mg

cafedrine INN, BAN

Cafergot tablets, suppositories R *migraine treatment; vasoconstrictor* [ergotamine tartrate; caffeine] 1•100 mg; 2•100 mg

Cafetrate suppositories R *migraine-specific vasoconstrictor* [ergotamine tartrate; caffeine] 2•100 mg

Caffedrine timed-release tablets, timed-release capsules OTC *CNS stimulant; analeptic* [caffeine] 200 mg

caffeine USP, BAN, JAN *CNS stimulant; diuretic; investigational (orphan) for apnea of prematurity*

caffeine, citrated NF

caffeine monohydrate [see: caffeine, citrated]

CAFP (cyclophosphamide, Adriamycin, fluorouracil, prednisone) *chemotherapy protocol*

**CAFTH (cyclophosphamide, Adriamycin, fluorouracil, tamoxifen, Halotestin)** *chemotherapy protocol*

**CAFVP (cyclophosphamide, Adriamycin, fluorouracil, vincristine, prednisone)** *chemotherapy protocol*

**'caine** *street drug slang* [see: cocaine; cocaine, crack]

**cakes** *street drug slang for round disks of crack* [see: cocaine, crack]

**Cal Carb-HD** powder OTC *calcium supplement* [calcium carbonate] 2.5 g/packet

**Caladryl** cream OTC *topical antihistamine; astringent; antipruritic/anesthetic* [diphenhydramine HCl; calamine] 1%•8% ⊡ Benadryl

**Caladryl** lotion OTC *topical poison ivy treatment* [calamine; pramoxine HCl; alcohol 2.2%] 8%•1%

**Caladryl** spray (discontinued 1994) OTC *topical antihistamine; astringent; antipruritic/anesthetic* [diphenhydramine HCl; calamine; alcohol 10%] 1%•8%

**Caladryl Clear** lotion OTC *topical poison ivy treatment* [pramoxine HCl; zinc acetate; alcohol 2%] 1%•0.1%

**Caladryl for Kids** cream OTC *topical poison ivy treatment* [calamine; pramoxine HCl] 8%•1%

**Cala-gen** lotion OTC *topical antihistamine; antipruritic/anesthetic* [diphenhydramine HCl; alcohol 2%] 1%

**Calamatum** spray OTC *topical poison ivy treatment* [calamine; zinc oxide; menthol; camphor; benzocaine]

**calamine** USP, JAN *topical protectant; astringent*

**Calamox** ointment OTC *topical poison ivy treatment* [calamine] 17 g/100 g ⊡ Camalox

**Calamycin** lotion OTC *topical antihistamine; astringent; anesthetic* [pyrilamine maleate; zinc oxide; calamine; benzocaine; chloroxylenol; alcohol 2%]

**Calan** film-coated tablets Ṛ *antianginal; antiarrhythmic; antihypertensive; calcium channel blocker* [verapamil HCl] 40, 80, 120 mg

**Calan SR** film-coated sustained-release tablets Ṛ *antihypertensive;*

*calcium channel blocker* [verapamil HCl] 120, 180, 240 mg

**Calcet** tablets OTC *dietary supplement* [calcium; vitamin D] 152.8 mg•100 IU

**Calcet Plus** tablets OTC *vitamin/calcium/iron supplement* [multiple vitamins; calcium; iron; folic acid] ±• 152.8•18•0.8 mg

**Calcibind** powder for oral solution Ṛ *antiurolithic to prevent stone formation in absorptive calciuria Type I* [cellulose sodium phosphate] 300 g bulk pack

**CalciCaps** tablets OTC *dietary supplement* [dibasic calcium phosphate; calcium gluconate; calcium carbonate; vitamin D] 125 mg (Ca)•60 mg (P)•67 IU

**CalciCaps with Iron** tablets OTC *dietary supplement* [dibasic calcium phosphate; calcium gluconate; calcium carbonate; vitamin D; ferrous gluconate] 125 mg (Ca)•60 mg (P)•67 IU•7 mg

**Calci-Chew** chewable tablets OTC *calcium supplement* [calcium carbonate] 1.25 g

**Calciday-667** tablets OTC *calcium supplement* [calcium carbonate] 667 mg

**calcidiol** [see: calcifediol]

**Calcidrine** syrup Ṛ *narcotic antitussive; expectorant* [codeine; calcium iodide; alcohol 6%] 8.4•152 mg/5 mL

**calcifediol** USAN, USP, INN *calcium regulator*

**calciferol** [now: ergocalciferol]

**Calciferol** tablets, IM injection Ṛ *vitamin deficiency therapy* [ergocalciferol (vitamin $D_2$)] 50 000 IU; 500 000 IU/mL

**Calciferol Drops** OTC *vitamin supplement* [ergocalciferol] 8000 IU/mL

**Calcijex** injection Ṛ *treatment of hypocalcemia in dialysis patients; decreases severity of psoriatic lesions* [calcitriol] 1, 2 μg/mL

**Calcilac** tablets (discontinued 1994) OTC *antacid* [calcium carbonate; glycine]

**Calcimar** intranasal spray (commercially available in Italy, Belgium, and Spain) Ṛ *investigational treat-*

*ment for postmenopausal osteoporosis* [calcitonin (salmon)]

**Calcimar** subcu or IM injection ℞ *calcium regulator for hypercalcemia, Paget's disease, and postmenopausal osteoporosis* [calcitonin (salmon)] 200 IU/mL

**Calci-Mix** capsules OTC *calcium supplement* [calcium carbonate] 1250 mg

**Calciparine** IV or deep subcu injection (discontinued 1995) ℞ *anticoagulant* [heparin calcium] 5000 U/dose

**calcipotriene** USAN *topical antipsoriatic* [also: calcipotriol]

**calcipotriol** INN, BAN *antipsoriatic* [also: calcipotriene]

**calcitonin (human)** USAN, INN, BAN, JAN *calcium regulator for symptomatic Paget's disease (osteitis deformans) (orphan)* ⏾ calcitriol

**calcitonin (salmon)** USAN, INN, BAN *calcium regulator for hypercalcemia, postmenopausal osteoporosis, and Paget's disease; orphan status withdrawn 1996*

**calcitonin salmon (synthesis)** JAN *synthetic analog of calcitonin (salmon); calcium regulator* [also: salcatonin]

**calcitonin salmon, recombinant** *investigational (Phase III) calcium regulator for hypercalcemia, postmenopausal osteoporosis, and Paget's disease*

**calcitriol** USAN, INN, BAN, JAN *calcium regulator* ⏾ calcitonin

**Calcitrol** ℞ *investigational antipsoriatic*

**calcium** *element (Ca)*

**calcium, oyster shell** [see: calcium carbonate]

**Calcium 600** tablets OTC *dietary supplement* [calcium carbonate] 600 mg

**Calcium 600 + D** tablets OTC *dietary supplement* [calcium; vitamin D] 600 mg•125 IU

**Calcium 600 with Vitamin D** tablets OTC *dietary supplement* [calcium; vitamin D] 600 mg•100 IU

**calcium acetate** USP, JAN *buffering agent for hyperphosphatemia of end-stage renal disease (orphan)*

**calcium aminacyl B-PAS (benzoyl para-aminosalicylate)** [see: benzoylpas calcium]

**calcium 4-aminosalicylate trihydrate** [see: aminosalicylate calcium]

**calcium amphomycin** [see: amphomycin]

**calcium antagonists** *a class of coronary vasodilators that inhibit cardiac muscle contraction and slow electrocardial conduction velocity* [also called: calcium channel blockers; slow channel blockers]

**calcium ascorbate** USP *vitamin C; antiscorbutic* 500 mg oral; 1652 mg/½ tsp. oral

**calcium benzamidosalicylate** INN, BAN *antibacterial; tuberculostatic* [also: benzoylpas calcium]

**calcium benzoyl p-aminosalicylate (B-PAS)** [see: benzoylpas calcium]

**calcium benzoylpas** [see: benzoylpas calcium]

**calcium bis-dioctyl sulfosuccinate** [see: docusate calcium]

**calcium bromide** JAN

**calcium carbimide** INN [also: cyanamide]

**calcium carbonate** USP *antacid; calcium replenisher; investigational (orphan) for hyperphosphatemia of end-stage renal disease* [also: precipitated calcium carbonate] 500, 600, 650, 1250 mg oral; 1250 mg/5 mL oral

**calcium carbonate, precipitated** [now: calcium carbonate]

**calcium carbophil** *bulk laxative*

**calcium caseinate** *dietary supplement; infant formula modifier*

**calcium channel blockers** *a class of coronary vasodilators that inhibit cardiac muscle contraction and slow electrocardial conduction velocity* [also called: calcium antagonists; slow channel blockers]

**calcium chloride** USP, JAN *calcium replenisher*

**calcium chloride Ca 45** USAN *radioactive agent*

**calcium chloride Ca 47** USAN *radioactive agent*

**calcium chloride dihydrate** [see: calcium chloride]

**calcium citrate** USP *calcium supplement*

**calcium citrate tetrahydrate** [see: calcium citrate]

**calcium clofibrate** INN

**calcium cyanamide** [see: calcium carbimide]

**calcium D-glucarate tetrahydrate** [see: calcium saccharate]

**calcium D-gluconate lactobionate monohydrate** [see: calcium glubionate]

**calcium dioctyl sulfosuccinate** [see: docusate calcium]

**calcium disodium edathamil** [see: edetate calcium disodium]

**calcium disodium edetate** JAN *heavy metal chelating agent* [also: edetate calcium disodium; sodium calcium edetate; sodium calciumedetate]

**Calcium Disodium Versenate** IM, IV, or subcu injection ℞ *lead chelation therapy; antidote to lead poisoning and lead encephalopathy* [edetate calcium disodium] 200 mg/mL

**calcium dobesilate** INN

**calcium doxybensylate** [see: calcium dobesilate]

**calcium edetate sodium** [see: edetate calcium disodium]

**calcium EDTA (ethylene diamine tetraacetic acid)** [see: edetate calcium disodium]

**calcium folinate** INN, BAN, JAN *antianemic; folate replenisher; antidote to folic acid antagonist* [also: leucovorin calcium]

**calcium glubionate** USAN, INN *calcium replenisher*

**calcium gluceptate** USP *calcium replenisher* [also: calcium glucoheptonate] 1100 mg/5 mL injection

**calcium glucoheptonate** INN, DCF *calcium replenisher* [also: calcium gluceptate]

**calcium gluconate (calcium D-gluconate)** USP *calcium replenisher; investigational (orphan) for hydrofluoric acid burns* 500, 650, 975, 1000 mg oral; 10% injection

**calcium glycerinophosphate** [see: calcium glycerophosphate]

**calcium glycerophosphate** NF, JAN

**calcium hopantenate** JAN

**calcium hydroxide** USP *astringent*

**calcium hydroxide phosphate** [see: calcium phosphate, tribasic]

**calcium hypophosphite** NF

**calcium iodide**

**calcium iododocosanoate** [see: iodobehenate calcium]

**calcium lactate** USP, JAN *calcium replenisher* 325, 650 mg oral

**calcium lactate hydrate** [see: calcium lactate]

**calcium lactate pentahydrate** [see: calcium lactate]

**calcium lactobionate** USP *calcium supplement*

**calcium lactobionate dihydrate** [see: calcium lactobionate]

**calcium lactophosphate** NF

**calcium L-aspartate** JAN

**calcium levofolinate** [see: levoleucovorin calcium]

**calcium levulate** [see: calcium levulinate]

**calcium levulinate** USP *calcium replenisher*

**calcium levulinate dihydrate** [see: calcium levulinate]

**calcium mandelate** USP

**calcium oxide** [see: lime]

**Calcium Oyster Shell** tablets (discontinued 1993) OTC *dietary supplement* [calcium carbonate]

**calcium pantothenate (calcium D-pantothenate)** USP, INN, JAN *vitamin $B_5$; enzyme cofactor* [also: pantothenic acid] 25, 100, 218, 250, 500, 545 mg oral

**calcium pantothenate, racemic (calcium DL-pantothenate)** USP *vitamin; enzyme cofactor*

**calcium para-aminosalicylate** JAN [also: aminosalicylate calcium]

**calcium phosphate, dibasic** USP, JAN *calcium replenisher; tablet base*

**calcium phosphate, monocalcium** [see: calcium phosphate, dibasic]

**calcium phosphate, tribasic** NF *calcium replenisher* [also: durapatite; hydroxyapatite]

**calcium polycarbophil** USAN, USP *bulk laxative*

**calcium polystyrene sulfonate** JAN

**calcium polysulfide & calcium thiosulfate** [see: lime, sulfurated]

**calcium saccharate** USP, INN *stabilizer*

**calcium silicate** NF *tablet excipient*

**calcium sodium ferriclate** INN *hematinic* [also: ferriclate calcium sodium]

**calcium stearate** NF, JAN *tablet and capsule lubricant*

**calcium sulfate** NF *tablet and capsule diluent*

**calcium tetracemine disodium** [see: edetate calcium disodium]

**calcium trisodium pentetate** INN, BAN *plutonium chelating agent* [also: pentetate calcium trisodium]

**calcium 10-undecenoate** [see: calcium undecylenate]

**calcium undecylenate** USAN *antifungal*

**calciumedetate sodium** [see: edetate calcium disodium]

**Calcort** (commercially available in Germany) Ŗ *investigational anti-inflammatory for rheumatoid arthritis and asthma* [deflazacort]

**CaldeCort** aerosol spray (discontinued 1997) OTC *topical corticosteroid* [hydrocortisone] 0.5%

**CaldeCort Anti-Itch; CaldeCort Light with Aloe** cream (discontinued 1997) OTC *topical corticosteroid* [hydrocortisone acetate] 0.5%

**Calderol** capsules Ŗ *increase serum calcium levels* [calcifediol] 20, 50 μg

**Caldesene** ointment OTC *moisturizer; emollient; astringent; antiseptic* [cod liver oil (vitamins A and D); zinc oxide; lanolin]

**Caldesene** powder OTC *topical antifungal* [calcium undecylenate] 10%

**caldiamide** INN *pharmaceutic aid* [also: caldiamide sodium]

**caldiamide sodium** USAN, BAN *pharmaceutic aid* [also: caldiamide]

**Calel D** tablets OTC *dietary supplement* [calcium carbonate; cholecalciferol] 500 mg•200 IU

**CALF (cyclophosphamide, Adriamycin, leucovorin [rescue], fluorouracil)** *chemotherapy protocol*

**CALF-E (cyclophosphamide, Adriamycin, leucovorin [rescue], flu-**

orouracil, ethinyl estradiol) *chemotherapy protocol*

**Calglycine** chewable tablets OTC *antacid* [calcium carbonate; glycine] 420•150 mg

**Cal-Guard** softgels OTC *calcium supplement* [calcium carbonate] 50 mg

**Calicylic Creme** (discontinued 1994) OTC *topical keratolytic; topical analgesic* [salicylic acid; trolamine] 10%• ²⁄

**California cornflakes** *street drug slang* [see: cocaine]

**California sunshine** *street drug slang* [see: LSD]

**californium** *element* (Cf)

**calioben** [see: calcium iodobehenate]

**Calmol 4** rectal suppositories OTC *emollient; astringent* [cocoa butter; zinc oxide] 80%•10%

**Calm-X** tablets OTC *anticholinergic; antiemetic; antivertigo agent; motion sickness preventative* [dimenhydrinate] 50 mg

**Calmylin** ⓒ oral solution OTC *antitussive; decongestant; expectorant* [dextromethorphan hydrobromide; pseudoephedrine HCl; guaifenesin] 3•6•20 mg/mL

**Calmylin #1** ⓒ syrup OTC *antihistamine* [dextromethorphan hydrobromide] 3 mg/mL

**Calmylin #2** ⓒ oral solution OTC *antitussive; decongestant* [dextromethorphan hydrobromide; pseudoephedrine HCl] 3•6 mg/mL

**Calmylin #4** ⓒ oral solution OTC *antitussive; antihistamine; expectorant* [dextromethorphan hydrobromide; diphenhydramine HCl; ammonium chloride] 2.5•3•25 mg/mL

**Calmylin Codeine** ⓒ oral solution Ŗ *narcotic antitussive; decongestant; expectorant* [codeine phosphate; pseudoephedrine HCl; guaifenesin] 0.66•6•20 mg/mL

**Calmylin Cough & Cold** ⓒ oral solution OTC *antitussive; decongestant; expectorant; analgesic* [dextromethorphan hydrobromide; pseudoephedrine HCl; guaifenesin; acetaminophen] 1•2•6.67•21.67 mg/mL

**Calmylin Expectorant** ⓒᴬᴺ syrup OTC *expectorant* [guaifenesin] 20 mg/mL

**Calmylin Pediatric** ⓒᴬᴺ syrup OTC *pediatric antitussive and decongestant* [dextromethorphan hydrobromide; pseudoephedrine HCl] 1.5•3 mg/mL

**calomel** NF

**Calphosan** IV injection ℞ *calcium replacement* [calcium glycerophosphate; calcium lactate] 50•50 mg/10 mL (0.08 mEq/mL)

**Calphron** tablets OTC *buffering agent for hyperphosphatemia in end-stage renal failure (orphan)* [calcium acetate] 667 mg

**Cal-Plus** tablets OTC *calcium supplement* [calcium carbonate] 1.5 g

**calteridol** INN *pharmaceutic aid* [also: calteridol calcium]

**calteridol calcium** USAN, BAN *pharmaceutic aid* [also: calteridol]

**Caltrate 600** film-coated tablets OTC *calcium supplement* [calcium carbonate] 1.5 g

**Caltrate 600 + D** tablets OTC *dietary supplement* [calcium carbonate; vitamin D] 600 mg•200 IU

**Caltrate 600 + Iron/Vitamin D** film-coated tablets OTC *dietary supplement* [calcium carbonate; ferrous fumarate; vitamin D] 600 mg•18 mg•125 IU

**Caltrate Jr.** chewable tablets OTC *calcium supplement* [calcium carbonate] 750 mg

**Caltrate Plus** tablets OTC *dietary supplement* [calcium carbonate; vitamin D; various minerals] 600 mg•200 IU•±

**Caltro** tablets OTC *dietary supplement* [calcium, vitamin D] 250 mg•125 IU

**calusterone** USAN, INN *antineoplastic*

**Calypte** test kit for professional use ℞ *urine test for HIV-1 antibodies*

**CAM (cyclophosphamide, Adriamycin, methotrexate)** *chemotherapy protocol*

**Cam red; Cam trip; Cambodian red** *street drug slang for high-potency marijuana from Cambodia* [see: marijuana]

**Cama Arthritis Pain Reliever** tablets OTC *analgesic; antipyretic; antiinflammatory; antirheumatic* [aspirin (buffered with magnesium oxide and aluminum hydroxide)] 500 mg

**Camalox** oral suspension (discontinued 1994) OTC *antacid* [aluminum hydroxide; magnesium hydroxide; calcium carbonate] 45•40•50 mg/mL

**Cam-Ap-Es** tablets (discontinued 1995) ℞ *antihypertensive* [hydrochlorothiazide; reserpine; hydralazine HCl] 15•0.1•25 mg

**camazepam** INN

**CAMB (Cytoxin, Adriamycin, methotrexate, bleomycin)** *chemotherapy protocol*

**cambendazole** USAN, INN, BAN *anthelmintic*

**came** *street drug slang* [see: cocaine]

**CAMELEON (cytosine arabinoside, methotrexate, Leukovorin, Oncovin)** *chemotherapy protocol*

**camellia oil** JAN

**CAMEO (cyclophosphamide, Adriamycin, methotrexate, etoposide, Oncovin)** *chemotherapy protocol*

**Cameo Oil** OTC *bath emollient*

**CAMF (cyclophosphamide, Adriamycin, methotrexate, folinic acid)** *chemotherapy protocol*

**camiglibose** USAN, INN *antidiabetic*

**camiverine** INN

**camonagrel** INN

**camostat** INN [also: camostat mesilate]

**camostat mesilate** JAN [also: camostat]

**CAMP (cyclophosphamide, Adriamycin, methotrexate, procarbazine HCl)** *chemotherapy protocol*

**Campath 1H** ℞ *investigational treatment for non-Hodgkin's lymphoma and rheumatoid arthritis*

**camphetamide** [see: camphotamide]

**Campho-Phenique** liquid, gel OTC *mild anesthetic; anti-infective; counterirritant* [camphor; phenol; eucalyptus oil] 10.8%•4.7%•≟

**Campho-Phenique Antibiotic Plus Pain Reliever** ointment OTC *topical antibiotic; local anesthetic* [polymyxin B sulfate; neomycin sulfate; bacitracin zinc; lidocaine] 5000 U•3.5 mg•500 U•40 mg per g

**camphor (*d*-camphor; *dl*-camphor)** USP, JAN *topical antipruritic; mild local anesthetic; counterirritant* [also: trans-π-oxocamphor]

**camphor, monobromated** USP

**camphorated opium tincture** [now: paregoric]

**camphorated parachlorophenol** [see: parachlorophenol, camphorated]

**camphoric acid** USP

**camphotamide** INN, DCF

**Camptosar** IV infusion ℞ *topoisomerase I inhibitor; antineoplastic for metastatic cervical, colon, and rectal cancers* [irinotecan HCl]

**camptothecin-11 (CPT-11)** [see: irinotecan]

**camsilate** INN *combining name for radicals or groups* [also: camsylate]

**camsylate** USAN, BAN *combining name for radicals or groups* [also: camsilate]

**camylofin** INN, DCF

**can** *street drug slang for 1 oz. of marijuana* [see: marijuana]

**Canadian black** *street drug slang* [see: marijuana]

**canamo** (Spanish for "hemp") *street drug slang* [see: marijuana]

**canappa** *street drug slang* [see: marijuana]

**canbisol** INN

**cancelled stick** *street drug slang for a marijuana cigarette* [see: marijuana]

**candicidin** USAN, USP, INN, BAN *polyene antifungal*

*Candida albicans* **skin test antigen** *diagnostic aid for diminished cellular immunity; test for HIV patients to assess TB antigen response*

**CandidaSure** *reagent slides for professional use* in vitro *diagnostic aid for Candida albicans in the vagina*

**Candin** *intradermal injection* ℞ *diagnostic aid for diminished cellular immunity; test for HIV patients to assess TB antigen response* [Candida albicans skin test antigen] 0.1 mL

**candocuronium iodide** INN

**candoxatril** USAN, INN, BAN *antihypertensive; investigational treatment for congestive heart failure*

**candoxatrilat** USAN, INN, BAN *antihypertensive*

**candy** *street drug slang for illegal drugs in general*

**candy C; candy cane; candycaine** *street drug slang* [see: cocaine]

**cannabinol** INN, BAN *antiemetic; antinauseant; a nonpsychoactive derivative of the Cannabis sativa plant*

**cannabis (Cannabis sativa)** *plant used to make the euphoric/hallucinogenic street drugs marijuana and hashish* [see also: marijuana; hashish]

**cannabis tea** *street drug slang* [see: marijuana]

**canrenoate potassium** USAN *aldosterone antagonist* [also: canrenoic acid; potassium canrenoate]

**canrenoic acid** INN, BAN *aldosterone antagonist* [also: canrenoate potassium; potassium canrenoate]

**canrenone** USAN, INN *aldosterone antagonist*

**cantharides** JAN

**cantharidin** *topical keratolytic*

**Cantharone** *liquid (discontinued 1994)* ℞ *topical keratolytic* [cantharidin] 0.7%

**Cantharone Plus** *liquid (discontinued 1994)* ℞ *topical keratolytic* [salicylic acid; podophyllum; cantharidin] 30%•2%•1%

**Cantil** *tablets* ℞ *treatment for peptic ulcer* [mepenzolate bromide] 25 mg

**CAO (cyclophosphamide, Adriamycin, Oncovin)** *chemotherapy protocol*

**CAP (cellulose acetate phthalate)** [q.v.]

**CAP (cyclophosphamide, Adriamycin, prednisone)** *chemotherapy protocol*

**cap; caps** *street drug slang* [see: cocaine, crack; LSD; heroin; psilocin; psilocybin]

**CAP; CAP-I (cyclophosphamide, Adriamycin, Platinol)** *chemotherapy protocol*

**CAP-II (cyclophosphamide, Adriamycin, high-dose Platinol)** *chemotherapy protocol*

**Capastat Sulfate** *powder for IM injection* ℞ *tuberculostatic* [capreomycin sulfate] 1 g/10 mL ⊘ Cepastat

**CAP-BOP (cyclophosphamide, Adriamycin, procarbazine, bleomycin, Oncovin, prednisone)** *chemotherapy protocol*

**capecitabine** USAN, INN *investigational (Phase II) antineoplastic for colorectal cancer*

**Capiscint** ℞ *investigational imaging agent for atherosclerotic plaque* [monoclonal antibodies]

**capital H** *street drug slang* [see: heroin]

**Capital with Codeine** oral suspension ℞ *narcotic analgesic* [codeine phosphate; acetaminophen] 12•120 mg/5 mL

**Capitrol** shampoo ℞ *antiseborrheic; antibacterial; antifungal* [chloroxine] 2% ⓡ captopril

**caplet** (dosage form) *capsule-shaped tablet*

**capmul 8210** [see: monoctanoin]

**capobenate sodium** USAN *antiarrhythmic*

**capobenic acid** USAN, INN *antiarrhythmic*

**Capoten** tablets ℞ *antihypertensive; angiotensin-converting enzyme (ACE) inhibitor* [captopril] 12.5, 25, 50, 100 mg

**Capozide 25/15; Capozide 25/25; Capozide 50/15; Capozide 50/25** tablets ℞ *antihypertensive* [captopril; hydrochlorothiazide] 25•15 mg; 25•25 mg; 50•15 mg; 50•25 mg

**CAPPr (cyclophosphamide, Adriamycin, Platinol, prednisone)** *chemotherapy protocol*

**capreomycin** INN, BAN *bactericidal antibiotic; tuberculostatic* [also: capreomycin sulfate]

**capreomycin sulfate** USAN, USP, JAN *bactericidal antibiotic; tuberculostatic* [also: capreomycin]

**capromab** INN *monoclonal antibody for diagnosis of prostate cancer* [also: capromab pendetide]

**capromab pendetide** USAN *monoclonal antibody for diagnosis of prostate cancer* [also: capromab]

**Capros** ℞ *investigational oral timed-release analgesic for severe pain*

**caproxamine** INN, BAN

**caps; cap** *street drug slang* [see: cocaine, crack; LSD; heroin; psilocin; psilocybin]

**capsaicin** *topical analgesic; counterirritant*

**capsicum oleoresin** *topical analgesic; counterirritant*

**Capsin** lotion OTC *topical analgesic* [capsaicin] 0.025%, 0.075%

**Capsulets** (trademarked form) *sustained-release caplet*

**captab** (dosage form) *capsule-shaped tablet*

**Captain Cody** *street drug slang* [see: codeine]

**captamine** INN *depigmentor* [also: captamine HCl]

**captamine HCl** USAN *depigmentor* [also: captamine]

**captodiame** INN, BAN

**captodiame HCl** [see: captodiame]

**captodiamine HCl** [see: captodiame]

**captopril** USAN, USP, INN, BAN, JAN *antihypertensive; angiotensin-converting enzyme (ACE) inhibitor* 12.5, 25, 50, 100 mg oral ⓡ Capitrol

**Captrix** cream OTC *topical analgesic* [capsaicin]

**capuride** USAN, INN *hypnotic*

**Capzasin-P** cream OTC *topical analgesic* [capsaicin] 0.025%

**caracemide** USAN, INN *antineoplastic*

**Carafate** tablets, oral suspension ℞ *treatment for duodenal ulcer* [sucralfate] 1 g; 1 g/10 mL

**caramel** NF *coloring agent*

**caramiphen** INN, BAN

**caramiphen edisylate**

**caramiphen HCl** [see: caramiphen]

**caraway oil** NF

**carazolol** INN, BAN

**carbachol** USP, INN, BAN, JAN *ophthalmic cholinergic; miotic for surgery; antiglaucoma agent* [also: carbacholine chloride]

**carbacholine chloride** DCF *ophthalmic cholinergic; miotic for surgery; antiglaucoma agent* [also: carbachol]

**carbacrylamine resins**

**carbadipimidine HCl** [see: carpipramine dihydrochloride]

**carbadox** USAN, INN, BAN *antibacterial*

**carbaldrate** INN

**carbamate choline chloride** [see: carbachol]

**carbamazepine** USAN, USP, INN, BAN, JAN *anticonvulsant; analgesic for trigeminal neuralgia* 100, 200 mg oral
**carbamide** [see: urea]
**carbamide peroxide** USP *topical dental anti-infective*
**N-carbamoylarsanilic acid** [see: carbarsone]
**carbamoylcholine chloride** [see: carbachol]
**O-carbamoylsalicylic acid lactam** [see: carsalam]
**carbamylcholine chloride** [see: carbachol]
**carbamylmethylcholine chloride** [see: bethanechol chloride]
**carbantel** INN *anthelmintic* [also: carbantel lauryl sulfate]
**carbantel lauryl sulfate** USAN *anthelmintic* [also: carbantel]
**carbaril** INN [also: carbaryl]
**carbarsone** USP, INN
**carbaryl** BAN [also: carbaril]
**carbasalate calcium** INN *analgesic* [also: carbaspirin calcium]
**carbaspirin calcium** USAN *analgesic* [also: carbasalate calcium]
**Carbastat** solution ℞ *direct-acting miotic for ophthalmic surgery* [carbachol] 0.01%
**carbazeran** USAN, INN *cardiotonic*
**carbazochrome** INN, JAN
**carbazochrome salicylate** INN
**carbazochrome sodium sulfonate** INN
**carbazocine** INN
**carbenicillin** INN, BAN *antibacterial* [also: carbenicillin disodium; carbenicillin sodium]
**carbenicillin disodium** USAN, USP *antibacterial* [also: carbenicillin; carbenicillin sodium]
**carbenicillin indanyl sodium** USAN, USP *bactericidal antibiotic* [also: carindacillin]
**carbenicillin phenyl sodium** USAN *antibacterial* [also: carfecillin]
**carbenicillin potassium** USAN *antibacterial*
**carbenicillin sodium** JAN *antibacterial* [also: carbenicillin disodium; carbenicillin]

**carbenoxolone** INN, BAN *glucocorticoid* [also: carbenoxolone sodium]
**carbenoxolone sodium** USAN *glucocorticoid* [also: carbenoxolone]
**carbenzide** INN
**carbesilate** INN *combining name for radicals or groups*
**carbetapentane citrate** NF [also: pentoxyverine]
**carbetapentane tannate**
**carbetimer** USAN, INN *antineoplastic*
**carbetocin** INN, BAN
**Carbex** tablets ℞ *antiparkinsonian* [selegiline HCl] 5 mg
**Carbex** tablets ℞ *antiparkinsonian (orphan)* [selegiline HCl] 5 mg
**carbidopa** USAN, USP, INN, BAN, JAN *decarboxylase inhibitor; antiparkinsonian (when used with levodopa)*
**carbidopa & levodopa** *antiparkinsonian* 10•100, 25•100, 25•250 mg oral
**carbifene** INN *analgesic* [also: carbiphene HCl; carbiphene]
**carbimazole** INN, BAN
**carbinoxamine** INN, BAN *antihistamine* [also: carbinoxamine maleate]
**Carbinoxamine Compound** syrup, pediatric drops ℞ *antitussive; decongestant; antihistamine* [dextromethorphan hydrobromide; pseudoephedrine HCl; carbinoxamine maleate] 15•60•4 mg/5 mL; 4•25•2 mg/mL
**carbinoxamine maleate** USP *antihistamine* [also: carbinoxamine]
**carbinoxamine maleate & pseudoephedrine HCl** *antihistamine; decongestant* 4•60 mg/5 mL oral; 2•25 mg/mL oral
**carbiphene** BAN *analgesic* [also: carbiphene HCl; carbifene]
**carbiphene HCl** USAN *analgesic* [also: carbifene; carbiphene]
**Carbiset** tablets ℞ *decongestant; antihistamine* [pseudoephedrine HCl; carbinoxamine maleate] 60•4 mg
**Carbiset-TR** timed-release tablets ℞ *decongestant; antihistamine* [pseudoephedrine HCl; carbinoxamine maleate] 120•8 mg
**Carbocaine** injection ℞ *injectable local anesthetic* [mepivacaine HCl] 1%, 1.5%, 2%, 3%

**Carbocaine with Neo-Cobefrin** injection ℞ *injectable local anesthetic* [mepivacaine HCl; levonordefrin] 2%•1:20 000

**carbocisteine** INN, BAN *mucolytic* [also: carbocysteine]

**carbocloral** USAN, INN, BAN *hypnotic*

**carbocromen** INN *coronary vasodilator* [also: chromonar HCl]

**carbocysteine** USAN *mucolytic* [also: carbocisteine]

**Carbodec** tablets, syrup ℞ *decongestant; antihistamine* [pseudoephedrine HCl; carbinoxamine maleate] 60•4 mg; 60•4 mg/5 mL

**Carbodec DM** syrup, pediatric drops ℞ *antitussive; decongestant; antihistamine* [dextromethorphan hydrobromide; pseudoephedrine HCl; carbinoxamine maleate] 15•60•4 mg/5 mL; 4•25•2 mg/mL

**Carbodec TR** timed-release tablets ℞ *decongestant; antihistamine* [pseudoephedrine HCl; carbinoxamine maleate] 120•8 mg

**carbodimid calcium** [see: calcium carbimide]

**carbofenotion** INN [also: carbophenothion]

**carbol-fuchsin solution (or paint)** USP *antifungal*

**carbolic acid** [see: phenol]

**carbolin** [see: carbachol]

**carbolonium bromide** BAN [also: hexcarbacholine bromide]

**carbomer** INN, BAN *emulsifying and suspending agent* [also: carbomer 910]

**carbomer 1342** NF *emulsifying and suspending agent*

**carbomer 910** USAN, NF *emulsifying and suspending agent* [also: carbomer]

**carbomer 934** USAN, NF *emulsifying and suspending agent*

**carbomer 934P** USAN, NF *emulsifying and suspending agent*

**carbomer 940** USAN, NF *emulsifying and suspending agent*

**carbomer 941** USAN, NF *emulsifying and suspending agent*

**carbomycin** INN

**carbon** *element* (C)

**carbon, activated**

**carbon dioxide ($CO_2$)** USP *respiratory stimulant*

**carbon tetrachloride** NF *solvent*

**carbonic acid, calcium salt** [see: calcium carbonate]

**carbonic acid, dilithium salt** [see: lithium carbonate]

**carbonic acid, dipotassium salt** [see: potassium carbonate]

**carbonic acid, disodium salt** [see: sodium carbonate]

**carbonic acid, magnesium salt** [see: magnesium carbonate]

**carbonic acid, monoammonium salt** [see: ammonium carbonate]

**carbonic acid, monopotassium salt** [see: potassium bicarbonate]

**carbonic acid, monosodium salt** [see: sodium bicarbonate]

**carbonic anhydrase inhibitors** *a class of diuretic agents that reduce the rate of aqueous humor formation, resulting in decreased intraocular pressure*

**carbonis detergens, liquor (LCD)** [see: coal tar]

**carbophenothion** BAN [also: carbofenotion]

**carboplatin** USAN, INN, BAN *alkylating antineoplastic for ovarian and other cancers*

**carboprost** USAN, INN, BAN *oxytocic*

**carboprost methyl** USAN *oxytocic*

**carboprost trometanol** BAN *oxytocic; prostaglandin-type abortifacient* [also: carboprost tromethamine]

**carboprost tromethamine** USAN, USP *oxytocic; prostaglandin-type abortifacient* [also: carboprost trometanol]

**Carboptic** Drop-Tainers (eye drops) ℞ *antiglaucoma agent; direct-acting miotic* [carbachol] 3%

**carboquone** INN

**carbose D** [see: carboxymethylcellulose sodium]

**carbovir** *investigational (orphan) for AIDS and symptomatic HIV*

**carboxyimamidate** [see: carbetimer]

**carboxymethylcellulose calcium** NF *tablet disintegrant*

**carboxymethylcellulose sodium** USP *suspending and viscosity-increasing* agent; *tablet excipient* [also: carmellose; carmellose sodium]

**carboxymethylcellulose sodium 12** NF *suspending and viscosity-increasing agent*

**carbromal** NF, INN

**carbubarb** INN

**carbubarbital** [see: carbubarb]

**carburazepam** INN

**carbutamide** INN, BAN

**carbuterol** INN, BAN *bronchodilator* [also: carbuterol HCl]

**carbuterol HCl** USAN *bronchodilator* [also: carbuterol]

**carcainium chloride** INN

**carcinoembryonic antigen (CEA)**

**cardamom seed** NF

**Cardec-DM** syrup, pediatric syrup, pediatric drops R *antitussive; decongestant; antihistamine* [dextromethorphan hydrobromide; pseudoephedrine HCl; carbinoxamine maleate] 15•60•4 mg/5 mL; 15•60•4 mg/5 mL; 4•25•2 mg/mL

**Cardec-S** syrup R *decongestant; antihistamine* [pseudoephedrine HCl; carbinoxamine maleate] 60•4 mg/5 mL

**Cardene** capsules R *antianginal; antihypertensive* [nicardipine HCl] 20, 30 mg

**Cardene I.V.** injection R *antihypertensive* [nicardipine HCl] 2.5 mg/mL

**Cardene QD** R *investigational once-daily antihypertensive* [nicardipine HCl]

**Cardene SR** sustained-release capsules R *antihypertensive* [nicardipine HCl] 30, 45, 60 mg

**cardiac glycosides** *a class of cardiovascular drugs that increase the force of cardiac contractions* [also called: digitalis glycosides]

**Cardiac T** test R *in vitro test for troponin T (indicator of cardiac damage) in whole blood*

**cardiamid** [see: nikethamide]

**Cardilate** oral or sublingual tablets (discontinued 1995) R *antianginal* [erythrityl tetranitrate] 10 mg

**Cardio-Green (CG)** powder for IV injection R *in vivo diagnostic aid for cardiac output, hepatic function, or ophthalmic angiography* [indocyanine green] 25, 50 mg

**Cardiolite** injection R *myocardial perfusion agent for cardiac SPECT imaging* [technetium Tc 99m sestamibi] 5 mL

**Cardi-Omega 3** capsules OTC *dietary supplement* [omega-3 fatty acids; multiple vitamins & minerals] 1000• ± mg

**cardioplegic solution (calcium chloride, magnesium chloride, potassium chloride, sodium chloride)** [q.v.]

**cardioprotective agents** *a class of potent intracellular chelating agents which protect the heart from the effects of doxorubicin*

**Cardioquin** tablets R *antiarrhythmic* [quinidine polygalacturonate] 275 mg

**Cardioxane** R *investigational adjunct to chemotherapy*

**Cardizem** IV injection, Lyo-Ject (prefilled syringe) R *calcium channel blocker for atrial fibrillation or paroxysmal supraventricular tachycardia (PSVT)* [diltiazem HCl] 5 mg/mL

**Cardizem** tablets R *antianginal; calcium channel blocker* [diltiazem HCl] 30, 60, 90, 120 mg

**Cardizem SR; Cardizem CD** sustained-release capsules R *antihypertensive; antianginal; calcium channel blocker* [diltiazem HCl] 60, 90, 120 mg; 120, 180, 240, 300 mg

**cardophyllin** [see: aminophylline]

**Cardura** tablets R *antihypertensive; antiadrenergic; treatment for benign prostatic hyperplasia* [doxazosin mesylate] 1, 2, 4, 8 mg

**carebastine** INN

**carena** [see: aminophylline]

**carfecillin** INN, BAN *antibacterial* [also: carbenicillin phenyl sodium]

**carfenazine** INN *antipsychotic* [also: carphenazine maleate; carphenazine]

**carfentanil** INN *narcotic analgesic* [also: carfentanil citrate]

**carfentanil citrate** USAN *narcotic analgesic* [also: carfentanil]

**carfimate** INN

**Carfin** tablets R *anticoagulant investigational (Phase III)* [warfarin sodium]

**carga** (Spanish for "weight" or "load") *street drug slang* [see: heroin]

**cargentos** [see: silver protein]

**cargutocin** INN

**Cariel** ℞ *investigational (Phase III) wound healing treatment*

**carindacillin** INN, BAN *antibacterial* [also: carbenicillin indanyl sodium]

**carisoprodol** USP, INN, BAN *skeletal muscle relaxant* 350 mg oral

**carmantadine** USAN, INN *antiparkinsonian*

**carmellose** INN *suspending agent; tablet excipient* [also: carboxymethylcellulose sodium; carmellose sodium]

**carmellose sodium** BAN *suspending agent; tablet excipient* [also: carboxymethylcellulose sodium; carmellose]

**carmetizide** INN

**carminomycin HCl** [now: carubicin HCl]

**carmofur** INN

**Carmol 10** lotion OTC *moisturizer; emollient; keratolytic* [urea] 10%

**Carmol 20** cream OTC *moisturizer; emollient; keratolytic* [urea] 20%

**Carmol HC** cream ℞ *topical corticosteroid; moisturizer; emollient* [hydrocortisone acetate; urea] 1%•10%

**carmoxirole** INN

**carmustine** USAN, INN, BAN *nitrosourea-type alkylating antineoplastic; polymer implant for recurrent malignant glioma (orphan)*

**Carnation Follow-Up; Carnation GoodStart** liquid, powder OTC *total or supplementary infant feeding*

**carnauba wax** [see: wax, carnauba]

**carne; carnie** (Spanish for "meat") *street drug slang* [see: heroin; cocaine]

**carnidazole** USAN, INN, BAN *antiprotozoal*

**carnitine** INN *vitamin B$_t$*

**L-carnitine** [see: levocarnitine]

**Carnitor** tablets, oral solution, IV injection or infusion ℞ *carnitine replenisher for deficiency of genetic origin (orphan); investigational (orphan) for secondary carnitine deficiency* [levocarnitine] 330 mg; 100 mg/mL; 500 mg/2.5 mL, 1 g/5 mL

**carocainide** INN

**β-carotene** [see: beta carotene]

**caroverine** INN

**caroxazone** USAN, INN *antidepressant*

**carperidine** INN, BAN

**carperone** INN

**carphenazine** BAN *antipsychotic* [also: carphenazine maleate; carfenazine]

**carphenazine maleate** USAN, USP *antipsychotic* [also: carfenazine; carphenazine]

**carpindolol** INN

**carpipramine** INN

**carpipramine dihydrochloride** [see: carpipramine]

**carpolene** [now: carbomer 934P]

**carprazidil** INN

**carprofen** USAN, INN, BAN *nonsteroidal anti-inflammatory drug (NSAID); analgesic; antipyretic*

**carpronium chloride** INN

**Carpuject** (trademarked delivery system) *prefilled cartridge-needle unit*

**Carpuject Smartpak** (trademarked delivery system) *prefilled cartridge-needle unit package*

**carrageenan** NF *suspending and viscosity-increasing agent*

**Carrie; Carrie Nation** *street drug slang* [see: cocaine]

**Carrisyn** ℞ *investigational (Phase I) antiviral/immunomodulator for AIDS* [acemannan]

**carsalam** INN, BAN

**carsatrin** INN *cardiotonic* [also: carsatrin succinate]

**carsatrin succinate** USAN *cardiotonic* [also: carsatrin]

**cartazolate** USAN, INN *antidepressant*

**carteolol** INN, BAN *antiadrenergic; topical antiglaucoma agent (β-blocker)* [also: carteolol HCl]

**carteolol HCl** USAN *antiadrenergic; topical antiglaucoma agent (β-blocker)* [also: carteolol]

**carticaine** BAN [also: articaine]

**Cartrix** (delivery system) *prefilled syringes*

**Cartrol** Filmtabs (film-coated tablets) OTC *antihypertensive; β-blocker* [carteolol HCl] 2.5, 5 mg

**cartucho** (Spanish for "cartridge") *street drug slang for a pack of marijuana cigarettes* [see: marijuana]

**cartwheels** *street drug slang* [see: amphetamines]

**carubicin** INN *antineoplastic* [also: carubicin HCl]

**carubicin HCl** USAN *antineoplastic* [also: carubicin]

**carumonam** INN, BAN *antibacterial* [also: carumonam sodium]

**carumonam sodium** USAN *antibacterial* [also: carumonam]

**carvedilol** USAN, INN, BAN, JAN *antianginal; antihypertensive; α- and β-blocker for congestive heart failure*

**carvotroline HCl** USAN *antipsychotic*

**Carwin** ℞ *investigational treatment for hypertension and congestive heart failure* [xamoterol]

**carzelesin** USAN *antineoplastic*

**carzenide** INN

**casanthranol** USAN, USP *laxative*

**cascara fluidextract, aromatic** USP *laxative*

**cascara sagrada** USP *stimulant laxative* 325 mg oral

**cascara sagrada fluid extract** *investigational (orphan) for oral drug overdose*

**cascarin** [see: casanthranol]

**Casec** powder OTC *protein supplement* [calcium caseinate]

**Casodex** film-coated tablets ℞ *antiandrogen for prostatic cancer* [bicalutamide] 50 mg

**Casper the ghost** *street drug slang* [see: cocaine, crack]

**cassia oil** [see: cinnamon oil]

**CAST (Color Allergy Screening Test)** reagent sticks for professional use *in vitro diagnostic aid for immunoglobulin E in serum*

**Castaderm** liquid OTC *topical antifungal; astringent; antiseptic* [resorcinol; boric acid; acetone; basic fuchsin; phenol; alcohol 9%]

**Castel Minus; Castel Plus** liquid OTC *topical antifungal* [resorcinol; acetone; basic fuchsin; alcohol 11.5%]

**Castellani Paint** solution (name changed to Castellani Paint Modified in 1996)

**Castellani Paint Modified** solution ℞ *topical antifungal; antibacterial* [basic fuchsin; phenol; resorcinol]

**Castellani's paint** [see: carbol-fuchsin solution]

**Castile soap**

**castor oil** USP *stimulant laxative*

**cat** *street drug slang* [see: methcathinone]

**CAT (cytarabine, Adriamycin, thioguanine)** *chemotherapy protocol*

**cat valium** *street drug slang* [see: ketamine HCl]

**Cataflam** tablets ℞ *nonsteroidal antiinflammatory drug (NSAID); antiarthritic; analgesic for primary dysmenorrhea* [diclofenac potassium] 50 mg

**catalase** *catalytic neutralizing agent and rinse for contact lenses*

**Catapres** tablets ℞ *antihypertensive* [clonidine HCl] 0.1, 0.2, 0.3 mg ⊠ Catarase; Combipres; Ser-Ap-Es

**Catapres-TTS-1; Catapres-TTS-2; Catapres-TTS-3** 7-day transdermal patch ℞ *antihypertensive* [clonidine HCl] 0.1 mg/day (2.5 mg); 0.2 mg/day (5 mg); 0.3 mg/day (7.5 mg)

**Catarase 1:5,000** ophthalmic solution ℞ *enzymatic zonulolytic for intracapsular lens extraction* [chymotrypsin] 300 U ⊠ Catapres

**Catarase 1:10,000** ophthalmic solution (discontinued 1993) ℞ *enzymatic zonulolytic for intracapsular lens extraction* [chymotrypsin] 150 U ⊠ Catapres

**Catatrol** ℞ *investigational bicyclic antidepressant; orphan status withdrawn 1994* [viloxazine]

**catgut suture** [see: absorbable surgical suture]

*Catha edulis* the plant from which cathinone, a naturally occurring stimulant, is derived [see also: cathinone; methcathinone]

**cathine** INN

**cathinone** INN *an extract of the Catha edulis plant, a naturally occurring stimulant* [see also: *Catha edulis*, methcathinone]

**cathomycin sodium** [see: novobiocin sodium]

**catnip** *street drug slang for a marijuana cigarette* [see: marijuana]

**Catrix** R investigational antineoplastic for breast, cervical, ovarian, uterine, and endometrial cancer

**Catrix Correction** cream OTC moisturizer; emollient

**CatVax** R investigational allergic desensitization to cats

**CAV (cyclophosphamide, Adriamycin, vinblastine)** chemotherapy protocol

**CAV (cyclophosphamide, Adriamycin, vincristine)** chemotherapy protocol [also: VAC]

**CAVe; CA-Ve (CCNU, Adriamycin, vinblastine)** chemotherapy protocol

**CAVE (cyclophosphamide, Adriamycin, vincristine, etoposide)** chemotherapy protocol

**Caverject** powder for intracavernosal injection, PenInject single-use autoinjector R vasodilator for erectile dysfunction [alprostadil] 5, 10, 20 μg/mL

**caviar** street drug slang [see: cocaine, crack]

**cavite all star** street drug slang [see: marijuana]

**CAVP16 (cyclophosphamide, Adriamycin, VP-16)** chemotherapy protocol

**C-B Time; C-B Time 500** timed-release tablets (discontinued 1995) OTC vitamin supplement [multiple B vitamins; vitamin C] ±•200 mg; ±•500 mg

**CBV (cyclophosphamide, BCNU, VePesid)** chemotherapy protocol

**CBV (cyclophosphamide, BCNU, VP-16-213)** chemotherapy protocol

**CC (carboplatin, cyclophosphamide)** chemotherapy protocol

**CC-Galactosidase** investigational (orphan) for Fabry's disease [alpha-galactosidase A]

**CCM (cyclophosphamide, CCNU, methotrexate)** chemotherapy protocol

**CCNU (chloroethyl-cyclohexyl-nitrosourea)** [see: lomustine]

**C-Crystals** crystals OTC vitamin supplement [vitamin C]

**CCV-AV (CCNU, cyclophosphamide, vincristine [alternates with] Adriamycin, vincristine)** chemotherapy protocol

**CCVPP (CCNU, cyclophosphamide, Velban, procarbazine, prednisone)** chemotherapy protocol

**CD (cytarabine, daunorubicin)** chemotherapy protocol

**CD4, human truncated 369 AA polypeptide** orphan status withdrawn 1996

**CD4, recombinant soluble human (rCD4)** investigational (Phase II, orphan) antiviral for AIDS

**CD4 immunoadhesin** [see: CD4 immunoglobulin G, recombinant human]

**CD4 immunoglobulin G, recombinant human** investigational (Phase I) antiviral for maternal/fetal transfer of HIV; investigational (orphan) for AIDS

**CD4-IgG** [see: CD4 immunoglobulin G, recombinant human]

**CD4-PE40** [see: alvircept sudotox]

**CD5-T lymphocyte immunotoxin** orphan status withdrawn 1997

**CD6-blocked ricin** investigational treatment for cutaneous T-cell lymphoma

**CD-18** investigational treatment for inflammatory disorders

**CD19** [see: anti-B4-blocked ricin]

**CD-33** [see: ricin (blocked) conjugated murine MCA myeloid cells]

**CD-40 ligand** investigational cytokine for rheumatoid arthritis, AIDS, and hyperimmunoglobulin M (HIM) syndrome

**CD-45 monoclonal antibodies** orphan status withdrawn 1996

**CdA (2-chloro-2'-deoxyadenosine)** [see: cladribine]

**CDC (carboplatin, doxorubicin, cyclophosphamide)** chemotherapy protocol

**CDDP; C-DDP (cis-diamminedichloroplatinum)** [see: cisplatin]

**CDDP/VP (CDDP, VePesid)** chemotherapy protocol

**CDE (cyclophosphamide, doxorubicin, etoposide)** chemotherapy protocol

**CDP-cholin** [see: citicoline]

**C-dust; C-game** street drug slang [see: cocaine]

**CEA (carcinoembryonic antigen)**

**CEAker** ℞ *orphan status withdrawn 1997* [indium In 111 murine anti-CEA MAb, type ZCE 025]

**CEA-Scan** powder for injection ℞ *imaging agent for detection of recurrent or metastatic colorectal cancer* [arcitumomab] 1.25 mg

**CEB (carboplatin, etoposide, bleomycin)** *chemotherapy protocol*

**Cebid** Timecelles (sustained-release capsules) OTC *vitamin supplement* [ascorbic acid] 500 mg

**CECA (cisplatin, etoposide, cyclophosphamide, Adriamycin)** *chemotherapy protocol*

**Cecil** *street drug slang* [see: cocaine]

**Ceclor** Pulvules (capsules), powder for oral suspension ℞ *cephalosporin-type antibiotic* [cefaclor] 250, 500 mg; 125, 187, 250, 375 mg/5 mL

**Ceclor CD** extended-release tablets ℞ *twice-daily cephalosporin-type antibiotic* [cefaclor] 375, 500 mg

**Ceclor SR** (pre-marketing name; released as Ceclor CD in 1996)

**Cecon** solution OTC *vitamin supplement* [vitamin C] 100 mg/mL

**Cedax** capsules, oral suspension ℞ *cephalosporin-type antibiotic for respiratory infections* [ceftibuten] 400 mg; 90, 180 mg/mL

**cedefingol** USAN *antipsoriatic; antineoplastic adjunct*

**cedelizumab** USAN *monoclonal antibody; prophylaxis of rejection of solid organ allograft; immunomodulator for autoimmune diseases*

**Cedilanid-D** IV or IM injection (discontinued 1993) ℞ *cardiac glycoside to increase cardiac output; antiarrhythmic* [deslanoside] 0.2 mg/mL

**CeeNu** capsules, dose pack ℞ *nitrosourea-type alkylating antineoplastic for brain tumors and Hodgkin's disease* [lomustine] 10, 40, 100 mg; 2 × 100 mg + 2 × 40 mg + 2 × 10 mg

**CEF (cyclophosphamide, epirubicin, fluorouracil)** *chemotherapy protocol*

**cefacetrile** INN *antibacterial* [also: cephacetrile sodium]

**cefacetrile sodium** [see: cephacetrile sodium]

**cefaclor** USAN, USP, INN, BAN, JAN *cephalosporin-type bactericidal antibiotic* 250, 500 mg oral; 125, 187, 250, 375 mg/5 mL oral suspension

**cefadroxil** USAN, USP, INN, BAN *bactericidal antibiotic* 125, 250, 500 mg/5 mL oral suspension

**cefadroxil monohydrate** *bactericidal antibiotic* 500, 1000 mg

**Cefadyl** powder for IV or IM injection (discontinued 1997) ℞ *cephalosporin-type antibiotic* [cephapirin sodium] 0.5, 1, 2, 4, 20 g

**cefalexin** INN, JAN *bactericidal antibiotic* [also: cephalexin]

**cefaloglycin** INN *antibacterial* [also: cephaloglycin]

**cefalonium** INN [also: cephalonium]

**cefaloram** INN [also: cephaloram]

**cefaloridine** INN *antibacterial* [also: cephaloridine]

**cefalotin** INN *bactericidal antibiotic* [also: cephalothin sodium; cephalothin]

**cefalotin sodium** [see: cephalothin sodium]

**cefamandole** USAN, INN *antibacterial* [also: cephamandole]

**cefamandole nafate** USAN, USP *bactericidal antibiotic* [also: cephamandole nafate]

**cefamandole sodium** USP *antibacterial*

**Cefanex** capsules (discontinued 1995) ℞ *cephalosporin-type antibiotic* [cephalexin monohydrate] 250, 500 mg

**cefaparole** USAN, INN *antibacterial*

**cefapirin** INN, BAN *antibacterial* [also: cephapirin sodium]

**cefapirin sodium** [see: cephapirin sodium]

**cefatrizine** USAN, INN, BAN *antibacterial*

**cefazaflur** INN *antibacterial* [also: cefazaflur sodium]

**cefazaflur sodium** USAN *antibacterial* [also: cefazaflur]

**cefazedone** INN, BAN

**cefazolin** USP, INN *systemic antibacterial* [also: cephazolin] ② cephalexin; cephalothin

**cefazolin sodium** USAN, USP *bactericidal antibiotic* [also: cephazolin

sodium] 0.25, 0.5, 1, 5, 10, 20 g
injection
**cefbuperazone** USAN, INN *antibacterial*
**cefcanel** INN
**cefcanel daloxate** INN
**cefdinir** USAN, INN *antibacterial*
**cefedrolor** INN
**cefempidone** INN, BAN
**cefepime** USAN, INN *antibacterial*
**cefepime HCl** USAN *cephalosporin-type antibiotic*
**cefetamet** USAN, INN *veterinary antibacterial*
**cefetecol** USAN, INN, BAN *antibacterial*
**cefetrizole** INN
**cefivitril** INN
**cefixime** USAN, USP, INN, BAN *bactericidal antibiotic*
**Cefizox** powder for IV or IM injection R *cephalosporin-type antibiotic* [ceftizoxime sodium] 0.5, 1, 2, 10 g
**cefmenoxime** INN *antibacterial* [also: cefmenoxime HCl]
**cefmenoxime HCl** USAN, USP *antibacterial* [also: cefmenoxime]
**cefmepidium chloride** INN
**cefmetazole** USAN, INN *antibacterial*
**cefmetazole sodium** USAN, USP, JAN *bactericidal antibiotic*
**cefminox** INN
**Cefobid** powder for IV or IM injection R *cephalosporin-type antibiotic* [cefoperazone sodium] 1, 2 g
**cefodizime** INN *investigational antibiotic*
**Cefol** Filmtabs (film-coated tablets) R *vitamin supplement* [multiple vitamins; folic acid] ± •0.5 mg
**cefonicid** INN, BAN *antibacterial* [also: cefonicid monosodium]
**cefonicid monosodium** USAN *antibacterial* [also: cefonicid]
**cefonicid sodium** USAN, USP *bactericidal antibiotic*
**cefoperazone** INN, BAN *antibacterial* [also: cefoperazone sodium]
**cefoperazone sodium** USAN, USP *bactericidal antibiotic* [also: cefoperazone]
**ceforanide** USAN, USP, INN, BAN *bactericidal antibiotic*
**Cefotan** powder or frozen premixed solution for IV or IM injection R

*cephalosporin-type antibiotic* [cefotetan disodium] 1, 2, 10 g
**cefotaxime** INN, BAN *antibacterial* [also: cefotaxime sodium] ② cefoxitin
**cefotaxime sodium** USAN, USP *bactericidal antibiotic* [also: cefotaxime]
**cefotetan** USAN, INN, BAN *antibacterial*
**cefotetan disodium** USAN, USP *bactericidal antibiotic*
**cefotiam** INN, BAN *antibacterial* [also: cefotiam HCl]
**cefotiam HCl** USAN *antibacterial* [also: cefotiam]
**cefoxazole** INN [also: cephoxazole]
**cefoxitin** USAN, INN, BAN *cephalosporin-type antibiotic* ② cefotaxime
**cefoxitin sodium** USAN, USP, BAN *cephalosporin-type antibiotic*
**cefpimizole** USAN, INN *antibacterial*
**cefpimizole sodium** USAN, JAN *antibacterial*
**cefpiramide** USAN, USP, INN *antibacterial*
**cefpiramide sodium** USAN, JAN *antibacterial*
**cefpirome** INN, BAN *antibacterial* [also: cefpirome sulfate]
**cefpirome sulfate** USAN, JAN *antibacterial* [also: cefpirome]
**cefpodoxime** INN, BAN *cephalosporin-type bactericidal antibiotic* [also: cefpodoxime proxetil]
**cefpodoxime proxetil** USAN, JAN *cephalosporin-type bactericidal antibiotic* [also: cefpodoxime]
**cefprozil** USAN, INN *bactericidal antibiotic*
**cefprozil monohydrate**
**cefquinome** INN, BAN *veterinary antibacterial*
**cefquinome sulfate** USAN *veterinary antibacterial*
**cefradine** INN *bactericidal antibiotic* [also: cephradine]
**Cefrom** R *investigational cephalosporin antibiotic* [cefpirome]
**cefrotil** INN
**cefroxadine** USAN, INN *antibacterial*
**cefsulodin** INN, BAN *antibacterial* [also: cefsulodin sodium]
**cefsulodin sodium** USAN *antibacterial* [also: cefsulodin]
**cefsumide** INN

**ceftazidime** USAN, USP, INN, BAN, JAN *bactericidal antibiotic*

**cefteram** INN

**ceftezole** INN

**ceftibuten** USAN, INN, BAN *antibacterial antibiotic*

**Ceftin** film-coated tablets, oral suspension ℞ *cephalosporin-type antibiotic* [cefuroxime axetil] 125, 250, 500 mg; 125 mg/5 mL

**ceftiofur** INN, BAN *veterinary antibacterial* [also: ceftiofur HCl]

**ceftiofur HCl** USAN *veterinary antibacterial* [also: ceftiofur]

**ceftiofur sodium** USAN *veterinary antibacterial*

**ceftiolene** INN

**ceftioxide** INN

**ceftizoxime** INN, BAN *bactericidal antibiotic* [also: ceftizoxime sodium] ▣ cefuroxime

**ceftizoxime sodium** USAN, USP *bactericidal antibiotic* [also: ceftizoxime]

**ceftriaxone** INN, BAN *bactericidal antibiotic* [also: ceftriaxone sodium]

**ceftriaxone sodium** USAN, USP *bactericidal antibiotic* [also: ceftriaxone]

**cefuracetime** INN, BAN

**cefuroxime** USAN, INN, BAN *cephalosporin-type antibiotic* ▣ ceftizoxime

**cefuroxime axetil** USAN, USP, BAN *cephalosporin-type antibiotic*

**cefuroxime pivoxetil** USAN *cephalosporin-type antibiotic*

**cefuroxime sodium** USP, BAN *cephalosporin-type antibiotic* 0.75, 1.5, 7.5 g injection

**cefuzonam** INN

**Cefzil** film-coated tablets, powder for oral suspension ℞ *cephalosporin-type antibiotic* [cefprozil] 250, 500 mg; 125, 250 mg/5 mL ▣ Kefzol

**Cefzon** (foreign name for U.S. product Omnicef)

**celecoxib** *investigational (Phase III) COX-2 inhibitor for osteoarthritis and rheumatoid arthritis*

**Celestone** tablets, syrup *glucocorticoids* [tamethasone] 0.6 mg; 0.6 mg/5 mL

**Celestone Phosphate** IV, IM injection ℞ *glucocorticoids* [betamethasone sodium phosphate] 4 mg/mL

**Celestone Soluspan** intrabursal, intra-articular, intralesional injection ℞ *glucocorticoids* [betamethasone sodium phosphate; betamethasone acetate] 3•3 mg/mL

**celiprolol** INN, BAN *antiadrenergic (β-receptor)* [also: celiprolol HCl]

**celiprolol HCl** USAN *antiadrenergic (β-receptor)* [also: celiprolol]

**cellacefate** INN *tablet-coating agent* [also: cellulose acetate phthalate; cellacephate]

**cellacephate** BAN *tablet-coating agent* [also: cellulose acetate phthalate; cellacefate]

**CellCept** capsules, film-coated tablets ℞ *immunosuppressant for renal transplants* [mycophenolate mofetil] 250 mg; 500 mg

**Cellufresh** eye drops OTC *ocular moisturizer/lubricant* [carboxymethylcellulose] 0.5%

**cellulase** USAN *digestive enzyme*

**cellulolytic enzyme** [see: cellulase]

**cellulose, absorbable** [see: cellulose, oxidized]

**cellulose, ethyl ester** [see: ethylcellulose]

**cellulose, hydroxypropyl methyl ether** [see: hydroxypropyl methylcellulose]

**cellulose, microcrystalline** NF *tablet and capsule diluent* [also: dispersible cellulose]

**cellulose, oxidized** USP *topical local hemostatic*

**cellulose, oxidized regenerated** USP *local hemostatic*

**cellulose, sodium carboxymethyl** [see: carboxymethylcellulose sodium]

**cellulose acetate** NF *tablet-coating agent; insoluble polymer membrane*

**cellulose acetate butyrate** [see: cabufocon A; cabufocon B]

**cellulose acetate dibutyrate** [see: porofocon A; porofocon B]

**cellulose acetate phthalate (CAP)** NF *tablet-coating agent* [also: cellacefate; cellacephate]

**cellulose carboxymethyl ether, sodium salt** [see: carboxymethylcellulose sodium]

**cellulose diacetate** [see: cellulose acetate]

**cellulose dihydrogen phosphate, disodium salt** [see: cellulose sodium phosphate]

**cellulose disodium phosphate** [see: cellulose sodium phosphate]

**cellulose ethyl ether** [see: ethylcellulose]

**cellulose gum, modified** [now: croscarmellose sodium]

**cellulose methyl ether** [see: methylcellulose]

**cellulose nitrate** [see: pyroxylin]

**cellulose sodium phosphate (CSP)** USAN, USP *antiurolithic to prevent stone formation in absorptive hypercalciuria Type I*

**cellulosic acid** [see: cellulose, oxidized]

**Celluvisc** solution OTC *ocular moisturizer/lubricant* [carboxymethylcellulose] 1%

**celmoleukin** INN *immunostimulant*

**Celontin** Kapseals (capsules) ℞ *anticonvulsant* [methsuximide] 150, 300 mg

**celucloral** INN, BAN

**Cel-U-Jec** IV, IM injection ℞ *glucocorticoids* [betamethasone sodium phosphate] 4 mg/mL

**CEM (cytosine arabinoside, etoposide, methotrexate)** *chemotherapy protocol*

**Cenafed** syrup OTC *nasal decongestant* [pseudoephedrine HCl] 30 mg/5 mL

**Cenafed** tablets (discontinued 1993) OTC *nasal decongestant* [pseudoephedrine HCl] 60 mg

**Cenafed Plus** tablets OTC *decongestant; antihistamine* [pseudoephedrine HCl; tripolidine HCl] 60•2.5 mg

**Cena-K** liquid ℞ *potassium supplement* [potassium chloride] 20, 40 mEq/15 mL

**Cenocort A-40** injection (discontinued 1994) ℞ *corticosteroid* [triamcinolone acetonide] 40 mg/mL

**Cenocort Forte** injection (discontinued 1994) ℞ *corticosteroid* [triamcinolone diacetate] 40 mg/mL

**Cenolate** IV, IM, or subcu injection ℞ *antiscorbutic* [sodium ascorbate] 562.5 mg/mL

**Centara** ℞ *investigational treatment for arthritis and multiple sclerosis; transplant rejection preventative* [priliximab]

**Center-Al** subcu or IM injection ℞ *allergenic sensitivity testing (subcu); allergenic desensitization therapy (IM)* [allergenic extracts, alum-precipitated]

**CenTNF** ℞ *investigational treatment for sepsis, rheumatoid arthritis and Crohn's disease* [anti-TNF (tumor necrosis factor)]

**CentoRx** (name changed to ReoPro upon its release in 1995)

**Centovir** *orphan status withdrawn 1994* [human IgM monoclonal antibody (C-58) to cytomegalovirus (CMV)]

**Centoxin** ℞ *investigational (orphan) for gram-negative bacteremia in endotoxin shock* [nebacumab]

**Centrafree** tablets OTC *antianemic* [ferrous fumarate; multiple vitamins]

**Centrax** capsules, tablets (discontinued 1995) ℞ *anxiolytic* [prazepam] 5, 10, 20 mg; 10 mg

**centrazene** [see: simtrazene]

**centrophenoxine** [see: meclofenoxate]

**Centrovite Advanced Formula** tablets (name changed to Cerovite Advanced Formula in 1995)

**Centrovite Jr.** tablets (name changed to Cerovite Jr. in 1995)

**Centrum** tablets OTC *antianemic* [ferrous fumarate; multiple vitamins]

**Centrum, Advanced Formula** liquid OTC *vitamin/mineral/iron supplement* [multiple vitamins & minerals; ferrous fumarate; biotin; alcohol 6.7%] ±•9•0.3 mg/15 mL

**Centrum, Advanced Formula** tablets OTC *vitamin/mineral/iron supplement* [multiple vitamins & minerals; ferrous fumarate; folic acid; biotin] ±•18 mg•0.4 mg•30 μg

**Centrum Jr. + Extra C; Centrum Jr. + Extra Calcium** chewable tablets OTC *vitamin/mineral/calcium/iron supplement* [multiple vitamins & minerals; calcium; iron; folic acid; biotin] ±•108•18•0.4•0.045 mg; ±•160•18•0.4•0.045 mg

**Centrum Jr. with Iron** tablets OTC *vitamin/mineral/iron supplement* [multiple vitamins & minerals; iron; folic acid; biotin] ⚕•18 mg•0.4 mg•45 μg

**Centrum Silver** tablets OTC *geriatric vitamin/mineral supplement* [multiple vitamins & minerals; folic acid; biotin] ⚕•400•30 μg

**Centura** ℞ *investigational treatment for multiple sclerosis* [monoclonal antibody IgG]

**Centurion A-Z** tablets (name changed to Multi-Vitamin Mineral with Beta-Carotene in 1995)

**Ceo-Two** suppository OTC *laxative* [sodium bicarbonate; potassium bitartrate]

**CEP (CCNU, etoposide, prednimustine)** *chemotherapy protocol*

**Cēpacol** mouthwash/gargle OTC *oral antiseptic* [cetylpyridinium chloride] 0.05%

**Cēpacol Anesthetic** troches OTC *topical oral anesthetic; antiseptic* [benzocaine; cetylpyridinium chloride] 10 mg•0.07%

**Cēpacol Throat** lozenges OTC *oral antiseptic* [cetylpyridinium chloride] 0.07%

**Cēpastat Sore Throat** lozenges OTC *topical antipruritic/counterirritant; mild local anesthetic* [phenol] 14.5, 29 mg ☑ Capastat

**cephacetrile sodium** USAN, USP *antibacterial* [also: cefacetrile]

**cephalexin** USAN, USP, BAN *bactericidal antibiotic* [also: cefalexin] ☑ cefazolin; cephalothin

**cephalexin HCl** USAN, USP *bactericidal antibiotic*

**cephalexin HCl monohydrate** *bactericidal antibiotic*

**cephalexin monohydrate** *bactericidal antibiotic* 250, 500, 1000 mg oral; 125, 250 mg/5 mL oral suspension

**cephaloglycin** USAN, USP, BAN *antibacterial* [also: cefaloglycin]

**cephalonium** BAN [also: cefalonium]

**cephaloram** BAN [also: cefaloram]

**cephaloridine** USAN, USP, BAN *antibacterial* [also: cefaloridine]

**cephalosporin N** [see: adicillin]

**cephalosporins** *a class of bactericidal antibiotics, divided into first-, second-, and third-generation cephalosporins*

**cephalothin** BAN *bactericidal antibiotic* [also: cephalothin sodium; cefalotin] ☑ cefazolin; cephalexin

**cephalothin sodium** USAN, USP *bactericidal antibiotic* [also: cefalotin; cephalothin] 1, 2 g/vial injection

**cephamandole** BAN *antibacterial* [also: cefamandole]

**cephamandole nafate** BAN *antibacterial* [also: cefamandole nafate]

**cephapirin sodium** USAN, USP *bactericidal antibiotic* [also: cefapirin] 0.5, 1, 2, 4, 20 g/vial injection ☑ cephradine

**cephazolin** BAN *systemic antibacterial* [also: cefazolin]

**cephazolin sodium** BAN *systemic antibacterial* [also: cefazolin sodium]

**cephoxazole** BAN [also: cefoxazole]

**cephradine** USAN, USP, BAN *bactericidal antibiotic* [also: cefradine] 250, 500 mg oral; 125, 250 mg/5 mL oral ☑ cephapirin

**Cephulac** syrup ℞ *prevent and treat portal-systemic encephalopathy* [lactulose] 10 g/15 mL

**Cepralan** ℞ *investigational antiarrhythmic* [cifenline]

**Ceprate SC** ℞ *investigational (Phase III) stem cell concentration/purification system for multiple myeloma and bone marrow transplants for breast cancer* [monoclonal antibodies]

**Ceptaz** powder for IV or IM injection ℞ *cephalosporin-type antibiotic* [ceftazidime pentahydrate] 1, 2, 10 g

**ceramide trihexosidase (CTH) & alpha-galactosidase A** *investigational (orphan) for Fabry's disease*

**ceranapril** *investigational once-daily ACE inhibitor for hypertension; investigational treatment for dementia*

**Cerebyx** IV or IM injection ℞ *hydantoin-type anticonvulsant; investigational (orphan) for grand mal status epilepticus* [fosphenytoin sodium (phenytoin sodium equivalent)] 75 (50) mg/mL

**CereCRIB** ℞ *investigational analgesic* [cellular implants]

**Ceredase** IV infusion ℞ *glucocerebrosidase enzyme replacement in Gaucher's disease type I (orphan); investigational*

*(orphan) for type II and III* [alglucerase] 10, 80 U/mL

**cerelose** [see: glucose]

**Cerespan** timed-release capsules (discontinued 1996) ℞ *peripheral vasodilator;smooth muscle relaxant for cerebral, myocardial, and peripheral ischemias* [papaverine HCl] 150 mg

**Cerestat** ℞ *investigational (Phase III) treatment for stroke and traumatic brain injury* [aptiganel HCl]

**Cerezyme** powder for IV infusion ℞ *enzyme replacement therapy for types I, II, and III Gaucher's disease (orphan)* [imiglucerase] 40 U/mL

**cerium** *element (Ce)*

**cerium oxalate** USP

**cerivastatin sodium** USAN *antihyperlipidemic; HMG-CoA reductase inhibitor*

**ceronapril** USAN, INN *antihypertensive*

**Cerose-DM** liquid OTC *antitussive; decongestant; antihistamine* [dextromethorphan hydrobromide; phenylephrine HCl; chlorpheniramine maleate; alcohol 2.4%] 15•10•4 mg/5 mL

**Cerovite; Cerovite Advanced Formula** tablets OTC *vitamin/mineral/iron supplement* [multiple vitamins & minerals; ferrous fumarate; folic acid; biotin] ±•18 mg•0.4 mg•30 μg

**Cerovite Jr.** tablets OTC *vitamin/mineral/iron supplement* [multiple vitamins & minerals; ferrous fumarate; folic acid; biotin] ±•18 mg•0.4 mg•45 μg

**Cerovite Senior** tablets OTC *geriatric vitamin/mineral supplement* [multiple vitamins and minerals; folic acid; biotin] ±•200•30 μg

**Certagen** film-coated tablets OTC *vitamin/mineral/iron supplement* [multiple vitamins & minerals; ferrous fumarate; folic acid; biotin] ±•18 mg•0.4 mg•30 μg

**Certagen** liquid OTC *vitamin/mineral/iron supplement* [multiple vitamins & minerals; iron; biotin; alcohol 6.6%] ±•9•0.3 mg

**Certagen Senior** tablets OTC *geriatric vitamin/mineral supplement* [multiple vitamins & minerals; folic acid; biotin] ±•200•30 μg

**CertaVite** tablets OTC *vitamin/mineral/iron supplement* [multiple vitamins & minerals; ferrous fumarate; folic acid; biotin] ±•18 mg•0.4 mg•30 μg

**Certa-Vite Golden** tablets OTC *geriatric vitamin/mineral supplement* [multiple vitamins & minerals; biotin] ±•30 μg

**Cerubidine** powder for IV injection (discontinued 1996) ℞ *antibiotic antineoplastic for multiple nonlymphocytic leukemias* [daunorubicin HCl] 20 mg

**ceruletide** USAN, INN, BAN *gastric secretory stimulant*

**ceruletide diethylamine** USAN *gastric secretory stimulant*

**Cerumenex** ear drops ℞ *agent to emulsify and disperse ear wax* [trolamine polypeptide oleate-condensate] 10%

**Cervene** injection ℞ *investigational treatment for stroke, benzodiazepine-induced hypotension, and opiate reversal* [nalmefene]

**Cervidil** vaginal insert ℞ *prostaglandin for cervical ripening at term* [dinoprostone] 10 mg

**cesium** *element (Cs)*

**cesium (131Cs) chloride** INN *radioactive agent* [also: cesium chloride Cs 131]

**cesium chloride Cs 131** USAN *radioactive agent* [also: cesium (131Cs) chloride]

**Ceta** liquid OTC *soap-free therapeutic skin cleanser*

**Ceta Plus** capsules ℞ *narcotic analgesic* [hydrocodone bitartrate; acetaminophen] 5•500 mg

**cetaben** INN *antihyperlipoproteinemic* [also: cetaben sodium]

**cetaben sodium** USAN *antihyperlipoproteinemic* [also: cetaben]

**Cetacaine** gel, liquid, ointment, aerosol ℞ *topical local anesthetic; antiseptic* [benzocaine; tetracaine HCl; butamben] 14%•2%•2%

**Cetacort** lotion ℞ *topical corticosteroid* [hydrocortisone] 0.25%, 0.5%

**cetalkonium** *antiseptic*

**cetalkonium chloride** USAN, INN, BAN *topical anti-infective*

**Cetamide** ophthalmic ointment ℞ *ophthalmic bacteriostatic* [sulfacetamide sodium] 10%

**cetamolol** INN *antiadrenergic (β-receptor)* [also: cetamolol HCl]

**cetamolol HCl** USAN *antiadrenergic (β-receptor)* [also: cetamolol]

**Cetaphil** cream, lotion OTC *soap-free therapeutic skin cleanser*

**Cetapred** ophthalmic ointment ℞ *ophthalmic topical corticosteroidal anti-inflammatory; bacteriostatic* [prednisolone acetate; sulfacetamide sodium] 0.25% • 10%

**cethexonium chloride** INN

**cetiedil** INN *peripheral vasodilator* [also: cetiedil citrate]

**cetiedil citrate** USAN *peripheral vasodilator; orphan status withdrawn 1993* [also: cetiedil]

**cetirizine** INN, BAN *antihistamine* [also: cetirizine HCl]

**cetirizine HCl** USAN *antihistamine* [also: cetirizine]

**cetobemidone** [see: ketobemidone]

**cetocycline** INN *antibacterial* [also: cetocycline HCl]

**cetocycline HCl** USAN *antibacterial* [also: cetocycline]

**cetofenicol** INN *antibacterial* [also: cetophenicol]

**cetohexazine** INN

**cetomacrogol 1000** INN, BAN

**cetophenicol** USAN *antibacterial* [also: cetofenicol]

**cetophenylbutazone** [see: kebuzone]

**cetostearyl alcohol** NF *emulsifying agent*

**cetotetrine HCl** [now: cetocycline HCl]

**cetotiamine** INN

**cetoxime** INN, BAN

**cetoxime HCl** [see: cetoxime]

**cetraxate** INN *GI antiulcerative* [also: cetraxate HCl]

**cetraxate HCl** USAN *GI antiulcerative* [also: cetraxate]

**cetrimide** INN, BAN

**cetrimonium bromide** INN *topical antiseptic* [also: cetrimonium chloride]

**cetrimonium chloride** BAN *topical antiseptic* [also: cetrimonium bromide]

**cetyl alcohol** NF *emulsifying and stiffening agent*

**cetyl esters wax** NF *stiffening agent*

**cetyldimethylbenzyl ammonium chloride** [see: cetalkonium chloride]

**cetylpyridinium chloride** USP, INN, BAN *topical antiseptic; preservative*

**cetyltrimethyl ammonium bromide**

**CEV (cyclophosphamide, etoposide, vincristine)** *chemotherapy protocol*

**Cevalin** IV, IM, or subcu injection ℞ *antiscorbutic* [ascorbic acid] 500 mg/mL

**Cevi-Bid** timed-release capsules OTC *vitamin supplement* [ascorbic acid] 500 mg

**Cevi-Fer** timed-release capsules ℞ *hematinic* [ferrous fumarate; ascorbic acid; folic acid] 20 • 300 • 1 mg

**Ce-Vi-Sol** drops OTC *vitamin supplement* [ascorbic acid; alcohol 5%] 35 mg/0.6 mL

**cevitamic acid** [see: ascorbic acid]

**cevitan** [see: ascorbic acid]

**ceylon gelatin** [see: agar]

**Cezin** capsules OTC *vitamin/mineral supplement* [multiple vitamins & minerals]

**Cezin-S** capsules ℞ *geriatric vitamin/mineral supplement* [multiple vitamins & minerals; folic acid] ± • 0.5 mg

**CF (carboplatin, fluorouracil)** *chemotherapy protocol*

**CF (cisplatin, fluorouracil)** *chemotherapy protocol*

**CFL (cisplatin, fluorouracil, leucovorin [rescue])** *chemotherapy protocol*

**CFM (cyclophosphamide, fluorouracil, mitoxantrone)** *chemotherapy protocol* [also: CNF; FNC]

**CFP (cyclophosphamide, fluorouracil, prednisone)** *chemotherapy protocol*

**CFPT (cyclophosphamide, fluorouracil, prednisone, tamoxifen)** *chemotherapy protocol*

**CFTR (cystic fibrosis transmembrane conductance regulator)** [q.v.]

**CG (Cardio-Green)** [q.v.]

**CG (chorionic gonadotropin)** [see: gonadotropin, chorionic]

**CGF (Control Gel Formula) dressing** [see: DuoDERM CGF]

**CGP 57701** ℞ *investigational penem antibiotic*

**CH1VPP; Ch1VPP (chlorambucil, vinblastine, procarbazine, prednisone)** *chemotherapy protocol*

**CHAD (cyclophosphamide, hexa-methylmelamine, Adriamycin, DDP)** *chemotherapy protocol*

**chalk** *street drug slang* [see: metham-phetamine HCl; amphetamines]

**chalk, precipitated** [see: calcium carbonate, precipitated]

**CHAMOCA (Cytoxan, hydroxy-urea, actinomycin D, methotrex-ate, Oncovin, calcium folinate, Adriamycin)** *chemotherapy protocol*

**champagne of drugs** *street drug slang* [see: cocaine HCl]

**chandoo; chandu** *street drug slang* [see: opium]

**CHAP (cyclophosphamide, Hexalen, Adriamycin, Platinol)** *chemotherapy protocol*

**CHAP (cyclophosphamide, hexa-methylmelamine, Adriamycin, Platinol)** *chemotherapy protocol*

**Chap Stick Medicated Lip Balm** stick, jar, squeezable tube OTC *counterirritant; moisturizer; protectant; emollient* [camphor; menthol; phenol] 1%•0.6%•0.5%

**charas** *street drug slang for marijuana from India* [see: marijuana]

**CharcoAid** oral suspension OTC *adsorbent antidote for poisoning* [activated charcoal] 15 g/120 mL, 30 g/150 mL

**CharcoAid 2000** oral liquid, granules OTC *adsorbent antidote for poisoning* [activated charcoal] 15 g/120 mL, 50 g/240 mL; 15 g

**charcoal** *gastric adsorbent/detoxicant; antiflatulent* 260 mg oral

**charcoal, activated** USP *general purpose antidote/adsorbent* 15, 30, 40, 120, 240 g, 208 mg/mL oral

**Charcoal Plus** enteric-coated tablets OTC *adsorbent; detoxicant* [activated charcoal] 200 mg

**CharcoCaps** capsules OTC *adsorbent; detoxicant; antiflatulent* [charcoal] 260 mg

**Chardonna-2** tablets ℞ *GI anticholinergic; sedative* [belladonna extract; phenobarbital] 15•15 mg

**charge** *street drug slang* [see: marijuana]

**Charley; Charlie** *street drug slang* [see: heroin; cocaine]

**chasing the dragon** *street drug slang for inhaling vapors of heroin or cocaine (powder or crack) heated on tinfoil* [see: heroin; cocaine; cocaine, crack]

**chasing the tiger** *street drug slang for smoking heroin* [see: heroin]

**chaulmosulfone** INN

**Chealamide** IV infusion ℞ *calcium-lowering agent; antiarrhythmic for digitalis toxicity* [edetate disodium] 150 mg/mL

**cheap basing** *street drug slang* [see: cocaine, crack]

**cheeba; cheeo** *street drug slang* [see: marijuana]

**chelafrin** [see: epinephrine]

**Chelated Magnesium** tablets OTC *magnesium supplement* [magnesium amino acid chelate] 500 mg

**Chelated Manganese** tablets OTC *manganese supplement* [manganese] 20, 50 mg

**chelating agents** *a class of agents that prevent bodily absorption and cause the excretion of substances such as heavy metals*

**chelen** [see: ethyl chloride]

**Chemet** capsules ℞ *heavy metal chelating agent for lead poisoning (orphan); investigational (orphan) for cystine kidney stones and mercury poisoning* [succimer] 100 mg

**chemical** *street drug slang* [see: cocaine, crack]

**Chemo-Pin** (trademarked form) *chemical-dispensing pin*

**Chemstrip 2 GP; Chemstrip 2 LN; Chemstrip 4 the OB; Chemstrip 6; Chemstrip 7; Chemstrip 8; Chemstrip 9; Chemstrip 10 with SG; Chemstrip uGK** reagent strips *in vitro diagnostic aid for multiple urine products*

**Chemstrip bG** reagent strips for home use OTC *in vitro diagnostic aid for blood glucose*

**Chemstrip K** reagent strips for professional use *in vitro diagnostic aid for acetone (ketones) in the urine*

**Chemstrip Micral** reagent strips for professional use *in vitro diagnostic aid for albumin (protein) in the urine*

**Chemstrip uG** reagent strips for home use OTC *in vitro diagnostic aid for urine glucose*

**chenic acid** [now: chenodiol]

**Chenix** tablets (discontinued 1994) ℞ *anticholelithogenic for radiolucent gallstones (orphan)* [chenodiol] 250 mg

**chenodeoxycholic acid** INN, BAN *anticholelithogenic* [also: chenodiol]

**chenodiol** USAN *anticholelithogenic for radiolucent gallstones (orphan)* [also: chenodeoxycholic acid]

**Cheracol Cough** syrup ℞ *narcotic antitussive; expectorant* [codeine phosphate; guaifenesin; alcohol 1.75%] 10•100 mg/5 mL

**Cheracol D Cough** liquid OTC *antitussive; expectorant* [dextromethorphan hydrobromide; guaifenesin; alcohol 4.75%] 10•100 mg/5 mL

**Cheracol Nasal** spray OTC *nasal decongestant* [oxymetazoline HCl] 0.05%

**Cheracol Plus** liquid OTC *antitussive; decongestant; antihistamine* [dextromethorphan hydrobromide; phenylpropanolamine HCl; chlorpheniramine maleate; alcohol 8%] 6.7•8.3•1.3 mg/5 mL

**Cheracol Sinus** sustained-action tablets (discontinued 1995) OTC *decongestant; antihistamine* [pseudoephedrine sulfate; dexbrompheniramine maleate] 120•6 mg

**Cheracol Sore Throat** spray OTC *topical antipruritic/counterirritant; mild local anesthetic* [phenol] 1.4%

**Cheralin Expectorant** liquid (discontinued 1994) OTC *expectorant* [potassium guaiacolsulfonate; ammonium chloride; antimony potassium tartrate; alcohol]

**Cheralin with Codeine** liquid (discontinued 1994) ℞ *narcotic antitussive; expectorant* [codeine phosphate; potassium guaiacolsulfonate; ammonium chloride; antimony potassium tartrate]

**Cherapas** tablets (discontinued 1993) ℞ *antihypertensive* [hydrochlorothiazide; reserpine; hydralazine HCl]

**cheroot** *street drug slang for a tobacco and/or marijuana cigar* [see: tobacco; marijuana]

**cherry juice** NF

**cherry menth** *street drug slang* [see: GHB]

**Chewable C** chewable tablets OTC *vitamin supplement* [sodium ascorbate & ascorbic acid] 100, 250, 300, 500 mg

**Chewable Multivitamins with Fluoride** tablets ℞ *pediatric vitamin supplement and dental caries preventative* [multiple vitamins; fluoride; folic acid] ±•1•0.3 mg

**Chewable Triple Vitamins with Fluoride** tablets ℞ *pediatric vitamin supplement and dental caries preventative* [vitamins A, C, and D; fluoride] 2500 IU•60 mg•400 IU•1 mg

**chewies** *street drug slang* [see: cocaine, crack]

**Chew-Vites** chewable tablets OTC *vitamin supplement* [multiple vitamins; folic acid]

**ChexUP; Chex-Up; CHEX-UP (cyclophosphamide, hexamethylmelamine, fluorouracil, Platinol)** *chemotherapy protocol*

**CHF (cyclophosphamide, hexamethylmelamine, fluorouracil)** *chemotherapy protocol*

**chiba chiba** *street drug slang for high-potency marijuana from Colombia* [see: marijuana]

**Chibroxin** Ocumeter (eye drops) ℞ *ophthalmic antibiotic* [norfloxacin] 3 mg/mL

**Chicago black; Chicago green** *street drug slang* [see: marijuana]

**chick** *street drug slang* [see: heroin]

**chicken powder** *street drug slang* [see: amphetamines]

**chicle** *street drug slang* [see: heroin]

**chief** *street drug slang* [see: LSD; mescaline]

**chieva** *street drug slang* [see: heroin]

**Chiggerex** ointment OTC *topical local anesthetic; counterirritant* [benzocaine; camphor; menthol] ≜

**Chigger-Tox** liquid OTC *topical local anesthetic* [benzocaine] ≟

**Children's Formula Cough** syrup OTC *pediatric antitussive and expectorant* [dextromethorphan hydrobromide; guaifenesin] 5•50 mg/5 mL

**chillifolinum** [see: quillifoline]

**chimeric (murine variable, human constant) MAb (C2B8) to CD20** [now: rituximab]

**chimeric A2 (human-murine) IgG monoclonal anti-TNF antibody (cA2)** *investigational (orphan) for Crohn's disease*

**chimeric L6 monoclonal antibodies** *investigational chemotherapy rescue agent*

**chimeric M-T412 (human-murine) IgG monoclonal anti-CD4** *orphan status withdrawn 1997* [now: priliximab]

**China cat** *street drug slang for high-potency heroin* [see: heroin]

**China girl; China town** *street drug slang* [see: fentanyl (citrate)]

**China white** *street drug slang for very pure heroin, fentanyl, or a fentanyl analog used as a heroin substitute* [see: heroin; fentanyl (citrate)]

**Chinese gelatin** [see: agar]

**Chinese isinglass** [see: chiniofon]

**Chinese molasses** *street drug slang* [see: opium]

**Chinese red** *street drug slang* [see: heroin]

**Chinese tobacco** *street drug slang* [see: opium]

**chinethazone** [see: quinethazone]

**chiniofon** NF, INN

**chip** *street drug slang* [see: heroin]

**chippy** *street drug slang* [see: cocaine]

**chips** *street drug slang for tobacco or marijuana cigarettes laced with PCP* [see: tobacco; marijuana; PCP]

**chira** *street drug slang* [see: marijuana]

**chitosan** [see: poliglusam]

**CHL + PRED (chlorambucil, prednisone)** *chemotherapy protocol*

**Chlamydiazyme** reagent kit for professional use *in vitro diagnostic aid for* Chlamydia trachomatis [solid phase enzyme immunoassay]

**Chlo-Amine** chewable tablets ℞ *antihistamine* [chlorpheniramine maleate] 2 mg

**chlophedianol** BAN *antitussive* [also: chlophedianol HCl; clofedanol]

**chlophedianol HCl** USAN *antitussive* [also: clofedanol; chlophedianol]

**chlophenadione** [see: clorindione]

**chloquinate** [see: cloquinate]

**Chlor-100** injection ℞ *antihistamine; anaphylaxis* [chlorpheniramine maleate] 100 mg/mL

**chloracyzine** INN

**Chlorafed** liquid OTC *decongestant; antihistamine* [pseudoephedrine HCl; chlorpheniramine maleate] 30•2 mg/5 mL

**Chlorafed; Chlorafed HS** Timecelles (sustained-release capsules) ℞ *decongestant; antihistamine* [pseudoephedrine HCl; chlorpheniramine maleate] 120•8 mg; 60•4 mg

**chloral betaine** USAN, NF, BAN *sedative* [also: cloral betaine]

**chloral hydrate** USP, BAN *hypnotic; sedative; also abused as a street drug* 500 mg oral; 250, 500 mg/5 mL oral

**chloral hydrate betaine** [see: chloral betaine]

**chloralformamide** USP

**chloralodol** INN [also: chlorhexadol]

**chloralose (α-chloralose)** INN

**chloralurethane** [see: carbocloral]

**chlorambucil** USP, INN, BAN *nitrogen mustard-type alkylating antineoplastic for multiple leukemias and lymphomas*

**chloramidobenzol** [see: clofenamide]

**chloramine** [now: chloramine-T]

**chloramine-T** NF [also: tosylchloramide sodium]

**chloramiphene** [see: clomiphene citrate]

**chloramphenicol** USP, INN, BAN, JAN *bacteriostatic antibiotic; antirickettsial* 250 mg oral; 5 mg/mL eye drops; 10 mg/g topical

**chloramphenicol palmitate** USP, JAN *antibacterial; antirickettsial* 150 mg/5 mL oral

**chloramphenicol pantothenate complex** USAN *antibacterial; antirick-*

*ettsial* [also: cloramfenicol pantotenate complex]

**chloramphenicol sodium succinate**
USP, JAN *antibacterial; antirickettsial*
100 mg/mL injection

**chloranautine** [see: dimenhydrinate]

**chlorarsen** [see: dichlorophenarsine
HCl]

**Chloraseptic** lozenges, throat spray
(discontinued 1994) OTC *topical anti-
pruritic/counterirritant; mild local anesthetic* [phenol] 32.5 mg; 1.4%

**Chloraseptic** mouthwash/gargle OTC
*topical antipruritic/counterirritant; mild
local anesthetic* [phenol] 1.4%

**Chloraseptic, Children's** lozenges
OTC *topical oral anesthetic* [benzo-
caine] 5 mg

**Chloraseptic, Children's** throat spray
OTC *topical antipruritic/counterirritant;
mild local anesthetic* [phenol] 0.5%

**Chloraseptic Sore Throat** lozenges
OTC *topical oral anesthetic; antipruritic/
counterirritant* [benzocaine; menthol]
6•10 mg

**Chlorate** tablets OTC *antihistamine*
[chlorpheniramine maleate] 4 mg

**chlorazanil** INN

**chlorazanil HCl** [see: chlorazanil]

**chlorazodin** INN [also: chloroazodin]

**chlorazone** [see: chloramine-T]

**chlorbenzoxamine** INN

**chlorbenzoxamine HCl** [see: chlor-
benzoxamine]

**chlorbetamide** INN, BAN

**chlorbutanol** [see: chlorobutanol]

**chlorbutin** [see: chlorambucil]

**chlorbutol** BAN *antimicrobial agent*
[also: chlorobutanol]

**chlorcinnazine** [see: clocinizine]

**chlorcyclizine** INN, BAN *antihistamine*
[also: chlorcyclizine HCl]

**chlorcyclizine HCl** USP *antihistamine*
[also: chlorcyclizine]

**chlordantoin** USAN, BAN *antifungal*
[also: clodantoin]

**chlordiazepoxide** USP, INN, BAN *anxiolytic; minor tranquilizer; alcohol
withdrawal therapy*

**chlordiazepoxide HCl** USAN, USP, BAN
*sedative; anxiolytic; sometimes abused
as a street drug* 5, 10, 25 mg oral

**chlordimorine** INN

**Chlordrine S.R.** sustained-release
capsules Ᵽ *decongestant; antihistamine* [pseudoephedrine HCl; chlorpheniramine maleate] 120•8 mg

**Chloresium** ointment, solution OTC
*vulnerary and deodorant for wounds,
burns, and ulcers* [chlorophyllin copper complex] 0.5%; 0.2%

**Chloresium** tablets OTC *systemic
deodorant for ostomy, breath, and body
odors* [chlorophyllin copper com-
plex] 14 mg

**chlorethate** [see: clorethate]

**chlorethyl** [see: ethyl chloride]

**chlorfenisate** [see: clofibrate]

**chlorfenvinphos** BAN [also: clofen-
vinfos]

**Chlorgest-HD** liquid (discontinued
1997) Ᵽ *narcotic antitussive; decongestant; antihistamine* [hydrocodone
bitartrate; phenylephrine HCl;
chlorpheniramine maleate] 1.67•5•
4 mg/5 mL

**chlorguanide HCl** [see: chloroguanide HCl]

**chlorhexadol** BAN [also: chloralodol]

**chlorhexidine** INN, BAN *antimicrobial*
[also: chlorhexidine gluconate]

**chlorhexidine gluconate** USAN *antimicrobial; investigational (orphan) for
oral mucositis in bone marrow transplant patients* [also: chlorhexidine]

**chlorhexidine HCl** USAN, BAN *topical
anti-infective*

**chlorhexidine phosphanilate** USAN
*antibacterial*

**chlorimiphenin** [see: imiclopazine]

**chlorimpiphenine** [see: imiclopazine]

**chlorinated & iodized peanut oil**
[see: chloriodized oil]

**chlorindanol** USAN *spermicide* [also:
clorindanol]

**chlorine** *element (Cl)*

**chloriodized oil** USP

**chlorisondamine chloride** INN, BAN

**chlorisondamone chloride** [see:
chlorisondamine chloride]

**chlormadinone** INN, BAN *progestin*
[also: chlormadinone acetate]

**chlormadinone acetate** USAN, NF
*progestin* [also: chlormadinone]

**chlormerodrin** NF, INN, BAN

**chlormerodrin (¹⁹⁷Hg)** INN *renal function test; radioactive agent* [also: chlormerodrin Hg 197]

**chlormerodrin Hg 197** USAN, USP *renal function test; radioactive agent* [also: chlormerodrin (¹⁹⁷Hg)]

**chlormerodrin Hg 203** USAN, USP *renal function test; radioactive agent*

**chlormeroprin** [see: chlormerodrin]

**chlormethazanone** [see: chlormezanone]

**chlormethiazole** BAN [also: clomethiazole]

**chlormethine** INN *nitrogen mustard-type alkylating antineoplastic* [also: mechlorethamine HCl; mustine; nitrogen mustard N-oxide HCl]

**chlormethylencycline** [see: clomocycline]

**chlormezanone** INN, BAN *mild anxiolytic*

**chlormidazole** INN, BAN

**chlornaphazine** INN

**chloroacetic acid** [see: monochloroacetic, dichloroacetic, or trichloroacetic acid]

**chloroazodin** USP [also: chlorazodin]

**5-chlorobenzoxazolinone** [see: chlorzoxazone]

**chlorobutanol** NF, INN *antimicrobial agent; preservative* [also: chlorbutol]

**8-chlorocamp** *investigational antineoplastic*

**chlorochine** [see: chloroquine]

**chlorocresol** USAN, NF, INN *antiseptic; disinfectant*

**2-chloro-2′-deoxyadenosine (CdA)** [now: cladribine]

**chlorodeoxylincomycin** [see: clindamycin]

**chloroethane** [see: ethyl chloride]

**chloroform** NF *solvent*

**chloroguanide HCl** USP [also: proguanil]

**chloroguanide triazine pamoate** [see: cycloguanil pamoate]

**chloro-iodohydroxyquinoline** [see: clioquinol]

**chlorolincomycin** [see: clindamycin]

**chloromethapyrilene citrate** [see: chlorothen citrate]

**Chloromycetin** cream (discontinued 1994) ℞ *broad-spectrum topical antibiotic* [chloramphenicol] 1%

**Chloromycetin** Kapseals (capsules) (discontinued 1996) ℞ *broad-spectrum bacteriostatic antibiotic* [chloramphenicol] 250 mg

**Chloromycetin** powder for eye drops, ophthalmic ointment ℞ *ophthalmic antibiotic* [chloramphenicol] 25 mg/15 mL; 10 mg/g

**Chloromycetin Hydrocortisone** powder for eye drops ℞ *ophthalmic topical corticosteroidal anti-inflammatory; broad-spectrum antibiotic* [hydrocortisone acetate; chloramphenicol] 0.5%•0.25%

**Chloromycetin Otic** ear drops ℞ *broad-spectrum antibiotic* [chloramphenicol] 0.5%

**Chloromycetin Palmitate** oral suspension (discontinued 1994) ℞ *broad-spectrum bacteriostatic antibiotic* [chloramphenicol palmitate] 150 mg/5 mL

**Chloromycetin Sodium Succinate** powder for IV injection ℞ *broad-spectrum bacteriostatic antibiotic* [chloramphenicol sodium succinate] 100 mg/mL

**p-chlorophenol** [see: parachlorophenol]

**chlorophenothane** NF [also: clofenotane; dicophane]

**chlorophenoxamide** [see: clefamide]

**chlorophenylmercury** [see: phenylmercuric chloride]

**chlorophyll, water soluble** [see: chlorophyllin]

**chlorophyllin** *vulnerary; deodorant for wounds and ulcers (topical); for ostomy, breath, and body odors (oral)* 20 mg oral

**chlorophyllin copper complex** USAN *deodorant for wounds and ulcers (topical); for ostomy, breath, and body odors (oral)*

**chloroprednisone** INN

**chloroprednisone acetate** [see: chloroprednisone]

**chloroprocaine** INN *local anesthetic* [also: chloroprocaine HCl]

**chloroprocaine HCl** USP *injectable local anesthetic* [also: chloroprocaine]

**Chloroptic** eye drops ℞ *ophthalmic antibiotic* [chloramphenicol] 5 mg/mL

**Chloroptic S.O.P.** ophthalmic ointment ℞ *ophthalmic antibiotic* [chloramphenicol] 10 mg/g

**chloropyramine** INN [also: halopyramine]

**chloropyrilene** INN, BAN [also: chlorothen citrate]

**chloroquine** USP, INN, BAN *antiamebic; antimalarial*

**chloroquine diphosphate** [see: chloroquine phosphate]

**chloroquine HCl** USP *amebicide; antimalarial* [also: chloroquine]

**chloroquine phosphate** USP, BAN *antimalarial; amebicide; lupus erythematosus suppressant* 250 mg oral

**chloroserpidine** INN

**Chloroserpine** tablets (discontinued 1995) ℞ *antihypertensive* [chlorothiazide; reserpine] 250•0.125 mg

**N-chlorosuccinimide** [see: succinchlorimide]

**chlorothen citrate** NF [also: chloropyrilene]

**chlorothenium citrate** [see: chlorothen citrate]

**chlorothenylpyramine** [see: chlorothen]

**chlorothiazide** USP, INN, BAN *diuretic; antihypertensive* 250, 500 mg oral

**chlorothiazide sodium** USAN, USP *diuretic; antihypertensive*

**chlorothymol** NF

**chlorotrianisene** USP, INN, BAN *estrogen for hormone replacement therapy or inoperable prostatic cancer*

**chloroxine** USAN *antiseborrheic*

**chloroxylenol** USP, INN, BAN *bacteriostatic*

**chlorozone** [see: chloramine-T]

**chlorpenthixol** [see: clopenthixol]

**Chlorphed-LA** nasal spray OTC *nasal decongestant* [oxymetazoline HCl] 0.05%

**Chlorphedrine SR** sustained-release capsules ℞ *decongestant; antihistamine* [pseudoephedrine HCl; chlorpheniramine maleate] 120•8 mg

**chlorphenamine** INN *antihistamine* [also: chlorpheniramine maleate; chlorpheniramine]

**chlorphenamine maleate** [see: chlorpheniramine maleate]

**chlorphenecyclane** [see: clofenciclan]

**chlorphenesin** INN, BAN *skeletal muscle relaxant* [also: chlorphenesin carbamate]

**chlorphenesin carbamate** USAN, JAN *skeletal muscle relaxant* [also: chlorphenesin]

**chlorphenindione** [see: clorindione]

**chlorpheniramine** BAN *antihistamine* [also: chlorpheniramine maleate; chlorphenamine] ⓔ chlorphentermine

**chlorpheniramine maleate** USP *antihistamine* [also: chlorphenamine; chlorpheniramine] 4, 8, 12 mg oral; 2 mg/5 mL oral; 100 mg/mL injection

**chlorpheniramine polistirex** USAN *antihistamine*

**chlorpheniramine tannate, pyrilamine tannate, and phenylephrine tannate** *antihistamine; decongestant* 8•25•25 mg oral

**chlorphenoctium amsonate** INN, BAN

**chlorphenotane** [see: chlorophenothane]

**chlorphenoxamine** INN, BAN [also: chlorphenoxamine HCl]

**chlorphenoxamine HCl** USP [also: chlorphenoxamine]

**chlorphentermine** INN, BAN *anorectic* [also: chlorphentermine HCl] ⓔ chlorpheniramine

**chlorphentermine HCl** USAN *anorectic* [also: chlorphentermine]

**chlorphenylindandione** [see: clorindione]

**chlorphthalidone** [see: chlorthalidone]

**Chlor-Pro** injection ℞ *antihistamine* [chlorpheniramine maleate] 10, 100 mg/mL

**chlorprocaine chloride** [see: chloroprocaine HCl]

**chlorproethazine** INN [also: chlorproethazine HCl]

**chlorproethazine HCl** [also: chlorproethazine]

**chlorproguanil** INN, BAN

**chlorproguanil HCl** [see: chlorproguanil]

**chlorpromazine** USP, INN, BAN *antiemetic; antipsychotic; antidopaminergic; intractable hiccough relief*

**chlorpromazine HCl** USP, BAN *antiemetic; antipsychotic; intractable hiccough relief* 10, 25, 50, 100, 200 mg oral; 10 mg/5 mL oral; 30, 100 mg/mL oral; 25 mg/mL injection

**chlorpropamide** USP, INN, BAN *sulfonylurea-type antidiabetic* 100, 250 mg oral

**chlorprophenpyridamine maleate** [see: chlorpheniramine maleate]

**chlorprothixene** USAN, USP, INN, BAN *antipsychotic*

**chlorprothixene HCl** *antipsychotic*

**chlorprothixene lactate** *antipsychotic*

**chlorpyrifos** BAN

**chlorquinaldol** INN, BAN

**Chlor-Rest** tablets OTC *decongestant; antihistamine* [phenylpropanolamine HCl; chlorpheniramine maleate] 18.7•2 mg

**Chlorspan-12** timed-release capsules ℞ *antihistamine* [chlorpheniramine maleate] 12 mg

**Chlortab-4** tablets (discontinued 1996) ℞ *antihistamine* [chlorpheniramine maleate] 4 mg

**Chlortab-8** timed-release tablets (discontinued 1996) ℞ *antihistamine* [chlorpheniramine maleate] 8 mg

**chlortalidone** INN *diuretic* [also: chlorthalidone]

**chlortetracycline** INN, BAN *antibacterial antibiotic; antiprotozoal* [also: chlortetracycline bisulfate]

**chlortetracycline bisulfate** USP *antibacterial; antiprotozoal* [also: chlortetracycline]

**chlortetracycline calcium**

**chlortetracycline HCl** USP, BAN *antibacterial antibiotic; antiprotozoal*

**chlorthalidone** USAN, USP, BAN *diuretic; antihypertensive* [also: chlortalidone] 25, 50, 100 mg oral

**chlorthenoxazin** BAN [also: chlorthenoxazine]

**chlorthenoxazine** INN [also: chlorthenoxazin]

**chlorthiazide** [see: chlorothiazide]

**chlortrianisestrol** [see: chlorotrianisene]

**Chlor-Trimeton** IV injection (discontinued 1997) OTC *antihistamine for anaphylaxis* [chlorpheniramine maleate] 10 mg/mL

**Chlor-Trimeton** Repetabs (repeataction tablets) (name changed to Chlor-Trimeton 12 Hour Allergy in 1993)

**Chlor-Trimeton** tablets, syrup OTC *antihistamine* [chlorpheniramine maleate] 4 mg; 2 mg/5 mL

**Chlor-Trimeton 4 Hour Relief** tablets OTC *decongestant; antihistamine* [pseudoephedrine sulfate; chlorpheniramine maleate] 60•4 mg

**Chlor-Trimeton 8 Hour Allergy; Chlor-Trimeton 12 Hour Allergy** timed-release tablets OTC *antihistamine* [chlorpheniramine maleate] 8 mg; 12 mg

**Chlor-Trimeton 12 Hour Relief** sustained-release tablets OTC *decongestant; antihistamine* [pseudoephedrine sulfate; chlorpheniramine maleate] 120•8 mg

**Chlor-Trimeton Allergy** tablets OTC *antihistamine* [chlorpheniramine maleate] 4 mg

**Chlor-Trimeton Allergy-Sinus** caplets OTC *decongestant; antihistamine; analgesic* [phenylpropanolamine HCl; chlorpheniramine maleate; acetaminophen] 12.5•2•500 mg

**Chlor-Trimeton Sinus** caplets (name changed to Chlor-Trimeton Allergy-Sinus in 1993)

**chlorzoxazone** USP, INN, BAN, JAN *skeletal muscle relaxant* 250, 500 mg oral

**chlosudimeprimylum** [see: clopamide]

**ChlVPP (chlorambucil, vinblastine, procarbazine, prednisone)** *chemotherapy protocol*

**ChlVPP/EVA (chlorambucil, vinblastine, procarbazine, prednisone, etoposide, vincristine, Adriamycin)** *chemotherapy protocol*

**CHO (cyclophosphamide, hydroxydaunomycin, Oncovin)** *chemotherapy protocol*

**CHO cells, recombinant** [see: CD4, human truncated]

**CHOB (cyclophosphamide, hydroxydaunomycin, Oncovin, bleomycin)** *chemotherapy protocol*

**chocolate** *street drug slang* [see: hashish; opium; amphetamines]

**chocolate chips** *street drug slang* [see: LSD]

**chocolate ecstasy** *street drug slang for crack made brown by adding chocolate milk powder during production* [see: cocaine, crack]

**CHOD (cyclophosphamide, hydroxydaunomycin, Oncovin, dexamethasone)** *chemotherapy protocol*

**Choice dm** oral liquid OTC *enteral nutritional therapy for abnormal glucose tolerance* [lactose-free formula] 240 mL

**Cholac** syrup ℞ *prevent and treat portal-systemic encephalopathy* [lactulose] 10 g/15 mL

**cholalic acid** [see: dehydrocholic acid]

**Cholan-HMB** tablets OTC *laxative; hydrocholeretic* [dehydrocholic acid] 250 mg

**Cholebrine** tablets ℞ *oral cholecystographic radiopaque agent* [iocetamic acid] 750 mg

**cholecalciferol** USP, BAN, JAN *vitamin $D_3$; antirachitic* [also: colecalciferol] 1000 IU oral

**Choledyl** tablets, pediatric syrup, elixir (discontinued 1996) ℞ *bronchodilator* [oxtriphylline] 100, 200 mg; 50 mg/5 mL; 100 mg/5 mL

**Choledyl SA** sustained-action tablets ℞ *bronchodilator* [oxtriphylline] 400, 600 mg

**cholera vaccine** USP *active bacterin for cholera (Vibrio cholerae)* 16 U/mL SC or IM injection

**cholesterin** [see: cholesterol]

**cholesterol** NF *emulsifying agent*

**cholestrin** [see: cholesterol]

**cholestyramine** BAN *bile salts ion-exchange resin; antihyperlipoproteinemic* [also: cholestyramine resin; colestyramine]

**cholestyramine resin** USP *bile salts ion-exchange resin; antihyperlipopro-*

*teinemic* [also: colestyramine; cholestyramine] 4 g powder for oral solution

**cholic acid** [see: dehydrocholic acid]

**Cholidase** tablets OTC *dietary lipotropic with vitamin supplementation* [choline; inositol; vitamins $B_6$, $B_{12}$, and E] 185•150•2.5•0.005•7.5 mg

**choline** *dietary lipotropic supplement* 250, 300, 500, 650 mg oral

**choline alfoscerate** INN

**choline bitartrate** NF 250 mg oral

**choline bromide hexamethylenedicarbamate** [see: hexacarbacholine bromide]

**choline chloride** INN *investigational (orphan) for choline deficiency of long-term parenteral nutrition*

**choline chloride acetate** [see: acetylcholine chloride]

**choline chloride carbamate** [see: carbachol]

**choline chloride succinate** [see: succinylcholine chloride]

**choline dihydrogen citrate** NF 650 mg oral

**choline gluconate** INN

**choline glycerophosphate** [see: choline alfoscerate]

**choline magnesium trisalicylate (choline salicylate + magnesium salicylate)** [q.v.] 500, 750, 1000 mg (293•362, 440•544, 587•725 mg) oral

**choline perchlorate, nitrate ester** [see: nitricholine perchlorate]

**choline salicylate** USAN, INN, BAN *analgesic; antipyretic; anti-inflammatory; antirheumatic*

**choline theophyllinate** INN, BAN *bronchodilator* [also: oxtriphylline]

**cholinergic agonists** *a class of agents that produce effects similar to those of the parasympathetic nervous system* [also called: parasympathomimetics]

**cholinesterase inhibitors** *a class of drugs which increase acetylcholine neurotransmitters, used as a cognition adjuvant in Alzheimer's dementia* [also called: acetylcholinesterase (AChE) inhibitors]

**Cholinoid** capsules OTC *dietary lipo-tropic with vitamin supplementation* [choline; inositol; multiple B vitamins; vitamin C; lemon bioflavonoids] 111•111•±•100•100 mg

**cholly** *street drug slang* [see: cocaine]

**Cholografin Meglumine** injection ℞ *parenteral cholecystographic and cholangiographic radiopaque agent* [iodipamide meglumine] 10.3%, 52%

**Choloxin** tablets ℞ *cholesterol-lowering antihyperlipidemic* [dextrothyroxine sodium] 2, 4 mg

**Cholybar** resin bar (discontinued 1994) ℞ *cholesterol-lowering antihyperlipidemic* [cholestyramine resin] 4 g

**chondodendron tomentosum** [see: tubocurarine chloride]

**chondroitin 4-sulfate** [see: danaparoid sodium]

**chondroitin 6-sulfate** [see: danaparoid sodium]

**chondroitin sulfate sodium** JAN

**chondroitinase** *investigational (orphan) for vitrectomy*

**Chooz** chewable tablets OTC *antacid* [calcium carbonate] 500 mg

**CHOP (cyclophosphamide, hydroxydaunomycin, Oncovin, prednisone)** *chemotherapy protocol*

**CHOP-BLEO (cyclophosphamide, hydroxydaunomycin, Oncovin, prednisone, bleomycin)** *chemotherapy protocol*

**CHOPE (cyclophosphamide, hydroxydaunomycin, Oncovin, prednisone, etoposide)** *chemotherapy protocol*

**CHOR (cyclophosphamide, hydroxydaunomycin, Oncovin, radiation therapy)** *chemotherapy protocol*

**chorals** *street drug slang for various CNS depressants*

**Chorex-5; Chorex-10** powder for IM injection ℞ *hormone for prepubertal cryptorchidism and hypogonadism; ovulation stimulant* [chorionic gonadotropin] 500 U/mL; 1000 U/mL

**Chorigon** powder for injection (discontinued 1995) ℞ *hormone for prepubertal cryptorchidism and hypogo-*
*nadism* [chorionic gonadotropin] 1000 U/mL

**chorionic gonadotrophin** [see: gonadotropin, chorionic]

**chorionic gonadotropin (CG)** [see: gonadotropin, chorionic]

**Choron-10** powder for IM injection ℞ *hormone for prepubertal cryptorchidism and hypogonadism; ovulation stimulant* [chorionic gonadotropin] 1000 U/mL

**CHP (chlorhexidine phosphanilate)** [q.v.]

**Chris; cris; Christina; Cristina** *street drug slang* [see: methamphetamine HCl]

**Christmas factor** [see: factor IX complex]

**Christmas rolls** *street drug slang for various CNS depressants*

**Christmas tree** *street drug slang for marijuana, various CNS depressants, or amphetamines* [see: marijuana; amphetamines]

**Christmas trees** *street drug slang for Dexamyl (dextroamphetamine sulfate + amobarbital; discontinued 1980) in green and clear capsules* [see: dextroamphetamine sulfate; amobarbital; amphetamines]

**Christy; Cristy** *street drug slang for smokable methamphetamine* [see: methamphetamine HCl]

**Chromagen** capsules ℞ *hematinic* [ferrous fumarate; cyanocobalamin; ascorbic acid; intrinsic factor concentrate] 66 mg•10 μg•250 mg•100 mg

**Chroma-Pak** IV injection ℞ *intravenous nutritional therapy* [chromic chloride hexahydrate] 20.5, 102.5 μg/mL

**chromargyre** [see: merbromin]

**chromated albumin** [see: albumin, chromated Cr 51 serum]

**Chromelin Complexion Blender** OTC *skin darkening agent for vitiligo and hypopigmented areas* [dihydroxyacetone] 5%

**chromic acid, disodium salt** [see: sodium chromate Cr 51]

**chromic chloride** USP *dietary chromium supplement* 4, 20 μg/mL injection

**chromic chloride Cr 51** USAN *radioactive agent*

**chromic chloride hexahydrate** [see: chromic chloride]

**chromic phosphate Cr 51** USAN *radioactive agent*

**chromic phosphate P 32** USAN, USP *antineoplastic; radioactive agent*

**chromium** *element (Cr)*

**Chromium Chloride** IV injection ℞ *intravenous nutritional therapy* [chromic chloride hexahydrate] 4 µg/mL

**chromium chloride** [see: chromic chloride Cr 51]

**chromium chloride hexahydrate** [see: chromic chloride]

**chromocarb** INN

**chromonar HCl** USAN *coronary vasodilator* [also: carbocromen]

**chronic** *street drug slang for marijuana or marijuana mixed with crack* [see: marijuana; cocaine, crack]

**Chronosule** (trademarked dosage form) *sustained-action capsule*

**Chronotab** (trademarked dosage form) *sustained-action tablet*

**Chronulac** syrup ℞ *laxative* [lactulose] 10 g/15 mL

**chrysazin** (*withdrawn from market by FDA*) [see: danthron]

**churus** *street drug slang* [see: marijuana]

**CHVP (cyclophosphamide, hydroxydaunomycin, VM-26, prednisone)** *chemotherapy protocol*

**Chymex** solution ℞ *in vivo pancreatic function test* [bentiromide] 500 mg/7.5 mL

**Chymodiactin** powder for intradiscal injection ℞ *enzyme for herniated nucleus pulposus* [chymopapain] 4 nKat

**chymopapain** USAN, INN, BAN *proteolytic enzyme for herniated lumbar discs*

**chymotrypsin** USP, INN, BAN *proteolytic enzyme; zonulolytic for intracapsular lens extraction*

**C.I. acid orange 24 monosodium salt (color index)** [see: resorcin brown]

**C.I. basic violet 3 (color index)** [see: gentian violet]

**C.I. basic violet 14 monohydrochloride (color index)** [see: fuchsin, basic]

**C.I. direct blue 53 tetrasodium salt (color index)** [see: Evans blue]

**C.I. mordant yellow 5, disodium salt (color index)** [see: olsalazine sodium]

**CI-980** *investigational antineoplastic mitotic inhibitor*

**CI-988** *investigational cholecystokinin-B receptor antagonist for obsessive-compulsive disorders (OCD)*

**CI-1020** *investigational antiviral for HIV*

**ciadox** INN

**ciamexon** INN, BAN

**cianergoline** INN

**cianidanol** INN

**cianidol** [see: cianidanol]

**cianopramine** INN

**ciapilome** INN

**Ciba Vision Cleaner for Sensitive Eyes** solution OTC *surfactant cleaning solution for soft contact lenses*

**Ciba Vision Saline** aerosol solution OTC *rinsing/storage solution for soft contact lenses* [preservative-free saline solution]

**Cibacalcin** subcu or IM injection (discontinued 1996) ℞ *calcium regulator for Paget's disease (osteitis deformans) (orphan)* [calcitonin (human)] 0.5 mg/vial

**Cibadrex** ℞ *investigational antihypertensive*

**Cibalith-S** syrup (discontinued 1994) ℞ *antipsychotic/antimanic* [lithium citrate] 8 mEq/5 mL

**CIBAs** *street drug slang for Doriden (glutethimide; discontinued 1990)* [see: glutethimide]

**cibenzoline** INN, BAN *antiarrhythmic* [also: cifenline]

**cibenzoline succinate** JAN *antiarrhythmic* [also: cifenline succinate]

**cicaprost** INN

**cicaprost clathrate** *investigational prostacyclin analog for metastatic tumors and cardiovascular disease*

**cicarperone** INN

**ciclacillin** INN, BAN *antibacterial* [also: cyclacillin]

**ciclactate** INN

**ciclafrine** INN *antihypotensive* [also: ciclafrine HCl]

**ciclafrine HCl** USAN *antihypotensive* [also: ciclafrine]

**ciclazindol** USAN, INN, BAN *antidepressant*

**cicletanine** USAN, INN, BAN *antihypertensive*

**ciclindole** INN *antidepressant* [also: cyclindole]

**cicliomenol** INN

**ciclobendazole** INN, BAN *anthelmintic* [also: cyclobendazole]

**ciclofenazine** INN *antipsychotic* [also: cyclophenazine HCl]

**ciclofenazine HCl** [see: cyclophenazine HCl]

**cicloheximide** INN *antipsoriatic* [also: cycloheximide]

**ciclonicate** INN

**ciclonium bromide** INN

**ciclopirox** USAN, INN, BAN *antifungal*

**ciclopirox olamine** USAN, USP, JAN *antifungal*

**ciclopramine** INN

**cicloprofen** USAN, INN, BAN *anti-inflammatory*

**cicloprolol** INN *antiadrenergic (β-receptor)* [also: cicloprolol HCl; cycloprolol]

**cicloprolol HCl** USAN *antiadrenergic (β-receptor)* [also: cicloprolol; cycloprolol]

**ciclosidomine** INN, BAN

**ciclosporin** INN *immunosuppressive* [also: cyclosporine; cyclosporin]

**ciclotate** INN *combining name for radicals or groups*

**ciclotizolam** INN, BAN

**ciclotropium bromide** INN

**cicloxilic acid** INN

**cicloxolone** INN, BAN

**cicortonide** INN

**cicrotoic acid** INN

**cid** *street drug slang* [see: LSD]

**cideferron** INN

**Cidex; Cidex-7; Cidex Plus 28** solution OTC *broad-spectrum antimicrobial* [glutaral] 2%; 2%; 3.2%

**cidofovir** USAN, INN *antiviral for AIDS-related cytomegalovirus retinitis*

**cidoxepin** INN *antidepressant* [also: cidoxepin HCl]

**cidoxepin HCl** USAN *antidepressant* [also: cidoxepin]

**cifenline** USAN *antiarrhythmic* [also: cibenzoline]

**cifenline succinate** USAN *antiarrhythmic* [also: cibenzoline succinate]

**cifostodine** INN

**cigarette paper** *street drug slang for a packet of heroin* [see: heroin]

**cigarrode cristal** *street drug slang* [see: PCP]

**ciglitazone** USAN, INN *antidiabetic*

**cignolin** [see: anthralin]

**ciheptolane** INN

**ciladopa** INN, BAN *antiparkinsonian; dopaminergic agent* [also: ciladopa HCl]

**ciladopa HCl** USAN *antiparkinsonian; dopaminergic agent* [also: ciladopa]

**cilansetron** INN *investigational treatment for irritable bowel syndrome*

**cilastatin** INN, BAN *enzyme inhibitor* [also: cilastatin sodium]

**cilastatin sodium** USAN, JAN *enzyme inhibitor* [also: cilastatin]

**cilazapril** USAN, INN, BAN, JAN *antihypertensive; ACE inhibitor*

**cilazaprilat** INN, BAN

**cilexetil** USAN *combining name for radicals or groups*

**ciliary neurotrophic factor** *investigational (orphan) for amyotrophic lateral sclerosis*

**ciliary neurotrophic factor, recombinant human** *orphan status withdrawn 1997*

**cilobamine** INN *antidepressant* [also: cilobamine mesylate]

**cilobamine mesylate** USAN *antidepressant* [also: cilobamine]

**cilofungin** USAN, INN *antifungal*

**ciloprost** [see: iloprost]

**cilostamide** INN

**cilostazol** INN

**Ciloxan** Drop-Tainers (eye drops) ℞ *ophthalmic antibiotic* [ciprofloxacin HCl] 3.5 mg/mL

**ciltoprazine** INN

**cilutazoline** INN

**cimaterol** USAN, INN *repartitioning agent*

**cimemoxin** INN

**cimepanol** INN

**cimetidine** USAN, USP, INN, BAN, JAN *treatment of GI ulcers; histamine H$_2$*

*antagonist* 200, 300, 400, 800 mg
oral 🔟 dimethicone

**cimetidine HCl** USAN *antagonist to
histamine H₂ receptors* 300 mg/5 mL
oral; 300 mg/2 mL injection

**cimetropium bromide** INN

**cimoxatone** INN

**cinalukast** USAN, INN *antiasthmatic*

**cinametic acid** INN

**cinamolol** INN

**cinanserin** INN *serotonin inhibitor* [also:
cinanserin HCl]

**cinanserin HCl** USAN *serotonin inhibitor* [also: cinanserin]

**cinaproxen** INN

**cincaine chloride** [see: dibucaine HCl]

**cinchocaine** INN, BAN *local anesthetic*
[also: dibucaine]

**cinchocaine HCl** BAN *local anesthetic*
[also: dibucaine HCl]

**cinchonidine sulfate** NF

**cinchonine sulfate** NF

**cinchophen** NF, INN, BAN

**cinecromen** INN

**cinepaxadil** INN

**cinepazet** INN, BAN *antianginal* [also:
cinepazet maleate]

**cinepazet maleate** USAN *antianginal*
[also: cinepazet]

**cinepazic acid** INN

**cinepazide** INN, BAN

**cinfenine** INN

**cinfenoac** INN, BAN

**cinflumide** USAN, INN *muscle relaxant*

**cingestol** USAN, INN *progestin*

**cinitapride** INN

**cinmetacin** INN

**cinnamaldehyde** NF

**cinnamaverine** INN

**cinnamedrine** USAN, INN *smooth muscle relaxant*

**cinnamedrine HCl** *smooth muscle relaxant*

**cinnamic aldehyde** [now: cinnamaldehyde]

**cinnamon** NF

**cinnamon oil** NF

**cinnarizine** USAN, INN, BAN *antihistamine*

**cinnarizine clofibrate** INN

**cinnofuradione** INN

**cinnofuron** [see: cinnofuradione]

**cinnopentazone** INN *anti-inflammatory* [also: cintazone]

**cinnopropazone** [see: apazone]

**Cinobac** capsules ℞ *urinary antibacterial* [cinoxacin] 250, 500 mg

**cinoctramide** INN

**cinodine HCl** USAN *veterinary antibacterial*

**cinolazepam** INN

**cinoquidox** INN

**cinoxacin** USAN, USP, INN, BAN *urinary antibacterial* 250, 500 mg oral

**cinoxate** USAN, USP, INN *ultraviolet screen*

**cinoxolone** INN, BAN

**cinoxopazide** INN

**cinperene** USAN, INN *antipsychotic*

**cinprazole** INN

**cinpropazide** INN

**cinromide** USAN, INN *anticonvulsant*

**cintazone** USAN *anti-inflammatory* [also: cinnopentazone]

**cintramide** INN *antipsychotic* [also: cintriamide]

**cintriamide** USAN *antipsychotic* [also: cintramide]

**cinuperone** INN

**cioteronel** USAN, INN *antiandrogen*

**cipamfylline** USAN *antiviral agent; tumor necrosis factor alpha inhibitor*

**cipionate** INN *combining name for radicals or groups* [also: cypionate]

**ciprafamide** INN

**Cipralan** ℞ *investigational antiarrhythmic* [cifenline succinate]

**Cipramil** ℞ *investigational treatment for depression and Alzheimer's disease* [citalopram]

**ciprazafone** INN

**ciprefadol** INN *analgesic* [also: ciprefadol succinate]

**ciprefadol succinate** USAN *analgesic* [also: ciprefadol]

**Cipro** film-coated tablets, Cystitis Pack (6 tablets), IV infusion ℞ *broad-spectrum fluoroquinolone-type antibiotic; investigational treatment for cystic fibrosis* [ciprofloxacin] 100, 250, 500, 750 mg; 100 mg; 200, 400 mg

**ciprocinonide** USAN, INN *adrenocortical steroid*

**ciprofibrate** USAN, INN, BAN *antihyperlipoproteinemic*

**ciprofloxacin** USAN, INN, BAN *broadspectrum bactericidal antibiotic; investigational treatment for cystic fibrosis*

**ciprofloxacin HCl** USAN, USP, JAN *broad-spectrum bactericidal antibiotic*

**cipropride** INN

**ciproquazone** INN

**ciproquinate** INN *coccidiostat for poultry* [also: cyproquinate]

**ciprostene** INN *platelet antiaggregatory agent* [also: ciprostene calcium]

**ciprostene calcium** USAN *platelet antiaggregatory agent* [also: ciprostene]

**ciproximide** INN *antipsychotic; antidepressant* [also: cyproximide]

**ciramadol** USAN, INN *analgesic*

**ciramadol HCl** USAN *analgesic*

**cirazoline** INN

**Circavite-T** tablets OTC *vitamin/mineral/iron supplement* [multiple vitamins & minerals; iron] $\pm$●12 mg

**circles** *street drug slang for Rohypnol (flunitrazepam; not marketed in the U.S.)* [see: Rohypnol; flunitrazepam]

**cirolemycin** USAN, INN *antineoplastic; antibacterial*

**cisapride** USAN, INN, BAN, JAN *peristaltic stimulant; treatment for nocturnal heartburn due to gastroesophageal reflux disease*

**cisatracurium besylate** USAN *nondepolarizing neuromuscular blocker*

**CISCA; CisCA** (cisplatin, cyclophosphamide, Adriamycin) *chemotherapy protocol*

**CISCA$_{II}$/VB$_{IV}$** (cisplatin, cyclophosphamide, Adriamycin, vinblastine, bleomycin) *chemotherapy protocol*

**cisclomiphene** [now: enclomiphene]

**cisconazole** USAN, INN *antifungal*

*cis*-**DDP (diamminedichloroplatinum)** [see: cisplatin]

*cis*-**diamminedichloroplatinum (DDP)** [see: cisplatin]

**cismadinone** INN

**cisplatin** USAN, USP, INN, BAN *alkylating antineoplastic for testicular, ovarian, and bladder cancer*

**cisplatin & epinephrine** *investigational (Phase II) injectable gel for inoperable primary liver cancer*

*cis*-**platinum** [now: cisplatin]

*cis*-**platinum II** [now: cisplatin]

**9-*cis*-retinoic acid** *investigational (Phase I/III) for AIDS-related Kaposi sarcoma; investigational (Phase III, orphan) for acute promyelocytic leukemia and proliferative vitreoretinopathy*

**13-*cis*-retinoic acid** [see: isotretinoin]

**cistinexine** INN

**citalopram** INN, BAN *investigational treatment for depression and Alzheimer's disease*

**Citanest Forte** injection ℞ *injectable local anesthetic for dental procedures* [prilocaine HCl; epinephrine] 4%● 1:200 000

**Citanest Plain** injection ℞ *injectable local anesthetic for dental procedures* [prilocaine HCl] 4%

**citatepine** INN

**citenamide** USAN, INN *anticonvulsant*

**citenazone** INN

**citicoline** INN, JAN *investigational (Phase III) oral treatment for ischemic stroke and head trauma* [also: citicoline sodium]

**citicoline & dizocilpine maleate** *investigational (Phase III) neuroprotective treatment for stroke*

**citicoline sodium** USAN *investigational (Phase III) oral treatment for ischemic stroke and head trauma* [also: citicoline]

**citiolone** INN, DCF

**Citra pH** oral solution OTC *antacid* [sodium citrate] 450 mg/5 mL

**Citracal** tablets OTC *calcium supplement* [calcium citrate] 900 mg

**Citracal 1500+D** tablets (discontinued 1993) OTC *dietary supplement* [calcium citrate; vitamin D]

**Citracal Caplets + D** OTC *dietary supplement* [calcium citrate; vitamin D] 315 mg●200 IU

**Citracal Liquitab** effervescent tablets OTC *calcium supplement* [calcium citrate] 23.76 mg

**Citralax** effervescent granules OTC *laxative* [magnesium citrate; magnesium sulfate]

**citrate dextrose** [see: ACD solution]
**citrate of magnesia** [see: magnesium citrate]
**citrate phosphate dextrose** [see: anticoagulant citrate phosphate dextrose solution]
**citrate phosphate dextrose adenine** [see: anticoagulant citrate phosphate dextrose adenine solution]
**citrated caffeine** [see: caffeine, citrated]
**citric acid** USP *pH adjusting agent*
**citric acid, glucono-delta-lactone & magnesium carbonate** *irrigant for renal and bladder apatite or struvite calculi (orphan)*
**citric acid, magnesium oxide & sodium carbonate** [see: Suby solution G]
**citrin** [see: bioflavonoids]
**Citrocarbonate** effervescent granules OTC *antacid* [sodium bicarbonate; sodium citrate] 780•1820 mg/dose
**Citro-Flav 200** capsules OTC *dietary supplement* [citrus bioflavonoids complex] 200 mg
**citrol** *street drug slang for high-potency marijuana from Nepal* [see: marijuana]
**Citrolith** tablets R *urinary alkalinizing agent* [potassium citrate; sodium citrate] 50•950 mg
**Citro-Nesia** solution (discontinued 1993) OTC *laxative* [magnesium citrate]
**Citrotein** powder, liquid OTC *enteral nutritional therapy* [lactose-free formula]
**citrovorum factor** [see: leucovorin calcium]
**Citrucel** powder OTC *bulk laxative* [methylcellulose] 2 g/tbsp.
**Citrucel Sugar Free** powder OTC *bulk laxative* [methylcellulose; phenylalanine] 2 g•52 mg per tbsp.
**citrus bioflavonoids** [see: bioflavonoids]
**Citrus-flav C 500** tablets OTC *dietary supplement* [vitamin C; citrus & acerola bioflavonoids; hesperidin; rutin] 200•250•40•10 mg
**CIVPP (chlorambucil, vinblastine, procarbazine, prednisone)** *chemotherapy protocol*
**cladribine** *antineoplastic for hairy-cell leukemia (orphan); investigational (orphan) for chronic lymphocytic leukemia and multiple sclerosis*
**Claforan** powder for IV or IM injection R *cephalosporin-type antibiotic* [cefotaxime sodium] 0.5, 1, 2, 10 g
**clamidoxic acid** INN, BAN
**clamoxyquin** BAN *antiamebic* [also: clamoxyquin HCl; clamoxyquine]
**clamoxyquin HCl** USAN *antiamebic* [also: clamoxyquine; clamoxyquin]
**clamoxyquine** INN *antiamebic* [also: clamoxyquin HCl; clamoxyquin]
**clanfenur** INN
**clanobutin** INN
**clantifen** INN
**claretin-12** [see: cyanocobalamin] ☒ Claritin; Clarityne
**clarithromycin** USAN, INN, BAN, JAN *macrolide antibacterial antibiotic*
**Claritin** tablets, RediTabs (rapidly disintegrating tablets), syrup R *nonsedating antihistamine; treatment for chronic urticaria* [loratadine] 10 mg; 10 mg; 1 mg/mL ☒ claretin; Clarityne
**Claritin-D** (name changed to Claritin-D 12 Hour in 1996)
**Claritin-D 12 Hour; Claritin-D 24 Hour** extended-release film-coated tablets R *decongestant; nonsedating antihistamine* [pseudoephedrine sulfate; loratadine] 120•5 mg; 240•10 mg
**clarity** *street drug slang* [see: MDMA]
**Clarityne** (Mexican name for U.S. product Claritin) ☒ claretin; Claritin
**clavulanate potassium** USAN, USP *β-lactamase inhibitor*
**clavulanate potassium & ticarcillin** [see: ticarcillin disodium]
**clavulanic acid** INN, BAN
**clavulanic acid & amoxicillin** [see: amoxicillin]
**clavulanic acid & ticarcillin** [see: ticarcillin disodium]
**clazolam** USAN, INN *minor tranquilizer*
**clazolimine** USAN, INN *diuretic*
**clazuril** USAN, INN, BAN *coccidiostat for pigeons*
**Clean-N-Soak** solution OTC *cleaning/soaking solution for hard contact lenses*
**Clear Away; Clear Away Plantar** (name changed to Dr. Scholl's Clear Away in 1994)

**Clear By Design** gel OTC *topical keratolytic for acne* [benzoyl peroxide] 2.5%

**Clear Eyes** eye drops OTC *topical ocular decongestant/vasoconstrictor* [naphazoline HCl] 0.012%

**Clear Eyes ACR** eye drops OTC *topical ocular decongestant; astringent* [naphazoline HCl; zinc sulfate] 0.012%•0.25%

**Clear Total Lice Elimination System** kit (shampoo + egg remover enzymes + nit comb) OTC *pediculicide* [pyrethrins; piperonyl butoxide] 0.3%•3%

**Clear Tussin 30** liquid OTC *antitussive; expectorant* [dextromethorphan hydrobromide; guaifenesin] 15•100 mg/5 mL

**Clearasil** cream, lotion OTC *topical keratolytic for acne* [benzoyl peroxide] 10%

**Clearasil Adult Care** cream OTC *topical acne treatment* [sulfur; resorcinol; alcohol 10%]

**Clearasil Adult Care Medicated Blemish Stick** (discontinued 1994) OTC *topical acne treatment* [sulfur; resorcinol; bentonite] 8%•1%•4%

**Clearasil Antibacterial Soap** bar OTC *medicated cleanser for acne* [triclosan]

**Clearasil Clearstick** liquid OTC *topical keratolytic for acne* [salicylic acid; alcohol 39%] 1.25%, 2%

**Clearasil Daily Face Wash** liquid OTC *antiseptic; disinfectant* [triclosan] 0.3%

**Clearasil Double Clear; Clearasil Double Textured** medicated pads OTC *topical keratolytic for acne* [salicylic acid; alcohol 40%] 1.25%, 2%; 2%

**Clearasil Medicated Astringent** liquid (name changed to Clearasil Medicated Deep Cleanser in 1994)

**Clearasil Medicated Deep Cleanser** liquid OTC *topical keratolytic cleanser for acne* [salicylic acid; alcohol 42%] 0.5%

**Clearblue** test kit for home use (discontinued 1995) OTC *in vitro diagnostic aid for urine pregnancy test*

**Clearblue Easy** test stick for home use OTC *in vitro diagnostic aid for urine pregnancy test*

**Clearly Cala-gel** OTC *topical antihistamine* [diphenhydramine HCl] ≜

**Clearplan Easy** test kit for home use OTC *in vitro diagnostic aid to predict ovulation time*

**Clearview Chlamydia** test for professional use *in vitro diagnostic aid for Chlamydia trachomatis* [color-label immunoassay]

**Clearview hCG** test kit for professional use (discontinued 1996) *in vitro diagnostic aid for urine pregnancy test*

**clebopride** USAN, INN *antiemetic*

**clefamide** INN, BAN

**clemastine** USAN, BAN *antihistamine*

**clemastine fumarate** USAN, USP, BAN *antihistamine* 1.34, 2.68 mg oral; 0.5 mg/5 mL oral

**clemeprol** INN, BAN

**clemizole** INN, BAN

**clemizole penicillin** INN, BAN

**clenbuterol** INN, BAN

**clenpirin** INN [also: clenpyrin]

**clenpyrin** BAN [also: clenpirin]

**Clens** solution (discontinued 1995) OTC *cleaning solution for hard contact lenses*

**clentiazem** INN *calcium channel antagonist* [also: clentiazem maleate]

**clentiazem maleate** USAN *calcium channel antagonist* [also: clentiazem]

**Cleocin** capsules ℞ *lincosamide-type antibiotic; investigational (orphan) for AIDS-related Pneumocystis carinii pneumonia* [clindamycin HCl] 75, 100, 300 mg ▣ bleomycin; Lincocin

**Cleocin** vaginal cream ℞ *lincosamide-type antibiotic* [clindamycin phosphate] 2%

**Cleocin Pediatric** granules for oral solution ℞ *lincosamide-type antibiotic* [clindamycin palmitate HCl] 75 mg/5 mL

**Cleocin Phosphate** IV infusion, IM injection ℞ *lincosamide-type antibiotic; investigational (orphan) for AIDS-related Pneumocystis carinii pneumonia* [clindamycin phosphate] 150 mg/mL

**Cleocin T** gel, topical solution, lotion, pads ℞ *topical antibiotic for acne* [clindamycin phosphate] 10 mg/mL

**Clerz 2** solution OTC *rewetting solution for hard or soft contact lenses*

**Clerz Drops** solution (discontinued 1993) OTC *rewetting solution for hard contact lenses*

**cletoquine** INN, BAN

**Clexane** (European name for U.S. product Lovenox)

**clibucaine** INN

**clicker** *street drug slang for a combination of crack and PCP* [see: cocaine, crack; PCP]

**clidafidine** INN

**clidanac** INN

**clidinium bromide** USAN, USP, INN, BAN *peptic ulcer adjunct*

**cliffhanger** *street drug slang* [see: PCP]

**Climara** transdermal patch ℞ *estrogen replacement therapy for postmenopausal disorders* [estradiol] 50, 100 µg/day

**climax** *street drug slang* [see: butyl nitrite; isobutyl nitrite; cocaine, crack; heroin]

**climazolam** INN

**climb** *street drug slang for a marijuana cigarette* [see: marijuana]

**climbazole** INN, BAN

**climiqualine** INN

**clinafloxacin HCl** USAN *quinolone antibacterial*

**Clinda-Derm** topical solution ℞ *topical antibiotic for acne* [clindamycin phosphate] 10 mg/mL

**clindamycin** USAN, INN, BAN *lincosamide bactericidal antibiotic; investigational (orphan) for AIDS-related Pneumocystis carinii pneumonia*

**clindamycin HCl** USP, BAN *lincosamide bactericidal antibiotic* 75, 150 mg oral

**clindamycin HCl & primaquine phosphate** *investigational (orphan) for AIDS-associated Pneumocystis carinii pneumonia*

**clindamycin palmitate HCl** USAN, USP *lincosamide bactericidal antibiotic*

**clindamycin phosphate** USAN, USP *lincosamide bactericidal antibiotic* 10 mg/mL topical; 150 mg/mL injection

**Clindex** capsules ℞ *GI anticholinergic; anxiolytic* [clidinium bromide; chlordiazepoxide HCl] 2.5•5 mg

**Clinipak** (trademarked packaging form) *unit dose package*

**Clinistix** reagent strips for home use OTC *in vitro diagnostic aid for urine glucose*

**Clinitest** reagent tablets for home use OTC *in vitro diagnostic aid for urine glucose*

**clinocaine HCl** [see: procaine HCl]

**clinofibrate** INN

**clinolamide** INN

**Clinoril** tablets ℞ *nonsteroidal anti-inflammatory drug (NSAID); antiarthritic; analgesic* [sulindac] 150, 200 mg

**Clinoxide** capsules (discontinued 1995) ℞ *GI anticholinergic; anxiolytic* [clidinium bromide; chlordiazepoxide HCl] 2.5•5 mg ⊡ clioxanide; Clipoxide

**clioquinol** USP, INN, BAN *topical antibacterial; antifungal*

**clioxanide** USAN, INN, BAN *anthelmintic* ⊡ Clinoxide

**clipoxamine** [see: cliropamine]

**Clipoxide** capsules (discontinued 1995) ℞ *GI anticholinergic; anxiolytic* [clidinium bromide; chlordiazepoxide HCl] 2.5•5 mg ⊡ Clinoxide

**cliprofen** USAN, INN *anti-inflammatory*

**clips** *street drug slang for rows of vials heat-sealed together*

**cliropamine** INN

**clobamine mesylate** [now: cilobamine mesylate]

**clobazam** USAN, INN, BAN *minor tranquilizer*

**clobedolum** [see: clonitazene]

**clobenoside** INN

**clobenzepam** INN

**clobenzorex** INN

**clobenztropine** INN

**clobetasol** INN, BAN *topical corticosteroidal anti-inflammatory* [also: clobetasol propionate]

**clobetasol propionate** USAN *topical corticosteroidal anti-inflammatory* [also: clobetasol] 0.05% topical

**clobetasone** INN, BAN *anti-inflammatory* [also: clobetasone butyrate]

**clobetasone butyrate** USAN *anti-inflammatory* [also: clobetasone]

**clobutinol** INN

**clobuzarit** INN, BAN

**clocanfamide** INN

**clocapramine** INN

**clociguanil** INN, BAN
**clocinizine** INN
**clocortolone** INN *topical corticosteroid* [also: clocortolone acetate]
**clocortolone acetate** USAN *topical corticosteroid* [also: clocortolone]
**clocortolone pivalate** USAN, USP *topical corticosteroid*
**clocoumarol** INN
**Clocream** cream OTC *moisturizer; emollient* [cod liver oil (vitamins A and E); cholecalciferol; vitamin A palmitate]
**clodacaine** INN
**clodanolene** USAN, INN *skeletal muscle relaxant*
**clodantoin** INN *antifungal* [also: chlordantoin]
**clodazon** INN *antidepressant* [also: clodazon HCl]
**clodazon HCl** USAN *antidepressant* [also: clodazon]
**Cloderm** cream ℞ *topical corticosteroid* [clocortolone pivalate] 0.1%
**clodoxopone** INN
**clodronic acid** USAN, INN, BAN *calcium regulator*
**clofazimine** USAN, INN, BAN *bactericidal; tuberculostatic; leprostatic (orphan)*
**clofedanol** INN *antitussive* [also: chlophedianol HCl; chlophedianol]
**clofedanol HCl** [see: chlophedianol HCl]
**clofenamic acid** INN
**clofenamide** INN
**clofenciclan** INN
**clofenetamine** INN
**clofenetamine HCl** [see: clofenetamine]
**clofenotane** INN [also: chlorophenothane; dicophane]
**clofenoxyde** INN
**clofenpyride** [see: nicofibrate]
**clofenvinfos** INN [also: chlorfenvinphos]
**clofeverine** INN
**clofexamide** INN
**clofezone** INN
**clofibrate** USAN, USP, INN, BAN *antihyperlipidemic*
**clofibric acid** INN

**clofibride** INN
**clofilium phosphate** USAN, INN *antiarrhythmic*
**clofinol** [see: nicofibrate]
**cloflucarban** USAN *disinfectant* [also: halocarban]
**clofluperol** INN, BAN *antipsychotic* [also: seperidol HCl]
**clofluperol HCl** [see: seperidol HCl]
**clofoctol** INN
**cloforex** INN
**clofurac** INN
**clogestone** INN, BAN *progestin* [also: clogestone acetate]
**clogestone acetate** USAN *progestin* [also: clogestone]
**cloguanamil** INN, BAN [also: cloguanamile]
**cloguanamile** BAN [also: cloguanamil]
**clomacran** INN, BAN *antipsychotic* [also: clomacran phosphate]
**clomacran phosphate** USAN *antipsychotic* [also: clomacran]
**clomegestone** INN *progestin* [also: clomegestone acetate]
**clomegestone acetate** USAN *progestin* [also: clomegestone]
**clometacin** INN
**clometerone** INN *antiestrogen* [also: clometherone]
**clometherone** USAN *antiestrogen* [also: clometerone]
**clomethiazole** INN [also: chlormethiazole]
**clometocillin** INN
**Clomid** tablets ℞ *ovulation stimulant* [clomiphene citrate] 50 mg
**clomide** [see: aklomide]
**clomifene** INN *gonad-stimulating principle; ovulation stimulant* [also: clomiphene citrate; clomiphene]
**clomifenoxide** INN
**clominorex** USAN, INN *anorectic*
**clomiphene** BAN *gonad-stimulating principle; ovulation stimulant* [also: clomiphene citrate; clomifene] ⊘ clonidine
**clomiphene citrate** USAN, USP *gonad-stimulating principle; ovulation stimulant* [also: clomifene; clomiphene] 50 mg oral

**clomipramine** INN, BAN *tricyclic antidepressant* [also: clomipramine HCl]

**clomipramine HCl** USAN *tricyclic antidepressant; used for obsessive-compulsive disorders* [also: clomipramine]

**clomocycline** INN, BAN

**clomoxir** INN

**Clomycin** ointment OTC *topical antibiotic; anesthetic* [polymyxin B sulfate; bacitracin; neomycin sulfate; lidocaine] 5000 U•500 U•3.5 mg•40 mg per g

**clonazepam** USAN, USP, INN, BAN *anticonvulsant; investigational (orphan) for hyperexplexia (startle disease)* 0.5, 1, 2 mg oral

**clonazoline** INN

**clonidine** USAN, INN, BAN *centrally acting antiadrenergic antihypertensive; adjunct to epidural opioid analgesics for severe cancer pain (orphan)* ⑨ clomiphene; Klonopin; quinidine

**clonidine HCl** USAN, USP, BAN *centrally acting antiadrenergic antihypertensive; adjunct to epidural opioid analgesics for severe cancer pain (orphan)* 0.1, 0.2, 0.3 mg oral

**clonitazene** INN, BAN

**clonitrate** USAN, INN *coronary vasodilator*

**clonixeril** USAN, INN *analgesic*

**clonixin** USAN, INN *analgesic*

**clopamide** USAN, INN, BAN *antihypertensive; diuretic*

**clopenthixol** USAN, INN, BAN *antipsychotic*

**cloperastine** INN

**cloperidone** INN *sedative* [also: cloperidone HCl]

**cloperidone HCl** USAN *sedative* [also: cloperidone]

**clophenoxate** [see: meclofenoxate]

**clopidogrel** INN *investigational preventative for stroke, myocardial ischemia, and peripheral artery disease*

**clopidol** USAN, INN, BAN *coccidiostat for poultry*

**clopimozide** USAN, INN *antipsychotic*

**clopipazan** INN *antipsychotic* [also: clopipazan mesylate]

**clopipazan mesylate** USAN *antipsychotic* [also: clopipazan]

**clopirac** USAN, INN, BAN *anti-inflammatory*

**cloponone** INN, BAN

**clopoxide** [see: chlordiazepoxide]

**clopoxide chloride** [see: chlordiazepoxide HCl]

**Clopra** tablets ℞ *antidopaminergic; antiemetic for chemotherapy; peristaltic* [metoclopramide monohydrochloride monohydrate] 10 mg

**cloprednol** USAN, INN, BAN *glucocorticoid*

**cloprostenol** INN, BAN *prostaglandin* [also: cloprostenol sodium]

**cloprostenol sodium** USAN *prostaglandin* [also: cloprostenol]

**cloprothiazole** INN

**cloquinate** INN, BAN

**cloquinozine** INN

**cloracetadol** INN

**cloral betaine** INN *sedative* [also: chloral betaine]

**cloramfenicol pantotenate complex** INN *antibacterial; antirickettsial* [also: chloramphenicol pantothenate complex]

**cloranolol** INN

**clorarsen** [see: dichlorophenarsine HCl]

**clorazepate dipotassium** USAN, USP *anxiolytic; minor tranquilizer; alcohol withdrawal relief* [also: dipotassium clorazepate] 3.75, 7.5, 15 mg oral

**clorazepate monopotassium** USAN *minor tranquilizer*

**clorazepic acid** BAN

**cloretate** INN *sedative; hypnotic* [also: clorethate]

**clorethate** USAN *sedative; hypnotic* [also: cloretate]

**clorexolone** USAN, INN, BAN *diuretic*

**clorgiline** INN [also: clorgyline]

**clorgyline** BAN [also: clorgiline]

**cloricromen** INN

**cloridarol** INN

**clorindanic acid** INN

**clorindanol** INN *spermaticide* [also: chlorindanol]

**clorindione** INN, BAN

**clormecaine** INN

**clorofene** INN *disinfectant* [also: clorophene]

**cloroperone** INN *antipsychotic* [also: cloroperone HCl]

**cloroperone HCl** USAN *antipsychotic* [also: cloroperone]

**clorophene** USAN *disinfectant* [also: clorofene]

**cloroqualone** INN

**clorotepine** INN

**Clorpactin WCS-90** powder for solution OTC *topical antimicrobial* [oxychlorosene sodium] 2 g

**Clorpactin XCB** powder for solution (discontinued 1994) OTC *topical antimicrobial* [oxychlorosene] 5 g

**clorprenaline** INN, BAN *adrenergic; bronchodilator* [also: clorprenaline HCl]

**clorprenaline HCl** USAN *adrenergic; bronchodilator* [also: clorprenaline]

**clorquinaldol** [see: chlorquinaldol]

**clorsulon** USAN, INN *antiparasitic; fasciolicide*

**clortermine** INN *anorectic* [also: clortermine HCl]

**clortermine HCl** USAN *anorectic* [also: clortermine]

**closantel** USAN, INN, BAN *anthelmintic*

**closilate** INN *combining name for radicals or groups* [also: closylate]

**closiramine** INN *antihistamine* [also: closiramine aceturate]

**closiramine aceturate** USAN *antihistamine* [also: closiramine]

**clostebol** INN [also: clostebol acetate]

**clostebol acetate** BAN [also: clostebol]

**clostridial collagenase** *investigational (orphan) for advanced Dupuytren's disease*

*Clostridium botulinum* **toxin** [see: botulinum toxin]

**closylate** USAN, BAN *combining name for radicals or groups* [also: closilate]

**clothiapine** USAN, BAN *antipsychotic* [also: clotiapine]

**clothixamide maleate** USAN *antipsychotic* [also: clotixamide]

**clotiapine** INN *antipsychotic* [also: clothiapine]

**clotiazepam** INN

**cloticasone** INN, BAN *anti-inflammatory* [also: cloticasone propionate]

**cloticasone propionate** USAN *anti-inflammatory* [also: cloticasone]

**clotioxone** INN

**clotixamide** INN *antipsychotic* [also: clothixamide maleate]

**clotixamide maleate** [see: clothixamide maleate]

**clotrimazole** USAN, USP, INN, BAN, JAN *broad-spectrum antifungal* 1% topical; 100 mg vaginal ⑫ co-trimoxazole

**clotrimidazole** *investigational (orphan) for sickle cell disease*

**cloud; cloud nine** *street drug slang* [see: cocaine, crack]

**clove oil** NF

**clovoxamine** INN

**cloxacepride** INN

**cloxacillin** INN, BAN *antibacterial* [also: cloxacillin benzathine]

**cloxacillin benzathine** USP *antibacterial* [also: cloxacillin]

**cloxacillin sodium** USAN, USP *bactericidal antibiotic* 250, 500 mg oral; 125 mg/5 mL oral

**Cloxapen** capsules ℞ *bactericidal antibiotic (penicillinase-resistant penicillin)* [cloxacillin sodium] 250, 500 mg

**cloxazolam** INN

**cloxestradiol** INN

**cloxifenol** [see: triclosan]

**cloximate** INN

**cloxiquine** INN *antibacterial* [also: cloxyquin]

**cloxotestosterone** INN

**cloxphendyl** [see: cloxypendyl]

**cloxypendyl** INN

**cloxyquin** USAN *antibacterial* [also: cloxiquine]

**clozapine** USAN, INN, BAN *sedative; antipsychotic for severe schizophrenia*

**Clozaril** tablets ℞ *antipsychotic* [clozapine] 25, 100 mg

**Clysodrast** powder for oral solution ℞ *laxative for pre-procedure bowel prep* [bisacodyl tannex] 2.5 g/packet

**C-Max** gradual-release tablets OTC *vitamin/mineral supplement* [various minerals; vitamin C] ± • 1 g

**CMC (carboxymethylcellulose) gum** [see: carboxymethylcellulose sodium]

**CMC (cyclophosphamide, methotrexate, CCNU)** *chemotherapy protocol*

**CMC-VAP (cyclophosphamide, methotrexate, CCNU, vincristine, Adriamycin, procarbazine)** *chemotherapy protocol*

**CMF (cyclophosphamide, methotrexate, fluorouracil)** *chemotherapy protocol*

**CMF/AV (cyclophosphamide, methotrexate, fluorouracil, Adriamycin, Oncovin)** *chemotherapy protocol*

**CMFAVP (cyclophosphamide, methotrexate, fluorouracil, Adriamycin, vincristine, prednisone)** *chemotherapy protocol*

**CMFP; CMF-P (cyclophosphamide, methotrexate, fluorouracil, prednisone)** *chemotherapy protocol*

**CMFPT (cyclophosphamide, methotrexate, fluorouracil, prednisone, tamoxifen)** *chemotherapy protocol*

**CMFPTH (cyclophosphamide, methotrexate, fluorouracil, prednisone, tamoxifen, Halotestin)** *chemotherapy protocol*

**CMFT (cyclophosphamide, methotrexate, fluorouracil, tamoxifen)** *chemotherapy protocol*

**CMFVAT (cyclophosphamide, methotrexate, fluorouracil, vincristine, Adriamycin, testosterone)** *chemotherapy protocol*

**CMFVP (cyclophosphamide, methotrexate, fluorouracil, vincristine, prednisone)** *chemotherapy protocol* [two dosing protocols: Cooper's protocol and SWOG protocol]

**CMH (cyclophosphamide, *m*-AMSA, hydroxyurea)** *chemotherapy protocol*

**C-MOPP (cyclophosphamide, mechlorethamine, Oncovin, procarbazine, prednisone)** *chemotherapy protocol*

**CMV (cisplatin, methotrexate, vinblastine)** *chemotherapy protocol*

**CMV-IGIV (cytomegalovirus immune globulin intravenous)** [see: globulin, immune]

**CN2 HCl** [see: mechlorethamine HCl]

**CNF (cyclophosphamide, Novantrone, fluorouracil)** *chemotherapy protocol* [also: CFM; FNC]

**CNOP (cyclophosphamide, Novantrone, Oncovin, prednisone)** *chemotherapy protocol*

**Co I (coenzyme I)** [see: nadide]

**Co Tinic** IM injection ℞ *antianemic* [ferrous gluconate; multiple B vitamins; procaine]

**$CO_2$ (carbon dioxide)** [q.v.]

**$^{57}Co$** [see: cobaltous chloride Co 57]

**$^{57}Co$** [see: cyanocobalamin Co 57]

**$^{58}Co$** [see: cyanocobalamin ($^{58}Co$)]

**$^{60}Co$** [see: cobaltous chloride Co 60]

**$^{60}Co$** [see: cyanocobalamin Co 60]

**coagulation factor IX (human)** [see: factor IX complex]

**coal tar** USP *topical antieczematic; antiseborrheic*

**COAP (cyclophosphamide, Oncovin, ara-C, prednisone)** *chemotherapy protocol*

**Co-Apap** tablets OTC *antitussive; decongestant; antihistamine; analgesic* [dextromethorphan hydrobromide; pseudoephedrine HCl; chlorpheniramine maleate; acetaminophen] 15•30•2•325 mg

**COAP-BLEO (cyclophosphamide, Oncovin, ara-C, prednisone, bleomycin)** *chemotherapy protocol*

**coast-to-coast** *street drug slang, a reference to truckers' use of amphetamines for long-distance runs* [see: amphetamines]

**COB (cisplatin, Oncovin, bleomycin)** *chemotherapy protocol*

**cobalamin concentrate** USP *vitamin $B_{12}$; hematopoietic*

**cobalt** *element* (Co)

**cobalt-labeled vitamin $B_{12}$** [see: cyanocobalamin Co 57 & Co 60]

**cobaltous chloride Co 57** USAN *radioactive agent*

**cobaltous chloride Co 60** USAN *radioactive agent*

**cobamamide** INN

**Cobex** IM or subcu injection (discontinued 1994) ℞ *antianemic; vitamin $B_{12}$ supplement* [cyanocobalamin] 100, 1000 μg/mL

**coca** *street drug slang* [see: cocaine]

**coca paste; cocaine paste** *street drug slang for a barely refined cocaine with adulterants* [see: cocaine]

**cocaine** USP, BAN *topical anesthetic for mucous membranes; widely abused as a street drug, derived from coca leaves* 4%, 10% topical

**cocaine, crack** *street drug made by converting cocaine HCl into a form that can be smoked, which causes a faster, more intense effect*

**cocaine HCl** USP *topical anesthetic for mucous membranes; widely abused as a street drug, derived from coca leaves* 135 mg oral; 4%, 10% topical

**Cocaine Viscous** topical solution ℞ *topical mucosal anesthesia* [cocaine] 4%, 10%

**cocarboxylase** INN [also: co-carboxylase]

**co-carboxylase** BAN [also: cocarboxylase]

**coccidioidin** USP *dermal coccidioidomycosis test*

**cocculin** [see: picrotoxin]

**cochornis** *street drug slang* [see: marijuana]

**cocktail** *street drug slang for a cigarette laced with cocaine, crack, or marijuana* [see: cocaine; cocaine, crack; marijuana]

**coco rocks** *street drug slang for dark brown crack made by adding chocolate pudding during production* [see: cocaine, crack]

**coco snow** *street drug slang for benzocaine used as a cutting agent for crack* [see: cocaine, crack; benzocaine]

**cocoa** NF

**cocoa butter** NF *suppository base; emollient/protectant*

**coconut** *street drug slang* [see: cocaine]

**cod liver oil** USP, BAN *vitamins A and D source; emollient/protectant*

**cod liver oil, nondestearinated** NF

**codactide** INN, BAN

**Codafed Expectorant** liquid (discontinued 1994) ℞ *narcotic antitussive; decongestant; expectorant* [codeine phosphate; pseudoephedrine HCl; guaifenesin; alcohol] ⊡ Codaphen

**Codamine** syrup, pediatric syrup ℞ *narcotic antitussive; decongestant* [hydrocodone bitartrate; phenylpropanolamine HCl] 5•25 mg/5 mL; 2.5•12.5 mg/5 mL

**Codaphen** tablets (discontinued 1993) ℞ *analgesic* [acetaminophen; codeine phosphate] ⊡ Codafed

**CODE (cisplatin, Oncovin, doxorubicin, etoposide)** *chemotherapy protocol*

**Codegest Expectorant** liquid ℞ *narcotic antitussive; decongestant; expectorant* [codeine phosphate; phenylpropanolamine HCl; guaifenesin] 10•12.5•100 mg/5 mL ⊡ Codehist

**Codehist DH** elixir ℞ *narcotic antitussive; decongestant; antihistamine* [codeine phosphate; pseudoephedrine HCl; chlorpheniramine maleate; alcohol 5.7%] 10•30•2 mg/5 mL ⊡ Codegest

**codehydrogenase I** [see: nadide]

**codeine** USP, BAN *antitussive; narcotic analgesic; sometimes abused as a street drug* ⊡ Kaodene

**codeine & acetaminophen** *narcotic analgesic* 15•300, 30•300, 60•300 mg oral; 12•30 mg/5 mL oral

**codeine phosphate** USP, BAN *antitussive; narcotic analgesic*

**codeine phosphate & guaifenesin** *antitussive; narcotic analgesic; expectorant* 10•300 mg oral; 10•100 mg/5 mL oral

**codeine polistirex** USAN *antitussive*

**codeine sulfate** USP *narcotic analgesic; antitussive* 15, 30, 60 mg oral; 30, 60 mg/mL injection

**codelcortone** [see: prednisolone]

**co-dergocrine mesylate** BAN *cognition adjuvant* [also: ergoloid mesylates]

**Codiclear DH** syrup ℞ *narcotic antitussive; expectorant* [hydrocodone bitartrate; guaifenesin] 5•100 mg/5 mL

**Codimal** capsules, film-coated tablets OTC *decongestant; antihistamine; analgesic* [pseudoephedrine HCl; chlorpheniramine maleate; acetaminophen] 30•2•325 mg

**Codimal A** injection (discontinued 1994) ℞ *antihistamine* [brompheniramine maleate] 10 mg/mL

**Codimal DH** syrup ℞ *narcotic antitussive; decongestant; antihistamine* [hydrocodone bitartrate; phenylephrine HCl; pyrilamine maleate] 1.66•5•8.33 mg/5 mL

**Codimal DM** syrup OTC *antitussive; decongestant; antihistamine* [dextromethorphan hydrobromide; phenylephrine HCl; pyrilamine maleate] 10•5•8.33 mg/5 mL

**Codimal Expectorant** liquid (discontinued 1994) OTC *decongestant; expectorant* [phenylpropanolamine HCl; guaifenesin] 25•100 mg/5 mL

**Codimal PH** syrup OTC *narcotic antitussive; decongestant; antihistamine* [codeine phosphate; phenylephrine HCl; pyrilamine maleate] 10•5•8.33 mg/5 mL

**Codimal-L.A.; Codimal-L.A. Half** extended-release capsules ℞ *decongestant; antihistamine* [pseudoephedrine HCl; chlorpheniramine maleate] 120•8 mg; 60•4 mg

**codorphone** [now: conorphone HCl]

**codoxime** USAN, INN *antitussive*

**Cody** *street drug slang* [see: codeine]

**coenzyme Q10** *investigational immune stimulant for AIDS; antioxidant; cardiac protectant*

**COF/COM (cyclophosphamide, Oncovin, fluorouracil + cyclophosphamide, Oncovin, methotrexate)** *chemotherapy protocol*

**coffee** *street drug slang* [see: LSD]

**caffeine** [see: caffeine]

**cofisatin** INN

**cofisatine** [see: cofisatin]

**cogazocine** INN

**Cogentin** tablets, IV or IM injection ℞ *anticholinergic; antiparkinsonian* [benztropine mesylate] 0.5, 1, 2 mg; 1 mg/mL

**Co-Gesic** tablets ℞ *narcotic analgesic* [hydrocodone bitartrate; acetaminophen] 5•500 mg

**Cognex** capsules ℞ *cholinesterase inhibitor; cognition adjuvant for Alz-heimer's dementia* [tacrine HCl] 10, 20, 30, 40 mg

**Co-Hist** tablets OTC *decongestant; antihistamine; analgesic* [pseudoephedrine HCl; chlorpheniramine maleate; acetaminophen] 30•2•325 mg

**coke** *street drug slang* [see: cocaine; cocaine, crack]

**cola** *street drug slang* [see: cocaine]

**Colabid** tablets ℞ *uricosuric for gout* [probenecid; colchicine]

**Colace** capsules, syrup, drops OTC *stool softener* [docusate sodium] 50, 100 mg; 60 mg/15 mL; 150 mg/15 mL

**colas** (Spanish for "tails") *street drug slang for flowering tops of marijuana plants* [see: marijuana]

**colaspase** BAN *antineoplastic for acute lymphocytic leukemia (ALL)* [also: asparaginase]

**Co-Lav** powder for oral solution ℞ *pre-procedure bowel evacuant* [polyethylene glycol-electrolyte solution (plus electrolytes)] 60 g/L

**Colax** tablets OTC *laxative; stool softener* [phenolphthalein; docusate sodium] 65•100 mg

**Colazide** ℞ *investigational (Phase III) gastrointestinal anti-inflammatory for ulcerative colitis* [balsalazide disodium]

**ColBenemid** tablets (discontinued 1997) ℞ *treatment for frequent, recurrent attacks of gouty arthritis* [probenecid; colchicine] 500•0.5 mg

**colchamine** [see: demecolcine]

**colchicine** USP, JAN *gout suppressant; orphan status withdrawn 1997* 0.5, 0.6 mg oral; 1 mg injection

**colchicine & probenecid** *treatment for frequent, recurrent attacks of gouty arthritis* 0.5•500 mg oral

**Cold & Allergy** elixir OTC *decongestant; antihistamine* [phenylpropanolamine HCl; brompheniramine maleate] 12.5•2 mg/5 mL

**cold cream** USP

**Cold Relief** tablets OTC *antitussive; decongestant; antihistamine; analgesic* [dextromethorphan hydrobromide; phenylpropanolamine HCl; chlorpheniramine maleate; acetaminophen] 10•12.5•2•325 mg

**Cold Symptoms Relief** tablets OTC
*antitussive; decongestant; antihista-*
*mine; analgesic* [dextromethorphan
hydrobromide; pseudoephedrine
HCl; chlorpheniramine maleate;
acetaminophen] 10•30•2•325 mg

**Cold-Gest** sustained-release capsules
OTC *decongestant; antihistamine*
[phenylpropanolamine HCl; chlorpheniramine maleate] 75•8 mg

**Coldloc** liquid ℞ *decongestant; expecto-*
*rant* [phenylpropanolamine HCl;
phenylephrine HCl; guaifenesin]
20•5•100 mg/5 mL

**Coldloc-LA** sustained-release caplets
℞ *decongestant; expectorant* [phenyl-
propanolamine HCl; guaifenesin]
75•600 mg

**Coldrine** tablets OTC *decongestant;*
*analgesic* [pseudoephedrine HCl;
acetaminophen] 30•325 mg

**colecalciferol** INN *vitamin D₃; antira-*
*chitic* [also: cholecalciferol]

**Colestid** tablets, granules ℞ *cholesterol-*
*lowering antihyperlipidemic* [colestipol
HCl] 1 g; 5 g/dose ⧉ colistin

**colestipol** INN, BAN *antihyperlipopro-*
*teinemic; bile acid sequestrant* [also:
colestipol HCl] ⧉ colistin

**colestipol HCl** USAN, USP *antihyper-*
*lipoproteinemic; bile acid sequestrant*
[also: colestipol]

**colestolone** USAN, INN *hypolipidemic*

**colestyramine** INN *bile salts ion-*
*exchange resin; antihyperlipoprotein-*
*emic* [also: cholestyramine resin;
cholestyramine]

**colestyramine resin** [see: cholestyramine resin]

**colextran** INN

**Colfed-A** sustained-release capsules ℞
*decongestant; antihistamine* [pseudo-
ephedrine HCl; chlorpheniramine
maleate] 120•8 mg

**colfenamate** INN

**colforsin** USAN, INN *antiglaucoma agent*

**colfosceril palmitate** USAN, INN, BAN
*pulmonary surfactant for hyaline mem-*
*brane disease and neonatal respiratory*
*distress syndrome (orphan); investiga-*
*tional (orphan) for ARDS*

**colfosceril palmitate & phosphati-**
**dylglycerol** *investigational (orphan) for*
*neonatal respiratory distress syndrome*

**coli** *street drug slang* [see: marijuana]

**coliflor tostada** (Spanish for "brown
or toasted cauliflower") *street drug
slang* [see: marijuana]

**colimecycline** INN

**colistimethate sodium** USAN, USP,
INN *bactericidal antibiotic* [also: colistin sulphomethate]

**colistin** INN, BAN *bactericidal antibiotic*
[also: colistin sulfate] ⧉ Colestid;
colestipol

**colistin methanesulfonate** [see: colistimethate sodium]

**colistin sulfate** USP *bactericidal antibi-*
*otic* [also: colistin]

**colistin sulphomethate** BAN *bactericidal*
*antibiotic* [also: colistimethate sodium]

**collagen** *ophthalmic implant to block
puncta and retain moisture*

**collagen, purified type II** *investiga-*
*tional (Phase III, orphan) oral treat-
ment for juvenile rheumatoid arthritis*

**collagenase** *topical proteolytic enzymes
for necrotic tissue debridement; investigational (orphan) for Peyronie's disease*

**collagenase, clostridial** [see: clostridial collagenase]

**Collastin Oil Free Moisturizer**
lotion OTC *moisturizer; emollient* [col-
lagen] ⧧

**collodion** USP *topical protectant*

**colloidal aluminum hydroxide** [see:
aluminum hydroxide gel]

**colloidal oatmeal** *demulcent*

**colloidal silicon dioxide** [see: silicon
dioxide, colloidal]

**Colloral** *investigational (Phase III,
orphan) oral treatment for juvenile
rheumatoid arthritis* [purified type II
collagen]

**Collyrium for Fresh Eyes** ophthalmic solution OTC *extraocular irrigating
solution* [sterile isotonic solution]

**Collyrium Fresh** eye drops OTC *topical
ocular decongestant/vasoconstrictor*
[tetrahydrozoline HCl] 0.05%

**ColoCare** test kit for home use OTC *in
vitro diagnostic aid for fecal occult blood*

**Colombian** *street drug slang* [see: marijuana]

**colony-stimulating factors** *a class of glycoproteins that stimulate the production of granulocytes and macrophages*

**Color Allergy Screening Test (CAST)** reagent assay tubes ℞ *in vitro diagnostic aid for immunoglobulin E in serum*

**Color Ovulation Test** kit for home use OTC *in vitro diagnostic aid to predict ovulation time*

**Colorado cocktail** *street drug slang* [see: marijuana]

**ColoScreen** slide test for professional use *in vitro diagnostic aid for fecal occult blood*

**Colovage** powder for oral solution ℞ *pre-procedure bowel evacuant* [polyethylene glycol-electrolyte solution]

**Col-Probenecid** tablets ℞ *treatment for frequent, recurrent attacks of gouty arthritis* [probenecid; colchicine] 500•0.5 mg

**Coltab Children's** tablets (discontinued 1993) OTC *pediatric decongestant and antihistamine* [phenylephrine HCl; chlorpheniramine maleate]

**colterol** INN *bronchodilator* [also: colterol mesylate]

**colterol mesylate** USAN *bronchodilator* [also: colterol]

**Columbo** *street drug slang* [see: PCP]

**Columbus black** *street drug slang* [see: marijuana]

**Coly-Mycin M** powder for IV or IM injection ℞ *bactericidal antibiotic* [colistimethate sodium] 150 mg

**Coly-Mycin S** powder for oral suspension (discontinued 1996) ℞ *bactericidal antibiotic* [colistin sulfate] 25 mg/5 mL

**Coly-Mycin S Otic** suspension ℞ *topical corticosteroidal anti-inflammatory; antibiotic* [hydrocortisone acetate; neomycin sulfate; colistin sulfate] 1%•4.71 mg•3 mg per mL

**Colyte** powder for oral solution ℞ *pre-procedure bowel evacuant* [polyethylene glycol-electrolyte solution]

**COM (cyclophosphamide, Oncovin, MeCCNU)** *chemotherapy protocol*

**COM (cyclophosphamide, Oncovin, methotrexate)** *chemotherapy protocol*

**COMA-A (cyclophosphamide, Oncovin, methotrexate/citrovorum factor, Adriamycin, ara-C)** *chemotherapy protocol*

**COMB (cyclophosphamide, Oncovin, MeCCNU, bleomycin)** *chemotherapy protocol*

**COMB (Cytoxin, Oncovin, methotrexate, bleomycin)** *chemotherapy protocol*

**Combi-patch** ℞ *investigational transdermal patch for hormone replacement therapy* [estrogen; progestin]

**Combipres 0.1; Combipres 0.2; Combipres 0.3** tablets ℞ *antihypertensive* [clonidine HCl; chlorthalidone] 0.1•15 mg; 0.2•15 mg; 0.3•15 mg ② Catapres

**Combistix** reagent strips *in vitro diagnostic aid for multiple urine products*

**Combivent** inhaler ℞ *bronchodilator for continued bronchospasm with COPD* [ipratropium bromide; albuterol sulfate] 18•103 μg/spray

**COMe (Cytoxin, Oncovin, methotrexate)** *chemotherapy protocol*

**comeback** *street drug slang for the benzocaine and mannitol used in the conversion of cocaine to crack* [see: cocaine; cocaine, crack]

**COMF (cyclophosphamide, Oncovin, methotrexate, fluorouracil)** *chemotherapy protocol*

**Comfort** eye drops OTC *topical ocular decongestant/vasoconstrictor* [naphazoline HCl] 0.03%

**Comfort Tears** eye drops OTC *ocular moisturizer/lubricant* [hydroxyethylcellulose]

**ComfortCare GP Wetting & Soaking** solution OTC *disinfecting/wetting/soaking solution for rigid gas permeable contact lenses*

**Comfortine** ointment OTC *moisturizer; emollient; astringent; antiseptic* [vitamins A and D; lanolin; zinc oxide]

**Comhist** tablets ℞ *decongestant; antihistamine* [phenylephrine HCl;

chlorpheniramine maleate; phenyltoloxamine citrate] 10•2•25 mg

**Comhist LA** long-acting capsules ℞ *decongestant; antihistamine* [phenylephrine HCl; chlorpheniramine maleate; phenyltoloxamine citrate] 20•4•50 mg

**COMLA (cyclophosphamide, Oncovin, methotrexate, leucovorin [rescue], ara-C)** *chemotherapy protocol*

**comosain** *investigational (orphan) for enzymatic debridement of severe burns*

**COMP (CCNU, Oncovin, methotrexate, procarbazine)** *chemotherapy protocol*

**COMP (cyclophosphamide, Oncovin, methotrexate, prednisone)** *chemotherapy protocol*

**Compazine** tablets, Spansules (capsules), IV or IM injection, suppositories, syrup ℞ *antiemetic; tranquilizer* [prochlorperazine maleate] 5, 10, 25 mg; 10, 15, 30 mg; 5 mg/mL; 2.5, 5, 25 mg; 5 mg/5 mL

**Compete** tablets OTC *vitamin/iron supplement* [multiple vitamins; ferrous gluconate; folic acid] ±•27•0.4 mg

**Compleat Modified Formula** closed system containers OTC *enteral nutritional therapy* [lactose-free formula]

**Compleat Modified Formula** ready-to-use liquid OTC *enteral nutritional therapy* [lactose-free formula]

**Compleat Regular Formula** ready-to-use liquid OTC *enteral nutritional therapy* [milk-based formula]

**complement receptor type I, soluble recombinant human** *investigational (orphan) for adult respiratory distress syndrome*

**Complete** solution OTC *rewetting solution for soft contact lenses*

**Complete All-in-One** solution OTC *cleaning/disinfecting/rinsing/storage solution for soft contact lenses*

**Complete Multi-Purpose** solution (name changed to Complete All-In-One in 1995)

**Complete Weekly Enzymatic Cleaner** effervescent tablets OTC *enzymatic cleaner for soft contact lenses* [subtilisin A]

**Complex 15 Face** cream OTC *moisturizer; emollient*

**Complex 15 Hand & Body** cream, lotion OTC *moisturizer; emollient*

**Comply** liquid OTC *enteral nutritional therapy* [lactose-free formula]

**compound 42** [see: warfarin]

**compound CB3025** [see: melphalan]

**compound E** [see: cortisone acetate]

**compound F** [see: hydrocortisone]

**compound insulin zinc suspension** INN *antidiabetic* [also: insulin zinc]

**compound orange spirit** [see: orange spirit, compound]

**compound Q** [see: trichosanthin]

**compound S** [see: zidovudine]

**compound solution of sodium chloride** INN *fluid and electrolyte replenisher* [also: Ringer's injection]

**compound solution of sodium lactate** INN *electrolyte and fluid replenisher; systemic alkalizer* [also: Ringer's injection, lactated]

**Compound W** liquid, gel OTC *topical keratolytic* [salicylic acid in collodion] 17%

**Compoz** gel caps OTC *antihistaminic sleep aid* [diphenhydramine HCl] 25 mg

**Compoz Nighttime Sleep Aid** tablets OTC *antihistaminic sleep aid* [diphenhydramine HCl] 50 mg

**compressible sugar** [see: sugar, compressible]

**Comtrex** caplets, tablets (name changed to Comtrex Multi-Symptom Cold & Flu Relief in 1995)

**Comtrex** liquid OTC *antitussive; decongestant; antihistamine; analgesic* [dextromethorphan hydrobromide; pseudoephedrine HCl; chlorpheniramine maleate; acetaminophen] 3.3•10•0.67•108.3 mg/5 mL

**Comtrex, Cough Formula** liquid OTC *antitussive; decongestant; expectorant; analgesic* [dextromethorphan hydrobromide; pseudoephedrine HCl; guaifenesin; acetaminophen; alcohol 20%] 7.5•15•50•125 mg/5 mL

**Comtrex, Day & Night** daytime caplets + nighttime tablets (discontinued 1995) OTC *antitussive; decongestant; analgesic; (antihistamine added nighttime)* [dextromethorphan hydrobromide; pseudoephedrine HCl; acetaminophen; (chlorpheniramine maleate added nighttime)] 15•30•500 mg daytime; 15•30•500•2 mg nighttime

**Comtrex Allergy-Sinus** caplets, tablets OTC *decongestant; antihistamine; analgesic* [pseudoephedrine HCl; chlorpheniramine maleate; acetaminophen] 30•2•500 mg

**Comtrex Hot Flu Relief** powder (discontinued 1995) OTC *antitussive; decongestant; antihistamine; analgesic* [dextromethorphan hydrobromide; pseudoephedrine HCl; chlorpheniramine maleate; acetaminophen] 20•60•4•500 mg/packet

**Comtrex Liqui-Gels** (liquid-filled capsules) OTC *antitussive; decongestant; antihistamine; analgesic* [dextromethorphan hydrobromide; phenylpropanolamine HCl; chlorpheniramine maleate; acetaminophen] 10•12.5•2•325, 15•12.5•2•500 mg

**Comtrex Multi-Symptom, Day & Night** daytime caplets + nighttime tablets (discontinued 1995) OTC *antitussive; decongestant; analgesic; (antihistamine added nighttime)* [dextromethorphan hydrobromide; pseudoephedrine HCl; acetaminophen; (chlorpheniramine maleate added nighttime)] 10•30•325 mg daytime; 10•30•325•2 mg nighttime

**Comtrex Multi-Symptom Cold & Flu Relief** tablets, caplets OTC *antitussive; decongestant; antihistamine; analgesic* [dextromethorphan hydrobromide; pseudoephedrine HCl; chlorpheniramine maleate; acetaminophen] 15•30•2•500 mg

**Comtrex Multi-Symptom Cold & Flu Relief Liqui-Gels** (capsules) OTC *antitussive; decongestant; antihistamine; analgesic* [dextromethorphan hydrobromide; phenylpropanolamine HCl; chlorpheniramine maleate; acetaminophen] 15•12.5•2•500 mg

**Comtrex Non-Drowsy** caplets OTC *antitussive; decongestant; analgesic* [dextromethorphan hydrobromide; pseudoephedrine HCl; acetaminophen] 15•30•500 mg

**Comvax** IM injection ℞ *infant (1½–15 months) vaccine for H. influenzae and hepatitis B* [Hemophilus b purified capsular polysaccharide; *Neisseria meningitidis* OMPC; hepatitis B surface antigen (recombinant)] 7.5•125•5 μg/0.5 mL

**Conceive Ovulation Predictor** 5-day test kit for professional use *in vitro diagnostic aid to predict ovulation time*

**Conceive Pregnancy** test kit for home use OTC *in vitro diagnostic aid for urine pregnancy test*

**Concentraid** nasal spray, intranasal pipets (discontinued 1994) ℞ *diabetes insipidus; hemophilia A; von Willebrand's disease* [desmopressin acetate]

**Concentrated Cleaner** solution OTC *cleaning solution for rigid gas permeable contact lenses*

**Conceptrol Contraceptive Inserts** vaginal suppositories OTC *spermicidal contraceptive* [nonoxynol 9] 150 mg

**Conceptrol Disposable Contraceptive** vaginal gel OTC *spermicidal contraceptive* [nonoxynol 9] 4%

**Condrin-LA** sustained-release capsules (discontinued 1995) ℞ *decongestant; antihistamine* [phenylpropanolamine HCl; chlorpheniramine maleate] 75•12 mg

**conductor** *street drug slang* [see: LSD]

**Condylox** solution, gel ℞ *topical antimitotic for external genital and perianal warts* [podofilox] 0.5%

**conessine** INN

**conessine hydrobromide** [see: conessine]

**Conex** lozenges (discontinued 1994) OTC *topical oral anesthetic; antiseptic* [benzocaine; cetylpyridinium chloride] 5•0.5 mg

**Conex** syrup OTC *decongestant; expectorant* [phenylpropanolamine HCl; guaifenesin] 12.5•100 mg/5 mL

**Conex D.A.** tablets (discontinued 1993) OTC *decongestant; antihistamine* [phenylpropanolamine HCl; chlorpheniramine maleate]

**Conex Plus** tablets (discontinued 1993) OTC *decongestant; antihistamine; analgesic* [phenylpropanolamine HCl; chlorpheniramine maleate; acetaminophen]

**Conex with Codeine** syrup ℞ *narcotic antitussive; decongestant; expectorant* [codeine phosphate; phenylpropanolamine HCl; guaifenesin] 10•12.5•100 mg/5 mL

**confectioner's sugar** [see: sugar, confectioner's]

**Confide** test kit for home use OTC *in vitro diagnostic aid for HIV in the blood*

**congazone sodium** [see: Congo red]

**Congespirin for Children** chewable tablets (discontinued 1995) OTC *decongestant; analgesic* [phenylephrine HCl; acetaminophen] 1.25•81 mg

**Congess JR** capsules ℞ *decongestant; expectorant* [pseudoephedrine HCl; guaifenesin] 60•125 mg

**Congess SR** sustained-release capsules ℞ *decongestant; expectorant* [pseudoephedrine HCl; guaifenesin] 120•250 mg

**Congestac** caplets OTC *decongestant; expectorant* [pseudoephedrine HCl; guaifenesin] 60•400 mg

**Congestant** tablets (name changed to Improved Congestant in 1995)

**Congestant D** tablets OTC *decongestant; antihistamine; analgesic* [phenylpropanolamine HCl; chlorpheniramine maleate; acetaminophen] 12.5•2•325 mg

**Congestion Relief** tablets OTC *nasal decongestant* [pseudoephedrine HCl] 30, 60 mg

**Congestion Relief, Children's** liquid OTC *nasal decongestant* [pseudoephedrine HCl] 30 mg/5 mL

**Congo red** USP

**conjugated estrogens** [see: estrogens, conjugated]

**conorfone** INN *analgesic* [also: conorphone HCl]

**conorfone HCl** [see: conorphone HCl]

**conorphone HCl** USAN *analgesic* [also: conorfone]

**CONPADRI; CONPADRI-I (cyclophosphamide, Oncovin, L-phenylalanine mustard, Adriamycin)** *chemotherapy protocol*

**Conray; Conray 30; Conray 43** injection ℞ *parenteral radiopaque agent* [iothalamate meglumine] 60%; 30%; 43%

**Conray 325; Conray 400** injection ℞ *parenteral radiopaque agent* [iothalamate sodium] 54.3%; 66.8%

**consensus interferon** *investigational antiviral for hepatitis C and antineoplastic*

**Consonar** ℞ *investigational reversible/selective MAO inhibitor, type A* [brofaromine]

**Constant-T** sustained-action tablets (discontinued 1994) ℞ *bronchodilator* [theophylline] 200, 300 mg

**Constene** ℞ *investigational treatment for constipation* [naloxone]

**Constilac** syrup ℞ *laxative* [lactulose] 10 g/15 mL

**Constulose** syrup ℞ *laxative* [lactulose] 10 g/15 mL

**Contac 12 Hour** sustained-release capsules, sustained-release caplets OTC *decongestant; antihistamine* [phenylpropanolamine HCl; chlorpheniramine maleate] 75•8 mg; 75•12 mg

**Contac Cough & Chest Cold** liquid OTC *antitussive; decongestant; expectorant; analgesic* [dextromethorphan hydrobromide; pseudoephedrine HCl; guaifenesin; acetaminophen; alcohol 10%] 5•15•50•125 mg/5 mL

**Contac Cough Formula** liquid (discontinued 1994) OTC *antitussive; expectorant* [dextromethorphan hydrobromide; guaifenesin]

**Contac Cough & Sore Throat** liquid OTC *antitussive; analgesic* [dextromethorphan hydrobromide; acetaminophen; alcohol 10%] 5•125 mg/5 mL

**Contac Day & Night Allergy/Sinus** daytime caplets + nighttime caplets OTC *decongestant; analgesic; (antihistamine/sleep aid added nighttime)* [pseudoephedrine HCl; acetaminophen; (diphenhydramine HCl added nighttime)] 60•650 mg daytime; 60•650•50 mg nighttime

**Contac Day & Night Cold & Flu** daytime caplets + nighttime caplets OTC *decongestant; analgesic; (antitussive added daytime; antihistamine/sleep aid added nighttime)* [pseudoephedrine HCl; acetaminophen; (dextromethorphan hydrobromide added daytime; diphenhydramine HCl added nighttime)] 60•650•30 mg daytime; 60•650•50 mg nighttime

**Contac Jr. Non-Drowsy Cold** liquid (discontinued 1994) OTC *pediatric antitussive, decongestant, and analgesic* [dextromethorphan hydrobromide; pseudoephedrine HCl; acetaminophen]

**Contac Non-Drowsy Formula Sinus** tablets, caplets (discontinued 1995) OTC *decongestant; analgesic; antipyretic* [pseudoephedrine HCl; acetaminophen] 30•500 mg

**Contac Severe Cold & Flu Formula** caplets (discontinued 1995) OTC *antitussive; decongestant; antihistamine; analgesic* [dextromethorphan hydrobromide; phenylpropanolamine HCl; chlorpheniramine maleate; acetaminophen] 15•12.5•2•500 mg

**Contac Severe Cold & Flu Hot Medicine** powder (discontinued 1995) OTC *antitussive; decongestant; antihistamine; analgesic* [dextromethorphan hydrobromide; pseudoephedrine HCl; chlorpheniramine maleate; acetaminophen] 20•60•4•650 mg/packet

**Contac Severe Cold & Flu Nighttime** liquid OTC *antitussive; decongestant; antihistamine; analgesic* [dextromethorphan hydrobromide; pseudoephedrine HCl; chlorpheniramine maleate; acetaminophen; alcohol 18.5%] 5•10•0.67•167 mg/5 mL

**Contac-C Cold Care Formula** ⒸⒶⓃ (U.S. product: Contac Severe Cold & Flu Formula) caplets OTC *antitussive; decongestant; antihistamine; analgesic* [dextromethorphan hydrobromide; phenylpropanolamine HCl; chlorpheniramine maleate; acetaminophen] 15•12.5•2•500 mg

**contact lens** *street drug slang* [see: LSD]

**conteben** [see: thioacetazone; thiacetazone]

**ConTE-Pak-4** IV injection ℞ *intravenous nutritional therapy* [multiple trace elements (metals)] ≛

**Contigen** urethral injection ℞ *treatment for stress urinary incontinence* [purified collagen implant]

**Contramid** ℞ *investigational (Phase III) controlled-release solid oral form of a racemic albuterol bronchodilator for asthma and COPD* [levalbuterol]

**Contrin** capsules ℞ *hematinic* [ferrous fumarate; cyanocobalamin; ascorbic acid; intrinsic factor concentrate; folic acid] 110 mg•15 μg•75 mg•240 mg•0.5 mg

**Control** timed-release capsules OTC *diet aid* [phenylpropanolamine HCl] 75 mg

**Control-L** liquid (discontinued 1993) OTC *lice treatment* [pyrethrins; piperonyl butoxide; petroleum distillate] 0.3%•3%• ≟

**ControlPak** (trademarked packaging form) *tamper-resistant unit-dose package*

**Contuss** liquid ℞ *decongestant; expectorant* [phenylpropanolamine HCl; phenylephrine HCl; guaifenesin; alcohol 5%] 20•5•100 mg/5 mL

**cookies** *street drug slang* [see: cocaine, crack]

**cooler** *street drug slang for a regular cigarette laced with a drug*

**coolie** *street drug slang for a regular cigarette laced with cocaine* [see: cocaine]

**Cooper's regimen** *chemotherapy protocol* [see: CMFVP]

**COP** [see: creatinolfosfate]

**COP (cyclophosphamide, Oncovin, prednisone)** *chemotherapy protocol*

**COP 1 (copolymer 1)** [see: glatiramer acetate]

**COPA (Cytoxin, Oncovin, prednisone, Adriamycin)** *chemotherapy protocol*

**COPA-BLEO (cyclophosphamide, Oncovin, prednisone, Adriamycin, bleomycin)** *chemotherapy protocol*

**COPAC (CCNU, Oncovin, prednisone, Adriamycin, cyclophosphamide)** *chemotherapy protocol*

**Copaxone** powder for subcu injection ℞ *immunomodulator for relapsing-remitting multiple sclerosis (orphan)* [glatiramer acetate] 20 mg

**COPB (cyclophosphamide, Oncovin, prednisone, bleomycin)** *chemotherapy protocol*

**COP-BLAM (cyclophosphamide, Oncovin, prednisone, bleomycin, Adriamycin, Matulane)** *chemotherapy protocol*

**COP-BLEO (cyclophosphamide, Oncovin, prednisone, bleomycin)** *chemotherapy protocol*

**Cope** tablets OTC *analgesic; antipyretic; anti-inflammatory; antacid* [aspirin; caffeine; magnesium hydroxide; aluminum hydroxide] 421•32•50•25 mg

**COPE (cyclophosphamide, Oncovin, Platinol, etoposide)** *chemotherapy protocol*

**Cophene No. 2** sustained-release capsules ℞ *decongestant; antihistamine* [pseudoephedrine HCl; chlorpheniramine maleate] 120•12 mg

**Cophene XP** liquid ℞ *narcotic antitussive; decongestant; expectorant* [hydrocodone bitartrate; pseudoephedrine HCl; guaifenesin; alcohol 12.5%] 5•60•200 mg/5 mL

**Cophene-B** subcu or IM injection ℞ *antihistamine; anaphylaxis* [brompheniramine maleate] 10 mg/mL

**Cophene-X** capsules ℞ *antitussive; decongestant; expectorant* [carbetapentane citrate; phenylephrine HCl; phenylpropanolamine HCl; potassium guaiacolsulfonate] 20•10•10•45 mg

**co-pilot** *street drug slang* [see: amphetamines]

**copolymer 1 (COP 1)** [see: glatiramer acetate]

**copovithane** BAN

**COPP (CCNU, Oncovin, procarbazine, prednisone)** *chemotherapy protocol*

**COPP (cyclophosphamide, Oncovin, procarbazine, prednisone)** *chemotherapy protocol*

**copper** *element (Cu)*

**copper chloride dihydrate** [see: cupric chloride]

**copper gluconate (copper D-gluconate)** USP *trace mineral supplement*

**copper sulfate pentahydrate** [see: cupric sulfate]

**copper 10-undecenoate** [see: copper undecylenate]

**copper undecylenate** USAN

**copperhead snake antivenin** [see: antivenin (Crotalidae) polyvalent]

**Co-Pyronil 2** Pulvules (capsules) OTC *decongestant; antihistamine* [pseudoephedrine HCl; chlorpheniramine maleate] 60•4 mg

**CoQ10** [see: coenzyme Q10]

**Coracin** ophthalmic ointment (discontinued 1995) ℞ *topical ophthalmic corticosteroidal anti-inflammatory; antibiotic* [hydrocortisone acetate; neomycin sulfate; bacitracin zinc; polymyxin B sulfate] 1%•0.5%•400 U/g•10 000 U/g

**coral** *street drug slang for various CNS depressants*

**coral snake antivenin** [see: antivenin (Micrurus fulvius)]

**corbadrine** INN *adrenergic; vasoconstrictor* [also: levonordefrin]

**Cordarone** tablets, IV infusion ℞ *antiarrhythmic for acute ventricular tachycardia and fibrillation (orphan)* [amiodarone HCl] 200 mg; 50 mg/mL

**Cordran** ointment, lotion, tape ℞ *topical corticosteroid* [flurandrenolide] 0.025%, 0.05%; 0.05%; 4 μg/cm²

**Cordran SP** cream ℞ *topical corticosteroid* [flurandrenolide] 0.025%, 0.05%

**Cordran-N** cream, ointment (discontinued 1993) ℞ *topical corticosteroid; antibiotic* [flurandrenolide; neomycin sulfate]

**Coreg** Tiltab (film-coated tablets) ℞ *antihypertensive; α- and β-blocker for congestive heart failure* [carvedilol] 3.125, 6.25, 12.5, 25 mg

**Corgard** tablets ℞ *antihypertensive; antianginal; β-blocker* [nadolol] 20, 40, 80, 120, 160 mg

**coriander oil** NF

**Coricidin** Demilets (chewable tablets) (discontinued 1993) OTC *pediatric decongestant, antihistamine and analgesic* [phenylpropanolamine HCl; chlorpheniramine maleate; acetaminophen]

**Coricidin** tablets OTC *antihistamine; analgesic* [chlorpheniramine maleate; acetaminophen] 2•325 mg

**Coricidin D; Coricidin Sinus Headache** tablets OTC *decongestant; antihistamine; analgesic* [phenylpropanolamine HCl; chlorpheniramine maleate; acetaminophen] 12.5•2•325 mg; 12.5•2•500 mg

**cork the air** *street drug slang for inhaling (snorting) cocaine* [see: cocaine]

**Corlopam** (commercially available overseas) ℞ *investigational vasodilator for severe hypertension and chronic renal failure* [fenoldopam]

**Cormax** ointment ℞ *topical corticosteroidal anti-inflammatory* [clobetasol propionate] 0.05%

**cormed** [see: nikethamide]

**cormetasone** INN *topical anti-inflammatory* [also: cormethasone acetate]

**cormetasone acetate** [see: cormethasone acetate]

**cormethasone acetate** USAN *topical anti-inflammatory* [also: cormetasone]

**Corn Huskers** lotion OTC *moisturizer; emollient*

**corn oil** NF *solvent; caloric replacement*

**corpus luteum extract** [see: progesterone]

**Corque** cream ℞ *topical corticosteroid; antifungal; antibacterial* [hydrocortisone; clioquinol] 1%•3%

**Correctol** tablets (discontinued 1996) OTC *laxative; stool softener* [yellow phenolphthalein; docusate sodium] 65•100 mg

**Correctol Extra Gentle** soft gel capsules OTC *stool softener* [docusate sodium] 100 mg

**Corrine** *street drug slang* [see: cocaine]

**Corsevin M** ℞ *investigational agent for coagulation disorders and unstable angina* [monoclonal antibodies]

**CortaGel** OTC *topical corticosteroid* [hydrocortisone] 1%

**Cortaid** cream, ointment OTC *topical corticosteroid* [hydrocortisone acetate] 1%

**Cortaid** lotion (discontinued 1997) OTC *topical corticosteroid* [hydrocortisone acetate] 1%

**Cortaid** pump spray OTC *topical corticosteroid* [hydrocortisone] 1%

**Cortaid Faststick** roll-on stick OTC *topical corticosteroid* [hydrocortisone; alcohol 55%] 1%

**Cortaid Intensive Therapy** cream OTC *topical corticosteroid* [hydrocortisone] 1%

**Cortaid with Aloe** cream, ointment OTC *topical corticosteroid* [hydrocortisone acetate] 0.5%

**Cortatrigen Modified** ear drops, otic suspension ℞ *topical corticosteroidal anti-inflammatory; antibiotic* [hydrocortisone; neomycin sulfate; polymyxin B sulfate] 1%•5 mg•10 000 U per mL

**Cort-Dome** cream ℞ *topical corticosteroid* [hydrocortisone] 0.5%, 1% ⧉ Cortone

**Cort-Dome** lotion (discontinued 1993) ℞ *topical corticosteroid* [hydrocortisone]

**Cort-Dome High Potency** rectal suppositories ℞ *topical corticosteroidal anti-inflammatory* [hydrocortisone acetate] 25 mg

**Cortef** tablets, oral suspension ℞ *glucocorticoids* [hydrocortisone] 5, 10, 20 mg; 10 mg/5 mL

**Cortef Feminine Itch** cream OTC *topical corticosteroid* [hydrocortisone acetate] 0.5%

**Cortenema** retention enema ℞ *ulcerative colitis* [hydrocortisone] 100 mg/60 mL ⧉ quart enema

**cortenil** [see: desoxycorticosterone acetate]

**cortexolone** [see: cortodoxone]

**Cortic** ear drops ℞ *topical corticosteroidal anti-inflammatory; topical anesthetic; bacteriostatic* [hydrocortisone; pramoxine HCl; chloroxylenol] 10•10•1 mg/mL

**Corticaine** anorectal cream (discontinued 1995) OTC *topical corticosteroidal anti-inflammatory; local anes-*

*thetic* [hydrocortisone acetate; dibucaine] 0.5%•0.5%

**Corticaine** cream OTC *topical corticosteroid* [hydrocortisone acetate] 0.5%

**corticorelin ovine triflutate** USAN, INN *corticotropin-releasing hormone; diagnostic aid for Cushing syndrome and adrenocortical insufficiency (orphan)*

**corticosteroids** *a class of anti-inflammatory drugs*

**corticotrophin** INN, BAN *adrenocorticotropic hormone; glucocorticoid; diagnostic aid* [also: corticotropin]

**corticotrophin-zinc hydroxide** INN *adrenocorticotropic hormone; glucocorticoid; diagnostic aid* [also: corticotropin zinc hydroxide]

**corticotropin** USP *adrenocorticotropic hormone; glucocorticoid; diagnostic aid* [also: corticotrophin] 40 U/vial injection

**corticotropin, repository** USP *adrenocorticotropic hormone; glucocorticoid; diagnostic aid*

**corticotropin tetracosapeptide** [see: cosyntropin]

**corticotropin zinc hydroxide** USP *adrenocorticotropic hormone; glucocorticoid; diagnostic aid* [also: corticotrophin-zinc hydroxide]

**Cortifoam** intrarectal foam aerosol ℞ *ulcerative proctitis* [hydrocortisone acetate] 90 mg/dose

**Cortin** cream ℞ *topical corticosteroid; antifungal; antibacterial* [hydrocortisone; clioquinol] ⊠ Cotrim

**cortisol** [see: hydrocortisone]

**cortisol 21-acetate** [see: hydrocortisone acetate]

**cortisol 21-butyrate** [see: hydrocortisone butyrate]

**cortisol 21-cyclopentanepropionate** [see: hydrocortisone cypionate]

**cortisol cyclopentylpropionate** [see: hydrocortisone cypionate]

**cortisol 21-valerate** [see: hydrocortisone valerate]

**cortisone** INN, BAN *glucocorticoid* [also: cortisone acetate] ⊠ Cortizone

**cortisone acetate** USP *glucocorticoid* [also: cortisone] 5, 10, 25 mg oral

**Cortisporin** cream ℞ *topical corticosteroid; antibiotic* [hydrocortisone acetate; neomycin sulfate; polymyxin B sulfate] 0.5%•0.5%•10 000 U per g

**Cortisporin** eye drop suspension ℞ *topical ophthalmic corticosteroidal anti-inflammatory; antibiotic* [hydrocortisone; neomycin sulfate; polymyxin B sulfate] 1%•0.35%•10 000 U per mL

**Cortisporin** ointment ℞ *topical corticosteroid; antibiotic* [hydrocortisone; neomycin sulfate; bacitracin zinc; polymyxin B sulfate] 1%•0.5%•400 U•5000 U per g

**Cortisporin** ophthalmic ointment ℞ *topical ophthalmic corticosteroidal anti-inflammatory; antibiotic* [hydrocortisone; neomycin sulfate; bacitracin zinc; polymyxin B sulfate] 1%•0.35%•400 U/g•10 000 U/g

**Cortisporin Otic** ear drops, otic suspension ℞ *topical corticosteroidal anti-inflammatory; antibiotic* [hydrocortisone; neomycin sulfate; polymyxin B sulfate] 1%•5 mg•10 000 U per mL

**cortisuzol** INN

**cortivazol** USAN, INN *glucocorticoid*

**Cortizone-5** ointment, cream OTC *topical corticosteroid* [hydrocortisone] 0.5%; 1% ⊠ cortisone

**Cortizone-10** ointment OTC *topical corticosteroid* [hydrocortisone] 1%

**cortodoxone** USAN, INN, BAN *anti-inflammatory*

**Cortone Acetate** tablets, intra-articular or intralesional injection ℞ *glucocorticoids* [cortisone acetate] 25 mg; 50 mg/mL ⊠ Cort-Dome

**Cortril** ointment (discontinued 1993) ℞ *topical corticosteroid* [hydrocortisone]

**Cortrosyn** powder for injection ℞ *multiple sclerosis; infantile spasms; diagnostic purposes* [cosyntropin] 0.25 mg

**Corvert** IV infusion ℞ *antiarrhythmic for atrial fibrillation/flutter* [ibutilide fumarate] 0.1 mg/mL

**Corzide 40/5; Corzide 80/5** tablets ℞ *antihypertensive* [nadolol; bendroflumethiazide] 40•5 mg; 80•5 mg

**cosa** (Spanish and Italian for "thing") *street drug slang* [see: marijuana]

**Cosmegen** powder for IV injection ℞ *antibiotic antineoplastic for melanomas, sarcomas, testicular and trophoblastic tumors* [dactinomycin] 0.5 mg

**cosmoline** [see: petrolatum]

**Cozmo's** *street drug slang* [see: PCP]

**cosyntropin** USAN *adrenocorticotropic hormone* [also: tetracosactide; tetracosactrin]

**cotarnine chloride** NF

**cotarnine HCl** [see: cotarnine chloride]

**Cotazym** capsules ℞ *digestive enzymes; antacid* [lipase; protease; amylase; calcium carbonate] 8000 U•30 000 U•30 000 U•25 mg

**Cotazym-S** capsules containing enteric-coated spheres ℞ *digestive enzymes* [lipase; protease; amylase] 5000•20 000•20 000 U

**'cotics** *street drug slang ("narcotics")* [see: heroin]

**cotinine** INN *antidepressant* [also: cotinine fumarate]

**cotinine fumarate** USAN *antidepressant* [also: cotinine]

**Cotridin** ⓒ syrup ℞ *narcotic antitussive; decongestant; antihistamine* [codeine phosphate; pseudoephedrine HCl; triprolidine HCl] 2•6•0.4 mg/mL

**Cotridin Expectorant** ⓒ oral solution ℞ *narcotic antitussive; decongestant; antihistamine* [codeine phosphate; pseudoephedrine HCl; triprolidine HCl; guaifenesin] 2•6•0.4•20 mg/mL

**Cotrim; Cotrim D.S.** tablets ℞ *anti-infective; antibacterial* [trimethoprim; sulfamethoxazole] 80•400 mg; 160•800 mg ☒ Cortin

**Cotrim IV** infusion (discontinued 1994) ℞ *anti-infective; antibacterial* [trimethoprim; sulfamethoxazole] 16•80 mg/mL

**Cotrim Pediatric** oral suspension ℞ *anti-infective; antibacterial* [trimethoprim; sulfamethoxazole] 40•200 mg/5 mL

**co-trimoxazole** BAN [also: trimethoprim + sulfamethoxazole] ☒ clotrimazole

**cotriptyline** INN

**cotton, purified** USP *surgical aid*

**cotton brothers** *street drug slang for a combination of cocaine, heroin, and morphine* [see: cocaine; heroin; morphine]

**cotton fever** *street drug slang for septicemia caused by injecting small amounts of cotton fiber with the drugs*

**cottonseed oil** NF *solvent*

**Co-Tuss V** liquid ℞ *narcotic antitussive; expectorant* [hydrocodone bitartrate; guaifenesin] 5•100 mg

**Cough** syrup OTC *antitussive; decongestant; expectorant* [dextromethorphan hydrobromide; phenylephrine HCl; guaifenesin] 10•5•100 mg/5 mL

**Cough Formula** liquid OTC *antitussive; antihistamine* [dextromethorphan hydrobromide; chlorpheniramine maleate; alcohol 10%] 15•2 mg/5 mL

**Cough Formula with Decongestant** liquid OTC *antitussive; decongestant* [dextromethorphan hydrobromide; pseudoephedrine HCl; alcohol 10%] 10•20 mg/5 mL

**Cough-X** lozenges OTC *antitussive; topical oral anesthetic* [dextromethorphan hydrobromide; benzocaine] 5•2 mg

**Coulter HIV-1 p24 Antigen Assay** test for professional use *in vitro diagnostic aid for HIV in the blood*

**Coumadin** tablets, powder for IV injection ℞ *coumarin-derivative anticoagulant* [warfarin sodium] 1, 2, 2.5, 3, 4, 5, 6, 7.5, 10 mg; 2 mg ☒ Kemadrin

**coumafos** INN [also: coumaphos]

**coumamycin** INN *antibacterial* [also: coumermycin]

**coumaphos** BAN [also: coumafos]

**coumarin** NF *anticoagulant; investigational (orphan) for renal cell carcinoma*

**coumarins** *a class of anticoagulants that interfere with vitamin K-dependent clotting factors*

**coumazoline** INN

**coumermycin** USAN *antibacterial* [also: coumamycin]

**coumermycin sodium** USAN *antibacterial*

**coumetarol** INN [also: cumetharol]

**courage pills** *street drug slang for heroin or various CNS depressants* [see: heroin]

**Covangesic** tablets OTC *decongestant; antihistamine; analgesic* [phenylpropanolamine HCl; phenylephrine HCl; chlorpheniramine maleate; pyrilamine maleate; acetaminophen] 12.5•7.5•2•12.5•275 mg

**covatin HCl** [see: captodiame HCl]

**Covera-HS** film-coated, extended-release tablets ℞ *antihypertensive; antianginal; calcium channel blocker* [verapamil HCl] 180, 240 mg

**COX-2 (cyclooxygenase-2) inhibitors** *a class of investigational anti-inflammatory drugs*

**Cozaar** film-coated tablets ℞ *antihypertensive; angiotensin II receptor antagonist* [losartan potassium] 25, 50 mg

**CP (chlorambucil, prednisone)** *chemotherapy protocol*

**CP (cyclophosphamide, Platinol)** *chemotherapy protocol*

**CP (cyclophosphamide, prednisone)** *chemotherapy protocol*

**CPA TR** extended-release capsules (discontinued 1993) ℞ *decongestant; antihistamine* [phenylpropanolamine HCl; chlorpheniramine maleate]

**CPB (cyclophosphamide, Platinol, BCNU)** *chemotherapy protocol*

**CPC (cyclophosphamide, Platinol, carboplatin)** *chemotherapy protocol*

**CPMBHFBVD**

**CPM (CCNU, procarbazine, methotrexate)** *chemotherapy protocol*

**CPOB (cyclophosphamide, prednisone, Oncovin, bleomycin)** *chemotherapy protocol*

**CPT-11 (camptothecin-11)** [see: irinotecan]

$^{51}$**Cr** [see: albumin, chromated Cr 51 serum]

$^{51}$**Cr** [see: chromic chloride Cr 51]

$^{51}$**Cr** [see: chromic phosphate Cr 51]

$^{51}$**Cr** [see: sodium chromate Cr 51]

**crack** *street drug slang* [see: cocaine, crack]

**crack back** *street drug slang for a combination of crack and marijuana* [see: cocaine, crack; marijuana]

**crack cooler** *street drug slang for crack soaked in a wine cooler* [see: cocaine, crack]

**crackers** *street drug slang* [see: cocaine, crack]

**crank** *street drug slang for various amphetamines, especially methamphetamine, or methcathinone* [see: amphetamines; methamphetamine HCl; methcathinone]

**crazy coke; crazy Eddie** *street drug slang* [see: PCP]

**crazy weed** *street drug slang* [see: marijuana]

**CRDS (curdlan sulfate)** [q.v.]

**cream and crimson** *street drug slang for Dalmane (flurazepam HCl), named for the white and red capsules* [see: Dalmane; flurazepam HCl]

**Creamy Tar** shampoo OTC *antiseborrheic; antipsoriatic; antipruritic; antibacterial* [coal tar] 7.32%

**creatinolfosfate** INN

**Creon** capsules containing enteric-coated microspheres ℞ *digestive enzymes* [pancreatin; lipase; protease; amylase] 300 mg•8000 U•13 000 U•30 000 U

**Creon 10; Creon 20** capsules containing enteric-coated microspheres ℞ *digestive enzymes* [lipase; amylase; protease] 10 000•33 200•37 500 U; 20 000•66 400•75 000 U

**Creon 25** capsules containing enteric-coated microspheres (discontinued 1994) ℞ *digestive enzymes* [lipase; amylase; protease; pancreatin] 25 000 U•74 700 U•62 500 U•300 mg

**creosote carbonate** USP

**Creo-Terpin** liquid OTC *antitussive* [dextromethorphan hydrobromide; alcohol 25%] 10 mg/15 mL

**cresol** NF *disinfectant*

**cresotamide** INN

**cresoxydiol** [see: mephenesin]

**crestomycin sulfate** [see: paromomycin sulfate]

**Cresylate** ear drops ℞ *antibacterial/antifungal* [m-cresyl acetate; alcohol; chlorobutanol] 25%•25%•1%

**cresylic acid** [see: cresol]

**crib** *street drug slang* [see: cocaine, crack]

**crilanomer** INN

**crilvastatin** USAN, INN *antihyperlipidemic*

**crimmie** *street drug slang for a regular cigarette laced with crack* [see: cocaine, crack]

**crink** *street drug slang* [see: methamphetamine HCl]

**Crinone 8%** gel ℞ *progestin replacement or supplementation for assisted reproductive technology (ART) treatment* [progesterone] 8%

**cripple** *street drug slang for a marijuana cigarette* [see: marijuana]

**cris; Chris; Cristina; Christina** *street drug slang* [see: methamphetamine HCl]

**crisnatol** INN *antineoplastic* [also: crisnatol mesylate]

**crisnatol mesylate** USAN *antineoplastic* [also: crisnatol]

**crisscross** *street drug slang* [see: amphetamines]

**Cristina; Christina; cris; Chris** *street drug slang* [see: methamphetamine HCl]

**Cristy; Christy** *street drug slang for smokable methamphetamine* [see: methamphetamine HCl]

**Criticare HN** ready-to-use liquid OTC *enteral nutritional therapy* [lactose-free formula]

**Crixivan** capsules ℞ *antiviral protease inhibitor for HIV* [indinavir sulfate] 200, 400 mg

**croak** *street drug slang for a combination of crack and methamphetamine* [see: cocaine, crack; methamphetamine HCl]

**crobefate** INN *combining name for radicals or groups*

**croconazole** INN

**crofilcon A** USAN *hydrophilic contact lens material*

**Crolom** eye drops ℞ *mast cell stabilizer; ocular antiallergic/antiviral for vernal keratoconjunctivitis (orphan)* [cromolyn sodium] 4%

**cromacate** INN *combining name for radicals or groups*

**cromakalim** INN, BAN

**Cro-Man-Zin** tablets OTC *mineral supplement* [chromium; manganese; zinc] 0.2•5•25 mg

**cromesilate** INN *combining name for radicals or groups*

**cromitrile** INN *antiasthmatic* [also: cromitrile sodium]

**cromitrile sodium** USAN *antiasthmatic* [also: cromitrile]

**cromoglicic acid** INN *prophylactic antiasthmatic* [also: cromolyn sodium; cromoglycic acid]

**cromoglycic acid** BAN *prophylactic antiasthmatic* [also: cromolyn sodium; cromoglicic acid]

**cromolyn sodium** USAN, USP *prophylactic antiasthmatic; treatment for mastocytosis and vernal keratoconjunctivitis (orphan)* [also: cromoglicic acid; cromoglycic acid] 20 mg/2 mL inhalation

**Cronassial** ℞ *orphan status withdrawn 1996* [gangliosides, sodium salts]

**cronetal** [see: disulfiram]

**cronidipine** INN

**crop** *street drug slang for low-quality heroin* [see: heroin]

**cropropamide** INN, BAN

**croscarmellose** INN *tablet disintegrant* [also: croscarmellose sodium]

**croscarmellose sodium** USAN, NF *tablet disintegrant* [also: croscarmellose]

**crosfumaril** [see: hemoglobin crosfumaril]

**crospovidone** NF *tablet excipient*

**cross tops** *street drug slang* [see: amphetamines]

**cross-linked carboxymethylcellulose sodium** [now: croscarmellose sodium]

**cross-linked carmellose sodium** [see: croscarmellose sodium]

**crossroads** *street drug slang* [see: amphetamines]

**CroTab** ℞ *investigational (orphan) treatment of Crotalidae snake bites* [antivenin (Crotalidae) polyvalent (ovine) Fab]

**crotaline antivenin** [see: antivenin (Crotalidae) polyvalent]

**crotamiton** USP, INN, BAN *scabicide*

**crotetamide** INN [also: crotethamide]

**crotethamide** BAN [also: crotetamide]

**crotoniazide** INN

**crotonylidenisoniazid** [see: crotoniazide]

**crotoxyfos** BAN

**crown crap** *street drug slang* [see: heroin]

**crude tuberculin** [see: tuberculin, old]

**Cruex** cream, aerosol powder OTC *topical antifungal* [undecylenic acid; zinc undecylenate] 20% total; 19% total

**Cruex** powder OTC *topical antifungal* [calcium undecylenate] 10%

**crufomate** USAN, INN, BAN *veterinary anthelmintic*

**crumbs** *street drug slang for tiny pieces of crack* [see: cocaine, crack]

**crunch and munch** *street drug slang* [see: cocaine, crack]

**'cruz** *street drug slang for opium from Veracruz, Mexico* [see: opium]

**crying weed** *street drug slang* [see: marijuana]

**cryofluorane** INN *aerosol propellant* [also: dichlorotetrafluoroethane]

**cryptenamine acetates**

**crypto** *street drug slang* [see: methamphetamine HCl]

**CryptoGAM** Rx *investigational treatment for cryptosporidiosis in immunocompromised patients*

**Crypto-LA** slide test for professional use *in vitro diagnostic aid for Cryptococcus neoformans antigens*

**cryptosporidium hyperimmune bovine colostrum IgG concentrate** *investigational (orphan) for cryptosporidium-induced diarrhea in AIDS*

**Cryptosporidium parvum bovine immunoglobulin concentrate** [see: bovine immunoglobulin concentrate]

**crystal** *street drug slang* [see: methamphetamine HCl; Desoxyn; amphetamines; PCP; cocaine]

**crystal; krystal; crystal joint; krystal joint** *street drug slang* [see: PCP]

**crystal joint** *street drug slang* [see: PCP]

**crystal meth** *street drug slang* [see: methamphetamine HCl]

**crystal tea; crystal T** *street drug slang* [see: LSD; PCP]

**crystal violet** [see: gentian violet]

**crystallized trypsin** [see: trypsin, crystallized]

**Crystamine** IM or subcu injection Rx *antianemic; vitamin $B_{12}$ supplement* [cyanocobalamin] 1000 μg/mL

**Crysti 12** IM or subcu injection (discontinued 1994) Rx *antianemic; vitamin $B_{12}$ supplement* [cyanocobalamin] 1000 μg/mL

**Crysti 1000** IM or subcu injection Rx *antianemic; vitamin $B_{12}$ supplement* [cyanocobalamin] 1000 μg/mL

**Crysticillin 300 A.S.; Crysticillin 600 A.S.** IM injection Rx *bactericidal antibiotic* [penicillin G procaine] 300 000 U/mL; 600 000 U/mL

**Crysti-Liver** IM injection (discontinued 1994) Rx *antianemic; vitamin supplement* [liver extracts; vitamin $B_{12}$; folic acid]

**Crystodigin** tablets Rx *cardiac glycoside to increase cardiac output; antiarrhythmic* [digitoxin] 0.05, 0.1 mg

**crystografin** [see: meglumine diatriazole]

**$^{131}$Cs** [see: cesium chloride Cs 131]

**C-Solve** OTC *lotion base*

**C-Solve 2** topical solution (discontinued 1994) Rx *topical antibiotic for acne* [erythromycin] 2%

**CSP (cellulose sodium phosphate)** [q.v.]

**CT (cisplatin, Taxol)** *chemotherapy protocol*

**CT (cytarabine, thioguanine)** *chemotherapy protocol*

**CTAB (cetyltrimethyl ammonium bromide)**

**CTCb (cyclophosphamide, thiotepa, carboplatin)** *chemotherapy protocol*

**CTH (ceramide trihexosidase)** [q.v.]

**C/T/S** topical solution Rx *topical antibiotic for acne* [clindamycin phosphate] 10 mg/mL

**Ctx-Plat (cyclophosphamide, Platinol)** *chemotherapy protocol*

**$^{64}$Cu** [see: cupric acetate Cu 64]

**cube; cubes** *street drug slang for morphine, LSD, marijuana tablets, or 1 oz. of any drug* [see: morphine; LSD; marijuana]

**culican** *street drug slang for high-potency marijuana from Mexico* [see: marijuana]

**Culturette 10 Minute Group A Strep ID** slide test for professional use *in vitro diagnostic test for Group A* streptococcal antigens in throat swabs [latex agglutination test]

**cumetharol** BAN [also: coumetarol]

**cupcakes** street drug slang [see: LSD]

**cupric acetate Cu 64** USAN radioactive agent

**cupric chloride** USP dietary copper supplement

**cupric sulfate** USP antidote to phosphorus; dietary copper supplement 0.4, 2 mg/mL injection

**Cuprimine** capsules ℞ metal chelating agent for rheumatoid arthritis, Wilson's disease, and cystinuria [penicillamine] 125, 250 mg

**cuprimyxin** USAN, INN veterinary antibacterial; antifungal

**cuproxoline** INN, BAN

**cura** (Spanish for "cure"; Italian for "care") street drug slang [see: heroin]

**curare** [see: tubocurarine chloride]

**curdlan sulfate (CRDS)** investigational (Phase I/II) antiviral for HIV

**Curel Moisturizing** cream, lotion (discontinued 1993) OTC moisturizer; emollient

**curium** element (Cm)

**Curosurf** ℞ investigational (orphan) for infant respiratory distress syndrome of prematurity [pulmonary surfactant replacement, porcine]

**curral** [see: diallybarbituric acid]

**Curretab** tablets ℞ progestin for secondary amenorrhea or abnormal uterine bleeding [medroxyprogesterone acetate] 10 mg

**Cūtar Bath Oil Emulsion** OTC antipsoriatic; antiseborrheic; antipruritic; emollient [coal tar] 7.5%

**cut-deck** street drug slang for heroin mixed with powdered milk [see: heroin]

**Cūtemol** cream OTC moisturizer; emollient [allantoin]

**Cuticura** ointment (discontinued 1995) OTC topical acne treatment [sulfur; phenol; oxyquinoline] 0.5%•0.1%•0.05%

**Cuticura Acne** cream (discontinued 1994) OTC topical keratolytic for acne [benzoyl peroxide] 5%

**Cuticura Medicated Soap** bar OTC therapeutic skin cleanser [triclocarban] 1%

**Cutivate** cream, ointment ℞ topical corticosteroidal anti-inflammatory [fluticasone propionate] 0.05%; 0.005%

**CV (cisplatin, VePesid)** chemotherapy protocol

**CVA (cyclophosphamide, vincristine, Adriamycin)** chemotherapy protocol

**CVA-BMP; CVA + BMP (cyclophosphamide, vincristine, Adriamycin, BCNU, methotrexate, procarbazine)** chemotherapy protocol

**CVAD; C-VAD (cyclophosphamide, vincristine, Adriamycin, dexamethasone)** chemotherapy protocol

**CVB (CCNU, vinblastine, bleomycin)** chemotherapy protocol

**CVBD (CCNU, bleomycin, vinblastine, dexamethasone)** chemotherapy protocol

**CVD (cisplatin, vinblastine, dacarbazine)** chemotherapy protocol

**CVEB (cisplatin, vinblastine, etoposide, bleomycin)** chemotherapy protocol

**CVI (carboplatin, VePesid, ifosfamide [with mesna rescue])** chemotherapy protocol [also: VIC]

**CVM (cyclophosphamide, vincristine, methotrexate)** chemotherapy protocol

**CVP (cyclophosphamide, vincristine, prednisone)** chemotherapy protocol

**CVPP (CCNU, vinblastine, procarbazine, prednisone)** chemotherapy protocol

**CVPP (cyclophosphamide, Velban, procarbazine, prednisone)** chemotherapy protocol

**CVPP-CCNU (cyclophosphamide, vinblastine, procarbazine, prednisone, CCNU)** chemotherapy protocol

**CY-1503** investigational (orphan) for post-ischemic pulmonary reperfusion edema

**CY-1787** investigational E-selectin blocker for sepsis

**CY-1899** investigational (orphan) for chronic active hepatitis B

**cyacetacide** INN [also: cyacetazide]

**cyacetazide** BAN [also: cyacetacide]

**CyADIC (cyclophosphamide, Adriamycin, DIC)** *chemotherapy protocol*

**cyamemazine** INN

**cyamepromazine** [see: cyamemazine]

**cyanamide** JAN [also: calcium carbimide]

**Cyanide Antidote Package** ℞ *emergency treatment of cyanide poisoning* [sodium nitrite; sodium thiosulfate; amyl nitrite inhalant] 300 mg•12.5 g•0.3 mL

**cyanoacetohydrazide** [see: cyacetazide]

**cyanocobalamin** USP, INN, BAN, JAN *vitamin B$_{12}$; hematopoietic* 25, 50, 100, 250, 500, 1000 μg oral; 100, 1000 μg/mL injection

**cyanocobalamin ($^{57}$Co)** INN *pernicious anemia test; radioactive agent* [also: cyanocobalamin Co 57]

**cyanocobalamin ($^{58}$Co)** INN

**cyanocobalamin ($^{60}$Co)** INN *pernicious anemia test; radioactive agent* [also: cyanocobalamin Co 60]

**cyanocobalamin Co 57** USAN, USP *pernicious anemia test; radioactive agent* [also: cyanocobalamin ($^{57}$Co)]

**cyanocobalamin Co 60** USAN, USP *pernicious anemia test; radioactive agent* [also: cyanocobalamin ($^{60}$Co)]

**Cyanoject** IM or subcu injection ℞ *antianemic; vitamin B$_{12}$ supplement* [cyanocobalamin] 1000 μg/mL

**cyclacillin** USAN, USP *antibacterial* [also: ciclacillin]

**cyclamate calcium** NF

**cyclamic acid** USAN, BAN *non-nutritive sweetener (banned in USA)*

**cyclamide** [see: glycyclamide]

**Cyclan** capsules (discontinued 1997) ℞ *peripheral vasodilator; vascular smooth muscle relaxant* [cyclandelate] 200, 400 mg

**cyclandelate** INN, BAN, JAN *peripheral vasodilator; vascular smooth muscle relaxant* 200, 400 mg oral

**cyclarbamate** INN, BAN

**cyclazocine** USAN, INN *analgesic*

**cyclazodone** INN

**cyclexanone** INN

**cyclic propylene carbonate** [see: propylene carbonate]

**cyclindole** USAN *antidepressant* [also: ciclindole]

**cycline; cyclones** *street drug slang* [see: PCP]

**Cyclinex-1** powder OTC *formula for infants with urea cycle disorders or gyrate atrophy*

**Cyclinex-2** powder OTC *enteral nutritional therapy for urea cycle disorders or gyrate atrophy* [essential amino acids]

**cycliramine** INN *antihistamine* [also: cycliramine maleate]

**cycliramine maleate** USAN *antihistamine* [also: cycliramine]

**cyclizine** USP, INN, BAN *antihistamine; antiemetic; anticholinergic; motion sickness relief*

**cyclizine HCl** USP, BAN *antiemetic*

**cyclizine lactate** USP, BAN *antinauseant*

**cyclobarbital** NF, INN [also: cyclobarbitone]

**cyclobarbital calcium** NF

**cyclobarbitone** BAN [also: cyclobarbital]

**cyclobendazole** USAN *anthelmintic* [also: ciclobendazole]

**cyclobenzaprine** INN *skeletal muscle relaxant* [also: cyclobenzaprine HCl]

**cyclobenzaprine HCl** USAN, USP *skeletal muscle relaxant* [also: cyclobenzaprine] 10 mg oral

**cyclobutoic acid** INN

**cyclobutyrol** INN

**cyclocarbothiamine** [see: cycotiamine]

**Cyclocort** ointment, cream, lotion ℞ *topical corticosteroid* [amcinonide] 0.1%

**cyclocoumarol** BAN

**cyclocumarol** [see: cyclocoumarol]

**α-cyclodextrin** [see: alfadex]

**Cyclofed Pediatric** syrup ℞ *pediatric narcotic antitussive, decongestant, and expectorant* [codeine phosphate; pseudoephedrine HCl; guaifenesin; alcohol 6%] 10•30•100 mg/5 mL

**cyclofenil** INN, BAN

**cyclofilcon A** USAN *hydrophilic contact lens material*

**cycloguanil embonate** INN, BAN *antimalarial* [also: cycloguanil pamoate]

**cycloguanil pamoate** USAN *antimalarial* [also: cycloguanil embonate]

**Cyclogyl** Drop-Tainers (eye drops) ℞ *cycloplegic; mydriatic* [cyclopentolate HCl] 0.5%, 1%, 2%

**cyclohexanehexol** [see: inositol]

**cyclohexanesulfamate dihydrate** [see: sodium cyclamate]

**cyclohexanesulfamic acid** *(banned in the USA)* [see: cyclamic acid]

**cycloheximide** USAN *antipsoriatic* [also: cicloheximide]

*p*-**cyclohexylhydratropic acid** [see: hexaprofen]

**N-cyclohexyllinoleamide** [see: clinolamide]

**4-cyclohexyloxybenzoate** [see: cyclomethycaine]

**1-cyclohexylpropyl carbamate** [see: procymate]

**N-cyclohexylsulfamic acid** *(banned in the USA)* [see: cyclamic acid]

**cyclomenol** INN

**cyclomethicone** NF *wetting agent*

**cyclomethycaine** INN, BAN *local anesthetic* [also: cyclomethycaine sulfate]

**cyclomethycaine sulfate** USP *local anesthetic* [also: cyclomethycaine]

**Cyclomydril** Drop-Tainers (eye drops) ℞ *cycloplegic; mydriatic* [cyclopentolate HCl; phenylephrine HCl] 0.2%•1%

**cyclones; cycline** *street drug slang* [see: PCP]

**cyclonium iodide** [see: oxapium iodide]

**cyclooxygenase-2 (COX-2) inhibitors** *a class of investigational anti-inflammatory drugs*

**cyclopentamine** INN, BAN [also: cyclopentamine HCl]

**cyclopentamine HCl** USP [also: cyclopentamine]

**cyclopentaphene** [see: cyclarbamate]

**cyclopenthiazide** USAN, INN, BAN *antihypertensive*

**cyclopentolate** INN, BAN *ophthalmic anticholinergic* [also: cyclopentolate HCl]

**cyclopentolate HCl** USP *ophthalmic anticholinergic; mydriatic; cycloplegic* [also: cyclopentolate] 1% eye drops

**8-cyclopentyl 1,3-dipropylxanthine** *investigational (orphan) for cystic fibrosis*

**cyclophenazine HCl** USAN *antipsychotic* [also: ciclofenazine]

**cyclophosphamide** USP, INN, BAN, JAN *nitrogen mustard-type alkylating antineoplastic; immunosuppressive*

**cycloplegics** *a class of drugs that paralyze the ciliary muscles of the eye*

**cyclopolydimethylsiloxane** [see: cyclomethicone]

**cyclopregnol** INN

**cycloprolol** BAN *antiadrenergic (β-receptor)* [also: cicloprolol HCl; cicloprolol]

**cyclopropane** USP, INN *inhalation general anesthetic*

**Cyclo-Prostin** ℞ *investigational (orphan) vasodilator for primary pulmonary hypertension* [epoprostenol]

**cyclopyrronium bromide** INN

**cycloserine** USP, INN, BAN, JAN *bacteriostatic; tuberculosis retreatment; investigational treatment for Alzheimer's disease*

**L-cycloserine** *investigational (orphan) for Gaucher's disease*

**Cyclospasmol** capsules (discontinued 1997) ℞ *peripheral vasodilator; vascular smooth muscle relaxant* [cyclandelate] 200, 400 mg

**Cyclospasmol** ⒸⒶⓃ film-coated tablets ℞ *peripheral vasodilator; vascular smooth muscle relaxant* [cyclandelate] 200 mg

**cyclosporin** BAN *immunosuppressive* [also: cyclosporine; ciclosporin]

**cyclosporin A** [now: cyclosporine]

**cyclosporine** USAN, USP *immunosuppressive for transplants; investigational (orphan) for Sjögren's keratoconjunctivitis sicca and corneal melting syndrome* [also: ciclosporin; cyclosporin]

**cyclothiazide** USAN, USP, INN, BAN *diuretic; antihypertensive*

**cyclovalone** INN

**cycobemin** [see: cyanocobalamin]

**cycotiamine** INN

**cycrimine** INN, BAN [also: cycrimine HCl]

**cycrimine HCl** USP [also: cycrimine]

**Cycrin** tablets ℞ *progestin for secondary amenorrhea or abnormal uterine bleeding* [medroxyprogesterone acetate] 2.5, 5, 10 mg

**cyfluthrin** BAN

**cyhalothrin** BAN

**cyheptamide** USAN, INN *anticonvulsant*

**cyheptropine** INN

**CyHOP (cyclophosphamide, Halotestin, Oncovin, prednisone)** *chemotherapy protocol*

**Cyklokapron** tablets, IV injection ℞ *systemic hemostatic; orphan status withdrawn 1996* [tranexamic acid] 500 mg; 100 mg/mL

**Cylert** tablets, chewable tablets ℞ *CNS stimulant for attention deficit hyperactivity disorders (ADHD)* [pemoline] 18.75, 37.5, 75 mg; 37.5 mg

**Cylex; Cylex Sugar-Free** throat lozenges OTC *topical oral anesthetic; antiseptic* [benzocaine; cetylpyridinium chloride] 15•5 mg

**Cylexin** ℞ *investigational (Phase III) adjunct to surgery for congenital heart defects in newborns*

**cymemoxine** [see: cimemoxin]

**cynarine** INN

**Cyomin** IM or subcu injection ℞ *antianemic; vitamin $B_{12}$ supplement* [cyanocobalamin] 1000 μg/mL

**cypenamine** INN, BAN *antidepressant* [also: cypenamine HCl]

**cypenamine HCl** USAN *antidepressant* [also: cypenamine]

**cypionate** USAN, BAN *combining name for radicals or groups* [also: cipionate]

**cypothrin** USAN *veterinary insecticide*

**cyprazepam** USAN, INN *sedative*

**cyprenorphine** INN, BAN

**cyprenorphine HCl** [see: cyprenorphine]

**cyprodemanol** [see: cyprodenate]

**cyprodenate** INN

**cyproheptadine** INN, BAN *antihistamine; antipruritic* [also: cyproheptadine HCl]

**cyproheptadine HCl** USP, JAN *antihistamine; antipruritic* [also: cyproheptadine] 4 mg oral; 2 mg/5 mL oral

**cyprolidol** INN *antidepressant* [also: cyprolidol HCl]

**cyprolidol HCl** USAN *antidepressant* [also: cyprolidol]

**cyproquinate** USAN *coccidiostat for poultry* [also: ciproquinate]

**cyproterone** INN, BAN *antiandrogen* [also: cyproterone acetate]

**cyproterone acetate** USAN *antiandrogen; orphan status withdrawn 1996* [also: cyproterone]

**cyproximide** USAN *antipsychotic; antidepressant* [also: ciproximide]

**cyren A** [see: diethylstilbestrol]

**cyren B** [see: diethylstilbestrol dipropionate]

**cyromazine** INN, BAN

**Cystadane** powder for oral solution ℞ *electrolyte replenisher for homocystinuria (orphan)* [betaine HCl] 1 g

**Cystagon** capsules ℞ *antiurolithic for nephropathic cystinosis (orphan)* [cysteamine bitartrate] 50, 150 mg

**cystamin** [see: methenamine]

**cysteamine** USAN, BAN *antiurolithic for nephropathic cystinosis (orphan)* [also: mercaptamine]

**cysteamine bitartrate** *antiurolithic for nephropathic cystinosis (orphan)*

**cysteamine HCl** USAN *antiurolithic*

**cysteine (L-cysteine)** INN *nonessential amino acid; investigational (orphan) for erythropoietic protoporphyria photosensitivity; symbols: Cys, C* [also: cysteine HCl]

**cysteine HCl (L-cysteine HCl)** USP *nonessential amino acid* [also: cysteine] 50 mg/mL injection

**L-cysteine HCl monohydrate** [see: cysteine HCl]

**Cystex** tablets ℞ *urinary anti-infective; analgesic; acidifier* [methenamine; sodium salicylate; benzoic acid] 162•162.5•32 mg

**cystic fibrosis gene, lipid/human DNA** *investigational (orphan) for cystic fibrosis*

**cystic fibrosis gene therapy** *investigational (orphan) for cystic fibrosis*

**cystic fibrosis transmembrane conductance regulator (CFTR)** *investigational (orphan) for cystic fibrosis*

**cystic fibrosis transmembrane conductance regulator, recombinant adenovirus (AdGV-CFTR)** *investigational (orphan) for cystic fibrosis*

**Cysticide** ℞ *orphan status withdrawn 1994* [praziquantel]

**cystine** (L-**cystine**) USAN *amino acid*

**Cysto-Conray; Cysto-Conray II** intracavitary instillation R radiopaque agent [iothalamate meglumine] 43%; 17.2%

**cystogen** [see: methenamine]

**Cystografin; Cystografin Dilute** intracavitary instillation R *cholecystographic radiopaque agent* [diatrizoate meglumine] 30%; 18%

**Cystospaz** tablets R *GI anticholinergic; antispasmodic* [hyoscyamine sulfate] 0.15 mg

**Cystospaz-M** timed-release capsules R *GI anticholinergic; antispasmodic* [hyoscyamine sulfate] 0.375 mg

**CYT-103-Y-90** *investigational antineoplastic for gastrointestinal and colorectal cancer; investigational (orphan) for ovarian cancer*

**CYT-356-In-111** *investigational imaging aid for prostatic cancer detection and staging*

**CYT-356-Y-90** *investigational antineoplastic for prostatic cancer*

**CYT-372-In-111** *investigational imaging aid for colorectal cancer detection and staging*

**CYTABOM (cytarabine, bleomycin, Oncovin, mechlorethamine)** *chemotherapy protocol*

**Cytadren** tablets R *adrenal steroid inhibitor; antisteroidal antineoplastic for corticotropin-producing tumors* [aminoglutethimide] 250 mg

**cytarabine** USAN, USP, INN, BAN *antimetabolic antineoplastic; antiviral* 100, 500, 1000 mg injection ② vidarabine

**cytarabine, depofoam encapsulated** *investigational (orphan) for neoplastic meningitis*

**cytarabine HCl** USAN *antiviral*

**CytoGam** IV infusion R *adjunct to kidney transplants from CMV seropositive donor to CMV seronegative recipient* [cytomegalovirus immune globulin, solvent/detergent treated] 50 mg/mL

**Cytolex** cream R *investigational (Phase III) topical antibacterial for impetigo and diabetic foot ulcers* [MSI-78 (code name—generic name not yet approved)] 1%

**cytomegalovirus immune globulin, human** *investigational (orphan) for primary cytomegalovirus of organ transplants in immunocompromised patients*

**cytomegalovirus immune globulin intravenous (CMV-IGIV)** [see: globulin, immune]

**cytomegalovirus immune globulin intravenous (CMV-IGIV) & ganciclovir sodium** *investigational (orphan) for cytomegalovirus pneumonia in bone marrow transplant patients*

**Cytomel** tablets R *thyroid hormone* [liothyronine sodium] 5, 25, 50 μg

**cytoprotective agents** *a class of drugs that provide prophylaxis against the side effects of antineoplastic agents*

**Cytosar-U** powder for subcu, intrathecal or IV injection R *antimetabolic antineoplastic for multiple leukemias* [cytarabine] 100, 500, 1000, 2000 mg

**cytosine arabinoside (ara-C)** [see: cytarabine]

**cytosine arabinoside HCl** [now: cytarabine HCl]

**Cytosol** liquid R *sterile irrigant* [physiological irrigating solution]

**Cytotec** tablets R *prevention of NSAID-induced gastric ulcers* [misoprostol] 100, 200 μg

**cytotoxic lymphocyte maturation factor** [see: interleukin-12]

**Cytovene** capsules R *antiviral for treatment of cytomegalovirus (CMV)* [ganciclovir] 250 mg

**Cytovene** powder for IV infusion R *antiviral for cytomegalovirus* [ganciclovir sodium] 500 mg/vial

**Cytoxan** tablets, powder for IV injection R *nitrogen mustard-type alkylating antineoplastic for multiple leukemias, lymphomas, blastomas, sarcomas and organ cancers* [cyclophosphamide] 25, 50 mg; 100 mg

**Cytra-2** solution R *urinary alkalizing agent* [sodium citrate; citric acid] 500•334 mg/5 mL

**Cytra-3** syrup R *urinary alkalinizing agent* [potassium citrate; sodium citrate; citric acid] 550•500•334 mg/5 mL

**Cytra-K** oral solution ℞ *urinary alkalizing agent* [potassium citrate; citric acid] 1100•334 mg/5 mL

**Cytra-LC** solution ℞ *urinary alkalizing agent* [potassium citrate; sodium citrate; citric acid] 550•500•334 mg/5 mL

**CY-VA-DACT (Cytoxin, vincristine, Adriamycin, dactinomycin)** *chemotherapy protocol*

**CYVADIC; CY-VA-DIC; CyVADIC (cyclophosphamide, vincristine, Adriamycin, DIC)** *chemotherapy protocol*

**D (vitamin D)** [q.v.]

**D-2.5-W; D-5-W; D-10-W; D-20-W; D-25-W; D-30-W; D-40-W; D-50-W; D-60-W; D-70-W** ℞ *intravenous nutritional therapy* [dextrose in water]

**D$_2$ (vitamin D$_2$)** [see: ergocalciferol]

**D$_3$ (vitamin D$_3$)** [see: cholecalciferol]

**d4T** [see: stavudine]

**D.A.** chewable tablets ℞ *decongestant; antihistamine; anticholinergic* [phenylephrine HCl; chlorpheniramine maleate; methscopolamine nitrate] 10•2•1.25 mg

**DA (daunorubicin, ara-C)** *chemotherapy protocol*

**D.A. II** tablets ℞ *decongestant; antihistamine; anticholinergic* [phenylephrine HCl; chlorpheniramine maleate; methscopolamine nitrate] 10•4•1.25 mg

**DAA (dihydroxyaluminum aminoacetate)** [q.v.]

**DAB$_{389}$ IL-2 fusion toxin** *investigational (Phase I/II, orphan) cytokine for cutaneous T-cell lymphoma*

**dacarbazine** USAN, USP, INN, BAN *alkylating antineoplastic for metastatic malignant melanoma and Hodgkin's disease* ⊠ Dicarbosil; procarbazine

**dacemazine** INN

**dacisteine** INN

**dacliximab** USAN, INN *immunosuppressant monoclonal antibody; investigational (Phase III, orphan) for kidney and bone marrow transplants*

**Dacriose** ophthalmic solution OTC *extraocular irrigating solution* [sterile isotonic solution]

**dactinomycin** USAN, USP, BAN *antibiotic antineoplastic* [also: actinomycin D]

**dacuronium bromide** INN, BAN

**DADDS (diacetyl diaminodiphenylsulfone)** [see: acedapsone]

**dagapamil** INN

**dagga** *street drug slang* [see: marijuana]

**Daily Care** ointment OTC *topical diaper rash treatment* [zinc oxide] 10%

**Daily Cleaner** solution (discontinued 1993) OTC *surfactant cleaning solution for soft contact lenses*

**Daily Vitamins** liquid OTC *vitamin supplement* [multiple vitamins] ≐

**Daily-Vite with Iron & Minerals** tablets OTC *vitamin/mineral/iron supplement* [multiple vitamins & minerals; iron; folic acid; biotin] ≐•18•0.4•≐ mg

**Dairy Ease** chewable tablets OTC *digestive aid for lactose intolerance* [lactase enzyme] 3300 U

**Daisy 2** test kit for home use (discontinued 1995) OTC *in vitro diagnostic aid for urine pregnancy test*

**Dakin solution** [see: sodium hypochlorite]

**Dakrina** eye drops OTC *ocular moisturizer/lubricant* [vitamin A palmitate; polyvinyl alcohol] 350 IU•0.6%

**DAL (daunorubicin, ara-C, L-asparaginase)** *chemotherapy protocol*

**Dalacin T** ℞ *investigational topical anti-acne agent*

**Dalalone** intra-articular, intralesional, soft tissue, or IM injection ℞ *glucocorticoids* [dexamethasone sodium phosphate] 4 mg/mL

**Dalalone D.P.** intra-articular, soft tissue, or IM injection R̥ *glucocorticoids* [dexamethasone acetate] 16 mg/mL

**Dalalone L.A.** intralesional, intra-articular, soft tissue, or IM injection R̥ *glucocorticoids* [dexamethasone acetate] 8 mg/mL

**dalanated insulin** [see: insulin, dalanated]

**dalbraminol** INN

**Dalcaine** injection (discontinued 1994) R̥ *injectable local anesthetic* [lidocaine HCl] 2%

**daledalin** INN *antidepressant* [also: daledalin tosylate]

**daledalin tosylate** USAN *antidepressant* [also: daledalin]

**dalfopristin** USAN, INN *streptogramin antibiotic bacteriostatic to gram-positive infections*

**dalfopristin & quinupristin** *two streptogramin antibiotics that are synergistically bactericidal to gram-positive infections; investigational (NDA filed) for pneumonia*

**Dalgan** IV, subcu or IM injection R̥ *narcotic agonist-antagonist analgesic* [dezocine] 5, 10, 15 mg/mL

**Dallergy** sustained-release capsules (discontinued 1994) R̥ *decongestant; antihistamine; anticholinergic* [phenylephrine HCl; chlorpheniramine maleate; methscopolamine nitrate] 20•8•2.5 mg

**Dallergy** tablets, sustained-release caplets, syrup R̥ *decongestant; antihistamine; anticholinergic* [phenylephrine HCl; chlorpheniramine maleate; methscopolamine nitrate] 10•4•1.25 mg; 20•8•2.5 mg; 10•2•0.625 mg/5 mL

**Dallergy-D** sustained-release capsules (discontinued 1994) OTC *decongestant; antihistamine* [pseudoephedrine HCl; chlorpheniramine maleate] 120•12 mg

**Dallergy-D** syrup OTC *decongestant; antihistamine* [phenylephrine HCl; chlorpheniramine maleate] 5•2 mg/5 mL

**Dallergy-JR** sustained-release capsules R̥ *pediatric decongestant and antihista-*mine [pseudoephedrine HCl; brompheniramine maleate] 60•6 mg

**Dalmane** capsules R̥ *sedative; hypnotic; sometimes abused as a street drug* [flurazepam HCl] 15, 30 mg ② Dialume

**dalteparin sodium** USAN, INN, BAN *a low molecular weight heparin-type anticoagulant and antithrombotic for prevention of deep vein thrombosis (DVT)*

**daltroban** USAN, INN *immunosuppressive*

**dama blanca** (Spanish for "white lady") *street drug slang* [see: cocaine]

**Damason-P** tablets R̥ *narcotic analgesic* [hydrocodone bitartrate; aspirin] 5•500 mg

**dambose** [see: inositol]

**dametralast** INN

**damotepine** INN

**D-Amp** capsules (discontinued 1997) R̥ *penicillin-type antibiotic* [ampicillin trihydrate] 500 mg

**danaparoid sodium** USAN, BAN *glycosaminoglycan anticoagulant and antithrombotic to prevent deep vein thrombosis (DVT)*

**danazol** USAN, USP, INN, BAN *anterior pituitary suppressant* 200 mg oral

**Danazol-NP** R̥ *investigational agent for endometriosis, menorrhagia and fibrocystic breast disease* [danazol nanoparticles]

**dance fever** *street drug slang* [see: fentanyl citrate]

**Danex** shampoo (discontinued 1994) OTC *antiseborrheic; antibacterial; antifungal* [pyrithione zinc] 1%

**daniquidone** BAN

**danitamon** [see: menadione]

**danitracen** INN

**Danocrine** capsules R̥ *androgen for endometriosis, fibrocystic breast disease, and hereditary angioedema* [danazol] 50, 100, 200 mg

**danofloxacin** INN *veterinary antibacterial* [also: danofloxacin mesylate]

**danofloxacin mesylate** USAN *veterinary antibacterial* [also: danofloxacin]

**danosteine** INN

**danthron** USP, BAN (*withdrawn from market by FDA*) [also: dantron] ② Dantrium

**Dantrium** capsules, powder for IV injection ℞ *skeletal muscle relaxant; orphan status withdrawn 1994* [dantrolene sodium] 25, 50, 100 mg; 20 mg/vial (0.32 mg/mL) ⊉ danthron

**dantrolene** USAN, INN, BAN *skeletal muscle relaxant*

**dantrolene sodium** USAN, BAN *skeletal muscle relaxant; orphan status withdrawn 1994*

**dantron** INN *(withdrawn from market by FDA)* [also: danthron]

**Dapa** tablets, capsules (discontinued 1997) OTC *analgesic; antipyretic* [acetaminophen] 325 mg; 500 mg

**Dapacin Cold** capsules OTC *decongestant; antihistamine; analgesic* [phenylpropanolamine HCl; chlorpheniramine maleate; acetaminophen] 12.5•2•325 mg

**dapiprazole** INN *α-adrenergic blocker; antiglaucoma agent; neuroleptic* [also: dapiprazole HCl]

**dapiprazole HCl** USAN *α-adrenergic blocker; miotic; neuroleptic* [also: dapiprazole]

**dapsone** USAN, USP, BAN *bactericidal; leprostatic; herpetiform dermatitis suppressant; investigational (orphan) for Pneumocystis carinii and toxoplasmosis*

**dapsone & trimethoprim** *investigational (orphan) for Pneumocystis carinii pneumonia*

**daptazole** [see: amiphenazole]

**daptomycin** USAN, INN, BAN *antibacterial*

**Daranide** tablets ℞ *carbonic anhydrase inhibitor; diuretic* [dichlorphenamide] 50 mg ⊉ Daraprim

**Daraprim** tablets ℞ *antimalarial; toxoplasmosis treatment adjunct* [pyrimethamine] 25 mg ⊉ Daranide

**Darbid** tablets (discontinued 1994) ℞ *anticholinergic; peptic ulcer treatment adjunct* [isopropamide iodide] 5 mg

**darenzepine** INN

**darglitazone sodium** USAN *oral hypoglycemic*

**Daricon** tablets ℞ *adjunctive therapy for peptic ulcer* [oxyphencyclimine HCl] 10 mg ⊉ Darvon

**darodipine** USAN, INN *antihypertensive; bronchodilator; vasodilator*

**Darvocet-N 50; Darvocet-N 100** tablets ℞ *narcotic analgesic* [propoxyphene napsylate; acetaminophen] 50•325 mg; 100•650 mg ⊉ Darvon-N

**Darvon** Pulvules (capsules) ℞ *narcotic analgesic* [propoxyphene HCl] 65 mg ⊉ Daricon

**Darvon Compound-65** Pulvules (capsules) ℞ *narcotic analgesic* [propoxyphene HCl; aspirin; caffeine] 65•389•32.4 mg

**Darvon-N** suspension (discontinued 1994) ℞ *narcotic analgesic* [propoxyphene napsylate] 10 mg/mL ⊉ Darvocet-N

**Darvon-N** tablets ℞ *narcotic analgesic* [propoxyphene napsylate] 100 mg

**Dasin** capsules (discontinued 1995) OTC *analgesic; antipyretic; anti-inflammatory; bronchodilator; emetic* [aspirin; caffeine; atropine sulfate; ipecac] 130•8•0.13•3 mg

**DAT (daunorubicin, ara-C, thioguanine)** *chemotherapy protocol* [also: DCT; TAD]

**date rape drug** *street drug slang for Rohypnol (flunitrazepam; not marketed in the U.S.)* [see: Rohypnol; flunitrazepam]

**Datelliptium** ℞ *investigational antineoplastic for breast cancer* [ellipticine]

**datelliptium chloride** INN

**Datril** tablets (discontinued 1993) OTC *analgesic; antipyretic* [acetaminophen] 500 mg

**daturine hydrobromide** [see: hyoscyamine hydrobromide]

**DATVP (daunorubicin, ara-C, thioguanine, vincristine, prednisone)** *chemotherapy protocol*

**daunomycin** [see: daunorubicin HCl]

**daunorubicin (DNR)** INN, BAN *antibiotic antineoplastic* [also: daunorubicin HCl] ⊉ doxorubicin

**daunorubicin citrate, liposomal** *antibiotic antineoplastic; treatment for advanced HIV-related Kaposi sarcoma (orphan)*

**daunorubicin HCl** USAN, USP, JAN *antibiotic antineoplastic* [also: daunorubicin] ⑨ doxorubicin

**DaunoXome** IV infusion ℞ *antibiotic antineoplastic for advanced AIDS-related Kaposi sarcoma (orphan)* [daunorubicin citrate, liposomal] 2 mg/mL

**DAV (daunorubicin, ara-C, VePesid)** *chemotherapy protocol*

**DAVA (desacetyl vinblastine amide)** [see: vindesine]

**DAVH (dibromodulcitol, Adriamycin, vincristine, Halotestin)** *chemotherapy protocol*

**davitamon** [see: menadione]

**dawamesk** *street drug slang* [see: marijuana]

**Dayalets** Filmtabs (film-coated tablets) OTC *vitamin supplement* [multiple vitamins; folic acid] ≛•0.4 mg

**Dayalets + Iron** Filmtabs (film-coated tablets) OTC *vitamin/iron supplement* [multiple vitamins; ferrous sulfate; folic acid] ≛•18•0.4 mg

**Daypro** film-coated caplets ℞ *nonsteroidal anti-inflammatory drug (NSAID) for osteoarthritis and rheumatoid arthritis* [oxaprozin] 600 mg

**DayQuil** LiquiCaps (soft gel capsules), liquid OTC *antitussive; decongestant; expectorant; analgesic* [dextromethorphan hydrobromide; pseudoephedrine HCl; guaifenesin; acetaminophen] 10•30•100•250 mg; 3.3•10•33.3•108.3 mg/5 mL

**DayQuil Allergy Relief 4 Hour** tablets OTC *decongestant; antihistamine* [phenylpropanolamine HCl; brompheniramine maleate] 25•4 mg

**DayQuil Allergy Relief 12 Hour** extended-release tablets OTC *decongestant; antihistamine* [phenylpropanolamine HCl; brompheniramine maleate] 75•12 mg

**DayQuil Sinus Pressure & Congestion Relief** caplets OTC *decongestant* [phenylpropanolamine HCl; guaifenesin] 25•200 mg

**DayQuil Sinus Pressure & Pain Relief** caplets OTC *decongestant; analgesic; antipyretic* [pseudoephedrine HCl; acetaminophen] 30•500 mg

**Dayto Himbin** tablets ℞ *no approved uses; sympatholytic; mydriatic; aphrodisiac* [yohimbine HCl] 5.4 mg

**Dayto Sulf** vaginal cream ℞ *broad-spectrum bacteriostatic* [sulfathiazole; sulfacetamide; sulfabenzamide] 3.42%•2.86%•3.7%

**Dayto-Anase** tablets (discontinued 1994) OTC *anti-inflammatory* [bromelains]

**Day-Vite** tablets (discontinued 1993) OTC *vitamin supplement* [multiple vitamins]

**dazadrol** INN *antidepressant* [also: dazadrol maleate]

**dazadrol maleate** USAN *antidepressant* [also: dazadrol]

**Dazamide** tablets ℞ *anticonvulsant; diuretic* [acetazolamide] 250 mg

**dazepinil** INN *antidepressant* [also: dazepinil HCl]

**dazepinil HCl** USAN *antidepressant* [also: dazepinil]

**dazidamine** INN

**dazmegrel** USAN, INN, BAN *thromboxane synthetase inhibitor*

**dazolicine** INN

**dazopride** INN *peristaltic stimulant* [also: dazopride fumarate]

**dazopride fumarate** USAN *peristaltic stimulant* [also: dazopride]

**dazoquinast** INN

**dazoxiben** INN, BAN *antithrombotic* [also: dazoxiben HCl]

**dazoxiben HCl** USAN *antithrombotic* [also: dazoxiben]

**DBED (dibenzylethylenediamine dipenicillin G)** [see: penicillin G benzathine]

**DBM (dibromomannitol)** [see: mitobronitol]

**DC** softgels OTC *stool softener* [docusate calcium] 240 mg

**DC (daunorubicin, cytarabine)** *chemotherapy protocol*

**D&C Brown No. 1 (drugs & cosmetics)** [see: resorcin brown]

**DCA (desoxycorticosterone acetate)** [q.v.]

**DCF (2'-deoxycoformycin)** [see: pentostatin]

**DCL (descarboethoxyloratadine)** [q.v.]

**DCL Hb (diaspirin crosslinked hemoglobin)** [q.v.]

**DCMP (daunorubicin, cytarabine, mercaptopurine, prednisone)** *chemotherapy protocol*

**DCPM (daunorubicin, cytarabine, prednisone, mercaptopurine)** *chemotherapy protocol*

**DCT (daunorubicin, cytarabine, thioguanine)** *chemotherapy protocol* [also: DAT; TAD]

**DCV (DTIC, CCNU, vincristine)** *chemotherapy protocol*

**DDAVP** tablets, nasal spray, rhinal tube, subcu or IV injection R̥ *pituitary antidiuretic hormone for hemophilia A, von Willebrand's disease (orphan), and nocturnal enuresis* [desmopressin acetate] 0.1, 0.2 mg; 10 μg/dose; 0.1 mg/mL; 4 μg/mL (0.1 mg=400 IU)

**DDAVP (1-deamino-8-D-arginine-vasopressin)** [see: desmopressin acetate]

**DDC; ddC (dideoxycytidine)** [see: zalcitabine]

***o,p′*-DDD** [now: mitotane]

**DDI; ddI (dideoxyinosine)** [see: didanosine]

**DDP; *cis*-DDP (diamminedichloroplatinum)** [see: cisplatin]

**DDS (diaminodiphenylsulfone)** [now: dapsone]

**DDT (dichlorodiphenyltrichloroethane)** [see: chlorophenothane]

**DDVP (dichlorovinyl dimethyl phosphate)** [see: dichlorvos]

**DEA (diethanolamine)** [q.v.]

**deacetyllanatoside C** [see: deslanoside]

**dead on arrival; DOA** *street drug slang* [see: heroin; PCP; cocaine, crack]

**deadly nightshade leaf** [see: belladonna extract]

**1-deamino-8-D-arginine-vasopressin (DDAVP)** [see: desmopressin acetate]

**deanil** INN *combining name for radicals or groups*

**deanol** BAN [also: deanol aceglumate]

**deanol aceglumate** INN [also: deanol]

**deanol acetamidobenzoate**

**3-deazaguanine** *investigational antineoplastic*

**deba** [see: barbital]

**deboxamet** INN

**Debrisan** beads, paste R̥ *debrider and cleanser for wet wounds* [dextranomer]

**debrisoquin sulfate** USAN *antihypertensive* [also: debrisoquine]

**debrisoquine** INN, BAN *antihypertensive* [also: debrisoquin sulfate]

**Debrox** ear drops OTC *agent to emulsify and disperse ear wax* [carbamide peroxide] 6.5%

**decadence** *street drug slang* [see: MDMA]

**Decaderm** gel (discontinued 1993) R̥ *topical corticosteroid* [dexamethasone] ☑ Decadron

**Decadron** tablets, elixir R̥ *glucocorticoids* [dexamethasone] 0.5, 0.75, 1.5, 4 mg; 0.5 mg/5 mL ☑ Decaderm; Percodan

**Decadron Phosphate** cream R̥ *topical corticosteroid* [dexamethasone sodium phosphate] 0.1%

**Decadron Phosphate** intra-articular, intralesional, soft tissue or IM injection R̥ *glucocorticoids* [dexamethasone sodium phosphate] 4 mg/mL

**Decadron Phosphate** IV injection R̥ *glucocorticoids* [dexamethasone sodium phosphate] 24 mg/mL

**Decadron Phosphate** Ocumeter (eye drops), ophthalmic ointment R̥ *ophthalmic topical corticosteroidal antiinflammatory* [dexamethasone sodium phosphate] 0.1%; 0.05%

**Decadron Phosphate** Respihaler, Turbinaire (name changed to Dexacort Phosphate in 1994)

**Decadron with Xylocaine** soft tissue injection R̥ *glucocorticoids* [dexamethasone sodium phosphate; lidocaine HCl] 4•10 mg/mL

**Decadron-LA** intralesional, intra-articular, soft tissue, or IM injection R̥ *glucocorticoids* [dexamethasone acetate] 8 mg/mL

**Deca-Durabolin** IM injection R̥ *anabolic steroid for anemia of renal insufficiency; sometimes abused as a street*

drug [nandrolone decanoate] 50, 100, 200 mg/mL

**Decagen** tablets OTC *vitamin/mineral/ iron supplement* [multiple vitamins & minerals; iron; folic acid; biotin] ± • 18 mg•0.4 mg•30 μg

**Decaject** intra-articular, intralesional, soft tissue, or IM injection ℞ *gluco- corticoids* [dexamethasone sodium phosphate] 4 mg/mL

**Decaject-L.A.** intralesional, intra- articular, soft tissue, or IM injection ℞ *glucocorticoids* [dexamethasone acetate] 8 mg/mL

**DECAL (dexamethasone, etopo- side, cisplatin, ara-C, L-asparagi- nase)** *chemotherapy protocol*

**decamethonium bromide** USP, INN [also: decamethonium iodide]

**decamethonium iodide** BAN [also: decamethonium bromide]

**Decapeptyl** injection ℞ *orphan status withdrawn 1996* [triptorelin pamoate]

**decapinol** [see: delmopinol]

**Decaspray** aerosol (discontinued 1996) ℞ *topical corticosteroid* [dexa- methasone] 0.04%

**decavitamin** USP

**Decholin** tablets OTC *laxative; hydro- choleretic* [dehydrocholic acid] 250 mg

**decicain** [see: tetracaine HCl]

**decil** INN *combining name for radicals or groups*

**decimemide** INN

**decitabine** USAN, INN, BAN *antineoplastic*

**decitropine** INN

**deck** *street drug slang for 1 to 15 g of her- oin; also known as a "bag"* [see: heroin]

**declaben** [now: lodelaben]

**declenperone** USAN, INN *veterinary sedative*

**Declomycin** capsules, film-coated tab- lets ℞ *broad-spectrum antibiotic* [deme- clocycline HCl] 150 mg; 150, 300 mg

**decloxizine** INN

**Decofed** syrup OTC *nasal decongestant* [pseudoephedrine HCl] 30 mg/5 mL

**Decohistine** elixir (discontinued 1993) OTC *decongestant; antihistamine* [phenylephrine HCl; chlorphenir- amine maleate]

**Decohistine DH** liquid ℞ *narcotic antitussive; decongestant; antihistamine* [codeine phosphate; pseudoephed- rine HCl; chlorpheniramine maleate; alcohol 5.8%] 10•30•2 mg/5 mL

**decominol** INN

**Deconamine** tablets, syrup ℞ *decon- gestant; antihistamine* [pseudoephed- rine HCl; chlorpheniramine male- ate] 60•4 mg; 30•2 mg/5 mL

**Deconamine CX** tablets, liquid ℞ *narcotic antitussive; decongestant; expectorant* [hydrocodone bitartrate; pseudoephedrine HCl; guaifenesin] 5•30•300 mg; 5•60•200 mg/5 mL

**Deconamine SR** sustained-release capsules ℞ *decongestant; antihista- mine* [pseudoephedrine HCl; chlor- pheniramine maleate] 120•8 mg

**Decongestabs** sustained-release tab- lets ℞ *decongestant; antihistamine* [phenylpropanolamine HCl; phenyl- ephrine HCl; chlorpheniramine maleate; phenyltoloxamine citrate] 40•10•5•15 mg

**Decongestant** sustained-release tab- lets ℞ *decongestant; antihistamine* [phenylpropanolamine HCl; phenyl- ephrine HCl; chlorpheniramine maleate; phenyltoloxamine citrate] 40•10•5•15 mg

**Decongestant** tablets OTC *decongves- tant; antihistamine; analgesic* [phenyl- ephrine HCl; chlorpheniramine mal- eate; acetaminophen] 5•2•325 mg

**Decongestant Expectorant** liquid ℞ *narcotic antitussive; decongestant; expectorant* [codeine phosphate; pseudoephedrine HCl; guaifenesin; alcohol 7.5%] 10•30•100 mg/5 mL

**Decongestant S.R.** sustained-release tablets (discontinued 1995) ℞ *decongestant; antihistamine* [phenyl- propanolamine HCl; phenylephrine HCl; chlorpheniramine maleate; phenyltoloxamine citrate] 40•10• 5•15 mg

**Deconhist L.A.** sustained-release tab- lets ℞ *decongestant; antihistamine; anticholinergic* [phenylpropanolamine HCl; phenylephrine HCl; chlor- pheniramine maleate; hyoscyamine sulfate; atropine sulfate; scopolamine hydrobromide] 50•25•8•0.19•0.04•0.01 mg

**Deconomed SR** sustained-release capsules ℞ *decongestant; antihistamine* [pseudoephedrine HCl; chlorpheniramine maleate] 120•8 mg

**Deconsal II** sustained-release tablets ℞ *decongestant; expectorant* [pseudoephedrine HCl; guaifenesin] 60•600 mg ▣ Deconal

**Deconsal Pediatric** syrup ℞ *narcotic antitussive; decongestant; expectorant* [codeine phosphate; pseudoephedrine HCl; guaifenesin; alcohol 6%] 10•30•100 mg ▣ Deconal

**Deconsal Sprinkle** sustained-release capsules ℞ *decongestant; expectorant* [phenylephrine HCl; guaifenesin] 10•300 mg ▣ Deconal

**decoquinate** USAN, INN, BAN *coccidiostat for poultry*

**Decotan** caplets (discontinued 1993) ℞ *decongestant; antihistamine* [phenylephrine tannate; chlorpheniramine tannate; pyrilamine tannate]

**dectaflur** USAN, INN *dental caries prophylactic*

**Decylenes** ointment OTC *topical antifungal* [undecylenic acid; zinc undecylenate]

**deditonium bromide** INN

**deeda** *street drug slang* [see: LSD]

**Deep-Down Rub** OTC *counterirritant* [methyl salicylate; menthol; camphor] 15%•5%•0.5%

**DEET (diethyltoluamide)** [q.v.]

**DeFed-60** tablets OTC *nasal decongestant* [pseudoephedrine HCl] 60 mg

**defenfluramine** *investigational obesity treatment*

**Defen-LA** sustained-release tablets ℞ *decongestant; expectorant* [pseudoephedrine HCl; guaifenesin] 60•600 mg

**deferoxamine** USAN, INN *iron-chelating agent* [also: desferrioxamine]

**deferoxamine HCl** USAN

**deferoxamine mesylate** USAN, USP *antidote to iron poisoning; iron-chelating agent* [also: desferrioxamine mesylate]

**defibrotide** INN, BAN *investigational (orphan) for thrombotic thrombocytopenic purpura*

**deflazacort** USAN, INN, BAN *anti-inflammatory; investigational treatment for rheumatoid arthritis and asthma*

**defosfamide** INN

**defungit sodium salt** [see: bensuldazic acid]

**Defy** eye drops ℞ *ophthalmic antibiotic* [tobramycin] 0.3%

**Degas** chewable tablets OTC *antiflatulent* [simethicone] 80 mg

**Degest 2** eye drops OTC *topical ocular decongestant/vasoconstrictor* [naphazoline HCl] 0.012%

**Dehist** subcu or IM injection ℞ *antihistamine; anaphylaxis* [brompheniramine maleate] 10 mg/mL

**Dehist** sustained-release capsules (discontinued 1994) OTC *decongestant; antihistamine* [phenylpropanolamine HCl; chlorpheniramine maleate] 75•8 mg

**dehydrated alcohol** [see: alcohol, dehydrated]

**dehydrex** *investigational (orphan) for recurrent corneal erosion*

**dehydroacetic acid** NF *preservative*

**dehydroandrosterone** [see: prasterone]

**dehydrocholate sodium** USP [also: sodium dehydrocholate]

**7-dehydrocholesterol, activated** [now: cholecalciferol]

**dehydrocholic acid** USP, INN, BAN, JAN *choleretic; laxative* 250 mg oral

**dehydrocholin** [see: dehydrocholic acid]

**dehydroemetine** INN, BAN, DCF *investigational anti-infective for amebiasis, amebic dysentery, and fascioliasis*

**dehydroepiandrosterone (DHEA)** *investigational (Phase I/II) immunomodulator for HIV; investigational (Phase III, orphan) for systemic lupus erythematosus (SLE)*

**dehydroepiandrosterone (DHEA) sulfate sodium** *investigational (orphan) for re-epithelialization of serious burns and skin graft donor sites*

**Del Aqua-5; Del Aqua-10** gel ℞ *topical keratolytic for acne* [benzoyl peroxide] 5%; 10%

**Delacort** lotion (discontinued 1993) OTC *topical corticosteroid* [hydrocortisone] ⃝ Delcort

**Deladiol-40** IM injection (discontinued 1996) ℞ *estrogen replacement therapy for postmenopausal disorders; antineoplastic for prostatic cancer* [estradiol valerate in oil] 40 mg/mL

**Deladumone** IM injection (discontinued 1995) ℞ *estrogen/androgen for menopausal vasomotor symptoms* [estradiol valerate; testosterone enanthate] 4•90 mg/mL

**delanterone** INN

**Delaprem** (commercially available in several foreign countries) ℞ *investigational tocolytic and bronchodilator* [hexoprenaline sulfate]

**delapril** INN *antihypertensive; angiotensin-converting enzyme inhibitor* [also: delapril HCl]

**delapril HCl** USAN *antihypertensive; angiotensin-converting enzyme inhibitor* [also: delapril]

**Delatest** IM injection (discontinued 1994) ℞ *androgen replacement for delayed puberty or breast cancer* [testosterone enanthate] 100 mg/mL

**Delatestryl** IM injection ℞ *androgen replacement for delayed puberty or breast cancer; sometimes abused as a street drug* [testosterone enanthate] 200 mg/mL

**delavirdine** INN *antiviral; non-nucleoside reverse transcriptase inhibitor for HIV-1* [also: delavirdine mesylate]

**delavirdine mesylate** USAN *antiviral; non-nucleoside reverse transcriptase inhibitor (NNRTI) for HIV-1* [also: delavirdine]

**delayed-release aspirin** [see: aspirin]

**Delcap** (trademarked dosage form) *unit dispensing cap*

**Delcort** cream OTC *topical corticosteroid* [hydrocortisone] 0.5%, 1% ⃝ Delcort

**delequamine HCl** USAN *α₂ adrenoreceptor antagonist for sexual dysfunction*

**delergotrile** INN

**Delestrogen** IM injection ℞ *estrogen replacement therapy for postmenopausal disorders; antineoplastic for prostatic cancer* [estradiol valerate in oil] 10, 20, 40 mg/mL

**delfantrine** INN

**delfaprazine** INN

**Delfen Contraceptive** vaginal foam OTC *spermicidal contraceptive* [nonoxynol 9] 12.5%

**delmadinone** INN, BAN *progestin; antiandrogen; antiestrogen* [also: delmadinone acetate]

**delmadinone acetate** USAN *progestin; antiandrogen; antiestrogen* [also: delmadinone]

**delmetacin** INN

**delmopinol** INN

**Del-Mycin** topical solution ℞ *topical antibiotic for acne* [erythromycin] 2%

**delnav** [see: dioxathion]

**delorazepam** INN

**deloxolone** INN

**m-delphene** [see: diethyltoluamide]

**delprostenate** INN, BAN

**Delsym** sustained-action liquid OTC *antitussive* [dextromethorphan polistirex] 30 mg/5 mL

**Delta-Cortef** tablets ℞ *glucocorticoids* [prednisolone] 5 mg

**deltacortone** [see: prednisone]

**Delta-D** tablets OTC *vitamin supplement* [cholecalciferol] 400 IU

**deltafilcon A** USAN *hydrophilic contact lens material*

**deltafilcon B** USAN *hydrophilic contact lens material*

**delta-1-hydrocortisone** [see: prednisolone]

**Deltalin** Gelseals (filled elastic capsules) (discontinued 1993) ℞ *vitamin deficiency therapy* [ergocalciferol] 50 000 IU

**Deltasone** tablets ℞ *glucocorticoids* [prednisone] 2.5, 5, 10, 20, 50 mg

**delta-9-tetrahydrocannabinol (THC)** [see: dronabinol]

**delta-9-THC (tetrahydrocannabinol)** [see: dronabinol]

**Delta-Tritex** cream, ointment ℞ *topical corticosteroid* [triamcinolone acetonide] 0.1%

160    Deltavac

**Deltavac** vaginal cream ℞ *bacteriostatic antibiotic; antiseptic; vulnerary* [sulfanilamide; aminacrine HCl; allantoin] 15%•0.2%•2%

**deltibant** USAN *bradykinin antagonist for treatment of systemic inflammatory response syndrome*

**deltra-stab** [see: prednisolone]

**delvaridine mesylate** *investigational (Phase III) reverse transcriptase inhibitor for HIV*

**Del-Vi-A** capsules ℞ *vitamin deficiency therapy* [vitamin A] 50 000 IU

**Demadex** tablets, IV injection ℞ *loop diuretic* [torsemide] 5, 10, 20, 100 mg; 10 mg/mL

**Demazin** Repetabs (repeat-action tablets), syrup OTC *decongestant; antihistamine* [phenylpropanolamine HCl; chlorpheniramine maleate] 25•4 mg; 12.5•2 mg/5 mL

**dembrexine** INN, BAN

**dembroxol** [see: dembrexine]

**demecarium bromide** USP, INN, BAN *antiglaucoma agent; reversible cholinesterase inhibitor miotic*

**demeclocycline** USP, BAN *antibacterial*

**demeclocycline HCl** USP, BAN *gram-negative and gram-positive bacteriostatic; antirickettsial*

**demecolcine** INN, BAN

**demecycline** USAN, INN *antibacterial*

**demegestone** INN

**demekastigmine bromide** [see: demecarium bromide]

**demelverine** INN

**Demerol HCl** tablets, syrup, IV or IM injection ℞ *narcotic analgesic; also abused as a street drug* [meperidine HCl] 50, 100 mg; 50 mg/5 mL; 50, 100 mg/mL

**demetacin** [see: delmetacin]

**11-demethoxyreserpine** [see: deserpidine]

**demethylchlortetracycline (DMCT)** [now: demeclocycline]

**demethylchlortetracycline HCl** [see: demeclocycline HCl]

**N-demethylcodeine** [see: norcodeine]

**demexiptiline** INN

**Demi-Regroton** tablets ℞ *antihypertensive* [chlorthalidone; reserpine] 25•0.125 mg

**demo** *street drug slang for a sample-size piece of crack* [see: cocaine, crack]

**democonazole** INN

**Demolin** liniment OTC *topical analgesic* [methyl salicylate; camphor; racemic menthol; mustard oil] ② Demulen

**demolish** *street drug slang* [see: cocaine, crack]

**demoxepam** USAN, INN *minor tranquilizer*

**demoxytocin** INN

**Demser** capsules ℞ *antihypertensive for pheochromocytoma* [metyrosine] 250 mg

**Demulen 1/35; Demulen 1/50** tablets ℞ *monophasic oral contraceptive* [ethynodiol diacetate; ethinyl estradiol] 1 mg•35 μg; 1 mg•50 μg ② Demerol; Demolin

**denatonium benzoate** USAN, NF, INN, BAN *alcohol denaturant; flavoring agent*

**denaverine** INN

**Denavir** cream ℞ *nucleoside analogue antiviral for herpes labialis* [penciclovir] 1%

**denbufylline** INN, BAN

**denipride** INN

**denofungin** USAN *antifungal; antibacterial*

**denopamine** INN

**Denorex** shampoo OTC *antiseborrheic; antipsoriatic; antipruritic; antibacterial* [coal tar; menthol; alcohol] 9%•1.5•7.5%; 12.5%•1.5%•10.4%

**denpidazone** INN

**Denquel** toothpaste OTC *tooth desensitizer* [potassium nitrate] 5%

**dental antiformin** [see: antiformin, dental]

**dental-type silica** [see: silica, dental-type]

**Dentipatch** transmucosal patch ℞ *mucous membrane anesthetic* [lidocaine HCl] 23, 46.1 mg

**Dent's Lotion-Jel** lotion/gel OTC *topical oral anesthetic* [benzocaine]

**Dent's Toothache Gum; Dent's Toothache Drops** OTC *topical oral anesthetic* [benzocaine]

**denyl sodium** [see: phenytoin sodium]

**denzimol** INN

**2'-deoxycoformycin (DCF)** [see: pentostatin]

**deoxycorticosterone acetate** [see: desoxycorticosterone acetate]

**deoxycorticosterone pivalate** [see: desoxycorticosterone pivalate]

**deoxycortolone pivalate** BAN *salt-regulating adrenocortical steroid* [also: desoxycorticosterone pivalate]

**deoxycortone** BAN *salt-regulating adrenocortical steroid* [also: desoxycorticosterone acetate; desoxycortone]

**2'-deoxycytidine** *investigational (orphan) host-protective agent in acute myelogenous leukemia*

**deoxyephedrine HCl** [see: methamphetamine HCl]

**12-deoxyerythromycin** [see: berythromycin]

**3'-deoxy-3-fluorodeoxythymidine** *investigational antiviral for AIDS (clinical trials discontinued 1994)*

**deoxynojirimycin (DNJ)** *investigational (Phase II) antiviral for AIDS and ARC*

**deoxyribonuclease, recombinant human (rhDNase)** [see: dornase alfa]

**deoxyribonucleic acid (DNA)**

**15-deoxyspergualin trihydrochloride** [now: gusperimus trihydrochloride]

**Depacin** capsules OTC *analgesic; antipyretic* [acetaminophen] 325 mg

**Depacin Cold Capsules** OTC *decongestant; antihistamine; analgesic* [phenylpropanolamine HCl; chlorpheniramine maleate; acetaminophen]

**Depacon** IV infusion R *anticonvulsant* [valproate sodium] 500 mg/5 mL

**Depakene** capsules R *anticonvulsant* [valproic acid] 250 mg

**Depakene** syrup R *anticonvulsant* [valproate sodium] 250 mg/5 mL

**Depakote** delayed-release tablets R *anticonvulsant; antipsychotic for manic episodes of a bipolar disorder; migraine prophylaxis* [divalproex sodium] 125, 250, 500 mg

**Depakote** sprinkle capsules R *anticonvulsant* [divalproex sodium] 125 mg

**depAndro 100; depAndro 200** IM injection R *androgen replacement for delayed puberty or breast cancer* [testosterone cypionate] 100 mg/mL; 200 mg/mL

**depAndrogyn** IM injection R *estrogen/androgen for menopausal vasomotor symptoms* [estradiol cypionate; testosterone cypionate] 2•50 mg/mL

**Depen** titratable tablets R *metal chelating agent for rheumatoid arthritis, Wilson's disease, and cystinuria* [penicillamine] 250 mg

**depepsen** [see: sodium amylosulfate]

**depGynogen** IM injection R *hormone replacement therapy for postmenopausal disorders* [estradiol cypionate in oil] 5 mg/mL

**Depitol** tablets R *anticonvulsant; analgesic for trigeminal neuralgia* [carbamazepine] 200 mg

**depMedalone 40; depMedalone 80** intralesional, soft tissue, and IM injection R *glucocorticoid; anti-inflammatory; immunosuppressant* [methylprednisolone acetate] 40 mg/mL; 80 mg/mL

**DepoCyt** R *investigational (NDA filed) treatment for neoplastic meningitis (NM) arising from solid tumors*

**Depo-Estradiol Cypionate** IM injection R *hormone replacement therapy for postmenopausal disorders* [estradiol cypionate in oil] 5 mg/mL

**DepoGen** IM injection R *hormone replacement therapy for postmenopausal disorders* [estradiol cypionate in oil] 5 mg/mL

**Depoject** intralesional, soft tissue, and IM injection R *glucocorticoid; anti-inflammatory; immunosuppressant* [methylprednisolone acetate] 40, 80 mg/mL

**Depo-Medrol** intralesional, soft tissue, and IM injection R *glucocorticoid; anti-inflammatory; immunosuppressant* [methylprednisolone acetate] 20, 40, 80 mg/mL

**Deponit** transdermal patch R *antianginal* [nitroglycerin] 16, 32 mg

**Depopred-40; Depopred-80** intralesional, soft tissue, and IM injection

R̥ *glucocorticoid; anti-inflammatory; immunosuppressant* [methylprednisolone acetate] 40 mg/mL; 80 mg/mL

**Depo-Provera** IM injection R̥ *hormonal adjunct for metastatic endometrial and renal carcinoma; long-term injectable contraceptive* [medroxyprogesterone acetate] 150, 400 mg/mL

**Depotest 100; Depotest 200** IM injection R̥ *androgen replacement for delayed puberty or breast cancer* [testosterone cypionate] 100 mg/mL; 200 mg/mL

**Depo-Testadiol** IM injection R̥ *estrogen/androgen for menopausal vasomotor symptoms* [estradiol cypionate; testosterone cypionate] 2•50 mg/mL

**Depotestogen** IM injection R̥ *estrogen/androgen for menopausal vasomotor symptoms* [estradiol cypionate; testosterone cypionate] 2•50 mg/mL

**Depo-Testosterone** IM injection R̥ *androgen replacement for delayed puberty or breast cancer; sometimes abused as a street drug* [testosterone cypionate] 100, 200 mg/mL

**depramine** INN [also: balipramine]

**Depranol** R̥ *investigational (orphan) for sickle cell disease* [OM 401 (code name—generic name not yet approved)]

**deprenyl (L-deprenyl)** [see: selegiline HCl]

**deprodone** INN, BAN

**Deproist Expectorant with Codeine** liquid R̥ *narcotic antitussive; decongestant; expectorant* [codeine phosphate; pseudoephedrine HCl; guaifenesin; alcohol 8.2%] 10•30•100 mg/5 mL

**Deprol** tablets (discontinued 1995) R̥ *psychotherapeutic agent* [meprobamate; benactyzine HCl] 400•1 mg

**deprostil** USAN, INN *gastric antisecretory*

**deptropine** INN, BAN

**deptropine citrate** [see: deptropine]

**Dequadin** lozenges *investigational sore throat emollient*

**dequalinium chloride** INN, BAN

**Dequasine** tablets OTC *dietary supplement* [multiple minerals & amino acids; vitamin C] ±•200 mg

**Deracyn SR** tablets R̥ *investigational antidepressant for panic disorder and anxiety* [adinazolam mesylate]

**Derifil** tablets OTC *systemic deodorant for ostomy, breath, and body odors* [chlorophyllin] 100 mg

**Derma Comb** cream R̥ *topical corticosteroid; antifungal* [triamcinolone acetonide; nystatin]

**Derma Viva** lotion OTC *moisturizer; emollient*

**Dermabase** OTC *cream base*

**Dermabet** cream R̥ *topical corticosteroid* [betamethasone valerate]

**Dermacoat** aerosol OTC *topical local anesthetic* [benzocaine] 4.5%

**Dermacort** cream, lotion R̥ *topical corticosteroid* [hydrocortisone] 1% ② DermiCort

**DermaFlex** gel OTC *topical local anesthetic* [lidocaine] 2.5%

**Dermagraft** R̥ *investigational skin substitute*

**Dermal-Rub** balm OTC *counterirritant* [methyl salicylate; camphor; racemic manthol; cajuput oil]

**Dermamycin** cream OTC *topical antihistamine* [diphenhydramine HCl] 2%

**Derma-Pax** lotion OTC *topical antihistamine; antiseptic; antipruritic* [pyrilamine maleate; chlorpheniramine maleate; alcohol 35%] 0.44%•0.06%

**Dermarest** gel OTC *topical antihistamine; antifungal* [diphenhydramine HCl; resorcinol] 2%•2%

**Dermarest Dricort Creme** OTC *topical corticosteroid* [hydrocortisone acetate] 1%

**Dermarest Plus** gel, spray OTC *topical antihistamine; counterirritant* [diphenhydramine HCl; menthol] 2%•1%

**Dermasept Antifungal** liquid spray OTC *antifungal; antiseptic; anesthetic; astringent* [tolnaftate; tannic acid; zinc chloride; benzocaine; methylbenzethonium HCl; undecylenic acid; alcohol 58.539%] 1.017%•6.098%•5.081%•2.032%•3.049%•5.081%

**Dermasil** lotion OTC *bath emollient*

**Derma-Smoothe/FS** oil R̥ *topical corticosteroid; emollient* [fluocinolone acetonide] 0.01%

**dermatan sulfate** [see: danaparoid sodium]

**dermatol** [see: bismuth subgallate]

**Dermatop** cream ℞ *topical corticosteroid* [prednicarbate] 0.1%

**Dermatophytin** shallow subcu or intradermal injection (discontinued 1996) ℞ *diagnosis and treatment of Trichophyton-induced skin infections* [Trichophyton extract] 5 mL (undiluted or 1:30)

**Dermatophytin "O"** shallow subcu or intradermal injection (discontinued 1996) ℞ *diagnosis and treatment of oidiomycin (Candida)-induced infections* [Candida albicans extract] 5 mL (undiluted or 1:100)

**Derm-Cleanse** liquid OTC *soap-free therapeutic skin cleanser*

**DermiCort** cream, lotion OTC *topical corticosteroid* [hydrocortisone] 🔊 Dermacort

**Dermol HC** anorectal cream, anorectal ointment ℞ *topical corticosteroidal anti-inflammatory* [hydrocortisone] 1%, 2.5%; 1%

**Dermolate Anti-Itch** cream OTC *topical corticosteroid* [hydrocortisone] 0.5%

**Dermolin** liniment OTC *counterirritant; topical antiseptic* [methyl salicylate; camphor; racemic menthol; mustard oil; alcohol 8%]

**Dermoplast** aerosol spray, lotion OTC *topical local anesthetic* [benzocaine; menthol] 20%•0.5%; 8%•0.5%

**Dermovan** OTC *cream base*

**Dermoxyl** gel (discontinued 1995) OTC *topical keratolytic for acne* [benzoyl peroxide] 2.5%, 5%, 10%

**Dermprotective Factor (DPF)** (trademarked ingredient) *aromatic syrup* [eriodictyon]

**Dermtex HC with Aloe** cream OTC *topical corticosteroid* [hydrocortisone] 0.5%

**Dermuspray** aerosol spray ℞ *topical enzyme for wound debridement* [trypsin; balsam Peru] 0.1•72.5 mg/0.82 mL

**derpanicate** INN

**DES (diethylstilbestrol)** [q.v.]

**desacetyl vinblastine amide (DAVA)** [see: vindesine]

**desacetyl-lanatoside C** [see: deslanoside]

**desaglybuzole** [see: glybuzole]

**desamino-oxytocin** [see: demoxytocin]

**desaspidin** INN

**descarboethoxyloratadine (DCL)** *investigational antihistamine for allergy*

**desciclovir** USAN, INN *antiviral*

**descinolone** INN *glucocorticoid* [also: descinolone acetonide]

**descinolone acetonide** USAN *glucocorticoid* [also: descinolone]

**Desenex** foam, soap OTC *topical antifungal* [undecylenic acid] 10%

**Desenex** powder, aerosol powder, ointment, cream OTC *topical antifungal* [undecylenic acid; zinc undecylenate] 25% total

**Desenex** spray liquid OTC *topical antifungal* [tolnaftate] 1%

**Desenex, Prescription Strength** cream OTC *topical antifungal* [clotrimazole] 1%

**Desenex, Prescription Strength** spray liquid, spray powder OTC *topical antifungal* [miconazole nitrate] 2%

**Desenex Antifungal** cream OTC *topical antifungal* [miconazole nitrate] 2%

**deserpidine** INN, BAN *antihypertensive; peripheral antiadrenergic; rauwolfia derivative* 🔊 desipramine

**Desert Pure Calcium** film-coated tablets OTC *calcium supplement* [calcium carbonate; vitamin D] 500 mg•125 IU

**Desferal** powder for IM, IV, or subcu injection ℞ *adjunct treatment for iron intoxication or overload* [deferoxamine mesylate] 500 mg 🔊 Disophrol

**desferrioxamine** BAN *iron-chelating agent* [also: deferoxamine]

**desferrioxamine mesylate** BAN *antidote to iron poisoning; iron-chelating agent* [also: deferoxamine mesylate]

**desflurane** USAN, INN *inhalation general anesthetic*

**desglugastrin** INN

**desipramine** INN, BAN *tricyclic antidepressant* [also: desipramine HCl] 🔊 deserpidine

**desipramine HCl** USAN, USP *tricyclic antidepressant* [also: desipramine] 10, 25, 50, 75, 100, 150 mg oral

**desirudin** USAN *anticoagulant; thrombin inhibitor*

**Desitin** ointment OTC *moisturizer; emollient; astringent; antiseptic* [cod liver oil; zinc oxide]

**Desitin with Zinc Oxide** powder OTC *topical diaper rash treatment* [zinc oxide; corn starch] 10%•88.2%

**deslanoside** USP, INN, BAN *cardiotonic; cardiac glycoside*

**deslorelin** USAN, INN *LHRH agonist; investigational (orphan) for central precocious puberty*

**desmethylmoramide** INN

**desmophosphamide** [see: defosfamide]

**desmopressin** INN, BAN *posterior pituitary antidiuretic hormone (ADH)* [also: desmopressin acetate]

**desmopressin acetate** USAN *posterior pituitary antidiuretic hormone for hemophilia A, von Willebrand's disease (orphan), and nocturnal enuresis* [also: desmopressin] 4 μg/mL injection

**desocriptine** INN

**Desogen** tablets R *monophasic oral contraceptive* [desogestrel; ethinyl estradiol] 0.15 mg•30 μg

**desogestrel** USAN, INN, BAN *progestin*

**desolone** [see: deprodone]

**desomorphine** INN, BAN

**desonide** USAN, INN, BAN *topical corticosteroidal anti-inflammatory* 0.05% topical

**DesOwen** ointment, cream, lotion R *topical corticosteroidal anti-inflammatory* [desonide] 0.05%

**desoximetasone** USAN, USP, INN *topical corticosteroidal anti-inflammatory* [also: desoxymethasone] 0.05%, 0.25% topical ② dexamethasone

**desoxycorticosterone acetate (DCA; DOCA)** USP *salt-regulating adrenocortical steroid* [also: desoxycortone; deoxycortone]

**desoxycorticosterone pivalate** USP *salt-regulating adrenocortical steroid* [also: deoxycortolone pivalate]

**desoxycorticosterone trimethylacetate** USP

**desoxycortone** INN *salt-regulating adrenocortical steroid* [also: desoxycorticosterone acetate; deoxycortone]

***l*-desoxyephedrine** *nasal decongestant*

**desoxyephedrine HCl** [see: methamphetamine HCl]

**desoxymethasone** BAN *topical corticosteroidal anti-inflammatory* [also: desoximetasone]

**Desoxyn** Gradumets (sustained-release tablets), tablets R *CNS stimulant; sometimes abused as a street drug* [methamphetamine HCl] 5, 10, 15 mg; 5 mg ② digitoxin; digoxin

**desoxyribonuclease** [see: fibrinolysin & desoxyribonuclease]

**Despec** controlled-release capsules (discontinued 1994) R *decongestant; expectorant* [guaifenesin; phenylpropanolamine HCl]

**Despec** liquid R *decongestant; expectorant* [phenylephrine HCl; phenylpropanolamine HCl; guaifenesin] 20•5•100 mg/5 mL

**Desquam-E; Desquam-E 5; Desquam-E 10** gel R *topical keratolytic for acne* [benzoyl peroxide] 2.5%; 5%; 10%

**Desquam-X 2.5** gel (discontinued 1995) R *topical keratolytic for acne* [benzoyl peroxide] 2.5%

**Desquam-X 5; Desquam-X 10** gel R *topical keratolytic for acne* [benzoyl peroxide] 5%; 10%

**Desquam-X 5 Wash; Desquam-X 10 Wash** liquid R *topical keratolytic for acne* [benzoyl peroxide] 5%; 10%

**de-Stat** solution (discontinued 1995) OTC *cleaning/soaking solution for hard contact lenses*

**de-Stat 3; de-Stat 4** solution OTC *cleaning/disinfecting/soaking solution for rigid gas permeable contact lenses*

**destradiol** [see: estradiol]

**63-desulfohirudin** [see: desirudin]

**Desyrel** film-coated tablets, Dividose (multiple-scored tablets) R *antidepressant* [trazodone HCl] 50, 100 mg; 150, 300 mg

**DET (diethyltryptamine)** [q.v.]

**detajmium bitartrate** INN

**Detane** gel OTC *topical local anesthetic* [benzocaine] 7.5%

**detanosal** INN

**Detect-A-Strep** slide tests for professional use *in vitro diagnostic aid for streptococcal antigens in throat swabs*

**Detecto-Seal** (trademarked packaging form) *tamper-resistant parenteral package*

**deterenol** INN *ophthalmic adrenergic* [also: deterenol HCl]

**deterenol HCl** USAN *ophthalmic adrenergic* [also: deterenol]

**detigon HCl** [see: chlophedianol HCl]

**detirelix** INN *luteinizing hormone-releasing hormone (LHRH) antagonist* [also: detirelix acetate]

**detirelix acetate** USAN *luteinizing hormone-releasing hormone (LHRH) antagonist* [also: detirelix]

**detomidine** INN, BAN *veterinary analgesic; sedative* [also: detomidine HCl]

**detomidine HCl** USAN *veterinary analgesic; sedative* [also: detomidine]

**detorubicin** INN

**detralfate** INN

**Detroit pink** *street drug slang* [see: PCP]

**detrothyronine** INN

**Detussin** liquid R *narcotic antitussive; decongestant* [hydrocodone bitartrate; pseudoephedrine HCl; alcohol 5%] 5•60 mg/5 mL

**Detussin Expectorant** liquid R *narcotic antitussive; decongestant; expectorant* [hydrocodone bitartrate; pseudoephedrine HCl; guaifenesin; alcohol] 5•60•200 mg/5 mL

**deuce** *street drug slang for heroin or $2 worth of drugs* [see: heroin]

**deuterium oxide** USAN *radioactive agent*

**devapamil** INN

**devazepide** USAN *cholecystokinin antagonist*

**devil's dandruff; devilsmoke** *street drug slang* [see: cocaine, crack]

**devil's dust** *street drug slang* [see: PCP]

**Devrom** chewable tablets OTC *systemic deodorizer for ostomy and incontinence odors* [bismuth subgallate] 200 mg

**dew; 'due** *street drug slang for marijuana or the resi**due** of oils left in a* pipe after smoking crack [see: marijuana; cocaine, crack]

**Dex4 Glucose** tablets OTC *glucose elevating agent* [glucose] ≗

**Dexacen LA-8** injection (discontinued 1994) R *corticosteroid* [dexamethasone acetate] 8 mg/mL

**Dexacen-4** injection (discontinued 1994) R *corticosteroid* [dexamethasone sodium phosphate]

**Dexacidin** eye drop suspension, ophthalmic ointment R *topical ophthalmic corticosteroidal anti-inflammatory; antibiotic* [dexamethasone; neomycin sulfate; polymyxin B sulfate] 0.1%•0.35%•10 000 U/mL; 0.1%•0.35%•10 000 U/g

**Dexacort Phosphate** Respihaler (oral inhalation aerosol) R *corticosteroid for bronchial asthma* [dexamethasone sodium phosphate] 84 µg/dose

**Dexacort Phosphate** Turbinaire (nasal inhalation aerosol) R *intranasal steroidal anti-inflammatory* [dexamethasone sodium phosphate; alcohol 2%] 84 µg/dose

**Dexafed Cough** syrup OTC *antitussive; decongestant; expectorant* [dextromethorphan hydrobromide; phenylephrine HCl; guaifenesin] 10•5•100 mg/5 mL

**Dexameth** tablets R *glucocorticoids* [dexamethasone] 0.5, 0.75, 1.5, 4 mg

**dexamethasone** USP, INN, BAN *corticosteroid* 0.25, 0.5, 0.75, 1, 1.5, 2, 4, 6 mg oral; 0.5 mg/5 mL oral; 0.5 mg/0.5 mL oral ▣ desoximetasone

**dexamethasone acefurate** USAN, INN *corticosteroid*

**dexamethasone acetate** USAN, USP, BAN *corticosteroid* 8 mg/mL injection

**dexamethasone dipropionate** USAN *corticosteroid*

**dexamethasone sodium phosphate** USP, BAN *corticosteroid* 0.05%, 0.1% eye drops; 4, 10 mg/mL injection

**dexamfetamine** INN *CNS stimulant* [also: dextroamphetamine; dexamphetamine]

**dexamisole** USAN, INN *antidepressant*

**dexamphetamine** BAN *CNS stimulant* [also: dextroamphetamine; dexamfetamine]

**Dexaphen S.A.** sustained-release tablets ℞ *decongestant; antihistamine* [pseudoephedrine sulfate; dexbrompheniramine maleate] 120•6 mg

**Dexasone** intra-articular, intralesional, soft tissue, or IM injection ℞ *glucocorticoids* [dexamethasone sodium phosphate] 4 mg/mL

**Dexasone L.A.** intralesional, intra-articular, soft tissue, or IM injection ℞ *glucocorticoids* [dexamethasone acetate] 8 mg/mL

**Dexasporin** eye drop suspension (discontinued 1995) ℞ *topical ophthalmic corticosteroidal anti-inflammatory; antibiotic* [dexamethasone; neomycin sulfate; polymyxin B sulfate] 0.1%•0.35%•10 000 U/mL

**Dexasporin** ophthalmic ointment ℞ *topical ophthalmic corticosteroidal anti-inflammatory; antibiotic* [dexamethasone; neomycin sulfate; polymyxin B sulfate] 0.1%•0.35%•10 000 U/g

**Dexatrim** extended-release tablets, timed-release capsules OTC *diet aid* [phenylpropanolamine HCl] 75 mg

**Dexatrim plus Vitamin C** timed-release capsules OTC *diet aid* [phenylpropanolamine HCl; vitamin C] 75•180 mg

**Dexatrim Plus Vitamins** timed-release caplets (diet aid) + caplets (vitamins) OTC *diet aid + vitamin/mineral/iron supplement* [(phenylpropanolamine HCl; vitamin C) + (multiple vitamins/minerals; iron; folic acid; biotin)] (75•60 mg) + (≜•18•0.4•0.03 mg)

**Dexatrim Pre-Meal** timed-release capsules OTC *diet aid* [phenylpropanolamine HCl] 25 mg

**dexbrompheniramine** INN, BAN *antihistamine* [also: dexbrompheniramine maleate]

**dexbrompheniramine maleate** USP *antihistamine* [also: dexbrompheniramine]

**Dexchlor** extended-release tablets ℞ *antihistamine* [dexchlorpheniramine maleate] 4, 6 mg

**dexchlorpheniramine** INN *antihistamine* [also: dexchlorpheniramine maleate]

**dexchlorpheniramine maleate** USP *antihistamine* [also: dexchlorpheniramine] 4, 6 mg oral

**dexclamol** INN *sedative* [also: dexclamol HCl]

**dexclamol HCl** USAN *sedative* [also: dexclamol]

**Dexedrine** Spansules (sustained-release capsules), tablets ℞ *amphetamine; CNS stimulant; widely abused as a street drug* [dextroamphetamine sulfate] 5, 10, 15 mg; 5 mg ② dextran

**dexetimide** USAN, INN, BAN *anticholinergic*

**dexetozoline** INN

**dexfenfluramine** INN, BAN *anorexiant; appetite suppressant; serotonin reuptake inhibitor* [also: dexfenfluramine HCl]

**dexfenfluramine HCl** USAN *anorexiant; appetite suppressant; serotonin reuptake inhibitor* [also: dexfenfluramine]

**DexFerrum** IV injection ℞ *hematinic* [iron dextran] 50 mg/mL

**dexibuprofen** INN *analgesic; cyclooxygenase inhibitor; anti-inflammatory* [also: dexibuprofen lysine]

**dexibuprofen lysine** USAN *analgesic; cyclooxygenase inhibitor; anti-inflammatory* [also: dexibuprofen]

**dexies** *street drug slang for Dexedrine (dextroamphetamine sulfate) or various other amphetamines, especially dextroamphetamine* [see: Dexedrine; dextroamphetamine sulfate; amphetamines]

**deximafen** USAN, INN *antidepressant*

**dexindoprofen** INN

**dexivacaine** USAN, INN *anesthetic*

**dexlofexidine** INN

**dexmedetomidine** USAN, INN, BAN *tranquilizer*

**dexnorgestrel acetime** [now: norgestimate]

**Dexone** intra-articular, intralesional, soft tissue, or IM injection ℞ *gluco-*

corticoids [dexamethasone sodium phosphate] 4 mg/mL

**Dexone** tablets ℞ *glucocorticoids* [dexamethasone] 0.5, 0.75, 1.5, 4 mg

**Dexone LA** intralesional, intra-articular, soft tissue, or IM injection ℞ *glucocorticoids* [dexamethasone acetate] 8 mg/mL

**dexormaplatin** USAN, INN *antineoplastic*

**dexoxadrol** INN *CNS stimulant; analgesic* [also: dexoxadrol HCl]

**dexoxadrol HCl** USAN *CNS stimulant; analgesic* [also: dexoxadrol]

**dexpanthenol** USAN, USP, INN, BAN *cholinergic; antipruritic; postoperative prophylaxis for paralytic ileus* 250 mg/mL injection

**dexpemedolac** USAN *analgesic*

**dexpropranolol HCl** USAN *antiarrhythmic; antiadrenergic (β-receptor)* [also: dexpropranolol]

**dexproxibutene** INN

**dexrazoxane** USAN, INN, BAN *cardioprotectant for doxorubicin-induced cardiomyopathy (orphan); chelates intracellular iron*

**dexsecoverine** INN

**dexsotalol HCl** USAN *class III antiarrhythmic*

**dextilidine** INN

**dextran** INN, BAN *blood flow adjuvant; plasma volume extender* [also: dextran 40] ⊚ Dexedrine; dextrin

**dextran, high molecular weight** [see: dextran 70]

**dextran, low molecular weight** [see: dextran 40]

**dextran 1** *monovalent hapten for prevention of dextran-induced anaphylactic reactions*

**dextran 40** USAN *blood flow adjuvant; plasma volume extender* [also: dextran] 10% injection

**dextran 70** USAN *plasma volume extender; viscosity-increasing agent* 6% injection

**dextran 75** USAN *plasma volume extender; viscosity-increasing agent* 6% injection

**dextran & deferoxamine** *investigational (orphan) for acute iron poisoning*

**dextran sulfate** *investigational (Phase II) antiviral for HIV and AIDS; investigational (orphan) for cystic fibrosis*

**dextran sulfate, sodium salt, aluminum complex** [see: detralfate]

**dextran sulfate sodium** *investigational (orphan) for AIDS*

**dextranomer** INN, BAN *wound debrider/cleanser*

**dextrates** USAN, NF *tablet binder and diluent*

**dextriferron** NF, INN, BAN

**dextrin** NF, BAN *suspending agent; tablet binder and diluent* ⊚ dextran

**dextroamphetamine** USAN *CNS stimulant; widely abused as a street drug, which causes strong psychic dependence* [also: dexamfetamine; dexamphetamine]

**dextroamphetamine phosphate** USP

**dextroamphetamine saccharate** *CNS stimulant*

**dextroamphetamine sulfate** USP *CNS stimulant; widely abused as a street drug, which causes psychic dependence* 5, 10, 15 mg oral

**dextrobrompheniramine maleate** [see: dexbrompheniramine maleate]

**dextrochlorpheniramine maleate** [see: dexchlorpheniramine maleate]

**dextrofemine** INN

**dextromethorphan** USP, INN, BAN *antitussive*

**dextromethorphan hydrobromide** USP, BAN *antitussive* 10 mg/5 mL oral

**dextromethorphan polistirex** USAN *antitussive*

**dextromoramide** INN, BAN

**dextromoramide tartrate** [see: dextromoramide]

**dextro-pantothenyl alcohol** [see: dexpanthenol]

**dextropropoxiphene chloride** [see: propoxyphene HCl]

**dextropropoxyphene** INN, BAN *narcotic analgesic* [also: propoxyphene HCl]

**dextropropoxyphene HCl** BAN [also: propoxyphene HCl]

**dextrorphan** INN, BAN *investigational glutamate receptor antagonist for neurodegenerative disorders*

**dextrorphan HCl** *treatment of cerebral ischemia*

**dextrose** USP *fluid and nutrient replenisher; parenteral antihypoglycemic*

**5% Dextrose and Electrolyte #48; 5% Dextrose and Electrolyte #75; 10% Dextrose and Electrolyte #48** IV infusion ℞ *intravenous nutritional/electrolyte therapy* [combined electrolyte solution; dextrose]

**dextrose excipient** NF *tablet excipient*

**50% Dextrose with Electrolyte Pattern A (or N)** IV infusion ℞ *intravenous nutritional/electrolyte therapy* [combined electrolyte solution; dextrose]

**50% Dextrose with Electrolyte Pattern B** IV infusion (discontinued 1994) ℞ *intravenous nutritional/electrolyte therapy* [combined electrolyte solution; dextrose]

**Dextrostat** tablets ℞ *amphetamine; CNS stimulant* [dextroamphetamine sulfate] 5 mg

**Dextrostix** reagent strips for home use OTC *in vitro diagnostic aid for blood glucose*

**dextrothyronine** [see: detrothyronine]

**dextrothyroxine** BAN *antihyperlipidemic* [also: dextrothyroxine sodium]

**dextrothyroxine sodium** USAN, USP, INN *antihyperlipidemic* [also: dextrothyroxine]

**dexverapamil** INN *investigational adjunct to chemotherapy*

**Dey-Dose** (delivery system) *nebulizer*

**Dey-Lute** (delivery system) *nebulizer*

**Dey-Pak Sodium Chloride 0.45% & 0.9%** solution OTC *for respiratory therapy and tracheal lavage* [sodium chloride] 0.45%; 0.9%

**Dey-Pak Sodium Chloride 3% & 10%** solution ℞ *for inducing sputum production for specimen collection* [sodium chloride] 3%; 10%

**Dey-Vial Sodium Chloride 0.9%** solution OTC *for respiratory therapy and tracheal lavage* [sodium chloride] 0.9%

**dezaguanine** USAN, INN *antineoplastic*

**dezaguanine mesylate** USAN *antineoplastic*

**dezinamide** *investigational antiepileptic*

**dezocine** USAN, INN *narcotic analgesic*

**d-Film** gel (discontinued 1993) OTC *cleaning gel for hard contact lenses*

**DFMO (difluoromethylornithine)** [see: eflornithine]

**DFMO (difluoromethylornithine) HCl** [see: eflornithine HCl]

**DFMO-MGBG (eflornithine, mitoguazone)** *chemotherapy protocol* [also see: DFMO; MGBG]

**DFP (diisopropyl flurophosphate)** [see: isoflurophate]

**DFV (DDP, fluorouracil, VePesid)** *chemotherapy protocol*

**DHA (docosahexaenoic acid)** [see: doconexent]

**DHAP (dexamethasone, high-dose ara-C, Platinol)** *chemotherapy protocol*

**DHC Plus** capsules ℞ *narcotic analgesic* [dihydrocodeine bitartrate; acetaminophen; caffeine] 16•356.4•30 mg

**DHE (dihydroergotamine)** [see: dihydroergotamine mesylate]

**D.H.E. 45** IV or IM injection ℞ *migraine prophylaxis or treatment* [dihydroergotamine mesylate] 1 mg/mL

**DHEA (dehydroepiandrosterone)** [q.v.]

**DHPG (dihydroxy propoxymethyl guanine)** [see: ganciclovir]

**DHS Tar** liquid shampoo, gel shampoo OTC *antiseborrheic; antipsoriatic; antipruritic; antibacterial* [coal tar] 0.5%

**DHS Zinc** shampoo OTC *antiseborrheic; antibacterial; antifungal* [pyrithione zinc] 2%

**DHT** tablets, Intensol (concentrated oral solution) ℞ *antihypocalcemic for tetany* [dihydrotachysterol] 0.125, 0.2, 0.4 mg; 0.2 mg/mL

**DHT (dihydrotachysterol)** [q.v.]

**DHT (dihydrotestosterone)** [see: androstanolone; stanolone]

**DI (doxorubicin, ifosfamide [with mesna rescue])** *chemotherapy protocol*

**Diaβeta (or DiaBeta)** tablets ℞ *sulfonylurea antidiabetic* [glyburide] 1.25, 2.5, 5 mg

**Diabetic Tussin** liquid OTC *antitussive; decongestant; expectorant* [dextromethorphan hydrobromide; phenylephrine HCl; guaifenesin] 10•5•100 mg/5 mL

**Diabetic Tussin DM** liquid OTC *antitussive; expectorant* [dextromethorphan hydrobromide; guaifenesin] 10•100 mg/5 mL

**Diabetic Tussin EX** liquid OTC *expectorant* [guaifenesin] 100 mg/5 mL

**Diabinese** tablets R *antidiabetic* [chlorpropamide] 100, 250 mg

**diacerein** INN

**diacetamate** INN, BAN

**diacetolol** INN, BAN *antiadrenergic (β-receptor)* [also: diacetolol HCl]

**diacetolol HCl** USAN *antiadrenergic (β-receptor)* [also: diacetolol]

**diacetoxyphenylisatin** [see: oxyphenisatin acetate]

**diacetoxyphenyloxindol** [see: oxyphenisatin acetate]

**diacetrizoate sodium** [see: diatrizoate sodium]

**diacetyl diaminodiphenylsulfone (DADDS)** [see: acedapsone]

**diacetylated monoglycerides** NF *plasticizer*

**diacetylcholine chloride** [see: succinylcholine chloride]

**diacetyl-dihydroxydiphenylisatin** [see: oxyphenisatin acetate]

**diacetyldioxphenylisatin** [see: oxyphenisatin acetate]

**diacetylmorphine HCl** USP (*heroin; banned in USA*) [also: diamorphine]

**diacetylmorphine salts** (*heroin; banned in USA*)

**diacetylsalicylic acid** [see: dipyrocetyl]

**diacetyltannic acid** [see: acetyltannic acid]

**diacetylthiamine** [see: acetiamine]

**Diachlor** tablets (discontinued 1993) R *diuretic* [chlorothiazide]

**diagniol** [see: sodium acetrizoate]

**diallybarbituric acid** [see: allobarbital]

**diallylbarbituric acid** [now: allobarbital]

**diallylnortoxiferene dichloride** [see: alcuronium chloride]

**diallymal** [see: allobarbital]

**Dialose** capsules (discontinued 1995) OTC *stool softener* [docusate potassium] 100 mg

**Dialose** tablets OTC *stool softener* [docusate sodium] 100 mg

**Dialose Plus** tablets, capsules OTC *laxative; stool softener* [yellow phenolphthalein; docusate sodium] 65•100 mg

**Dialpak** (trademarked packaging form) *patient compliance package*

**Dialume** capsules R *antacid* [aluminum hydroxide gel] 500 mg ☒ Dalmane

**Dialyte Pattern LM** solution R *peritoneal dialysis solution* [multiple electrolytes; dextrose] 1.5%• ☀, 2.5%• ☀, 4.5%• ☀

**diamba; djamba** *street drug slang* [see: marijuana]

**dia-mer-sulfonamides (sulfadiazine & sulfamerazine)** [q.v.]

**diamethine** [see: dimethyltubocurarinium chloride; dimethyltubocurarine]

**diamfenetide** INN [also: diamphenethide]

**Diamine T.D.** timed-release tablets R *antihistamine* [brompheniramine maleate] 8, 12 mg

**diaminedipenicillin G** [see: penicillin G benzathine]

**diaminodiphenylsulfone (DDS)** [now: dapsone]

**3,4-diaminopyridine** *investigational (orphan) for Lambert-Eaton myasthenic syndrome*

**cis-diamminedichloroplatinum (DDP)** [see: cisplatin]

**diammonium phosphate** [see: ammonium phosphate]

**diamocaine** INN, BAN *local anesthetic* [also: diamocaine cyclamate]

**diamocaine cyclamate** USAN *local anesthetic* [also: diamocaine]

**diamorphine** BAN (*heroin; banned in USA*) [also: diacetylmorphine HCl]

**Diamox** powder for IV injection R *anticonvulsant; diuretic* [acetazolamide sodium] 500 mg

**Diamox** tablets, Sequels (sustained-release capsules) R *anticonvulsant; diuretic* [acetazolamide] 125, 250 mg; 500 mg

**diamphenethide** BAN [also: diamfenetide]

**diampromide** INN, BAN

**diampron** [see: amicarbalide]

**diamthazole** BAN [also: dimazole]

**diamthazole dihydrochloride** [see: diamthazole]

**Dianeal; Dianeal 137** solution (discontinued 1996) ℞ *investigational (orphan) nutritional supplement for continuous ambulatory peritoneal dialysis patients* [multiple electrolytes; dextrose] ≛•1.5%, ≛•4.25%

**diapamide** USAN *diuretic; antihypertensive* [also: tiamizide]

**Diaparene Baby** cream OTC *topical diaper rash treatment*

**Diaparene Cornstarch Baby** powder OTC *topical diaper rash treatment* [corn starch; aloe]

**Diaparene Cradol** liquid (discontinued 1994) OTC *antimicrobial hair dressing* [methylbenzethonium chloride] 0.07%

**Diaparene Diaper Rash** ointment OTC *topical diaper rash treatment* [zinc oxide]

**Diaparene Medicated** powder, cream (discontinued 1993) OTC *topical diaper rash treatment* [methylbenzethonium chloride]

**Diaparene Peri-Anal Medicated** ointment (discontinued 1993) OTC *topical diaper rash treatment* [methylbenzethonium chloride; zinc oxide]

**Diaper Guard** ointment OTC *topical diaper rash treatment* [dimethicone; vitamins A, D, and E; zinc oxide] 1%•≛•≛

**Diaper Rash** ointment OTC *topical diaper rash treatment* [zinc oxide]

**diaphene** [see: dibromsalan]

**diaphenylsulfone** [see: dapsone]

**Diapid** nasal spray ℞ *pituitary antidiuretic hormone for diabetes insipidus* [lypressin] 50 U/mL

**Diaqua** tablets (discontinued 1993) ℞ *diuretic; antihypertensive* [hydrochlorothiazide]

**Diar-Aid** tablets OTC *antidiarrheal; GI adsorbent* [loperamide HCl] 2 mg

**diarbarone** INN

**Diascan** reagent strips for home use OTC *in vitro diagnostic aid for blood glucose*

**Diasorb** tablets, liquid OTC *antidiarrheal; GI adsorbent* [activated attapulgite] 750 mg; 750 mg/5 mL

**diaspirin crosslinked hemoglobin (DCL Hb)** *investigational blood substitute*

**Diastat** viscous solution for rectal administration ℞ *investigational (orphan) for acute repetitive seizures* [diazepam]

**Diastix** reagent strips for home use OTC *in vitro diagnostic aid for urine glucose*

**diathymosulfone** INN

**diatrizoate meglumine** USP *GI radiopaque medium* [also: meglumine diatrizoate] 76% injection

**diatrizoate methylglucamine** [see: diatrizoate meglumine]

**diatrizoate sodium** USP *GI radiopaque medium* [also: sodium amidotrizoate; sodium diatrizoate]

**diatrizoate sodium I 125** USAN *radioactive agent*

**diatrizoate sodium I 131** USAN *radioactive agent*

**diatrizoic acid** USAN, USP, BAN *radiopaque medium* [also: amidotrizoic acid]

**Diatrol** tablets OTC *antacid; antidiarrheal* [calcium carbonate; pectin]

**diaveridine** USAN, INN, BAN *antibacterial*

**diazacholesterol dihydrochloride** [see: azacosterol HCl]

**Diazemuls** ⒸⒶⓃ emulsified IV or IM injection ℞ *sedative; anxiolytic; skeletal muscle relaxant; anticonvulsant adjunct* [diazepam] 5 mg/mL

**diazepam** USAN, USP, INN, BAN, JAN *anxiolytic; sedative; skeletal muscle relaxant; investigational (orphan) for acute repetitive seizures; also abused as a street drug* 2, 5, 10 mg oral; 1, 5 mg/mL oral; 5 mg/mL injection

**diazinon** BAN [also: dimpylate]

**diaziquone** USAN, INN *antineoplastic; orphan status withdrawn 1994*

**diazoxide** USAN, USP, INN, BAN *emergency antihypertensive; glucose-elevating agent*

**dibasic calcium phosphate** [see: calcium phosphate, dibasic]

**dibasic potassium phosphate** [see: potassium phosphate, dibasic]

**dibasic sodium phosphate** [see: sodium phosphate, dibasic] dibasol [see: bendazol]

dibazol [see: bendazol]

dibekacin INN, BAN

dibemethine INN

dibencil [see: penicillin G benzathine]

dibencozide [see: cobamamide]

**Dibent** IM injection ℞ *gastrointestinal antispasmodic* [dicyclomine HCl] 10 mg/mL

dibenthiamine [see: bentiamine]

dibenzathione [see: sulbentine]

dibenzepin INN, BAN *antidepressant* [also: dibenzepin HCl]

dibenzepin HCl USAN *antidepressant* [also: dibenzepin]

dibenzodiazepines *a class of antipsychotic agents*

dibenzothiazine [see: phenothiazine]

dibenzothiophene USAN *keratolytic*

dibenzoxazepines *a class of antipsychotic agents*

dibenzoyl peroxide [see: benzoyl peroxide]

dibenzoylthiamin [see: bentiamine]

dibenzthion [see: sulbentine]

dibenzylethylenediamine dipenicillin G (DBED) [see: penicillin G benzathine]

**Dibenzyline** capsules ℞ *antihypertensive for pheochromocytoma* [phenoxybenzamine HCl] 10 mg

**N,N-dibenzylmethylamine** [see: dibemethine]

dibromodulcitol [see: mitolactol]

dibromohydroxyquinoline [see: broxyquinoline]

dibromomannitol (DBM) [see: mitobronitol]

dibromopropamidine BAN [also: dibrompropamidine]

dibrompropamidine INN [also: dibromopropamidine]

dibromsalan USAN, INN *disinfectant*

dibrospidium chloride INN

dibucaine USP *topical local anesthetic* [also: cinchocaine] 1% topical

dibucaine HCl USP *local anesthetic* [also: cinchocaine HCl]

dibudinate INN *combining name for radicals or groups*

dibunate INN *combining name for radicals or groups*

dibuprol INN

dibupyrone INN, BAN

dibusadol INN

dibutoline sulfate

**DIC (dimethyl imidazole carboxamide)** [see: dacarbazine]

**Dical** CapTabs (capsule-shaped tablets) OTC *dietary supplement* [dibasic calcium phosphate; vitamin D] 117 mg (Ca)•90 mg (P)•133 IU

dicalcium phosphate [see: calcium phosphate, dibasic]

**Dical-D** tablets, chewable wafers OTC *dietary supplement* [dibasic calcium phosphate; vitamin D] 117 mg (Ca)•90 mg (P)•133 IU; 232 mg (Ca)•180 mg (P)•200 IU

dicarbine INN

**Dicarbosil** chewable tablets OTC *antacid* [calcium carbonate] 500 mg ⊡ dacarbazine

dicarfen INN

dichlofenthion BAN

dichloralantipyrine [see: dichloralphenazone]

dichloralphenazone (chloral hydrate + phenazone) BAN *mild sedative*

dichloralpyrine [see: dichloralphenazone]

dichloramine-T NF

dichloranilino imidazol [see: clonidine HCl]

dichloren [see: mechlorethamine HCl]

dichlorisone INN

dichlorisone acetate [see: dichlorisone]

dichlormethazanone [see: dichlormezanone]

dichlormezanone INN

dichloroacetate sodium *orphan status withdrawn 1996*

dichloroacetic acid *strong keratolytic/cauterant* ⊡ Bichloracetic acid

dichlorodifluoromethane NF *aerosol propellant*

dichlorodiphenyl trichloroethane (DDT) [see: chlorophenothane]

dichlorometaxylenol [see: dichloroxylenol]

dichloromethane [see: methylene chloride]

dichlorophen INN, BAN

**dichlorophenarsine** INN, BAN [also: dichlorophenarsine HCl]

**dichlorophenarsine HCl** USP [also: dichlorophenarsine]

**dichlorotetrafluoroethane** NF *aerosol propellant* [also: cryofluorane]

**dichlorovinyl dimethyl phosphate (DDVP)** [see: dichlorvos]

**dichloroxylenol** INN, BAN

**dichlorphenamide** USP, BAN *carbonic anhydrase inhibitor* [also: diclofenamide]

**dichlorvos** USAN, INN, BAN *anthelmintic*

**dichysterol** [see: dihydrotachysterol]

**diciferron** INN

**dicirenone** USAN, INN *hypotensive; aldosterone antagonist*

**Dick test (scarlet fever streptococcus toxin)**

**diclazuril** USAN, INN, BAN *coccidiostat for poultry; investigational for cryptosporidiosis in AIDS*

**diclofenac** INN, BAN *antiarthritic; nonsteroidal anti-inflammatory drug (NSAID); analgesic* [also: diclofenac potassium] 25, 50, 75 mg oral

**diclofenac potassium** USAN *antiarthritic; nonsteroidal anti-inflammatory drug (NSAID); analgesic* [also: diclofenac]

**diclofenac potassium & hyaluronate sodium** *investigational (Phase III) topical treatment for actinic keratosis; clinical trials as a topical analgesic discontinued 1996*

**diclofenac sodium** USAN, JAN *antiarthritic; analgesic; nonsteroidal anti-inflammatory drug (NSAID); ocular treatment for cataract extraction* 25, 50, 75 mg oral

**diclofenamide** INN *carbonic anhydrase inhibitor* [also: dichlorphenamide]

**diclofensine** INN

**diclofibrate** [see: simfibrate]

**diclofurime** INN

**diclometide** INN

**diclonixin** INN

**dicloralurea** USAN, INN *veterinary food additive*

**dicloxacillin** USAN, INN, BAN *antibacterial*

**dicloxacillin sodium** USAN, USP, BAN *bactericidal antibiotic* 250, 500 mg oral

**dicobalt edetate** INN, BAN

**dicolinium iodide** INN

**dicophane** BAN [also: chlorophenothane; clofenotane]

**dicoumarin** [see: dicumarol]

**dicoumarol** INN *coumarin-derivative anticoagulant* [also: dicumarol]

**dicresulene** INN

**DTIC-ACTD; DICT-ACT-D (DTIC, actinomycin D)** *chemotherapy protocol*

**dicumarol** USAN, USP *coumarin-derivative anticoagulant* [also: dicoumarol] 25 mg oral ☒ Demerol

**dicyclomine** BAN *anticholinergic* [also: dicyclomine HCl; dicycloverine]

**dicyclomine HCl** USP *GI antispasmodic; anticholinergic* [also: dicycloverine; dicyclomine] 10, 20 mg oral; 10 mg/5 mL oral; 10 mg/mL injection

**dicycloverine** INN *anticholinergic* [also: dicyclomine HCl; dicyclomine]

**dicycloverine HCl** [see: dicyclomine HCl]

**dicysteine** [see: cystine]

**didanosine** USAN, INN, BAN *antiviral for AIDS*

**didehydrodideoxythymidine** [see: stavudine]

**Di-Delamine** gel, spray OTC *topical antihistamine; bacteriostatic* [diphenhydramine HCl; tripelennamine HCl] 1%•0.5%•

**2′,3′-dideoxyadenosine** *orphan status withdrawn 1994*

**dideoxycytidine (DDC; ddC)** [see: zalcitabine]

**dideoxyinosine (DDI; ddI)** [see: didanosine]

**Didrex** tablets ℞ *anorexiant* [benzphetamine HCl] 25, 50 mg

**Didrocal** ℞ *investigational treatment for osteoporosis* [etidronate]

**Didro-Kit** (Italian name for U.S. product Didronel)

**Didronel** IV infusion ℞ *bisphosphonate bone resorption suppressant for hypercalcemia of malignancy (orphan)* [etidronate disodium] 300 mg/amp

**Didronel** tablets ℞ *bisphosphonate bone resorption suppressant for Paget's dis-*

*ease and heterotopic ossification* [etidronate disodium] 200, 400 mg

**didrovaltrate** INN

**didroxane** [see: dichlorophen]

**dieldrin** INN, BAN

**diemal** [see: barbital]

**dienestrol** USP, INN *estrogen* [also: dienoestrol]

**dienoestrol** BAN *estrogen* [also: dienestrol]

**dienogest** INN

**Diet Ayds** candy OTC *decrease taste perception of sweetness* [benzocaine] 6 mg

**diet pills** *street drug slang* [see: amphetamines]

**dietamiphylline** [see: etamiphyllin]

**dietamiverine HCl** [see: bietamiverine HCl]

**diethadione** INN, BAN

**diethanolamine** NF *alkalizing agent*

**diethazine** INN, BAN

**diethazine HCl** [see: diethazine]

**diethyl phthalate** NF *plasticizer*

**diethylamine *p*-aminobenzenestibonate** [see: stibosamine]

**3-diethylaminobutyranilide** [see: octacaine]

**diethylbarbiturate monosodium** [see: barbital sodium]

**diethylbarbituric acid** [see: barbital]

**diethylcarbamazine** INN, BAN *anthelmintic for Bancroft's filariasis, onchocerciasis, tropical eosinophilia, and loiasis* [also: diethylcarbamazine citrate]

**diethylcarbamazine citrate** USP *anthelmintic for Bancroft's filariasis, onchocerciasis, tropical eosinophilia, and loiasis* [also: diethylcarbamazine]

**diethylcarbamazine dihydrogen citrate** [see: diethylcarbamazine citrate]

**diethyldithiocarbamate** *investigational (Phase II/III, orphan) immunomodulator for HIV and AIDS*

**diethyldixanthogen** [see: dixanthogen]

**diethylenediamine citrate** [see: piperazine citrate]

**diethylenetriaminepentaacetic acid (DTPA)** [see: pentetic acid]

**N,N-diethyllysergamide** [see: lysergide]

**diethylmalonylurea** [see: barbital]

**diethylmalonylurea sodium** [see: barbital sodium]

**N,N-diethylnicotinamide** [see: nikethamide]

**diethylpropion** BAN *anorexiant* [also: diethylpropion HCl; amfepramone] 75 mg oral

**diethylpropion HCl** USP *anorexiant; CNS stimulant* [also: amfepramone; diethylpropion] 25 mg oral

**diethylstilbestrol (DES)** USP, INN *estrogen for inoperable breast and prostate cancer* [also: stilboestrol] 1, 5 mg oral

**diethylstilbestrol diphosphate** USP *antineoplastic; estrogen* [also: fosfestrol]

**diethylstilbestrol dipropionate** NF

***p*-diethylsulfamoylbenzoic acid** [see: etebenecid; ethebenecid]

**diethylthiambutene** INN, BAN

**diethyltoluamide (DEET)** USP, BAN *arthropod repellent*

**diethyltryptamine (DET)** *a hallucinogenic street drug closely related to dimethyltryptamine (DMT), but prepared synthetically*

**N,N-diethylvanillamide** [see: ethamivan]

**dietifen** INN

**dietroxine** [see: diethadione]

**Dieutrim T.D.** timed-release capsules OTC *diet aid; decrease perception of sweetness* [phenylpropanolamine HCl; benzocaine] 75•9 mg

**diexanthogen** [see: dixanthogen]

**difebarbamate** INN

**difemerine** INN [also: difemerine HCl]

**difemerine HCl** [also: difemerine]

**difemetorex** INN

**difenamizole** INN

**difencloxazine** INN

**difencloxazine HCl** [see: difencloxazine]

**difenidol** INN *antiemetic; antivertigo* [also: diphenidol]

**difenoximide** INN *antiperistaltic* [also: difenoximide HCl]

**difenoximide HCl** USAN *antiperistaltic* [also: difenoximide]

**difenoxin** USAN, INN, BAN *antiperistaltic*

**difenoxin HCl** *antiperistaltic*

**difetarsone** INN, BAN

**difeterol** INN

**Differin** gel ℞ *synthetic retinoid analog for acne* [adapalene] 0.1%

**diflorasone** INN, BAN *topical corticosteroidal anti-inflammatory* [also: diflorasone diacetate]

**diflorasone diacetate** USAN, USP *topical corticosteroidal anti-inflammatory* [also: diflorasone]

**difloxacin** INN *anti-infective; DNA gyrase inhibitor* [also: difloxacin HCl]

**difloxacin HCl** USAN *anti-infective; DNA gyrase inhibitor* [also: difloxacin]

**difluanazine** INN *CNS stimulant* [also: difluanine HCl]

**difluanazine HCl** [see: difluanine HCl]

**difluanine HCl** USAN *CNS stimulant* [also: difluanazine]

**Diflucan** tablets, powder for oral suspension, IV infusion ℞ *systemic antifungal* [fluconazole] 50, 100, 150, 200 mg; 10, 40 mg/mL; 2 mg/mL

**diflucortolone** USAN, INN, BAN *glucocorticoid*

**diflucortolone pivalate** USAN *glucocorticoid*

**diflumidone** INN, BAN *anti-inflammatory* [also: diflumidone sodium]

**diflumidone sodium** USAN *anti-inflammatory* [also: diflumidone]

**diflunisal** USAN, USP, INN, BAN *anti-inflammatory; analgesic; antipyretic; antiarthritic; antirheumatic* 250, 500 mg oral

**difluoromethylornithine (DFMO)** [see: eflornithine]

**difluoromethylornithine HCl** [see: eflornithine HCl]

**difluprednate** USAN, INN *anti-inflammatory*

**difolliculin** [see: estradiol benzoate]

**diftalone** USAN, INN *anti-inflammatory*

**digalloyl trioleate** USAN

**Di-Gel** liquid OTC *antacid; antiflatulent* [aluminum hydroxide; magnesium hydroxide; simethicone] 200•200•20 mg/5 mL

**Di-Gel, Advanced Formula** chewable tablets OTC *antacid; antiflatulent* [magnesium hydroxide; calcium carbonate; simethicone] 128•280•20 mg

**Digepepsin** dual-coated tablets ℞ *digestive enzymes* [pancreatin; pepsin; bile salts] 300•250•150 mg

**Digestozyme** tablets ℞ *digestive enzymes; laxative* [pancreatin; pepsin; dehydrocholic acid] 300•250•25 mg

**Digibind** powder for IV injection ℞ *antidote to digoxin/digitoxin overdose (orphan); investigational (orphan) for other cardiac glycoside intoxication* [digoxin immune Fab (ovine)] 38 mg/vial

**Digidote** ℞ *antidote to digoxin/digitoxin overdose (orphan); investigational (orphan) for other cardiac glycoside intoxication* [digoxin immune Fab (ovine)]

**digitalis** USP *cardiotonic*

**digitalis glycosides** *a class of cardiovascular drugs that increase the force of cardiac contractions* [also called: cardiac glycosides]

**digitoxin** USP, INN, BAN *cardiotonic; cardiac glycoside* ⚤ Desoxyn; digoxin

**digitoxin, acetyl** [see: acetyldigitoxin]

**α-digitoxin monoacetate** [see: acetyldigitoxin]

**digitoxoside** [see: digitoxin]

**digolil** INN *combining name for radicals or groups*

**digoxin** USP, INN, BAN *cardiotonic; cardiac glycoside* 0.125, 0.25, 0.5 mg oral, 0.05 mg/mL oral, 0.15 mg/mL injection ⚤ Desoxyn; digitoxin

**digoxin antibody** [see: digoxin immune Fab]

**digoxin immune Fab (ovine)** *antidote to digoxin/digitoxin intoxication (orphan); investigational (orphan) for other cardiac glycoside intoxication*

**dihematoporphyrin ethers** *orphan status withdrawn 1996*

**dihexyverine** INN *anticholinergic* [also: dihexyverine HCl]

**dihexyverine HCl** USAN *anticholinergic* [also: dihexyverine]

**Dihistine** elixir (discontinued 1993) OTC *decongestant; antihistamine* [phenylephrine HCl; chlorpheniramine maleate]

**Dihistine DH** liquid OTC *narcotic antitussive; decongestant; antihistamine* [codeine phosphate; pseudoephedrine HCl; chlorpheniramine maleate; alcohol] 10•30•2 mg/5 mL

**Dihistine Expectorant** liquid ℞ *narcotic antitussive; decongestant; expectorant* [codeine phosphate; pseudoephedrine HCl; guaifenesin; alcohol] 10•30•100 mg/5 mL

**dihydan soluble** [see: phenytoin sodium]

**dihydralazine** INN, BAN

**dihydralazine sulfate** [see: dihydralazine]

**5,6-dihydro-5-azacytidine** *investigational (orphan) for malignant mesothelioma*

**dihydrobenzthiazide** [see: hydrobentizide]

**dihydrocodeine** INN, BAN *analgesic* [also: dihydrocodeine bitartrate]

**dihydrocodeine bitartrate** USP *analgesic* [also: dihydrocodeine]

**dihydrocodeinone bitartrate** [see: hydrocodone bitartrate]

**dihydroergocornine** [see: ergoloid mesylates]

**dihydroergocristine** [see: ergoloid mesylates]

**dihydroergocryptine** [see: ergoloid mesylates]

**dihydroergotamine (DHE)** INN, BAN *antiadrenergic; anticoagulant; ergot alkaloid for rapid control of migraines* [also: dihydroergotamine mesylate; dihydroergotamine mesilate]

**dihydroergotamine mesilate** JAN *antiadrenergic; anticoagulant; ergot alkaloid for rapid control of migraines* [also: dihydroergotamine mesylate; dihydroergotamine]

**dihydroergotamine mesylate** USAN, USP *antiadrenergic; anticoagulant; ergot alkaloid for rapid control of migraines* [also: dihydroergotamine; dihydroergotamine mesilate]

**dihydroergotamine methanesulfonate** [see: dihydroergotamine mesylate]

**dihydroergotoxine mesylate** [now: ergoloid mesylates]

**dihydroergotoxine methanesulfonate** [now: ergoloid mesylates]

**dihydroethaverine** [see: drotaverine]

**dihydrofollicular hormone** [see: estradiol]

**dihydrofolliculine** [see: estradiol]

**dihydrogenated ergot alkaloids** [now: ergoloid mesylates]

**dihydrohydroxycodeinone** [see: oxycodone]

**dihydrohydroxycodeinone HCl** [see: oxycodone HCl]

**6-dihydro-6-iminopurine** [see: adenine]

**dihydroindolones** *a class of antipsychotic agents*

**dihydroisoperparine** [see: drotaverine]

**dihydromorphinone HCl** [now: hydromorphone HCl]

**dihydroneopine** [see: dihydrocodeine bitartrate]

**dihydropyridines** *a class of calcium channel blockers*

**dihydrostreptomycin (DST)** INN *antibacterial* [also: dihydrostreptomycin sulfate]

**dihydrostreptomycin sulfate** USP *antibacterial* [also: dihydrostreptomycin]

**dihydrostreptomycin-streptomycin** [see: streptoduocin]

**dihydrotachysterol (DHT)** USP, INN, BAN, JAN *calcium regulator; vitamin* $D_1$ 0.125, 0.2, 0.4 mg oral; 0.2 mg/mL oral

**dihydrotestosterone (DHT)** *investigational (orphan) for AIDS-wasting syndrome* [see: androstanolone; stanolone]

**dihydrotheelin** [see: estradiol]

**dihydroxy(stearato)aluminum** [see: aluminum monostearate]

**dihydroxy propoxymethyl guanine (DHPG)** [see: gancyclovir]

**dihydroxyacetone** *skin darkener for vitiligo and hypopigmented areas*

**dihydroxyaluminum aminoacetate (DAA)** USP *antacid*

**dihydroxyaluminum sodium carbonate** USP *antacid*

**dihydroxyanthranol** [see: anthralin]

**dihydroxyanthraquinone** *(withdrawn from market)* [see: danthron]

**24,25-dihydroxycholecalciferol** *investigational (orphan) for uremic osteodystrophy*

**1,25-dihydroxycholecalciferol** [see: calcitriol]

**dihydroxyestrin** [see: estradiol]

**dihydroxyfluorane** [see: fluorescein]

**dihydroxyphenylalanine (DOPA)** [see: levodopa]

**dihydroxyphenylisatin** [see: oxyphenisatin acetate]

**dihydroxyphenyloxindol** [see: oxyphenisatin acetate]

**dihydroxyprogesterone acetophenide** [see: algestone acetophenide]

**dihydroxypropyl theophylline** [see: dyphylline]

**diiodobuphenine** [see: bufeniode]

**diiodohydroxyquin** [now: iodoquinol]

**diiodohydroxyquinoline** INN, BAN *antiamebic* [also: iodoquinol]

**diisopromine** INN

**diisopromine HCl** [see: diisopromine]

**diisopropanolamine** NF *alkalizing agent*

**diisopropyl flurophosphate (DFP)** [see: isoflurophate]

**diisopropyl flurophosphonate** [see: isoflurophate]

**diisopropyl phosphorofluoridate** [see: isoflurophate]

**2,6-diisopropylphenol** [see: propofol]

**Dilacor XR** sustained-release capsules ℞ *antihypertensive; antianginal; calcium channel blocker* [diltiazem HCl] 120, 180, 240 mg

**Dilantin** Infatabs (chewable tablets) ℞ *hydantoin-type anticonvulsant* [phenytoin] 50 mg ⊡ Dilaudid

**Dilantin** IV or IM injection (discontinued 1996) ℞ *hydantoin-type anticonvulsant* [phenytoin sodium] 50 mg/mL

**Dilantin** Kapseals (capsules) ℞ *hydantoin-type anticonvulsant* [phenytoin sodium] 30, 100 mg

**Dilantin Oros** ℞ *investigational controlled-release form of Dilantin* [osmotic phenytoin]

**Dilantin with Phenobarbital** Kapseals (capsules) (discontinued 1996) ℞ *hydantoin-type anticonvulsant; sedative* [phenytoin sodium; phenobarbital] 100•16, 100•32 mg

**Dilantin-30 Pediatric** oral suspension (discontinued 1996) ℞ *hydantoin-type anticonvulsant* [phenytoin] 30 mg/5 mL

**Dilantin-125** oral suspension ℞ *hydantoin-type anticonvulsant* [phenytoin] 125 mg/5 mL

**Dilatrate-SR** sustained-release capsules ℞ *antianginal* [isosorbide dinitrate] 40 mg

**Dilaudid** tablets, subcu or IM injection, suppositories ℞ *narcotic analgesic; widely abused as a street drug* [hydromorphone HCl] 2, 4, 8 mg; 1, 2, 4 mg/mL; 3 mg ⊡ Dilantin

**Dilaudid Cough** syrup ℞ *narcotic antitussive; expectorant* [hydromorphone HCl; guaifenesin; alcohol 5%] 1• 100 mg/5 mL

**Dilaudid-5** oral liquid ℞ *narcotic analgesic* [hydromorphone HCl] 5 mg/5 mL

**Dilaudid-HP** subcu or IM injection ℞ *narcotic analgesic* [hydromorphone HCl] 10 mg/mL (250 mg/vial)

**dilazep** INN

**dilevalol** INN, BAN *antihypertensive; antiadrenergic (β-receptor)* [also: dilevalol HCl]

**dilevalol HCl** USAN, JAN *antihypertensive; antiadrenergic (β-receptor)* [also: dilevalol]

**dilithium carbonate** [see: lithium carbonate]

**dillys** *street drug slang* [see: Dilaudid; hydromorphone HCl]

**dilmefone** INN

**Dilocaine** injection ℞ *injectable local anesthetic* [lidocaine HCl] 1%, 2%

**Dilor** tablets, elixir, IM injection ℞ *bronchodilator* [dyphylline] 200 mg; 160 mg/15 mL; 250 mg/mL

**Dilor 400** tablets ℞ *bronchodilator* [dyphylline] 400 mg

**Dilor-G** tablets, liquid ℞ *antiasthmatic; bronchodilator; expectorant* [dyphylline; guaifenesin] 200•200 mg; 300•300 mg/15 mL

**diloxanide** INN, BAN, DCF

**diloxanide furoate** *investigational antiinfective for amebiasis (available only from the Centers for Disease Control and Prevention)*

**diltiazem** INN, BAN *coronary vasodilator; calcium channel blocker; antianginal; antihypertensive* [also: diltiazem HCl]

**diltiazem HCl** USAN, USP, JAN *coronary vasodilator; calcium channel blocker; antianginal; antihypertensive* [also: diltiazem] 30, 60, 90, 120 mg oral; 5 mg/mL injection

**diltiazem malate** USAN *antihypertensive*

**diluted acetic acid** [see: acetic acid, diluted]

**diluted alcohol** [see: alcohol, diluted]

**diluted hydrochloric acid** [see: hydrochloric acid, diluted]

**diluted sodium hypochlorite** [see: sodium hypochlorite, diluted]

**dimabefylline** INN

**Dimacid** chewable tablets (discontinued 1994) OTC *antacid* [calcium carbonate; magnesium carbonate]

**Dimacol** caplets OTC *antitussive; decongestant; expectorant* [dextromethorphan hydrobromide; pseudoephedrine HCl; guaifenesin] 10•30•100 mg ⑨ dimercaprol

**dimantine** INN *anthelmintic* [also: dymanthine HCl]

**dimantine HCl** INN [also: dymanthine HCl]

**Dimaphen** tablets, Release-Tabs (timed-release tablets), elixir OTC *decongestant; antihistamine* [phenylpropanolamine HCl; brompheniramine maleate] 25•4 mg; 75•12 mg; 12.5•2 mg/5 mL

**Dimaphen S.A.** sustained-release tablets (discontinued 1993) ℞ *decongestant; antihistamine* [phenylpropanolamine HCl; phenylephrine HCl; brompheniramine maleate]

**dimazole** INN [also: diamthazole]

**dimazole dihydrochloride** [see: dimazole; diamthazole]

**dimba** *street drug slang for marijuana from West Africa* [see: marijuana]

**dime** *street drug slang for $10 worth of crack* [see: cocaine, crack]

**dime store high** *street drug slang for glue sniffing*

**dimecamine** INN

**dimecolonium iodide** INN

**dimecrotic acid** INN

**dimedrol** [see: diphenhydramine HCl]

**dimefadane** USAN, INN *analgesic*

**dimefilcon A** USAN *hydrophilic contact lens material*

**dimefline** INN, BAN *respiratory stimulant* [also: dimefline HCl]

**dimefline HCl** USAN *respiratory stimulant* [also: dimefline]

**dimefocon A** USAN *hydrophobic contact lens material*

**dimekolin** [see: dimecolonium iodide]

**dimelazine** INN

**dimelin** [see: dimecolonium iodide]

**dimemorfan** INN

**dimenhydrinate** USP, INN, BAN *antiemetic; anticholinergic; antivertigo; motion sickness prophylaxis* 50 mg oral; 12.5 mg/4 mL oral; 50 mg/mL injection ⑨ diphenhydramine

**dimenoxadol** INN [also: dimenoxadole]

**dimenoxadole** BAN [also: dimenoxadol]

**dimepheptanol** INN, BAN

**dimepranol** INN *immunomodulator* [also: dimepranol acedoben]

**dimepranol acedoben** USAN *immunomodulator* [also: dimepranol]

**dimepregnen** INN, BAN

**dimepropion** BAN [also: metamfepramone]

**dimeprozan** INN

**dimeprozinum** [see: dimeprozan]

**dimercaprol** USP, INN *antidote to arsenic, gold and mercury poisoning; lead poisoning adjunct; chelating agent* ⑨ Dimacol

**dimercaptopropanol** [see: dimercaprol]

**2,3-dimercaptosuccinic acid (DMSA)** [see: succimer]

**dime's worth** *street drug slang for the amount of heroin needed to cause death* [see: heroin]

**dimesna** INN

**dimesone** INN, BAN

**Dimetabs** tablets ℞ *anticholinergic; antiemetic; antivertigo agent; motion sickness preventative* [dimenhydrinate] 50 mg ⑨ Dimetane; Dimetapp

**dimetacrine** INN

**dimetamfetamine** INN

**Dimetane** elixir (discontinued 1996) OTC *antihistamine* [brompheniramine maleate] 2 mg/5 mL ⑨ Dimetabs

**Dimetane** Extentabs (long-acting tablets) OTC *antihistamine* [brompheniramine maleate] 12 mg ℞ Dimetabs

**Dimetane** tablets (name changed to Dimetapp Allergy in 1994)

**Dimetane Decongestant** caplets, elixir OTC *decongestant; antihistamine* [phenylephrine HCl; brompheniramine maleate] 10•4 mg; 5•2 mg/5 mL

**Dimetane-DC Cough** syrup ℞ *narcotic antitussive; decongestant; antihistamine* [codeine phosphate; phenylpropanolamine HCl; brompheniramine maleate; alcohol 0.95%] 10•12.5•2 mg/5 mL

**Dimetane-DX Cough** syrup ℞ *antitussive; decongestant; antihistamine* [dextromethorphan hydrobromide; pseudoephedrine HCl; brompheniramine maleate; alcohol 0.95%] 10• 30•2 mg/5 mL

**Dimetapp** tablets, Extentabs (long-acting tablets), elixir OTC *decongestant; antihistamine* [phenylpropanolamine HCl; brompheniramine maleate] 25•4 mg; 75•12 mg; 12.5• 2 mg/5 mL ℞ Dimetabs

**Dimetapp 4-Hour Liqui-Gels** (liquid-filled capsules) OTC *decongestant; antihistamine* [phenylpropanolamine HCl; brompheniramine maleate] 25•4 mg

**Dimetapp Allergy** tablets OTC *antihistamine* [brompheniramine maleate] 4 mg

**Dimetapp Cold & Allergy** chewable tablets, quick-dissolve tablets OTC *pediatric decongestant and antihistamine* [phenylpropanolamine HCl; brompheniramine maleate] 6.25•1 mg

**Dimetapp Cold & Flu** caplets OTC *decongestant; antihistamine; analgesic* [phenylpropanolamine HCl; brompheniramine maleate; acetaminophen] 12.5•2•500 mg

**Dimetapp DM** elixir OTC *antitussive; decongestant; antihistamine* [dextromethorphan hydrobromide; phenylpropanolamine HCl; brompheniramine maleate] 10•12.5•2 mg/5 mL

**Dimetapp Sinus** caplets OTC *decongestant; analgesic* [pseudoephedrine HCl; ibuprofen] 30•200 mg

**dimethadione** USAN, INN *anticonvulsant*

**dimethazan**

**dimethazine** [see: mebolazine]

**dimethicone** USAN, NF, BAN *lubricant and hydrophobing agent; soft tissue prosthetic aid* [also: dimeticone] ℞ cimetidine

**dimethicone 350** USAN *soft tissue prosthetic aid*

**dimethindene** BAN *antihistamine* [also: dimethindene maleate; dimetindene]

**dimethindene maleate** USP *antihistamine* [also: dimetindene; dimethindene]

**dimethiodal sodium** INN

**dimethisoquin** BAN [also: dimethisoquin HCl; quinisocaine]

**dimethisoquin HCl** USAN [also: quinisocaine; dimethisoquin]

**dimethisterone** USAN, NF, INN, BAN *progestin*

**dimetholizine** INN

**dimethothiazine** BAN *serotonin inhibitor* [also: fonazine mesylate; dimetotiazine]

**dimethoxanate** INN, BAN

**dimethoxanate HCl** [see: dimethoxanate]

**2,5-dimethoxy-4-methylamphetamine (DOM)** *a hallucinogenic street drug derived from amphetamine, popularly called STP*

**dimethoxyphenyl penicillin sodium** [see: methicillin sodium]

**dimethpyridene maleate** [see: dimethindene maleate]

**dimethyl ketone** [see: acetone]

**dimethyl phthalate** USP

**dimethyl polysiloxane** [see: dimethicone]

**dimethyl sulfoxide (DMSO)** USAN, USP, INN *solvent; topical anti-inflammatory for symptomatic relief of interstitial cystitis; investigational (orphan) for traumatic brain coma* [also: dimethyl sulphoxide]

**dimethyl sulphoxide** BAN *topical anti-inflammatory; solvent* [also: dimethyl sulfoxide]

**dimethyl triazeno imidazole carboxamide (DIC; DTIC)** [see: dacarbazine]

**dimethylaminophenazone** [see: aminopyrine]

**dimethylcysteine** [see: penicillamine]

**dimethylglycine HCl**

**dimethylhexestrol** [see: methestrol]

**1,5-dimethylhexylamine** [see: octodrine]

**5,5-dimethyl-2,4-oxazolidinedione (DMO)** [see: dimethadione]

**dimethyloxyquinazine** [see: antipyrine]

**o,α-dimethylphenethylamine** [see: ortetamine]

**dimethylsiloxane polymers** [see: dimethicone]

**dimethylthiambutene** INN, BAN

**dimethyltryptamine (DMT)** *hallucinogenic street drug derived from a plant native to South America and the West Indies*

**dimethyltubocurarine** BAN [also: dimethyltubocurarinium chloride]

**dimethyltubocurarine iodide** [see: metocurine iodide]

**dimethyltubocurarinium chloride** INN [also: dimethyltubocurarine]

**dimethylxanthine** [see: theophylline]

**dimeticone** INN *lubricant and hydrophobing agent; soft tissue prosthetic aid* [also: dimethicone]

**dimetindene** INN *antihistamine* [also: dimethindene maleate; dimethindene]

**dimetindene maleate** [see: dimethindene maleate]

**dimetipirium bromide** INN

**dimetofrine** INN

**dimetotiazine** INN *serotonin inhibitor* [also: fonazine mesylate; dimethothiazine]

**dimetridazole** INN, BAN

**dimevamide** INN

**dimevamide sulfate** [see: dimevamide]

**diminazene** INN, BAN

**dimoxamine HCl** USAN *memory adjuvant*

**dimoxaprost** INN

**dimoxyline** INN

**dimpylate** INN [also: diazinon]

**dinaline** INN

**Dinate** IV or IM injection ℞ *anticholinergic; antiemetic; antivertigo agent;*

*motion sickness preventative* [dimenhydrinate] 50 mg/mL

**dinazafone** INN

**ding** *street drug slang* [see: marijuana]

**diniprofylline** INN

**dinitolmide** INN, BAN

**dinitrotoluamide** [see: dinitolmide]

**dinkie dow** *street drug slang* [see: marijuana]

**dinoprost** USAN, INN, BAN *oxytocic; prostaglandin*

**dinoprost trometamol** BAN *oxytocic; prostaglandin* [also: dinoprost tromethamine]

**dinoprost tromethamine** USAN *oxytocic; prostaglandin-type abortifacient* [also: dinoprost trometamol]

**dinoprostone** USAN, INN, BAN *oxytocic; prostaglandin-type abortifacient; cervical ripening agent*

**dinsed** USAN, INN *coccidiostat for poultry*

**Diocto** liquid, syrup OTC *stool softener* [docusate sodium] 150 mg/15 mL; 60 mg/15 mL

**Diocto-C** syrup OTC *stimulant laxative; stool softener* [casanthranol; docusate sodium] 30•60 mg/15 mL

**Diocto-K** capsules OTC *stool softener* [docusate potassium] 100 mg

**Diocto-K Plus** capsules OTC *laxative; stool softener* [casanthranol; docusate potassium] 30•100 mg

**Dioctolose Plus** capsules OTC *laxative; stool softener* [casanthranol; docusate potassium] 30•100 mg

**dioctyl calcium sulfosuccinate** [now: docusate calcium]

**dioctyl potassium sulfosuccinate** [now: docusate potassium]

**dioctyl sodium sulfosuccinate (DSS)** [now: docusate sodium]

**Diodex** ⒸⒶⓃ (U.S. product: Decadron Phosphate) eye drops ℞ *ophthalmic topical corticosteroidal anti-inflammatory* [dexamethasone sodium phosphate] 0.1%

**diodone** INN [also: iodopyracet]

**Dioeze** capsules OTC *stool softener* [docusate sodium] 250 mg

**diohippuric acid I 125** USAN *radioactive agent*

**diohippuric acid I 131** USAN *radioactive agent*

**diolamine** USAN, INN *combining name for radicals or groups*

**diolostene** [see: methandriol]

**dionin** [see: ethylmorphine HCl]

**Dionosil Oily** suspension for intratracheal use ℞ *radiopaque agent* [propyliodone in peanut oil] 60%

**diophyllin** [see: aminophylline]

**diosmin** INN

**Diostate D** tablets OTC *dietary supplement* [calcium; phosphorus; vitamin D] 114 mg•88 mg•133 IU

**diotyrosine I 125** USAN *radioactive agent*

**diotyrosine I 131** USAN *radioactive agent*

**Dioval XX; Dioval 40** IM injection ℞ *estrogen replacement therapy for postmenopausal disorders; antineoplastic for prostatic cancer* [estradiol valerate in oil] 20 mg/mL; 40 mg/mL

**Diovan** capsules ℞ *antihypertensive; angiotensin II receptor antagonist* [valsartan] 80, 160 mg

**dioxadilol** INN

**dioxadrol** INN *antidepressant* [also: dioxadrol HCl]

**dioxadrol HCl** USAN *antidepressant* [also: dioxadrol]

**d-dioxadrol HCl** [see: dexoxadrol HCl]

**dioxamate** INN, BAN

**dioxaphetyl butyrate** INN, BAN

**dioxathion** BAN [also: dioxation]

**dioxation** INN [also: dioxathion]

**dioxethedrin** INN

**dioxethedrin HCl** [see: dioxethedrin]

**dioxifedrine** INN

**dioxindol** [see: oxyphenisatin acetate]

**dioxyanthranol** [see: anthralin]

**dioxyanthraquinone** (*withdrawn from market*) [see: danthron]

**dioxybenzone** USAN, USP, INN *ultraviolet screen*

**dip** *street drug slang* [see: cocaine, crack]

**dipalmitoylphosphatidylcholine (DPPC)** [see: colfosceril palmitate]

**diparcol HCl** [see: diethazine HCl]

**dipegyl** [see: niacinamide]

**dipenicillin G** [see: penicillin G benzathine]

**dipenine bromide** BAN [also: diponium bromide]

**Dipentum** capsules ℞ *anti-inflammatory for ulcerative colitis* [olsalazine sodium] 250 mg

**diperodon** USP, INN, BAN *topical anesthetic*

**diperodon HCl** *topical anesthetic*

**diphemanil methylsulfate** USP *anticholinergic* [also: diphemanil metilsulfate; diphemanil methylsulphate]

**diphemanil methylsulphate** BAN *anticholinergic* [also: diphemanil methylsulfate; diphemanil metilsulfate]

**diphemanil metilsulfate** INN *anticholinergic* [also: diphemanil methylsulfate; diphemanil methylsulphate]

**Diphen Cough Syrup** OTC *antihistamine; antitussive* [diphenhydramine HCl, alcohol 5%] 12.5 mg/5 mL

**Diphenacen-50** injection (discontinued 1994) ℞ *antihistamine* [diphenhydramine HCl] 50 mg/mL

**diphenadione** USP, INN, BAN

**diphenan** INN

**diphenatil** [see: diphemanil methylsulfate]

**diphenchloxazine HCl** [see: difencloxazine HCl]

**diphenesenic acid** [see: xenyhexenic acid]

**Diphenhist** Captabs (capsule-shaped tablets), elixir OTC *antihistamine; motion sickness preventative; sleep aid; antiparkinsonian* [diphenhydramine HCl] 25 mg; 12.5 mg/5 mL

**diphenhydramine** INN, BAN *antihistamine; anticholinergic; antiparkinsonian; motion sickness relief* [also: diphenhydramine citrate] ⑫ dimenhydrinate

**diphenhydramine citrate** USP *antihistamine; anticholinergic; antiparkinsonian; motion sickness relief* [also: diphenhydramine]

**diphenhydramine HCl** USP, BAN *antihistamine; antitussive; motion sickness prevention; sleep aid* 25, 50 mg oral; 12.5 mg/5 mL oral; 10, 50 mg/mL injection

**diphenhydramine theoclate** [see: dimenhydrinate]

**diphenidol** USAN, BAN *antiemetic; antivertigo* [also: difenidol]

**diphenidol HCl** USAN *antiemetic*

**diphenidol pamoate** USAN *antiemetic*
**diphenmethanil methylsulfate** [see: diphemanil methylsulfate]
**diphenoxylate** INN, BAN *antiperistaltic* [also: diphenoxylate HCl]
**diphenoxylate HCl** USP *antiperistaltic* [also: diphenoxylate]
**diphenylacetylindandione** [see: diphenadione]
**diphenylalkylamines** *a class of calcium channel blockers*
**Diphenylan Sodium** capsules ℞ *anticonvulsant* [phenytoin sodium] 30, 100 mg ☑ Diphenylin
**diphenylbutazone** [see: phenylbutazone]
**diphenylbutylpiperidines** *a class of antipsychotic agents*
**diphenylhydantoin** [now: phenytoin]
**diphenylhydantoin sodium** [now: phenytoin sodium]
**diphenylisatin** [see: oxyphenisatin]
**diphenylpyraline** INN, BAN *antihistamine* [also: diphenylpyraline HCl]
**diphenylpyraline HCl** USP *antihistamine* [also: diphenylpyraline]
**diphetarsone** [see: difetarsone]
**diphexamide iodomethylate** [see: buzepide metiodide]
**diphosphonic acid** [see: etidronic acid]
**diphosphopyridine nucleotide (DPN)** [now: nadide]
**diphosphoric acid, tetrasodium salt** [see: sodium pyrophosphate]
**diphosphothiamin** [see: co-carboxylase]
**diphoxazide** INN
**diphtheria antitoxin** USP *passive immunizing agent* [also: diphtheria toxoid] 500 U/mL injection
**diphtheria equine antitoxin** *investigational passive immunizing agent (available only from the Centers for Disease Control and Prevention)*
**diphtheria & tetanus toxoids, adsorbed (DT; Td)** USP *active immunizing agent* 2•2, 2•5, 2•10, 6.6•5, 7.5•7.5, 10•5, 12.5•5, 15•10 LfU/0.5 mL injection
**diphtheria & tetanus toxoids & acellular pertussis vaccine (DTaP)** *active immunizing agent*

**diphtheria & tetanus toxoids & pertussis vaccine (DTP)** USP *active immunizing agent*
**diphtheria & tetanus toxoids & whole-cell pertussis vaccine (DTwP)** *active immunizing agent* 6.5•5•4, 10•5.5•4 LfU/0.5 mL injection
**diphtheria toxin, diagnostic** [now: diphtheria toxin for Schick test]
**diphtheria toxin, inactivated diagnostic** [now: Schick test control]
**diphtheria toxin for Schick test** USP *dermal diphtheria immunity test*
**diphtheria toxoid** USP *active immunizing agent* [also: diphtheria antitoxin]
**diphtheria toxoid, adsorbed** USP *active immunizing agent* 15 LfU/0.5 mL injection
**dipipanone** INN, BAN
**dipipanone HCl** [see: dipipanone]
**dipiproverine** INN
**dipiproverine HCl** [see: dipiproverine]
**dipivalyl epinephrine (DPE)** [now: dipivefrin]
**dipivefrin** USAN *ophthalmic adrenergic* [also: dipivefrine]
**dipivefrin HCl** USP *topical antiglaucoma agent* 0.1% eye drops
**dipivefrine** INN, BAN *ophthalmic adrenergic* [also: dipivefrin]
**diponium bromide** INN [also: dipenine bromide]
**dipotassium carbonate** [see: potassium carbonate]
**dipotassium clorazepate** INN *anxiolytic; minor tranquilizer; alcohol withdrawal relief* [also: clorazepate dipotassium]
**dipotassium hydrogen phosphate** [see: potassium phosphate, dibasic]
**dipotassium phosphate** [see: potassium phosphate, dibasic]
**dipotassium pyrosulfite** [see: potassium metabisulfite]
**dipper** *street drug slang* [see: PCP]
**diprafenone** INN
**diprenorphine** INN, BAN
**Diprivan** emulsion for IV ℞ *general anesthetic* [propofol] 10 mg/mL
**diprobutine** INN, BAN
**diprofene** INN

**diprogulic acid** INN

**diproleandomycin** INN

**Diprolene** ointment, gel, lotion R℞ *topical corticosteroid* [augmented betamethasone diprorionate] 0.05%

**Diprolene AF** cream R℞ *topical corticosteroid* [augmented betamethasone diprorionate] 0.05%

**diprophylline** INN, BAN *bronchodilator* [also: dyphylline]

**dipropylacetic acid** [see: valproic acid]

**2-dipropylaminoethyl diphenylthioacetate** [see: diprofene]

**1,1-dipropylbutylamine** [see: diprobutine]

**diproqualone** INN

**Diprosone** ointment, cream, lotion, aerosol R℞ *topical corticosteroid* [betamethasone diprorionate] 0.05%; 0.05%; 0.05%; 0.1%

**diproteverine** INN, BAN

**diprothazine** [see: dimelazine]

**diprotrizoate sodium** USP [also: sodium diprotrizoate]

**diproxadol** INN

**dipyridamole** USAN, USP, INN, BAN *coronary vasodilator; antiplatelet agent* 25, 50, 75 mg oral

**dipyrithione** USAN, INN *antibacterial; antifungal*

**dipyrocetyl** INN

**dipyrone** USAN, BAN *analgesic; antipyretic* [also: metamizole sodium]

**Dirame** R℞ *investigational narcotic analgesic for moderate to severe pain* [propiram]

**Direct LDL Cholesterol Test** kit *investigational diagnostic aid*

**dirithromycin** USAN, INN, BAN *macrolide antibacterial antibiotic*

**dirt** *street drug slang* [see: heroin]

**dirt grass** *street drug slang for inferior-quality marijuana* [see: marijuana]

**dirty basing** *street drug slang* [see: cocaine, crack]

**disaccharide tripeptide glycerol dipalmitoyl** *investigational (orphan) for pulmonary and hepatic metastases of colorectal adenocarcinoma*

**Disalcid** film-coated tablets, capsules R℞ *analgesic; antipyretic; anti-inflam-*

*matory; antirheumatic* [salsalate] 500, 750 mg; 500 mg

**disalicylic acid** [see: salsalate]

**Disanthrol** capsules OTC *laxative; stool softener* [casanthranol; docusate sodium] 30•100 mg

**disco biscuits** *street drug slang for Quaalude (methaqualone; discontinued 1983) or other CNS depressants* [see: methaqualone]

**Dis-Co Pack** (trademarked packaging form) *unit-dose package*

**Disinfecting Solution** OTC *chemical disinfecting solution for soft contact lenses*

**disiquonium chloride** USAN, INN *antiseptic*

**Disket** (trademarked dosage form) *dispersible tablet*

**Dismutec** *investigational free-radical scavenger to prevent irreversible brain damage after head trauma* [pegorgotein]

**Disobrom** sustained-release tablets R℞ *decongestant; antihistamine* [pseudoephedrine sulfate; dexbrompheniramine maleate] 120•6 mg

**disobutamide** USAN, INN *antiarrhythmic*

**disodium carbenicillin** [see: carbenicillin disodium]

**disodium carbonate** [see: sodium carbonate]

**disodium cefotetan** [see: cefotetan disodium]

**disodium chromate** [see: sodium chromate]

**disodium clodronate** *investigational (orphan) for hypercalcemia of malignancy*

**disodium clodronate tetrahydrate** *investigational (orphan) for increased bone resorption due to malignancy*

**disodium cromoglycate (DSC; DSCG)** [see: cromolyn sodium]

**disodium dihydrogen methylenediphosphonate** [see: medronate disodium]

**disodium edathamil** [see: edathamil disodium]

**disodium edetate** BAN *metal-chelating agent* [also: edetate disodium]

**disodium ethylenediamine tetraacetate** [see: edetate disodium]

**disodium hydrogen phosphate** [see: sodium phosphate]

**disodium hydrogen phosphate heptahydrate** [see: sodium phosphate, dibasic]

**disodium hydrogen phosphate hydrate** [see: sodium phosphate, dibasic]

**(disodium) methylene diphosphonate (MDP)** [now: medronate disodium]

**disodium phosphate** [see: sodium phosphate, dibasic]

**disodium phosphate heptahydrate** [see: sodium phosphate]

**disodium phosphonoacetate monohydrate** [see: fosfonet sodium]

**disodium phosphorofluoridate** [see: sodium monofluorophosphate]

**disodium pyrosulfite** [see: sodium metabisulfite]

**disodium silibinin dihemisuccinate** *orphan status withdrawn 1997*

**disodium sulfate decahydrate** [see: sodium sulfate]

**disodium thiosulfate pentahydrate** [see: sodium thiosulfate]

**disofenin** USAN, INN, BAN *carrier agent in diagnostic tests*

**disogluside** INN

**Disolan** capsules OTC *laxative; stool softener* [phenolphthalein; docusate sodium] 65•100 mg

**Disolan Forte** capsules OTC *laxative; stool softener* [casanthranol; sodium carboxymethylcellulose; docusate sodium] 30•400•100 mg

**Disonate** capsules, syrup, liquid OTC *stool softener* [docusate sodium] 100, 240 mg; 60 mg/15 mL; 150 mg/15 mL

**Disophrol** tablets, Chronotabs (sustained-action tablets) OTC *decongestant; antihistamine* [pseudoephedrine sulfate; dexbrompheniramine maleate] 60•2 mg; 120•6 mg ☒ Desferal; disoprofol; Stilphostrol

**Disoplex** capsules OTC *laxative; stool softener* [sodium carboxymethylcellulose; docusate sodium] 400•100 mg

**disoprofol** [see: propofol] ☒ Disophrol

**disopromine HCl** [see: diisopromine HCl]

**disopyramide** USAN, INN, BAN *antiarrhythmic*

**disopyramide phosphate** USAN, USP, BAN *antiarrhythmic* 100, 150 mg oral

**Disotate** IV infusion ℞ *calcium-lowering agent; antiarrhythmic for digitalis toxicity* [edetate disodium] 150 mg/mL

**disoxaril** USAN, INN *antiviral*

**Di-Spaz** capsules, IM injection ℞ *gastrointestinal antispasmodic* [dicyclomine HCl] 10 mg; 10 mg/mL

**Dispenserpak** (trademarked packaging form) *unit-of-use package*

**dispersible cellulose** BAN *tablet and capsule diluent* [also: cellulose, microcrystalline]

**Dispertab** (trademarked dosage form) *delayed-release tablet*

**Dispette** (trademarked delivery system) *disposable pipette*

**Dispos-a-Med** (trademarked delivery form) *solution for inhalation*

**distaquaine** [see: penicillin V]

**distigmine bromide** INN, BAN

**disulergine** INN

**disulfamide** INN [also: disulphamide]

**disulfiram** USP, INN, BAN *deterrent to alcohol consumption* 250, 500 mg oral

**disulfurous acid, dipotassium salt** [see: potassium metabisulfite]

**disulfurous acid, disodium salt** [see: sodium metabisulfite]

**disulphamide** BAN [also: disulfamide]

**disuprazole** INN

**Dital** slow-release capsules ℞ *anorexiant* [phendimetrazine tartrate] 105 mg

**ditazole** INN

**ditch; ditch weed** *street drug slang for inferior-quality marijuana from Mexico or any low-potency marijuana that grows wild* [see: marijuana]

**ditekiren** USAN *antihypertensive; renin inhibitor*

**ditercalinium chloride** INN

**dithiazanine** BAN [also: dithiazanine iodide]

**dithiazanine iodide** USP, INN [also: dithiazanine]

**dithranol** INN, BAN *antipsoriatic* [also: anthralin]

**D.I.T.I.-2** vaginal cream ℞ *bacteriostatic antibiotic; antiseptic; vulnerary* [sul-

fanilamide; aminacrine HCl; allan-
toin] 15%•0.2%•2%

**ditiocarb sodium** INN

**ditiomustine** INN

**ditolamide** INN

**ditophal** INN, BAN

**Ditropan** tablets, syrup ℞ *urinary antispasmodic for neurogenic bladder* [oxy-
butynin chloride] 5 mg; 5 mg/5 mL
🖫 Intropin

**Diucardin** tablets ℞ *diuretic; antihypertensive* [hydroflumethiazide] 50 mg

**Diulo** tablets (discontinued 1993) ℞
*diuretic; antihypertensive* [metolazone]

**Diupres-250; Diupres-500** tablets
(discontinued 1996) ℞ *antihypertensive* [chlorothiazide; reserpine] 250•
0.125 mg; 500•0.125 mg

**Diurese** tablets ℞ *diuretic; antihypertensive* [trichlormethiazide] 4 mg

**diuretics** *a class of agents that stimulate
increased excretion of urine*

**Diurigen** tablets ℞ *diuretic* [chlorothi-
azide] 500 mg

**Diuril** tablets, oral suspension ℞
*diuretic* [chlorothiazide] 250, 500 mg;
250 mg/5 mL

**Diutensen-R** tablets ℞ *antihypertensive* [methyclothiazide; reserpine]
2.5•0.1 mg 🖫 Salutensin

**divabuterol** INN

**divalproex sodium** USAN *anticonvulsant; antipsychotic for manic episodes;
migraine prophylaxis* [also: valproate
semisodium; semisodium valproate]

**divanilliden cyclohexanone** [see:
cyclovalone]

**divaplon** INN

**Divide-Tab** (trademarked dosage
form) *scored tablet*

**Dividose** (trademarked dosage form)
*multiple-scored tablets*

**diviminol** [see: viminol]

**divinyl ether** [see: vinyl ether]

**divinyl oxide** [see: vinyl ether]

**dixamone bromide** [see: methantheline bromide]

**dixanthogen** INN

**dixarit** [see: clonidine]

**Dizac** injection ℞ *anxiolytic; premedica-
tion to anesthesia* [diazepam] 5 mg/mL

**dizatrifone** INN

**Dizmiss** chewable tablets OTC *anticholinergic; antivertigo agent; motion sickness
preventative* [meclizine HCl] 25 mg

**dizocilpine** INN *neuroprotective;
NMDA (N-methyl-D-aspartate)
antagonist* [also: dizocilpine maleate]

**dizocilpine maleate** USAN *neuroprotective; NMDA (N-methyl-D-aspartate) antagonist* [also: dizocilpine]

**dizocilpine maleate & citicoline**
*investigational (Phase III) neuroprotec-
tive treatment for stroke*

**Dizymes** enteric-coated tablets (discontinued 1994) OTC *digestive
enzymes* [pancreatin; lipase; protease;
amylase] 250 mg•6750 U•41 250
U•43 750 U

**djamba; diamba** *street drug slang* [see:
marijuana]

**D-Lay** (trademarked dosage form)
*timed-release tablet*

**DM Cough Syrup** OTC *antitussive*
[dextromethorphan hydrobromide]

**DMC (dactinomycin, methotrex-
ate, cyclophosphamide)** *chemotherapy protocol*

**DMCT (demethylchlortetracy-
cline)** [see: demeclocycline]

**DML** lotion OTC *moisturizer; emollient*

**DML Forte** cream OTC *moisturizer;
emollient*

**DMO (dimethyl oxazolidinedione)**
[see: dimethadione]

**DMP 266** *investigational (Phase I) antiviral non-nucleoside reverse transcriptase inhibitor for HIV*

**DMP 728** *investigational antiplatelet
agent for angina, heart attack, and
stroke*

**DMP 777** *investigational (orphan) for
management for cystic fibrosis lung disease*

**DMP-504** *investigational (Phase III)
hydrogel bile acid sequestrant (BAS)
for lowering serum cholesterol*

**DMSA (dimercaptosuccinic acid)**
[see: succimer]

**DMSO (dimethyl sulfoxide)** [q.v.]

**DMT (dimethyltryptamine)**

**DMT (dimethyltryptamine)** *street
drug* [q.v.]

**DNA (deoxyribonucleic acid)**

**DNA polymerase** [see: reverse transcriptase inhibitors; non-nucleoside reverse transcriptase inhibitors]

**DNase (recombinant human deoxyribonuclease I)** [see: dornase alfa]

**DNJ (deoxynojirimycin)** [q.v.]

**DNR (daunorubicin)** [q.v.]

**do a joint** *street drug slang for smoking marijuana* [see: marijuana]

**do a line** *street drug slang for inhaling (snorting) powdered cocaine* [see: cocaine]

**DOA; dead on arrival** *street drug slang* [see: heroin; PCP; cocaine, crack]

**Doak Tar** bath oil, lotion, shampoo OTC *topical antipsoriatic; antiseborrheic; antiseptic* [coal tar] 0.8%; 2%; 1.2%, 3%

**Doak Tar Distillate** liquid OTC *topical antipsoriatic; antiseborrheic; antiseptic* [coal tar] 40%

**Doak Tar Oil** liquid OTC *topical antipsoriatic; antiseborrheic; antiseptic* [coal tar] 2%

**Doan's Pills** caplets OTC *analgesic; antirheumatic* [magnesium salicylate] 325, 500 mg

**Doan's P.M.** caplets OTC *analgesic; antirheumatic; antihistaminic sleep aid* [magnesium salicylate; diphenhydramine HCl] 500•25 mg

**DOAP (daunorubicin, Oncovin, ara-C, prednisone)** *chemotherapy protocol*

**dobupride** INN

**dobutamine** USAN, INN, BAN *cardiotonic; vasopressor for shock* ② dopamine

**dobutamine HCl** USAN, USP, BAN *cardiotonic; vasopressor for shock* 12.5 mg/mL injection

**dobutamine lactobionate** USAN *cardiotonic*

**dobutamine tartrate** USAN *cardiotonic*

**Dobutrex** IV infusion ℞ *vasopressor for cardiac shock* [dobutamine] 12.5 mg/mL

**DOCA (desoxycorticosterone acetate)** [q.v.]

**docarpamine** INN

**docebenone** USAN, INN *5-lipoxygenase inhibitor*

**docetaxel** USAN, INN *antineoplastic for breast cancer; investigational for ovarian and lung cancers; analog to paclitaxel*

**doconazole** USAN, INN *antifungal*

**doconexent** INN *omega-3 marine triglyceride*

**docosahexaenoic acid (DHA)** [see: doconexent]

**docosil** INN *combining name for radicals or groups*

**Doctar** shampoo OTC *antiseborrheic; antipsoriatic; antipruritic; antibacterial* [coal tar] 0.5%

**doctor** *street drug slang* [see: MDMA]

**Docucal-P** softgels OTC *laxative; stool softener* [phenolphthalein; docusate calcium] 65•60 mg

**docusate calcium** USAN, USP *stool softener* 240 mg oral

**docusate potassium** USAN, USP *stool softener*

**docusate sodium** USAN, USP, BAN *stool softener; surfactant/wetting agent* [also: sodium dioctyl sulfosuccinate] 50, 100, 250 mg oral; 50, 60 mg/15 mL oral;

**dodecafluoropentane** [see: perflenapent]

**dodeclonium bromide** INN

**2-dodecylisoquinolinium bromide** [see: lauryl isoquinolinium bromide]

**dofamium chloride** INN, BAN

**dofetilide** USAN, INN, BAN *antiarrhythmic; potassium channel blocker*

**dofosfate** INN *combining name for radicals or groups*

**dog food** *street drug slang* [see: heroin]

**dogie; doojee** *street drug slang* [see: heroin]

**DOK** capsules, syrup, liquid OTC *stool softener* [docusate sodium] 100, 250 mg; 60 mg/15 mL; 150 mg/15 mL

**Dolacet** capsules ℞ *narcotic analgesic* [hydrocodone bitartrate; acetaminophen] 5•500 mg

**Dolanex** elixir (discontinued 1997) OTC *analgesic; antipyretic* [acetaminophen] 325 mg/5 mL

**dolantal** [see: meperidine HCl]

**dolantin** [see: meperidine HCl]

**dolasetron** INN *antiemetic; antimigraine* [also: dolasetron mesylate]

**dolasetron mesylate** USAN *antiemetic; antimigraine* [also: dolasetron]

**Dolene** capsules ℞ *narcotic analgesic* [propoxyphene HCl; acetaminophen] 65 mg

**Dolfen** tablets ℞ *narcotic analgesic* [hydrocodone bitartrate; acetaminophen]

**doliracetam** INN

**dollies** *street drug slang for methadone (from the brand name Dolophine)* [see: Dolophine HCl; methadone HCl]

**dolls** *street drug slang for various CNS depressants*

**Dolobid** film-coated tablets ℞ *analgesic; antiarthritic; antirheumatic; antiinflammatory; antipyretic* [diflunisal] 250, 500 mg

**Dolomite** tablets OTC *mineral supplement* [calcium; magnesium] 130•78 mg

**Dolophine HCl** tablets, subcu or IM injection ℞ *narcotic analgesic; narcotic addiction detoxicant; often abused as a street drug* [methadone HCl] 5, 10 mg; 10 mg/mL

**Dolorac** cream OTC *topical analgesic* [capsaicin] 0.025%

**dolosal** [see: meperidine HCl]

**Dolsed** sugar-coated tablets ℞ *urinary anti-infective; analgesic; antispasmodic; acidifier* [methenamine; phenyl salicylate; atropine sulfate; methylene blue; hyoscyamine sulfate; benzoic acid] 40.8•18.1•0.03•5.4•0.03•4.5 mg

**dolvanol** [see: meperidine HCl]

**DOM (2,5-dimethoxy-4-methylamphetamine)** *a hallucinogenic street drug derived from amphetamine, popularly called STP*

**domazoline** INN *anticholinergic* [also: domazoline fumarate]

**domazoline fumarate** USAN *anticholinergic* [also: domazoline]

**Domeboro** powder packets, effervescent tablets OTC *astringent wet dressing (modified Burow solution)* [aluminum sulfate; calcium acetate]

**Domeboro Otic** [see: Otic Domeboro]

**Dome-Paste** medicated gauze bandage OTC *protection and support of extremities* [zinc oxide; calamine; gelatin]

**domes** *street drug slang* [see: LSD]

**domestic** *street drug slang for locally grown marijuana* [see: marijuana]

**domestrol** [see: diethylstilbestrol]

**domex** *street drug slang for a combination of PCP and MDMA* [see: PCP; MDMA]

**domibrom** [see: domiphen bromide]

**dominoes** *street drug slang* [see: amphetamines]

**domiodol** USAN, INN *mucolytic*

**domiphen bromide** USAN, BAN *topical anti-infective*

**domipizone** INN

**Dommanate** IV or IM injection (discontinued 1994) ℞ *anticholinergic; antiemetic; antivertigo agent; motion sickness preventative* [dimenhydrinate] 50 mg/mL ☑ Dramanate

**Domol Bath and Shower Oil** OTC *bath emollient*

**domoprednate** INN

**domoxin** INN

**domperidone** USAN, INN, BAN, JAN *antiemetic*

**don jem** *street drug slang* [see: marijuana]

**Dona Juana; Dona Juanita** *street drug slang* [see: marijuana]

**Donatussin** drops ℞ *pediatric decongestant, antihistamine, and expectorant* [phenylephrine HCl; chlorpheniramine maleate; guaifenesin] 2•1•20 mg/mL

**Donatussin** syrup ℞ *antitussive; decongestant; antihistamine; expectorant* [dextromethorphan hydrobromide; phenylephrine HCl; chlorpheniramine maleate; guaifenesin] 7.5•10•2•100 mg/5 mL

**Donatussin DC** syrup ℞ *narcotic antitussive; decongestant; expectorant* [hydrocodone bitartrate; phenylephrine HCl; guaifenesin] 2.5•7.5•50 mg/5 mL

**Dondril** tablets (discontinued 1993) OTC *decongestant; antihistamine; antitussive* [phenylephrine HCl; chlorpheniramine maleate; dextromethorphan hydrobromide]

**donepezil HCl** *reversible acetylcholinesterase (AChE) inhibitor; cognition adjuvant for Alzheimer's dementia*

**donetidine** USAN, INN, BAN *antagonist to histamine H₂ receptors*

**Donnagel** chewable tablets, liquid OTC *antidiarrheal; GI adsorbent* [attapulgite] 600 mg; 600 mg/15 mL ☒ Donnatal

**Donnagel-PG** liquid (discontinued 1993) ℞ *GI adsorbent; not generally regarded as safe and effective as an antidiarrheal* [opium; kaolin; pectin; hyoscyamine sulfate; atropine sulfate; scopolamine hydrobromide]

**Donnamar** tablets ℞ *anticholinergic; antispasmodic* [hyoscyamine sulfate] 0.125 mg

**Donnamor** elixir (discontinued 1995) ℞ *GI anticholinergic; sedative* [atropine sulfate; scopolamine hydrobromide; hyoscyamine hydrobromide; phenobarbital] 0.0194•0.0065•0.1037•16.2 mg/5 mL

**Donnapectolin-PG** liquid (discontinued 1994) ℞ *GI adsorbent; not generally regarded as safe and effective as an antidiarrheal* [opium; kaolin; pectin; hyoscyamine sulfate; atropine sulfate; scopolamine hydrobromide]

**Donnapine** tablets (discontinued 1995) ℞ *GI anticholinergic; sedative* [atropine sulfate; scopolamine hydrobromide; hyoscyamine hydrobromide; phenobarbital] 0.0194•0.0065•0.1037•16.2 mg

**Donna-Sed** elixir ℞ *anticholinergic; sedative* [atropine sulfate; scopolamine hydrobromide; hyoscyamine hydrobromide; phenobarbital] 0.0194•0.0065•0.1037•16.2 mg/5 mL

**Donnatal** capsules & tablets, elixir, Extentabs (extended-release tablets) ℞ *GI anticholinergic; sedative* [atropine sulfate; scopolamine hydrobromide; hyoscyamine sulfate; phenobarbital] 0.0194•0.0065•0.1037•16.2 mg; 0.0194•0.0065•0.1037•16.2 mg/5 mL; 0.0582•0.0195•0.3111•48.6 mg ☒ Donnagel

**Donnatal No. 2** tablets ℞ *anticholinergic; sedative* [atropine sulfate; scopolamine hydrobromide; hyoscyamine sulfate; phenobarbital] 0.0194•0.0065•0.1037•32.4 mg

**Donnazyme** tablets ℞ *digestive enzymes* [pancreatin; lipase; protease; amylase] 500 mg•1000 U•12 500 U•12 500 U ☒ Entozyme

**doobie** street drug slang [see: marijuana]

**doojee; dogie** street drug slang [see: heroin]

**dooley** street drug slang [see: heroin]

**doors** street drug slang for Doriden (glutethimide; discontinued 1990) [see: glutethimide]

**doors and fours** street drug slang for Doriden (glutethimide; discontinued 1990) and codeine [see: glutethimide; codeine]

**DOPA (dihydroxyphenylalanine)** [see: levodopa]

**L-dopa** [see: levodopa]

**dopamantine** USAN, INN *antiparkinsonian*

**dopamine** INN, BAN *adrenergic* [also: dopamine HCl] ☒ dobutamine; Dopram

**dopamine D₁-receptor antagonist** *investigational antipsychotic*

**dopamine HCl** USAN, USP *adrenergic; vasopressor for shock* [also: dopamine] 40, 80, 160 mg/mL injection

**dopamine HCl in 5% dextrose** *adrenergic; vasopressor for shock* 80, 160, 320 mg/100 mL injection

**dopaminergics** *a class of antiparkinsonian agents that affect the dopamine neurotransmitters in the brain*

**Dopar** capsules ℞ *antiparkinsonian* [levodopa] 100, 250, 500 mg ☒ Dopram

**Dopastat** IV (discontinued 1994) ℞ *vasopressor used in shock* [dopamine HCl] 40 mg/mL

**dope** street drug slang for heroin, marijuana, or any other street drug [see: heroin; marijuana]

**dope smoke** street drug slang [see: marijuana]

**dopexamine** USAN, INN, BAN *cardiovascular agent*

**dopexamine HCl** USAN, BAN *cardiovascular agent*

**dopium** street drug slang [see: opium]

**Dopram** IV injection or infusion ℞ *CNS stimulant; analeptic; adjunct to* *postanesthesia "stir-up"* [doxapram HCl] 20 mg/mL ② dopamine; Dopar

**dopropidil** INN

**doqualast** INN

**doradilla** *street drug slang* [see: marijuana]

**Doral** tablets ℞ *sedative; hypnotic* [quazepam] 7.5, 15 mg

**dorastine** INN *antihistamine* [also: dorastine HCl]

**dorastine HCl** USAN *antihistamine* [also: dorastine]

**Dorcol Children's Cold Formula** liquid OTC *pediatric decongestant and antihistamine* [pseudoephedrine HCl; chlorpheniramine maleate] 15•1 mg/5 mL

**Dorcol Children's Cough** syrup OTC *pediatric antitussive, decongestant, and expectorant* [dextromethorphan hydrobromide; pseudoephedrine HCl; guaifenesin] 5•15•50 mg/5 mL

**Dorcol Children's Decongestant** liquid OTC *nasal decongestant* [pseudoephedrine HCl] 15 mg/5 mL

**Dorcol Children's Fever & Pain Reducer** liquid (discontinued 1997) OTC *analgesic; antipyretic* [acetaminophen] 160 mg/5 mL

**Dorcol Pediatric Cold Formula** liquid (name changed to Dorcol Children's Cold Formula in 1993)

**doreptide** INN

**doretinel** USAN, INN *antikeratinizing agent*

**Dormarex** capsules (discontinued 1993) OTC *antihistaminic sleep aid* [pyrilamine maleate]

**Dormarex 2** tablets OTC *antihistaminic sleep aid; motion sickness preventative* [diphenhydramine HCl] 50 mg

**dormethan** [see: dextromethorphan hydrobromide]

**Dormin** caplets, capsules OTC *antihistaminic sleep aid* [diphenhydramine HCl] 25 mg

**dormiral** [see: phenobarbital]

**dormonal** [see: barbital]

**dornase alfa** *reduces respiratory viscoelasticity of sputum in cystic fibrosis (orphan)*

**Doryx** capsules ℞ *tetracycline-type antibiotic* [doxycycline hyclate] 100 mg

**dorzolamide HCl** USAN *carbonic anhydrase inhibitor for glaucoma*

**DOS** softgels OTC *stool softener* [docusate sodium] 100, 250 mg

**Dosalax** syrup OTC *laxative* [senna concentrate; alcohol 7%] ②

**Dosa-Trol Pack** (trademarked dosage form) *unit-of-use package*

**Dosepak** (trademarked dosage form) *unit-of-use package*

**dosergoside** INN

**Dosette** (trademarked dosage form) *injectable unit-of-use system (vials, ampules, syringes, etc.)*

**Dospan** (trademarked form) *controlled-release tablets*

**Dostinex** tablets ℞ *dopamine agonist for hyperprolactinemia; investigational treatment for Parkinson's disease and gynecologic disorders* [cabergoline] 0.5 mg

**dosulepin** INN *antidepressant* [also: dothiepin HCl; dothiepin; dosulepin HCl]

**dosulepin HCl** JAN *antidepressant* [also: dothiepin HCl; dosulepin; dothiepin]

**dotarizine** INN

**dotefonium bromide** INN

**dothiepin** BAN *antidepressant* [also: dothiepin HCl; dosulepin; dosulepin HCl]

**dothiepin HCl** USAN *antidepressant* [also: dosulepin; dothiepin; dosulepin HCl]

**dots** *street drug slang* [see: LSD]

**doub** *street drug slang for a $20 piece of crack* [see: cocaine, crack]

**double bubble** *street drug slang* [see: cocaine]

**double cross** *street drug slang* [see: amphetamines]

**double dome** *street drug slang* [see: LSD]

**Double Ice ArthriCare** [see: ArthriCare, Double Ice]

**double rock** *street drug slang for crack diluted with procaine* [see: cocaine, crack; procaine]

**double trouble** *street drug slang for Dexamyl (dextroamphetamine sulfate + amobarbital; discontinued 1980)* [see: dextroamphetamine sulfate; amobarbital]

**double trouble** *street drug slang for Tuinal (amobarbital sodium + secobarbital sodium) or other CNS depressants* [see: Tuinal; amobarbital sodium; secobarbital sodium]

**double yoke** *street drug slang* [see: cocaine, crack]

**Double-Action Toothache Kit** *tablets + liquid* OTC *analgesic; topical oral anesthetic* [(acetaminophen) + (benzocaine; alcohol 74%)] (325 mg) + ( ≗ )

**dove** *street drug slang for a $35 piece of crack* [see: cocaine, crack]

**Dover's powder** *street drug slang* [see: opium]

**Dovonex** *cream, ointment, scalp solution* R *topical antipsoriatic* [calcipotriene] 0.005%

**down; downer; downies** *street drug slang for various CNS depressants*

**down and dirty** *street drug slang for Quaalude (methaqualone; discontinued 1983)* [see: methaqualone]

**doxacurium chloride** USAN, INN, BAN *nondepolarizing neuromuscular blocker; muscle relaxant; adjunct to anesthesia*

**doxaminol** INN

**doxapram** INN, BAN *respiratory stimulant* [also: doxapram HCl]

**doxapram HCl** USAN, USP *respiratory stimulant; analeptic* [also: doxapram] 20 mg/mL injection

**doxaprost** USAN, INN *bronchodilator*

**doxate** [see: docusate sodium]

**doxazosin** INN, BAN *antihypertensive; $\alpha_1$-adrenergic blocker* [also: doxazosin mesylate]

**doxazosin mesylate** USAN *antihypertensive; $\alpha_1$-adrenergic blocker* [also: doxazosin]

**doxefazepam** INN

**doxenitoin** INN

**doxepin** INN, BAN *tricyclic antidepressant* [also: doxepin HCl] ▢ Doxidan

**doxepin HCl** USAN, USP *tricyclic antidepressant; anxiolytic; topical antipruritic* [also: doxepin] 10, 25, 50, 75, 100, 150 mg oral; 10 mg/mL oral

**doxibetasol** INN [also: doxybetasol]

**Doxidan** *capsules* OTC *laxative; stool softener* [phenolphthalein; docusate calcium] 65•60 mg ▢ doxepin

**doxifluridine** INN *investigational antineoplastic*

**Doxil** *IV injection* R *antibiotic antineoplastic for Kaposi sarcoma; investigational for metastatic breast cancer* [doxorubicin HCl (liposomal formulation)] 20 mg/vial

**Doxinate** *capsules, solution (discontinued 1994)* OTC *stool softener* [docusate sodium] 240 mg; 50 mg/mL

**doxofylline** USAN, INN *bronchodilator*

**doxorubicin** USAN, INN, BAN *antibiotic antineoplastic* ▢ daunorubicin

**doxorubicin HCl** USP *antibiotic antineoplastic* 10, 20, 50 mg, 2 mg/mL injection

**doxpicodin HCl** [now: doxpicomine HCl]

**doxpicomine** INN *analgesic* [also: doxpicomine HCl]

**doxpicomine HCl** USAN *analgesic* [also: doxpicomine]

**Dox-SL** R *investigational antineoplastic for AIDS-related Kaposi sarcoma, leukemia, breast and ovarian cancers* [liposome formulation of doxorubicin]

**Doxy 100; Doxy 200** *powder for IV injection* R *tetracycline-type antibiotic* [doxycycline hyclate] 100 mg; 200 mg

**Doxy Caps** *capsules* R *tetracycline-type antibiotic* [doxycycline hyclate] 100 mg

**doxybetasol** BAN [also: doxibetasol]

**Doxychel Hyclate** *capsules, tablets, powder for IV injection* R *tetracycline-type antibiotic* [doxycycline hyclate] 50, 100 mg; 50, 100 mg; 100, 200 mg

**doxycycline** USAN, USP, INN, BAN *bacteriostatic; antirickettsial; malaria prophylaxis*

**doxycycline calcium** USP *antibacterial; antiprotozoal*

**doxycycline fosfatex** USAN, BAN *antibacterial*

**doxycycline hyclate** USP *antibacterial* 50, 100 mg oral; 100, 200 mg/vial injection

**doxylamine** INN, BAN *antihistamine* [also: doxylamine succinate]

**doxylamine succinate** USP *antihistamine; sleep aid* [also: doxylamine]

**Doxysom Nighttime Sleep-Aid** tablets (discontinued 1993) OTC *antihistaminic sleep aid* [doxylamine succinate]

**DPE (dipivalyl epinephrine)** [now: dipivefrin]

**DPF** [see: Dermprotective Factor]

**DPN (diphosphopyridine nucleotide)** [now: nadide]

**DPPC (dipalmitoylphosphatidylcholine)** [see: colfosceril palmitate]

**Dr. Caldwell Senna Laxative** liquid OTC *laxative* [senna concentrate] 33.3 mg/mL

**Dr. Dermi-Heal** ointment OTC *vulnerary; antipruritic; astringent* [allantoin; zinc oxide; balsam Peru] 1%• ? • ?

**Dr. Scholl's Advanced Pain Relief Corn Removers; Dr. Scholl's Callus Removers; Dr Scholl's Clear Away; Dr. Scholl's Corn Removers** medicated discs OTC *topical keratolytic* [salicylic acid in a rubber-based vehicle] 40%

**Dr. Scholl's Athlete's Foot** powder, spray powder, spray liquid OTC *topical antifungal* [tolnaftate] 1%

**Dr. Scholl's Clear Away OneStep; Dr. Scholl's OneStep Corn Removers** medicated strips OTC *topical keratolytic* [salicylic acid in a rubber-based vehicle] 40%

**Dr. Scholl's Corn/Callus Remover** liquid OTC *topical keratolytic* [salicylic acid in flexible collodion] 17%

**Dr. Scholl's Cracked Heel Relief** cream OTC *topical local anesthetic; antiseptic* [lidocaine HCl; benzalkonium chloride] 2%•0.13%

**Dr. Scholl's Moisturizing Corn Remover Kit** medicated discs + cushions + moisturizing cream OTC *topical keratolytic* [salicylic acid in a rubber-based vehicle] 40%

**Dr. Scholl's Tritin** powder, spray powder OTC *topical antifungal* [tolnaftate] 1%

**Dr. Scholl's Wart Remover Kit** liquid + adhesive pads OTC *topical keratolytic* [salicylic acid in flexible collodion] 17%

**draf weed; drag weed** *street drug slang* [see: marijuana]

**draflazine** USAN *cardioprotectant*

**dragée** (French for "sugar plum") *a sugar-coated pill or medicated confection* [pronounced "drah zhá"]

**Dramamine** IV or IM injection (discontinued 1994) ℞ *antinauseant; antiemetic; antivertigo agent; motion sickness preventative* [dimenhydrinate] 50 mg/mL

**Dramamine** liquid ℞ *antinauseant; antiemetic; antivertigo agent; motion sickness preventative* [dimenhydrinate] 15.62 mg/5 mL

**Dramamine** tablets, chewable tablets, liquid OTC *antinauseant; antiemetic; antivertigo agent; motion sickness preventative* [dimenhydrinate] 50 mg; 50 mg; 12.5 mg/4 mL

**Dramamine, Children's** liquid OTC *antinauseant; antiemetic; antivertigo agent; motion sickness preventative* [dimenhydrinate; alcohol 5%] 12.5 mg/5 mL

**Dramamine II** tablets OTC *anticholinergic; antihistamine; antivertigo agent; motion sickness preventative* [meclizine HCl] 25 mg

**Dramanate** IV or IM injection ℞ *antinauseant; antiemetic; antivertigo agent; motion sickness preventative* [dimenhydrinate] 50 mg/mL ⓘ Dommanate

**dramarin** [see: dimenhydrate]

**dramedilol** INN

**Dramilin** IV or IM injection ℞ *antinauseant; antiemetic; antivertigo agent; motion sickness preventative* [dimenhydrinate] 50 mg/mL

**Dramocen** IV or IM injection (discontinued 1994) ℞ *antinauseant; antiemetic; antivertigo agent; motion sickness preventative* [dimenhydrinate] 50 mg/mL

**Dramoject** IV or IM injection (discontinued 1996) ℞ *antinauseant; antiemetic; antivertigo agent; motion sickness preventative* [dimenhydrinate] 50 mg/mL

**dramyl** [see: dimenhydrate]

**draquinolol** INN

**drazidox** INN

**dream** *street drug slang* [see: cocaine]

**dream gum; dream stick; dreams** *street drug slang* [see: opium]

**dreamer** *street drug slang* [see: morphine]

**dreck** *street drug slang* [see: heroin]

**Drepanol** Ŗ *investigational (orphan) for prophylactic treatment of sickle cell disease* [OM 401 (code name—generic name not yet approved)]

**dribendazole** USAN, INN *anthelmintic*

**dricol** [see: amidephrine]

**Dri/Ear** ear drops OTC *antibacterial/antifungal* [boric acid] 2.75%

**dried aluminum hydroxide gel** [see: aluminum hydroxide gel, dried]

**dried basic aluminum carbonate** [see: aluminum carbonate, basic]

**dried ferrous sulfate** [see: ferrous sulfate, dried]

**dried yeast** [see: yeast, dried]

**drinidene** USAN, INN *analgesic*

**drink** *street drug slang* [see: PCP]

**Drisdol** capsules Ŗ *vitamin deficiency therapy* [ergocalciferol] 50 000 IU

**Drisdol Drops** OTC *vitamin supplement* [ergocalciferol] 8000 IU/mL

**Dristan** nasal spray OTC *nasal decongestant; antihistamine* [phenylephrine HCl; pheniramine maleate] 0.5%•0.2%

**Dristan 12-Hr.** nasal spray OTC *nasal decongestant* [oxymetazoline HCl] 0.05%

**Dristan Advanced Formula** tablets (name changed to Dristan Cold Multi-Symptom Formula in 1993)

**Dristan Allergy** caplets (discontinued 1995) OTC *decongestant; antihistamine* [pseudoephedrine HCl; brompheniramine maleate] 60•4 mg

**Dristan Cold** caplets OTC *decongestant; analgesic; antipyretic* [pseudoephedrine HCl; acetaminophen] 30•500 mg

**Dristan Cold, Maximum Strength** caplets OTC *decongestant; antihistamine; analgesic* [pseudoephedrine HCl; brompheniramine maleate; acetaminophen] 30•2•500 mg

**Dristan Cold & Flu** powder (discontinued 1995) OTC *antitussive; decongestant; antihistamine; analgesic* [dextromethorphan hydrobromide; pseudoephedrine HCl; chlorpheniramine maleate; acetaminophen] 20•60•4•500 mg/packet

**Dristan Cold Multi-Symptom Formula** tablets OTC *decongestant; antihistamine; analgesic* [phenylephrine HCl; chlorpheniramine maleate; acetaminophen] 5•2•325 mg

**Dristan Decongestant** inhaler (discontinued 1993) OTC *nasal decongestant* [propylhexedrine; camphor; eucalyptol; menthol]

**Dristan Juice Mix-In** powder (discontinued 1995) OTC *antitussive; decongestant; analgesic* [dextromethorphan hydrobromide; pseudoephedrine HCl; acetaminophen] 20•60•500 mg/packet

**Dristan Long Lasting** nasal spray (name changed to Dristan 12-Hr. in 1994)

**Dristan Saline Spray** OTC *nasal moisturizer* [sodium chloride (saline)]

**Dristan Sinus** caplets OTC *decongestant; analgesic* [pseudoephedrine HCl; ibuprofen] 30•200 mg

**Dristan-AF** tablets (discontinued 1993) OTC *decongestant; antihistamine; analgesic* [phenylephrine HCl; chlorpheniramine maleate; acetaminophen; caffeine]

**Drithocreme; Drithocreme HP 1%; Dritho-Scalp** cream Ŗ *topical antipsoriatic* [anthralin] 0.1%, 0.25%, 0.5%; 1%; 0.5%

**Drixomed** sustained-release tablets Ŗ *decongestant; antihistamine* [pseudoephedrine sulfate; dexbrompheniramine maleate] 120•6 mg

**Drixoral** syrup OTC *decongestant; antihistamine* [pseudoephedrine sulfate; brompheniramine maleate] 30•2 mg/5 mL

**Drixoral Allergy Sinus; Drixoral Cold & Flu** extended-release tablets OTC *decongestant; antihistamine; analgesic* [pseudoephedrine sulfate; dexbrompheniramine maleate; acetaminophen] 60•3•500 mg

**Drixoral Cold & Allergy** sustained-action tablets OTC *decongestant; antihis-

*tamine* [pseudoephedrine sulfate; dexbrompheniramine maleate] 120•6 mg

**Drixoral Cough & Congestion Liquid Caps** (capsules) OTC *antitussive; decongestant* [dextromethorphan hydrobromide; pseudoephedrine HCl] 30•60 mg

**Drixoral Cough Liquid Caps** (liquid-filled capsules) OTC *antitussive* [dextromethorphan hydrobromide] 30 mg

**Drixoral Cough & Sore Throat Liquid Caps** (liquid-filled capsules) OTC *antitussive; analgesic* [dextromethorphan hydrobromide; acetaminophen] 15•325 mg

**Drixoral Non-Drowsy Formula** extended-release tablets OTC *nasal decongestant* [pseudoephedrine sulfate] 120 mg

**Drixoral Plus** extended-release tablets (name changed to Drixoral Cold & Flu in 1993)

**Drixoral Sinus** extended-release tablets (name changed to Drixoral Allergy Sinus in 1994)

**Drize** sustained-release capsules Ŗ *decongestant; antihistamine* [phenylpropanolamine HCl; chlorpheniramine maleate] 75•12 mg

**drobuline** USAN, INN *antiarrhythmic*

**drocarbil** NF

**drocinonide** USAN, INN *anti-inflammatory*

**droclidinium bromide** INN

**drocode** [see: dihydrocodeine]

**drofenine** INN

**droloxifene** INN *investigational (Phase III) antineoplastic for breast cancer; investigational (Phase III) antiestrogen for postmenopausal osteoporosis*

**droloxifene citrate** USAN *antineoplastic; antiestrogen*

**drometrizole** USAN, INN *ultraviolet screen*

**dromostanolone propionate** USAN, USP *antineoplastic* [also: drostanolone]

**dronabinol** USAN, USP, INN *antiemetic for chemotherapy; appetite stimulant in AIDS patients (orphan)*

**drop chalk** [see: calcium carbonate]

**Drop-Dose** (trademarked delivery system) *prefilled eye drop dispenser*

**dropempine** INN

**droperidol** USAN, USP, INN, BAN *general anesthetic; antipsychotic*

**Dropperettes** (delivery system) *prefilled droppers*

**droprenilamine** USAN, INN *coronary vasodilator*

**dropropizine** INN, BAN

**Drop-Tainers** (trademarked dosage form) *prefilled eye drop dispenser*

**drostanolone** INN, BAN *antineoplastic* [also: dromostanolone propionate]

**drotaverine** INN

**drotebanol** INN, BAN

**Drotic** ear drops Ŗ *topical corticosteroidal anti-inflammatory; antibiotic* [hydrocortisone; neomycin sulfate; polymyxin B sulfate] 1%•5 mg• 10 000 U per mL

**drowsy high** *street drug slang for various CNS depressants*

**droxacin** INN *antibacterial* [also: droxacin sodium]

**droxacin sodium** USAN *antibacterial* [also: droxacin]

**droxicainide** INN

**droxicam** INN

**droxidopa** INN

**droxifilcon A** USAN *hydrophilic contact lens material*

**droxinavir HCl** USAN *antiviral; HIV-1 protease inhibitor*

**droxypropine** INN, BAN

**drug store dope** *street drug slang* [see: morphine]

**Dry Eye Therapy** eye drops OTC *ocular moisturizer/lubricant* [glycerin] 0.3%

**Dry Eyes** eye drops OTC *ocular moisturizer/lubricant* [polyvinyl alcohol] 1.4%

**Dry Eyes** ophthalmic ointment OTC *ocular moisturizer/lubricant* [white petrolatum; mineral oil]

**dry high** *street drug slang* [see: marijuana]

**Dryox 2.5; Dryox 5; Dryox 10; Dryox 20** gel OTC *topical keratolytic for acne* [benzoyl peroxide] 2.5%; 5%; 10%; 20%

**Dryox 10S 5; Dryox 20S 10** gel OTC *topical keratolytic for acne* [benzoyl peroxide; sulfur] 10%•5%; 20%•10%

**Dryox Wash 5; Dryox Wash 10** liquid OTC *topical keratolytic for acne* [benzoyl peroxide] 5%; 10%

**Drysol** solution ℞ *astringent for hyperhidrosis* [aluminum chloride] 20%

**Drytergent** liquid OTC *soap-free therapeutic skin cleanser*

**Drytex** lotion OTC *topical keratolytic cleanser for acne* [salicylic acid; acetone; isopropyl alcohol] ≟•10%•40%

**DSC; DSCG (disodium cromoglycate)** [see: cromolyn sodium]

**DSMC Plus** capsules OTC *laxative; stool softener* [casanthranol; docusate potassium] 30•100 mg

**D-S-S** capsules OTC *stool softener* [docusate sodium] 100 mg

**DSS (dioctyl sodium sulfosuccinate)** [now: docusate sodium]

**D-S-S Plus** capsules (discontinued 1997) OTC *laxative; stool softener* [casanthranol; docusate sodium] 30•100 mg

**DST (dihydrostreptomycin)** [q.v.]

**DT; Td (diphtheria & tetanus [toxoids])** *the designation DT or TD denotes the pediatric vaccine; Td denotes the adult vaccine* [see: diphtheria & tetanus toxoids, adsorbed]

**DTaP (diphtheria & tetanus [toxoids] & acellular pertussis [vaccine])** [q.v.]

**DTC 101** *investigational antineoplastic for neoplastic meningitis*

**DTIC (dimethyl triazeno imidazole carboxamide)** [see: dacarbazine]

**DTIC-Dome** IV injection ℞ *alkylating antineoplastic for metastatic malignant melanoma and Hodgkin's disease* [dacarbazine] 10 mg/mL

**DTP (diphtheria & tetanus [toxoids] & pertussis [vaccine])** [q.v.]

**DTPA (diethylenetriaminepentaacetic acid)** [see: pentetic acid]

**DTPA (diethylenetriaminepentaacetic acid) technetium ($^{99m}$Tc), human serum albumin** [see: technetium Tc 99m pentetate]

**DTwP (diphtheria & tetanus [toxoids] & whole-cell pertussis [vaccine])** [q.v.]

**Duadacin** capsules OTC *decongestant; antihistamine; analgesic* [phenylpropanolamine HCl; chlorpheniramine maleate; acetaminophen] 12.5•2•325 mg

**duazomycin** USAN, INN *antineoplastic*

**duazomycin A** [see: duazomycin]

**duazomycin B** [see: azotomycin]

**duazomycin C** [see: ambomycin]

**ducodal** [see: oxycodone]

**duct** *street drug slang* [see: cocaine]

**'due; dew** *street drug slang for marijuana or the residue of oils left in a pipe after smoking crack* [see: marijuana; cocaine, crack]

**duji** *street drug slang* [see: heroin]

**Dulcagen** enteric-coated tablets OTC *stimulant laxative* [bisacodyl] 5 mg

**Dulcagen** suppositories OTC *stimulant laxative* [bisacodyl] 10 mg

**Dulcet** (trademarked dosage form) *chewable tablet*

**Dulcolax** enteric-coated tablets OTC *stimulant laxative* [bisacodyl] 5 mg

**Dulcolax** suppositories OTC *stimulant laxative* [bisacodyl] 10 mg

**Dulcolax Bowel Prep Kit** 4 enteric-coated tablets + 1 suppository OTC *pre-procedure bowel evacuant* [bisacodyl] 5 mg; 10 mg

**Dull-C** powder OTC *vitamin supplement* [ascorbic acid] 4 g/tsp.

**dulofibrate** INN

**duloxetine** INN *antidepressant* [also: duloxetine HCl]

**duloxetine HCl** USAN *antidepressant* [also: duloxetine]

**dulozafone** INN

**dummy dust** *street drug slang* [see: PCP]

**dumorelin** INN

**duneryl** [see: phenobarbital]

**Duocet** tablets ℞ *narcotic analgesic* [hydrocodone bitartrate; acetaminophen] 5•500 mg

**Duo-Cyp** IM injection ℞ *estrogen/androgen for menopausal vasomotor symptoms* [estradiol cypionate; testosterone cypionate] 2•50 mg/mL

**DuoDerm CGF; DuoDerm Extra Thin; DuoDerm Hydroactive** adhesive dressings OTC *occlusive wound dressing* [hydrocolloid gel]

**DuoDerm Hydroactive** paste, granules OTC *wound dressing* [hydrocolloid gel] 30 g; 5 g

**DuoFilm** liquid OTC *topical keratolytic* [salicylic acid in flexible collodion] 17%

**DuoFilm** transdermal patch OTC *topical keratolytic* [salicylic acid in a rubber-based vehicle] 40%

**duo-Flow** solution (discontinued 1993) OTC *cleaning and soaking solution for hard contact lenses*

**Duolube** ophthalmic ointment (discontinued 1993) OTC *ocular moisturizer/lubricant*

**Duo-Medihaler** inhalation aerosol ℞ *bronchodilator* [isoproterenol HCl; phenylephrine bitartrate] 0.16•0.24 mg/dose

**duometacin** INN

**duomycin** [see: chlortetracycline HCl]

**duoperone** INN *neuroleptic* [also: duoperone fumarate]

**duoperone fumarate** USAN *neuroleptic* [also: duoperone]

**DuoPlant** gel ℞ *topical keratolytic* [salicylic acid in flexible collodion] 17%

**duotal** [see: guaiacol carbonate]

**Duo-Trach Kit** pre-filled syringe with cannula ℞ *injectable local anesthetic* [lidocaine HCl] 4%

**Duotrate; Duotrate 45** sustained-release capsules (discontinued 1995) ℞ *antianginal* [pentaerythritol tetranitrate] 30 mg; 45 mg

**Duphalac** syrup ℞ *laxative* [lactulose] 10 g/15 mL

**Duplex** liquid OTC *soap-free therapeutic skin cleanser* [sodium lauryl sulfate] 15%

**Duplex T** shampoo OTC *antiseborrheic; antipsoriatic; antipruritic; antibacterial* [coal tar] 10%

**duponol** [see: sodium lauryl sulfate]

**dupracetam** INN

**Durabolin** IM injection ℞ *anabolic steroid for metastatic breast cancer in women; also abused as a street drug* [nandrolone phenpropionate] 25, 50 mg/mL

**Duracaps** (dosage form) *sustained-release capsules*

**DURAcare** solution (discontinued 1995) OTC *surfactant cleaning solution for soft contact lenses*

**DURAcare II** solution OTC *surfactant cleaning solution for soft contact lenses*

**Duracid** chewable tablets (discontinued 1994) OTC *antacid* [aluminum hydroxide; magnesium carbonate; calcium carbonate] 175•175•325 mg

**Duraclon** continuous epidural infusion ℞ *central analgesic; adjunct to opioid analgesics for severe cancer pain* [clonidine HCl] 100 µg/mL

**Duract** capsules ℞ *long-acting nonsteroidal anti-inflammatory drug (NSAID); analgesic; antipyretic* [bromfenac sodium] 25 mg

**Duradyne** tablets (discontinued 1994) OTC *analgesic; antipyretic; anti-inflammatory* [acetaminophen; aspirin; caffeine] 180•230•15 mg

**Duradyne DHC** tablets (discontinued 1994) ℞ *narcotic analgesic* [hydrocodone bitartrate; acetaminophen]

**Dura-Estrin** IM injection (discontinued 1996) ℞ *hormone replacement therapy for postmenopausal disorders* [estradiol cypionate in oil] 5 mg/mL

**Duragen-20; Duragen-40** IM injection (discontinued 1996) ℞ *estrogen replacement therapy for postmenopausal disorders; antineoplastic for prostatic cancer* [estradiol valerate in oil] 20 mg/mL; 40 mg/mL

**Duragesic-25; Duragesic-50; Duragesic-75; Duragesic-100** transdermal patch ℞ *narcotic analgesic* [fentanyl] 25 µg/hr.; 50 µg/hr.; 75 µg/hr.; 100 µg/hr.

**Dura-Gest** capsules ℞ *decongestant; expectorant* [phenylephrine HCl; phenylpropanolamine HCl; guaifenesin] 45•5•200 mg

**Duralex** sustained-release capsules ℞ *decongestant; antihistamine* [pseudoephedrine HCl; chlorpheniramine maleate] 120•8 mg

**Duralone-40; Duralone-80** intralesional, soft tissue, and IM injection ℞ *glucocorticoid; anti-inflammatory; immunosuppressant* [methylprednisolone acetate] 40 mg/mL; 80 mg/mL

**Duralutin** IM injection (discontinued 1996) ℞ *progestin for amenorrhea, metrorrhagia, and dysfunctional uterine*

*bleeding* [hydroxyprogesterone caproate in oil] 250 mg/mL

**Duramist Plus** nasal spray OTC *nasal decongestant* [oxymetazoline HCl] 0.05%

**Duramorph** IV, subcu or IM injection R *narcotic analgesic; preoperative sedative and anxiolytic* [morphine sulfate] 0.5, 1 mg/mL

**Duranest; Duranest MPF** injection R *injectable local anesthetic* [etidocaine HCl] 1%

**Duranest; Duranest MPF** injection R *injectable local anesthetic* [etidocaine HCl; epinephrine] 1%•1:200 000, 1.5%•1:200 000

**Duranest HCl** injection (name changed to Duranest in 1995)

**durapatite** USAN *prosthetic aid* [also: calcium phosphate, tribasic; hydroxyapatite]

**DuraSite** (delivery system) *polymer-based eye drops*

**Dura-Tab** (trademarked dosage form) *sustained-release tablet*

**Dura-Tap/PD** prolonged-action capsule R *pediatric decongestant and antihistamine* [pseudoephedrine HCl; chlorpheniramine maleate] 60•4 mg

**Duratears Naturale** ophthalmic ointment OTC *ocular moisturizer/lubricant* [white petrolatum; mineral oil; lanolin]

**Duratest 100; Duratest 200** IM injection R *androgen replacement for delayed puberty or breast cancer* [testosterone cypionate] 100 mg/mL; 200 mg/mL

**Duratestrin** IM injection R *estrogen/androgen for menopausal vasomotor symptoms* [estradiol cypionate; testosterone cypionate] 2•50 mg/mL

**Durathate-200** IM injection R *androgen replacement for delayed puberty or breast cancer* [testosterone enanthate] 200 mg/mL

**Duration** nasal spray OTC *nasal decongestant* [oxymetazoline HCl] 0.05%

**Duratuss** long-acting film-coated tablets R *decongestant; expectorant* [pseudoephedrine HCl; guaifenesin] 120•600 mg

**Duratuss HD** elixir R *narcotic antitussive; decongestant; expectorant* [hydrocodone bitartrate; pseudoephedrine HCl; guaifenesin] 2.5•30•100 mg/5 mL

**Duratuss-G** film-coated tablets R *expectorant* [guaifenesin] 1.2 g

**Dura-Vent** long-acting tablets R *decongestant; expectorant* [phenylpropanolamine HCl; guaifenesin] 75•600 mg

**Dura-Vent/A** continuous-release capsule R *decongestant; antihistamine* [phenylpropanolamine HCl; chlorpheniramine maleate] 75•10 mg

**Dura-Vent/DA** sustained-release tablets R *decongestant; antihistamine; anticholinergic* [phenylephrine HCl; chlorpheniramine maleate; methscopolamine nitrate] 20•8•2.5 mg

**Duricef** capsules, tablets R *cephalosporin-type antibiotic* [cefadroxil monohydrate] 500 mg; 1000 mg

**Duricef** oral suspension R *cephalosporin-type antibiotic* [cefadroxil] 125, 250, 500 mg/5 mL

**durog; duros** street drug slang [see: marijuana]

**dust** street drug slang for heroin, cocaine, PCP, or marijuana mixed with various other substances [see: heroin; cocaine; PCP; marijuana]

**dust joint; dust of angels; dusted parsley** street drug slang [see: PCP]

**dusting** street drug slang for a combination of marijuana and PCP, heroin, or other powdered street drug [see: marijuana; PCP; heroin]

**dusting powder, absorbable** USP *surgical glove lubricant*

**dusty roads** street drug slang for a combination of cocaine and PCP for smoking [see: cocaine; PCP]

**Dutonin** (British name for U.S. product Serzone)

**Duvoid** tablets R *cholinergic urinary stimulant for postsurgical and postpartum urinary retention* [bethanechol chloride] 10, 25, 50 mg

**DV** vaginal cream (discontinued 1996) R *estrogen replacement therapy for postmenopausal disorders* [dienestrol] 0.01%

**DVB (DDP, vindesine, bleomycin)** *chemotherapy protocol*

**DVP (daunorubicin, vincristine, prednisone)** *chemotherapy protocol*

**DVPL-ASP (daunorubicin, vincristine, prednisone, L-asparaginase)** *chemotherapy protocol*

**Dwelle** eye drops OTC *ocular moisturizer/lubricant*

**Dyazide** capsules R *diuretic; antihypertensive* [triamterene; hydrochlorothiazide] 37.5•25 mg ② Thiacide; thiazides

**Dycill** capsules R *bactericidal antibiotic (penicillinase-resistant penicillin)* [dicloxacillin sodium] 250, 500 mg

**dyclocaine** BAN *topical anesthetic* [also: dyclonine HCl; dyclonine]

**Dyclone** solution R *anesthetic prior to upper GI and respiratory endoscopies* [dyclonine HCl] 0.5%, 1%

**dyclonine** INN *topical anesthetic* [also: dyclonine HCl; dyclocaine]

**dyclonine HCl** USP *topical anesthetic* [also: dyclonine; dyclocaine]

**dydrogesterone** USAN, USP, INN, BAN *progestin*

**Dyflex-200** tablets (discontinued 1996) R *bronchodilator* [dyphylline] 200 mg

**Dyflex-400** tablets (discontinued 1993) R *bronchodilator* [dyphylline] 400 mg

**Dyflex-G** tablets R *antiasthmatic; expectorant* [dyphylline; guaifenesin] 200•200 mg

**dyflos** BAN *antiglaucoma agent; irreversible cholinesterase inhibitor miotic* [also: isoflurophate]

**dylate** [see: clonitrate]

**Dyline-GG** tablets, liquid R *antiasthmatic; bronchodilator; expectorant* [dyphylline; guaifenesin] 200•200 mg; 300•300 mg/15 mL

**dymanthine HCl** USAN *anthelmintic* [also: dimantine HCl]

**Dymelor** tablets R *sulfonylurea-type antidiabetic* [acetohexamide] 250, 500 mg ② Demerol; Pamelor

**Dymenate** IV or IM injection R *antinauseant; antiemetic; antivertigo; motion sickness preventative* [dimenhydrinate] 50 mg/mL

**Dynabac** enteric-coated tablets R *once-daily macrolide antibiotic for respiratory and dermatological infections* [dirithromycin] 250 mg

**Dynacin** capsules R *tetracycline-type antibiotic* [minocycline HCl] 50, 100 mg

**DynaCirc** capsules R *antihypertensive; dihydropyridine calcium channel blocker* [isradipine] 2.5, 5 mg

**DynaCirc CR** controlled-release tablets R *once-daily antihypertensive; dihydropyridine calcium channel blocker* [isradipine] 5, 10 mg

**dynacoryl** [see: nikethamide]

**Dynafed; Dynafed Plus** tablets OTC *decongestant; analgesic; antipyretic* [pseudoephedrine HCl; acetaminophen] 30•500 mg

**Dynafed Asthma Relief** tablets OTC *decongestant; expectorant* [ephedrine HCl; guaifenesin] 25•200 mg

**Dynafed E.X.** tablets OTC *analgesic; antipyretic* [acetaminophen] 500 mg

**Dynafed IB** tablets OTC *nonsteroidal anti-inflammatory drug (NSAID); antiarthritic; analgesic* [ibuprofen] 200 mg

**Dynafed Jr., Children's** chewable tablets OTC *analgesic; antipyretic* [acetaminophen] 80 mg

**Dynafed Pseudo** tablets OTC *nasal decongestant* [pseudoephedrine HCl] 60 mg

**Dyna-Hex Skin Cleanser; Dyna-Hex 2 Skin Cleanser** liquid OTC *broad-spectrum antimicrobial; germicidal* [chlorhexidine gluconate; alcohol 4%] 4%; 2%

**dynamine** *investigational (orphan) for Lambert-Eaton myasthenic syndrome and Charcot-Marie-Tooth disease*

**dynamite** *street drug slang for a combination of heroin and cocaine* [see: heroin; cocaine]

**Dynapen** capsules, powder for oral suspension R *bactericidal antibiotic (penicillinase-resistant penicillin)* [dicloxacillin sodium] 125, 250, 500 mg; 62.5 mg/5 mL

**dynarsan** [see: acetarsone]

**dyno; dyno-pure** *street drug slang* [see: heroin]

**Dynospheres M-035** ℞ *investigational imaging agent for MRI* [ferristene]

**dyphylline** USP *bronchodilator* [also: diprophylline] 200, 400 mg oral

**Dyphylline-GG** elixir OTC *antiasthmatic; bronchodilator; expectorant* [dyphylline; guaifenesin] 100•100 mg/15 mL

**Dyprotex** pads OTC *topical diaper rash treatment* [zinc oxide; dimethicone] 40%•2.5%

**Dyrenium** capsules ℞ *potassium-sparing diuretic* [triamterene] 50, 100 mg ⑨ Pyridium

**Dyrexan-OD** sustained-release capsules ℞ *anorexiant* [phendimetrazine tartrate] 105 mg

**Dysport** ℞ *blepharospasm and strabismus of dystonia (orphan); investigational (orphan) for pediatric cerebral palsy and cervical dystonia* [botulinum toxin, type A]

**dysprosium** *element (Dy)*

**DZAPO (daunorubicin, azacitidine, ara-C, prednisone, Oncovin)** *chemotherapy protocol*

**E5** ℞ *investigational agent for gram-negative sepsis* [H65-RTA monoclonal antibody]

**E-200; E-400; E-1000** softgels OTC *vitamin supplement* [vitamin E] 147 mg; 400 IU; 1000 IU

**E-2020** *investigational cholinesterase inhibitor for Alzheimer's disease*

**E5 MAb** [now: edobacomab]

**Eaase** capsules (discontinued 1993) OTC *dietary supplement* [multiple amino acids, vitamins, and minerals]

**EACA (epsilon-aminocaproic acid)** [see: aminocaproic acid]

**EAP (etoposide, Adriamycin, Platinol)** *chemotherapy protocol*

**Ear-Dry** ear drops OTC *antibacterial/antifungal* [boric acid] 2.75%

**Ear-Eze** ear drops ℞ *topical corticosteroidal anti-inflammatory; antibiotic* [hydrocortisone; neomycin sulfate; polymyxin B sulfate] 1%•5 mg•10 000 U per mL

**EarSol** ear drops OTC *antiseptic* [alcohol] 44%

**EarSol-HC** ear drops OTC *topical corticosteroidal anti-inflammatory; antiseptic* [hydrocortisone; alcohol 44%] 1%

**earth** *street drug slang for a marijuana cigarette* [see: marijuana]

**earthnut oil** [see: peanut oil]

**easing powder** *street drug slang* [see: opium]

**Easprin** enteric-coated delayed-release tablets ℞ *analgesic; antipyretic; anti-inflammatory; antirheumatic* [aspirin] 975 mg

**eastside player** *street drug slang* [see: cocaine, crack]

**easy lay** *street drug slang* [see: GHB]

**EasyClean/GP Weekly Enzymatic Cleaner** solution (discontinued 1993) OTC *cleaning solution for rigid gas permeable lenses*

**E-Base** delayed-release enteric-coated caplets and tablets ℞ *macrolide antibiotic* [erythromycin] 333, 500 mg

**ebastine** USAN, INN *antihistamine*

**ebiratide** INN

**ebrotidine** INN

**ebselen** INN

**EC (etoposide, carboplatin)** *chemotherapy protocol*

**ecadotril** USAN, INN *antihypertensive*

**ecarazine** [see: todralazine]

**ecastolol** INN

**Ecee Plus** tablets OTC *vitamin/mineral supplement* [vitamins C and E; zinc sulfate; magnesium sulfate] 100•165•80•70 mg

**ECHO (etoposide, cyclophosphamide, hydroxydaunomycin, Oncovin)** *chemotherapy protocol*

**EchoGen** emulsion ℞ *investigational (Phase III) ultrasound contrast agent for stress cardiography and transrectal prostate imaging* [perflenapent; perflisopent] 85%•15%

**echothiophate iodide** USP *antiglaucoma agent; irreversible cholinesterase inhibitor miotic* [also: ecothiopate iodide]

**Echovist** intracoronary injection ℞ *ultrasound contrast agent; investigational for gynecologic uses* [galactose]

**ecipramidil** INN

**eclanamine** INN *antidepressant* [also: eclanamine maleate]

**eclanamine maleate** USAN *antidepressant* [also: eclanamine]

**eclazolast** USAN, INN *antiallergic; mediator release inhibitor*

**EC-Naprosyn** enteric-coated delayed-release tablets ℞ *nonsteroidal anti-inflammatory drug (NSAID); antiarthritic; analgesic* [naproxen] 375, 500 mg

**ecogramostim** BAN

**E-Complex-600** capsules OTC *dietary supplement* [vitamin E] 600 IU

**ecomustine** INN

**econazole** USAN, INN, BAN *antifungal*

**econazole nitrate** USAN, USP, BAN *antifungal*

**Econo B & C** caplets OTC *vitamin supplement* [multiple B vitamins; vitamin C] ≜•300 mg

**Econopred; Econopred Plus** Drop-Tainers (eye drop suspension) ℞ *ophthalmic topical corticosteroidal anti-inflammatory* [prednisolone acetate] 0.125%; 1%

**ecostigmine iodide** [see: echothiophate iodide]

**ecothiopate iodide** INN, BAN *antiglaucoma agent; irreversible cholinesterase inhibitor miotic* [also: echothiophate iodide]

**Ecotrin** enteric-coated tablets, enteric-coated caplets OTC *analgesic; antipyretic; anti-inflammatory; antiarthritic* [aspirin] 325, 500 mg ② Edecrin

**Ecotrin Adult Low Strength** enteric-coated tablets OTC *analgesic; antipyretic; anti-inflammatory; antiarthritic* [aspirin] 81 mg

**ecstasy; ex; X** *street drug slang* [see: MDMA]

**ectylurea** BAN

**Ed A-Hist** long-acting capsules, liquid ℞ *decongestant; antihistamine* [phenylephrine HCl; chlorpheniramine maleate] 20•8 mg; 10•4 mg/5 mL

**edamine** [see: ethylenediamine]

**EDAP (etoposide, dexamethasone, ara-C, Platinol)** *chemotherapy protocol*

**edathamil** [now: edetate calcium disodium]

**edathamil calcium disodium** [now: edetate calcium disodium]

**edathamil disodium** [now: edetate disodium]

**edatrexate** USAN, INN *antineoplastic; methotrexate analog*

**Edecrin** tablets ℞ *loop diuretic* [ethacrynic acid] 25, 50 mg ② Ecotrin; Ethaquin

**Edecrin Sodium** powder for IV injection ℞ *loop diuretic* [ethacrynate sodium] 50 mg

**edelfosine** INN

**edetate calcium disodium** USAN, USP *heavy metal chelating agent for lead poisoning* [also: sodium calcium edetate; sodium calciumedetate; calcium disodium edetate]

**edetate dipotassium** USAN *chelating agent*

**edetate disodium** USP *chelating agent; preservative; antioxidant* [also: disodium edetate] 150 mg/mL injection

**edetate sodium** USAN *chelating agent*

**edetate trisodium** USAN *chelating agent*

**edetic acid** NF, INN, BAN *chelating agent*

**edetol** USAN, INN *alkalizing agent*

**Edex** injection ℞ *vasodilator for erectile dysfunction* [alprostadil] 5, 10, 20, 40 µg/mL

**edifolone** INN *antiarrhythmic* [also: edifolone acetate]

**edifolone acetate** USAN *antiarrhythmic* [also: edifolone]

**edisilate** INN *combining name for radicals or groups* [also: edisylate]

**edisylate** USAN, BAN *combining name for radicals or groups* [also: edisilate]

**edithamil** [see: edetate ...]

**edobacomab** USAN *antiendotoxin monoclonal antibody for gram-negative sepsis; clinical trials discontinued 1997*

**edogestrone** INN, BAN

**edoxudine** USAN, INN *antiviral*

**edrecolomab** USAN *monoclonal antibody; antineoplastic adjuvant*

**edrofuradene** [see: nifurdazil]

**Edronax** (commercially available in England) Ŗ *investigational (Phase III) fast-acting antidepressant* [reboxetine]

**edrophone chloride** [see: edrophonium chloride]

**edrophonium chloride** USP, INN, BAN *antidote to curare; myasthenia gravis diagnostic aid*

**Ed-Spaz** tablets Ŗ *anticholinergic; antispasmodic* [hyoscyamine sulfate] 0.125 mg

**EDTA (ethylenediaminetetraacetic acid)** [see: edetate disodium]

**EDTA calcium** [see: edetate calcium disodium]

**ED-TLC; ED Tuss HC** liquid Ŗ *narcotic antitussive; decongestant; antihistamine* [hydrocodone bitartrate; phenylephrine HCl; chlorpheniramine maleate] 1.67•5•2 mg/5 mL; 2.5•10•4 mg/5 mL

**E.E.S.** granules for oral suspension Ŗ *macrolide antibiotic* [erythromycin ethylsuccinate] 200 mg/5 mL

**EES (erythromycin ethylsuccinate)** [q.v.]

**E.E.S. 200** oral suspension Ŗ *macrolide antibiotic* [erythromycin ethylsuccinate] 200 mg/5 mL

**E.E.S. 400** film-coated tablets, oral suspension Ŗ *macrolide antibiotic* [erythromycin ethylsuccinate] 400 mg; 400 mg/5 mL

**Efamol PMS** soft gel capsules OTC *dietary supplement* [multiple vitamins & amino acids]

**efaroxan** INN, BAN

**Efed II** capsules OTC *decongestant* [phenylpropanolamine HCl]

**efegatran sulfate** USAN *antithrombotic*

**efetozole** INN

**Effer-K** effervescent tablets Ŗ *potassium supplement* [potassium bicarbonate; potassium citrate] 25 mEq

**Effer-Syllium** effervescent powder (replaced by Mylanta Natural Fiber Supplement in 1994)

**Effervescent Potassium** effervescent tablets Ŗ *potassium supplement* [potassium bicarbonate; potassium citrate] 25 mEq

**Effexor** tablets Ŗ *antidepressant* [venlafaxine] 25, 37.5, 50, 75, 100 mg

**Effexor SR** Ŗ *investigational once-daily antidepressant* [venlafaxine]

**Efidac/24** extended-release tablets OTC *nasal decongestant* [pseudoephedrine HCl] 240 mg

**Efidac/24 Chlorpheniramine** extended-release tablets OTC *antihistamine* [chlorpheniramine maleate] 16 mg

**Eflone** eye drop suspension Ŗ *ophthalmic topical corticosteroidal anti-inflammatory* [fluorometholone acetate] 0.1%

**eflornithine** INN, BAN *antineoplastic; antiprotozoal* [also: eflornithine HCl]

**eflornithine HCl** USAN *antineoplastic; antiprotozoal; treatment for Trypanosoma brucei gambiense infection (orphan)* [also: eflornithine]

**efloxate** INN

**eflumast** INN

**Efodine** ointment OTC *broad-spectrum antimicrobial* [povidone-iodine] 1%

**EFP (etoposide, fluorouracil, Platinol)** *chemotherapy protocol*

**Efricon Expectorant** liquid Ŗ *narcotic antitussive; decongestant; antihistamine; expectorant* [codeine phosphate; phenylephrine HCl; chlorpheniramine maleate; ammonium chloride; potassium guaiacolsulfonate; sodium citrate]

**efrotomycin** USAN, INN, BAN *veterinary growth stimulant*

**Efudex** cream, topical solution Ŗ *antimetabolic antineoplastic for actinic keratoses and basal cell carcinomas* [fluorouracil] 5%; 2%, 5%

**egg** *street drug slang* [see: cocaine, crack]

**egtazic acid** USAN, INN *pharmaceutic aid*

**EHDP (ethane hydroxydiphosphonate)** [see: etidronate disodium]

**Ehrlich 594** [see: acetarsone]

**Ehrlich 606** [see: arsphenamine]

**eicosapentaenoic acid (EPA)** [see: icosapent]

**eight ball** *street drug slang for heroin or 1/8 oz. of any drug* [see: heroin]

**8 in 1 (Medrol, vincristine, CCNU, procarbazine, hydroxyurea, cisplatin, ara-C, cyclophosphamide)** *chemotherapy protocol*

**8 in 1 (Medrol, vincristine, CCNU, procarbazine, hydroxyurea, cisplatin, ara-C, dacarbazine)** *chemotherapy protocol*

**eighth** *street drug slang* [see: heroin]

**8-MOP** capsules ℞ *to increase tolerance to sunlight and enhance pigmentation* [methoxsalen] 10 mg

**einsteinium** *element (Es)*

**eIPV (enhanced, inactivated polio vaccine)** [see: poliovirus vaccine, enhanced inactivated]

**el diablillo** (Spanish for "the little devil") *street drug slang for a combination of marijuana, cocaine, heroin, and PCP* [see: marijuana; cocaine; heroin; PCP]

**el diablo** (Spanish for "the devil") *street drug slang for a combination of marijuana, cocaine, and heroin* [see: marijuana; cocaine; heroin]

**elantrine** USAN, INN *anticholinergic*

**elanzepine** INN

**Elase** powder, ointment ℞ *topical enzyme for biochemical debridement* [fibrinolysin; desoxyribonuclease] 25•15 000 U; 1•666.6 U/g

**Elase-Chloromycetin** ointment ℞ *topical enzyme for biochemical debridement; antibiotic* [fibrinolysin; desoxyribonuclease; chloramphenicol] 1 U•666.6 U•10 mg per g

**elastofilcon A** USAN *hydrophilic contact lens material*

**Elavil** film-coated tablets, IM injection ℞ *tricyclic antidepressant* [amitriptyline HCl] 10, 25, 50, 75, 100, 150 mg; 10 mg/mL ⍰ Aldoril; Enovil; Equanil; Mellaril

**elbanizine** INN

**elcatonin** INN, JAN *investigational (orphan) intrathecal treatment of intractable pain*

**eldacimibe** USAN *antihyperlipidemic; antiatherosclerotic; AcylCoA transferase (ACAT) inhibitor*

**Eldecort** cream (discontinued 1995) ℞ *topical corticosteroid* [hydrocortisone] 2.5%

**Eldepryl** capsules ℞ *antiparkinsonian (orphan)* [selegiline HCl] 5 mg

**Eldercaps** capsules ℞ *vitamin/mineral supplement* [multiple vitamins & minerals; folic acid] ±•1 mg

**Eldertonic** liquid OTC *vitamin/mineral supplement* [multiple B vitamins & minerals; alcohol 13.5%] ±

**eldexomer** INN

**Eldisine** ℞ *investigational antineoplastic for leukemia, melanoma, breast and lung cancers* [vindesine sulfate]

**Eldopaque; Eldopaque-Forte** cream OTC *hyperpigmentation bleaching agent; sunscreen* [hydroquinone in a sunblock base] 2%; 4%

**Eldoquin** lotion (discontinued 1993) OTC *hyperpigmentation bleaching agent* [hydroquinone] 2%

**Eldoquin; Eldoquin-Forte Sunbleaching** cream OTC *hyperpigmentation bleaching agent* [hydroquinone] 2%; 4%

**electric Kool Aid** *street drug slang* [see: LSD]

**electrocortin** [see: aldosterone]

**eledoisin** INN

**elephant; elephant tranquilizer** *street drug slang* [see: PCP]

**ELF (etoposide, leucovorin [rescue], fluorouracil)** *chemotherapy protocol*

**elfazepam** USAN, INN *veterinary appetite stimulant*

**elgodipine** INN

**Elimite** cream ℞ *pediculicide; scabicide* [permethrin] 5%

**eliprodil** INN *investigational treatment for ischemic stroke*

**Elixomin** elixir ℞ *bronchodilator* [theophylline] 80 mg/15 mL

**Elixophyllin** capsules, elixir ℞ *bronchodilator* [theophylline] 100, 200 mg; 80 mg/15 mL

**Elixophyllin GG** liquid ℞ *antiasthmatic; bronchodilator; expectorant*

[theophylline; guaifenesin] 100•100 mg/15 mL

**Elixophyllin SR** timed-release capsules (discontinued 1994) ℞ *bronchodilator* [theophylline] 125, 250 mg

**Elixophyllin-KI** elixir ℞ *antiasthmatic; bronchodilator; expectorant* [theophylline; potassium iodide] 80•130 mg/15 mL

**ellagic acid** INN

**Elliott's B solution** *investigational (orphan) intrathecal chemotherapy diluent*

**ellipticine** *investigational antineoplastic for breast cancer*

**elliptinium acetate** INN, BAN

**Elmiron** capsules ℞ *urinary tract anti-inflammatory and analgesic for interstitial cystitis (orphan)* [pentosan polysulfate sodium] 100 mg

**elmustine** INN

**elnadipine** INN

**Elobromol** ℞ *investigational antineoplastic* [mitolactol]

**Elocon** ointment, cream, lotion ℞ *topical corticosteroid* [mometasone furoate] 0.1%

**E-Lor** film-coated tablets (discontinued 1995) ℞ *narcotic analgesic* [propoxyphene HCl; acetaminophen] 65•650 mg

**elsamitrucin** USAN, INN *antineoplastic*

**Elspar** powder for IV or IM injection ℞ *antineoplastic adjunct for acute lymphocytic leukemia* [asparaginase] 10 000 IU

**eltanolone** INN *investigational IV anesthetic*

**eltenac** INN

**eltoprazine** INN

**Eltroxin** tablets ℞ *thyroid hormone* [levothyroxine sodium] 50, 75, 100, 125, 150, 200, 300 μg

**elucaine** USAN, INN *gastric anticholinergic*

**Elyzol Dentalgel** ℞ *investigational treatment for periodontitis*

**elziverine** INN

**EMA (estramustine L-alanine)** [q.v.]

**EMA 86 (etoposide, mitoxantrone, ara-C)** *chemotherapy protocol*

**EMACO (etoposide, methotrexate, actinomycin D, cyclophospha-** mide, **Oncovin)** *chemotherapy protocol*

**embalming fluid** *street drug slang* [see: PCP]

**embinal** [see: barbital sodium]

**embonate** INN, BAN *combining name for radicals or groups* [also: pamoate]

**embramide** INN, BAN

**embramine HCl** [see: embramine]

**Embutane** ℞ *veterinary anesthetic; veterinary euthanasia* [embutramide]

**embutramide** USAN, INN, BAN *veterinary anesthetic; veterinary euthanasia*

**Emcyt** capsules ℞ *hormonal chemotherapy for metastatic or progressive prostatic carcinoma* [estramustine phosphate sodium] 140 mg

**Emecheck** liquid OTC *antinauseant; antiemetic* [phosphorated carbohydrate solution (glucose, fructose, and phosphoric acid)]

**emedastine** INN *antihistamine; antiallergic; antiasthmatic* [also: emedastine difumarate]

**emedastine difumarate** USAN, JAN *antihistamine; antiallergic; antiasthmatic* [also: emedastine]

**emepronium bromide** INN, BAN

**emepronium carrageenate** BAN

**Emergent-Ez Kit** ℞ *carry-kit for medical personnel* [multiple drugs and devices for emergencies] ⚕

**Emersal** emulsion ℞ *topical antipsoriatic; antiseborrheic* [ammoniated mercury; salicylic acid] 5%•2.5%

**Emete-con** IV or IM injection (discontinued 1994) ℞ *post-anesthesia antiemetic* [benzoquinamide HCl] 50 mg/vial

**emetine** BAN *antiamebic* [also: emetine HCl] ⊡ Emetrol

**emetine bismuth iodide** [see: emetine HCl]

**emetine HCl** USP *amebicide* [also: emetine]

**Emetrol** solution OTC *antinauseant; antiemetic* [phosphorated carbohydrate solution (fructose, dextrose, and orthophosphoric acid)] ⊡ emetine

**Emgel** gel ℞ *topical antibiotic for acne* [erythromycin] 2%

**emigliate** INN, BAN

**emilium tosilate** INN *antiarrhythmic* [also: emilium tosylate]

**emilium tosylate** USAN *antiarrhythmic* [also: emilium tosilate]

**Eminase** powder for IV injection ℞ *thrombolytic enzyme for acute myocardial infarction* [anistreplase] 30 U/vial

**Emitasol** intranasal ℞ *investigational anti-emetic for chemotherapy* [metoclopramide HCl]

**Emko; Emko Pre-Fil** vaginal foam OTC *spermicidal contraceptive* [nonoxynol 9] 8%

**Emla** cream ℞ *topical local anesthetic* [lidocaine; prilocaine] 2.5%•2.5%

**Emollia** lotion OTC *moisturizer; emollient*

**emollients** *a class of dermatological agents that soften and soothe the skin*

**emonapride** INN

**emopamil** INN

**emorfazone** INN

**Empirin** tablets OTC *analgesic; antipyretic; anti-inflammatory; antirheumatic* [aspirin] 325 mg

**Empirin with Codeine No. 3 & No. 4** tablets ℞ *narcotic analgesic; sometimes abused as a street drug* [codeine phosphate; aspirin] 30•325 mg; 60•325 mg

**emsel** *street drug slang; a pronunciation of the brand name MS/L (morphine sulfate liquid)* [see: MS/L; morphine sulfate]

**emtryl** [see: dimetridazole]

**emulsifying wax** [see: wax, emulsifying]

**Emulsoil** emulsion OTC *stimulant laxative* [castor oil] 95%

**E-Mycin** enteric-coated tablets ℞ *macrolide antibiotic* [erythromycin] 250, 333 mg

**emylcamate** INN, BAN

**Enable** ℞ *investigational anti-inflammatory for rheumatoid arthritis and osteoarthritis* [tenidap]

**Enablex** (foreign name for U.S. product Enable)

**enadoline** INN *analgesic* [also: enadoline HCl]

**enadoline HCl** USAN *analgesic; investigational (orphan) for severe head injury* [also: enadoline]

**enalapril** INN, BAN *antihypertensive; angiotensin-converting enzyme (ACE) inhibitor* [also: enalapril maleate]

**enalapril maleate** USAN, USP *antihypertensive; angiotensin-converting enzyme (ACE) inhibitor* [also: enalapril]

**enalaprilat** USAN, USP, INN, BAN *antihypertensive; angiotensin-converting enzyme inhibitor*

**enalkiren** USAN, INN *antihypertensive; renin inhibitor*

**enallynymal sodium** [see: methohexital sodium]

**enantate** INN *combining name for radicals or groups* [also: enanthate]

**enanthate** USAN, USP, BAN *combining name for radicals or groups* [also: enantate]

**enbucrilate** INN, BAN

**encainide** INN, BAN *antiarrhythmic* [also: encainide HCl]

**encainide HCl** USAN *antiarrhythmic* [also: encainide]

**Encare** vaginal suppositories OTC *spermicidal contraceptive* [nonoxynol 9] 2.27%

**En-Cebrin** Pulvules (capsules) OTC *vitamin/mineral/iron supplement* [multiple vitamins & minerals; iron]

**enciprazine** INN, BAN *minor tranquilizer* [also: enciprazine HCl]

**enciprazine HCl** USAN *minor tranquilizer* [also: enciprazine]

**enclomifene** INN [also: enclomiphene]

**enclomiphene** USAN [also: enclomifene]

**encyprate** USAN, INN *antidepressant*

**End Lice** liquid OTC *pediculicide* [pyrethrins; piperonyl butoxide] 0.3%•3%

**Endafed** sustained-release capsules ℞ *decongestant; antihistamine* [pseudoephedrine HCl; brompheniramine maleate] 120•12 mg

**Endagen-HD** liquid ℞ *narcotic antitussive; decongestant; antihistamine* [hydrocodone bitartrate; phenylephrine HCl; chlorpheniramine maleate] 1.67•5•2 mg/5 mL

**Endal** timed-release tablets ℞ *decongestant; expectorant* [phenylephrine HCl; guaifenesin] 20•300 mg ⧫ Intal

**Endal Expectorant** syrup ℞ *narcotic antitussive; decongestant; expectorant* [codeine phosphate; phenylpropanolamine HCl; guaifenesin; alcohol 5%] 10•12.5•100 mg/5 mL

**Endal-HD; Endal-HD Plus** liquid ℞ *narcotic antitussive; decongestant; antihistamine* [hydrocodone bitartrate; phenylephrine HCl; chlorpheniramine maleate] 1.7•5•2 mg/5 mL; 2.5•5•2 mg/5 mL

**Endep** film-coated tablets (discontinued 1996) ℞ *tricyclic antidepressant* [amitriptyline HCl] 10, 50, 75, 100, 150 mg

**endiemal** [see: metharbital]

**endixaprine** INN

**endo** *street drug slang* [see: marijuana]

**endobenzyline bromide**

**endocaine** [see: pyrrocaine]

**EndoCRIB** ℞ *investigational treatment for type II diabetes* [cellular implants]

**endolate** [see: meperidine HCl]

**Endolor** capsules ℞ *analgesic; antipyretic; sedative* [acetaminophen; caffeine; butalbital] 325•40•50 mg

**endomide** INN

**endomycin**

**endralazine** INN, BAN *antihypertensive* [also: endralazine mesylate]

**endralazine mesylate** USAN *antihypertensive* [also: endralazine]

**Endrate** IV infusion ℞ *calcium-lowering agent; antiarrhythmic for digitalis toxicity* [edetate disodium] 150 mg/mL

**endrisone** INN *topical ophthalmic anti-inflammatory* [also: endrysone]

**endrysone** USAN *topical ophthalmic anti-inflammatory* [also: endrisone]

**Enduret** (trademarked dosage form) *prolonged-action tablet*

**Enduron** tablets ℞ *diuretic; antihypertensive* [methyclothiazide] 5 mg ⧫ Imuran; Inderal

**Enduronyl; Enduronyl Forte** tablets ℞ *antihypertensive* [methyclothiazide; deserpidine] 5•0.25 mg; 5•0.5 mg ⧫ Inderal

**Enecat** concentrated suspension ℞ *GI contrast radiopaque agent* [barium sulfate] 5%

**enefexine** INN

**Ener-B** nasal gel OTC *vitamin supplement* [cyanocobalamin] 400 µg

**energizer** *street drug slang* [see: PCP]

**enestebol** INN

**Enfamil** liquid, powder OTC *total or supplementary infant feeding*

**Enfamil Human Milk Fortifier** powder OTC *supplement to breast milk*

**Enfamil Next Step** liquid, powder OTC *total or supplementary infant feeding*

**Enfamil Premature Formula** liquid OTC *total or supplementary infant feeding*

**Enfamil with Iron** liquid, powder OTC *total or supplementary infant feeding*

**enfenamic acid** INN

**enflurane** USAN, USP, INN, BAN *inhalation general anesthetic*

**Engerix-B** adult IM injection, pediatric IM injection ℞ *active immunizing agent for hepatitis B and hepatitis D* [hepatitis B virus vaccine, recombinant] 20 µg/mL, 10 µg/0.5 mL

**englitazone** INN *antidiabetic* [also: englitazone sodium]

**englitazone sodium** USAN *antidiabetic* [also: englitazone]

**enhanced, inactivated polio vaccine (eIPV)** [see: poliovirus vaccine, enhanced inactivated]

**enhexymal** [see: hexobarbital]

**eniclobrate** INN

**enilconazole** USAN, INN, BAN *antifungal*

**enilospirone** INN

**enisoprost** USAN, INN *antiulcerative; orphan status withdrawn 1996*

**enisoprost & cyclosporine** *orphan status withdrawn 1996*

**Enisyl** tablets OTC *dietary amino acid supplement* [L-lysine] 334, 500 mg

**Enlon** IV or IM injection ℞ *myasthenia gravis treatment; antidote to curare-type overdose* [edrophonium chloride] 10 mg/mL

**Enlon Plus** IV or IM injection ℞ *muscle stimulant; neuromuscular blocker antagonist* [edrophonium chloride; atropine sulfate] 10•0.14 mg

**enloplatin** USAN, INN *antineoplastic*

**ENO** powder (discontinued 1994) oTc *antacid* [sodium tartrate; sodium citrate] 1620•1172 mg/dose

**enocitabine** INN

**enofelast** USAN, INN *antiasthmatic*

**enolicam** INN *anti-inflammatory; antirheumatic* [also: enolicam sodium]

**enolicam sodium** USAN *anti-inflammatory; antirheumatic* [also: enolicam]

**Enomine** capsules ℞ *decongestant; expectorant* [phenylpropanolamine HCl; phenylephrine HCl; guaifenesin] 45•5•200 mg

**Enovid** tablets (discontinued 1997) ℞ *progestin for hypermenorrhea or endometriosis* [mestranol; norethynodrel] 75 μg•5 mg; 150 μg•9.85 mg

**Enovil** IM injection (discontinued 1996) ℞ *tricyclic antidepressant* [amitriptyline HCl] 10 mg/mL ② Elavil

**enoxacin** USAN, INN, BAN, JAN *antibacterial*

**enoxamast** INN

**enoxaparin** BAN *a low molecular weight heparin-type anticoagulant and antithrombotic* [also: enoxaparin sodium]

**enoxaparin sodium** USAN, INN *a low molecular weight heparin-type anticoagulant and antithrombotic* [also: enoxaparin]

**enoximone** USAN, INN, BAN *cardiotonic*

**enoxolone** INN, BAN

**enphenemal** [see: mephobarbital]

**enpiprazole** INN, BAN

**enpiroline** INN *antimalarial* [also: enpiroline phosphate]

**enpiroline phosphate** USAN *antimalarial* [also: enpiroline]

**enprazepine** INN

**enprofen** [now: furaprofen]

**enprofylline** USAN, INN *bronchodilator*

**enpromate** USAN, INN *antineoplastic*

**enprostil** USAN, INN, BAN *investigational antisecretory and antiulcerative for acute peptic ulcers*

**enramycin** INN

**Enrich Liquid with Fiber** (discontinued 1994) oTc *enteral nutritional therapy* [lactose-free formula] 8 oz., 1 qt. ready-to-use

**enrofloxacin** USAN, INN, BAN *veterinary antibacterial*

**Enseal** (trademarked dosage form) *enteric-coated tablet*

**Ensure** liquid, powder oTc *enteral nutritional therapy* [lactose-free formula]

**Ensure** pudding oTc *enteral nutritional therapy* [milk-based formula] 150 g

**Ensure High Protein** ready-to-use liquid oTc *enteral nutritional therapy* [lactose-free formula] 237 mL

**Ensure HN; Ensure with Fiber** ready-to-use liquid oTc *enteral nutritional therapy* [lactose-free formula]

**Ensure Plus; Ensure Plus HN** liquid oTc *enteral nutritional therapy* [lactose-free formula]

**E.N.T.** sustained-release tablets (discontinued 1997) ℞ *decongestant; antihistamine* [phenylpropanolamine HCl; brompheniramine maleate] 75•12 mg

**EN-tab** (trademarked dosage form) *enteric-coated tablet*

**enteramine** [see: serotonin]

**Entero-Test; Entero-Test Pediatric** string capsules for professional use *in vitro diagnostic aid for GI disorders*

**Entertainer's Secret Throat Relief** spray oTc *saliva substitute*

**Entex** capsules, liquid ℞ *decongestant; expectorant* [phenylephrine HCl; phenylpropanolamine HCl; guaifenesin] 5•45•200 mg; 5•20•100 mg/5 mL

**Entex LA** long-acting tablets ℞ *decongestant; expectorant* [phenylpropanolamine HCl; guaifenesin] 75•400 mg

**Entex PSE** prolonged-action tablets ℞ *decongestant; expectorant* [pseudoephedrine HCl; guaifenesin] 60•120 mg

**Entocort** ⒸⒶⓃ tablets for rectal suspension ℞ *steroidal anti-inflammatory for bowel disease* [budesonide]

**Entozyme** tablets (discontinued 1994) ℞ *digestive enzymes* [pancreatin; lipase; protease; amylase] 300 mg•600 U•7500 U•7500 U ② Donnazyme

**Entri-Pak** (dosage form) *liquid-filled pouch*

**Entrition; Entrition RDA** Entri-Pak (liquid-filled pouch) (discontinued 1994) OTC *enteral nutritional therapy* [lactose-free formula]

**Entrition 0.5** liquid OTC *enteral nutritional therapy* [lactose-free formula]

**Entrition Half-Strength** (name changed to Entrition 0.5 in 1994)

**Entrition HN** Entri-Pak (liquid-filled pouch) OTC *enteral nutritional therapy* [lactose-free formula]

**Entrobar** suspension R *GI contrast radiopaque agent* [barium sulfate] 50%

**entsufon** INN *detergent* [also: entsufon sodium]

**entsufon sodium** USAN *detergent* [also: entsufon]

**Entuss Expectorant** liquid R *narcotic antitussive; expectorant* [hydrocodone bitartrate; potassium guaiacolsulfonate] 5•300 mg/5 mL

**Entuss Expectorant** tablets R *narcotic antitussive; expectorant* [hydrocodone bitartrate; guaifenesin] 5•300 mg

**Entuss-D** liquid R *narcotic antitussive; decongestant* [hydrocodone bitartrate; pseudoephedrine HCl] 5•30 mg/5 mL

**Entuss-D** tablets R *narcotic antitussive; decongestant; expectorant* [hydrocodone bitartrate; pseudoephedrine HCl; guaifenesin] 5•30•300 mg

**Entuss-D Jr.** liquid R *pediatric narcotic antitussive, decongestant, and expectorant* [hydrocodone bitartrate; pseudoephedrine HCl; guaifenesin; alcohol 5%] 2.5•30•100 mg/5 mL

**Enuclene** eye drops OTC *cleaning, wetting and lubricating agent for artificial eyes* [tyloxapol] 0.25%

**Enulose** syrup R *prevent and treat portal-systemic encephalopathy* [lactulose] 10 g/15 mL

**enviomycin** INN

**enviradene** USAN, INN *antiviral*

**Enviro-Stress** slow-release tablets OTC *vitamin/mineral supplement* [multiple vitamins & minerals; folic acid] ≛•0.4 mg

**enviroxime** USAN, INN *antiviral*

**Enzone** cream R *topical corticosteroid; local anesthetic* [hydrocortisone acetate; pramoxine HCl] 1%•1%

**Enzymatic Cleaner for Extended Wear** tablets OTC *enzymatic cleaner for soft contact lenses* [pork pancreatin]

**Enzyme** chewable tablets OTC *digestive enzymes* [amylase; protease; lipase; cellulase] 30•6•2•25 mg

**EP (etoposide, Platinol)** *chemotherapy protocol*

**EPA** capsules OTC *dietary supplement* [omega-3 fatty acids] 1000 mg

**EPA (eicosapentaenoic acid)** [see: icosapent]

**epalrestat** INN *investigational treatment for diabetic neuropathy*

**epanolol** INN, BAN

**eperisone** INN

**epervudine** INN

**ephedrine** USP, BAN *bronchodilator; nasal decongestant; vasopressor for shock* ⚕ Appedrine; aprindine

**ephedrine HCl** USP, BAN *bronchodilator; nasal decongestant; vasopressor for shock*

**ephedrine sulfate** USP *bronchodilator; nasal decongestant; vasopressor for acute hypotensive shock* [also: ephedrine sulphate] 25, 50 mg oral; 25, 50 mg/mL injection

**ephedrine sulphate** BAN *bronchodilator; nasal decongestant* [also: ephedrine sulfate]

**ephedrine tannate**

**ephedrone** *street drug slang* [see: methcathinone]

**Epi-C** concentrated suspension R *GI contrast radiopaque agent* [barium sulfate] 150%

**epicainide** INN

**epicillin** USAN, INN, BAN *antibacterial*

**epicriptine** INN

**Epiderm** balm (discontinued 1994) OTC *counterirritant; topical antiseptic* [methyl salicylate; menthol; alcohol]

**epidermal growth factor, human** *investigational (orphan) for acceleration of corneal regeneration*

**epiestriol** INN [also: epioestriol]

**Epifoam** aerosol foam R *topical corticosteroid; local anesthetic* [hydrocortisone acetate; pramoxine] 1%•1%

**Epifrin** eye drops R *antiglaucoma agent* [epinephrine HCl] 0.5%, 1%, 2% ⚕ epinephrine; EpiPen

**EpiLeukin** ℞ *investigational (Phase III) treatment for malignant melanoma*

**epilin** [see: dietifen]

**E-Pilo-1; E-Pilo-2; E-Pilo-4; E-Pilo-6** eye drops ℞ *antiglaucoma agent* [pilocarpine HCl; epinephrine bitartrate] 1%•1%; 2%•1%; 4%•1%; 6%•1%

**E-Pilo-3** eye drops (discontinued 1995) ℞ *antiglaucoma agent* [pilocarpine HCl; epinephrine bitartrate] 3%•1%

**Epilyt** lotion concentrate OTC *moisturizer; emollient*

**epimestrol** USAN, INN, BAN *anterior pituitary activator*

**Epinal** eye drops ℞ *antiglaucoma agent* [epinephryl borate] 0.5%, 1% ⊡ Epitol

**epinastine** INN

**epinephran** [see: epinephrine]

**epinephrine** USP, INN *vasoconstrictor; bronchodilator; topical antiglaucoma agent; vasopressor for shock* [also: adrenaline] 1:10 000 (0.1 mg/mL) injection ⊡ Epifrin

**epinephrine bitartrate** USP *bronchodilator; ophthalmic adrenergic; topical antiglaucoma agent*

**epinephrine borate** *topical antiglaucoma agent*

**epinephrine & cisplatin** *investigational (Phase II) injectable gel for inoperable primary liver cancer*

**epinephrine HCl** *nasal decongestant; topical antiglaucoma agent; vasopressor for shock* 0.1% eye drops; 1:1000, 1:2000, 1:10 000 (1, 0.5, 0.1 mg/mL) injection

**Epinephrine Pediatric** subcu injection ℞ *bronchodilator for bronchial asthma or bronchospasm; vasopressor for shock* [epinephrine HCl] 1:100 000 (0.01 mg/mL)

**epinephryl borate** USAN, USP *adrenergic; topical antiglaucoma agent*

**epioestriol** BAN [also: epiestriol]

**EpiPen; EpiPen Jr.** auto-injector (automatic IM injection device) ℞ *emergency treatment of anaphylaxis; vasopressor for shock* [epinephrine] 1:1000 (1 mg/mL); 1:2000 (0.5 mg/mL) ⊡ Epifrin

**epipropidine** USAN, INN *antineoplastic*

**epirizole** USAN, INN *analgesic; antiinflammatory*

**epiroprim** INN

**epirubicin** INN, BAN *antibiotic antineoplastic* [also: epirubicin HCl]

**epirubicin HCl** USAN, JAN *antibiotic antineoplastic* [also: epirubicin]

**epitetracycline HCl** USP *antibacterial*

**epithiazide** USAN, BAN *antihypertensive; diuretic* [also: epitizide]

**epithioandrostanol** [see: epitiostanol]

**epitiostanol** INN

**epitizide** INN *antihypertensive; diuretic* [also: epithiazide]

**Epitol** tablets ℞ *anticonvulsant; analgesic for trigeminal neuralgia* [carbamazepine] 200 mg ⊡ Epinal

**Epivir** film-coated tablets, oral solution ℞ *nucleoside reverse transcriptase inhibitor antiviral for HIV; investigational (Phase III) for hepatitis B* [lamivudine] 150 mg; 10 mg/mL

**eplerenone** USAN *aldosterone receptor antagonist for congestive heart failure, hypertension, and cirrhosis*

**EPlus** tablets OTC *vitamin supplement* [multiple vitamins; lemon bioflavonoids]

**EPO (epoetin alfa)** [q.v.]

**EPOCH (etoposide, prednisone, Oncovin, cyclophosphamide, Halotestin)** *chemotherapy protocol*

**epoetin alfa (EPO)** USAN, INN, BAN, JAN *hematinic for anemia of chronic renal failure, HIV, and chemotherapy (orphan); to reduce blood transfusions in surgery*

**epoetin beta** USAN, INN, BAN, JAN *antianemic; hematinic; investigational (orphan) for anemia of end-stage renal disease*

**Epogen** IV or subcu injection ℞ *stimulates RBC production; for anemia of chronic renal failure, HIV, or chemotherapy (orphan)* [epoetin alfa] 2000, 3000, 4000, 10 000, 20 000 U/mL

**epoprostenol** USAN, INN *platelet aggregation inhibitor; investigational (orphan) vasodilator for primary pulmonary hypertension*

**epoprostenol & prostacyclin** *orphan status withdrawn 1994*

**epoprostenol sodium** USAN, BAN *platelet aggregation inhibitor; vasodilator; antihypertensive*

**epostane** USAN, INN, BAN *interceptive*

**epoxytropine tropate methylbromide** [see: methscopolamine bromide]

**Eppy/N ½% eye drops** (discontinued 1994) ℞ *antiglaucoma agent* [epinephrine borate] 0.5%

**Eppy/N 1%; Eppy/N 2% eye drops** (discontinued 1995) ℞ *antiglaucoma agent* [epinephrine borate] 1%; 2%

**eprazinone** INN

**Eprex** ℞ *investigational (orphan) hematinic for anemia of AIDS and ARC* [epoetin alfa]

**eprinomectin** USAN *veterinary antiparasitic*

**epristeride** USAN *alpha reductase inhibitor for benign prostatic hypertrophy*

**Epromate tablets** (discontinued 1995) ℞ *analgesic; antipyretic; anti-inflammatory; anxiolytic* [aspirin; meprobamate] 325•200 mg

**eprosartan** USAN *antihypertensive (angiotensin II blocker)*

**eprosartan mesylate** USAN *antihypertensive (angiotensin II blocker)*

**eprovafen** INN

**eproxindine** INN

**eprozinol** INN

**epsikapron** [see: aminocaproic acid]

**epsilon-aminocaproic acid (EACA)** [see: aminocaproic acid]

**epsiprantel** INN, BAN

**Epsom salt** [see: magnesium sulfate]

**e.p.t. Quick Stick** test stick for home use OTC *in vitro diagnostic aid for urine pregnancy test*

**eptaloprost** INN

**eptamestrol** [see: etamestrol]

**eptaprost** [see: eptaloprost]

**eptastatin sodium** [see: pravastatin sodium]

**eptastigmine** INN *investigational treatment for Alzheimer's disease*

**eptazocine** INN

**Equagesic tablets** ℞ *analgesic; antipyretic; anti-inflammatory; anxiolytic* [aspirin; meprobamate] 325•200 mg

**Equalactin chewable tablets** OTC *bulk laxative; antidiarrheal* [calcium polycarbophil] 500 mg

**Equanil tablets** ℞ *anxiolytic* [meprobamate] 200, 400 mg ⧈ Elavil

**Equazine M tablets** (discontinued 1995) ℞ *analgesic; antipyretic; anti-inflammatory; anxiolytic* [aspirin; meprobamate] 325•200 mg

**Equilet chewable tablets** OTC *antacid* [calcium carbonate] 500 mg

**equilin** USP *estrogen*

**Equipoise** *brand name for boldenone undecylenate, a veterinary anabolic steroid abused as a street drug*

**Eramycin film-coated tablets** ℞ *macrolide antibiotic* [erythromycin stearate] 250 mg

**erbium** *element (Er)*

**erbulozole** USAN, INN *antineoplastic adjunct*

**erbumine** USAN, INN, BAN *combining name for radicals or groups*

**Ercaf tablets** ℞ *migraine-specific vasoconstrictor* [ergotamine tartrate; caffeine] 1•100 mg

**erdosteine** INN

**Ergamisol tablets** ℞ *antineoplastic adjuvant for colon cancer* [levamisole HCl] 50 mg

**ergocalciferol** USP, INN, BAN, JAN *vitamin D₂; antirachitic* 50 000 IU oral

**ergoloid mesylates** USAN, USP *cognition adjuvant for age-related mental capacity decline* [also: co-dergocrine mesylate] 0.5, 1 mg oral

**Ergomar sublingual tablets** ℞ *agent for migraine; vasoconstrictor* [ergotamine tartrate] 2 mg

**ergometrine** INN, BAN *oxytocic* [also: ergonovine maleate]

**ergonovine maleate** USP *oxytocic* [also: ergometrine]

**Ergoset tablets** ℞ *investigational (Phase III) dopamine agonist for hypoglycemic control in type 2 diabetes; investigational (Phase II/III) treatment for clinical obesity*

**Ergostat sublingual tablets** (discontinued 1996) ℞ *migraine-specific vasoconstrictor* [ergotamine tartrate] 2 mg

**ergosterol, activated** [see: ergocalciferol]

**ergot alkaloids** [see: ergoloid mesylates]

**ergotamine** INN, BAN *migraine-specific analgesic* [also: ergotamine tartrate]

**ergotamine tartrate** USP *migraine-specific analgesic* [also: ergotamine]

**Ergotrate Maleate** IM or IV injection ℞ *prevention of postpartum and postabortal hemorrhage* [ergonovine maleate] 0.2 mg/mL

**Ergotrate Maleate** tablets (discontinued 1995) ℞ *prevention of postpartum and postabortal hemorrhage* [ergonovine maleate] 0.2 mg

**ericolol** INN

**Eridium** tablets (discontinued 1996) ℞ *urinary analgesic* [phenazopyridine HCl] 100 mg

**eriodictyon** NF

**eritrityl tetranitrate** INN *coronary vasodilator* [also: erythrityl tetranitrate]

**erizepine** INN

**E-R-O Ear Drops** OTC *agent to emulsify and disperse ear wax* [carbamide peroxide] 6.5%

**erocainide** INN

**ersofermin** USAN, INN *wound healing agent; transglutaminase inhibitor for the treatment of scar tissue*

**Erwinase** ℞ *investigational (orphan) antineoplastic for acute lymphocytic leukemia* [erwinia L-asparaginase]

**erwinia L-asparaginase** *investigational (orphan) antineoplastic for acute lymphocytic leukemia*

**ERYC** delayed-release capsules containing enteric-coated pellets ℞ *macrolide antibiotic* [erythromycin] 250 mg ☒ ara-C

**Erycette** topical solution ℞ *topical antibiotic for acne* [erythromycin] 2% ☒ Aricept

**EryDerm 2%** topical solution ℞ *topical antibiotic for acne* [erythromycin] 2%

**Erygel** gel ℞ *topical antibiotic for acne* [erythromycin; alcohol 92%] 2%

**Erymax** topical solution ℞ *topical antibiotic for acne* [erythromycin] 2%

**EryPed** chewable tablets, granules for oral suspension, drops ℞ *macrolide antibiotic* [erythromycin ethylsuccinate] 200 mg; 400 mg/5 mL; 100 mg/2.5 mL

**EryPed 200; EryPed 400** oral suspension ℞ *macrolide antibiotic* [erythromycin ethylsuccinate] 200 mg/5 mL; 400 mg/5 mL

**Ery-Sol** topical solution (discontinued 1995) ℞ *topical antibiotic for acne* [erythromycin] 2%

**Ery-Tab** enteric-coated delayed-release tablets ℞ *macrolide antibiotic* [erythromycin] 250, 333, 500 mg

**erythorbic acid**

**Erythra-Derm** topical solution ℞ *topical antibiotic for acne* [erythromycin] 2%

**erythrityl tetranitrate** USAN, USP *coronary vasodilator; antianginal* [also: eritrityl tetranitrate]

**Erythrocin Stearate** Filmtabs (film-coated tablets) ℞ *antibiotic* [erythromycin stearate] 250, 500 mg

**erythrol tetranitrate** [now: erythrityl tetranitrate]

**erythromycin** USP, INN, BAN *macrolide bactericidal/bacteriostatic antibiotic* 250, 333, 500 mg oral; 2% topical; 5 mg/g topical ☒ clarithromycin

**erythromycin 2′-acetate octadecanoate** [see: erythromycin acistrate]

**erythromycin 2′-acetate stearate** [see: erythromycin acistrate]

**erythromycin acistrate** USAN, INN *antibacterial*

**erythromycin B** [see: berythromycin]

**erythromycin estolate** USAN, USP, BAN *macrolide bactericidal/bacteriostatic antibiotic* 250 mg oral; 125, 250 mg/5 mL oral

**erythromycin ethyl succinate** BAN *antibacterial* [also: erythromycin ethylsuccinate]

**erythromycin ethylcarbonate** USP

**erythromycin ethylsuccinate (EES)** USP *macrolide bactericidal/bacteriostatic antibiotic* [also: erythromycin ethyl succinate] 400 mg oral; 200, 400 mg/5 mL oral;

**erythromycin gluceptate** USP *antibacterial*

**erythromycin glucoheptonate** [see: erythromycin gluceptate]

**erythromycin lactobionate** USP *macrolide bactericidal/bacteriostatic antibiotic* 500, 1000 mg/vial injection

**erythromycin lauryl sulfate, propionyl** [now: erythromycin estolate]

**erythromycin monoglucoheptonate** [see: erythromycin gluceptate]

**erythromycin octadecanoate** [see: erythromycin stearate]

**erythromycin 2′-propanoate** [see: erythromycin propionate]

**erythromycin propionate** USAN *antibacterial*

**erythromycin 2′-propionate dodecyl sulfate** [see: erythromycin estolate]

**erythromycin propionate lauryl sulfate** [now: erythromycin estolate]

**erythromycin salnacedin** USAN *antibiotic for acne vulgaris*

**erythromycin stearate** USP, BAN *macrolide bactericidal/bacteriostatic antibiotic* 250, 500 mg oral

**erythromycin stinoprate** INN

**erythropoietin, recombinant human (rEPO)** [see: epoetin alfa; epoetin beta]

**erythrosine sodium** USP *dental disclosing agent*

**Eryzole** granules for oral suspension ℞ *antibiotic* [erythromycin ethylsuccinate; sulfisoxazole acetyl] 200•600 mg/5 mL

**esafloxacin** INN

**esaprazole** INN

**esculamine** INN

**eseridine** INN

**eserine** [see: physostigmine]

**Eserine Salicylate** eye drops (discontinued 1995) ℞ *antiglaucoma agent; reversible cholinesterase inhibitor miotic* [physostigmine salicylate] 0.5%

**Eserine Sulfate** ophthalmic ointment ℞ *antiglaucoma agent; reversible cholinesterase inhibitor miotic* [physostigmine sulfate] 0.25%

**esflurbiprofen** INN, BAN

**Esgic** tablets, capsules ℞ *analgesic; antipyretic; sedative* [acetaminophen; caffeine; butalbital] 325•40•50 mg

**Esgic-Plus** tablets ℞ *analgesic; antipyretic; sedative* [acetaminophen; caffeine; butalbital] 500•40•50 mg

**ESHAP (etoposide, Solu-Medrol, high-dose ara-C, Platinol)** *chemotherapy protocol*

**ESHAP-MINE (alternating cycles of ESHAP and MINE)** *chemotherapy protocol*

**Esidrix** tablets ℞ *diuretic; antihypertensive* [hydrochlorothiazide] 25, 50, 100 mg ℞ Lasix

**esilate** INN *combining name for radicals or groups* [also: esylate]

**Esimil** tablets ℞ *antihypertensive* [hydrochlorothiazide; guanethidine monosulfate] 25•10 mg ℞ Estinyl; Isomil

**Eskalith** capsules, tablets ℞ *antipsychotic* [lithium carbonate] 300 mg

**Eskalith CR** controlled-release tablets ℞ *antipsychotic* [lithium carbonate] 450 mg

**esmolol** INN, BAN *antiadrenergic (β-receptor)* [also: esmolol HCl]

**esmolol HCl** USAN *antiadrenergic (β-receptor)* [also: esmolol]

**E-Solve** OTC *lotion base*

**E-Solve 2** topical solution (discontinued 1994) ℞ *topical antibiotic for acne vulgaris* [erythromycin]

**esorubicin** INN *antineoplastic* [also: esorubicin HCl]

**esorubicin HCl** USAN *antineoplastic* [also: esorubicin]

**Esotérica Dry Skin Treatment** lotion OTC *moisturizer; emollient*

**Esotérica Facial; Esotérica Fortified; Esotérica Sunscreen** cream OTC *hyperpigmentation bleaching agent; sunscreen* [hydroquinone; padimate O; oxybenzone] 2%•3.3%•2.5%

**Esotérica Regular; Esotérica Sensitive Skin Formula** cream OTC *hyperpigmentation bleaching agent* [hydroquinone] 2%; 1.5%

**Esotérica Soap** OTC *bath emollient*

**esperamycin** *investigational antineoplastic*

**Espotabs** tablets OTC *laxative* [yellow phenolphthalein] 97.2 mg

**esproquin HCl** USAN *adrenergic* [also: esproquine]

**esproquine** INN *adrenergic* [also: esproquin HCl]

**esrar** *street drug slang for a mixture of marijuana and tobacco* [see: marijuana]

**essence** *street drug slang* [see: MDMA]

**Estar** gel OTC *topical antipsoriatic; anti-seborrheic* [coal tar] 5%

**estazolam** USAN, INN *hypnotic* 1, 2 mg oral

**Ester-C Plus** capsules OTC *dietary supplement* [vitamin C; calcium; various bioflavonoids; rutin] 500•62•45•5 mg

**Ester-C Plus, Extra Potency** tablets OTC *dietary supplement* [vitamin C; calcium; various bioflavonoids; rutin] 1000•125•250•25 mg

**Ester-C Plus Multi-Mineral** capsules OTC *dietary supplement* [vitamin C; multiple minerals; various bioflavonoids; rutin] 425• ± •75•5 mg

**esterified estrogens** [see: estrogens, esterified]

**esterifilcon A** USAN *hydrophilic contact lens material*

**estilben** [see: diethylstilbestrol dipropionate]

**Estinyl** tablets ℞ *hormone for estrogen replacement therapy or inoperable prostatic and breast cancer* [ethinyl estradiol] 0.02, 0.05, 0.5 mg ⊡ Esimil

**Estivin II** eye drops (discontinued 1995) OTC *topical ocular decongestant/vasoconstrictor* [naphazoline HCl] 0.012%

**estolate** INN *combining name for radicals or groups*

**estomycin sulfate** [see: paromomycin sulfate]

**Estrace** tablets ℞ *estrogen replacement for postmenopausal disorders; antineoplastic for prostatic and breast cancer* [estradiol] 0.5, 1, 2 mg

**Estrace** vaginal cream ℞ *topical estrogen replacement for postmenopausal disorders* [estradiol] 0.1 mg/g

**Estra-D** IM injection (discontinued 1996) ℞ *hormone replacement therapy for postmenopausal disorders* [estradiol cypionate in oil] 5 mg/mL

**Estraderm** transdermal patch ℞ *estrogen replacement therapy for postmenopausal disorders* [estradiol] 50, 100 μg/day ⊡ Estradurin

**estradiol** USP, INN *estrogen* [also: oestradiol] 0.5, 1, 2 mg oral

**estradiol benzoate** USP, INN, JAN [also: oestradiol benzoate]

**estradiol 17-cyclopentanepropionate** [see: estradiol cypionate]

**estradiol cypionate** USP *estrogen for hormone replacement therapy* 5 mg/mL injection (in oil)

**estradiol dipropionate** NF, JAN

**estradiol enanthate** USAN *estrogen*

**estradiol 17-heptanoate** [see: estradiol enanthate]

**Estradiol L.A.; Estradiol L.A. 20; Estradiol L.A. 40** IM injection (discontinued 1994) ℞ *estrogen replacement therapy; antineoplastic for prostatic cancer* [estradiol valerate] 10 mg/mL; 20 mg/mL; 40 mg/mL

**estradiol monobenzoate** [see: estradiol benzoate]

**estradiol 17-nicotinate 3-propionate** [see: estrapronicate]

**estradiol phosphate polymer** [see: polyestradiol phosphate]

**estradiol 17-undecanoate** [see: estradiol undecylate]

**estradiol undecylate** USAN, INN *estrogen*

**estradiol valerate** USP, INN, JAN *estrogen replacement; hormonal antineoplastic for prostatic carcinoma* [also: oestradiol valerate] 10, 20, 40 mg/mL IM injection

**Estradurin** powder for IM injection (discontinued 1993) ℞ *hormonal therapy for inoperable progressing prostatic cancer* [polyestradiol phosphate] 40 mg ⊡ Estraderm

**Estra-L 20; Estra-L 40** IM injection ℞ *estrogen replacement therapy for postmenopausal disorders; antineoplastic for prostatic cancer* [estradiol valerate in oil] 20 mg/mL; 40 mg/mL

**estramustine** USAN, INN, BAN *antineoplastic*

**estramustine L-alanine (EMA)** *investigational antineoplastic for advanced prostatic cancer*

**estramustine phosphate sodium** USAN, BAN, JAN *hormonal antineoplastic for prostate cancer*

**estrapronicate** INN

**Estratab** tablets ℞ *estrogen replacement therapy; hypogonadism; inoperable prostatic and breast cancer* [esterified

estrogens] 0.3, 0.625, 1.25, 2.5 mg
② Ethatab

**Estratest; Estratest H.S.** sugar-coated tablets ℞ *estrogen/androgen for menopausal vasomotor symptoms* [esterified estrogens; methyltestosterone] 1.25•2.5 mg; 0.625•1.25 mg

**Estra-Testrin** IM injection (discontinued 1995) ℞ *estrogen/androgen for menopausal vasomotor symptoms* [estradiol valerate; testosterone enanthate] 4•90 mg/mL

**estrazinol** INN *estrogen* [also: estrazinol hydrobromide]

**estrazinol hydrobromide** USAN *estrogen* [also: estrazinol]

**Estrinex** ℞ *investigational (orphan) antiestrogen for metastatic carcinoma of the breast and desmoid tumors* [toremifene]

**Estring** vaginal ring ℞ *three-month therapy for postmenopausal urogenital symptoms* [estradiol] 2 mg (7.5 μg/day)

**estriol** USP *estrogen* [also: estriol succinate; oestriol succinate]

**estriol succinate** INN *estrogen* [also: estriol; oestriol succinate]

**estrobene** [see: diethylstilbestrol]

**estrobene DP** [see: diethylstilbestrol dipropionate]

**Estro-Cyp** IM injection ℞ *hormone replacement therapy for postmenopausal disorders* [estradiol cypionate in oil] 5 mg/mL

**estrofurate** USAN, INN *estrogen*

**Estrogenic Substance Aqueous** IM injection ℞ *estrogen replacement therapy; antineoplastic for prostatic and breast cancer* [estrone and other estrogens] 2 mg/mL

**estrogenic substances, conjugated** [see: estrogens, conjugated]

**estrogenine** [see: diethylstilbestrol]

**estrogens** *a class of female sex hormones that includes estradiol, estrone, and estriol, also used as an antineoplastic*

**estrogens, conjugated** USP, JAN *estrogen*

**estrogens, esterified** USP *estrogen*

**Estroject-L.A.** IM injection (discontinued 1995) ℞ *hormone for estrogen replacement therapy* [estradiol cypionate in oil] 5 mg/mL

**estromenin** [see: diethylstilbestrol]

**estrone** USP, INN *estrogen* [also: oestrone]

**Estrone 5** IM injection ℞ *estrogen replacement therapy; antineoplastic for prostatic and breast cancer* [estrone] 5 mg/mL

**Estrone Aqueous** IM injection ℞ *estrogen replacement therapy; antineoplastic for prostatic and breast cancer* [estrone] 2, 5 mg/mL

**estrone hydrogen sulfate** [see: estrone sodium sulfate]

**estrone sodium sulfate**

**Estronol** injection (discontinued 1993) ℞ *estrogen replacement therapy; antineoplastic for prostatic and breast cancer* [estrone] 2 mg/mL

**Estronol-LA** injection (discontinued 1993) ℞ *estrogen* [estradiol cypionate]

**Estrophasic** (trademarked/patented dosing regimen) *gradual estrogen intake with steady progestin intake*

**estropipate** USP *estrogen replacement therapy for postmenopausal disorders* 0.75, 1.5, 3 mg oral

**Estrostep 21** tablets (21-day, 21-tablet stepped regimen) ℞ *triphasic oral contraceptive* [norethindrone acetate; ethinyl estradiol] 5 × 1 mg•20 μg, 7 × 1 mg•30 μg, 9 × 1 mg•35 μg

**Estrostep Fe** tablets (28-day, 28-tablet stepped regimen) ℞ *triphasic oral contraceptive with iron* [norethindrone acetate; ethinyl estradiol; ferrous fumerate] 5 × 1 mg•20 μg•75 mg, 7 × 1 mg•30 μg•75 mg, 9 × 1 mg•35 μg•75 mg, 7 × 0•0•75 mg (iron only)

**Estrovis** tablets (discontinued 1996) ℞ *hormone replacement therapy for postmenopausal disorders* [quinestrol] 100 μg

**estufa** (Spanish for "stove") *street drug slang* [see: heroin]

**esuprone** INN

**esylate** USAN, BAN *combining name for radicals or groups* [also: esilate]

**ET** *street drug slang* [see: alpha-ethyltryptamine]

**etabenzarone** INN

**etabonate** USAN, INN *combining name for radicals or groups*

**etacepride** INN

**etacrynic acid** INN, JAN *loop diuretic* [also: ethacrynic acid]

**etafedrine** INN, BAN *adrenergic* [also: etafedrine HCl]

**etafedrine HCl** USAN *adrenergic* [also: etafedrine]

**etafenone** INN

**etafilcon A** USAN *hydrophilic contact lens material*

**etamestrol** INN

**etaminile** INN

**etamiphyllin** INN [also: etamiphylline]

**etamiphyllin methesculetol** [see: metescufylline]

**etamiphylline** BAN [also: etamiphyllin]

**etamivan** INN *central and respiratory stimulant* [also: ethamivan]

**etamocycline** INN

**etamsylate** INN *hemostatic* [also: ethamsylate]

**etanidazole** USAN, INN *antineoplastic; hypoxic cell radiosensitizer*

**etanterol** INN

**etaperazine** [see: perphenazine]

**etaqualone** INN

**etarotene** USAN, INN *keratolytic*

**etasuline** INN

**etazepine** INN

**etazolate** INN *antipsychotic* [also: etazolate HCl]

**etazolate HCl** USAN *antipsychotic* [also: etazolate]

**etebenecid** INN [also: ethebenecid]

**etenzamide** BAN [also: ethenzamide]

**eterobarb** USAN, INN, BAN *anticonvulsant*

**etersalate** INN

**ethacridine** INN [also: ethacridine lactate; acrinol] ⊡ ethacrynic

**ethacridine lactate** [also: ethacridine; acrinol]

**ethacrynate sodium** USAN, USP *diuretic*

**ethacrynic acid** USAN, USP, BAN *loop diuretic* [also: etacrynic acid] ⊡ ethacridine

**ethambutol** INN, BAN *bacteriostatic; primary tuberculostatic* [also: ethambutol HCl]

**ethambutol HCl** USAN, USP *bacteriostatic; primary tuberculostatic* [also: ethambutol]

**ethamivan** USAN, USP, BAN *central and respiratory stimulant* [also: etamivan]

**Ethamolin** IV injection ℞ *sclerosing agent for bleeding esophageal varices (orphan)* [ethanolamine oleate] 5%

**ethamsylate** USAN, BAN *hemostatic* [also: etamsylate]

**ethanol** JAN *topical anti-infective/antiseptic; astringent; solvent; a widely abused "legal street drug" used to produce euphoria* [also: alcohol]

**ethanol, dehydrated** JAN *antidote* [also: alcohol, dehydrated]

**ethanolamine oleate** USAN *sclerosing agent for bleeding esophageal varices (orphan)* [also: monoethanolamine oleate]

**ethanolamines** *a class of antihistamines*

**Ethaquin** tablets (discontinued 1996) ℞ *peripheral vasodilator* [ethaverine HCl] 100 mg ⊡ Edecrin

**Ethatab** tablets (discontinued 1996) ℞ *peripheral vasodilator* [ethaverine HCl] 100 mg ⊡ Estratab

**ethaverine** INN *peripheral vasodilator*

**ethaverine HCl** *peripheral vasodilator* [see: ethaverine]

**Ethavex-100** tablets (discontinued 1996) ℞ *peripheral vasodilator* [ethaverine HCl] 100 mg

**ethchlorvynol** USP, INN, BAN *sedative; hypnotic*

**ethebenecid** BAN [also: etebenecid]

**ethenzamide** INN, JAN [also: etenzamide]

**ether** USP *inhalation anesthetic*

**ethiazide** INN, BAN

**ethidium bromide** [see: homidium bromide]

**ethinamate** USP, INN, BAN *sedative; hypnotic* ⊡ ethionamide

**ethinyl estradiol** USP *estrogen for hormone replacement therapy or breast and prostate cancer; investigational (orphan) for Turner syndrome* [also: ethinylestradiol; ethinyloestradiol]

**ethinylestradiol** INN *estrogen* [also: ethinyl estradiol; ethinyloestradiol]

**ethinyloestradiol** BAN *estrogen* [also: ethinyl estradiol; ethinyloestradiol]

**ethiodized oil** USP *radiopaque medium*

**ethiodized oil ($^{131}$I)** INN *antineoplastic; radioactive agent* [also: ethiodized oil I 131]

**ethiodized oil I 131** USAN *antineoplastic; radioactive agent* [also: ethiodized oil ($^{131}$I)]

**Ethiodol** intracavitary instillation ℞ *hysterosalpingographic and lymphographic contrast medium* [ethiodized oil] 100% ⧉ ethynodiol

**ethiofos** *(previously used USAN)* [now: amifostine]

**ethionamide** USAN, USP, INN, BAN *bacteriostatic; tuberculosis retreatment* ⧉ ethinamate

**ethisterone** NF, INN, BAN

**Ethmozine** film-coated tablets ℞ *antiarrhythmic* [moricizine HCl] 200, 250, 300 mg

**ethodryl** [see: diethylcarbamazine citrate]

**ethoglucid** BAN [also: etoglucid]

**ethoheptazine** BAN [also: ethoheptazine citrate]

**ethoheptazine citrate** NF, INN [also: ethoheptazine]

**ethohexadiol** USP

**ethomoxane** INN, BAN

**ethomoxane HCl** [see: ethomoxane]

**Ethon** tablets (discontinued 1993) ℞ *diuretic; antihypertensive* [methyclothiazide]

**ethonam nitrate** USAN *antifungal* [also: etonam]

**ethopabate** BAN

**ethopropazine** BAN *antiparkinsonian* [also: ethopropazine HCl; profenamine]

**ethopropazine HCl** USP *antiparkinsonian; anticholinergic* [also: profenamine; ethopropazine]

**ethosalamide** BAN [also: etosalamide]

**ethosuximide** USAN, USP, INN, BAN *anticonvulsant* 250 mg/5 mL oral

**ethotoin** USP, INN, BAN *hydantoin-type anticonvulsant*

**ethoxarutine** [see: ethoxazorutoside]

**ethoxazene HCl** USAN *analgesic* [also: etoxazene]

**ethoxazorutoside** INN

**ethoxyacetanilide** *(withdrawn from market)* [see: phenacetin]

**o-ethoxybenzamide** [see: ethenzamide; etenzamide]

**ethoxzolamide** USP

**Ethrane** liquid for vaporization ℞ *inhalation general anesthetic* [enflurane]

**ethybenztropine** USAN, BAN *anticholinergic* [also: etybenzatropine]

**ethyl acetate** NF *solvent*

**ethyl alcohol (EtOH; ETOH)** [now: alcohol; ethanol]

**ethyl aminobenzoate (ethyl *p*-aminobenzoate)** JAN *topical anesthetic; nonprescription diet aid* [also: benzocaine]

**ethyl 2-benzimidazolecarbamate** [see: lobendazole]

**ethyl N-benzylcyclopropanecarbamate** [see: encyprate]

**ethyl biscoumacetate** NF, INN, BAN

**ethyl biscumacetate** [see: ethyl biscoumacetate]

**ethyl carbamate** [now: urethane]

**ethyl carfluzepate** INN

**ethyl cartrizoate** INN

**ethyl chloride** USP *topical local anesthetic; topical vapo-coolant*

**ethyl dibunate** USAN, INN, BAN *antitussive*

**ethyl dirazepate** INN

**ethyl ether** [see: ether]

**ethyl *p*-fluorophenyl sulfone** [see: fluoresone]

**ethyl *p*-hydroxybenzoate** [see: ethylparaben]

**ethyl loflazepate** INN

**ethyl nitrite** NF

**ethyl oleate** NF *vehicle*

**ethyl oxide** [see: ether]

**ethyl vanillin** NF *flavoring agent*

**ethylcellulose** NF *tablet binder*

**ethylchlordiphene** [see: etofamide]

**ethyldicoumarol** [see: ethyl biscoumacetate]

**ethylene** NF *inhalation general anesthesia*

**ethylene distearate** [see: glycol distearate]

**ethylenediamine** USP, JAN

**ethylenediaminetetraacetate** [see: edetate disodium]

**ethylenediaminetetraacetic acid (EDTA)** [see: edetate disodium]

**N,N-ethylenediarsanilic acid** [see: difetarsone]

**ethylenedinitrilotetraacetate disodium** [see: edetate disodium]

**ethylestrenol** USAN, INN *anabolic steroid; also abused as a street drug* [also: ethyloestrenol; ethylnandrol]

**ethylhexanediol** [see: ethohexadiol]

**2-ethylhexyl diphenyl phosphate** [see: octicizer]

**ethylhydrocupreine HCl** NF

**ethylmethylthiambutene** INN, BAN

**ethylmorphine** BAN [also: ethylmorphine HCl]

**ethylmorphine HCl** NF [also: ethylmorphine]

**ethylnandrol** JAN *anabolic steroid; also abused as a street drug* [also: ethylestrenol; ethyloestrenol]

**ethylnorepinephrine HCl** USP *bronchodilator*

**ethyloestradiol** BAN *estrogen* [also: ethinyl estradiol]

**ethyloestrenol** BAN *anabolic steroid; also abused as a street drug* [also: ethylestrenol; ethylnandrol]

**ethylpapaverine HCl** [see: ethaverine HCl]

**ethylparaben** NF *antifungal agent*

**ethylphenacemide** [see: pheneturide]

**ethylstibamine** [see: stibosamine]

**2-ethylthioisonicotinamide** [see: ethionamide]

**ethynerone** USAN, INN *progestin*

**ethynodiol** BAN *progestin* [also: ethynodiol diacetate; etynodiol] ⑨ Ethiodol

**ethynodiol diacetate** USAN, USP *progestin* [also: etynodiol; ethynodiol]

**Ethyol** powder for IV infusion ℞ *chemoprotective agent for cisplatin and paclitaxel chemotherapy (orphan); investigational (orphan) for cyclophosphamide rescue* [amifostine] 500 mg/vial

**ethypicone** INN

**ethypropymal sodium** [see: probarbital sodium]

**etibendazole** USAN, INN *anthelmintic*

**eticlopride** INN

**eticyclidine** INN

**etidocaine** USAN, INN, BAN *injectable local anesthetic*

**etidocaine HCl** *injectable local anesthetic*

**etidronate disodium** USAN, USP *bisphosphonate bone resorption suppressant for Paget's disease, heterotopic ossification and hypercalcemia of malignancy*

**etidronate monosodium**

**etidronate sodium** (*this term used only when the form of sodium cannot be more accurately identified*)

**etidronate tetrasodium**

**etidronate trisodium**

**etidronic acid** USAN, INN, BAN *calcium regulator*

**etifelmine** INN

**etifenin** USAN, INN, BAN *diagnostic aid*

**etifoxin** BAN [also: etifoxine]

**etifoxine** INN [also: etifoxin]

**etilamfetamine** INN

**etilefrine** INN

**etilefrine pivalate** INN

**etintidine** INN *antagonist to histamine* $H_2$ *receptors* [also: etintidine HCl]

**etintidine HCl** USAN *antagonist to histamine* $H_2$ *receptors* [also: etintidine]

**etiocholanedione** *investigational (orphan) for aplastic anemia and Prader-Willi syndrome*

**etipirium iodide** INN

**etiproston** INN

**etiracetam** INN

**etiroxate** INN

**etisazole** INN, BAN

**etisomicin** INN, BAN

**etisulergine** INN

**etizolam** INN

**etobedolum** [see: etonitazene]

**etocarlide** INN

**etocrilene** INN *ultraviolet screen* [also: etocrylene]

**etocrylene** USAN *ultraviolet screen* [also: etocrilene]

**etodolac** USAN, INN, BAN *antiarthritic; nonsteroidal anti-inflammatory drug (NSAID); analgesic* [also: etodolic acid] 400 mg oral

**etodolic acid** INN *antiarthritic; nonsteroidal anti-inflammatory drug (NSAID); analgesic* [also: etodolac]

**etodroxizine** INN

**etofamide** INN

**etofenamate** USAN, INN, BAN *analgesic; anti-inflammatory*

**etofenprox** INN
**etofibrate** INN
**etoformin** INN *antidiabetic* [also: etoformin HCl]
**etoformin HCl** USAN *antidiabetic* [also: etoformin]
**etofuradine** INN
**etofylline** INN
**etofylline clofibrate** INN *antihyperlipoproteinemic* [also: theofibrate]
**etoglucid** INN [also: ethoglucid]
**EtOH; ETOH (ethyl alcohol)** [now: alcohol]
**etolorex** INN
**etolotifen** INN
**etoloxamine** INN
**etomidate** USAN, INN, BAN *rapid-acting nonbarbiturate general anesthetic; hypnotic*
**etomidoline** INN
**etomoxir** INN
**etonam** INN *antifungal* [also: ethonam nitrate]
**etonam nitrate** [see: ethonam nitrate]
**etonitazene** INN, BAN
**etonogestrel** USAN, INN *progestin*
**etoperidone** INN *antidepressant* [also: etoperidone HCl]
**etoperidone HCl** USAN *antidepressant* [also: etoperidone]
**etophylate** [see: acepifylline]
**Etopophos** powder for IV injection ℞ *antineoplastic for testicular and small cell lung cancers* [etoposide phosphate diethanolate] 119.3 mg/vial
**etoposide** USAN, INN, BAN *antineoplastic* 20, 30 mg/mL injection
**etoposide phosphate** USAN *antineoplastic*
**etoprindole** INN
**etoprine** USAN *antineoplastic*
**etorphine** INN, BAN
**etosalamide** INN [also: ethosalamide]
**etoxadrol** INN *anesthetic* [also: etoxadrol HCl]
**etoxadrol HCl** USAN *anesthetic* [also: etoxadrol]
**etoxazene** INN *analgesic* [also: ethoxazene HCl]
**etoxazene HCl** [see: ethoxazene HCl]
**etoxeridine** INN, BAN
**etozolin** USAN, INN *diuretic*

**etrabamine** INN
**Etrafon; Etrafon 2–10; Etrafon-A; Etrafon-Forte** tablets ℞ *antipsychotic; antidepressant* [perphenazine; amitriptyline HCl] 2•25 mg; 2•10 mg; 4•10 mg; 4•25 mg
**etretin** [see: acitretin]
**etretinate** USAN, INN, BAN, JAN *systemic antipsoriatic*
**etryptamine** INN, BAN *CNS stimulant* [also: etryptamine acetate]
**etryptamine acetate** USAN *CNS stimulant* [also: etryptamine]
**ETS-2%** topical solution (name changed to Erythra-Derm in 1994)
**etybenzatropine** INN *anticholinergic* [also: ethybenztropine]
**etymemazine** INN
**etymemazine HCl** [see: etymemazine]
**etynodiol** INN *progestin* [also: ethynodiol diacetate; ethynodiol]
**etyprenaline** [see: isoetharine]
**eucaine HCl** NF
**Eucalyptamint** ointment, gel OTC *counterirritant; topical antiseptic* [menthol; eucalyptus oil] 16%•⅔; 8%•⅔
**eucalyptol** USAN *topical bacteriostatic antiseptic/germicidal*
**eucalyptus oil** NF *topical antiseptic*
**eucatropine** INN, BAN *ophthalmic anticholinergic* [also: eucatropine HCl]
**eucatropine HCl** USP *ophthalmic anticholinergic* [also: eucatropine]
**Eucerin** cream, lotion OTC *moisturizer; emollient*
**Eucerin** OTC *cream base*
**Eucerin Cleansing** lotion (discontinued 1994) OTC *cleanser; moisturizer; emollient*
**Eucerin Plus** lotion OTC *moisturizer; emollient* [sodium lactate; urea] 5%•5%
**eucodal** [see: oxycodone]
**Eudal-SR** sustained-release tablets ℞ *decongestant; expectorant* [pseudoephedrine HCl; guaifenesin] 120•400 mg
**euflavine** [see: acriflavine]
**Euflex** Ⓒᴬᴺ (U.S. product: Eulexin) tablets ℞ *adjunctive hormonal chemotherapy for metastatic prostatic cancer* [flutamide] 250 mg

**eugenol** USP *dental analgesic*

**eukadol** [see: oxycodone]

**Eulexin** capsules ℞ *adjunctive hormonal chemotherapy for metastatic prostatic cancer* [flutamide] 125 mg

**euprocin** INN *topical anesthetic* [also: euprocin HCl]

**euprocin HCl** USAN *topical anesthetic* [also: euprocin]

**euquinine** [see: quinine ethylcarbonate]

**Eurax** cream, lotion ℞ *scabicide; antipruritic* [crotamiton] 10% ☑ Serax; Urex

**europium** *element (Eu)*

**EVA (etoposide, vinblastine, Adriamycin)** *chemotherapy protocol*

**Evac-Q-Kit** oral solution + 2 tablets + 2 suppositories OTC *pre-procedure bowel evacuant* [Evac-Q-Mag (q.v.); Evac-Q-Tabs (q.v.); Evac-Q-Sert (q.v.)] ☑ Evac-Q-Kwik

**Evac-Q-Kwik** suppositories OTC *laxative* [bisacodyl] 10 mg ☑ Evac-Q-Kit

**Evac-Q-Kwik Kit** oral solution + 2 tablets + 1 suppository OTC *pre-procedure bowel evacuant* [Evac-Q-Mag (q.v.); Evac-Q-Tabs (q.v.); Evac-Q-Kwik suppository (q.v.)]

**Evac-Q-Mag** carbonated oral solution OTC *laxative* [magnesium citrate; citric acid; potassium citrate]

**Evac-Q-Sert** suppositories OTC *laxative* [sodium bicarbonate; potassium bitartrate]

**Evac-Q-Tabs** tablets OTC *laxative* [phenolphthalein] 130 mg

**Evac-U-Gen** chewable tablets OTC *laxative* [yellow phenolphthalein] 97.2 mg

**Evac-U-Lax** chewable wafers OTC *laxative* [phenolphthalein] 80 mg

**Evalose** syrup ℞ *laxative* [lactulose] 10 g/15 mL

**evandamine** INN

**Evans blue** USP *blood volume test* [also: azovan blue] 5 mL injection

**Eve** *street drug slang* [see: MDMA]

**Everone 100** IM injection (discontinued 1994) ℞ *androgen replacement for delayed puberty or breast cancer* [testosterone enanthate] 100 mg/mL

**Everone 200** IM injection ℞ *androgen replacement for delayed puberty or*

*breast cancer* [testosterone enanthate] 200 mg/mL

**E-Vista** IM injection (discontinued 1997) ℞ *anxiolytic* [hydroxyzine HCl] 50 mg/mL

**E-Vitamin** ointment OTC *emollient* [vitamin E] 30 mg/g

**E-Vitamin Succinate** capsules OTC *vitamin supplement* [vitamin E] 165, 330 mg

**E-VMAC (escalated methotrexate, vinblastine, Adriamycin, cisplatin)** *chemotherapy protocol*

**E-VMAC (escalated methotrexate, vinblastine, Adriamycin, cyclophosphamide)** *chemotherapy protocol*

**ex; X; extasy** *street drug slang, from "ecstasy"* [see: MDMA]

**Exact** liquid OTC *topical keratolytic cleanser for acne* [salicylic acid] 2%

**Exact** vanishing cream OTC *topical keratolytic for acne* [benzoyl peroxide] 5%

**exalamide** INN

**exametazime** USAN, INN, BAN *regional cerebral perfusion imaging aid*

**exaprolol** INN *antiadrenergic (β-receptor)* [also: exaprolol HCl]

**exaprolol HCl** USAN *antiadrenergic (β-receptor)* [also: exaprolol]

**Excedrin** caplets, tablets, geltabs OTC *analgesic; antipyretic; anti-inflammatory* [acetaminophen; aspirin; caffeine] 250•250•65 mg

**Excedrin, Aspirin Free** caplets, geltabs OTC *analgesic; antipyretic* [acetaminophen; caffeine] 500•65 mg

**Excedrin, Sinus** tablets, caplets OTC *decongestant; analgesic; antipyretic* [pseudoephedrine HCl; acetaminophen] 30•500 mg

**Excedrin Dual, Aspirin Free** film-coated caplets OTC *analgesic; antipyretic; antacid* [acetaminophen; calcium carbonate; magnesium carbonate; magnesium oxide] 500•111•64•30 mg

**Excedrin IB** tablets, caplets (discontinued 1995) OTC *nonsteroidal anti-inflammatory drug (NSAID); antiarthritic; analgesic* [ibuprofen] 200 mg

**Excedrin P.M.** liquid, liquigels OTC *antihistaminic sleep aid; analgesic* [diphenhydramine HCl; acetaminophen] 50•1000 mg/30 mL; 25•500 mg

**Excedrin P.M.** tablets, caplets OTC *antihistaminic sleep aid; analgesic* [diphenhydramine citrate; acetaminophen] 38•500 mg

**Excegran** ℞ *investigational anticonvulsant* [zonisamide]

**Excita Extra** premedicated condom OTC *spermicidal/barrier contraceptive* [nonoxynol 9] 8%

**Exelderm** cream (discontinued 1993) ℞ *topical antifungal* [sulconazole nitrate] 1%

**Exelderm** solution ℞ *topical antifungal* [sulconazole nitrate] 1%

**exemestane** INN *investigational (orphan) hormonal antineoplastic for advanced breast cancer*

**exepanol** INN

**Exgest LA** long-acting tablets ℞ *decongestant; expectorant* [phenylpropanolamine HCl; guaifenesin] 75•400 mg

**Exidine Skin Cleanser; Exidine-2 Scrub; Exidine-4 Scrub** liquid OTC *broad-spectrum antimicrobial; germicidal* [chlorhexidine gluconate; alcohol 4%] 4%; 2%; 4%

**exifone** INN

**exiproben** INN

**Ex-Lax** chocolated chewable tablets OTC *laxative* [yellow phenolphthalein] 90 mg

**Ex-Lax Extra Gentle Pills** tablets OTC *laxative; stool softener* [phenolphthalein; docusate sodium] 65•75 mg

**Ex-Lax Gentle Nature** tablets OTC *laxative* [sennosides] 20 mg

**Ex-Lax Maximum Relief; Ex-Lax Unflavored** tablets OTC *laxative* [yellow phenolphthalein] 135 mg; 90 mg

**Exna** tablets ℞ *diuretic; antihypertensive* [benzthiazide] 50 mg

**Exocaine Medicated Rub; Exocaine Plus Rub** OTC *counterirritant* [methyl salicylate] 25%; 30%

**Exocaine Odor Free Creme** (discontinued 1993) OTC *topical analgesic* [trolamine salicylate] 10%

**Exosurf** ℞ *orphan status withdrawn 1997* [colfosceril palmitate]

**Exosurf Neonatal** powder for injection, intratracheal suspension ℞ *pulmonary surfactant for hyaline membrane disease and respiratory distress syndrome (orphan)* [colfosceril palmitate] 108 mg

**Exovir-HZ** gel ℞ *investigational treatment for recurrent genital herpes*

**expectorants** *a class of drugs that promote the ejection of mucus from the respiratory tract*

**Expidet** (trademarked dosage form) *fast-dissolving dose*

**Exsel** lotion/shampoo ℞ *antiseborrheic; antifungal* [selenium sulfide] 2.5%

**exsiccated sodium arsenate** [see: sodium arsenate, exsiccated]

**Extencap** (trademarked dosage form) *extended-release capsule*

**extended insulin zinc** [see: insulin zinc, extended]

**Extendryl** chewable tablets, syrup ℞ *decongestant; antihistamine; anticholinergic* [phenylephrine HCl; chlorpheniramine maleate; methscopolamine nitrate] 10•2•1.25 mg; 10•2•1.25 mg/5 mL

**Extendryl JR** sustained-release capsules ℞ *pediatric decongestant, antihistamine, and anticholinergic* [phenylephrine HCl; chlorpheniramine maleate; methscopolamine nitrate] 10•4•1.25 mg

**Extendryl SR** sustained-release capsules ℞ *decongestant; antihistamine; anticholinergic* [phenylephrine HCl; chlorpheniramine maleate; methscopolamine nitrate] 20•8•2.5 mg

**Extentab** (trademarked dosage form) *extended-release tablet*

**Extra Action Cough** syrup OTC *antitussive; expectorant* [dextromethorphan hydrobromide; guaifenesin; alcohol 1.4%] 10•100 mg/5 mL

**"Extra Strength"** products [see under product name]

**Extreme Cold Formula** caplets (discontinued 1993) OTC *decongestant; antihistamine; analgesic; antitussive* [phenylpropanolamine HCl; chlorpheniramine maleate; acetaminophen; dextromethorphan hydrobromide]

**Eye Drops** OTC *topical ocular deconges-tant/vasoconstrictor* [tetrahydrozoline HCl] 0.05%

**Eye Irrigating Solution** OTC *extraocular irrigating solution* [sterile isotonic solution]

**Eye Irrigating Wash** OTC *extraocular irrigating solution* [sterile isotonic solution]

**eye opener** *street drug slang* [see: cocaine, crack; amphetamines]

**Eye Scrub** solution OTC *eyelid cleanser for blepharitis or contact lenses*

**Eye Stream** ophthalmic solution OTC *extraocular irrigating solution* [sterile isotonic solution]

**Eye Wash** ophthalmic solution OTC *extraocular irrigating solution* [sterile isotonic solution]

**Eye-Lube-A** eye drops OTC *ocular moisturizer/lubricant* [glycerin] 0.25%

**Eye-Sed** eye drops OTC *ophthalmic astringent* [zinc sulfate] 0.25%

**Eyesine** eye drops OTC *topical ocular decongestant/vasoconstrictor* [tetrahydrozoline HCl] 0.05%

**EZ Detect** test kit for home use OTC *in vitro diagnostic aid for fecal occult blood*

**EZ Detect** test kit for home use (discontinued 1995) OTC *in vitro diagnostic aid for urine occult blood*

**EZ Detect Strep-A** swab test for professional use (discontinued 1995) *in vitro diagnostic aid for streptococci*

**Ezide** tablets ℞ *diuretic; antihypertensive* [hydrochlorothiazide] 50 mg

**1 + 1-F Creme** ℞ *topical corticosteroid; antifungal; antibacterial; local anesthetic* [hydrocortisone; clioquinol; pramoxine] 1%•3%•1%

**$^{18}$F** [see: fludeoxyglucose F 18]

**$^{18}$F** [see: sodium fluoride F 18]

**FABRase** ℞ *investigational (orphan) for Fabry's disease* [alpha-galactosidase A]

**FAC (fluorouracil, Adriamycin, cyclophosphamide)** *chemotherapy protocol*

**FAC-LEV (fluorouracil, Adriamycin, Cytoxin, levamisole)** *chemotherapy protocol*

**FAC-M (fluorouracil, Adriamycin, cyclophosphamide, methotrexate)** *chemotherapy protocol*

**Fact Plus** test kit for home use OTC *in vitro diagnostic aid for urine pregnancy test*

**factor II (prothrombin)**

**factor III** [see: thromboplastin]

**factor VIIa, recombinant, DNA origin** *investigational (orphan) for hemophilia A and B and von Willebrand's disease*

**factor VIII** [see: antihemophilic factor]

**factor VIII (rDNA)** BAN *blood coagulating factor*

**factor VIII fraction** BAN *blood coagulating factor*

**factor IX complex** USP *hemostatic; antihemophilic for hemophilia B (orphan)* [also: factor IX fraction]

**factor IX fraction** BAN *hemostatic; antihemophilic* [also: factor IX complex]

**factor XIII (plasma-derived)** *investigational (orphan) for congenital factor XIII deficiency*

**factor XIII, recombinant** *orphan status withdrawn 1996*

**factor VIII SQ, recombinant** *investigational (orphan) for long-term hemophilia A treatment or for surgical procedures*

**Factrel** powder for subcu or IV injection ℞ *gonadotropin releasing hormone* [gonadorelin HCl] 100, 500 μg

**fadrozole** INN *antineoplastic; aromatase inhibitor* [also: fadrozole HCl]

**fadrozole HCl** USAN *antineoplastic; aromatase inhibitor* [also: fadrozole]

**fairy dust** *street drug slang* [see: heroin]

**fake STP** *street drug slang* [see: PCP]

**falintolol** INN

**falipamil** INN

**Fallbrook redhair** *street drug slang for marijuana from Fallbrook, California* [see: marijuana]

**FAM (fluorouracil, Adriamycin, mitomycin)** *chemotherapy protocol*

**FAM-CF (fluorouracil, Adriamycin, mitomycin, citrovorum factor)** *chemotherapy protocol*

**famciclovir** USAN, INN, BAN *antiviral for herpes simplex and zoster*

**FAME; FAMe (fluorouracil, Adriamycin, MeCCNU)** *chemotherapy protocol*

**Family Tabs** tablets (discontinued 1995) OTC *vitamin supplement* [multiple vitamins; folic acid] $\triangleq \bullet 0.4$ mg

**Familytabs with Calcium, Iron & Zinc** tablets (discontinued 1995) OTC *vitamin/mineral supplement* [multiple vitamins; calcium carbonate; ferrous fumarate; zinc oxide]

**Familytabs with Iron** tablets (discontinued 1995) OTC *vitamin/iron supplement* [multiple vitamins; iron]

**famiraprinium chloride** INN

**FAMMe (fluorouracil, Adriamycin, mitomycin, MeCCNU)** *chemotherapy protocol*

**famotidine** USAN, USP, INN, BAN *treatment of GI ulcers; histamine $H_2$ antagonist*

**famotine** INN *antiviral* [also: famotine HCl]

**famotine HCl** USAN *antiviral* [also: famotine]

**famous dimes** *street drug slang* [see: cocaine, crack]

**fampridine** USAN, INN *investigational (orphan) for multiple sclerosis*

**famprofazone** INN, BAN

**FAM-S (fluorouracil, Adriamycin, mitomycin, streptozocin)** *chemotherapy protocol*

**FAMTX (fluorouracil, Adriamycin, methotrexate [with leucovorin rescue])** *chemotherapy protocol*

**Famvir** film-coated tablets Ɽ *antiviral for acute herpes zoster and genital herpes* [famciclovir] 125, 250, 500 mg

**fananserin** USAN *antipsychotic; antischizophrenic; dopamine $D_2$ and serotonin 5-$HT_2$ receptor antagonist*

**fanetizole** INN, BAN *immunoregulator* [also: fanetizole mesylate]

**fanetizole mesylate** USAN *immunoregulator* [also: fanetizole]

**Fansidar** tablets Ɽ *antimalarial* [sulfadoxine; pyrimethamine] 500•25 mg

**fantasia** *street drug slang* [see: dimethyltryptamine]

**fanthridone** BAN *antidepressant* [also: fantridone HCl; fantridone]

**fantridone** INN *antidepressant* [also: fantridone HCl; fanthridone]

**fantridone HCl** USAN *antidepressant* [also: fantridone; fanthridone]

**FAP (fluorouracil, Adriamycin, Platinol)** *chemotherapy protocol*

**Farbee with Vitamin C** caplets OTC *vitamin supplement* [multiple B vitamins; vitamin C] $\triangleq \bullet 300$ mg

**Fareston** Ɽ *antiestrogen antineoplastic for estrogen-receptive tumors, such as breast cancer in postmenopausal women* [toremifene citrate]

**Farmorubicin** (available in Canada as Pharmorubicin) Ɽ *investigational antibiotic antineoplastic for multiple myeloma, leukemia, lymphoma and other tumors* [epirubicin HCl]

**farnesil** INN *combining name for radicals or groups*

**fasiplon** INN

**Faspak** (trademarked form) *flexible plastic bag*

**Fastin** capsules Ɽ *amphetamine-type anorectic* [phentermine HCl] 30 mg

**Fast-Trak** (trademarked delivery system) *quick-loading syringe*

**fat, hard** NF *suppository base*

**fat bags** *street drug slang* [see: cocaine, crack]

**fat emulsion, intravenous** *parenteral essential fatty acid replacement*

**Father John's Medicine Plus** liquid OTC *antitussive; decongestant; antihistamine; expectorant* [dextromethorphan hydrobromide; phenylephrine HCl; chlorpheniramine maleate; guaifenesin; ammonium chloride] 7.5•2.5•1•30•83.3 mg/5 mL

**fatty** *street drug slang for a marijuana cigarette* [see: marijuana]

**fazadinium bromide** INN, BAN

**fazarabine** USAN, INN *antineoplastic*

**5-FC (5-fluorocytosine)** [see: flucytosine]

**FCAP (fluorouracil, cyclophosphamide, Adriamycin, Platinol)** *chemotherapy protocol*

**FCE (fluorouracil, cisplatin, etoposide)** *chemotherapy protocol*

**F-CL (fluorouracil, leucovorin calcium [rescue])** *chemotherapy protocol* [also: FU/LV]

**FCP (fluorouracil, cyclophosphamide, prednisone)** *chemotherapy protocol*

**FD&C Red No. 2 (Food, Drug & Cosmetic Act)** [see: amaranth]

**FD&C Red No. 3 (Food, Drug & Cosmetic Act)** [see: erythrosine sodium]

**18FDG (fludeoxyglucose)** [see: fludeoxyglucose F 18]

**Fe50 (or Fe50)** caplets OTC *hematinic* [ferrous sulfate] 160 mg (50 mg Fe)

**59Fe** [see: ferric chloride Fe 59]

**59Fe** [see: ferric citrate (59Fe)]

**59Fe** [see: ferrous citrate Fe 59]

**59Fe** [see: ferrous sulfate Fe 59]

**febantel** USAN, INN, BAN *veterinary anthelmintic*

**febarbamate** INN

**febuprol** INN

**febuverine** INN

**FEC (fluorouracil, epirubicin, cyclophosphamide)** *chemotherapy protocol*

**feclemine** INN

**feclobuzone** INN

**FED (fluorouracil, etoposide, DDP)** *chemotherapy protocol*

**Fedahist** tablets OTC *decongestant; antihistamine* [pseudoephedrine HCl; chlorpheniramine maleate] 60•4 mg

**Fedahist** Timecaps (timed-release capsules), Gyrocaps (extended-release capsules) R *decongestant; antihistamine* [pseudoephedrine HCl; chlorpheniramine maleate] 120•8 mg; 65•10 mg

**Fedahist Decongestant** syrup (discontinued 1994) OTC *decongestant; antihistamine* [pseudoephedrine HCl; chlorpheniramine maleate] 30•2 mg/5 mL

**Fedahist Expectorant** pediatric drops (discontinued 1995) OTC *decongestant; expectorant* [pseudoephedrine HCl; guaifenesin] 7.5•40 mg/mL

**Fedahist Expectorant** syrup OTC *decongestant; expectorant* [pseudoephedrine HCl; guaifenesin] 20•200 mg/5 mL

**fedotozine** INN *investigational kappa selective opioid agonist for irritable bowel syndrome*

**fedrilate** INN

**Feen-A-Mint** chocolated chewable tablets OTC *laxative* [yellow phenolphthalein] 65 mg

**Feen-A-Mint** tablets, chewable tablets, gum OTC *laxative* [yellow phenolphthalein] 97.2 mg

**Feen-A-Mint Pills** tablets OTC *laxative; stool softener* [phenolphthalein; docusate sodium] 65•100 mg

**feenies** *street drug slang* [see: phenobarbital]

**Feiba VH Immuno** IV injection or drip R *antihemophilic to correct factor VIII deficiency and coagulation deficiency* [anti-inhibitor coagulant complex, vapor heated and freeze-dried] (each bottle is labeled with dosage)

**felbamate** USAN, INN *antiepileptic; investigational (orphan) for Lennox-Gastaut syndrome*

**Felbamyl** (name changed to Felbatol upon marketing release in 1994)

**Felbatol** tablets, oral suspension (the FDA and the manufacturer recommend discontinuing use due to adverse side effects) R *anticonvulsant; investigational (orphan) for Lennox-Gastaut syndrome; investigational neuroprotectant* [felbamate] 400, 600 mg; 600 mg/5 mL

**felbinac** USAN, INN, BAN *anti-inflammatory*

**Feldene** capsules R *nonsteroidal anti-inflammatory drug (NSAID); antiarthritic* [piroxicam] 10, 20 mg

**Feldene Melt** R *investigational instantaneously dissolving form* [piroxicam]

**felipyrine** INN

**felodipine** USAN, INN, BAN *vasodilator; antihypertensive; calcium channel blocker*

**felypressin** USAN, INN, BAN *vasoconstrictor*

**Fem-1** tablets OTC *analgesic; anti-inflammatory; diuretic* [acetaminophen; pamabrom] 500•25 mg

**Femara** film-coated tablets ℞ *hormonal antineoplastic/aromatase inhibitor for advanced breast cancer in postmenopausal women* [letrozole] 2.5 mg

**Femaston** ℞ *investigational treatment for menopausal symptoms* [estrogen; progestogen]

**FemCal** tablets OTC *calcium supplement* [calcium carbonate; vitamin D; multiple minerals] 250 mg•100 IU• ±

**FemCare** vaginal cream, tablets (discontinued 1996) OTC *antifungal* [clotrimazole] 1%; 100 mg

**Femcet** capsules ℞ *analgesic; antipyretic; sedative* [acetaminophen; caffeine; butalbital] 325•40•50 mg

**Fem-Etts** tablets (discontinued 1997) OTC *analgesic; anti-inflammatory; diuretic* [acetaminophen; pamabrom] 325•25 mg

**Femicine** vaginal suppositories OTC *for vaginal irritations, itching, and burning* [pulsatilla 28x]

**Femidine Douche** solution (discontinued 1995) OTC *antiseptic/germicidal; vaginal cleanser and deodorizer* [povidone-iodine]

**Femilax** tablets OTC *laxative; stool softener* [phenolphthalein; docusate sodium] 65•100 mg

**Feminique Disposable Douche** solution OTC *antiseptic/antifungal; vaginal cleanser and deodorizer; acidity modifier* [sodium benzoate; sorbic acid; lactic acid]

**Feminique Disposable Douche** solution OTC *vaginal cleanser and deodorizer; acidity modifier* [vinegar (acetic acid)]

**Feminone** tablets (discontinued 1993) ℞ *estrogen deficiency; inoperable prostatic and breast cancer* [ethinyl estradiol]

**Femiron** tablets OTC *hematinic* [ferrous fumarate] 63 mg

**Femiron Multi-Vitamins and Iron** tablets OTC *vitamin/iron supplement* [multiple vitamins; ferrous fumarate; folic acid] ± •20•0.4 mg

**Femizol-M** vaginal cream OTC *antifungal* [miconazole nitrate] 2%

**femoxetine** INN

**FemPatch** transdermal patch ℞ *estrogen replacement therapy for postmenopausal disorders* [estradiol] 25 μg/day

**Femstat** vaginal cream (discontinued 1995) ℞ *antifungal* [butoconazole nitrate] 2%

**Femstat 3; FemStat One** vaginal cream in prefilled applicator OTC *antifungal* [butoconazole nitrate] 2%

**Femstat Prefill** (prefilled applicator) (discontinued 1993) ℞ *antifungal* [butoconazole nitrate]

**fenabutene** INN

**fenacetinol** INN

**fenaclon** INN

**fenadiazole** INN

**fenaftic acid** INN

**fenalamide** USAN, INN *smooth muscle relaxant*

**fenalcomine** INN

**fenamifuril** INN

**fenamisal** INN *antibacterial; tuberculostatic* [also: phenyl aminosalicylate]

**fenamole** USAN, INN *anti-inflammatory*

**fenaperone** INN

**fenarsone** [see: carbarsone]

**fenasprate** [see: benorilate]

**fenbendazole** USAN, INN, BAN *anthelmintic*

**fenbenicillin** INN [also: phenbenicillin]

**fenbufen** USAN, INN, BAN *anti-inflammatory*

**fenbutrazate** INN [also: phenbutrazate]

**fencamfamin** INN, BAN

**fencamfamin HCl** [see: fencamfamin]

**fencarbamide** INN *anticholinergic* [also: phencarbamide]

**fenchlorphos** BAN *systemic insecticide* [also: ronnel; fenclofos]

**fencilbutirol** USAN, INN *choleretic*

**fenclexonium metilsulfate** INN

**fenclofenac** USAN, INN, BAN *anti-inflammatory*

**fenclofos** INN *systemic insecticide* [also: ronnel; fenchlorphos]

**fenclonine** USAN, INN *serotonin inhibitor*

**fenclorac** USAN, INN *anti-inflammatory*

**fenclozic acid** INN, BAN

**fendiline** INN

**fendizoate** INN *combining name for radicals or groups*

**fendosal** USAN, INN, BAN *anti-inflammatory*

**feneritrol** INN

**Fenesin** sustained-release tablets ℞ *expectorant* [guaifenesin] 600 mg

**Fenesin DM** tablets ℞ *antitussive; expectorant* [dextromethorphan hydrobromide; guaifenesin] 30•600 mg

**fenestrel** USAN, INN *estrogen*

**fenethazine** INN

**fenethylline** BAN *CNS stimulant* [also: fenethylline HCl; fenetylline]

**fenethylline HCl** USAN *CNS stimulant* [also: fenetylline; fenethylline]

**fenetradil** INN

**fenetylline** INN *CNS stimulant* [also: fenethylline HCl; fenethylline]

**fenflumizole** INN

**fenfluramine** INN, BAN *anorexiant; CNS depressant* [also: fenfluramine HCl]

**fenfluramine HCl** USAN *anorexiant; CNS depressant* [also: fenfluramine]

**fenfluthrin** INN, BAN

**fengabine** USAN, INN, BAN *mood regulator*

**fenharmane** INN

**fenimide** USAN, INN, BAN *antipsychotic*

**feniodium chloride** INN

**fenipentol** INN

**fenirofibrate** INN

**fenisorex** USAN, INN, BAN *anorectic*

**fenleuton** USAN *5-lipoxygenase inhibitor*

**fenmetozole** INN *antidepressant; narcotic antagonist* [also: fenmetozole HCl]

**fenmetozole HCl** USAN *antidepressant; narcotic antagonist* [also: fenmetozole]

**fenmetramide** USAN, INN, BAN *antidepressant*

**fennel oil** NF

**fennies; phennies** *street drug slang* [see: phenobarbital]

**fenobam** USAN, INN *sedative*

**fenocinol** INN

**fenoctimine** INN *gastric antisecretory* [also: fenoctimine sulfate]

**fenoctimine sulfate** USAN *gastric antisecretory* [also: fenoctimine]

**fenofibrate** INN, BAN *antihyperlipidemic for hypertriglyceridemia*

**fenoldopam** INN, BAN *antihypertensive; dopamine agonist* [also: fenoldopam mesylate]

**fenoldopam mesylate** USAN *antihypertensive; dopamine agonist* [also: fenoldopam]

**fenoprofen** USAN, INN, BAN *nonsteroidal anti-inflammatory drug (NSAID); analgesic*

**fenoprofen calcium** USAN, USP, BAN *antiarthritic; nonsteroidal anti-inflammatory drug (NSAID); analgesic* 200, 300, 600 mg oral

**feno's; pheno's** *street drug slang* [see: phenobarbital]

**fenoterol** USAN, INN, BAN *bronchodilator* [also: fenoterol hydrobromide]

**fenoterol hydrobromide** JAN *bronchodilator* [also: fenoterol]

**fenoverine** INN

**fenoxazol** [see: pemoline]

**fenoxazoline** INN

**fenoxazoline HCl** [see: fenoxazoline]

**fenoxedil** INN

**fenoxypropazine** INN [also: phenoxypropazine]

**fenozolone** INN

**fenpentadiol** INN

**fenperate** INN

**fenpipalone** USAN, INN *anti-inflammatory*

**fenpipramide** INN, BAN

**fenpiprane** INN, BAN

**fenpiprane HCl** [see: fenpiprane]

**fenpiverinium bromide** INN

**fenprinast** INN *bronchodilator; antiallergic* [also: fenprinast HCl]

**fenprinast HCl** USAN *bronchodilator; antiallergic* [also: fenprinast]

**fenproporex** INN

**fenprostalene** USAN, INN, BAN *luteolysin*

**fenquizone** USAN, INN *diuretic*

**fenretinide** USAN, INN *investigational (Phase III) retinoid cancer chemopreventative*

**fenspiride** INN *bronchodilator; antiadrenergic (α-receptor)* [also: fenspiride HCl]

**fenspiride HCl** USAN *bronchodilator; antiadrenergic (α-receptor)* [also: fenspiride]

**fentanyl** INN, BAN *narcotic agonist analgesic; also abused as a street drug* [also: fentanyl citrate]

**fentanyl citrate** USAN, USP, JAN *narcotic agonist analgesic; also abused as a street drug* [also: fentanyl] 0.05 mg/mL injection

**Fentanyl Oralet** lozenges ℞ *narcotic analgesic* [fentanyl] 100, 200, 300, 400 μg

**fenthion** BAN

**fentiazac** USAN, INN, BAN *anti-inflammatory*

**fenticlor** USAN, INN, BAN *topical anti-infective*

**fenticonazole** INN, BAN *antifungal* [also: fenticonazole nitrate]

**fenticonazole nitrate** USAN *antifungal* [also: fenticonazole]

**fentonium bromide** INN

**fenyramidol** INN *analgesic; skeletal muscle relaxant* [also: phenyramidol HCl]

**fenyripol** INN *skeletal muscle relaxant* [also: fenyripol HCl]

**fenyripol HCl** USAN *skeletal muscle relaxant* [also: fenyripol]

**Feocyte** prolonged-action tablets ℞ *hematinic* [ferrous fumarate, ferrous gluconate, and ferrous sulfate; desiccated liver; vitamins B₆, B₁₂, and C; folic acid] 110 mg•15 mg•2 mg•50 μg•100 mg•0.8 mg

**Fe-O.D.** timed-release tablets OTC *hematinic* [ferrous fumarate; ascorbic acid] 100•500 mg

**Feosol** elixir OTC *hematinic* [ferrous sulfate] 220 mg/5 mL ☑ Feostat; Fer-In-Sol; Festal

**Feosol** tablets, timed-release capsules OTC *hematinic* [ferrous sulfate, dried] 200 mg; 159 mg

**Feostat** chewable tablets, suspension, drops OTC *hematinic* [ferrous fumarate] 100 mg; 100 mg/5 mL; 45 mg/0.6 mL ☑ Feosol

**fepentolic acid** INN
**fepitrizol** INN
**fepradinol** INN
**feprazone** INN, BAN

**fepromide** INN
**feprosidnine** INN

**Ferancee** chewable tablets OTC *hematinic* [ferrous fumarate; vitamin C] 67•150 mg

**Ferancee-HP** film-coated tablets OTC *hematinic* [ferrous fumarate; vitamin C] 110•600 mg

**Feratab** tablets OTC *hematinic* [ferrous sulfate] 300 mg

**Fer-gen-sol** drops OTC *hematinic* [ferrous sulfate] 75 mg/0.6 mL

**Fergon** tablets, elixir OTC *hematinic* [ferrous gluconate] 320 mg; 300 mg/5 mL

**Fergon Plus** caplets (discontinued 1995) ℞ *hematinic* [ferrous gluconate; vitamin B₁₂ with intrinsic factor concentrate; ascorbic acid] 58 mg•0.5 U•75 mg

**Feridex** IV injection ℞ *contrast agent for MRI of the liver* [ferumoxides] (11.2 mg iron)

**Fer-In-Sol** capsules (discontinued 1997) OTC *hematinic* [ferrous sulfate, dried] 190 mg ☑ Feosol

**Fer-In-Sol** drops, syrup OTC *hematinic* [ferrous sulfate] 75 mg/0.6 mL; 90 mg/5 mL

**Fer-Iron** drops OTC *hematinic* [ferrous sulfate] 75 mg/0.6 mL

**fermium** *element (Fm)*

**Ferocyl** sustained-release tablets OTC *hematinic* [ferrous fumarate; docusate sodium] 150•100 mg

**Fero-Folic-500** controlled-release Filmtabs (film-coated tablets) ℞ *hematinic* [ferrous sulfate; ascorbic acid; folic acid] 105•500•0.8 mg

**Fero-Grad-500** controlled-release Filmtabs (film-coated tablets) OTC *hematinic* [ferrous sulfate; sodium ascorbate] 105•500 mg

**Fero-Gradumet** timed-release Filmtabs (film-coated tablets) OTC *hematinic* [ferrous sulfate] 525 mg

**Ferospace** capsules OTC *hematinic* [ferrous sulfate] 250 mg

**Ferotrinsic** capsules ℞ *hematinic* [ferrous fumarate; cyanocobalamin; ascorbic acid; intrinsic factor concentrate; folic acid] 110 mg•15 μg•75•240 mg•0.5 mg

**Ferralet** tablets OTC *hematinic* [ferrous gluconate] 320 mg

**Ferralet Plus** tablets OTC *hematinic* [ferrous gluconate; cyanocobalamin; ascorbic acid; folic acid] 46 mg•25 μg•400 mg•0.8 mg

**Ferralet S.R.** sustained-release tablets OTC *hematinic* [ferrous gluconate] 320 mg

**Ferralyn** Lanacaps (timed-release capsules) OTC *hematinic* [ferrous sulfate, dried] 250 mg

**Ferra-TD** timed-release capsules OTC *hematinic* [ferrous sulfate, dried] 250 mg

**Ferretts** tablets (discontinued 1997) OTC *hematinic* [ferrous fumarate] 325 mg

**ferric ammonium citrate** NF

**ferric ammonium sulfate**

**ferric cacodylate** NF

**ferric chloride**

**ferric chloride Fe 59** USAN *radioactive agent*

**ferric citrate ($^{59}$Fe)** INN

**ferric citrochloride** NF

**ferric fructose** USAN, INN *hematinic*

**ferric glycerophosphate** NF

**ferric hypophosphite** NF

**ferric oxide** NF *coloring agent*

**ferric oxide, red** NF

**ferric oxide, yellow** NF

**ferric pyrophosphate, soluble** NF

**ferric subsulfate** NF

**ferricholinate** [see: ferrocholinate]

**ferriclate calcium sodium** USAN *hematinic* [also: calcium sodium ferriclate]

**ferristene** USAN *paramagnetic imaging agent for MRI*

**Ferrixan** ℞ *investigational contrast medium for MRI of the liver*

**Ferro Dok TR** timed-release capsules OTC *hematinic* [ferrous fumarate; docusate sodium] 150•100 mg

**ferrocholate** [see: ferrocholinate]

**ferrocholinate** INN

**Ferro-Docusate T.R.** timed-release capsules OTC *hematinic* [ferrous fumarate; docusate sodium] 150•100 mg

**Ferro-DSS S.R.** timed-release capsules OTC *hematinic* [ferrous fumarate; docusate sodium] 150•100 mg

**Ferromar** sustained-release caplets OTC *hematinic* [ferrous fumarate; vitamin C] 201.5•200 mg

**ferropolimaler** INN

**Ferro-Sequels** timed-release tablets OTC *hematinic* [ferrous fumarate] 50 mg

**ferrotrenine** INN

**ferrous citrate Fe 59** USAN, USP *radioactive agent*

**ferrous fumarate** USP *hematinic (33% elemental iron)* 200, 325 mg oral

**ferrous gluconate** USP *hematinic (11.6% elemental iron)* 300, 325 mg oral

**ferrous lactate** NF

**ferrous sulfate** USP *hematinic (20% elemental iron)* 250, 325 mg oral; 220 mg/5 mL oral; 75 mg/0.6 mL oral

**ferrous sulfate, dried** USP *antianemic*

**ferrous sulfate, exsiccated** [see: ferrous sulfate, dried]

**ferrous sulfate Fe 59** USAN *radioactive agent*

**Fertinex** subcu injection ℞ *ovulation stimulant* [urofollitropin] 75, 150 IU

**Fertinorm HP** (commercially available in Europe) ℞ *investigational infertility therapy*

**fertirelin** INN, BAN *veterinary gonadotropin-releasing hormone* [also: fertirelin acetate]

**fertirelin acetate** USAN *veterinary gonadotropin-releasing hormone* [also: fertirelin]

**ferumoxides** USAN *diagnostic aid for magnetic resonance imaging of the liver*

**ferumoxsil** USAN *diagnostic aid for magnetic imaging*

**Fetal Fibronectin Test** kit for professional use *in vitro diagnostic aid for fetal fibronectin in vaginal secretions at 24–34 weeks, a predictor of preterm delivery*

**fetal neural cells** [see: porcine fetal neural cells]

**fetoxilate** INN *smooth muscle relaxant* [also: fetoxylate HCl; fetoxylate]

**fetoxylate** BAN *smooth muscle relaxant* [also: fetoxylate HCl; fetoxilate]

**fetoxylate HCl** USAN *smooth muscle relaxant* [also: fetoxilate; fetoxylate]

**Feverall, Children's; Infant's Feverall; Junior Feverall** suppositories OTC *analgesic; antipyretic* [acetaminophen] 120 mg; 80 mg; 325 mg

**Feverall, Children's; Junior Feverall** Sprinkle Caps (powder) OTC *analgesic; antipyretic* [acetaminophen] 80 mg; 160 mg ☒ Fiberall

**fexicaine** INN, DCF

**fexinidazole** INN

**fexofenadine HCl** USAN *nonsedating antihistamine*

**fezatione** INN

**fezolamine** INN *antidepressant* [also: fezolamine fumarate]

**fezolamine fumarate** USAN *antidepressant* [also: fezolamine]

**FGF-4 (fibroblast growth factor-4)** [q.v.]

**FGN-1** *investigational (Phase III, orphan) for familial adenomatous polyposis (FAP; also known as adenomatous polyposis coli, or APC)*

**fiacitabine (FIAC)** USAN, INN *antiviral; investigational (Phase I/II) for HIV and AIDS*

**fialuridine (FIAU)** USAN, INN *antiviral; investigational (Phase II) for HIV; investigational (orphan) for chronic active hepatitis B*

**Fiberall** chewable tablets OTC *bulk laxative; antidiarrheal* [calcium polycarbophil] 1250 mg ☒ Feverall

**Fiberall** powder, wafers OTC *laxative* [psyllium hydrophilic mucilloid] 3.4 g/tsp.; 3.4 g

**FiberCon** film-coated tablets OTC *bulk laxative; antidiarrheal* [calcium polycarbophil] 500 mg

**Fiberlan** liquid OTC *enteral nutritional therapy* [lactose-free formula]

**Fiber-Lax** tablets OTC *bulk laxative; antidiarrheal* [calcium polycarbophil] 625 mg

**FiberNorm** tablets OTC *bulk laxative; antidiarrheal* [calcium polycarbophil] 625 mg

**fibracillin** INN

**Fibrad** powder OTC *oral dietary fiber supplement* [pea, oat and sugar beet fiber] 7 g total fiber per serving

**fibrin** INN

**fibrinase** [see: factor XIII]

**fibrinogen ($^{125}$I)** INN [also: fibrinogen I 125]

**fibrinogen, human** USP *investigational (orphan) to control bleeding in fibrinogen-deficient patients*

**fibrinogen I 125** USAN *vascular patency test; radioactive agent* [also: fibrinogen ($^{125}$I)]

**fibrinoligase** [see: factor XIII]

**fibrinolysin, human** INN [also: plasmin]

**fibrinolysin & desoxyribonuclease** *topical enzymes for necrotic tissue debridement*

**fibrin-stabilizing factor (FSF)** [see: factor XIII]

**Fibriscint** ℞ *investigational imaging aid for deep venous thrombosis* [antifibrin monoclonal antibodies]

**fibroblast growth factor, basic (bFGF)** [see: ersofermin]

**fibroblast growth factor-4 (FGF-4)** *investigational vulnerary*

**fibroblast interferon** [now: interferon beta]

**Fibrogammin P** ℞ *investigational (orphan) for congenital factor XIII deficiency* [factor XIII (plasma-derived)]

**fibronectin** *investigational (orphan) for nonhealing corneal ulcers or epithelial defects*

**fields** street drug slang [see: LSD]

**50% Dextrose with Electrolyte Pattern A (or N)** IV infusion ℞ *intravenous nutritional/electrolyte therapy* [combined electrolyte solution; dextrose]

**50% Dextrose with Electrolyte Pattern B** IV infusion (discontinued 1994) ℞ *intravenous nutritional/electrolyte therapy* [combined electrolyte solution; dextrose]

**fifty-one; one-fifty-one** street drug slang [see: cocaine, crack]

**filaminast** USAN *selective phosphodiesterase IV inhibitor for asthma*

**filenadol** INN

**filgrastim** USAN, INN, BAN *hematopoietic stimulant; investigational (orphan) for severe chronic neutropenia; investigational (Phase III, orphan) cytokine for CMV retinitis of AIDS*

**filgrastim & methionyl stem cell factor, recombinant human** *investigational (orphan) adjunct to myelosuppressive or myeloablative therapy*

**Filibon** tablets (discontinued 1995) OTC *vitamin/calcium/iron supplement* [multiple vitamins; calcium; iron; folic acid] ≛•125•18•0.4 mg

**Filibon F.A.; Filibon Forte** tablets (discontinued 1995) ℞ *vitamin/calcium/iron supplement* [multiple vitamins; calcium; iron; folic acid] ≛• 250•45•1 mg; 300•45•1 mg

**filipin** USAN, INN *antifungal*

**Filmix** ℞ *investigational (orphan) neurosonographic contrast medium for intracranial tumors* [microbubble contrast agent]

**Filmlok** (trademarked dosage form) *film-coated tablet*

**Filmseal** (trademarked dosage form) *film-coated tablet*

**Filmtabs** (trademarked dosage form) *film-coated tablets*

**FIME (fluorouracil, ICRF-159, MeCCNU)** *chemotherapy protocol*

**Finac** lotion OTC *topical acne treatment* [salicylic acid; isopropyl alcohol] 2%•22.5%

**Finajet; Finaplix** *brand names for trenbolone acetate, a European veterinary anabolic steroid abused as a street drug*

**finasteride** USAN, INN, BAN *antineoplastic; androgen hormone inhibitor for benign prostatic hypertension; investigational (Phase III) for androgenic alopecia*

**fine stuff** *street drug slang* [see: marijuana]

**finger** *street drug slang for a marijuana cigarette or a stick-shaped piece of hashish* [see: marijuana; hashish]

**Fiogesic** tablets OTC *decongestant; antihistamine; analgesic* [phenylpropanolamine HCl; pheniramine maleate; pyrilamine maleate; aspirin]

**Fiorgen PF** tablets ℞ *analgesic; antipyretic; anti-inflammatory; sedative* [aspirin; caffeine; butalbital] 325•40•50 mg

**Fioricet** tablets ℞ *analgesic; antipyretic; sedative* [acetaminophen; caffeine; butalbital] 325•40•50 mg ② Lorcet

**Fioricet with Codeine** capsules ℞ *narcotic analgesic; sedative* [codeine phosphate; acetaminophen; caffeine; butalbital] 30•325•40•50 mg

**Fiorinal** tablets, capsules ℞ *analgesic; antipyretic; anti-inflammatory; sedative* [aspirin; caffeine; butalbital] 325•40•50 mg ② Florinef

**Fiorinal with Codeine** capsules ℞ *narcotic analgesic; sedative* [codeine phosphate; aspirin; caffeine; butalbital] 30•325•40•50 mg

**Fiorpap** tablets ℞ *analgesic; antipyretic; sedative* [acetaminophen; caffeine; butalbital] 325•40•50 mg

**fipexide** INN

**fir** *street drug slang* [see: marijuana]

**fire** *street drug slang for a combination of crack and methamphetamine* [see: cocaine, crack; methamphetamine HCl]

**fire ant venom allergenic extract** *investigational (orphan) skin test and immunotherapy for fire ant reactions*

**First Choice** reagent strips for home use OTC *in vitro diagnostic aid for blood glucose*

**first line** *street drug slang* [see: morphine]

**First Response** test stick for home use OTC *in vitro diagnostic aid for urine pregnancy test*

**First Response Ovulation Predictor** test kit for home use OTC *in vitro diagnostic aid to predict ovulation time*

**fisalamine** [see: mesalamine]

**fish scales** *street drug slang* [see: cocaine, crack]

**5 + 2 protocol (cytarabine, daunorubicin)** *chemotherapy protocol*

**5 + 2 protocol (cytarabine, mitoxantrone)** *chemotherapy protocol*

**5% Alcohol and 5% Dextrose in Water; 10% Alcohol and 5% Dextrose in Water** IV infusion ℞ *for caloric replacement and rehydration* [alcohol; dextrose] 5%•5%; 10%•5%

**5 Benzagel; 10 Benzagel** gel ℞ *keratolytic for acne* [benzoyl peroxide] 5%; 10%

**5% Dextrose and Electrolyte #48; 5% Dextrose and Electrolyte #75; 10% Dextrose and Electrolyte #48** IV infusion ℞ *intravenous nutritional/electrolyte therapy* [combined electrolyte solution; dextrose]

**5% Travert and Electrolyte No. 2; 10% Travert and Electrolyte No. 2** IV infusion ℞ *intravenous nutritional/electrolyte therapy* [combined electrolyte solution; invert sugar (50% dextrose + 50% fructose)]

**520C9x22** [see: bispecific antibody 520C9x22]

**5A8 MAb to CD4** *investigational (orphan) for post-exposure prophylaxis to occupational HIV exposure*

**5-HT₃ (hydroxytryptamine) receptor antagonists** *a class of antiemetic and antinauseant agents used primarily after emetogenic cancer chemotherapy*

**fives** *street drug slang* [see: amphetamine]

**fizzies** *street drug slang* [see: methadone]

**FK-037** *investigational cephalosporin antibiotic*

**FK-143** *investigational T5 alpha reductase inhibitor for benign prostatic hypertrophy*

**FK-176** *investigational treatment for pollakiuria*

**FK-224** *investigational neurokinin antagonist*

**FK-366** *investigational aldose reductase inhibitor for diabetic neuropathy and diabetic cataracts*

**FK-409** *investigational vasodilator for angina*

**FK-453** *investigational adenosine A₁ receptor antagonist for acute renal failure*

**FK-480** *investigational cholecystokinin antagonist for pancreatitis*

**FK-508** *investigational treatment for Alzheimer's senile dementia*

**FK-565** *investigational (Phase I) immunomodulator for cancer and HIV*

**FK-613** *investigational antihistamine for asthma, allergic rhinitis, and urticaria*

**FK-739** *investigational angiotensin II antagonist for hypertension*

**FK-780** *investigational treatment for hyperglycemia, hyperinsulinemia, and diabetes-related hirsutism*

**FK-906** *investigational renin inhibitor for hypertension*

**FK-1052** *investigational 5-HT₃ and 5-HT₄ dual antagonist for irritable bowel syndrome*

**FK-3311** *investigational nonsteroidal anti-inflammatory and analgesic*

**FL (flutamide, leuprolide acetate)** *chemotherapy protocol*

**FLAC (fluorouracil, leucovorin [rescue], Adriamycin, cyclophosphamide)** *chemotherapy protocol*

**Flagyl** film-coated tablets, capsules ℞ *antibiotic; antiprotozoal; amebicide* [metronidazole] 250, 500 mg; 375 mg

**Flagyl IV** powder for injection ℞ *antibiotic; antiprotozoal; amebicide* [metronidazole HCl] 500 mg

**Flagyl IV RTU** (ready-to-use) injection ℞ *antibiotic; antiprotozoal; amebicide* [metronidazole] 500 mg/100 mL

**flake; flakes** *street drug slang* [see: cocaine; PCP]

**flamenol** INN

**flamethrowers** *street drug slang for cigarette laced with cocaine and heroin* [see: cocaine; heroin]

**Flanders Buttocks** ointment OTC *topical diaper rash treatment* [zinc oxide; balsam Peru]

**FLAP (fluorouracil, leucovorin [rescue], Adriamycin, Platinol)** *chemotherapy protocol*

**Flarex** Drop-Tainers (eye drop suspension) ℞ *ophthalmic topical corticosteroidal anti-inflammatory* [fluorometholone acetate] 0.1%

**flash** *street drug slang for glue (for sniffing) or LSD* [see: petroleum distillate inhalants; LSD]

**flat blues** *street drug slang* [see: LSD]

**flat chunks** *street drug slang for crack cut with benzocaine* [see: cocaine, crack]

**Flatulex** drops OTC *antiflatulent* [simethicone] 40 mg/0.6 mL

**Flatulex** tablets OTC *adsorbent; detoxicant; antiflatulent* [activated charcoal; simethicone] 250•80 mg

**flavamine** INN

**flavine** [see: acriflavine HCl]

**flavodic acid** INN

**flavodilol** INN *antihypertensive* [also: flavodilol maleate]

**flavodilol maleate** USAN *antihypertensive* [also: flavodilol]

**flavonoid** [see: troxerutin]

**Flavons-500** tablets OTC *dietary supplement* [citrus bioflavonoids and hesperidin complex] 500 mg

**Flavorcee** chewable tablets OTC *vitamin supplement* [ascorbic acid] 100, 250, 500 mg

**flavoxate** INN, BAN *smooth muscle relaxant; urinary antispasmodic* [also: flavoxate HCl]

**flavoxate HCl** USAN *smooth muscle relaxant; urinary antispasmodic* [also: flavoxate]

**Flaxedil** IV (discontinued 1996) ℞ *neuromuscular blocker* [gallamine triethiodide] 20 mg/mL ② Flexeril

**flazalone** USAN, INN, BAN *anti-inflammatory*

**FLe (fluorouracil, levamisole)** *chemotherapy protocol*

**flea powder** *street drug slang for low-purity heroin* [see: heroin]

**flecainide** INN, BAN *antiarrhythmic* [also: flecainide acetate]

**flecainide acetate** USAN *antiarrhythmic* [also: flecainide]

**Fleet Babylax** rectal liquid OTC *hyperosmolar laxative* [glycerin] 4 mL/dose

**Fleet Bisacodyl Enema; Fleet Bisacodyl Prep** rectal liquid OTC *stimulant laxative* [bisacodyl] 10 mg/30 mL; 10 mg/packet

**Fleet Enema** rectal liquid OTC *saline laxative* [monobasic sodium phosphate; dibasic sodium phosphate] 7•19 g/118 mL

**Fleet Flavored Castor Oil** emulsion OTC *stimulant laxative* [castor oil] 67%

**Fleet Laxative** enteric-coated tablets OTC *stimulant laxative* [bisacodyl] 5 mg

**Fleet Laxative** suppositories OTC *stimulant laxative* [bisacodyl] 10 mg

**Fleet Medicated Wipes** cleansing pads OTC *moisturizer and cleanser for external rectal/vaginal areas; astringent; antiseptic; antifungal* [hamamelis water; glycerin; alcohol] 50%•10%•7%

**Fleet Mineral Oil Enema** rectal liquid OTC *lubricant laxative* [mineral oil]

**Fleet Pain Relief** anorectal wipes OTC *topical local anesthetic* [pramoxine HCl; glycerin] 1%•12%

**Fleet Phospho-Soda** oral solution OTC *buffered saline laxative* [monobasic sodium phosphate; dibasic sodium phosphate] 18•48 g/100 mL

**Fleet Prep Kits No. 1 to No. 6** OTC *pre-procedure bowel evacuant* [other Fleet products in combination kits]

**Fleet Relief** anorectal ointment (discontinued 1995) OTC *hemorrhoidal astringent; protectant* [zinc oxide; white petrolatum; mineral oil]

**Fleet Relief Anesthetic Hemorrhoidal** ointment (discontinued 1995) OTC *topical local anesthetic* [pramoxine HCl] 1%

**FLEP (fluorouracil, leucovorin, etoposide, Platinol)** *chemotherapy protocol*

**flerobuterol** INN

**fleroxacin** USAN, INN *antibacterial*

**flesinoxan** INN *investigational antidepressant and anxiolytic*

**flestolol** INN *antiadrenergic (β-receptor)* [also: flestolol sulfate]

**flestolol sulfate** USAN *antiadrenergic (β-receptor)* [also: flestolol]

**fletazepam** USAN, INN, BAN *skeletal muscle relaxant*

**Fletcher's Castoria** liquid OTC *laxative* [senna concentrate] 33.3 mg/mL

**Flex-all 454** gel OTC *topical antipruritic; counterirritant; topical local anesthetic* [menthol; methyl salicylate] 16%• ²

**Flexaphen** capsules ℞ *skeletal muscle relaxant; analgesic* [chlorzoxazone; acetaminophen] 250•300 mg

**Flex-Care Especially for Sensitive Eyes** solution OTC *chemical disinfecting solution for soft contact lenses* [note: soft contact indication different from RGP contact indication for same product]

**Flex-Care Especially for Sensitive Eyes** solution OTC *disinfecting/wetting/soaking solution for rigid gas permeable contact lenses* [note: RGP contact indication different from soft contact indication for same product]

**Flexeril** film-coated tablets ℞ *skeletal muscle relaxant* [cyclobenzaprine HCl] 10 mg ⌺ Flaxedil

**Flexoject** IV or IM injection ℞ *skeletal muscle relaxant* [orphenadrine citrate] 30 mg/mL

**Flexon** IV or IM injection ℞ *skeletal muscle relaxant* [orphenadrine citrate] 30 mg/mL

**FlexPack HP** test for professional use *diagnostic aid for serum IgG antibodies to H. pylori (for peptic ulcers)*

**Flintstones Children's; Flintstones Plus Calcium; Flintstones Plus Extra C Children's** chewable tablets OTC *vitamin supplement* [multiple vitamins; folic acid] ⩲•0.3 mg

**Flintstones Complete** chewable tablets OTC *vitamin/mineral/iron supplement* [multiple vitamins & minerals; iron; folic acid; biotin] ⩲•18 mg•0.4 mg•40 μg

**Flintstones Plus Iron** chewable tablets OTC *vitamin/iron supplement* [multiple vitamins; iron; folic acid] ⩲•15•0.3 mg

**Flixonase** (foreign name for U.S. product Flonase)

**Flixotide** (foreign name for U.S. product Flovent)

**Flo-Coat** suspension ℞ *GI contrast radiopaque agent* [barium sulfate] 100%

**floctafenine** USAN, INN, BAN *analgesic*

**Flolan** IV infusion ℞ *platelet aggregation inhibitor; investigational (orphan) vasodilator for primary pulmonary hypertension* [epoprostenol] 0.5, 1.5 mg

**Flomax** capsules ℞ *selective $\alpha_1$ antagonist for benign prostatic hypertrophy (BPH)* [tamsulosin HCl] 0.4 mg

**flomoxef** INN

**Flonase** nasal spray ℞ *intranasal steroidal anti-inflammatory* [fluticasone propionate] 50 μg/dose

**Flo-Pack** (trademarked packaging form) *vial for IV drip*

**flopropione** INN

**florantyrone** INN, BAN

**flordipine** USAN, INN *antihypertensive*

**floredil** INN

**floretione** [see: fluoresone]

**florfenicol** USAN, INN, BAN *veterinary antibacterial*

**Florical** capsules, tablets OTC *calcium supplement* [calcium carbonate; sodium fluoride] 364•8.3 mg

**Florida snow** *street drug slang for cocaine or a cocaine look-alike* [see: cocaine]

**Florida Sunburn Relief** lotion OTC *antipruritic; counterirritant* [benzyl alcohol; phenol; camphor; menthol] 3%•0.4%•0.2%•0.15%

**florifenine** INN

**Florinef Acetate** tablets ℞ *adrenocortical insufficiency in Addison's disease* [fludrocortisone acetate] 0.1 mg ⌺ Fiorinal

**Florone** cream, ointment ℞ *topical corticosteroidal anti-inflammatory* [diflorasone diacetate] 0.05%

**Florone E** cream ℞ *topical corticosteroidal anti-inflammatory; emollient* [diflorasone diacetate] 0.05%

**floropipamide** [now: pipamperone]

**floropipeton** [see: propyperone]

**Floropryl** ophthalmic ointment (discontinued 1995) ℞ *antiglaucoma agent; irreversible cholinesterase inhibitor miotic* [isoflurophate] 0.025%

**Florvite** drops ℞ *pediatric vitamin supplement and dental caries preventative* [multiple vitamins; sodium fluoride] ⩲•0.25, ⩲•0.5 mg/mL

**Florvite; Florvite Half Strength** chewable tablets ℞ *pediatric vitamin supplement and dental caries preventative* [multiple vitamins; sodium fluoride; folic acid] ⩲•1•0.3 mg; ⩲•0.5•0.3 mg

**Florvite + Iron** drops ℞ *pediatric vitamin/iron supplement and dental caries preventative* [multiple vitamins & minerals; sodium fluoride; ferrous sulfate] ⩲•0.25•10, ⩲•0.5•10 mg/mL

**Florvite + Iron; Half Strength Florvite + Iron** chewable tablets ℞ *pediatric vitamin/iron supplement and dental caries preventative* [multiple vitamins & minerals; sodium fluoride; ferrous sulfate; folic acid] ⩲•1•12•0.3 mg; ⩲•0.5•12•0.3 mg

**flosequinan** USAN, INN, BAN *antihypertensive; vasodilator*

**flotrenizine** INN

**Flovent** metered dose inhaler ℞ *corticosteroidal antiasthmatic* [fluticasone propionate] 44, 110, 220 μg/inhalation

**floverine** INN

**flower; flower tops** *street drug slang* [see: marijuana]

**floxacillin** USAN *antibacterial* [also: flucloxacillin]

**floxacrine** INN

**Floxin** film-coated tablets, UroPak (3-day supply), IV injection ℞ *broad-spectrum fluoroquinolone-type antibiotic* [ofloxacin] 200, 300, 400 mg; 6 tablets × 200 mg; 200, 400 mg

**floxuridine** USAN, USP, INN *antiviral; antimetabolic antineoplastic* 100 mg/mL injection; 500 mg/vial injection

**FLT (fluorothymidine)** [q.v.]

**Flu, Cold & Cough Medicine** powder for oral solution OTC *antitussive; decongestant; antihistamine; analgesic* [dextromethorphan hydrobromide; pseudoephedrine HCl; chlorpheniramine maleate; acetaminophen] 20•60•4•500 mg/packet

**fluacizine** INN

**flualamide** INN

**fluanisone** INN, BAN

**fluazacort** USAN, INN *anti-inflammatory*

**flubanilate** INN *CNS stimulant* [also: flubanilate HCl]

**flubanilate HCl** USAN *CNS stimulant* [also: flubanilate]

**flubendazole** USAN, INN, BAN *antiprotozoal*

**flubenisolone** [see: betamethasone]

**flubepride** INN

**flubuperone** [see: melperone]

**flucarbril** INN

**flucetorex** INN

**flucindole** USAN, INN *antipsychotic*

**fluciprazine** INN

**fluclorolone acetonide** INN, BAN *glucocorticoid* [also: flucloronide]

**flucloronide** USAN *glucocorticoid* [also: fluclorolone acetonide]

**flucloxacillin** INN, BAN *antibacterial* [also: floxacillin]

**fluconazole** USAN, INN, BAN *broad-spectrum systemic fungistatic*

**flucrilate** INN *tissue adhesive* [also: flucrylate]

**flucrylate** USAN *tissue adhesive* [also: flucrilate]

**flucytosine** USAN, USP, INN, BAN *fungicidal*

**fludalanine** USAN, INN *antibacterial*

**Fludara** powder for IV injection ℞ *antimetabolic antineoplastic for chronic lymphocytic leukemia and non-Hodgkin's lymphoma (orphan)* [fludarabine phosphate] 50 mg

**fludarabine** INN *antimetabolic antineoplastic* [also: fludarabine phosphate]

**fludarabine phosphate** USAN *antimetabolic antineoplastic for chronic lymphocytic leukemia and non-Hodgkin's lymphoma (orphan)* [also: fludarabine]

**fludazonium chloride** USAN, INN *topical anti-infective*

**fludeoxyglucose ($^{18}$F)** INN *diagnostic aid; radioactive agent* [also: fludeoxyglucose F 18]

**fludeoxyglucose F 18** USAN, USP *diagnostic aid; radioactive agent* [also: fludeoxyglucose ($^{18}$F)]

**fludiazepam** INN

**fludorex** USAN, INN *anorectic; antiemetic*

**fludoxopone** INN

**fludrocortisone** INN, BAN *salt-regulating adrenocortical steroid; mineralocorticoid* [also: fludrocortisone acetate]

**fludrocortisone acetate** USP *salt-regulating adrenocortical steroid; mineralocorticoid* [also: fludrocortisone]

**fludroxicortide** [see: flurandrenolide]

**fludroxycortide** INN *topical corticosteroid* [also: flurandrenolide; flurandrenolone]

**flufenamic acid** USAN, INN, BAN *anti-inflammatory*

**flufenisal** USAN, INN *analgesic*

**flufosal** INN

**flufylline** INN

**flugestone** INN, BAN *progestin* [also: flurogestone acetate]

**flugestone acetate** [see: flurogestone acetate]

**Fluimucil** ℞ *investigational (Phase I) immunomodulator for AIDS/HIV* [acetylcysteine]

**Flu-Imune** IM injection (discontinued 1994) ℞ *flu vaccine* [influenza purified surface antigen] 90 μg/mL

**fluindarol** INN

**fluindione** INN

**Flumadine** film-coated tablets, syrup ℞ *antiviral; prophylaxis and treatment for influenza A virus* [rimantadine HCl] 100 mg; 50 mg/5 mL

**flumazenil** USAN, INN, BAN *benzodiazepine antagonist/antidote*

**flumazepil** [see: flumazenil]

**flumecinol** INN *investigational (orphan) for neonatal hyperbilirubinemia*

**flumedroxone** INN, BAN

**flumequine** USAN, INN, BAN *antibacterial*

**flumeridone** USAN, INN, BAN *antiemetic*

**flumetasone** INN *glucocorticoid* [also: flumethasone]

**flumethasone** USAN, BAN *glucocorticoid* [also: flumetasone]

**flumethasone pivalate** USAN, USP, BAN *glucocorticoid*

**flumethiazide** INN, BAN

**flumethrin** BAN

**flumetramide** USAN, INN *skeletal muscle relaxant*

**flumexadol** INN

**flumezapine** USAN, INN, BAN *antipsychotic; neuroleptic*

**fluminorex** USAN, INN *anorectic*

**flumizole** USAN, INN *anti-inflammatory*

**flumoxonide** USAN, INN *adrenocortical steroid*

**flunamine** INN

**flunarizine** INN, BAN *vasodilator; investigational (orphan) for alternating hemiplegia* [also: flunarizine HCl]

**flunarizine HCl** USAN *vasodilator* [also: flunarizine]

**flunidazole** USAN, INN *antiprotozoal*

**flunisolide** USAN, USP, INN, BAN *corticosteroid inhalant for asthma; intranasal steroid*

**flunisolide acetate** USAN *anti-inflammatory*

**flunitrazepam** USAN, INN, BAN, JAN *benzodiazepine sedative and hypnotic; also abused as a "date rape" street drug*

**flunixin** USAN, INN, BAN *anti-inflammatory; analgesic*

**flunixin meglumine** USAN *anti-inflammatory; analgesic*

**flunoprost** INN

**flunoxaprofen** INN

**fluocinolide** [now: fluocinonide]

**fluocinolone** BAN *topical corticosteroid* [also: fluocinolone acetonide]

**fluocinolone acetonide** USAN, USP, INN *topical corticosteroid* [also: fluocinolone] 0.01%, 0.025% topical

**fluocinonide** USAN, USP, INN, BAN *topical corticosteroid* 0.05% topical

**fluocortin** INN *anti-inflammatory* [also: fluocortin butyl]

**fluocortin butyl** USAN, BAN *anti-inflammatory* [also: fluocortin]

**fluocortolone** USAN, INN, BAN *glucocorticoid*

**fluocortolone caproate** USAN *glucocorticoid*

**Fluogen** IM injection, Steri-Vials, Steri-Dose (disposable syringes) ℞ *flu vaccine* [influenza split-virus vaccine] 0.5 mL/dose

**Fluonex** cream ℞ *topical corticosteroid* [fluocinonide] 0.05%

**Fluonid** topical solution ℞ *topical corticosteroid* [fluocinolone acetonide] 0.01%

**fluopromazine** BAN *antipsychotic* [also: triflupromazine]

**Fluoracaine** eye drops ℞ *topical ophthalmic anesthetic; corneal disclosing agent* [proparacaine HCl; fluorescein sodium] 0.5%•0.25%

**fluoracizine** [see: fluacizine]

**fluorescein** USP, BAN, JAN *corneal trauma indicator*

**fluorescein, soluble** [now: fluorescein sodium]

**fluorescein sodium** USP, BAN, JAN *corneal trauma indicator* 2% eye drops

**fluorescein sodium & proparacaine HCl** *corneal disclosing agent; topical ophthalmic anesthetic* 0.25%•0.5%

**Fluorescite** IV injection ℞ *corneal disclosing agent* [fluorescein sodium] 10%, 25%

**Fluoresoft** eye drops ℞ *diagnostic aid in fitting contact lenses* [fluorexon] 0.35%

**fluoresone** INN

**Fluorets** ophthalmic strips OTC *corneal disclosing agent* [fluorescein sodium] 1 mg

**fluorexon** *diagnosis and fitting aid for contact lenses*

**fluorhydrocortisone acetate** [see: fludrocortisone acetate]

**Fluoride** tablets OTC *dental caries preventative* [sodium fluoride] 2.21 mg

**Fluoride Loz** lozenges R *dental caries preventative* [sodium fluoride] 2.21 mg

**Fluorigard** oral rinse OTC *topical dental caries preventative* [sodium fluoride; alcohol 6%] 0.05%

**Fluori-Methane** spray R *topical vapocoolant anesthetic* [trichloromonofluoromethane; dichlorodifluoromethane] 85%•15%

**fluorine** *element (F)*

**fluorine F 18 fluorodeoxyglucose** [see: fludeoxyglucose F 18]

**Fluorinse** oral rinse R *topical dental caries preventative* [sodium fluoride] 0.2%

**Fluor-I-Strip; Fluor-I-Strip A.T.** ophthalmic strips R *corneal disclosing agent* [fluorescein sodium] 9 mg; 1 mg

**Fluoritab** chewable tablets, drops R *dental caries preventative* [sodium fluoride] 1.1, 2.2 mg; 0.55 mg/drop

**fluormethylprednisolone** [see: dexamethasone]

**5-fluorocytosine (5-FC)** [see: flucytosine]

**fluorodeoxyglucose F 18** [see: fludeoxyglucose F 18]

**fluorometholone** USP, INN, BAN *glucocorticoid; ophthalmic anti-inflammatory*

**fluorometholone acetate** USAN *anti-inflammatory*

**Fluor-Op** eye drop suspension R *ophthalmic topical corticosteroidal anti-inflammatory* [fluorometholone] 0.1%

**Fluoroplex** cream, topical solution R *antimetabolic antineoplastic for actinic keratoses and basal cell carcinomas* [fluorouracil] 1%

**fluoroquinolones** *a class of synthetic, broad-spectrum, antimicrobial, bactericidal antibiotics*

**fluorosalan** USAN *disinfectant* [also: flusalan]

**fluorothymidine (FLT)** *investigational (Phase II) antiviral for HIV and AIDS*

**fluorouracil (5-FU)** USAN, USP, INN, BAN *antimetabolic antineoplastic* 50 mg/mL injection

**fluorouracil & interferon alfa-2a** *investigational (orphan) for esophageal and advanced colorectal carcinoma*

**fluorouracil & leucovorin** *investigational (orphan) for metastatic adenocarcinoma of colon and rectum*

**fluoruridine deoxyribose** [see: floxuridine]

**Fluosol** emulsion for intracoronary perfusion (discontinued 1995) R *myocardial oxygenation during PTCA* [intravascular perfluorochemical (PFC) emulsion] 20%

**fluostigmine** [see: isoflurophate]

**Fluothane** liquid for vaporization R *inhalation general anesthetic* [halothane]

**fluotracen** INN *antipsychotic; antidepressant* [also: fluotracen HCl]

**fluotracen HCl** USAN *antipsychotic; antidepressant* [also: fluotracen]

**fluoxetine** USAN, INN, BAN *antidepressant*

**fluoxetine HCl** USAN *selective serotonin reuptake inhibitor (SSRI) for depression, obsessive-compulsive disorder, and bulimia nervosa*

**fluoximesterone** [see: fluoxymesterone]

**Flu-Oxinate** eye drops R *topical ophthalmic anesthetic; corneal disclosing agent* [benoxinate HCl; fluorescein sodium] 0.4%•0.25%

**fluoxiprednisolone** [see: triamcinolone]

**fluoxymesterone** USP, INN, BAN *oral androgen* 10 mg oral

**fluparoxan** INN, BAN *antidepressant; investigational treatment for male sexual dysfunction* [also: fluparoxan HCl]

**fluparoxan HCl** USAN *antidepressant; investigational treatment for male sexual dysfunction* [also: fluparoxan]

**flupenthixol** BAN [also: flupentixol]

**flupentixol** INN [also: flupenthixol]

**fluperamide** USAN, INN *antiperistaltic*

**fluperlapine** INN

**fluperolone** INN, BAN *glucocorticoid* [also: fluperolone acetate]

**fluperolone acetate** USAN *glucocorticoid* [also: fluperolone]

**fluphenazine** INN, BAN *antipsychotic* [also: fluphenazine enanthate]

**fluphenazine decanoate** *antipsychotic; prolonged parenteral neuroleptic therapy* 25 mg/mL injection

**fluphenazine enanthate** USP *antipsychotic; prolonged parenteral neuroleptic therapy* [also: fluphenazine]

**fluphenazine HCl** USP, BAN *antipsychotic* 1, 2.5, 5, 10 mg oral; 2.5 mg/mL injection

**flupimazine** INN

**flupirtine** INN, BAN *analgesic* [also: flupirtine maleate]

**flupirtine maleate** USAN *analgesic* [also: flupirtine]

**flupranone** INN

**fluprazine** INN

**fluprednidene** INN, BAN

**fluprednisolone** USAN, NF, INN, BAN *glucocorticoid*

**fluprednisolone valerate** USAN *glucocorticoid*

**fluprofen** INN, BAN

**fluprofylline** INN

**fluproquazone** USAN, INN, BAN *analgesic*

**fluprostenol** INN, BAN *prostaglandin* [also: fluprostenol sodium]

**fluprostenol sodium** USAN *prostaglandin* [also: fluprostenol]

**fluquazone** USAN, INN *anti-inflammatory*

**Flura** tablets ℞ *dental caries preventative* [sodium fluoride] 2.2 mg

**fluracil** [see: fluorouracil]

**fluradoline** INN *analgesic* [also: fluradoline HCl]

**fluradoline HCl** USAN *analgesic* [also: fluradoline]

**Flura-Drops** ℞ *dental caries preventative* [sodium fluoride] 0.55 mg/drop

**Flura-Loz** lozenges ℞ *dental caries preventative* [sodium fluoride] 2.2 mg

**flurandrenolide** USAN, USP *topical corticosteroid* [also: fludroxycortide; flurandrenolone] 0.05% topical

**flurandrenolone** BAN *topical corticosteroid* [also: flurandrenolide; fludroxycortide]

**flurantel** INN

**Flurate** eye drops ℞ *topical ophthalmic anesthetic; corneal disclosing agent* [benoxinate HCl; fluorescein sodium] 0.4%•0.25%

**flurazepam** INN, BAN *anticonvulsant; hypnotic; muscle relaxant; sedative; also abused as a street drug* [also: flurazepam HCl]

**flurazepam HCl** USAN, USP *anticonvulsant; hypnotic; muscle relaxant; sedative; also abused as a street drug* [also: flurazepam] 15, 30 mg oral

**flurbiprofen** USAN, USP, INN, BAN *antiarthritic; nonsteroidal anti-inflammatory drug (NSAID); analgesic* 50, 100 mg oral

**flurbiprofen sodium** USP *prostaglandin synthesis inhibitor; antimiotic; ocular nonsteroidal anti-inflammatory drug (NSAID)* 0.03% eye drops

**Fluress** eye drops ℞ *topical ophthalmic anesthetic; corneal disclosing agent* [benoxinate HCl; fluorescein sodium] 0.4%•0.25%

**fluretofen** USAN, INN *anti-inflammatory; antithrombotic*

**flurfamide** [now: flurofamide]

**flurithromycin** INN

**flurocitabine** USAN, INN *antineoplastic*

**Fluro-Ethyl** aerosol spray ℞ *topical refrigerant anesthetic* [ethyl chloride; dichlorotetrafluoroethane] 25%•75%

**flurofamide** USAN, INN *urease enzyme inhibitor*

**flurogestone acetate** USAN *progestin* [also: flugestone]

**Flurosyn** ointment, cream ℞ *topical corticosteroid* [fluocinolone acetonide] 0.025%; 0.01, 0.025%

**flurothyl** USAN, USP, BAN *CNS stimulant* [also: flurotyl]

**flurotyl** INN *CNS stimulant* [also: flurothyl]

**fluroxene** USAN, NF, INN *inhalation anesthetic*

**fluroxyspiramine** [see: spiramide]

**flusalan** INN *disinfectant* [also: fluorosalan]

**FluShield** IM injection, Tubex (cartridge-needle unit) ℞ *flu vaccine* [influenza purified split-virus vaccine] 0.5 mL/dose

**flusoxolol** INN, BAN

**fluspiperone** USAN, INN *antipsychotic*

**fluspirilene** USAN, INN, BAN *antipsychotic*

**flutamide** USAN, INN, BAN *antineoplastic; antiandrogen hormone for prostatic carcinoma*

**flutazolam** INN

**flutemazepam** INN

**Flutex** ointment, cream ℞ *topical corticosteroid* [triamcinolone acetonide] 0.025%, 0.1%, 0.5%

**flutiazin** USAN, INN *veterinary anti-inflammatory*

**fluticasone** INN, BAN *topical corticosteroidal anti-inflammatory* [also: fluticasone propionate]

**fluticasone propionate** USAN *topical corticosteroidal anti-inflammatory* [also: fluticasone]

**flutizenol** INN

**flutomidate** INN

**flutonidine** INN

**flutoprazepam** INN

**flutrimazole** INN

**flutroline** USAN, INN *antipsychotic*

**flutropium bromide** INN

**fluvastatin** INN, BAN *antihyperlipidemic for hypercholesterolemia; HMG-CoA reductase inhibitor* [also: fluvastatin sodium]

**fluvastatin sodium** USAN *antihyperlipidemic for hypercholesterolemia; HMG-CoA reductase inhibitor* [also: fluvastatin]

**Fluvirin** IM injection, prefilled syringes ℞ *flu vaccine* [influenza purified surface antigen] 0.5 mL/dose

**fluvoxamine** INN, BAN *selective serotonin reuptake inhibitor (SSRI) for depression and obsessive-compulsive disorder* [also: fluvoxamine maleate]

**fluvoxamine maleate** USAN *selective serotonin reuptake inhibitor (SSRI) for depression and obsessive-compulsive disorder; investigational (Phase III) for panic disorder* [also: fluvoxamine]

**fluzinamide** USAN, INN *anticonvulsant*

**Fluzone** IM injection, prefilled syringes ℞ *flu vaccine* [influenza split-virus or whole-virus vaccine] 0.5 mL/dose

**fluzoperine** INN

**fly agaric** *street drug slang* [see: Amanita muscaria mushrooms]

**Flying Saucers** *street drug slang* [see: morning glory seeds]

**FML; FML Forte** eye drop suspension ℞ *ophthalmic topical corticosteroidal anti-inflammatory* [fluorometholone] 0.1%; 0.25%

**FML S.O.P.** ophthalmic ointment ℞ *ophthalmic topical corticosteroidal anti-inflammatory* [fluorometholone] 0.1%

**FML-S** eye drop suspension ℞ *ophthalmic topical corticosteroidal anti-inflammatory; bacteriostatic* [fluorometholone; sulfacetamide sodium] 0.1%•10%

**FMS (fluorouracil, mitomycin, streptozocin)** *chemotherapy protocol*

**FMV (fluorouracil, MeCCNU, vincristine)** *chemotherapy protocol*

**FNC (fluorouracil, Novantrone, cyclophosphamide)** *chemotherapy protocol* [also: CFM; CNF]

**FNM (fluorouracil, Novantrone, methotrexate)** *chemotherapy protocol*

**FOAM (fluorouracil, Oncovin, Adriamycin, mitomycin)** *chemotherapy protocol*

**Foamicon** chewable tablets OTC *antacid* [aluminum hydroxide; magnesium trisilicate] 80•20 mg

**focofilcon A** USAN *hydrophilic contact lens material*

**fo-do-nie** *street drug slang* [see: opium]

**Foille** spray OTC *topical local anesthetic; antiseptic* [benzocaine; chloroxylenol] 5%•0.63%

**Foille Medicated First Aid** ointment, aerosol spray OTC *topical local anesthetic; antiseptic* [benzocaine; chloroxylenol] 5%•0.1%; 5%•0.6%

**Foille Plus** aerosol spray OTC *topical local anesthetic; antiseptic* [benzocaine; chloroxylenol; alcohol 57.33%] 5%•0.6%

**FoilleCort** cream (discontinued 1993) OTC *topical corticosteroid* [hydrocortisone acetate]

**Folabee** IM injection (discontinued 1994) ℞ *antianemic; vitamin supplement* [liver extracts; vitamin B$_{12}$; folic acid]

**folacin** [see: folic acid] Ⓡ Fulvicin

**folate** [see: folic acid]

**folate sodium** USP

**folescutol** INN

**Folex PFS** powder for IV or IM injection ℞ *antimetabolic antineoplastic for multiple leukemias; systemic antipsoriatic; antirheumatic* [methotrexate sodium] 25 mg/mL

**folic acid** USP, INN, BAN *vitamin B$_c$; vitamin M; hematopoietic* 0.4, 0.8, 1 mg oral; 5 mg/mL injection

**folinate-SF calcium** [see: leucovorin calcium]

**folinic acid** [see: leucovorin calcium]

**follicle-stimulating hormone (FSH)** BAN [also: menotropins]

**follidrin** [see: estradiol benzoate]

**follotropin** [see: menotropins]

**Follow-Up** [see: Carnation Follow-Up]

**Follutein** powder for IM injection (discontinued 1995) ℞ *hormone for prepubertal cryptorchidism and hypogonadism; ovulation stimulant* [chorionic gonadotropin] 1000 U/mL

**Foltrin** capsules ℞ *hematinic* [ferrous fumarate; cyanocobalamin; ascorbic acid; intrinsic factor concentrate; folic acid] 110 mg•15 μg•75 mg•240 mg•0.5 mg

**Folvite** IM injection ℞ *antianemic* [folic acid] 5 mg/mL

**Folvite** tablets (discontinued 1993) ℞ *antianemic* [folic acid]

**fomepizole** USAN, INN *antidote; investigational (orphan) alcohol dehydrogenase inhibitor for methanol or ethylene glycol poisoning*

**FOMI; FOMi (fluorouracil, Oncovin, mitomycin)** *chemotherapy protocol*

**fomidacillin** INN, BAN

**fominoben** INN [also: fominoben HCl]

**fominoben HCl** JAN [also: fominoben]

**fomivirsen** *investigational (Phase III) antisense drug for CMV retinitis*

**fomocaine** INN, BAN

**fonatol** [see: diethylstilbestrol]

**fonazine mesylate** USAN *serotonin inhibitor* [also: dimetotiazine; dimethothiazine]

**fontarsol** [see: dichlorophenarsine HCl]

**foo foo dust; foo foo stuff** *street drug slang* [see: cocaine; heroin]

**foolish powder** *street drug slang* [see: cocaine; heroin]

**footballs** *street drug slang for Dilaudid (hydromorphone HCl) or Biphetamine (dextroamphetamine + amphetamine; discontinued 1979)* [see: Dilaudid; hydromorphone HCl; amphetamines]

**fopirtoline** INN

**Foradil** ℞ *investigational long-acting antiasthmatic*

**Forane** liquid for vaporization ℞ *inhalation general anesthetic* [isoflurane]

**forasartan** USAN *antihypertensive; CHF treatment; angiotensin II receptor antagonist*

**forfenimex** INN

**formaldehyde solution** USP *disinfectant*

**Formalyde-10** spray ℞ *for hyperhidrosis and bromhidrosis* [formaldehyde] 10%

**formebolone** INN, BAN

**formetamide** [see: formetorex]

**formetorex** INN

**formidacillin** [see: fomidacillin]

**forminitrazole** INN, BAN

**formocortal** USAN, INN, BAN *glucocorticoid*

**formoterol** INN

**Formula 44** syrup (name changed to Vicks Dry Hacking Cough in 1994)

**Formula 44 Cough Control Disks; Formula 44 Cough Silencers** lozenges OTC *antitussive; topical oral anesthetic* [dextromethorphan hydrobromide; benzocaine] 5•1.25 mg; 2.5•1 mg

**Formula 44 Non-Drowsy Cold & Cough** LiquiCaps (capsules) (name changed to Vicks 44 Non-Drowsy Cold & Cough in 1994)

**Formula 44 Pediatric** syrup (name changed to Vicks Pediatric 44d Dry Hacking Cough and Head Congestion in 1994)

**Formula 44D Cough & Decongestant** liquid (name changed to Vicks

Formula 44D Cough & Decongestant in 1994)

**Formula 44d Cough & Decongestant, Pediatric** liquid (name changed to Vicks Pediatric Formula 44d Cough & Decongestant in 1994)

**Formula 44D Cough & Head Congestion** liquid (name changed to Vicks 44D Cough & Head Congestion in 1994)

**Formula 44E** liquid (name changed to Vicks 44E in 1994)

**Formula 44e, Pediatric** liquid (name changed to Vicks Pediatric Formula 44e in 1994)

**Formula 44M Cold, Flu & Cough LiquiCaps** (capsules) (name changed to Vicks 44M Cold, Flu & Cough LiquiCaps in 1994)

**Formula 44M Cough and Cold** liquid (discontinued 1994) OTC *antitussive; decongestant; antihistamine; analgesic* [dextromethorphan hydrobromide; pseudoephedrine HCl; chlorpheniramine maleate; acetaminophen; alcohol]

**Formula 44m Multi-Symptom Cough and Cold, Pediatric** liquid (name changed to Vicks Pediatric Formula 44m Multi-Symptom Cough & Cold in 1994)

**Formula 405** cleansing bar OTC *therapeutic skin cleanser*

**Formula B** tablets ℞ *vitamin supplement* [multiple B vitamins; vitamin C; folic acid] ± •500•0.5 mg

**Formula B Plus** tablets ℞ *vitamin/mineral/iron supplement* [multiple vitamins & minerals; ferrous fumarate; folic acid; biotin] ± •27•0.8•0.15 mg

**Formula Q** capsules (discontinued 1996) OTC *prevention and treatment of nocturnal leg cramps* [quinine sulfate] 65 mg

**Formula VM-2000** tablets OTC *dietary supplement* [multiple vitamins, minerals, and amino acids; iron; folic acid; biotin] ± •5 mg•0.2 mg•50 μg

**4′-formylacetanilide thiosemicarbazone** [see: thioacetazone; thiacetazone]

**forskolin** [see: colforsin]

**Forta Cereal** (discontinued 1993) OTC *oral nutritional supplement*

**Forta Drink** powder OTC *enteral nutritional therapy* [lactose-free formula]

**Forta Shake** powder OTC *enteral nutritional therapy* [milk-based formula]

**Fortaz** powder for IV or IM injection ℞ *cephalosporin-type antibiotic* [ceftazidime] 0.5, 1, 2, 6 g

**Forte L.I.V.** IM injection ℞ *antianemic* [ferrous gluconate; multiple B vitamins; procaine]

**Fortel Home Ovulation Test** kit for home use (discontinued 1995) OTC *in vitro diagnostic aid to predict ovulation time*

**Fortel Midstream** test stick for professional use *in vitro diagnostic aid for urine pregnancy test*

**Fortel Plus** test kit for home use OTC *in vitro diagnostic aid for urine pregnancy test*

**Fortical** injection ℞ *investigational (Phase III) calcium regulator for hypercalcemia, Paget's disease, and postmenopausal osteoporosis* [calcitonin salmon, recombinant]

**fortimicin A** [now: astromicin sulfate]

**40 winks** capsules OTC *antihistaminic sleep aid* [diphenhydramine HCl] 50 mg

**forwards** *street drug slang* [see: amphetamines]

**Fosamax** tablets ℞ *bisphosphonate bone resorption inhibitor for postmenopausal osteoporosis and Paget's disease* [alendronate sodium] 10, 40 mg

**fosarilate** USAN, INN *antiviral*

**fosazepam** USAN, INN, BAN *hypnotic*

**foscarnet sodium** USAN, INN, BAN *antiviral for cytomegalovirus (CMV) and various herpes viruses (HSV-1, HSV-2)*

**Foscavir** IV injection ℞ *antiviral for cytomegalovirus (CMV) retinitis and herpes simplex virus (HSV) infections in immunocompromised patients* [foscarnet sodium] 24 mg/mL

**Foscavir** topical ℞ *investigational (Phase I) antiviral for herpes simplex infections in AIDS* [foscarnet sodium]

**foscolic acid** INN

**fosenazide** INN

**fosenopril sodium** [see: fosinopril sodium]

**fosfestrol** INN, BAN *antineoplastic; estrogen* [also: diethylstilbestrol diphosphate]

**fosfocreatinine** INN

**fosfomycin** USAN, INN, BAN *antibacterial* [also: fosfomycin calcium; fosfomycin sodium]

**fosfomycin calcium** JAN *antibacterial* [also: fosfomycin; fosfomycin sodium]

**fosfomycin sodium** JAN *antibacterial* [also: fosfomycin; fosfomycin calcium]

**fosfomycin tromethamine** USAN *broad-spectrum bactericidal antibiotic for urinary tract infections*

**fosfonet sodium** USAN, INN *antiviral*

**fosfosal** INN

**Fosfree** tablets OTC *vitamin/iron supplement* [multiple vitamins; iron] $\pm$•29 mg

**fosinopril** INN, BAN *antihypertensive; angiotensin-converting enzyme (ACE) inhibitor* [also: fosinopril sodium]

**fosinopril sodium** USAN *antihypertensive; angiotensin-converting enzyme (ACE) inhibitor* [also: fosinopril]

**fosinoprilat** USAN, INN *antihypertensive*

**fosmenic acid** INN

**fosmidomycin** INN

**fosphenytoin** INN *hydantoin-type anticonvulsant* [also: fosphenytoin sodium]

**fosphenytoin sodium** USAN *hydantoin-type anticonvulsant; investigational (orphan) for grand mal status epilepticus* [also: fosphenytoin]

**fospirate** USAN, INN *veterinary anthelmintic*

**fosquidone** USAN, INN, BAN *antineoplastic*

**fostedil** USAN, INN *vasodilator; calcium channel blocker*

**Fostex** cleansing bar OTC *topical keratolytic for acne* [benzoyl peroxide] 10% ® pHisoHex

**Fostex 5% BPO** gel (discontinued 1994) OTC *topical keratolytic for acne* [benzoyl peroxide] 5%

**Fostex 10% BPO** gel OTC *topical keratolytic for acne* [benzoyl peroxide] 10%

**Fostex 10% BPO** tinted cream (discontinued 1994) OTC *topical keratolytic for acne* [benzoyl peroxide] 10%

**Fostex 10% BPO** wash (name changed to Fostex 10% Wash in 1994)

**Fostex 10% Wash** liquid OTC *topical keratolytic for acne* [benzoyl peroxide] 10%

**Fostex Acne Cleansing** cream OTC *topical keratolytic for acne* [salicylic acid] 2%

**Fostex Acne Medication Cleansing** bar OTC *medicated cleanser for acne* [salicylic acid] 2%

**Fostex Medicated Cleansing Shampoo** OTC *antiseborrheic; keratolytic* [sulfur; salicylic acid] 2%•2%

**Fostex Medicated Cover-Up** cream (discontinued 1994) OTC *antibacterial and exfoliant for acne* [sulfur] 2%

**fostriecin** INN *antineoplastic* [also: fostriecin sodium]

**fostriecin sodium** USAN *antineoplastic* [also: fostriecin]

**Fostril** lotion OTC *topical acne treatment* [sulfur; zinc oxide]

**fotemustine** INN, BAN

**Fototar** cream OTC *topical antipsoriatic; antiseborrheic* [coal tar] 2%

**fotretamine** INN

**Fouchet's reagent (solution)**

**four doors** *street drug slang for a combination of Doriden (glutethimide; discontinued 1990) and codeine* [see: glutethimide; codeine]

**4 Hair** softgel capsules OTC *vitamin/mineral/iron supplement* [multiple vitamins & minerals; iron; folic acid; biotin] $\pm$•2.5•33.3•0.25 mg

**4 Nails** softgel capsules OTC *vitamin/mineral/calcium/iron supplement* [multiple vitamins & minerals; calcium; iron; folic acid; biotin] $\pm$•167•3•0.333•0.0083 mg

**4-Way Cold** tablets (discontinued 1995) OTC *decongestant; antihistamine; analgesic* [phenylpropanolamine HCl; chlorpheniramine maleate; acetaminophen] 12.5•2•325 mg

**4-Way Fast Acting** nasal spray OTC *nasal decongestant; antihistamine* [phenylephrine HCl; naphazoline

HCl; pyrilamine maleate] 0.5%•
0.05%•0.2%

**4-Way Long Lasting** nasal spray OTC *nasal decongestant* [oxymetazoline HCl] 0.05%

**four ways** *street drug slang for a combination of LSD, methamphetamine, strychnine, and STP* [see: LSD; methamphetamine HCl; strychnine; STP]

**403U** *investigational antidepressant*

**4197X-RA** *investigational cataract preventative*

**447C** *investigational ACAT inhibitor to reduce serum cholesterol*

**4MRTA** *investigational antineoplastic for T-cell malignancies*

**Fourneau 309** (available only from the Centers for Disease Control) ℞ *investigational anti-infective for trypanosomiasis and onchocerciasis* [suramin sodium]

**fours** *street drug slang* [see: Tylenol with Codeine No. 4; Empirin with Codeine No. 4; codeine]

**FPL64170** *investigational treatment for psoriasis and ulcerative colitis*

**FPL67085** *investigational treatment for acute thrombotic events*

**frabuprofen** INN

**Fractar** (trademarked ingredient) OTC *antipsoriatic; antiseborrheic* [crude coal tar]

**Fragmin** subcu injection ℞ *anticoagulant/antithrombotic for prevention of deep vein thrombosis (DVT) after abdominal surgery* [dalteparin sodium] 2500, 5000 anti-Xa IU/0.2 mL (16, 32 mg/0.2 mL)

**fraho; frajo** *street drug slang* [see: marijuana]

**framycetin** INN, BAN

**francium** *element (Fr)*

**FreAmine III 3% (8.5%) with Electrolytes** IV infusion ℞ *total parenteral nutrition (8.5% only); peripheral parenteral nutrition (both)* [multiple essential and nonessential amino acids & electrolytes]

**FreAmine III 8.5%; FreAmine III 10%** IV infusion ℞ *total parenteral nutrition; peripheral parenteral nutri-*

*tion* [multiple essential and nonessential amino acids]

**FreAmine HBC 6.9%** IV infusion ℞ *nutritional therapy for high metabolic stress* [multiple branched-chain essential and nonessential amino acids; electrolytes]

**Free & Clear** shampoo OTC *soap-free therapeutic cleanser*

**Freedavite** tablets OTC *vitamin/mineral/iron supplement* [multiple vitamins & minerals; ferrous fumarate] ≛•10 mg

**Freedox** solution ℞ *investigational lazaroid for subarachnoid hemorrhage, ischemic stroke, spinal cord and head injury* [tirilazad mesylate]

**freeze** *street drug slang* [see: cocaine]

**Freezone** liquid OTC *topical keratolytic* [salicylic acid in a collodion-like vehicle] 13.6%

**French blue** *street drug slang* [see: amphetamine]

**French fries; fries; fry** *street drug slang* [see: cocaine, crack]

**frentizole** USAN, INN, BAN *immunoregulator*

**fresh** *street drug slang* [see: PCP]

**friend** *street drug slang* [see: fentanyl]

**fries; French fries; fry** *street drug slang* [see: cocaine, crack]

**frio** (Spanish for "cold") *street drug slang for marijuana laced with PCP* [see: marijuana; PCP]

**Frisco special; Frisco speedball** *street drug slang for a combination of cocaine, heroin, and LSD* [see: cocaine; heroin; LSD]

**Frisium** ℞ *investigational benzodiazepine-type tranquilizer; anxiolytic* [clobazam]

**Friskie powder** *street drug slang* [see: cocaine]

**Frone** (commercially available in Europe, Asia, and Latin America) ℞ *investigational treatment for multiple sclerosis, herpes, leukemia, cervical neoplasia and hepatitis* [natural beta interferon]

**fronepidil** INN

**froxiprost** INN

**fructose (D-fructose)** USP *nutrient; caloric replacement* [also: levulose]

**Fruity Chews** chewable tablets OTC *vitamin supplement* [multiple vitamins; folic acid] ≚•0.3 mg

**Fruity Chews with Iron** chewable tablets OTC *vitamin/iron supplement* [multiple vitamins; iron; folic acid] ≚•12•0.3 mg

**frusemide** BAN *diuretic* [also: furosemide]

**fry; fries; French fries** *street drug slang* [see: cocaine, crack]

**fry daddy** *street drug slang for a regular or marijuana cigarette laced with crack* [see: marijuana; cocaine, crack]

**FS Shampoo** ℞ *topical corticosteroid; antiseborrheic* [fluocinolone acetonide] 0.01%

**FSF (fibrin-stabilizing factor)** [see: factor XIII]

**FSH (follicle-stimulating hormone)** [see: menotropins]

**ftalofyne** INN *veterinary anthelmintic* [also: phthalofyne]

**ftaxilide** INN

**ftivazide** INN

**ftormetazine** INN

**ftorpropazine** INN

**Fu** *street drug slang* [see: marijuana]

**5-FU (5-fluorouracil)** [see: fluorouracil]

**fubrogonium iodide** INN

**fuchsin, basic** USP *topical antibacterial/ antifungal*

**Fucidin** *investigational topical antibacterial for impetigo and folliculitis* [fusidate sodium]

**FUDR** powder for IV injection ℞ *antimetabolic antineoplastic for brain, breast, head, neck, liver, gallbladder, and bile duct cancer* [floxuridine] 500 mg

**FUDR; FUdR (5-fluorouracil deoxyribonucleoside)** [see: floxuridine]

**fuel** *street drug slang for PCP or marijuana mixed with insecticides* [see: PCP; marijuana]

**Ful-Glo** ophthalmic strips ℞ *corneal disclosing agent* [fluorescein sodium] 0.6 mg

**fulmicoton** [see: pyroxylin]

**FU/LV (fluorouracil, leucovorin calcium [rescue])** *chemotherapy protocol* [also: F-CL]

**Fulvicin P/G** tablets ℞ *systemic antifungal* [griseofulvin (ultramicrosize)] 125, 165, 250, 330 mg ⧆ folacin; Furacin

**Fulvicin U/F** tablets ℞ *systemic antifungal* [griseofulvin (microsize)] 250, 500 mg

**FUM (fluorouracil, methotrexate)** *chemotherapy protocol*

**fumagillin** INN, BAN

**fumaric acid** NF *acidifier*

**Fumasorb** tablets OTC *hematinic* [ferrous fumarate] 200 mg

**Fumatinic** sustained-release capsules ℞ *hematinic* [ferrous fumarate; cyanocobalamin; ascorbic acid; folic acid] 90 mg•15 μg•100 mg•1 mg

**Fumerin** sugar-coated tablets OTC *hematinic* [ferrous fumarate] 195 mg

**Fumide** tablets (discontinued 1993) ℞ *loop diuretic* [furosemide]

**fumo d'Angola** (Spanish for "Angola smoke") *street drug slang* [see: marijuana]

**fumoxicillin** USAN, INN *antibacterial*

**Funduscein-10; Funduscein-25** IV injection ℞ *corneal disclosing agent* [fluorescein sodium] 10%; 25%

**Fungatin** cream OTC *topical antifungal* [tolnaftate]

**fungicidin** [see: nystatin]

**fungimycin** USAN *antifungal*

**Fungi-Nail** liquid OTC *topical antifungal; keratolytic; anesthetic* [resorcinol; salicylic acid; chloroxylenol; benzocaine; alcohol 50%] 1%•2%•2%•0.5%

**Fungizone** cream, lotion, ointment ℞ *topical antifungal* [amphotericin B] 3%

**Fungizone** oral solution ℞ *systemic antifungal* [amphotericin B] 100 mg/mL

**Fungizone** oral suspension ("swish and swallow") ℞ *antifungal for oral candidiasis* [amphotericin B] 100 mg/mL

**Fungizone** powder for IV infusion ℞ *systemic antifungal* [amphotericin B deoxycholate] 50 mg/vial

**Fungoid** cream, tincture ℞ *topical antifungal* [miconazole nitrate] 2%

**Fungoid** solution ℞ *topical antifungal* [clotrimazole] 1%

**Fungoid** solution (became OTC and name changed to Fungoid AF in

1997) ℞ *topical antifungal* [undecylenic acid] 25%

**Fungoid AF** solution OTC *topical antifungal* [undecylenic acid] 25%

**Fungoid-HC** cream ℞ *topical corticosteroid; antipruritic; antifungal; antibacterial* [miconazole nitrate; hydrocortisone] 2%•1%

**fungus** *street drug slang, a reference to the source (mushrooms)* [see: psilocybin]

**funk** *street drug slang* [see: marijuana]

**funny stuff** *street drug slang* [see: marijuana]

**fuprazole** INN

**furacilin** [see: nitrofurazone]

**Furacin** topical solution, cream ℞ *broad-spectrum antibacterial for adjunctive burn therapy* [nitrofurazone] 0.2% ⑨ Fulvicin

**Furacin Soluble Dressing** ointment ℞ *broad-spectrum antibacterial for adjunctive burn therapy* [nitrofurazone] 2%

**furacrinic acid** INN, BAN

**Furadantin** oral suspension ℞ *urinary bacteriostatic* [nitrofurantoin] 25 mg/5 mL

**Furadantin** tablets (discontinued 1993) ℞ *urinary bacteriostatic* [nitrofurantoin] 50, 100 mg

**furafylline** INN

**Furalan** tablets ℞ *urinary bacteriostatic* [nitrofurantoin] 50, 100 mg

**furalazine** INN

**furaltadone** INN, BAN

**Furamide** (available only from the Centers for Disease Control) ℞ *investigational anti-infective for amebiasis* [diloxanide furoate]

**Furanite** tablets ℞ *urinary bacteriostatic* [nitrofurantoin] 50, 100 mg

**furaprofen** USAN, INN *anti-inflammatory*

**furazabol** INN

**furazolidone** USP, INN, BAN *bactericidal; antiprotozoal (Trichomonas); antidiarrheal*

**furazolium chloride** USAN, INN *antibacterial*

**furazolium tartrate** USAN *antibacterial*

**furbucillin** INN

**furcloprofen** INN

**furegrelate** INN *thromboxane synthetase inhibitor* [also: furegrelate sodium]

**furegrelate sodium** USAN *thromboxane synthetase inhibitor* [also: furegrelate]

**furethidine** INN, BAN

**furfenorex** INN

**furfuryltrimethylammonium iodide** [see: furtrethonium iodide]

**furidarone** INN

**furmethoxadone** INN

**furobufen** USAN, INN *anti-inflammatory*

**furodazole** USAN, INN *anthelmintic*

**furofenac** INN

**furomazine** INN

**Furomide M.D.** injection (discontinued 1993) ℞ *loop diuretic* [furosemide]

**furosemide** USAN, USP, INN, JAN *loop diuretic* [also: frusemide] 20, 40, 80 mg oral; 10 mg/mL oral; 40 mg/5 mL oral; 10 mg/mL injection

**furostilbestrol** INN

**furoxicillin** [see: fumoxicillin]

**Furoxone** tablets, liquid ℞ *antibacterial* [furazolidone] 100 mg; 50 mg/15 mL

**fursalan** USAN, INN *disinfectant*

**fursultiamine** INN

**furterene** INN

**furtrethonium iodide** INN

**furtrimethonium iodide** [see: furtrethonium iodide]

**Furtulon** (commercially available in Japan and Korea) ℞ *investigational antineoplastic* [doxifluridine]

**fusafungine** INN, BAN

**fusidate sodium** USAN *antibacterial*

**fusidic acid** USAN, INN, BAN *antibacterial*

**fusidic acid, sodium salt** [see: fusidate sodium]

**FUVAC (5-FU, vinblastine, Adriamycin, cyclophosphamide)** *chemotherapy protocol*

**fuzlocillin** INN, BAN

**fytic acid** INN

**FZ (flutamide, Zoladex)** *chemotherapy protocol*

**G; gee** *street drug slang* [see: paregoric; opium]

**⁶⁷Ga** [see: gallium citrate Ga 67]

**gabapentin** USAN, INN *anticonvulsant; investigational (orphan) for amyotrophic lateral sclerosis*

**Gabbromicina** ℞ *investigational (orphan) for tuberculosis, Mycobacterium avium complex, and visceral leishmaniasis* [aminosidine]

**gabexate** INN

**Gabitril** *investigational anticonvulsant* [tiagabine HCl]

**gaboxadol** INN

**gadobenate dimeglumine** USAN *MRI diagnostic aid* [also: gadobenic acid]

**gadobenic acid** INN *MRI diagnostic aid* [also: gadobenate dimeglumine]

**gadobutrol** INN *investigational aid for MRI*

**gadodiamide** USAN, INN, BAN *diagnostic aid for magnetic imaging*

**gadolinium** *element (Gd)*

**gadopenamide** INN

**gadopentetate dimeglumine** USAN *radiopaque medium* [also: gadopentetic acid]

**gadopentetic acid** INN, BAN *diagnostic aid* [also: gadopentetate dimeglumine]

**gadoteric acid** INN

**gadoteridol** USAN, INN, BAN *diagnostic aid for magnetic imaging*

**gadoversetamide** USAN, INN *paramagnetic MRI contrast agent for brain, head, and spine*

**gaffel** *street drug slang for fake cocaine* [see: cocaine]

**gagers; gaggers** *street drug slang* [see: methcathinone]

**gaiactamine** [see: guaiactamine]

**gaietamine** [see: guaiactamine]

**galamustine** INN

**galantamine** INN

**galantamine hydrobromide**

**galanthamine** [see: galantamine]

**Galardin** ℞ *investigational (orphan) treatment for corneal ulcers* [matrix metalloproteinase inhibitor]

**galdansetron** INN, BAN *antiemetic* [also: galdansetron HCl]

**galdansetron HCl** USAN *antiemetic* [also: galdansetron]

**gallamine** BAN *neuromuscular blocker* [also: gallamine triethiodide]

**gallamine triethiodide** USP, INN *neuromuscular blocker; muscle relaxant* [also: gallamine]

**gallamone triethiodide** [see: gallamine triethiodide]

**gallic acid** NF

**gallic acid, bismuth basic salt** [see: bismuth subgallate]

**gallium** *element (Ga)*

**gallium (⁶⁷Ga) citrate** INN *radiopaque medium; radioactive agent* [also: gallium citrate Ga 67]

**gallium citrate Ga 67** USAN, USP *radiopaque medium; radioactive agent* [also: gallium (⁶⁷Ga) citrate]

**gallium nitrate** USAN *bone resorption inhibitor for hypercalcemia of malignancy (orphan)*

**gallium nitrate nonahydrate** [see: gallium nitrate]

**gallopamil** INN, BAN

**galloping horse** *street drug slang* [see: heroin]

**gallotannic acid** [see: tannic acid]

**gallstone solubilizing agents** *a class of drugs that dissolve gallstones*

**galosemide** INN

**galtifenin** INN

**Galzin** capsules ℞ *investigational (orphan) copper blocking/complexing agent for Wilson's disease* [zinc acetate] 25, 50 mg

**Gamastan** IM injection (discontinued 1996) ℞ *passive immunizing agent* [immune globulin] 2, 10 mL ☒ Garamycin

**gamfexine** USAN, INN *antidepressant*

**Gamimune N** IV infusion ℞ *passive immunizing agent for HIV, pediatric HIV, ITP, and BMT; investigational (orphan) for myocarditis and juvenile rheumatoid arthritis* [immune globulin] 5%, 10%

**gamma benzene hexachloride** [now: lindane]

**gamma globulin** [see: globulin, immune]

**gamma hydroxybutyrate (GHB)** *a CNS depressant used as an anesthetic in some countries, produced and abused as a "date rape" street drug in the U.S.* [the sodium salt is medically known as sodium oxybate]

**Gammagard** powder for IV infusion (discontinued 1994; replaced by Gammagard S/D) ℞ *passive immunizing agent* [immune globulin]

**Gammagard S/D** freeze-dried powder for IV infusion ℞ *passive immunizing agent for HIV, idiopathic thrombocytopenic purpura (ITP), and B-cell chronic lymphocytic leukemia* [immune globulin, solvent/detergent treated] 50 mg/mL

**gamma-hydroxybutyrate sodium** [see: sodium oxybate]

**gamma-linolenic acid (GLA)** *investigational (orphan) for juvenile rheumatoid arthritis*

**gammaphos** [now: ethiofos]

**Gammar** IM injection (discontinued 1996) ℞ *immunizing agent* [immune globulin] 2, 10 mL

**Gammar-IV** powder for IV infusion (replaced with Gammar-P IV in 1996; P is for "pasteurized") ℞ *immunizing agent* [immune globulin] 5%

**Gammar-P IV** powder for IV infusion ℞ *passive immunizing agent and immunomodulator for HIV* [immune globulin, pasteurized] 5%

**gamma-vinyl GABA (gamma-aminobutyric acid)** [see: vigabatrin]

**gamolenic acid** INN, BAN

**gamot** *street drug slang* [see: heroin]

**Gamulin Rh** IM injection ℞ *obstetric Rh factor immunity suppressant* [Rh$_0$(D) immune globulin] 300 μg

**ganaxolone** *neuroactive steroid; investigational (orphan) for infantile spasms; investigational (Phase II) for migraine*

**ganciclovir** USAN, INN, BAN *antiviral; investigational (Phase I/II) for HIV prophylaxis; investigational (orphan) ocular implant for cytomegalovirus retinitis* [also: ganciclovir sodium]

**ganciclovir sodium** USAN *antiviral* [also: ganciclovir]

**ganga; gange; ganja; Ghana; ghanja; gunga; gungeon** *street drug slang* [see: marijuana]

**ganglefene** INN

**gangliosides, sodium salts** *orphan status withdrawn 1996*

**gangster** *street drug slang* [see: marijuana]

**ganirelix** INN *gonad-stimulating principle* [also: ganirelix acetate]

**ganirelix acetate** USAN *gonad-stimulating principle* [also: ganirelix]

**Ganite** IV infusion ℞ *bisphosphonate bone resorption inhibitor for hypercalcemia of malignancy (orphan)* [gallium nitrate] 25 mg/mL

**gank** *street drug slang for fake crack* [see: cocaine, crack]

**Gantanol** oral suspension (discontinued 1994) ℞ *broad-spectrum bacteriostatic* [sulfamethoxazole] 500 mg/5 mL ⍰ Gantrisin

**Gantanol** tablets ℞ *broad-spectrum sulfonamide bacteriostatic* [sulfamethoxazole] 500 mg

**Gantrisin** eye drops (discontinued 1995) ℞ *ophthalmic bacteriostatic* [sulfisoxazole diolamine] 4% ⍰ Gantanol

**Gantrisin** pediatric suspension (discontinued 1996) ℞ *broad-spectrum bacteriostatic* [sulfisoxazole acetyl] 500 mg/5 mL

**Gantrisin** syrup (discontinued 1994) ℞ *broad-spectrum bacteriostatic* [sulfisoxazole acetyl] 500 mg/5 mL

**Gantrisin** tablets (discontinued 1996) ℞ *broad-spectrum bacteriostatic* [sulfisoxazole] 500 mg

**gapicomine** INN

**gapromidine** INN

**Garamicina** (Mexican name for U.S. product Garamycin)

**Garamycin** cream, ointment ℞ *topical antibiotic* [gentamicin sulfate] 0.1% ⍰ Gamastan; kanamycin; Terramycin

**Garamycin** eye drops, ophthalmic ointment ℞ *ophthalmic antibiotic* [gentamicin sulfate] 3 mg/mL; 3 mg/g

**Garamycin** IV or IM injection, intrathecal injection ℞ *aminoglycoside-*

type antibiotic [gentamicin sulfate] 40 mg/mL; 2 mg/mL

**Garamycin Pediatric** IV or IM injection R *aminoglycoside-type antibiotic* [gentamicin sulfate] 10 mg/mL

**garbage rock** *street drug slang* [see: cocaine, crack]

**Gardrin** R *investigational treatment for acute peptic ulcers* [enprostil]

**Garfield; Garfield Plus Extra C** chewable tablets OTC *vitamin supplement* [multiple vitamins; folic acid] ±•0.3 mg

**Garfield Complete with Minerals** chewable tablets OTC *vitamin/mineral/iron supplement* [multiple vitamins & minerals; iron; folic acid; biotin] ±•18•0.4•0.04 mg

**Garfield Plus Iron** chewable tablets OTC *vitamin/iron supplement* [multiple vitamins; iron; folic acid] ±•15•0.3 mg

**gas** *street drug slang* [see: nitrous oxide]

**gas gangrene antitoxin, pentavalent**

**gas gangrene antitoxin, polyvalent** [see: gas gangrene antitoxin, pentavalent]

**Gas Permeable Daily Cleaner** solution OTC *cleaning solution for rigid gas permeable contact lenses*

**Gas Permeable Wetting and Soaking** solution (discontinued 1993) OTC *disinfecting/wetting/soaking solution for rigid gas permeable contact lenses*

**Gas Relief** chewable tablets, drops OTC *antiflatulent* [simethicone] 80, 125 mg; 40 mg/0.6 mL

**Gas-Ban** tablets OTC *antacid; antiflatulent* [calcium carbonate; simethicone] 300•40 mg

**Gas-Ban DS** liquid OTC *antacid; antiflatulent* [aluminum hydroxide; magnesium hydroxide; simethicone] 400•400•40 mg/5 mL

**gash** *street drug slang* [see: marijuana]

**gasper; gasper stick** *street drug slang for a marijuana cigarette* [see: marijuana]

**gastric mucin** BAN

**Gastrimmune** R *investigational (Phase III) synthetic peptide vaccine for gastrointestinal cancers*

**Gastroccult** slide test for professional use *in vitro diagnostic aid for gastric occult blood*

**Gastrocrom** capsules R *bronchodilator for bronchial asthma; mastocytosis treatment (orphan)* [cromolyn sodium] 100 mg

**Gastrografin** solution R *GI contrast radiopaque agent* [diatrizoate meglumine; diatrizoate sodium] 66%•10%

**Gastromark** oral suspension R *investigational bowel imaging agent for MRI* [ferumoxsil]

**Gastronol** R *investigational antiulcerative* [proglumide]

**Gastrosed** drops, tablets R *anticholinergic* [hyoscyamine sulfate] 0.125 mg/mL; 0.125 mg

**Gastro-Test** string capsules for professional use *in vitro diagnostic aid for GI disorders*

**Gastrozepine** R *investigational antiulcerative* [pirenzepine HCl]

**Gas-X** chewable tablets, softgels OTC *antiflatulent* [simethicone] 80, 125 mg; 125 mg

**gato** (Spanish for "cat") *street drug slang* [see: heroin]

**gauge; gauge butt** *street drug slang* [see: marijuana]

**gaultheria oil** [see: methyl salicylate]

**gauze, absorbent** USP *surgical aid*

**gauze, petrolatum** USP *surgical aid*

**gauze bandage** [see: bandage, gauze]

**Gaviscon** liquid OTC *antacid* [aluminum hydroxide; magnesium carbonate] 31.7•119.3 mg/5 mL

**Gaviscon; Gaviscon-2** chewable tablets OTC *antacid* [aluminum hydroxide; magnesium trisilicate] 80•20 mg; 160•40 mg

**Gaviscon Relief Formula** chewable tablets, liquid OTC *antacid* [aluminum hydroxide; magnesium carbonate] 160•105 mg; 254•237.5 mg/5 mL

**G-CSF (granulocyte colony-stimulating factor)** [see: filgrastim]

**gedocarnil** INN *investigational treatment of central nervous system disorders*

**gee; G** *street drug slang* [see: paregoric; opium]

**Gee-Gee** tablets OTC *expectorant* [guai-fenesin] 200 mg

**geek** *street drug slang for combination of crack and marijuana* [see: cocaine, crack; marijuana]

**gefarnate** INN, BAN

**gelatin** NF *encapsulating, suspending, binding and coating agent*

**gelatin film, absorbable** USP *topical local hemostatic*

**gelatin powder, absorbable** *topical local hemostatic*

**gelatin solution, special intravenous** [see: polygeline]

**gelatin sponge, absorbable** USP *topical local hemostatic*

**gelcaps** (dosage form) *soft gelatin capsules*

**Gelfilm; Gelfilm Ophthalmic** ℞ *topical local hemostat for surgery* [absorbable gelatin film]

**Gelfoam** powder ℞ *topical local hemostat for surgery* [absorbable gelatin powder] ② Ger-O-Foam

**Gelfoam** sponge, packs, dental packs, prostatectomy cones ℞ *topical local hemostat for surgery* [absorbable gelatin sponge] ② Ger-O-Foam

**Gel-Kam** gel ℞ *topical dental caries preventative* [stannous fluoride] 0.4%

**Gelpirin** tablets OTC *analgesic; antipyretic; anti-inflammatory* [acetaminophen; aspirin, buffered; caffeine] 125•240•32 mg

**Gelpirin-CCF** tablets OTC *decongestant; antihistamine; analgesic; expectorant* [phenylpropanolamine HCl; chlorpheniramine maleate; acetaminophen; guaifenesin] 12.5•1•325•25 mg

**Gelseal** (trademarked dosage form) *soft gelatin capsule*

**gelsolin, recombinant human** *investigational (orphan) for respiratory symptoms of cystic fibrosis and bronchiectasis*

**Gel-Tin** gel OTC *topical dental caries preventative* [stannous fluoride] 0.4%

**Gelusil** chewable tablets OTC *antacid; antiflatulent* [aluminum hydroxide; magnesium hydroxide; simethicone] 200•200•25 mg

**Gelusil** liquid (discontinued 1996) OTC *antacid; antiflatulent* [aluminum hydroxide; magnesium hydroxide; simethicone] 200•200•25 mg/5 mL

**Gelusil-II** chewable tablets, liquid (discontinued 1994) OTC *antacid; antiflatulent* [aluminum hydroxide; magnesium hydroxide; simethicone] 400•400•30 mg; 80•80•6 mg/mL

**GEM 91** *investigational (phase I) antiviral for HIV*

**gemazocine** INN

**gemcadiol** USAN, INN *antihyperlipoproteinemic*

**gemcitabine** USAN, INN,BAN *antineoplastic*

**gemcitabine HCl** USAN *antineoplastic for pancreatic cancer*

**Gemcor** film-coated tablets ℞ *antihyperlipidemic agent (cholesterol-lowering)* [gemfibrozil] 600 mg

**gemeprost** USAN, INN, BAN *prostaglandin*

**gemfibrozil** USAN, USP, INN, BAN *antihyperlipidemic for hypertriglyceridemia and coronary heart disease* 600 mg oral

**Gemnisyn** tablets (discontinued 1994) OTC *analgesic; antipyretic; anti-inflammatory* [acetaminophen; aspirin] 325•325 mg

**Gemzar** powder for IV infusion ℞ *antineoplastic for advanced or metastatic pancreatic cancer; investigational for lung cancer* [gemcitabine HCl] 20 mg/mL

**Genabid** timed-release capsules (discontinued 1997) ℞ *peripheral vasodilator; smooth muscle relaxant for cerebral, myocardial, and peripheral ischemias* [papaverine HCl] 150 mg

**Genac** tablets OTC *decongestant; antihistamine* [pseudoephedrine HCl; triprolidine HCl] 60•2.5 mg

**Genacol** tablets OTC *antitussive; decongestant; antihistamine; analgesic* [dextromethorphan hydrobromide; phenylpropanolamine HCl; chlorpheniramine maleate; acetaminophen] 10•30•2•325 mg

**Genagesic** tablets (discontinued 1995) ℞ *narcotic analgesic* [propoxyphene HCl; acetaminophen] 65•650 mg

**Genahist** capsules, tablets, elixir ℞ *antihistamine; motion sickness preven-*

tative; sleep aid; antiparkinsonian [diphenhydramine HCl] 25 mg; 25 mg; 12.5 mg/5 mL

**Genalac** chewable tablets (discontinued 1994) OTC antacid [calcium carbonate; glycine]

**Gen-Allerate** tablets OTC antihistamine [chlorpheniramine maleate] 4 mg

**Genamin Cold** syrup OTC decongestant; antihistamine [phenylpropanolamine HCl; chlorpheniramine maleate] 6.25•1 mg/5 mL

**Genapap** tablets, caplets OTC analgesic; antipyretic [acetaminophen] 325, 500 mg; 500 mg

**Genapap, Children's** chewable tablets, elixir OTC analgesic; antipyretic [acetaminophen] 80 mg; 160 mg/5 mL

**Genapap, Infants'** drops OTC analgesic; antipyretic [acetaminophen] 100 mg/mL

**Genapax** medicated tampons (discontinued 1994) R antifungal [gentian violet]

**Genaphed** tablets OTC nasal decongestant [pseudoephedrine HCl] 30 mg

**Genasal** nasal spray OTC nasal decongestant [oxymetazoline HCl] 0.05%

**Genasoft Plus** softgels OTC laxative; stool softener [casanthranol; docusate sodium] 30•100 mg

**Genaspor** cream OTC topical antifungal [tolnaftate] 1%

**Genatap** elixir OTC decongestant; antihistamine [phenylpropanolamine HCl; brompheniramine maleate] 12.5•2 mg/5 mL ⓓ Genapap

**Genaton** chewable tablets OTC antacid [aluminum hydroxide; magnesium trisilicate] 80•20 mg

**Genaton** liquid OTC antacid [aluminum hydroxide; magnesium carbonate] 31.7•137.3 mg/5 mL

**Genaton, Extra Strength** chewable tablets OTC antacid [aluminum hydroxide; magnesium carbonate] 160•105 mg

**Genatuss** syrup OTC expectorant [guaifenesin; alcohol 3.5%] 100 mg/5 mL

**Genatuss DM** syrup OTC antitussive; expectorant [dextromethorphan hydrobromide; guaifenesin] 10•100 mg/5 mL

**Gen-bee with C** caplets OTC vitamin supplement [multiple B vitamins; vitamin C] ≛•300 mg

**Gencalc 600** film-coated tablets OTC calcium supplement [calcium carbonate] 1.5 g

**GenCept** tablets (discontinued 1994) R oral contraceptive [norethindrone; ethinyl estradiol]

**Gencold** sustained-release capsules OTC decongestant; antihistamine [phenylpropanolamine HCl; chlorpheniramine maleate] 75•8 mg

**Gendecon** tablets OTC decongestant; antihistamine; analgesic [phenylephrine HCl; chlorpheniramine maleate; acetaminophen] 5•2•325 mg

**Gendex 75** IV infusion R plasma volume expander for shock due to hemorrhage, burns, or surgery [dextran 75] 6%

**Gen-D-Phen** syrup (discontinued 1994) OTC antihistamine; antitussive [diphenhydramine HCl; alcohol 5%] 12.5 mg/5 mL

**Genebs** tablets, caplets OTC analgesic; antipyretic [acetaminophen] 325, 500 mg; 500 mg

**Generet-500** timed-release tablets OTC hematinic [ferrous sulfate; multiple B vitamins; sodium ascorbate] 105•≛•500 mg ⓓ Gentap

**Generix-T** tablets OTC vitamin/mineral/iron supplement [multiple vitamins & minerals; iron] ≛•15 mg

**GenESA System** R investigational (NDA filed) stress test for coronary artery disease, with a computer-controlled delivery system [arbutamine]

**Genevax-HIV** R investigational (Phase I/II) vaccine for HIV

**Genex** capsules (discontinued 1993) OTC decongestant; analgesic [phenylpropanolamine HCl; acetaminophen]

**Geneye** eye drops OTC topical ocular decongestant/vasoconstrictor [tetrahydrozoline HCl] 0.05%

**Geneye AC Allergy Formula** eye drops (discontinued 1997) OTC topical ocular decongestant; astringent [tetrahydrozoline HCl; zinc sulfate] 0.05%•0.25%

**Geneye Extra** eye drops OTC *topical ocular decongestant/vasoconstrictor; emollient* [tetrahydrozoline HCl; PEG 400] 0.05%•1%

**Genite** liquid OTC *antitussive; decongestant; antihistamine; analgesic* [dextromethorphan hydrobromide; pseudoephedrine HCl; doxylamine succinate; acetaminophen; alcohol 25%] 5•10•1.25•167 mg/5 mL

**Gen-K** powder ℞ *potassium supplement* [potassium chloride] 20 mEq/packet

**genophyllin** [see: aminophylline]

**Genoptic** eye drops ℞ *ophthalmic antibiotic* [gentamicin sulfate] 3 mg/mL

**Genoptic S.O.P.** ophthalmic ointment ℞ *ophthalmic antibiotic* [gentamicin sulfate] 3 mg/g

**Genora 0.5/35; Genora 1/35** tablets ℞ *monophasic oral contraceptive* [norethindrone; ethinyl estradiol] 0.5 mg•35 μg; 1 mg•35 μg

**Genora 1/50** tablets ℞ *monophasic oral contraceptive* [norethindrone; mestranol] 1 mg•50 μg

**Genotonorm** (name changed to Genotropin upon marketing release in 1995)

**Genotropin** powder for subcu injection ℞ *growth hormone for congenital or renal-induced growth failure (orphan); investigational (orphan) for severe burns* [somatropin] 1.5, 5.8 mg (4, 15 IU) per mL

**Genpril** film-coated tablets, film-coated caplets OTC *nonsteroidal anti-inflammatory drug (NSAID); antiarthritic; analgesic* [ibuprofen] 200 mg

**Genprin** tablets OTC *analgesic; antipyretic; anti-inflammatory; antirheumatic* [aspirin] 325 mg

**Gensan** tablets OTC *analgesic; antipyretic; anti-inflammatory* [aspirin; caffeine] 400•32 mg

**Gentab-LA** long-acting tablets (discontinued 1994) ℞ *decongestant; expectorant* [phenylpropanolamine HCl; guaifenesin]

**Gentacidin** eye drops, ophthalmic ointment ℞ *ophthalmic antibiotic* [gentamicin sulfate] 3 mg/mL; 3 mg/g

**Gentak** eye drops, ophthalmic ointment ℞ *ophthalmic antibiotic* [gentamicin sulfate] 3 mg/mL; 3 mg/g

**gentamicin** BAN *aminoglycoside bactericidal antibiotic* [also: gentamicin sulfate] ⑨ Jenamicin; kanamycin

**gentamicin liposome** *investigational (orphan) for disseminated Mycobacterium avium-intracellulare infection*

**gentamicin sulfate** USAN, USP *aminoglycoside bactericidal antibiotic* [also: gentamicin] 3 mg/mL eye drops; 3 mg/g topical; 0.1% topical; 10, 40 mg/mL injection

**gentamicin-impregnated polymethyl methacrylate (PMMA) beads** *investigational (orphan) for chronic osteomyelitis*

**gentian violet** USP *topical anti-infective/antifungal* [also: methylrosanilinium chloride]

**gentisic acid ethanolamide** NF *complexing agent*

**Gentlax** granules OTC *laxative* [senna concentrate] 326 mg/tsp.

**Gentlax S** tablets OTC *laxative; stool softener* [docusate sodium; sennosides] 50•8.6 mg

**Gentran 40** IV injection ℞ *plasma volume expander for shock due to hemorrhage, burns, or surgery* [dextran 40] 10%

**Gentran 70** IV infusion ℞ *plasma volume expander for shock due to hemorrhage, burns, or surgery* [dextran 70] 6%

**Gentran 75** IV infusion (discontinued 1996) ℞ *plasma volume expander for shock due to hemorrhage, burns, or surgery* [dextran 75] 6%

**Gentrasul** eye drops, ophthalmic ointment (discontinued 1993) ℞ *ophthalmic antibiotic* [gentamicin]

**Gentz** anorectal wipes (discontinued 1995) OTC *topical local anesthetic; astringent* [pramoxine HCl; alcloxa; hamamelis water; propylene glycol] 1%•0.2%•50%•10%

**Genvite** tablets OTC *antianemic* [ferrous fumarate; multiple vitamins]

**Gen-Xene** tablets ℞ *anxiolytic; minor tranquilizer; anticonvulsant adjunct* [chlorazepate dipotassium] 3.75, 7.5, 15 mg

**Geocillin** film-coated tablets ℞ *extended-spectrum penicillin-type antibiotic* [carbenicillin indanyl sodium] 382 mg

**George smack** *street drug slang* [see: heroin]

**Georgia home boy** *street drug slang (acronym)* [see: GHB]

**gepefrine** INN

**gepirone** INN *tranquilizer; anxiolytic; antidepressant* [also: gepirone HCl]

**gepirone HCl** USAN *tranquilizer; anxiolytic; antidepressant* [also: gepirone]

**2-geranylhydroquinone** [see: geroquinol]

**Geravim** elixir OTC *vitamin/mineral supplement* [multiple B vitamins & minerals] ±

**Geravite** elixir OTC *geriatric vitamin supplement* [multiple B vitamins] ±

**Gerber Baby Formula with Iron** liquid, powder (discontinued 1997) OTC *total or supplementary infant feeding*

**Gerber Baby Low Iron Formula** liquid, powder OTC *total or supplementary infant feeding*

**Gerber Soy Formula** liquid (discontinued 1997) OTC *hypoallergenic infant formula* [soy protein formula]

**Gerber Soy Formula** powder OTC *hypoallergenic infant formula* [soy protein formula]

**Geref** powder for IV injection ℞ *pituitary diagnostic aid; investigational (orphan) for growth hormone deficiency, anovulation, and AIDS-related weight loss* [sermorelin acetate] 50 μg

**Geridium** tablets (discontinued 1997) ℞ *urinary analgesic* [phenazopyridine HCl] 100, 200 mg

**Gerimal** sublingual tablets, tablets ℞ *for age-related mental capacity decline* [ergoloid mesylates] 0.5, 1 mg; 1 mg

**Gerimed** film-coated tablets OTC *geriatric vitamin/mineral supplement* [multiple vitamins & minerals] ±

**Geriot** film-coated tablets OTC *hematinic; vitamin/mineral supplement* [carbonyl iron; multiple vitamins & minerals; folic acid; biotin] 50 mg•±•0.4 mg•45 μg

**Geriplex-FS** Kapseals (capsules) (discontinued 1995) OTC *geriatric dietary supplement* [multiple vitamins & minerals] ±

**Geritol Complete** tablets OTC *vitamin/mineral/iron supplement* [multiple vitamins & minerals; ferrous fumarate; folic acid; biotin] ±•18 mg•0.4 mg•45 μg

**Geritol Extend** caplets OTC *vitamin/mineral/iron supplement* [multiple vitamins & minerals; ferrous fumarate; folic acid] ±•10•0.2 mg

**Geritol Tonic** liquid OTC *hematinic* [ferric pyrophosphate; multiple B vitamins; alcohol 12%] 18•± mg/15 mL

**Geritonic** liquid OTC *hematinic* [ferric ammonium citrate; liver fraction 1; multiple B vitamins and minerals; alcohol 20%] 105•375•± mg/15 mL

**Gerivite** liquid OTC *geriatric vitamin/mineral supplement* [multiple B vitamins & minerals; alcohol 18%] ±

**Gerivites** tablets OTC *hematinic; vitamin/mineral supplement* [ferrous sulfate; multiple vitamins and minerals; folic acid] 50•±•0.4 mg

**Germanin** (available only from the Centers for Disease Control) ℞ *investigational anti-infective for trypanosomiasis and onchocerciasis* [suramin sodium]

**germanium** *element* (Ge)

**germicides** *a class of agents that destroy micro-organisms* [compare to: antiseptics]

**geroquinol** INN

**Geroton Forte** liquid OTC *geriatric vitamin/mineral supplement* [multiple B vitamins & minerals; alcohol 13.5%] ±

**gesarol** [see: chlorophenothane]

**gestaclone** USAN, INN *progestin*

**gestadienol** INN

**gestanin** [see: allyloestrenol]

**Gesterol 50** IM injection (discontinued 1994) ℞ *progestin for amenorrhea* *or functional uterine bleeding* [progesterone] 50 mg/mL

**Gesterol L.A. 250** IM injection (discontinued 1994) ℞ *progestin for amenorrhea, metrorrhagia, and dysfunctional uterine bleeding* [hydroxyprogesterone caproate in oil] 250 mg/mL

**gestodene** USAN, INN, BAN *progestin*

**gestonorone caproate** USAN, INN *progestin* [also: gestronol]

**gestrinone** USAN, INN *progestin*

**gestronol** BAN *progestin* [also: gestonorone caproate]

**get your own** *street drug slang* [see: cocaine]

**Gets-It** liquid OTC *topical keratolytic* [salicylic acid; zinc chloride; alcohol 28%]

**gevotroline** INN *antipsychotic* [also: gevotroline HCl]

**gevotroline HCl** USAN *antipsychotic* [also: gevotroline]

**Gevrabon** liquid OTC *vitamin/mineral supplement* [multiple B vitamins & minerals; alcohol 18%] ±

**Gevral** tablets OTC *vitamin/mineral/iron supplement* [multiple vitamins & minerals; ferrous fumarate; folic acid] ± • 18 mg•0.4 mg

**Gevral Protein** powder OTC *oral protein supplement* [calcium caseinate; sucrose]

**Gevral T** film-coated tablets (discontinued 1995) OTC *vitamin/mineral/iron supplement* [ferrous fumarate; multiple vitamins & minerals; folic acid] 27• ± •0.4 mg

**GG-Cen** capsules OTC *expectorant* [guaifenesin] 200 mg

**Ghana; ghanja; ganga; gange; ganja; gunga; gungeon** *street drug slang* [see: marijuana]

**GHB (gamma hydroxybutyrate)** *a CNS depressant used as an anesthetic in some countries, produced and abused as a "date rape" street drug in the U.S.* [the sodium salt is medically known as sodium oxybate]

**ghost** *street drug slang* [see: LSD]

**GHRF; GH-RF (growth hormone-releasing factor)** [q.v.]

**GI gin** *street drug slang for an elixir of terpin hydrate and codeine (disapproved in 1991)* [see: terpin hydrate; codeine]

**gift of the sun** *street drug slang* [see: cocaine]

**giggle weed; giggle smoke** *street drug slang* [see: marijuana]

**gimmie** *street drug slang for a combination of crack and marijuana* [see: cocaine, crack; marijuana]

**gin** *street drug slang* [see: cocaine]

**giparmen** INN

**giractide** INN

**girisopam** INN

**girl** *street drug slang* [see: cocaine, cocaine, crack; heroin]

**girlfriend** *street drug slang* [see: cocaine]

**gitalin** NF [also: gitalin amorphous]

**gitalin amorphous** INN [also: gitalin]

**gitaloxin** INN

**gitoformate** INN

**gitoxin 16-formate** [see: gitaloxin]

**gitoxin pentaacetate** [see: pengitoxin]

**GLA (gamma-linolenic acid)**

**glacial acetic acid** [see: acetic acid, glacial]

**glad stuff** *street drug slang* [see: cocaine]

**glafenine** INN, DCF, JAN

**Glandosane** oral spray OTC *saliva substitute*

**glaphenine** [see: glafenine]

**glass** *street drug slang* [see: amphetamines]

**glassines** *street drug slang, from the type of translucent glazed paper in which heroin is sold* [see: heroin]

**glatiramer acetate** *immunomodulator for relapsing-remitting multiple sclerosis (orphan)* [formerly known as copolymer 1]

**Glauber salt** [see: sodium sulfate]

**glaucarubin**

**Glaucon** Drop-Tainers (eye drops) ℞ *antiglaucoma agent* [epinephrine HCl] 1%, 2%

**GlaucTabs** tablets ℞ *carbonic anhydrase inhibitor; diuretic* [methazolamide] 25, 50 mg

**Glaxal** cream OTC *investigational moisturizing cream base*

**glaze, pharmaceutical** NF *tablet-coating agent*

**glaziovine** INN

**glemanserin** USAN, INN *anxiolytic*

**gleptoferron** USAN, INN, BAN *veterinary hematinic*

**Gliadel** wafers ℞ *nitrosourea-type alkylating antineoplastic cerebral implants for excised brain tumors (orphan)* [carmustine in a polifeprosan 20 carrier] 7.7 mg

**gliamilide** USAN, INN *antidiabetic*

**glibenclamide** INN, BAN *sulfonylurea-type antidiabetic* [also: glyburide]

**glibornuride** USAN, INN, BAN *antidiabetic*

**glibutimine** INN

**glicaramide** INN

**glicetanile** INN *antidiabetic* [also: glicetanile sodium]

**glicetanile sodium** USAN *antidiabetic* [also: glicetanile]

**gliclazide** INN, BAN

**glicondamide** INN

**glidazamide** INN

**gliflumide** USAN, INN *antidiabetic*

**glimepiride** USAN, INN, BAN *sulfonylurea-type antidiabetic*

**glipentide** [see: glisentide]

**glipizide** USAN, INN, BAN *sulfonylurea-type antidiabetic* 5, 10 mg oral

**gliquidone** INN, BAN

**glisamuride** INN

**glisentide** INN

**glisindamide** INN

**glisolamide** INN

**glisoxepide** INN, BAN

**glo** *street drug slang* [see: cocaine, crack]

**globin zinc insulin** INN [also: insulin, globin zinc]

**globulin, aerosolized pooled immune** *orphan status withdrawn 1994*

**globulin, immune** USP *passive immunizing agent for HIV, ITP, B-cell CLL, and BMT; investigational (orphan) for myocarditis and juvenile rheumatoid arthritis*

**globulin, immune human serum** [now: globulin, immune]

**Glossets** (trademarked form) *sublingual or rectal administration*

**gloxazone** USAN, INN, BAN *veterinary anaplasmodastat*

**gloximonam** USAN, INN *antibacterial*

**glucagon** USP, INN, BAN *antidiabetic; glucose elevating agent* 1, 10 mg/vial injection

**Glucagon Emergency Kit** Hyporets (prefilled disposable syringes) ℞ *emergency treatment for hypoglycemic crisis* [glucagon; lactose] 1•49 mg/mL

**glucalox** INN [also: glycalox]

**glucametacin** INN

**D-glucaric acid, calcium salt tetrahydrate** [see: calcium saccharate]

**gluceptate** USAN, USP, INN, BAN *combining name for radicals or groups*

**gluceptate sodium** USAN *pharmaceutic aid*

**Glucerna** ready-to-use liquid OTC *enteral nutritional therapy for abnormal glucose tolerance*

**D-glucitol** [see: sorbitol]

**D-glucitol hexanicotinate** [see: sorbinicate]

**Glucobay** (commercially available in Europe and Japan) ℞ *investigational antidiabetic* [acarbose]

**β-glucocerebrosidase, macrophage-targeted** [see: alglucerase]

**glucocerebrosidase, recombinant retroviral vector** *investigational (orphan) enzyme replacement for types I, II, or III Gaucher's disease*

**glucocerebrosidase-β-glucosidase** [see: alglucerase]

**glucocorticoids** *a class of adrenal cortical steroids that modify the body's immune response*

**Glucofilm** reagent strips for home use OTC *in vitro diagnostic aid for blood glucose*

**glucoheptonic acid, calcium salt** [see: calcium gluceptate]

**Glucometer Encore; Glucometer Elite** reagent strips for home use OTC *in vitro diagnostic aid for blood glucose*

**D-gluconic acid, calcium salt** [see: calcium gluconate]

**D-gluconic acid, magnesium salt** [see: magnesium gluconate]

**D-gluconic acid, monopotassium salt** [see: potassium gluconate]

**D-gluconic acid, monosodium salt** [see: sodium gluconate]

**Glucophage** film-coated tablets ℞ *biguanide antidiabetic* [metformin HCl] 500, 850 mg

**β-ᴅ-glucopyranuronamide** [see: glucuronamide]

**glucosamine** USAN, INN *pharmaceutic aid*

**ᴅ-glucose** [see: dextrose]

**glucose, liquid** NF *tablet binder and coating agent; antihypoglycemic* ⊡ Glutose

**Glucose & Ketone Urine Test** reagent strips (discontinued 1995) *in vitro diagnostic aid for multiple urine products*

**ᴅ-glucose monohydrate** [see: dextrose]

**glucose oxidase**

**glucose polymers** *caloric replacement*

**Glucose-40** ophthalmic ointment ℞ *corneal edema-reducing agent* [glucose] 40%

**Glucostix** reagent strips for home use OTC *in vitro diagnostic aid for blood glucose*

**glucosulfamide** INN

**glucosulfone** INN

**glucosylceramidase** [see: alglucerase]

**Glucotrol** tablets ℞ *sulfonylurea-type antidiabetic* [glipizide] 5, 10 mg

**Glucotrol XL** extended-release tablets ℞ *sulfonylurea-type antidiabetic* [glipizide] 5, 10 mg

**glucurolactone** INN

**glucuronamide** INN, BAN

**Glukor** powder for IM injection (discontinued 1995) ℞ *hormone for prepubertal cryptorchidism and hypogonadism; ovulation stimulant* [chorionic gonadotropin] 200 U/mL

**glunicate** INN

**gluside** [see: saccharin]

**gluside, soluble** [see: saccharin sodium]

**glusoferron** INN

**glutamic acid (ʟ-glutamic acid)** USAN, INN *nonessential amino acid; symbols: Glu, E* 340, 500 mg oral

**glutamic acid HCl** *gastric acidifier*

**glutamine (ʟ-glutamine)** *nonessential amino acid; symbols: Gln, Q* [see: levoglutamide]

**glutamine & somatropin** *investigational (orphan) for GI malabsorption due to short bowel syndrome*

**glutaral** USAN, USP, INN *disinfectant*

**glutaraldehyde** [see: glutaral]

**Glutarex-1** powder OTC *formula for infants with glutaric aciduria type I*

**Glutarex-2** powder OTC *enteral nutritional therapy for glutaric aciduria type I*

**glutasin** [see: glutamic acid HCl]

**ʟ-glutathione, reduced** *investigational (orphan) for AIDS-related cachexia*

**glutaurine** INN

**glutethimide** USP, INN, BAN *sedative; sometimes abused as a street drug* 250, 500 mg oral

**Glutofac** tablets OTC *vitamin/mineral supplement* [multiple vitamins & minerals] ±

**Glutose** gel OTC *glucose elevating agent* [glucose] 40% ⊡ glucose

**Glyate** syrup OTC *expectorant* [guaifenesin; alcohol 3.5%] 100 mg/5 mL

**glyburide** USAN *sulfonylurea-type antidiabetic* [also: glibenclamide] 1.25, 2.5, 5 mg oral

**glybutamide** [see: carbutamide]

**glybuthiazol** INN

**glybuthizol** [see: glybuthiazol]

**glybuzole** INN

**glycalox** BAN [also: glucalox]

**glycerides oleiques polyoxyethylenes** [see: peglicol 5 oleate]

**glycerin** USP *humectant; solvent; osmotic diuretic; laxative; emollient/protectant* [also: glycerol]

**glycerol** INN *humectant; solvent; osmotic diuretic; laxative; emollient/protectant; monoctanoin component D* [also: glycerin]

**glycerol, iodinated** USAN, BAN *(disapproved for use as an expectorant in 1991)*

**glycerol 1-decanoate** *monoctanoin component B* [see: monoctanoin]

**glycerol 1,2-dioctanoate** *monoctanoin component C* [see: monoctanoin]

**glycerol 1-octanoate** *monoctanoin component A* [see: monoctanoin]

**glycerol phosphate, manganese salt** [see: manganese glycerophosphate]

**glyceryl behenate** NF *tablet and capsule lubricant*

**glyceryl borate** [see: boroglycerin]

**glyceryl guaiacolate** [now: guaifenesin]

**glyceryl monostearate** NF *emulsifying agent*

**glyceryl triacetate** [now: triacetin]

**glyceryl trierucate** *investigational (orphan) for adrenoleukodystrophy* [also: glyceryl trioleate]

**glyceryl trinitrate** BAN *coronary vasodilator* [also: nitroglycerin]

**glyceryl trioleate** *investigational (orphan) for adrenoleukodystrophy* [also: glyceryl trierucate]

**glycerylaminophenaquine** [see: glafenine]

**Glyceryl-T** capsules, liquid ℞ *antiasthmatic; bronchodilator; expectorant* [theophylline; guaifenesin] 150•90 mg; 150•90 mg/15 mL

**glycinato dihydroxyaluminum hydrate** [see: dihydroxyaluminum aminoacetate]

**glycine** USP, INN *nonessential amino acid; urologic irrigant; symbols: Gly, G* [also: aminoacetic acid] 1.5%

**glycine aluminum-zirconium complex** [see: aluminum zirconium tetrachlorohydrex gly; aluminum zirconium trichlorohydrex gly]

**glyclopyramide** INN

**glycobiarsol** USP, INN [also: bismuth glycollylarsanilate]

**glycocholate sodium** [see: sodium glycocholate]

**glycocoll** [see: glycine]

**Glycofed** tablets OTC *decongestant; expectorant* [pseudoephedrine HCl; guaifenesin] 30•100 mg

**glycol distearate** USAN *thickening agent*

**glycolic acid** *mild exfoliant and keratolytic*

*p*-**glycolophenetidide** [see: fenacetinol]

**glycopeptides** *a class of antibiotic antineoplastics*

**glycophenylate** [see: mepenzolate bromide]

**glycopyrrolate** USAN, USP *peptic ulcer adjunct* [also: glycopyrronium bromide] 0.2 mg/mL injection

**glycopyrrone bromide** [see: glycopyrrolate]

**glycopyrronium bromide** INN, BAN *anticholinergic* [also: glycopyrrolate]

**glycosides, cardiac** *a class of cardiovascular drugs that increase the force of cardiac contractions* [also called: digitalis glycosides]

**Glycotuss** tablets OTC *expectorant* [guaifenesin] 100 mg ⃞ Glytuss

**Glycotuss-dM** tablets OTC *antitussive; expectorant* [dextromethorphan hydrobromide; guaifenesin] 10•100 mg

**glycyclamide** INN, BAN

**glycyrrhetinic acid** [see: enoxolone]

**glycyrrhiza** NF

**glydanile sodium** [now: glicetanile sodium]

**glyhexamide** USAN, INN *antidiabetic*

**glyhexylamide** [see: metahexamide]

**Glylorin** ℞ *investigational (orphan) for congenital primary ichthyosis* [monolaurin]

**glymidine** BAN *antidiabetic* [also: glymidine sodium]

**glymidine sodium** USAN, INN *antidiabetic* [also: glymidine]

**glymol** [see: mineral oil]

**Glynase** PresTabs (micronized tablets) ℞ *sulfonylurea antidiabetic* [glyburide] 1.5, 3, 6 mg

**glyoctamide** USAN, INN *antidiabetic*

**Gly-Oxide** oral solution OTC *oral antiinflammatory/anti-infective* [carbamide peroxide] 10%

**glyparamide** USAN *antidiabetic*

**glyphylline** [see: dyphylline]

**glypinamide** INN

**Glypressin** ℞ *investigational treatment for epistaxis; investigational (orphan) for bleeding esophageal ulcers* [terlipressin]

**glyprothiazol** INN

**glyprothizol** [see: glyprothiazol]

**Glyset** tablets ℞ *antidiabetic agent for type 2 diabetes; α-glucosidase inhibitor that delays the digestion of dietary carbohydrates* [miglitol] 25, 50, 100 mg

**glysobuzole** INN [also: isobuzole]

**Glytuss** film-coated tablets OTC *expectorant* [guaifenesin] 200 mg ⃞ Glycotuss

**GM 6001** *orphan status withdrawn 1994*

**GM-CSF (granulocyte-macrophage colony-stimulating factor)** [see: regramostim; sargramostim; molgramostim]

**GMK** *investigational (Phase III) GM2 ganglioside protein vaccine for malignant melanoma*

**G-myticin** cream, ointment ℞ *topical antibiotic* [gentamicin sulfate] 1 mg

**God's drug** *street drug slang* [see: morphine]

**God's flesh** *street drug slang* [see: psilocybin; psilocin]

**God's medicine** *street drug slang* [see: opium]

**Go-Evac** powder for oral solution ℞ *pre-procedure bowel evacuant* [polyethylene glycol-electrolyte solution (plus electrolytes)] 59 g/L

**go-fast** *street drug slang* [see: methcathinone]

**gold** *element (Au)*

**gold** *street drug slang* [see: marijuana; cocaine, crack]

**gold Au 198** USAN, USP *antineoplastic; liver imaging aid; radioactive agent*

**gold sodium thiomalate** USP *antirheumatic (50% gold)* [also: sodium aurothiomalate] 50 mg/mL injection

**gold sodium thiosulfate** NF [also: sodium aurotiosulfate]

**gold star** *street drug slang* [see: marijuana]

**gold thioglucose** [see: aurothioglucose]

**golden dragon** *street drug slang* [see: LSD]

**golden girl** *street drug slang* [see: heroin]

**golden leaf** *street drug slang for very high quality marijuana* [see: marijuana]

**golf ball** *street drug slang* [see: cocaine, crack]

**golpe** *street drug slang* [see: heroin]

**GoLYTELY** powder for oral solution ℞ *pre-procedure bowel evacuant* [polyethylene glycol-electrolyte solution]

**goma** (Spanish for "rubber") *street drug slang for morphine, opium, or black tar heroin* [see: morphine; opium; black tar heroin]

**gonacrine** [see: acriflavine]

**gonadorelin** INN, BAN *gonad-stimulating principle* [also: gonadorelin acetate]

**gonadorelin acetate** USAN *gonad-stimulating principle for hypothalamic amenorrhea (orphan)* [also: gonadorelin]

**gonadorelin HCl** USAN *gonad-stimulating principle*

**gonadotrophin, chorionic** INN, BAN *gonad-stimulating principle* [also: gonadotropin, chorionic]

**gonadotrophin, serum** INN

**gonadotropin, chorionic** USP *gonad-stimulating principle* [also: gonadotrophin, chorionic] 500, 1000, 2000 U/mL injection

**gonadotropin, serum** [see: gonadotrophin, serum]

**gonadotropin-releasing hormone analogs** *a class of hormonal antineoplastics*

**gonadotropins** *a class of hormones that stimulate the ovaries, including follicle-stimulating hormone and luteinizing hormone*

**Gonak** ophthalmic solution OTC *gonioscopic examination aid* [hydroxypropyl methylcellulose] 2.5% ☒ Gonic

**Gonal-F** ℞ *investigational fertility stimulant* [recombinant human follicle-stimulating hormone (rhFSH)]

**gondola** *street drug slang* [see: opium]

**gong** *street drug slang* [see: marijuana; opium]

**Gonic** powder for IM injection ℞ *hormone for prepubertal cryptorchidism and hypogonadism; ovulation stimulant* [chorionic gonadotropin] 1000 U/mL ☒ Gonak

**Gonioscopic Prism Solution** Drop-Tainers (eye drops) OTC *agent for bonding gonioscopic prisms to eye* [hydroxyethyl cellulose]

**Goniosol** ophthalmic solution OTC *gonioscopic examination aid* [hydroxypropyl methylcellulose] 2.5%

**Gonodecten Test Kit** tube test for professional use (discontinued 1995) *in vitro diagnostic aid for Neisseria gonorrhoeae*

**Gonozyme Diagnostic** reagent kit for professional use *in vitro diagnostic aid for Neisseria gonorrhoeae*

**goob** *street drug slang* [see: methcathinone]

**good** *street drug slang* [see: PCP]

**good and plenty** *street drug slang* [see: heroin]

**good butt** *street drug slang for a marijuana cigarette* [see: marijuana]

**good giggles** *street drug slang* [see: marijuana]

**good H** *street drug slang* [see: heroin]

**goodfellas** *street drug slang* [see: fentanyl]

**GoodStart** [see: Carnation GoodStart]

**Goody's Headache** powder OTC *analgesic; antipyretic; anti-inflammatory* [acetaminophen; aspirin; caffeine] 250•520•32.5 mg/dose

**goof butt** *street drug slang for a marijuana cigarette* [see: marijuana]

**goofball** *street drug slang for barbiturates or a combination of cocaine and heroin* [see: barbiturates; cocaine; heroin]

**goofers** *street drug slang* [see: barbiturates]

**goofies** *street drug slang* [see: LSD]

**goon; goon dust** *street drug slang* [see: PCP]

**gooney birds** *street drug slang* [see: LSD]

**Gordobalm** OTC *counterirritant; topical antiseptic* [methyl salicylate; menthol; camphor; alcohol 16%]

**Gordochom** solution ℞ *topical antifungal; antiseptic* [undecylenic acid; chloroxylenol] 25%•3%

**Gordofilm** liquid ℞ *topical keratolytic* [salicylic acid in flexible collodion] 16.7%

**Gordogesic Creme** OTC *counterirritant* [methyl salicylate] 10%

**Gordon's Urea 40%** cream ℞ *for removal of dystrophic nails* [urea] 40%

**'goric** *street drug slang, from "paregoric"* [see: paregoric; opium]

**gorilla biscuits; gorilla tabs** *street drug slang* [see: PCP]

**gorilla pills** *street drug slang for barbiturate sleeping pills* [see: barbiturates]

**Gormel Creme** OTC *moisturizer; emollient; keratolytic* [urea] 20%

**goserelin** USAN, INN, BAN *hormonal antineoplastic for prostate and breast cancer; luteinizing hormone-releasing hormone (LHRH) agonist* [also: goserelin acetate]

**goserelin acetate** JAN *hormonal antineoplastic for prostate and breast cancer; luteinizing hormone-releasing hormone (LHRH) agonist* [also: goserelin]

**gossypol** *investigational (orphan) for adrenal cortex cancer*

**govafilcon A** USAN *hydrophilic contact lens material*

**gp100 adenoviral gene therapy** *investigational (orphan) for metastatic melanoma*

**gp120 (glycoprotein)** *investigational (Phase III) antiviral vaccine for HIV prophylaxis* [also: AIDS vaccine]

**gp160 (glycoprotein)** *investigational (orphan) antiviral (therapeutic, Phase II) and vaccine (preventative, Phase I) for HIV and AIDS*

**GPIIb/IIIa receptor inhibitors** *a class of antiplatelet/antithrombotic agents for unstable angina*

**GP-500** tablets ℞ *decongestant; expectorant* [pseudoephedrine HCl; guaifenesin] 120•500 mg

**GR 85478** *investigational antiviral*

**Gradumet** (trademarked dosage form) *controlled-release tablet*

**gram** *street drug slang* [see: hashish]

**gramicidin** USP, INN *antibacterial antibiotic*

**gramicidin S** INN

**granisetron** USAN, INN, BAN *antiemetic*

**granisetron HCl** USAN $5\text{-}HT_3$ *receptor antagonist; antiemetic and antinauseant for chemotherapy*

**Granocyte** ℞ *investigational treatment for chemotherapy-induced neutropenia* [lenograstim]

**Granulderm** aerosol spray ℞ *topical enzyme for wound debridement* [trypsin; balsam Peru] 0.1•72.5 mg/0.82 mL

**Granulex** aerosol spray ℞ *topical enzyme for wound debridement* [trypsin; balsam Peru] 0.1•72.5 mg/0.82 mL

**granulocyte colony-stimulating factor (G-CSF), recombinant** [see: filgrastim]

**granulocyte-macrophage colony-stimulating factor (GM-CSF)** [see: regramostim; sargramostim; molgramostim]

**GranuMed** aerosol spray ℞ *topical enzyme for wound debridement* [trypsin; balsam Peru] 0.1•72.5 mg/0.82 mL

**grape parfait** *street drug slang* [see: LSD]

**grass; grass brownies** *street drug slang* [see: marijuana]

**grata** (Spanish for "pleasing") *street drug slang* [see: marijuana]

**gravel** *street drug slang* [see: cocaine, crack]

**gravy** *street drug slang* [see: heroin]

**great bear** *street drug slang* [see: fentanyl]

**great tobacco** *street drug slang* [see: opium]

**green** *street drug slang for inferior-quality marijuana, PCP, or ketamine* [see: marijuana; PCP; ketamine HCl]

**green double domes; green single domes** *street drug slang* [see: LSD]

**green goddess** *street drug slang* [see: marijuana]

**green gold** *street drug slang* [see: cocaine]

**green leaves; green tea** *street drug slang* [see: PCP]

**green single domes; green double domes** *street drug slang* [see: LSD]

**green soap** [see: soap, green]

**green wedge** *street drug slang* [see: LSD]

**greens and clears** *street drug slang for Dexamyl (dextroamphetamine sulfate + amobarbital; discontinued 1980), named for the capsule color* [see: dextroamphetamine sulfate; amobarbital]

**greeter** *street drug slang* [see: marijuana]

**grefa; grifa; griff; griffa; griffo** *street drug slang* [see: marijuana]

**grepafloxacin** INN

**grepafloxacin HCl** USAN *antibacterial*

**Greta** *street drug slang* [see: marijuana]

**grey shields** *street drug slang* [see: LSD]

**GRF1-44** *investigational (Phase III) human growth hormone releasing factor in slow-release implant form for growth disorders*

**grievous bodily harm** *street drug slang* [see: GHB]

**grifa; grefa; griff; griffa; griffo** *street drug slang* [see: marijuana]

**G-riffic** *street drug slang* [see: GHB]

**Grifulvin V** tablets, oral suspension Ŗ *systemic antifungal* [griseofulvin (microsize)] 250, 500 mg; 125 mg/5 mL

**Grisactin; Grisactin 250** capsules (discontinued 1996) Ŗ *systemic antifungal* [griseofulvin (microsize)] 125 mg; 250 mg

**Grisactin 500** tablets Ŗ *systemic antifungal* [griseofulvin (microsize)] 500 mg

**Grisactin Ultra** tablets Ŗ *systemic antifungal* [griseofulvin (ultramicrosize)] 125, 250, 330 mg

**griseofulvin** USP, INN, BAN *fungistatic* 165, 330 mg oral

**Gris-PEG** film-coated tablets Ŗ *systemic antifungal* [griseofulvin (ultramicrosize)] 125, 250 mg

**grit** *street drug slang* [see: cocaine, crack]

**groceries** *street drug slang* [see: cocaine, crack]

**grocery store high** *street drug slang* [see: nitrous oxide]

**g-rock** *street drug slang for one gram of crack* [see: cocaine, crack]

**groovy lemon** *street drug slang for a yellow LSD tablet* [see: LSD]

**growth hormone, human (hGH)** [see: somatropin]

**growth hormone, human recombinant (rhGH) with insulin-like growth factor, human recombinant (rhIGF)** *investigational (Phase II) cytokine for AIDS wasting syndrome*

**growth hormone-releasing factor (GHRF; GH-RF)** *investigational (orphan) for inadequate endogenous growth hormone in children*

**GS 393** *investigational (Phase I/II) antiviral for HIV* [PMEA]

**GS 504** *investigational treatment for peripheral retinitis due to cytomegalovirus*

**G-strophanthin** [see: ouabain]

**guabenxan** INN

**guacetisal** INN

**guafecainol** INN

**guaiac**

**guaiacol** NF

**guaiacol carbonate** NF

**guaiacol glyceryl ether** [see: guaifenesin]

**guaiactamine** INN

**guaiapate** USAN, INN *antitussive*

**guaiazulene soluble** [see: sodium gualenate]

**guaietolin** INN

**Guaifed** syrup OTC *decongestant; expectorant* [pseudoephedrine HCl; guaifenesin] 30•200 mg

**Guaifed** timed-release capsules Ŗ *decongestant; expectorant* [pseudoephedrine HCl; guaifenesin] 120•250 mg

**Guaifed-PD** timed-release capsules ℞ *pediatric decongestant and expectorant* [pseudoephedrine HCl; guaifenesin] 60•300 mg

**guaifenesin** USAN, USP, INN *expectorant* [also: guaiphenesin] 100 mg/5 mL oral ⊡ guanfacine

**guaifenesin & codeine phosphate** *expectorant; antitussive; narcotic analgesic* 300•10 mg oral; 100•10 mg/5 mL oral

**Guaifenesin DAC** liquid ℞ *narcotic antitussive; decongestant; expectorant* [codeine phosphate; pseudoephedrine HCl; guaifenesin; alcohol 1.9%] 10•30•100 mg

**Guaifenex** liquid ℞ *decongestant; expectorant* [phenylpropanolamine HCl; phenylephrine HCl; guaifenesin] 20•5•100 mg/5 mL

**Guaifenex DM** extended-release tablets ℞ *antitussive; expectorant* [dextromethorphan hydrobromide; guaifenesin] 30•600 mg

**Guaifenex LA** extended-release tablets ℞ *expectorant* [guaifenesin] 600 mg

**Guaifenex PPA 75** extended-release tablets ℞ *decongestant; expectorant* [phenylpropanolamine HCl; guaifenesin] 75•600 mg

**Guaifenex PSE 60; Guaifenex PSE 120** extended-release tablets ℞ *decongestant; expectorant* [pseudoephedrine HCl; guaifenesin] 60•600 mg; 120•600 mg

**guaifylline** INN *bronchodilator; expectorant* [also: guaithylline]

**GuaiMAX-D** extended-release tablets ℞ *decongestant; expectorant* [pseudoephedrine HCl; guaifenesin] 120•600 mg

**guaimesal** INN

**Guaipax** sustained-release tablets ℞ *decongestant; expectorant* [phenylpropanolamine HCl; guaifenesin] 75•400 mg

**guaiphenesin** BAN *expectorant* [also: guaifenesin]

**guaisteine** INN

**Guaitab** tablets OTC *decongestant; expectorant* [pseudoephedrine HCl; guaifenesin] 60•400 mg

**guaithylline** USAN *bronchodilator; expectorant* [also: guaifylline]

**Guaivent** capsules ℞ *decongestant; expectorant* [pseudoephedrine HCl; guaifenesin] 120•250 mg

**Guaivent PD** capsules ℞ *pediatric decongestant and expectorant* [pseudoephedrine HCl; guaifenesin] 60•300 mg

**Guai-Vent/PSE** sustained-release tablets ℞ *decongestant; expectorant* [pseudoephedrine HCl; guaifenesin] 120•600 mg

**guamecycline** INN, BAN

**guanabenz** USAN, INN *centrally acting antiadrenergic antihypertensive*

**guanabenz acetate** USAN, USP, JAN *centrally acting antiadrenergic antihypertensive* 4, 8 mg oral

**guanacline** INN, BAN *antihypertensive* [also: guanacline sulfate]

**guanacline sulfate** USAN *antihypertensive* [also: guanacline]

**guanadrel** INN *antihypertensive* [also: guanadrel sulfate]

**guanadrel sulfate** USAN, USP *antihypertensive* [also: guanadrel]

**guanatol HCl** [see: chloroguanide HCl]

**guanazodine** INN

**guancidine** INN *antihypertensive* [also: guancydine]

**guancydine** USAN *antihypertensive* [also: guancidine]

**guanethidine** INN, BAN *antihypertensive* [also: guanethidine monosulfate] ⊡ guanidine

**guanethidine monosulfate** USAN, USP *antihypertensive; investigational (orphan) for reflex sympathetic dystrophy and causalgia* [also: guanethidine]

**guanethidine sulfate** USAN, USP, JAN *antihypertensive*

**guanfacine** INN, BAN *antihypertensive; antiadrenergic* [also: guanfacine HCl] ⊡ guaifenesin

**guanfacine HCl** USAN *antihypertensive; antiadrenergic* [also: guanfacine] 1, 2 mg oral

**guanidine HCl** *cholinergic muscle stimulant* 125 mg oral ⊡ guanethidine

**guanisoquin sulfate** USAN *antihypertensive* [also: guanisoquine]

**guanisoquine** INN *antihypertensive* [also: guanisoquin sulfate]

**guanoclor** INN, BAN *antihypertensive* [also: guanoclor sulfate]

**guanoclor sulfate** USAN *antihypertensive* [also: guanoclor]

**guanoctine** INN *antihypertensive* [also: guanoctine HCl]

**guanoctine HCl** USAN *antihypertensive* [also: guanoctine]

**guanoxabenz** USAN, INN *antihypertensive*

**guanoxan** INN, BAN *antihypertensive* [also: guanoxan sulfate]

**guanoxan sulfate** USAN *antihypertensive* [also: guanoxan]

**guanoxyfen** INN *antihypertensive; antidepressant* [also: guanoxyfen sulfate]

**guanoxyfen sulfate** USAN *antihypertensive; antidepressant* [also: guanoxyfen]

**guar gum** NF *tablet binder and disintegrant*

**guaranine** [see: caffeine]

**GuiaCough CF** liquid OTC *antitussive; decongestant; expectorant* [dextromethorphan hydrobromide; phenylpropanolamine HCl; guaifenesin; alcohol 4.75%] 10•12.5•100 mg/5 mL

**GuiaCough PE** syrup OTC *decongestant; expectorant* [pseudoephedrine HCl; guaifenesin; alcohol 1.4%] 30•100 mg/5 mL

**Guiafenesin-DAC** syrup (discontinued 1993) ℞ *narcotic antitussive; decongestant; expectorant* [codeine phosphate; pseudoephedrine HCl; guaifenesin; alcohol]

**Guiaphed** elixir (discontinued 1993) OTC *antiasthmatic; bronchodilator; decongestant; expectorant; sedative* [theophylline; ephedrine sulfate; guaifenesin; phenobarbital]

**Guiatuss** syrup OTC *expectorant* [guaifenesin] 100 mg/5 mL ⊡ Guiatussin

**Guiatuss AC** syrup ℞ *narcotic antitussive; expectorant* [codeine phosphate; guaifenesin; alcohol] 10•100 mg/5 mL

**Guiatuss CF** liquid OTC *antitussive; decongestant; expectorant* [dextromethorphan hydrobromide; phenylpropanolamine HCl; guaifenesin; alcohol 4.75%] 10•12.5•100 mg/5 mL

**Guiatuss DAC** liquid ℞ *narcotic antitussive; decongestant; expectorant* [codeine phosphate; pseudoephedrine HCl; guaifenesin; alcohol] 10•30•100 mg/5 mL

**Guiatuss DM** liquid OTC *antitussive; expectorant* [dextromethorphan hydrobromide; guaifenesin] 10•100 mg/5 mL

**Guiatuss PE** liquid OTC *decongestant; expectorant* [pseudoephedrine HCl; guaifenesin; alcohol 1.4%] 30•100 mg/5 mL

**Guiatussin DAC** syrup ℞ *narcotic antitussive; decongestant; expectorant* [codeine phosphate; pseudoephedrine HCl; guaifenesin; alcohol 1.6%] 10•30•100 mg/5 mL ⊡ Guiatuss

**Guiatussin with Codeine Expectorant** liquid ℞ *narcotic antitussive; expectorant* [codeine phosphate; guaifenesin; alcohol 3.5%] 10•100 mg/5 mL

**Guiatussin with Dextromethorphan** liquid OTC *antitussive; expectorant* [dextromethorphan hydrobromide; guaifenesin; alcohol 1.4%] 15•100 mg/5 mL

**Guipax** tablets ℞ *decongestant; expectorant* [phenylpropanolamine HCl; guaifenesin]

**gum; guma** *street drug slang for opium refined for smoking* [see: opium]

**gum arabic** [see: acacia]

**gum senegal** [see: acacia]

**guncotton, soluble** [see: pyroxylin]

**gunga; gungeon; ganga; gange; ganja; Ghana; ghanja** *street drug slang* [see: marijuana]

**gungeon; gungun** *street drug slang for potent Jamaican marijuana* [see: marijuana]

**gunny; gunnysack** *street drug slang, a reference to sacks made with hemp fiber* [see: marijuana]

**gusperimus** INN *immunosuppressant; investigational (orphan) for acute renal graft rejection* [also: gusperimus trihydrochloride; gusperimus HCl]

**gusperimus HCl** JAN *immunosuppressant* [also: gusperimus trihydrochloride; gusperimus]

**gusperimus trihydrochloride** USAN *immunosuppressant* [also: gusperimus; gusperimus HCl]

**Gustase** tablets OTC *digestive enzymes* [amylase; protease; cellulase] 30•6•2 mg

**Gustase Plus** tablets ℞ *digestive enzymes; sedative* [amylase; protease; cellulase; homatropine methylbromide; phenobarbital] 30•6•2•2.5•8 mg

**gutta percha** USP *dental restoration agent*

**gutter glitter** *street drug slang for cocaine or illegal drugs in general* [see: cocaine]

**G-Well** lotion, shampoo ℞ *scabicide; pediculicide* [lindane] 1%

**Gynecort 5** cream (discontinued 1997) OTC *topical corticosteroid* [hydrocortisone acetate] 0.5%

**Gynecort 10** (name changed to Gynecort Female Creme in 1997)

**Gynecort Female Creme** cream OTC *topical corticosteroid* [hydrocortisone acetate] 1%

**Gyne-Lotrimin** vaginal cream, vaginal tablets, combination pack (vaginal tablets + cream) OTC *antifungal* [clotrimazole] 1%; 100 mg

**Gyne-Lotrimin 3** vaginal tablets, combination pack (vaginal tablets + cream) OTC *antifungal* [clotrimazole] 100 mg; 1%

**Gyne-Moistrin** vaginal gel OTC *lubricant* [propylene glycol]

**gynergon** [see: estradiol]

**Gyne-Sulf** vaginal cream ℞ *broad-spectrum bacteriostatic* [sulfathiazole; sulfacetamide; sulfabenzamide] 3.42%•2.86%•3.7%

**gynoestryl** [see: estradiol]

**Gynogen L.A. "20"** IM injection ℞ *estrogen replacement therapy for postmenopausal disorders; antineoplastic for prostatic cancer* [estradiol valerate in oil] 20 mg/mL

**Gynogen L.A. "40"** IM injection (discontinued 1996) ℞ *estrogen replacement therapy for postmenopausal disorders; antineoplastic for prostatic cancer* [estradiol valerate in oil] 40 mg/mL

**Gynol II Contraceptive** vaginal gel, vaginal jelly OTC *spermicidal contraceptive (for use with a diaphragm)* [nonoxynol 9] 2%; 3%

**Gynovite Plus** tablets OTC *vitamin/mineral/calcium/iron supplement* [multiple vitamins & minerals; calcium; iron; folic acid; biotin] ≗•83•3•0.067•≗ mg

**Gy-Pak** (trademarked packaging form) *unit-of-issue package*

**Gyrocap** (trademarked dosage form) *timed-release capsule*

**gyve** *street drug slang for a marijuana cigarette* [see: marijuana]

**H₁ blockers** *a class of antihistamines* [also called: histamine $H_1$ antagonists]

**²H (deuterium)** [see: deuterium oxide]

**H₂ blockers** *a class of gastrointestinal antisecretory agents* [also called: histamine $H_2$ antagonists]

**H₂¹⁵O** [see: water O 15]

**³H (tritium)** [see: tritiated water]

**Habitrol** transdermal patch ℞ *smoking deterrent; nicotine withdrawal aid* [nicotine] 17.5, 35, 52.5 mg

**hache** *street drug slang* [see: heroin]

**hachimycin** INN, BAN

**HAD (hexamethylmelamine, Adriamycin, DDP)** *chemotherapy protocol*

**hafnium** *element (Hf)*

**hail** *street drug slang* [see: cocaine, crack]

**Hair Booster Vitamin** tablets OTC *vitamin/mineral/iron supplement* [multiple B vitamins & minerals; iron; folic acid] ≗•18•0.4 mg

**hairy** *street drug slang* [see: heroin]

**halarsol** [see: dichlorophenarsine HCl]

**halazepam** USAN, USP, INN, BAN *anxiolytic; sedative*

**halazone** USP, INN *disinfectant; water purifier*

**Halazone** tablets (discontinued 1996) OTC *water purifier*

**Hal-C** ℞ *investigational coating agent for abdominal procedures* [hyaluronic acid]

**halcinonide** USAN, USP, INN, BAN *topical corticosteroidal anti-inflammatory*

**Halcion** tablets ℞ *sedative; hypnotic* [triazolam] 0.125, 0.25 mg

**Haldol** oral concentrate, IM injection ℞ *antipsychotic; control manifestations of Tourette syndrome* [haloperidol lactate] 2 mg/mL; 5 mg/mL ⊡ Halenol; Halog

**Haldol** tablets ℞ *antipsychotic; control manifestations of Tourette syndrome* [haloperidol] 0.5, 1, 2, 5, 10, 20 mg

**Haldol Decanoate 50; Haldol Decanoate 100** long-acting IM injection ℞ *antipsychotic* [haloperidol decanoate] 50 mg/mL; 100 mg/mL

**Halenol, Children's** liquid OTC *analgesic; antipyretic* [acetaminophen] 160 mg/5 mL

**Halercol** capsules OTC *vitamin supplement* [multiple vitamins]

**haletazole** INN [also: halethazole]

**halethazole** BAN [also: haletazole]

**Haley's M-O** liquid OTC *laxative* [magnesium hydroxide; mineral oil] 900 mg•3.75 mL per 15 mL

**Hal-F** *investigational resorbable film for abdominal surgery* [hyaluronic acid]

**half moon** *street drug slang* [see: mescaline]

**half track** *street drug slang* [see: cocaine, crack]

**Halfan** (approved by the FDA but not marketed by the manufacturer) ℞ *antimalarial (orphan)* [halofantrine HCl]

**Halfprin; Halfprin 81** enteric-coated tablets OTC *analgesic; antipyretic; anti-inflammatory; antirheumatic* [aspirin] 165 mg; 81 mg

**Hal-G** *investigational gel to prevent adhesions in minor surgery* [hyaluronic acid]

**Hall's Mentho-Lyptus** lozenges (discontinued 1994) OTC *antipruritic/counterirritant; mild local anesthetic; antiseptic* [menthol; eucalyptus oil]

**Hall's Plus** lozenges OTC *antipruritic/counterirritant; mild local anesthetic; antiseptic* [menthol] 10 mg

**Hall's Sugar Free Mentho-Lyptus** lozenges OTC *antipruritic/counterirritant; mild local anesthetic; antiseptic* [menthol; eucalyptus oil] 5•2.8, 6•2.8 mg

**halobetasol propionate** USAN *topical corticosteroidal anti-inflammatory* [also: ulobetasol]

**halocarban** INN *disinfectant* [also: cloflucarban]

**halocortolone** INN

**halocrinic acid** [see: brocrinat]

**Halodrin** tablets (discontinued 1994) ℞ *estrogen/androgen for menopausal vasomotor symptoms* [ethinyl estradiol; fluoxymesterone] 0.02•1 mg

**halofantrine** INN, BAN *antimalarial* [also: halofantrine HCl]

**halofantrine HCl** USAN *antimalarial (orphan)* [also: halofantrine]

**Halofed** syrup (discontinued 1993) OTC *nasal decongestant* [pseudoephedrine HCl]

**Halofed** tablets OTC *nasal decongestant* [pseudoephedrine HCl] 30, 60 mg

**halofenate** USAN, INN, BAN *antihyperlipoproteinemic; uricosuric*

**halofuginone** INN, BAN *antiprotozoal* [also: halofuginone hydrobromide]

**halofuginone hydrobromide** USAN *antiprotozoal* [also: halofuginone]

**Halog** ointment, cream, solution ℞ *topical corticosteroidal anti-inflammatory* [halcinonide] 0.1%; 0.025%, 0.1%; 0.1% ⊡ Haldol

**Halog-E** cream ℞ *topical corticosteroidal anti-inflammatory; emollient* [halcinonide] 0.1%

**halometasone** INN

**halonamine** INN

**halopemide** USAN, INN *antipsychotic*

**halopenium chloride** INN, BAN

**haloperidol** USAN, USP, INN, BAN *antidyskinetic for Tourette's disease; antipsychotic* 0.5, 1, 2, 5, 10, 20 mg oral

**haloperidol decanoate** USAN, BAN *antipsychotic*

**haloperidol lactate** *antidyskinetic for Tourette's disease; antipsychotic* 2 mg/mL oral; 5 mg/mL injection

**halopone chloride** [see: halopenium chloride]

**halopredone** INN *topical anti-inflammatory* [also: halopredone acetate]

**halopredone acetate** USAN *topical anti-inflammatory* [also: halopredone]

**haloprogesterone** USAN, INN *progestin*

**haloprogin** USAN, USP, INN, JAN *antibacterial; antifungal*

**halopyramine** BAN [also: chloropyramine]

**Halotestin** tablets ℞ *androgenic hormone for male hypogonadism and female breast cancer* [fluoxymesterone] 2, 5, 10 mg ② Halotex; Halotussin

**Halotex** cream, solution ℞ *topical antifungal* [haloprogin] 1% ② Halotestin

**halothane** USP, INN, BAN *inhalation general anesthetic*

**Halotussin** syrup OTC *expectorant* [guaifenesin; alcohol 3.5%] 100 mg/5 mL ② Halotestin

**Halotussin-DM** liquid, sugar-free liquid OTC *antitussive; expectorant* [dextromethorphan hydrobromide; guaifenesin] 10•100 mg/5 mL

**haloxazolam** INN

**haloxon** INN, BAN

**halquinol** BAN *topical anti-infective* [also: halquinols]

**halquinols** USAN *topical anti-infective* [also: halquinol]

**Hal-S** *investigational synovial fluid replacement for arthroscopic surgery of meniscal tear* [hyaluronic acid]

**Haltran** tablets OTC *nonsteroidal anti-inflammatory drug (NSAID); antiarthritic; analgesic* [ibuprofen] 200 mg

**HAM (hexamethylmelamine, Adriamycin, melphalan)** *chemotherapy protocol*

**HAM (hexamethylmelamine, Adriamycin, methotrexate)** *chemotherapy protocol*

**hamamelis water** *astringent*

**hamburger helper** *street drug slang* [see: cocaine, crack]

**hamycin** USAN, INN *antifungal*

**hanhich** *street drug slang* [see: marijuana]

**hanyak** *street drug slang for smokable speed* [see: amphetamines]

**happy cigarette** *street drug slang for a marijuana cigarette* [see: marijuana]

**happy dust; happy powder; happy trails** *street drug slang* [see: cocaine]

**hard candy** *street drug slang* [see: heroin]

**hard fat** [see: fat, hard]

**hard line; hard rock** *street drug slang* [see: cocaine, crack]

**hard on; heart on** *street drug slang* [see: amyl nitrite]

**hard stuff** *street drug slang* [see: heroin; opium]

**hardware** *street drug slang* [see: isobutyl nitrite]

**Harry; Harry Jones** *street drug slang* [see: heroin]

**hash** *street drug slang* [see: hashish; marijuana]

**hashish** *euphoric/hallucinogenic street drug made from the resin of the flowering tops of the cannabis plant*

**hats** *street drug slang* [see: LSD]

**have a dust; haven dust** *street drug slang* [see: cocaine]

**Havrix** IM injection, prefilled syringe ℞ *immunization against hepatitis A virus (HAV)* [hepatitis A vaccine, inactivated] 720 ELISA units (EL.U.)/0.5 mL (pediatric), 1440 EL.U./mL (adult)

**Hawaiian** *street drug slang for very high potency marijuana* [see: marijuana]

**Hawaiian sunshine** *street drug slang* [see: LSD]

**Hawaiian Tropic Cool Aloe with I.C.E.** gel OTC *topical local anesthetic; counterirritant* [lidocaine; menthol] ² • ²

**hawk** *street drug slang* [see: LSD]

**hay** *street drug slang* [see: marijuana]

**hay butt** *street drug slang for a marijuana cigarette* [see: marijuana]

**Hayfebrol** liquid OTC *decongestant; antihistamine* [pseudoephedrine HCl; chlorpheniramine maleate] 30•2 mg/5 mL

**haze** *street drug slang* [see: LSD]

**Hazel** *street drug slang* [see: heroin]

**H-BIG** IM injection ℞ *hepatitis B immunizing agent* [hepatitis B immune globulin] 4, 5 mL

**H-BIG** IV injection *investigational (orphan) prophylaxis against hepatitis B reinfection in liver transplant patients* [hepatitis B immune globulin]

**HBIG (hepatitis B immune globulin)** [q.v.]

**HBY097** *investigational (Phase II) antiviral non-nucleoside reverse transcriptase inhibitor for HIV*

**1% HC** ointment ℞ *topical corticosteroid* [hydrocortisone] 1%

**HC (hydrocortisone)** [q.v.]

**4-HC (4-hydroperoxycyclophosphamide)** [q.v.]

**HC Derma-Pax** liquid OTC *topical corticosteroid; antihistamine; antiseptic* [hydrocortisone; pyrilamine maleate; chlorpheniramine maleate; chlorobutanol] 0.5%•0.44%•0.06%•25%

**HCA (hydrocortisone acetate)** [q.v.]

**H-CAP (hexamethylmelamine, cyclophosphamide, Adriamycin, Platinol)** *chemotherapy protocol*

**H-caps** *street drug slang* [see: heroin]

**hCG (human chorionic gonadotropin)** [see: gonadotropin, chorionic]

**HCG-nostick** test kit for professional use (discontinued 1995) *in vitro diagnostic aid for urine pregnancy test* [sol particle immunoassay (SPIA)]

**HCP-30** *Investigational (Phase I) vaccine for HIV*

**HCT (hydrochlorothiazide)** [q.v.]

**HCTZ (hydrochlorothiazide)** [q.v.]

**HD 85** suspension ℞ *GI contrast radiopaque agent* [barium sulfate] 85%

**HD 200 Plus** powder for suspension ℞ *GI contrast radiopaque agent* [barium sulfate] 98%

**HDCV (human diploid cell vaccine)** [see: rabies vaccine]

**HDMTX (high-dose methotrexate [with leucovorin rescue])** *chemotherapy protocol*

**HDMTX-CF (high-dose methotrexate, citrovorum factor)** *chemotherapy protocol*

**HDMTX/LV (high-dose methotrexate, leucovorin [rescue])** *chemotherapy protocol*

**HDPEB (high-dose PEB protocol)** *chemotherapy protocol* [see: PEB]

**HD-VAC (high-dose [methotrexate], vinblastine, Adriamycin, cisplatin)** *chemotherapy protocol*

**head drugs** *street drug slang* [see: amphetamines]

**Head & Shoulders** cream shampoo, lotion shampoo OTC *antiseborrheic; antibacterial; antifungal* [pyrithione zinc] 1%

**Head & Shoulders Dry Scalp** shampoo OTC *antiseborrheic; antibacterial; antifungal* [pyrithione zinc] 1%

**Head & Shoulders Intensive Treatment Dandruff Shampoo** OTC *antiseborrheic* [selenium sulfide] 1%

**headlights** *street drug slang* [see: LSD]

**Healon; Healon GV** intraocular injection ℞ *viscoelastic agent for ophthalmic surgery* [hyaluronate sodium] 10 mg/mL; 14 mg/mL

**Healon Yellow** intraocular injection ℞ *viscoelastic agent for ophthalmic surgery; corneal disclosing agent* [sodium hyaluronate; fluorescein sodium] 10•0.005 mg/mL

**heart on; hard on** *street drug slang* [see: amyl nitrite]

**Heartline** enteric-coated tablets OTC *analgesic; antipyretic; anti-inflammatory; antirheumatic* [aspirin] 81 mg

**hearts** *street drug slang* [see: amphetamines]

**heaven and hell** *street drug slang* [see: PCP]

**heaven dust** *street drug slang* [see: cocaine; heroin]

**Heavenly Blue** *street drug slang for LSD or a variety of psychedelic morning glory seeds* [see: LSD; morning glory seeds]

**heavy liquid petrolatum** [see: mineral oil]

**heavy stuff** *street drug slang* [see: cocaine; heroin]

**heavy water ($D_2O$)** [see: deuterium oxide]

**Heb Cream Base** OTC *cream base*

**hedaquinium chloride** INN, BAN

**"hedgehog" proteins** *a class of novel human proteins that induce the formation of regenerative tissue*

**Heet Liniment** OTC *counterirritant; topical antiseptic* [methyl salicylate; camphor; capsaicin; alcohol 70%] 15%•3.6%•0.025%

**Heet Spray** (discontinued 1994) OTC *counterirritant; topical antiseptic* [methyl salicylate; camphor; menthol; methyl nicotinate; alcohol] 25%•3%•3%•1%

**hefilcon A** USAN *hydrophilic contact lens material*

**hefilcon B** USAN *hydrophilic contact lens material*

**hefilcon C** USAN *hydrophilic contact lens material*

**Helen** *street drug slang* [see: heroin]

**helenien** [see: xantofyl palmitate]

**helicon** [see: aspirin]

**Helidac** 14-day dose-pack ℞ *combination treatment for active duodenal ulcer with H. pylori infection* [bismuth subsalicylate (chewable tablets); metronidazole (tablets); tetracycline HCl (capsules)] 262.4 mg; 250 mg; 500 mg

**heliomycin** INN

**Helistat** sponge ℞ *hemostasis adjunct during surgery* [absorbable collagen hemostatic sponge]

**helium** USP *diluent for gases; element* (He)

**Helixate** powder for IV injection ℞ *antihemophilic to correct coagulation deficiency* [antihemophilic factor VIII, recombinant] 250, 500, 1000 IU

**hell dust** *street drug slang* [see: heroin]

**Hem Fe** capsules (discontinued 1996) ℞ *hematinic* [ferrous fumarate; cyanocobalamin; ascorbic acid; docusate sodium] 100 mg•5 μg•125 mg•25 mg

**HEMA (2-hydroxyethyl methacrylate)** *contact lens material*

**Hemabate** IM injection ℞ *prostaglandin-type abortifacient; for postpartum uterine bleeding* [carboprost tromethamine] 250 μg/mL

**Hema-Check** slide tests for home use OTC *in vitro diagnostic aid for fecal occult blood*

**Hema-Combistix** reagent strips *in vitro diagnostic aid for multiple urine products*

**He-man** *street drug slang* [see: fentanyl; isobutyl nitrite]

**Hemaspan** timed-release tablets OTC *hematinic* [ferrous fumarate; vitamin C; docusate sodium] 110•200•20 mg

**HemAssist** *investigational (Phase III) blood substitute for perfusion deficit disorders and blood loss from severe trauma* [hemoglobin crosfumaril]

**Hemastix** reagent strips for professional use *in vitro diagnostic aid for urine occult blood*

**Hematest** reagent tablets for professional use *in vitro diagnostic aid for fecal occult blood*

**hematinics** *a class of iron-containing agents for the prevention and treatment of iron-deficiency anemia*

**hematopoietics** *a class of antianemic agents that promote the formation of red blood cells*

**heme arginate** *investigational (orphan) for acute symptomatic porphyria and myelodysplastic syndrome*

**HemeSelect Collection** kit for home use *in vitro diagnostic aid for fecal occult blood* [for use with HemeSelect Reagent kit]

**HemeSelect Reagent** kit for professional use *in vitro diagnostic aid for fecal occult blood* [for use with HemeSelect Collection kit]

**Hemet Rectal** ointment (discontinued 1993) OTC *topical anesthetic; vasoconstrictor; astringent* [diperodon HCl; pyrilamine maleate; phenylephrine HCl; bismuth subcarbonate; zinc oxide] 0.25%•0.1%•0.25%• 0.2%•5%

**Hemex** ℞ *investigational (orphan) for acute porphyric syndromes* [hemin; zinc mesoporphyrin]

**hemiacidrin** [see: citric acid, glucono-delta-lactone & magnesium carbonate]

**hemin** *enzyme inhibitor for acute intermittent porphyria (AIP), porphyria variegata, and hereditary coproporphyria (orphan)*

**hemin & zinc mesoporphyrin** *investigational (orphan) for acute porphyric syndromes*

**Hemocaine** anorectal ointment (discontinued 1995) OTC *topical anesthetic; vasoconstrictor; astringent* [diperodon HCl; pyrilamine maleate; phenylephrine HCl; bismuth subcarbonate; zinc oxide] 0.25%•0.1%•0.25%•0.2%•5%

**Hemoccult** slide tests for professional use, test tape for professional use *in vitro diagnostic aid for fecal occult blood*

**Hemoccult II** slide tests for professional use *in vitro diagnostic aid for fecal occult blood*

**Hemoccult II Dispenserpak; Hemoccult II Dispenserpak Plus** slide tests for home use OTC *in vitro diagnostic aid for fecal occult blood*

**Hemoccult SENSA; Hemoccult II SENSA** slide tests for professional use *in vitro diagnostic aid for fecal occult blood*

**Hemocitrate** *investigational (orphan) agent for leukapheresis procedures* [sodium citrate]

**Hemocyte** IM injection (discontinued 1995) ℞ *hematinic* [ferrous gluconate; multiple B vitamins; procaine HCl] 3 mg/mL•≛•2%

**Hemocyte** tablets OTC *hematinic* [ferrous fumarate] 324 mg

**Hemocyte Plus** elixir ℞ *hematinic* [polysaccharide iron complex; multiple B vitamins and minerals; folic acid] 12•≛•0.33 mg

**Hemocyte Plus** tablets ℞ *hematinic* [ferrous fumarate; multiple B vitamins and minerals; sodium ascorbate; folic acid] 106•≛•200•1 mg

**Hemocyte-F** tablets ℞ *hematinic* [ferrous fumarate; folic acid] 106•1 mg

**Hemocyte-V** IM injection (discontinued 1995) ℞ *hematinic* [ferrous gluconate; multiple B vitamins] 3.6•≛ mg/mL

**Hemofil M** IV injection ℞ *antihemophilic to correct coagulation deficiency* [antihemophilic factor VIII] 10, 20, 30 mL

**hemoglobin crosfumaril** USAN *investigational (Phase III) blood substitute for perfusion deficit disorders and blood loss due to severe trauma*

**Hemokine** *investigational progenitor cell stimulator for neutropenia and thrombocytopenia* [muplestim]

**Hemonyne** IV infusion ℞ *antihemophilic to correct factor IX deficiency (Christmas disease)* [coagulation factors II, VII, IX, and X, heat treated] 20, 40 mL

**Hemopad** fiber ℞ *topical hemostatic aid in surgery* [microfibrillar collagen hemostat]

**Hemophilus b conjugate vaccine** *active bacterin for Haemophilus influenzae type b*

**Hemopure; Hemopure 2** ℞ *investigational blood substitute*

**Hemorid for Women** cream OTC *topical local anesthetic; vasoconstrictor* [pramoxine HCl; phenylephrine HCl] 1%•0.25%

**Hemorid for Women** lotion OTC *emollient/protectant* [mineral oil; petrolatum; glycerin]

**Hemorid for Women** rectal suppositories OTC *astringent; topical vasoconstrictor* [zinc oxide; phenylephrine HCl] 11%•0.25%

**Hemorrhoidal HC** rectal suppositories ℞ *topical corticosteroidal anti-inflammatory* [hydrocortisone acetate] 25 mg

**hemostatics** *a class of therapeutic blood modifiers that arrest the flow of blood*

**Hemotene** fiber ℞ *topical hemostatic aid in surgery* [microfibrillar collagen hemostat] 1 g

**hemp** *street drug slang* [see: marijuana]

**Hem-Prep** anorectal ointment, rectal suppositories OTC *temporary relief of hemorrhoidal symptoms; topical vasoconstrictor; astringent* [phenylephrine HCl; zinc oxide] 0.025%•11%; 0.25%•11%

**Hemril** Uniserts (rectal suppositories) OTC *temporary relief of hemorrhoidal symptoms* [bismuth subgallate; bismuth resorcin compound; benzyl benzoate; peruvian balsam; zinc oxide] 2.25%•1.75%•1.2%•1.8%•11%

**Hemril-HC** Uniserts (suppositories) R *topical corticosteroidal anti-inflammatory; antipruritic* [hydrocortisone acetate] 25 mg

**heneicosafluorotripropylamine** [see: perfluamine]

**Henry** *street drug slang* [see: heroin]

**Henry VIII** *street drug slang* [see: cocaine]

**HEOD (hexachloro-epoxy-octahydro-dimethanonaththalene)** [see: dieldrin]

**Hepandrin** R *anabolic steroid; investigational (orphan) for Turner syndrome, growth and puberty delay, AIDS wasting, and alcoholic hepatitis* [oxandrolone]

**heparin** BAN *anticoagulant; antithrombotic* [also: heparin calcium]

**heparin, 2-0-desulfated** *investigational (orphan) for cystic fibrosis*

**heparin calcium** USP *anticoagulant; antithrombotic* [also: heparin]

**Heparin Lock Flush** solution R *IV flush for catheter patency (not therapeutic)* [heparin sodium] 10, 100 U/mL

**heparin sodium** USP, INN, BAN *anticoagulant; antithrombotic* 1000, 2000, 2500, 5000, 7500, 10 000, 20 000, 40 000 U/mL injection

**heparin sodium & sodium chloride 0.45%** *anticoagulant; antithrombotic* 12 500 U•250 mL, 25 000 U•250 mL, 25 000 U•500 mL

**heparin sodium & sodium chloride 0.9%** *anticoagulant; antithrombotic* 1000 U•500 mL, 2000 U•1000 mL

**heparin sulfate** [see: danaparoid sodium]

**heparin whole blood** [see: blood, whole]

**heparin-binding neurotrophic factor** *investigational protectant for nerve calls*

**HepatAmine** IV infusion R *nutritional therapy for hepatic failure and hepatic encephalopathy* [multiple branched-chain essential and nonessential amino acids; electrolytes]

**Hepatic-Aid II Instant Drink** powder OTC *enteral nutritional treatment for chronic liver disease* [branched chain amino acids]

**hepatitis A and B combination vaccine** *investigational immunizing agent*

**hepatitis A vaccine, inactivated** *active immunizing agent for the hepatitis A virus (HAV)*

**hepatitis B immune globulin (HBIG)** USP *passive immunizing agent; investigational (orphan) prophylaxis against hepatitis B reinfection in liver transplant patients*

**hepatitis B surface antigen** [see: hepatitis B virus vaccine, inactivated]

**hepatitis B virus vaccine, inactivated** USP *active immunizing agent for hepatitis B and hepatitis D*

**Hep-B-Gammagee** IM injection (discontinued 1996) R *hepatitis B immunizing agent* [hepatitis B immune globulin] 5 mL

**Hepfomin-R** IM injection (discontinued 1994) R *antianemic; vitamin supplement* [liver extracts; vitamin $B_{12}$; folic acid]

**Hep-Forte** capsules OTC *geriatric dietary supplement* [multiple vitamins & food products; folic acid; biotin] ±•60•²⁄ µg

**Hep-Lock; Hep-Lock U/P** solution R *IV flush for catheter patency (not therapeutic)* [heparin sodium] 10, 100 U/mL

**HEPP (H-chain** [see: pentigetide]

**hepronicate** INN

**hepsulfam** *investigational antineoplastic*

**heptabarb** INN [also: heptabarbitone]

**heptabarbital** [see: heptabarb; heptabarbitone]

**heptabarbitone** BAN [also: heptabarb]

**Heptalac** syrup R *laxative* [lactulose] 10 g/15 mL

**heptaminol** INN, BAN

**heptaminol HCl** [see: heptaminol]

**2-heptanamine** [see: tuaminoheptane]

**2-heptanamine sulfate** [see: tuaminoheptane sulfate]

**heptaverine** INN

**heptolamide** INN

**Heptuna Plus** capsules (discontinued 1995) ℞ *hematinic* [ferrous sulfate; multiple B vitamins; multiple minerals; vitamin C; intrinsic factor concentrate] 100• ± • ± •150•25 mg

**hepzidine** INN

**Her** *street drug slang* [see: cocaine]

**HER2 humanized MAb** *investigational antineoplastic for breast and ovarian cancer*

**herb; herba** ("herbaje" is Spanish for "grass") *street drug slang* [see: marijuana]

**Herb and Al** *street drug slang for a combination of marijuana and alcohol* [see: alcohol; marijuana]

**Herbal Laxative** tablets OTC *laxative* [senna leaves; cascara sagrada bark] 125•20 mg

**herms** *street drug slang* [see: PCP]

**hero; heroina; heroine; hero of the underworld** *street drug slang* [see: heroin]

**heroin** *potent narcotic analgesic street drug which is highly addictive; banned in the USA* [medically known as diacetylmorphine HCl and diamorphine]

**heroin HCl** (*banned in the USA*) [see: diacetylmorphine HCl]

**Herpecin-L** lip balm OTC *vulnerary; sunblock* [allantoin; padimate O]

**herpes simplex virus gene** *investigational (orphan) for primary and metastatic brain tumors*

**Herpetrol** tablets OTC *dietary supplement; claimed to prevent and treat herpes simplex infections* [L-lysine; multiple vitamins; zinc]

**Herplex** eye drops (discontinued 1997) ℞ *ophthalmic antiviral* [idoxuridine] 0.1%

**Herrick Lacrimal Plug** ℞ *blocks the puncta and caniculus to eliminate tear loss in keratitis sicca* [silicone plug]

**HES (hydroxyethyl starch)** [see: hetastarch]

**Hespan** IV infusion ℞ *plasma volume expander for shock due to hemorrhage, burns, surgery* [hetastarch] 6 g/100 mL ⍰ Histatan

**hesperidin**

**hesperidin methyl chalcone** [see: bioflavonoids]

**hessle** *street drug slang* [see: heroin]

**hetacillin** USAN, USP, INN, BAN *antibacterial*

**hetacillin potassium** USAN, USP *antibacterial*

**hetaflur** USAN, INN, BAN *dental caries prophylactic*

**hetastarch** USAN, BAN *plasma volume extender* [also: hydroxyethylstarch]

**heteronium bromide** USAN, INN, BAN *anticholinergic*

**Hetrazan** tablets (available for compassionate use only) ℞ *anthelmintic for Bancroft's filariasis, onchocerciasis, tropical eosinophilia, and loiasis* [diethylcarbamazine citrate] 50 mg

**hexaammonium molybdate tetrahydrate** [see: ammonium molybdate]

**Hexabrix** injection ℞ *parenteral radiopaque agent* [ioxaglate meglumine; ioxaglate sodium] 39.3%•19.6%

**HexaCAF; Hexa-CAF (hexamethylmelamine, cyclophosphamide, amethopterin, fluorouracil)** *chemotherapy protocol*

**hexacarbacholine bromide** INN [also: carbolonium bromide]

**hexachlorane** [see: lindane]

**hexachlorocyclohexane** [see: lindane]

**hexachlorophane** BAN *topical anti-infective; detergent* [also: hexachlorophene]

**hexachlorophene** USP, INN *topical anti-infective; detergent* [also: hexachlorophane]

**hexacyclonate sodium** INN

**hexacyprone** INN

**hexadecanoic acid, methylethyl ester** [see: isopropyl palmitate]

**hexadecanol** [see: cetyl alcohol]

**hexadecylamine hydrofluoride** [see: hetaflur]

**hexadecylpyridinium chloride** [see: cetylpyridinium chloride]

**hexadecyltrimethylammonium bromide** [see: cetrimonium bromide]

**hexadecyltrimethylammonium chloride** [see: cetrimonium chloride]

**2,4-hexadienoic acid, potassium salt** [see: potassium sorbate]

**hexadiline** INN

**hexadimethrine bromide** INN, BAN

**hexadiphane** [see: prozapine]

**Hexadrol** tablets, elixir ℞ *glucocorticoids* [dexamethasone] 1.5, 4 mg; 0.5 mg/5 mL ⧉ Hexalol

**Hexadrol Phosphate** intra-articular, intralesional, soft tissue, or IM injection ℞ *glucocorticoids* [dexamethasone sodium phosphate] 4, 10, 20 mg/mL

**hexadylamine** [see: hexadiline]

**hexafluorenium bromide** USAN, USP *skeletal muscle relaxant; succinylcholine synergist* [also: hexafluronium bromide]

**hexafluorodiethyl ether** [see: flurothyl]

**hexaflurone bromide** [see: hexafluorenium bromide]

**hexafluronium bromide** INN *skeletal muscle relaxant; succinylcholine synergist* [also: hexafluorenium bromide]

**Hexalen** capsules ℞ *antineoplastic for advanced ovarian adenocarcinoma (orphan)* [altretamine] 50 mg ⧉ Hexalol

**Hexalol** sugar-coated tablets (discontinued 1994) ℞ *urinary anti-infective; analgesic; antispasmodic; acidifier* [methenamine; phenyl salicylate; atropine sulfate; methylene blue; hyoscyamine; benzoic acid] 40.8•18.1•0.03•5.4•0.03•4.5 mg ⧉ Hexadrol; Hexalen

**hexamarium bromide** [see: distigmine bromide]

**hexametazime** BAN

**hexamethone bromide** [see: hexamethonium bromide]

**hexamethonium bromide** INN, BAN

**hexamethylenamine** [now: methenamine]

**hexamethylenamine mandelate** [see: methenamine mandelate]

**hexamethylenetetramine** [see: methenamine]

**hexamethylmelamine (HMM; HXM)** [see: altretamine]

**hexamidine** INN

**hexamine hippurate** BAN *urinary antibacterial* [also: methenamine hippurate]

**hexamine mandelate** [see: methenamine mandelate]

**hexapradol** INN

**hexaprofen** INN, BAN

**hexapropymate** INN, BAN

**hexasonium iodide** INN

**Hexastat** capsules ℞ *antineoplastic for ovarian adenocarcinoma (orphan)* [altretamine]

**hexavitamin** USP

**Hexavitamin** tablets OTC *vitamin supplement* [multiple vitamins] ±

**hexcarbacholine bromide** INN [also: carbolonium bromide]

**hexedine** USAN, INN *antibacterial*

**hexemal** [see: cyclobarbital]

**hexestrol** NF, INN

**hexetidine** BAN

**hexicide** [see: lindane]

**hexinol** [see: cyclomenol]

**hexobarbital** USP, INN

**hexobarbital sodium** NF

**hexobendine** USAN, INN, BAN *vasodilator*

**hexocyclium methylsulfate** *peptic ulcer adjunct* [also: hexocyclium metilsulfate; hexocyclium methylsulphate]

**hexocyclium methylsulphate** BAN [also: hexocyclium methylsulfate; hexocyclium metilsulfate]

**hexocyclium metilsulfate** INN [also: hexocyclium methylsulfate; hexocyclium methylsulphate]

**hexoprenaline** INN, BAN *tocolytic; bronchodilator* [also: hexoprenaline sulfate]

**hexoprenaline sulfate** USAN, JAN *tocolytic; bronchodilator* [also: hexoprenaline]

**hexopyrimidine** [see: hexetidine]

**hexopyrrolate** [see: hexopyrronium bromide]

**hexopyrronium bromide** INN

**Hextend** ℞ *investigational (Phase III) blood plasma volume expander for surgical blood loss*

**hexydaline** [see: methenamine mandelate]

**hexylcaine** INN *local anesthetic* [also: hexylcaine HCl]

**hexylcaine HCl** USP *local anesthetic* [also: hexylcaine]

**hexylene glycol** NF *humectant; solvent*
**hexylresorcinol** USP *anthelmintic; topical antiseptic*
**1-hexyltheobromine** [see: pentifylline]
**H-F Gel** ℞ *investigational (orphan) for hydrofluoric acid burns* [calcium gluconate]
**hFSH (human follicle-stimulating hormone)** [now: menotropins]
**HFZ (homofenazine)** [q.v.]
**¹⁹⁷Hg** [see: chlormerodrin Hg 197]
**¹⁹⁷Hg** [see: merisoprol acetate Hg 197]
**¹⁹⁷Hg** [see: merisoprol Hg 197]
**²⁰³Hg** [see: chlormerodrin Hg 203]
**²⁰³Hg** [see: merisoprol acetate Hg 203]
**hGH (human growth hormone)** [see: somatropin]
**HGP-30** *investigational (Phase I) vaccine for HIV*
**H-H-R** tablets (discontinued 1993) ℞ *antihypertensive* [hydralazine HCl; hydrochlorothiazide; reserpine]
**hi speeds; high speed** *street drug slang* [see: amphetamines]
**hibenzate** INN *combining name for radicals or groups* [also: hybenzate]
**Hibiclens** sponge/brush OTC *broad-spectrum antimicrobial; germicidal* [chlorhexidine gluconate; alcohol 4%] 4%
**Hibiclens Antiseptic/AntiMicrobial Skin Cleanser** liquid OTC *broad-spectrum antimicrobial; germicidal* [chlorhexidine gluconate; alcohol 4%] 4%
**Hibistat Germicidal Hand Rinse** liquid OTC *broad-spectrum antimicrobial; germicidal* [chlorhexidine gluconate; alcohol 70%] 0.5%
**Hibistat Towelette** OTC *broad-spectrum antimicrobial; germicidal* [chlorhexidine gluconate; alcohol 70%] 0.5%
**HibTITER** IM injection ℞ *Haemophilus influenzae type b (HIB) vaccine* [Hemophilus b conjugate vaccine] 0.5 mL
**Hi-Cal VM** nutrition bar OTC *enteral nutritional therapy for HIV and AIDS*
**Hi-Cor 1.0; Hi-Cor 2.5** cream ℞ *topical corticosteroid* [hydrocortisone] 1%; 2.5%
**HIDA (hepatoiminodiacetic acid)** [see: lidofenin]
**HiDAC (high-dose ara-C)** *chemotherapy protocol*

**high molecular weight dextran** [see: dextran 70]
**High Potency N-Vites** tablets OTC *vitamin supplement* [multiple B vitamins; vitamin C] ± •500 mg
**High Potency Tar** gel shampoo OTC *antiseborrheic; antipsoriatic; antipruritic; antibacterial* [coal tar] 25%
**hikori** *street drug slang* [see: mescaline]
**hikuli** *street drug slang* [see: mescaline]
**Him** *street drug slang* [see: heroin]
**Hinkley** *street drug slang* [see: PCP]
**hioxifilcon A** USAN *hydrophilic contact lens material*
**Hipotest** tablets OTC *dietary supplement* [multiple vitamins, minerals, and food products; calcium; iron; biotin] ± •53.5•50•0.001 mg
**Hi-Po-Vites** tablets OTC *dietary supplement* [multiple vitamins, minerals, and food products; iron; folic acid; biotin] ± •6•0.4•1 mg
**Hiprex** tablets ℞ *urinary bactericidal* [methenamine hippurate] 1 g
**hiropon** *street drug slang for smokable methamphetamine* [see: methamphetamine HCl]
**hirudin, recombinant** *investigational anticoagulant and antithrombotic*
**Hirulog** ℞ *investigational agent for DVT and unstable angina, and to prevent reocclusion in MI and angioplasty* [bivalirudin]
**Hismanal** tablets ℞ *nonsedating antihistamine* [astemizole] 10 mg
**Hismanal-D** ℞ *investigational antihistamine/decongestant combination* [astemizole; pseudoephedrine HCl]
**Histagesic Modified** tablets OTC *decongestant; antihistamine; analgesic* [phenylephrine HCl; chlorpheniramine maleate; acetaminophen] 10•4•324 mg
**Histaject** subcu or IM injection (discontinued 1996) ℞ *antihistamine; anaphylaxis* [brompheniramine maleate] 10 mg/mL
**Histalet** syrup ℞ *decongestant; antihistamine* [pseudoephedrine HCl; chlorpheniramine maleate] 45•3 mg/5 mL
**Histalet Forte** tablets ℞ *decongestant; antihistamine* [phenylpropanolamine

HCl; phenylephrine HCl; chlorpheniramine maleate; pyrilamine maleate] 50•10•4•25 mg

**Histalet X** tablets, syrup ℞ *decongestant; expectorant* [pseudoephedrine HCl; guaifenesin] 120•400 mg; 45•200 mg/5 mL

**Histamic** sustained-release capsules ℞ *decongestant; antihistamine* [phenylpropanolamine HCl; phenylephrine HCl; chlorpheniramine maleate; phenyltoloxamine citrate]

**histamine dihydrochloride** USAN

**histamine H₁ antagonists** *a class of antihistamines* [also called: H₁ blockers]

**histamine H₂ antagonists** *a class of antihistamines* [also called: H₂ blockers]

**histamine phosphate** USP *gastric secretory stimulant; diagnostic aid for pheochromocytoma*

**histantin** [see: chlorcyclizine HCl]

**histapyrrodine** INN

**Histatab Plus** tablets OTC *decongestant; antihistamine* [phenylephrine HCl; chlorpheniramine maleate] 5•2 mg

**Histatime Forte** tablets (discontinued 1993) ℞ *decongestant; antihistamine* [phenylpropanolamine HCl; phenylephrine HCl; chlorpheniramine maleate; pyrilamine maleate] ⃞ Histatan

**Hista-Vadrin** tablets ℞ *decongestant; antihistamine* [phenylpropanolamine HCl; phenylephrine HCl; chlorpheniramine maleate] 40•5•6 mg

**Histerone 50** IM injection (discontinued 1994) ℞ *androgen replacement for delayed puberty or breast cancer* [testosterone] 50 mg/mL

**Histerone 100** IM injection ℞ *androgen replacement for delayed puberty or breast cancer* [testosterone] 100 mg/mL

**histidine (L-histidine)** USAN, USP, INN *amino acid (essential in infants and in renal failure, nonessential otherwise); symbols: His, H*

**histidine monohydrochloride** NF

**495-L-histidineglucosylceramidase** [see: imiglucerase]

**Histine DM** syrup ℞ *antitussive; decongestant; antihistamine* [dextromethorphan hydrobromide; phenyl-

propanolamine HCl; brompheniramine maleate] 10•12.5•2 mg/5 mL

**Histinex HC** syrup ℞ *narcotic antitussive; decongestant; antihistamine* [hydrocodone bitartrate; phenylephrine HCl; chlorpheniramine maleate] 2•5•2 mg/5 mL

**Histinex PV** syrup ℞ *narcotic antitussive; decongestant; antihistamine* [hydrocodone bitartrate; pseudoephedrine HCl; chlorpheniramine maleate] 2.5•30•2 mg/5 mL

**Histodrix** sustained-release tablets (discontinued 1993) OTC *decongestant; antihistamine* [pseudoephedrine sulfate; dexbrompheniramine maleate]

**Histolyn-CYL** intradermal injection ℞ *diagnostic aid for histoplasmosis* [histoplasmin (mycelial derivative)] 1:100

**histoplasmin** USP *dermal histoplasmosis test; Histoplasma capsulatum cultures in mycelial or yeast lysate form* 1:100 injection (yeast lysate form)

**Histor-D** syrup ℞ *decongestant; antihistamine* [phenylephrine HCl; chlorpheniramine maleate; alcohol 2%] 5•2 mg/5 mL

**Histor-D** Timecelles (sustained-release capsules) (discontinued 1995) ℞ *decongestant; antihistamine; anticholinergic* [phenylephrine HCl; chlorpheniramine maleate; methscopolamine nitrate] 20•8•2.5 mg

**Histosal** tablets OTC *decongestant; antihistamine; analgesic* [phenylpropanolamine HCl; pyrilamine maleate; acetaminophen; caffeine] 20•12.5•324•30 mg

**histrelin** USAN, INN *LHRH agonist; investigational (orphan) for acute intermittent porphyria, hereditary coproporphyria, and variegate porphyria*

**histrelin acetate** *LHRH agonist; central precocious puberty treatment (orphan)*

**Histussin D** oral liquid ℞ *narcotic antitussive; decongestant* [hydrocodone bitartrate; pseudoephedrine HCl] 5•60 mg/5 mL

**Histussin HC** syrup ℞ *narcotic antitussive; decongestant; antihistamine* [hydrocodone bitartrate; phenylephrine HCl; chlorpheniramine maleate] 2.5•5•2 mg/5 mL

**hit** *street drug slang for crack or a marijuana cigarette* [see: cocaine, crack; marijuana]

**HIV immune globulin (HIVIG)** [see: human immunodeficiency virus immune globulin]

**HIV immunotherapeutic (HIV-IT)** *investigational (Phase II/III) gene therapy for HIV infection*

**HIV protease inhibitors** *a class of antivirals that block HIV replication*

**HIV vaccine** [see: AIDS vaccine]

**HIV-1 LA test** [see: Recombigen HIV-1 LA]

**HIV-1 peptide vaccine** *investigational (Phase I) vaccine for HIV*

**HIVAB HIV-1 EIA; HIVAB HIV-1/ HIV-2 EIA; HIVAB HIV-2 EIA** reagent kit for professional use *in vitro diagnostic aid for HIV antibodies* [enzyme immunoassay (EIA)]

**HIVAG-1** reagent kit for professional use *in vitro diagnostic aid for HIV antibodies* [enzyme immunoassay (EIA)]

**Hi-Value III; Hi-Value V** ℞ *investigational in vitro diagnostic aid for glucose levels*

**Hi-Vegi-Lip** tablets OTC *digestive enzymes* [pancreatin; lipase; protease; amylase] 2400 mg•4800 U•60 000 U•60 000 U

**Hivid** film-coated tablets ℞ *antiviral for advanced HIV infection and AIDS (orphan)* [zalcitabine] 0.375, 0.75 mg

**HIV-IG** ℞ *investigational (Phase III, orphan) immunomodulator for AIDS and maternal/fetal HIV transfer* [HIV immune globulin]

**HIV-neutralizing antibodies** *orphan status withdrawn 1997*

**HMB (homatropine methylbromide)** [q.v.]

**HMDP (hydroxymethylene diphosphonate)** [see: oxidronic acid]

**hMG (human menopausal gonadotropin)** [see: menotropins]

**HMG-CoA (3-hydroxy-3-methylglutaryl-coenzyme A) reductase inhibitors** *a class of antihyperlipi-*demics that reduce serum LDL, VLDL, and triglycerides, but increase HDL

**HMM (hexamethylmelamine)** [see: altretamine]

**HMS** eye drop suspension ℞ *ophthalmic topical corticosteroidal anti-inflammatory* [medrysone] 1%

**HN₂ (nitrogen mustard)** [see: mechlorethamine HCl]

**hNGF (human nerve growth factor)** [see: nerve growth factor]

**HNK-20** *investigational (Phase III) monoclonal antibody for respiratory syncytial virus (RSV) infections in infants*

**HOAP-BLEO (hydroxydaunomycin, Oncovin, ara-C, prednisone, bleomycin)** *chemotherapy protocol*

**hocus** *street drug slang* [see: marijuana; opium]

**hog** *street drug slang* [see: PCP]

**Hold DM; Children's Hold** lozenges OTC *antitussive* [dextromethorphan hydrobromide] 5 mg

**holmium** *element* (Ho)

**homarylamine** INN

**homatropine** BAN *ophthalmic anticholinergic* [also: homatropine hydrobromide]

**homatropine hydrobromide** USP *ophthalmic anticholinergic; cycloplegic; mydriatic* [also: homatropine] 5% eye drops

**homatropine methylbromide** USP, INN, BAN *GI anticholinergic/antispasmodic*

**hombre** (Spanish for "man") *street drug slang* [see: heroin]

**hombrecitos** (Spanish for "little men") *street drug slang* [see: psilocybin]

**Home Access; Home Access Express** test kit for home use OTC *in vitro diagnostic aid for HIV in the blood*

**homegrown** *street drug slang* [see: marijuana]

**homer** *street drug slang for freebase cocaine* [see: cocaine, crack]

**homidium bromide** INN, BAN

**Hominex-1** powder OTC *formula for infants with homocystinuria or hypermethioninemia*

**Hominex-2** powder OTC *enteral nutritional therapy for homocystinuria or hypermethioninemia*

**homochlorcyclizine** INN, BAN

**homofenazine (HFZ)** INN

**homomenthyl salicylate** [now: homosalate]

**homopipramol** INN

**homosalate** USAN, INN *ultraviolet screen*

**4-homosulfanilamide** [see: mafenide]

**homprenorphine** INN, BAN

**honey blunts** *street drug slang for marijuana cigars sealed with honey* [see: marijuana]

**honey oil** *street drug slang* [see: ketamine HCl]

**hong-yen** *street drug slang for heroin in pill form* [see: heroin]

**hooch** *street drug slang* [see: marijuana]

**hooter** *street drug slang* [see: cocaine; marijuana]

**HOP (hydroxydaunomycin, Oncovin, prednisone)** *chemotherapy protocol*

**hop; hops** *street drug slang for opium* [see: opium]

**hopantenic acid** INN

**hoquizil** INN *bronchodilator* [also: hoquizil HCl]

**hoquizil HCl** USAN *bronchodilator* [also: hoquizil]

**horning** *street drug slang for powdered cocaine or heroin* [see: cocaine; heroin]

**horse** *street drug slang* [see: heroin]

**horse heads** *street drug slang* [see: amphetamines]

**horse tracks; horse tranquilizer** *street drug slang* [see: PCP]

**hot dope** *street drug slang* [see: heroin]

**hot heroin** *street drug slang for poisoned heroin to give to a police informant* [see: heroin]

**hot ice** *street drug slang for smokable methamphetamine* [see: methamphetamine HCl]

**hot stick** *street drug slang for a marijuana cigarette* [see: marijuana]

**hotcakes** *street drug slang* [see: cocaine, crack]

**How do you like me now?** *street drug slang* [see: cocaine, crack]

**hows** *street drug slang* [see: morphine]

**H.P. Acthar Gel** IM or subcu injectable gel ℞ *steroid* [repository corticotropin] 40, 80 U/mL

**HPA-23** *orphan status withdrawn 1994*

**HPMCP (hydroxypropyl methylcellulose phthalate)** [q.v.]

**HPMPC (3-hydroxy-2-phosphonomethoxypropyl cytosine [dihydrate])** [see: cidofovir]

**H-R Lubricating** vaginal jelly OTC *lubricant* [hydroxypropyl methylcellulose]

**HRT** ℞ *investigational hormone replacement therapy for osteoporosis* [norethindrone acetate; ethinyl estradiol]

**5-HT (5-hydroxytryptamine)** [see: serotonin]

**HT (human thrombin)** [see: thrombin]

**HT; 3-HT (3-hydroxytyramine)** [see: dopamine]

**H-Tuss-D** liquid ℞ *narcotic antitussive; decongestant* [hydrocodone bitartrate; pseudoephedrine HCl; alcohol 5%] 5•60 mg/5 mL

**HU-211** *investigational antiglaucoma agent*

**hubba; hubbas; Hubba, I am back** *street drug slang* [see: cocaine, crack]

**hug drug; huggers** *street drug slang* [see: MDMA]

**Hulk Hogan Complete Multi-Vitamins** chewable tablets (discontinued 1993) OTC *vitamin/mineral supplement* [multiple vitamins & minerals; folic acid; biotin]

**Hulk Hogan Multi-Vitamins Plus Extra C** chewable tablets (discontinued 1993) OTC *vitamin supplement* [multiple vitamins; folic acid]

**Hulk Hogan Multi-Vitamins Plus Iron** chewable tablets (discontinued 1993) OTC *vitamin/iron supplement* [multiple vitamins; iron; folic acid]

**Humalog** subcu injection, prefilled syringe cartridges ℞ *insulin analog for diabetes* [human insulin lispro (rDNA)] 100 U/mL; 1.5 mL

**human acid alpha-glucosidase** *investigational (orphan) for glycogen storage disease type II*

**human albumin** [see: albumin, human]

**human amniotic fluid-derived surfactant** [see: surfactant, human amniotic fluid derived]

**human antihemophilic factor** [see: antihemophilic factor]

**human chorionic gonadotropin (hCG)** [see: gonadotropin, chorionic]

**human complement receptor** [see: complement receptor type I, soluble recombinant human]

**human cytomegalovirus immune globulin** [see: cytomegalovirus immune globulin, human]

**human diploid cell vaccine (HDCV)** [see: rabies vaccine]

**human epidermal growth factor** [see: epidermal growth factor, human]

**human fibrinogen** [see: fibrinogen, human]

**human fibrinolysin** [see: fibrinolysin, human]

**human follicle-stimulating hormone (hFSH)** [now: menotropins]

**human growth hormone (hGH)** JAN *growth hormone* [also: somatropin]

**human growth hormone, recombinant (rhGH)** *orphan status withdrawn 1993* [see: somatropin]

**human growth hormone releasing factor** [see: growth hormone-releasing factor]

**human IgM MAb (C-58) to cytomegalovirus (CMV)** *orphan status withdrawn 1994*

**human immunodeficiency virus (HIV-1) immune globulin (HIVIG)** *investigational (Phase III, orphan) immunomodulator for AIDS and maternal/fetal HIV transfer*

**human insulin** [see: insulin, human]

**human luteinizing hormone, recombinant & menotropins** *investigational (orphan) for chronic anovulation due to hypogonadotropic hypogonadism*

**human menopausal gonadotropin (hMG)** [see: menotropins]

**human nerve growth factor (hNGF)** [see: nerve growth factor]

**human respiratory syncytial virus immune globulin** [see: respiratory syncytial virus immune globulin, human]

**human serum albumin diethylene-triaminepentaacetic acid (DTPA) technetium ($^{99m}$Tc)** JAN *radioactive agent* [also: technetium Tc 99m pentetate]

**human superoxide dismutase (SOD)** [see: superoxide dismutase, human]

**Human Surf** *orphan status withdrawn 1994* [surfactant, human amniotic fluid derived]

**human T-cell inhibitor** [see: muromonab-CD3]

**human T-cell lymphotrophic virus type III (HTLV-III)** [now: human immunodeficiency virus (HIV)]

**Human T-Lymphotropic Virus Type I EIA** *reagent kit for professional use in vitro diagnostic aid for HTLV I antibody in serum or plasma* [enzyme immunoassay (EIA)]

**Humate-P** IV injection ℞ *antihemophilic; investigational (orphan) for von Willebrand's disease* [antihemophilic factor VIII] ?

**Humatin** capsules ℞ *aminoglycoside-type antibiotic; amebicide* [paromomycin sulfate] 250 mg

**Humatrope** powder for subcu or IM injection ℞ *growth hormone for congenital or renal-induced growth failure (orphan); investigational (orphan) for severe burns* [somatropin] 5 mg (15 IU) per vial

**Humegon** powder for IM injection ℞ *ovulation stimulant for women; spermatogenesis stimulant for men* [menotropins] 75, 150 IU

**Humibid DM** sustained-release tablets ℞ *antitussive; expectorant* [dextromethorphan hydrobromide; guaifenesin] 30•600 mg

**Humibid DM Sprinkle** sustained-release capsules ℞ *antitussive; expectorant* [dextromethorphan hydrobromide; guaifenesin] 15•300 mg

**Humibid L.A.** sustained-release tablets ℞ *expectorant* [guaifenesin] 600 mg

**Humibid Sprinkle** sustained-release capsules ℞ *expectorant* [guaifenesin] 300 mg

**HuMist** nasal mist OTC *nasal moisturizer* [sodium chloride (saline)] 0.65%

**Humorphan H.P.** (name changed to Numorphan HP in 1996)

**Humorsol** Ocumeter (eye drops) Ṛ *antiglaucoma agent; reversible cholinesterase inhibitor miotic* [demecarium bromide] 0.125%, 0.25%

**Humulin 30/70** ⓒⒶⓃ (U.S. product: Humulin 70/30) subcu injection, prefilled syringe cartridges OTC *antidiabetic* [insulin; isophane insulin] 100 U/mL; 1.5 mL

**Humulin 50/50** subcu injection (prefilled cartridges available in Canada) OTC *antidiabetic* [isophane human insulin (rDNA); human insulin (rDNA)] 100 U/mL; 1.5 mL

**Humulin 70/30** subcu injection, prefilled syringe cartridges OTC *antidiabetic* [isophane human insulin (rDNA); human insulin (rDNA)] 100 U/mL; 1.5 mL

**Humulin BR** subcu injection (discontinued 1994) OTC *antidiabetic* [buffered human insulin (recombinant)] 100 U/mL

**Humulin L** subcu injection OTC *antidiabetic* [human insulin zinc (rDNA)] 100 U/mL

**Humulin N** subcu injection, prefilled syringe cartridges OTC *antidiabetic* [isophane human insulin (rDNA)] 100 U/mL; 1.5 mL

**Humulin R** ⓒⒶⓃ (U.S. product: Regular Iletin I) subcu injection OTC *antidiabetic* [human insulin (recombinant)] 100 U/mL; 1.5 mL

**Humulin U Ultralente** subcu injection OTC *antidiabetic* [extended human insulin zinc (rDNA)] 100 U/mL

**Humulin-U** ⓒⒶⓃ (U.S. product: Humulin U Ultralente) subcu injection OTC *antidiabetic* [extended insulin zinc] 100 U/mL

**hunter** *street drug slang* [see: cocaine]

**Hurricaine** spray, liquid, gel OTC *mucous membrane anesthetic* [benzocaine] 20%

**HVS 1+2** solution (discontinued 1994) OTC *oral antibacterial* [benzalkonium chloride]

**HXM (hexamethylmelamine)** [see: altretamine]

**Hyacne** Ṛ *investigational (Phase III) acne treatment*

**Hyal-ct 1101** *investigational antineoplastic for basal cell carcinoma*

**hyalosidase** INN, BAN

**hyaluronate sodium** USAN, JAN *veterinary synovitis agent; ophthalmic surgical aid; investigational (Phase III) treatment for osteoarthritis and TMJ syndrome* [also: hyaluronic acid]

**hyaluronate sodium & diclofenac potassium** *investigational (Phase III) topical treatment for actinic keratosis; clinical trials as a topical analgesic discontinued 1996*

**hyaluronic acid** BAN *veterinary synovitis agent; ophthalmic surgical aid; investigational (Phase III) treatment for osteoarthritis and TMJ syndrome* [also: hyaluronate sodium]

**hyaluronidase** USP, INN, BAN *dispersion aid; absorption facilitator*

**hyaluronoglucosaminidase** [see: hyalosidase]

**hyamate** [see: buramate]

**Hyanalgese-D** Ṛ *investigational (Phase III) topical analgesic; clinical trials discontinued 1996* [hyaluronate sodium; diclofenac potassium]

**hyatari** *street drug slang* [see: mescaline]

**hybenzate** USAN *combining name for radicals or groups* [also: hibenzate]

**Hybolin Decanoate-50; Hybolin Decanoate-100** IM injection Ṛ *anabolic steroid for anemia of renal insufficiency* [nandrolone decanoate] 50 mg/mL; 100 mg/mL

**Hybolin Improved** IM injection Ṛ *anabolic steroid for metastatic breast cancer in women* [nandrolone phenpropionate] 50 mg/mL

**Hybri-CEAker** *orphan status withdrawn 1997* [indium In 111 altumomab pentetate]

**Hycamtin** powder for IV injection Ṛ *topoisomerase I inhibitor; antineoplastic for ovarian cancer* [topotecan HCl] 4 mg/vial

**hycanthone** USAN, INN *antischistosomal*

**hycanthone mesylate**

**hyclate** INN *combining name for radicals or groups*

**HycoClear Tuss** syrup ℞ *narcotic antitussive; expectorant* [hydrocodone bitartrate; guaifenesin] 5•100 mg/5 mL

**Hycodan** tablets, syrup ℞ *narcotic antitussive; GI anticholinergic/antispasmodic* [hydrocodone bitartrate; homatropine methylbromide] 5•1.5 mg; 5•1.5 mg/5 mL ⊡ Hycomine; Vicodin

**Hycomine** syrup, pediatric syrup ℞ *narcotic antitussive; decongestant* [hydrocodone bitartrate; phenylpropanolamine HCl] 5•25 mg/5 mL; 2.5•12.5 mg/5 mL ⊡ Byclomine; Hycodan; Vicodin

**Hycomine Compound** tablets ℞ *narcotic antitussive; decongestant; antihistamine; analgesic* [hydrocodone bitartrate; phenylephrine HCl; chlorpheniramine maleate; acetaminophen; caffeine] 5•10•2•250•30 mg

**Hycort** cream, ointment ℞ *topical corticosteroid* [hydrocortisone] 1%

**Hycotuss Expectorant** syrup ℞ *narcotic antitussive; expectorant* [hydrocodone bitartrate; guaifenesin; alcohol 10%] 5•100 mg/5 mL

**hydantoins** *a class of anticonvulsants*

**Hydeltrasol** IV, IM injection ℞ *glucocorticoid* [prednisolone sodium phosphate] 20 mg/mL

**Hydeltra-T.B.A.** intra-articular, intralesional, or soft tissue injection (discontinued 1997) ℞ *glucocorticoid* [prednisolone tebutate] 20 mg/mL

**Hydergine** sublingual tablets, tablets, liquid ℞ *for age-related mental capacity decline* [ergoloid mesylates] 0.5, 1 mg; 1 mg; 1 mg/mL ⊡ Hydramine

**Hydergine LC** liquid capsules ℞ *for age-related mental capacity decline* [ergoloid mesylates] 1 mg

**hydracarbazine** INN

**hydralazine** INN, BAN *antihypertensive; peripheral vasodilator* [also: hydralazine HCl]

**hydralazine HCl** USP, JAN *antihypertensive; peripheral vasodilator* [also: hydralazine] 10, 25, 50, 100 mg oral; 20 mg/mL injection

**hydralazine polistirex** USAN *antihypertensive*

**Hydramine** syrup, elixir (discontinued 1994) ℞ *antitussive* [diphenhydramine HCl] 12.5 mg/5 mL ⊡ Bydramine; Hydergine; Hydramyn; Hytramyn

**Hydramyn** syrup ℞ *antihistamine; antitussive* [diphenhydramine HCl; alcohol 5%] 12.5 mg/5 mL ⊡ Hydramine; Hytramyn

**Hydrap-ES** tablets ℞ *antihypertensive* [hydrochlorothiazide; reserpine; hydralazine HCl] 15•0.1•25 mg

**hydrargaphen** INN, BAN

**hydrastine** USP

**hydrastine HCl** USP

**hydrastinine HCl** NF

**Hydrate** IV or IM injection ℞ *antinauseant; antiemetic; antivertigo; motion sickness preventative* [dimenhydrinate] 50 mg/mL

**Hydrazide 25/25; Hydrazide 50/50** capsules (discontinued 1995) ℞ *antihypertensive* [hydrochlorothiazide; hydralazine HCl] 25•25 mg; 50•50 mg

**hydrazinecarboximidamide monohydrochloride** [see: pimagedine HCl]

**hydrazinoxane** [see: domoxin]

**Hydrea** capsules ℞ *antineoplastic for melanoma, ovarian carcinoma, and myelocytic leukemia; investigational (orphan) for sickle cell anemia* [hydroxyurea] 500 mg

**Hydrex** tablets (discontinued 1993) ℞ *diuretic; antihypertensive* [benzthiazide]

**Hydrisalic** gel (discontinued 1994) ℞ *topical keratolytic* [salicylic acid] 6%

**Hydrisea** lotion OTC *moisturizer; emollient* [Dead Sea salts]

**Hydrisinol** cream, lotion OTC *moisturizer; emollient*

**Hydro Cobex** IM injection ℞ *antianemic; vitamin $B_{12}$ supplement* [hydroxocobalamin] 1000 μg/mL

**hydrobentizide** INN

**Hydrobexan** IM injection (discontinued 1995) ℞ *antianemic; vitamin $B_{12}$ supplement* [hydroxocobalamin] 1000 μg/mL

**hydrobutamine** [see: butidrine]

**Hydrocare Cleaning and Disinfecting** solution OTC *chemical disinfecting solution for soft contact lenses*

**Hydrocare Preserved Saline** solution OTC *rinsing/storage solution for soft contact lenses* [preserved saline solution]

**Hydrocet** capsules Ɍ *narcotic analgesic* [hydrocodone bitartrate; acetaminophen] 5•500 mg

**Hydro-Chlor** tablets (discontinued 1993) Ɍ *diuretic; antihypertensive* [hydrochlorothiazide]

**hydrochloric acid** NF *acidifying agent*

**hydrochloric acid, diluted** NF *acidifying agent*

**hydrochlorothiazide (HCT; HCTZ)** USP, INN, BAN *diuretic; antihypertensive* 25, 50, 100 mg oral; 50 mg/5 mL oral; 100 mg/mL oral

**hydrocholeretics** *a class of gastrointestinal drugs that exert laxative effects and increase volume and water content of bile actions*

**Hydrocil Instant** powder OTC *bulk laxative* [psyllium hydrophilic mucilloid] 3.5 g/scoop or packet

**hydrocodone** INN, BAN *antitussive* [also: hydrocodone bitartrate]

**hydrocodone bitartrate** USAN, USP *antitussive* [also: hydrocodone]

**Hydrocodone Compound** syrup Ɍ *narcotic antitussive; GI anticholinergic/antispasmodic* [hydrocodone bitartrate; homatropine hydrobromide] 5•1.5 mg/5 mL

**Hydrocodone CP; Hydrocodone HD** oral liquid Ɍ *narcotic antitussive; decongestant; antihistamine* [hydrocodone bitartrate; phenylephrine HCl; chlorpheniramine maleate] 2.5•5•2 mg/5 mL; 1.67•5•2 mg/5 mL

**Hydrocodone GF** syrup Ɍ *narcotic antitussive; expectorant* [hydrocodone bitartrate; guaifenesin] 5•100 mg/5 mL

**Hydrocodone PA** syrup, pediatric syrup Ɍ *narcotic antitussive; decongestant* [hydrocodone bitartrate; phenylpropanolamine HCl] 5•25 mg/5 mL; 2.5•12.5 mg/5 mL

**hydrocodone polistirex** USAN *antitussive*

**hydrocolloid gel** *dressings for wet wounds*

**Hydrocort** cream Ɍ *topical corticosteroid* [hydrocortisone] 2.5%

**hydrocortamate** INN

**hydrocortamate HCl** [see: hydrocortamate]

**hydrocortisone (HC)** USP, INN, BAN *corticosteroid* 5, 10, 20 mg oral; 0.5%, 1%, 2.5% topical

**hydrocortisone aceponate** INN

**hydrocortisone acetate (HCA)** USP, BAN *corticosteroid* 25, 50 mg/mL injection

**hydrocortisone buteprate** USAN *corticosteroid*

**hydrocortisone butyrate** USAN, USP, BAN *topical corticosteroid*

**hydrocortisone cyclopentylpropionate** [see: hydrocortisone cypionate]

**hydrocortisone cypionate** USP *glucocorticoid*

**hydrocortisone hemisuccinate** USP *adrenocortical steroid*

**hydrocortisone sodium phosphate** USP, BAN *glucocorticoid*

**hydrocortisone sodium succinate** USP, BAN *glucocorticoid*

**hydrocortisone valerate** USAN, USP *topical corticosteroid*

**Hydrocortone** tablets Ɍ *glucocorticoids* [hydrocortisone] 10, 20 mg

**Hydrocortone Acetate** intralesional, intra-articular, or soft tissue injection Ɍ *glucocorticoids* [hydrocortisone acetate] 25, 50 mg/mL

**Hydrocortone Phosphate** IV, subcu, or IM injection Ɍ *glucocorticoids* [hydrocortisone sodium phosphate] 50 mg/mL

**Hydrocream Base** OTC *cream base*

**Hydro-Crysti 12** IM injection Ɍ *antianemic; vitamin $B_{12}$ supplement* [hydroxocobalamin] 1000 µg/mL

**HydroDIURIL** tablets Ɍ *diuretic; antihypertensive* [hydrochlorothiazide] 25, 50, 100 mg

**hydrofilcon A** USAN *hydrophilic contact lens material*

**hydroflumethiazide** USP, INN, BAN *antihypertensive; diuretic* 50 mg oral

**hydrofluoric acid** *dental caries prophylactic*

**hydrogen** *element (H)*

**hydrogen peroxide** USP *topical antiinfective*

**hydrogen tetrabromoaurate** [see: bromauric acid]

**hydrogenated ergot alkaloids** [now: ergoloid mesylates]

**hydrogenated vegetable oil** [see: vegetable oil, hydrogenated]

**Hydrogesic** capsules ℞ *narcotic analgesic* [hydrocodone bitartrate; acetaminophen] 5•500 mg

**hydromadinone** INN

**Hydromal** tablets (discontinued 1993) ℞ *diuretic; antihypertensive* [hydrochlorothiazide]

**Hydromet** syrup ℞ *narcotic antitussive; GI anticholinergic/antispasmodic* [hydrocodone bitartrate; homatropine methylbromide] 5•1.5 mg/5 mL

**hydromorphinol** INN, BAN

**hydromorphone** INN, BAN *narcotic analgesic; widely abused as a street drug* [also: hydromorphone HCl]

**hydromorphone HCl** USP *narcotic analgesic; widely abused as a street drug* [also: hydromorphone] 2, 4 mg oral; 1, 2, 3, 4, 10 mg/mL injection

**hydromorphone sulfate**

**Hydromox** tablets ℞ *diuretic; antihypertensive* [quinethazone] 50 mg

**Hydropane** syrup (name changed to Hydrocodone Compound in 1995)

**Hydro-Par** tablets ℞ *diuretic; antihypertensive* [hydrochlorothiazide] 25, 50 mg

**Hydropel** ointment OTC *skin protectant* [silicone; hydrophobic starch derivative] 30%•10%

**4-hydroperoxycyclophosphamide (4-HC)** *orphan status withdrawn 1994*

**Hydrophed** tablets ℞ *antiasthmatic; bronchodilator; decongestant; anxiolytic* [theophylline; ephedrine sulfate; hydroxyzine HCl] 130•25•10 mg

**Hydrophilic** OTC *ointment base*

**hydrophilic ointment** [see: ointment, hydrophilic]

**hydrophilic petrolatum** [see: petrolatum, hydrophilic]

**Hydropine; Hydropine H.P.** tablets (discontinued 1993) ℞ *antihypertensive* [hydroflumethiazide; reserpine] ⓓ Hydropane; Hydrophen

**Hydropres-25** tablets (discontinued 1996) ℞ *antihypertensive* [hydrochlorothiazide; reserpine] 25•0.125 mg

**Hydropres-50** tablets ℞ *antihypertensive* [hydrochlorothiazide; reserpine] 50•0.125 mg

**hydroquinone** USP *hyperpigmentation bleaching agent* 3%, 4% topical

**Hydro-Serp** tablets ℞ *antihypertensive* [hydrochlorothiazide; reserpine] 50•0.125 mg

**Hydroserpine #1; Hydroserpine #2** tablets ℞ *antihypertensive* [hydrochlorothiazide; reserpine] 25•0.125 mg; 50•0.125 mg

**Hydrosine 25, Hydrosine 50** tablets ℞ *antihypertensive* [hydrochlorothiazide; reserpine]

**HydroStat IR** tablets ℞ *narcotic analgesic* [hydromorphone HCl] 1, 2, 3, 4 mg

**Hydro-T** tablets (discontinued 1993) ℞ *diuretic; antihypertensive* [hydrochlorothiazide]

**hydrotalcite** INN, BAN

**HydroTex** cream ℞ *topical corticosteroid* [hydrocortisone] 0.5%

**HydroTex** ointment (discontinued 1993) ℞ *topical corticosteroid* [hydrocortisone]

**Hydroxacen** injection (discontinued 1994) ℞ *anxiolytic; antihistamine* [hydroxyzine HCl] 50 mg/mL

**hydroxamethocaine** BAN [also: hydroxytetracaine]

**hydroxidione sodium succinate** [see: hydroxydione sodium succinate]

**hydroxindasate** INN

**hydroxindasol** INN

**hydroxizine chloride** [see: hydroxyzine HCl]

**hydroxocobalamin** USAN, USP, INN, BAN, JAN *vitamin $B_{12}$; hematopoietic* [also: hydroxocobalamin acetate] 1 mg/mL injection

**hydroxocobalamin acetate** JAN *vitamin $B_{12}$; hematopoietic* [also: hydroxocobalamin]

**hydroxocobalamin & sodium thiosulfate** *investigational (orphan) for severe acute cyanide poisoning*

**hydroxocobemine** [see: hydroxocobalamin]

**3-hydroxy-2-phosphonomethoxypropyl cytosine (HPMPC) dihydrate** [see: cidofovir]

**N-hydroxyacetamide** [see: acetohydroxamic acid]

**4′-hydroxyacetanilide** [see: acetaminophen]

**4′-hydroxyacetanilide salicylate** [see: acetaminosalol]

**hydroxyamfetamine** INN *ophthalmic adrenergic; mydriatic* [also: hydroxyamphetamine hydrobromide; hydroxyamphetamine]

**hydroxyamphetamine** BAN *ophthalmic adrenergic; mydriatic* [also: hydroxyamphetamine hydrobromide; hydroxyamfetamine]

**hydroxyamphetamine hydrobromide** USP *ophthalmic adrenergic/vasoconstrictor; mydriatic* [also: hydroxyamfetamine; hydroxyamphetamine]

**hydroxyapatite** BAN *prosthetic aid* [also: durapatite; calcium phosphate, tribasic]

**2-hydroxybenzamide** [see: salicylamide]

**2-hydroxybenzoic acid** [see: salicylic acid]

**o-hydroxybenzyl alcohol** [see: salicyl alcohol]

**hydroxybutanedioic acid** [see: malic acid]

**4-hydroxybutanoic acid, sodium salt** [see: sodium oxybate]

**hydroxybutyrate sodium, gamma** [see: sodium oxybate]

**hydroxycarbamide** INN *antineoplastic* [also: hydroxyurea]

**hydroxychloroquine** INN, BAN *antimalarial; lupus erythematosus suppressant* [also: hydroxychloroquine sulfate]

**hydroxychloroquine sulfate** USP *antimalarial; antirheumatic; lupus erythematosus suppressant* [also: hydroxychloroquine] 200 mg oral

**25-hydroxycholecalciferol** [see: calcifediol]

**hydroxycincophene** [see: oxycinchophen]

**hydroxydaunomycin** [see: doxorubicin]

**14-hydroxydihydromorphine** [see: hydromorphinol]

**hydroxydione sodium succinate** INN, BAN

**hydroxyethyl cellulose** NF *suspending and viscosity-increasing agent; ophthalmic aid*

**2-hydroxyethyl methacrylate (HEMA)** *contact lens material*

**hydroxyethyl starch (HES)** [see: hetastarch]

**hydroxyethylstarch** JAN *plasma volume extender* [also: hetastarch]

**hydroxyhexamide**

**hydroxylapatite** [see: durapatite; calcium phosphate, tribasic]

**hydroxymagnesium aluminate** [see: magaldrate]

**hydroxymesterone** [see: medrysone]

**hydroxymethylene diphosphonate (HMDP)** [see: oxidronic acid]

**hydroxymethylgramicidin** [see: methocidin]

**N-hydroxynaphthalimide diethyl phosphate** [see: naftalofos]

**hydroxypethidine** INN, BAN

**hydroxyphenamate** USAN *minor tranquilizer* [also: oxyfenamate]

**hydroxyprocaine** INN, BAN

**hydroxyprogesterone** INN, BAN *progestin* [also: hydroxyprogesterone caproate]

**hydroxyprogesterone caproate** USP, INN, JAN *progestin for amenorrhea, metrorrhagia, and dysfunctional uterine bleeding* [also: hydroxyprogesterone] 125, 250 mg/mL IM injection (in oil)

**2-hydroxypropanoic acid, calcium salt, hydrate** [see: calcium lactate]

**hydroxypropyl cellulose** NF *topical protectant; emulsifying and coating agent* [also: hydroxypropylcellulose]

**hydroxypropyl methylcellulose** USP *suspending and viscosity-increasing agent; ophthalmic surgical aid* [also: hypromellose; hydroxypropylmethylcellulose]

**hydroxypropyl methylcellulose 1828** USP

**hydroxypropyl methylcellulose phthalate (HPMCP)** NF *tablet-coating agent* [also: hydroxypropylmethylcellulose phthalate]

**hydroxypropyl methylcellulose phthalate 200731** NF *tablet-coating agent*

**hydroxypropyl methylcellulose phthalate 220824** NF *tablet-coating agent*

**hydroxypropylcellulose** JAN *topical protectant; emulsifying and coating agent* [also: hydroxypropyl cellulose]

**hydroxypropylmethylcellulose** JAN *suspending and viscosity-increasing agent; ophthalmic surgical aid* [also: hydroxypropyl methylcellulose; hypromellose]

**hydroxypropylmethylcellulose phthalate** JAN *tablet-coating agent* [also: hydroxypropyl methylcellulose phthalate]

**hydroxypyridine tartrate** INN

**hydroxyquinoline** *topical antiseptic*

**4′-hydroxysalicylanilide** [see: osalmid]

**hydroxystearin sulfate** NF

**hydroxystenozole** INN

**hydroxystilbamidine** INN, BAN *antileishmanial* [also: hydroxystilbamidine isethionate]

**hydroxystilbamidine isethionate** USP *antileishmanial* [also: hydroxystilbamidine]

**hydroxysuccinic acid** [see: malic acid]

**hydroxytetracaine** INN [also: hydroxamethocaine]

**hydroxytoluic acid** INN, BAN

**5-hydroxytryptamine (5-HT)** [see: serotonin]

**5-hydroxytryptamine$_3$ (5-HT$_3$) receptor antagonists** *a class of antinauseant and antiemetic agents used primarily after emetogenic cancer chemotherapy*

**hydroxytryptophan** [see: L-5 hydroxytryptophan]

**3-hydroxytyramine (HT; 3-HT)** [see: dopamine]

**hydroxyurea** USAN, USP, BAN *antineoplastic; investigational (orphan) for* sickle cell anemia [also: hydroxycarbamide] 500 mg oral

**hydroxyzine** INN, BAN *anxiolytic; minor tranquilizer; antihistamine; antipruritic* [also: hydroxyzine HCl]

**hydroxyzine HCl** USP *anxiolytic; minor tranquilizer; antihistamine; antipruritic* [also: hydroxyzine] 10, 25, 50 mg oral; 10 mg/5 mL oral; 25, 50 mg/mL injection

**hydroxyzine pamoate** USP *minor tranquilizer* 25, 50, 100 mg oral

**Hydrozide-50** tablets (discontinued 1993) ℞ *diuretic; antihypertensive* [hydrochlorothiazide]

**hy-Flow** solution (discontinued 1993) OTC *wetting solution for hard contact lenses*

**Hygenic Cleansing** anorectal pads OTC *moisturizer and cleanser for external rectal/vaginal areas; astringent* [witch hazel] 50%

**Hygroton** tablets ℞ *diuretic; antihypertensive* [chlorthalidone] 25, 50, 100 mg ② Regroton

**Hylidone** tablets (discontinued 1993) ℞ *antihypertensive* [chlorthalidone]

**Hyliver Plus** IM injection (discontinued 1994) ℞ *antianemic; vitamin supplement* [liver extracts; vitamin B$_{12}$; folic acid]

**Hylorel** tablets ℞ *antihypertensive* [guanadrel sulfate] 10, 25 mg

**Hylutin** IM injection ℞ *progestin for amenorrhea, metrorrhagia, and dysfunctional uterine bleeding* [hydroxyprogesterone caproate in oil] 250 mg/mL

**hymecromone** USAN, INN *choleretic*

**hyoscine hydrobromide** BAN *GI antispasmodic; prevent motion sickness; cycloplegic; mydriatic* [also: scopolamine hydrobromide]

**hyoscine methobromide** BAN *anticholinergic* [also: methscopolamine bromide]

**hyoscyamine (L-hyoscyamine)** USP, BAN *anticholinergic*

**hyoscyamine hydrobromide** USP *anticholinergic*

**hyoscyamine sulfate** USP *GI anticholinergic/antispasmodic* [also: hyoscyamine sulphate] 0.375 mg oral; 0.125 mg/mL oral

**hyoscyamine sulphate** BAN GI *anticholinergic/antispasmodic* [also: hyoscyamine sulfate]

**Hyosophen** tablets, elixir ℞ *GI anticholinergic; sedative* [atropine sulfate; scopolamine hydrobromide; hyoscyamine hydrobromide; phenobarbital] 0.0194•0.0065•0.1037•16.2 mg; 0.0194•0.0065•0.1037•16.2 mg/5 mL

**Hypaque Meglumine** injection ℞ *parenteral radiopaque agent* [diatrizoate meglumine] 30%, 60%

**Hypaque Sodium** injection ℞ *GI contrast radiopaque agent* [diatrizoate sodium] 20%, 25%, 50%

**Hypaque Sodium** solution, powder ℞ *GI contrast radiopaque agent* [diatrizoate sodium] 41.66%; 100%

**Hypaque-Cysto** intracavitary instillation ℞ *cholecystographic radiopaque agent* [diatrizoate meglumine] 30%

**Hypaque-M 75; Hypaque-M 90; Hypaque-76** injection ℞ *parenteral radiopaque agent* [diatrizoate meglumine; diatrizoate sodium] 50%•25%; 60%•30%; 66%•10%

**Hyperab** IM injection ℞ *rabies prophylaxis* [rabies immune globulin] 150 IU/mL

**HyperGAM+CF** ℞ *investigational vaccine for Pseudomonas aeruginosa lung infections associated with cystic fibrosis* [polyclonal antibodies]

**HyperHep** IM injection ℞ *hepatitis B immunizing agent* [hepatitis B immune globulin] 0.5, 1, 5 mL ② Hyper-Tet; Hyperstat

**hypericin** *investigational (Phase I) antiviral for HIV and AIDS*

**Hyperlyte; Hyperlyte CR; Hyperlyte R** IV admixture ℞ *intravenous electrolyte therapy* [combined electrolyte solution]

**Hypermune RSV** ℞ *preventative for respiratory syncytial virus (RSV) infections in high-risk infants (orphan)* [respiratory syncytial virus immune globulin (RSV-IG)]

**Hyperstat** IV injection ℞ *antihypertensive for hypertensive emergencies* [diazoxide] 15 mg/mL ② Hyper-Tet; HyperHep; Nitrostat

**Hyper-Tet** IM injection ℞ *tetanus immunizing agent* [tetanus immune globulin] 250 U ② HyperHep; Hyperstat

**Hypervax** ℞ *investigational anti-infective for renal dialysis patients* [Staphylococcus aureus vaccine]

**Hy-Phen** tablets ℞ *narcotic analgesic* [hydrocodone bitartrate; acetaminophen] 5•500 mg

**hyphylline** [see: dyphylline]

**hypnogene** [see: barbital]

**hypochlorous acid, sodium salt** [see: sodium hypochlorite]

**β-hypophamine** [see: vasopressin]

**α-hypophamine** [see: oxytocin]

**hypophosphorous acid** NF *antioxidant*

**Hyporet** (trademarked delivery system) *prefilled disposable syringe*

**HypoTears** ophthalmic ointment OTC *ocular moisturizer/lubricant* [white petrolatum; mineral oil]

**HypoTears; HypoTears PF** eye drops OTC *ocular moisturizer/lubricant* [polyvinyl alcohol] 1%

**HypoTears PF** ophthalmic ointment (discontinued 1993) OTC *ocular moisturizer/lubricant*

**HypRho-D; HypRho-D Mini-Dose** IM injection ℞ *obstetric Rh factor immunity suppressant* [$Rh_0(D)$ immune globulin] 300 μg; 50 μg

**Hyprogest 250** IM injection ℞ *progestin for amenorrhea, metrorrhagia, and dysfunctional uterine bleeding* [hydroxyprogesterone caproate in oil] 250 mg/mL

**hyprolose** [see: hydroxypropyl cellulose]

**hypromellose** INN, BAN *suspending and viscosity-increasing agent* [also: hydroxypropyl methylcellulose; hydroxypropylmethylcellulose]

**Hyrexin-50** injection ℞ *antihistamine; motion sickness preventative; sleep aid; antiparkinsonian* [diphenhydramine HCl] 50 mg/mL

**Hyskon** uterine infusion ℞ *hysteroscopy aid* [dextran 70; dextrose] 32%•10%

**Hysone** cream OTC *topical corticosteroid; antifungal; antibacterial* [hydrocortisone; clioquinol] 10•30 mg/g

**Hytakerol** capsules, oral solution ℞ *vitamin deficiency therapy* [dihydrotachysterol] 0.125 mg; 0.25 mg/mL

**Hytinic** capsules OTC *hematinic* [polysaccharide-iron complex] 150 mg

**Hytinic** IM injection ℞ *hematinic* [ferrous gluconate; multiple B vitamins; procaine HCl] 3 mg/mL• ± •2%

**Hytone** cream, lotion, ointment ℞ *topical corticosteroid* [hydrocortisone] 1%, 2.5%; 1%, 2.5%; 2.5% ⊡ Vytone

**Hytone 1%** ointment, spray ℞ *topical corticosteroid* [hydrocortisone] 1%

**Hytrin** soft capsules ℞ *antihypertensive; antiadrenergic; treatment for benign prostatic hyperplasia* [terazosin HCl] 1, 2, 5, 10 mg

**Hytrin** ⒸⒶⓃ tablets ℞ *antihypertensive; antiadrenergic; treatment for benign prostatic hyperplasia* [terazosin HCl] 1, 2, 5, 10 mg

**Hytuss** tablets OTC *expectorant* [guaifenesin] 100 mg

**Hytuss 2X** capsules OTC *expectorant* [guaifenesin] 200 mg

**Hyzaar** film-coated tablets ℞ *antihypertensive; angiotensin II blocker; diuretic* [losartan potassium; hydrochlorothiazide] 50•12.5 mg

**Hyzine-50** IM injection ℞ *anxiolytic* [hydroxyzine HCl] 50 mg/mL

# I

**I am back** *street drug slang* [see: cocaine, crack]

$^{123}$**I** [see: iodohippurate sodium I 123]

$^{123}$**I** [see: sodium iodide I 123]

$^{125}$**I** [see: albumin, iodinated I 125 serum]

$^{125}$**I** [see: diatrizoate sodium I 125]

$^{125}$**I** [see: diohippuric acid I 125]

$^{125}$**I** [see: diotyrosine I 125]

$^{125}$**I** [see: fibrinogen I 125]

$^{125}$**I** [see: insulin I 125]

$^{125}$**I** [see: iodohippurate sodium I 125]

$^{125}$**I** [see: iodopyracet I 125]

$^{125}$**I** [see: iomethin I 125]

$^{125}$**I** [see: iothalamate sodium I 125]

$^{125}$**I** [see: liothyronine I 125]

$^{125}$**I** [see: oleic acid I 125]

$^{125}$**I** [see: povidone I 125]

$^{125}$**I** [see: rose bengal sodium I 125]

$^{125}$**I** [see: sodium iodide I 125]

$^{125}$**I** [see: thyroxine I 125]

$^{125}$**I** [see: triolein I 125]

$^{131}$**I** [see: albumin, aggregated iodinated I 131 serum]

$^{131}$**I** [see: albumin, iodinated I 131 serum]

$^{131}$**I** [see: diatrizoate sodium I 131]

$^{131}$**I** [see: diohippuric acid I 131]

$^{131}$**I** [see: diotyrosine I 131]

$^{131}$**I** [see: ethiodized oil I 131]

$^{131}$**I** [see: insulin I 131]

$^{131}$**I** [see: iodipamide sodium I 131]

$^{131}$**I** [see: iodoantipyrine I 131]

$^{131}$**I** [see: iodocholesterol I 131]

$^{131}$**I** [see: iodohippurate sodium I 131]

$^{131}$**I** [see: iodopyracet I 131]

$^{131}$**I** [see: iomethin I 131]

$^{131}$**I** [see: iothalamate sodium I 131]

$^{131}$**I** [see: iotyrosine I 131]

$^{131}$**I** [see: liothyronine I 131]

$^{131}$**I** [see: macrosalb ($^{131}$I)]

$^{131}$**I** [see: oleic acid I 131]

$^{131}$**I** [see: povidone I 131]

$^{131}$**I** [see: rose bengal sodium I 131]

$^{131}$**I** [see: sodium iodide I 131]

$^{131}$**I** [see: thyroxine I 131]

$^{131}$**I** [see: tolpovidone I 131]

$^{131}$**I** [see: triolein I 131]

**Iamin** ℞ *investigational treatment for peptic ulcers, surgical wound repair, and bone healing* [peptide copper compound]

**ibacitabine** INN

**ibafloxacin** USAN, INN, BAN *antibacterial*

**ibazocine** INN

**IBC (isobutyl cyanoacrylate)** [see: bucrylate]

**Iberet; Iberet-500** controlled-release Filmtabs (film-coated tablets) OTC *hematinic* [ferrous sulfate; multiple B vitamins; sodium ascorbate] 105•±•150 mg; 105•±•500 mg

**Iberet; Iberet-500** liquid OTC *hematinic* [ferrous sulfate; multiple B vitamins] 78.75•± mg/15 mL

**Iberet-Folic-500** controlled-release Filmtabs (film-coated tablets) ℞ *hematinic* [ferrous sulfate; multiple B vitamins; sodium ascorbate; folic acid] 105•±•500•0.8 mg

**ibopamine** USAN, INN, BAN *peripheral dopaminergic agent; vasodilator*

**ibrotal** [see: ibrotamide]

**ibrotamide** INN

**Ibu** film-coated tablets ℞ *nonsteroidal anti-inflammatory drug (NSAID); antiarthritic; analgesic* [ibuprofen] 400, 600, 800 mg

**ibudilast** INN

**ibufenac** USAN, INN, BAN *analgesic; anti-inflammatory*

**Ibuprin** tablets OTC *nonsteroidal anti-inflammatory drug (NSAID); antiarthritic; analgesic* [ibuprofen] 200 mg

**ibuprofen** USAN, USP, INN, BAN *antiarthritic; nonsteroidal anti-inflammatory drug (NSAID); analgesic; investigational (orphan) IV treatment for patent ductus arteriosus* 200, 300, 400, 600, 800 mg oral; 100 mg/5 mL oral

**ibuprofen aluminum** USAN *anti-inflammatory*

**ibuprofen piconol** USAN *topical anti-inflammatory*

**Ibuprohm** caplets, tablets OTC *nonsteroidal anti-inflammatory drug (NSAID); antiarthritic; analgesic* [ibuprofen] 200 mg

**Ibuprohm** tablets ℞ *nonsteroidal anti-inflammatory drug (NSAID); antiarthritic; analgesic* [ibuprofen] 400 mg

**ibuproxam** INN

**Ibu-Tab** film-coated tablets (discontinued 1996) OTC *nonsteroidal anti-inflammatory drug (NSAID); antiarthritic; analgesic* [ibuprofen] 200 mg

**Ibu-Tab** film-coated tablets (discontinued 1996) ℞ *nonsteroidal anti-inflammatory drug (NSAID); antiarthritic; analgesic* [ibuprofen] 400, 600, 800 mg

**ibuterol** INN

**ibutilide** INN *antiarrhythmic* [also: ibutilide fumarate]

**ibutilide fumarate** USAN *antiarrhythmic for atrial fibrillation/flutter* [also: ibutilide]

**ibuverine** INN

**ibylcaine chloride** [see: butethamine HCl]

**ICAPS** timed-release tablets OTC *vitamin/mineral supplement* [multiple vitamins & minerals] ±

**ICAPS Plus** tablets OTC *vitamin/mineral supplement* [multiple vitamins & minerals] ±

**icatibant acetate** USAN *antiasthmatic*

**ice** *street drug slang* [see: cocaine; amphetamines; MDMA; methamphetamine HCl; PCP]

**ICE (ifosfamide [with mesna rescue], carboplatin, etoposide)** *chemotherapy protocol* [also: MICE]

**ice cube** *street drug slang* [see: cocaine, crack]

**ichthammol** USP, BAN *topical anti-infective* 10%, 20%

**icing** *street drug slang* [see: cocaine]

**iclazepam** INN

**icopezil maleate** USAN *acetylcholinesterase inhibitor; cognition adjuvant for Alzheimer's disease*

**icosapent** INN *omega-3 marine triglyceride*

**icospiramide** INN

**icotidine** USAN *antagonist to histamine $H_1$ and $H_2$ receptors*

**ictasol** USAN *disinfectant*

**Ictotest** reagent tablets for professional use *in vitro diagnostic aid for bilirubin in the urine*

**Icy Hot** balm, cream, stick OTC *counterirritant* [methyl salicylate; menthol] 29%•7.6%; 30%•10%; 30%•10%

**Idamycin** powder for IV injection ℞ *antibiotic antineoplastic for acute myelogenous and other leukemias (orphan); investigational (orphan) for pediatric use* [idarubicin HCl] 5, 10, 20 mg

**Idamycin PFS** powder for IV injection
℞ *antibiotic antineoplastic for acute
myelogenous and other leukemias
(orphan); investigational (orphan) for
pediatric use* [idarubicin HCl] 1 mg/mL

**Idarac** ℞ *investigational nonsteroidal
anti-inflammatory drug (NSAID);
analgesic* [floctafenine]

**idarubicin** INN, BAN *antibiotic antineoplastic* [also: idarubicin HCl]

**idarubicin HCl** USAN, INN *antibiotic
antineoplastic; orphan status withdrawn 1996* [also: idarubicin]

**idaverine** INN

**idazoxan** INN, BAN

**idebenone** INN *investigational treatment
for Alzheimer's disease*

**IDEC-CE9.1** *investigational (Phase III)
anti-CD4 antibody for rheumatoid
arthritis* [also: SB-210396]

**idenast** INN

**Identi-Dose** (trademarked dosage
form) *unit dose package*

**idiot pills** *street drug slang* [see: barbi-
turates]

**idoxifene** USAN *antihormone antineoplastic; osteoporosis treatment; estrogen
receptor antagonist for hormone
replacement therapy*

**idoxuridine (IDU)** USAN, USP, INN,
BAN, JAN *ophthalmic antiviral; investigational (orphan) for nonparenchyma-
tous sarcomas*

**idralfidine** INN

**idrobutamine** [see: butidrine]

**idrocilamide** INN

**idropranolol** INN

**IDU (idoxuridine)** [q.v.]

**IE (ifosfamide [with mesna rescue],
etoposide)** *chemotherapy protocol*

**ifenprodil** INN

**ifetroban** USAN *antithrombotic; anti-
ischemic; antivasospastic*

**ifetroban sodium** USAN *antithrombotic; anti-ischemic; antivasospastic*

**Ifex** powder for IV injection ℞ *nitrogen mustard-type alkylating antineoplastic for testicular cancer (orphan);
investigational (orphan) for bone and
soft tissue sarcomas* [ifosfamide] 1, 3 g

**IFN (interferon)** [q.v.]

**IFN-alpha 2 (interferon alfa-2)** [see:
interferon alfa-2b, recombinant]

**ifosfamide** USAN, USP, INN, BAN *nitrogen mustard-type alkylating antineoplastic for testicular cancer (orphan);
investigational (orphan) for bone and
soft tissue sarcomas*

**IfoVP (ifosfamide [with mesna res-
cue], VePesid)** *chemotherapy protocol*

**ifoxetine** INN

**IG (immune globulin)** [see: globulin, immune]

**IgE pentapeptide** [see: pentigetide]

**Igef** ℞ *investigational treatment for
growth hormone receptor impairment
(Laron syndrome)* [recombinant
human insulin-like growth factor]

**IGF-1 (insulin-like growth factor-
1)** [q.v.]

**IgG 1** [see: immunoglobulin G 1]

**IGIV (immune globulin intrave-
nous)** [see: globulin, immune]

**Ikorel** ℞ *investigational treatment for
angina and congestive heart failure*
[nicorandil]

**IL-1, IL-2, etc.** [see: interleukin-1,
interleukin-2, etc.]

**IL-1R (interleukin-1 receptor)** [q.v.]

**IL-2 (interleukin-2)** [see: aldesleukin;
teceleukin; celmoleukin]

**IL-2 fusion toxin** *investigational
(Phase I/II) agent for HIV; investigational antipsoriatic*

**IL-4R (interleukin-4 receptor)** [q.v.]

**ilepcimide** USAN, INN *anticonvulsant;
investigational (orphan) for drug-resistant generalized tonic-clonic epilepsy*

**Iletin** (U.S. products) [see under: Regular, NPH, Lente, Semilente, and
Ultralente]

**Iletin** Ⓒ (U.S. product: Lente Iletin I)
subcu injection OTC *antidiabetic*
[insulin zinc (beef-pork)] 100 U/mL

**Iletin** Ⓒ (U.S. product: Regular Iletin
I) subcu injection OTC *antidiabetic*
[insulin (beef-pork)] 100 U/mL

**Iletin NPH** Ⓒ (U.S. product: NPH
Iletin I) subcu injection OTC *antidiabetic* [insulin (beef-pork)] 100 U/mL

**Iletin II** Ⓒ (U.S. product: Lente
Iletin II) subcu injection OTC *antidiabetic* [insulin zinc (pork)] 100 U/mL

**Iletin II** Ⓒᴬᴺ (U.S. product: Regular Iletin II) subcu injection oᴛc *antidiabetic* [insulin (pork)] 100 U/mL

**Iletin II NPH** Ⓒᴬᴺ (U.S. product: NPH Iletin II) subcu injection oᴛc *antidiabetic* [insulin (pork)] 100 U/mL

**ilmofosine** USAN, INN *antineoplastic*

**ilonidap** USAN, INN *anti-inflammatory*

**Ilopan** IM injection, IV infusion ℞ *postoperative ileus prophylactic* [dexpanthenol] 250 mg/mL

**Ilopan-Choline** tablets ℞ *antiflatulent for splenic flexure syndrome* [dexpanthenol; choline bitartrate] 50•25 mg

**iloperidone** USAN, INN *investigational (Phase III) antipsychotic for schizophrenia*

**iloprost** INN, BAN *prostacyclin analog for cardiovascular disorders; orphan status withdrawn 1996*

**Ilosone** tablets, Pulvules (capsules), oral suspension ℞ *macrolide antibiotic* [erythromycin estolate] 500 mg; 250 mg; 125, 250 mg/5 mL 🔲 inosine

**Ilotycin** ophthalmic ointment ℞ *ophthalmic antibiotic* [erythromycin] 5 mg/g

**Ilotycin Gluceptate** injection ℞ *macrolide antibiotic* [erythromycin gluceptate] 33.33 mg/mL

**Ilozyme** tablets ℞ *digestive enzymes* [lipase; protease; amylase] 11 000•30 000•30 000 U

**I-L-X** elixir oᴛc *hematinic* [ferrous gluconate; liver concentrate 1:20; multiple B vitamins] 70•98•± mg/15 mL

**I-L-X B₁₂** caplets oᴛc *hematinic* [carbonyl iron; desiccated liver; multiple B vitamins; ascorbic acid] 37.5•130•±•120 mg

**I-L-X B₁₂** elixir oᴛc *hematinic* [ferric ammonium citrate; liver fraction 1; multiple B vitamins] 102•98•± mg/15 mL

**imafen** INN *antidepressant* [also: imafen HCl]

**imafen HCl** USAN *antidepressant* [also: imafen]

**Imagent BP** ℞ *investigational imaging agent for CT and ultrasound scans of the liver and spleen*

**Imagent GI** oral liquid ℞ *oral GI contrast agent for MRI and x-ray imaging* [perflubron] 200 mL

**Imagent LN** ℞ *investigational lymph node imaging agent for CT scans*

**Imagent US** ℞ *investigational imaging agent for ultrasound procedures*

**imanixil** INN

**imazodan** INN *cardiotonic* [also: imazodan HCl]

**imazodan HCl** USAN *cardiotonic* [also: imazodan]

**imcarbofos** USAN, INN *veterinary anthelmintic*

**imciromab** INN *antimyosin monoclonal antibody* [also: imciromab pentetate]

**imciromab pentetate** USAN, BAN *antimyosin monoclonal antibody; investigational (orphan) diagnostic aid for cardiac transplant rejection* [also: imciromab]

**Imdur** extended-release tablets ℞ *angina preventative* [isosorbide mononitrate] 30, 120 mg

**imexon** INN *investigational (orphan) for multiple myeloma*

**IMF (ifosfamide [with mesna rescue], methotrexate, fluorouracil)** *chemotherapy protocol*

**imiclopazine** INN

**imidapril** INN, BAN

**imidazole carboxamide** [see: dacarbazine]

**imidazole salicylate** INN

**imidecyl iodine** USAN *topical anti-infective*

**imidocarb** INN, BAN *antiprotozoal (Babesia)* [also: imidocarb HCl]

**imidocarb HCl** USAN *antiprotozoal (Babesia)* [also: imidocarb]

**imidoline** INN *antipsychotic* [also: imidoline HCl]

**imidoline HCl** USAN *antipsychotic* [also: imidoline]

**imidurea** NF *antimicrobial*

**imiglucerase** USAN, INN *glucocerebrosidase enzyme replacement for types I, II, and III Gaucher's disease (orphan)*

**Imigran** (foreign name for U.S. product Imitrex)

**imiloxan** INN *antidepressant* [also: imiloxan HCl]

**imiloxan HCl** USAN *antidepressant* [also: imiloxan]

**iminophenimide** INN

**iminostilbene** [see: carbamazepine]

**imipemide** [now: imipenem]

**imipenem** USAN, USP, INN, BAN, JAN *thienamycin-type bactericidal antibiotic*

**imipramine** INN, BAN *tricyclic antidepressant* [also: imipramine HCl] ⑨ Imferon; Norpramin; trimipramine

**imipramine HCl** USP *tricyclic antidepressant; treatment of childhood enuresis* [also: imipramine] 10, 25, 50 mg oral ⑨ Imferon; Norpramin; trimipramine

**imipramine pamoate** *tricyclic antidepressant* ⑨ Imferon; Norpramin; trimipramine

**imipraminoxide** INN

**imiquimod** USAN, INN *immunomodulator for external genital and perianal warts*

**imirestat** INN

**Imitrex** film-coated tablets ℞ *vascular serotonin agonist to relieve migraine attacks and cluster headaches* [sumatriptan succinate] 25, 50 mg (100 mg available in Canada)

**Imitrex** subcu injection in vials, prefilled syringes, or STATdose kits (two prefilled syringes) ℞ *vascular serotonin agonist to relieve migraine attacks and cluster headaches* [sumatriptan succinate] 12 mg/mL

**ImmTher** ℞ *investigational (orphan) for pulmonary and hepatic metastases of colorectal adenocarcinoma* [disaccharide tripeptide glycerol dipalmitoyl]

**Immun-Aid** powder OTC *enteral nutritional therapy for immunocompromised patients*

**immune globulin (IG)** [see: globulin, immune]

**immune globulin intramuscular** [see: globulin, immune]

**immune globulin intravenous (IGIV)** [see: globulin, immune]

**immune globulin intravenous pentetate** USAN *radiodiagnostic imaging agent for inflammation and infection* [also: indium In 111 IGIV pentetate]

**immune serum globulin (ISG)** [see: globulin, immune]

**Immuneron** ℞ *investigational antiinfective for granulomatous disease, rheumatoid arthritis, and venereal warts* [interferon gamma]

**Immunex CRP** test kit for professional use *in vitro diagnostic aid for C-reactive protein (CRP) in blood to diagnose inflammatory conditions* [latex agglutination test]

**Immuno-C** ℞ *investigational (Phase II, orphan) treatment of cryptosporidiosis in immunocompromised patients* [bovine whey protein concentrate]

**immunoglobulin G 1 (mouse monoclonal 7E11-C5.3 antihuman prostatic carcinoma cell) disulfide** [see: capromab pendetide]

**immunoglobulin G 1 (mouse monoclonal ZCE025 antihuman antigen CEA) disulfide** [see: indium In 111 altumomab pentetate; altumomab]

**immunosuppressives** *a class of drugs used to suppress the immune response, used primarily after organ transplantation surgery*

**Immunovir** ℞ *investigational treatment for HIV infection* [isoprinosine]

**Immupath** ℞ *orphan status withdrawn 1997* [HIV-neutralizing antibodies]

**ImmuRAID-AFP** ℞ *investigational (orphan) for diagnostic aid for AFP-producing tumors, hepatoblastoma, and hepatocellular carcinoma* [technetium Tc 99m murine MAb to human alpha-fetoprotein (AFP)]

**ImmuRAID-CEA** ℞ *investigational monoclonal antibody-based diagnostic aid for colorectal cancer*

**ImmuRAID-hCG** ℞ *investigational (orphan) for diagnostic aid for hCG-producing tumors* [technetium Tc 99m murine MAb to human chorionic gonadotropin (hCG)]

**ImmuRAID-LL2** ℞ *investigational (orphan) for diagnostic aid for B-cell leukemias, non-Hodgkin's lymphomas, and AIDS-related lymphomas* [technetium Tc 99m bectumomab]

**ImmuRAID-MN3** ℞ *investigational monoclonal antibody-based diagnostic aid for infectious diseases*

**ImmuRAIT-CEA** ℞ *investigational treatment for colorectal cancer* [iodine I 131 murine MAb IgG]

**ImmuRAIT-LL2** ℞ *investigational (orphan) treatment for B-cell leukemia and lymphoma* [iodine I 131 murine MAb IgG₂a to B cell]

**Imodium** capsules ℞ *antidiarrheal* [loperamide HCl] 2 mg

**Imodium A-D** caplets, liquid OTC *antidiarrheal* [loperamide HCl] 1 mg; 1 mg/5 mL

**Imogam** IM injection ℞ *rabies prophylaxis* [rabies immune globulin] 150 IU/mL (300 IU/mL available in Canada)

**imolamine** INN, BAN

**Imovane** ⒸⒶⓃ tablets ℞ *sedative; hypnotic* [zopiclone] 7.5 mg

**Imovax** intradermal (ID) injection, IM injection ℞ *rabies prophylaxis* [rabies vaccine (HDCV)] 0.25 IU/0.1 mL; 2.5 IU/mL

**imoxiterol** INN

**impacarzine** INN

**Impact** ready-to-use liquid OTC *enteral nutritional therapy* [lactose-free formula]

**Impact Rubella** slide test for professional use *in vitro diagnostic aid for detection of rubella virus antibodies in serum* [latex agglutination test]

**IMPE** [see: etipirium iodide]

**impromidine** INN, BAN *gastric secretion indicator* [also: impromidine HCl]

**impromidine HCl** USAN *gastric secretion indicator* [also: impromidine]

**improsulfan** INN

**Improved Analgesic** ointment OTC *counterirritant* [methyl salicylate; menthol] 18.3%•16%

**Improved Congestant** tablets OTC *antihistamine; analgesic* [chlorpheniramine maleate; acetaminophen] 2•325 mg

**Imreg-1** ℞ *investigational (Phase III) immunomodulator for HIV*

**Imreg-2** ℞ *investigational immunomodulator for AIDS (clinical trials discontinued 1994)*

**imuracetam** INN

**Imuran** IV injection ℞ *immunosuppressant for organ transplantation and rheumatoid arthritis* [azathioprine sodium] 100 mg ⊠ Enduron; Imferon

**Imuran** tablets ℞ *immunosuppressant for organ transplantation and rheumatoid arthritis* [azathioprine] 50 mg

**Imuthiol** ℞ *investigational (Phase II/III, orphan) immunomodulator for HIV and AIDS* [diethyldithiocarbamate]

**Imuvert** ℞ *investigational antineoplastic for breast and ovarian cancers; investigational (orphan) for primary brain malignancies* [Serratia marcescens extract (polyribosomes)]

¹¹¹**In** [see: indium In 111 altumomab pentetate]

¹¹¹**In** [see: indium In 111 imciromab pentetate]

¹¹¹**In** [see: indium In 111 murine anti-CEA monoclonal antibody]

¹¹¹**In** [see: indium In 111 murine monoclonal antibody]

¹¹¹**In** [see: indium In 111 oxyquinoline]

¹¹¹**In** [see: indium In 111 pentetate]

¹¹¹**In** [see: indium In 111 pentetreotide]

¹¹¹**In** [see: indium In 111 satumomab pendetide]

¹¹¹**In** [see: pentetate indium disodium In 111]

¹¹³ᵐ**In** [see: indium chlorides In 113m]

**inactivated mumps vaccine** [see: mumps virus vaccine, inactivated]

**inactivated poliomyelitis vaccine (IPV)** [see: poliovirus vaccine, inactivated]

**inactivated poliovirus vaccine (IPV)** [see: poliovirus vaccine, inactivated]

**inaperisone** INN

**Inapsine** IV or IM injection ℞ *general anesthetic* [droperidol] 2.5 mg/mL

**in-betweens** *street drug slang* [see: amphetamines]

**Inca message** *street drug slang* [see: cocaine]

**incentive** *street drug slang* [see: cocaine]

**Incremin with Iron** syrup (discontinued 1995) OTC *hematinic* [ferric pyrophosphate; multiple B vitamins; lysine; alcohol 0.75%] 90• ≟ •900 mg/15 mL

**Incystene** ℞ *investigational oral treatment for interstitial cystitis and stroke* [nalmefene]

**indacrinic acid** [see: indacrinone]

**indacrinone** USAN, INN *antihypertensive; diuretic*

**indalpine** INN, BAN

**indanazoline** INN

**indandione** *anticoagulant*

**indandiones** *a class of anticoagulants that interfere with vitamin K-dependent clotting factors*

**indanidine** INN

**indanorex** INN

**indapamide** USAN, INN, BAN *antihypertensive; diuretic* 2.5 mg oral

**indatraline** INN

**indecainide** INN *antiarrhythmic* [also: indecainide HCl]

**indecainide HCl** USAN *antiarrhythmic* [also: indecainide]

**indeloxazine** INN *antidepressant* [also: indeloxazine HCl]

**indeloxazine HCl** USAN *antidepressant* [also: indeloxazine]

**indenolol** INN, BAN

**Inderal** tablets, IV injection ℞ *antianginal; antihypertensive; migraine preventative* [propranolol HCl] 10, 20, 40, 60, 80 mg; 1 mg/mL ② Enduron; Enduronyl; Inderide

**Inderal LA** long-acting capsules ℞ *antianginal; antihypertensive; migraine preventative* [propranolol HCl] 60, 80, 120, 160 mg

**Inderide 40/25; Inderide 80/25** tablets ℞ *antihypertensive* [propranolol HCl; hydrochlorothiazide] 40•25 mg; 80•25 mg ② Inderal

**Inderide LA 80/50; Inderide LA 120/50; Inderide LA 160/50** long-acting capsules ℞ *antihypertensive* [propranolol HCl; hydrochlorothiazide] 80•50 mg; 120•50 mg; 160•50 mg

**Indian boy; Indian hay; Indian hemp** *street drug slang* [see: marijuana]

**Indiana** *street drug slang* [see: mescaline]

**Indiana ditchweed** *street drug slang for low-potency wild marijuana that grows wild from seeds originally bred for hemp rope* [see: marijuana]

**Indiana hay** *street drug slang* [see: marijuana]

**Indica** *street drug slang for a species of cannabis found in hot climates* [see: cannabis]

**indigo carmine** BAN *cystoscopy aid* [also: indigotindisulfonate sodium]

**indigotindisulfonate sodium** USP *cystoscopy aid* [also: indigo carmine]

**indinavir sulfate** USAN *investigational antiviral; HIV-1 protease inhibitor*

**indium** *element* (In)

**indium ($^{111}$In) diethylenetriamine pentaacetate** JAN *radionuclide cisternography aid; radioactive agent* [also: indium In 111 pentetate]

**indium chlorides In 113m** USAN, USP *radioactive agent*

**indium In 111 altumomab pentetate** USAN *radiodiagnostic monoclonal antibody for colorectal carcinoma; anticarcinoembryonic antigen; orphan status withdrawn 1997* [also: altumomab]

**indium In 111 antimelanoma antibody XMMME-0001-DTPA** [see: antimelanoma antibody]

**indium In 111 CYT-103** [now: indium In 111 satumomab pendetide]

**indium In 111 IGIV pentetate** *radiodiagnostic imaging agent for inflammation and infection* [also: immune globulin intravenous pentetate]

**indium In 111 imciromab pentetate** *radioactive diagnostic aid for cardiac imaging*

**indium In 111 murine anti-CEA MAb type ZCE 025** *orphan status withdrawn 1997*

**indium In 111 murine MAb (2B8-MXDTPA) & Y-90 murine MAb (2B8-MXDTPA)** *investigational (orphan) for non-Hodgkin's B-cell lymphoma*

**indium In 111 murine MAb B72.3** *orphan status withdrawn 1994*

**indium In 111 murine MAb Fab to myosin** [now: imciromab pentetate]

**indium In 111 oxyquinoline** USAN, USP *radioactive agent; diagnostic aid*

**indium In 111 pentetate** USP *radionuclide cisternography aid; radio-*

*active agent* [also: indium ($^{111}$In) diethylenetriamine pentaacetate]

**indium In 111 pentetreotide** USAN *tumor imaging agent for SPECT scans*

**indium In 111 satumomab pende-tide** USAN *radiodiagnostic monoclonal antibody for ovarian (orphan) and colo-rectal carcinoma* [also: satumomab]

**Indo; Indonesian bud** *street drug slang* [see: marijuana; opium]

**indobufen** INN

**indocate** INN

**Indochron E-R** extended-release tablets ℞ *nonsteroidal anti-inflammatory drug (NSAID); antiarthritic; analgesic* [indomethacin] 75 mg

**Indocin** capsules, oral suspension, suppositories ℞ *nonsteroidal anti-inflammatory drug (NSAID); antiarthritic; analgesic* [indomethacin] 25, 50 mg; 25 mg/5 mL; 50 mg ℞ Lincocin; Minocin

**Indocin I.V.** powder for IV injection ℞ *prostaglandin synthesis inhibitor for patent ductus arteriosus* [indomethacin sodium trihydrate] 1 mg

**Indocin SR** sustained-release capsules ℞ *nonsteroidal anti-inflammatory drug (NSAID); antiarthritic; analgesic* [indomethacin] 75 mg

**indocyanine green** USP, JAN *cardiac output test; hepatic function test; ophthalmic angiography*

**indolapril** INN *antihypertensive* [also: indolapril HCl]

**indolapril HCl** USAN *antihypertensive* [also: indolapril]

**indolidan** USAN, INN, BAN *cardiotonic*

**indometacin** INN, JAN *nonsteroidal anti-inflammatory drug (NSAID); antiarthritic; analgesic* [also: indomethacin]

**indometacin farnecil** JAN *nonsteroidal anti-inflammatory drug (NSAID); antiarthritic; analgesic* [also: indomethacin]

**indomethacin** USAN, USP, BAN *nonsteroidal anti-inflammatory drug (NSAID); antiarthritic; analgesic* [also: indometacin; indometacin farnecil] 25, 50, 75 mg oral; 25 mg/5 mL oral

**indomethacin sodium** USAN *anti-inflammatory*

**indomethacin sodium trihydrate** *neonatal closure of patent ductus arteriosus*

**indopanolol** INN

**indopine** INN

**indoprofen** USAN, INN, BAN *analgesic; anti-inflammatory*

**indoramin** USAN, INN, BAN *antihypertensive*

**indoramin HCl** USAN, BAN *antihypertensive*

**indorenate** INN *antihypertensive* [also: indorenate HCl]

**indorenate HCl** USAN *antihypertensive* [also: indorenate]

**indoxole** USAN, INN *antipyretic; anti-inflammatory*

**indriline** INN *CNS stimulant* [also: indriline HCl]

**indriline HCl** USAN *CNS stimulant* [also: indriline]

**inductin** [see: diphoxazide]

**Infalyte** oral solution OTC *electrolyte replacement* [sodium, potassium, and chloride electrolytes]

**Infanrix** IM injection ℞ *immunization against diphtheria, tetanus, and pertussis* [diphtheria & tetanus toxoids & acellular pertussis vaccine (DTaP)] 25 Lf•10 Lf•25 μg per 0.5 mL

**Infasurf** ℞ *investigational (orphan) for respiratory failure in premature infants* [surface active extract of saline lavage of bovine lungs]

**Infatab** (trademarked dosage form) *pediatric chewable tablet*

**Infectrol** eye drop suspension, ophthalmic ointment (discontinued 1993) ℞ *topical ophthalmic corticosteroidal anti-inflammatory; antibiotic* [dexamethasone; neomycin sulfate; polymyxin B sulfate]

**InFeD** IV injection ℞ *hematinic* [iron dextran] 50 mg/mL

**Infergen** ℞ *investigational treatment for hepatitis C* [consensus interferon] placebo

**Inflamase Mild; Inflamase Forte** eye drops ℞ *ophthalmic topical corticosteroidal anti-inflammatory* [prednisolone sodium phosphate] 0.125%; 1%

**influenza purified split-virus vaccine** *subcategory of influenza virus vaccine*

**influenza purified surface antigen** *subcategory of influenza virus vaccine*

**influenza split-virus vaccine** *subcategory of influenza virus vaccine*

**influenza subvirion vaccine** [see: influenza split-virus vaccine]

**influenza vaccine, intranasal** *investigational (Phase III) delivery form for the vaccine*

**influenza virus vaccine** USP *active immunizing agent for influenza*

**influenza whole-virus vaccine** *subcategory of influenza virus vaccine*

**infraRUB** cream OTC *counterirritant* [methyl salicylate; menthol] 35%•10%

**Infumorph 200; Infumorph 500** concentrate for continuous microinfusion ℞ *narcotic analgesic; intraspinal microinfusion for intractable chronic pain (orphan)* [morphine sulfate] 10 mg/mL (200 mg/vial); 25 mg/mL (500 mg/vial)

**INH (isonicotinic acid hydrazide)** [see: isoniazid]

**Inhal-Aid** (trademarked form) *portable inhalation device*

**inhalants** *a class of street drugs that include nitrous oxide, volatile nitrites, and petroleum distillates* [see: nitrous oxide; volatile nitrites; petroleum distillate inhalants]

**Inhibace** (commercially available in Latin America) ℞ *antihypertensive; ACE inhibitor (approved by the FDA, but not being marketed by the manufacturer)* [cilazapril]

**Inhibace Plus** ℞ *investigational antihypertensive* [cilazapril; hydrochlorothiazide]

**inicarone** INN

**Inject-all** (trademarked delivery system) *prefilled disposable syringe*

**Inlay-Tab** (trademarked dosage form) *tablets with contrasting inlay*

**InnoGel Plus** gel packs + comb OTC *pediculicide* [pyrethrins; piperonyl butoxide technical] 0.3%•3%

**Innovar** injection ℞ *narcotic analgesic; major tranquilizer* [fentanyl citrate; droperidol] 0.05•2.5 mg/mL

**Inocor** IV injection ℞ *vasodilator for congestive heart failure* [amrinone lactate] 5 mg/mL

**inocoterone** INN *anti-acne* [also: inocoterone acetate]

**inocoterone acetate** USAN *anti-acne* [also: inocoterone]

**inosine** INN, JAN ② Ilosone

**inosine pranobex** BAN, JAN *investigational antiviral/immunomodulator for AIDS; investigational (orphan) for subacute sclerosing panencephalitis*

**inosiplex** [now: inosine pranobex]

**inositol** NF *dietary lipotropic supplement* 250, 500, 650 mg oral

**inositol niacinate** USAN *peripheral vasodilator* [also: inositol nicotinate]

**inositol nicotinate** INN, BAN *peripheral vasodilator* [also: inositol niacinate]

**inotropes** *a class of drugs that affect the force or energy of muscle contractions*

**Inpersol; Inpersol-LM** solution (discontinued 1996) ℞ *peritoneal dialysis solution* [multiple electrolytes; dextrose] ≜•1.5%, ≜•2.5%, ≜•4.5%

**inprochone** [see: inproquone]

**inproquone** INN, BAN

**INSH (isonicotinoyl-salicylidenehydrazine)** [see: salinazid]

**InspirEase** (trademarked form) *portable inhalation device*

**Insta-Glucose** gel OTC *glucose elevating agent* [glucose] 40%

**instant Zen** *street drug slang* [see: LSD]

**Insulatard NPH** subcu injection (discontinued 1994) OTC *antidiabetic* [isophane insulin (pork)]

**Insulatard NPH Human** subcu injection (discontinued 1994) OTC *antidiabetic* [isophane insulin (human semisynthetic)]

**insulin** USP *antidiabetic* ② inulin

**insulin, biphasic** INN, BAN

**insulin, dalanated** USAN, INN *antidiabetic*

**insulin, globin zinc** USP [also: globin zinc insulin]

**insulin, human** USAN, USP, INN, BAN *antidiabetic*

**insulin, isophane** USP, INN *antidiabetic* [also: isophane insulin]

**insulin, neutral** USAN *antidiabetic* [also: neutral insulin]

**insulin, NPH (neutral protamine Hagedorn)** [see: insulin, isophane]

**insulin, protamine zinc (PZI)** USP *antidiabetic* [also: protamine zinc insulin]

**insulin argine** INN

**insulin defalan** INN

**insulin I 125** USAN *radioactive agent*

**insulin I 131** USAN *radioactive agent*

**insulin lispro** USAN *antidiabetic*

**Insulin Reaction** gel OTC *glucose elevating agent* [glucose] 40%

**insulin zinc** USP, BAN *antidiabetic* [also: compound insulin zinc suspension]

**insulin zinc, extended** USP *antidiabetic* [also: insulin zinc suspension (crystalline)]

**insulin zinc, prompt** USP *antidiabetic* [also: insulin zinc suspension (amorphous)]

**insulin zinc suspension (amorphous)** INN, BAN *antidiabetic* [also: insulin zinc, prompt]

**insulin zinc suspension (crystalline)** INN, BAN *antidiabetic* [also: insulin zinc, extended]

**insulin-like growth factor-1, recombinant human (rhIGF)** [now: mecasermin]

**insulinotropin** *investigational blood glucose regulating agent*

**Intal** capsules for inhalation (discontinued 1995) R̟ *bronchodilator for bronchial asthma and bronchospasm* [cromolyn sodium] 20 mg ⊡ Endal

**Intal** solution for nebulization, aerosol spray R̟ *bronchodilator for bronchial asthma and bronchospasm* [cromolyn sodium] 20 mg/ampule; 800 μg/dose ⊡ Endal

**Integrelin** injection R̟ *investigational (Phase III) antithrombotic for unstable angina* [intrifiban]

**Intensol** (trademarked form) *concentrated oral solution*

**α-2-interferon** [see: interferon alfa-2b, recombinant]

**interferon, fibroblast** [now: interferon beta]

**interferon, leukocyte** [now: interferon alfa-n3]

**interferon α2b** [see: interferon alfa-2b]

**interferon αA** [see: interferon alfa-2a]

**interferon alfa** JAN

**interferon alfa (BALL-1)** JAN

**interferon alfa-2a (IFN-αA)** USAN, INN, BAN, JAN *antineoplastic/antiviral for Kaposi sarcoma (orphan); investigational (orphan) for chronic myelogenous leukemia and renal cell carcinoma*

**interferon alfa-2a & fluorouracil** *investigational (orphan) for esophageal carcinoma and advanced colorectal cancer*

**interferon alfa-2a & teceleukin** *investigational (orphan) for metastatic renal cell carcinoma and metastatic malignant melanoma*

**interferon alfa-2b (IFN-α2)** USAN, INN, BAN *antineoplastic for various cancers and AIDS-related Kaposi sarcoma (orphan); antiviral for hepatitis*

**interferon alfa-n1** USAN, INN, BAN *antineoplastic; investigational (Phase III) cytokine for HIV; investigational (orphan) for human papillomavirus in severe respiratory papillomatosis*

**interferon alfa-n3** USAN *antineoplastic; antiviral; investigational (Phase III) cytokine for HIV, AIDS, ARC, and hepatitis C*

**interferon beta (IFN-B)** BAN, JAN *antineoplastic; antiviral; immunomodulator; investigational (orphan) for malignant melanoma, renal cell carcinoma, and Kaposi sarcoma*

**interferon beta-1a** USAN *immunomodulator for relapsing multiple sclerosis (orphan); investigational (orphan) for non-A, non-B hepatitis and brain tumors*

**interferon beta-1b** USAN *immunomodulator for relapsing-remitting multiple sclerosis (orphan); investigational (Phase II/III) for AIDS; investigational (Phase III) for atopic dermatitis*

**interferon gamma-1a** JAN

**interferon gamma-1b** USAN, INN, BAN *antineoplastic; antiviral; immunoregulator for chronic granulomatous disease (orphan); investigational (orphan) for renal cell carcinoma*

**interferon gamma-2a** [see: interferon gamma-1b]

**α-interferons** [see: interferon alfa-n1 and -n3]

**interleukin-1 alpha, recombinant
human** *orphan status withdrawn 1996*
**interleukin-1 beta** *investigational antineoplastic for melanoma*
**interleukin-1 receptor (IL-1R)**
*investigational treatment for rheuma-
toid arthritis, sepsis, GVH disease,
AML, asthma, and allergy*
**interleukin-1 receptor, soluble** *investigational (Phase I) antiviral for HIV*
**interleukin-1 receptor antagonist,
recombinant human** [now:
anakinra]
**interleukin-2, liposome-encapsu-
lated recombinant** *orphan status
withdrawn 1997*
**interleukin-2, recombinant (IL-2)**
[see: aldesleukin; teceleukin; celmo-
leukin]
**interleukin-2 PEG** [see: PEG-inter-
leukin-2]
**interleukin-3, recombinant human**
*investigational HIV drug and adjunct
to bone marrow transplants; orphan
status withdrawn 1996*
**interleukin-3, recombinant human
& sargramostim** *orphan status withdrawn 1996*
**interleukin-4 (IL-4)** *investigational
immunomodulator for life-threatening
immunodeficiency diseases and cancer*
**interleukin-4 receptor (IL-4R)**
*investigational treatment for allergy,
asthma, transplant rejection, and infectious disease*
**interleukin-6 mutein** *investigational
treatment for thrombocytopenia*
**interleukin-7 (IL-7)** *investigational
antineoplastic and lymphocyte stimulant*
**interleukin-9 (IL-9)** *investigational
treatment for anemia and red blood cell
disorders*
**interleukin-10 (IL-10)** *investigational
immunomodulator for solid tumors,
organ transplants, and autoimmune
disorders*
**interleukin-11 (IL-11)** *investigational
biological response modifier for cancer
chemotherapy and bone marrow transplantation*
**interleukin-11, recombinant
human (rhIL-11)** *investigational*

*adjunct to chemotherapy for breast can-
cer; investigational (orphan) prophylaxis for thrombocytopenia of chemotherapy* [now: oprelvekin]
**interleukin-12 (IL-12)** *investigational
(Phase I) immunomodulator for HIV*
**interleukin-2 receptor (IL-2R)
fusion protein** *investigational (Phase
III) for cutaneous T-cell lymphoma
(CTCL); investigational (Phase II) for
other lymphomas and leukemias*
**interleukin-6, recombinant human
(rhIL-6)** *investigational (Phase III)
bone marrow/platelet stimulant adjunct
for chemotherapy*
**intermedine** INN
**Interquim** ℞ *investigational treatment
for stroke and head trauma* [citicoline
sodium]
**intoplicine** INN *investigational antineoplastic*
**IntraDose** injectable gel ℞ *investigational (Phase II) antineoplastic for
inoperable primary liver cancer* [cis-
platin; epinephrine]
**Intralipid 10%; Intralipid 20%** IV
infusion ℞ *nutritional therapy* [intra-
venous fat emulsion]
**IntraSite** gel OTC *wound dressing* [graft
T starch copolymer] 2%
**intravascular perfluorochemical
emulsion** *synthetic blood oxygen carrier for PTCA*
**intravenous fat emulsion** [see: fat
emulsion, intravenous]
**intravenous immunoglobulin
(IVIG)** *investigational IV solution of
concentrated antibodies for AIDS*
**intrazole** USAN, INN *anti-inflammatory*
**intrifiban** GPIIb/IIIa receptor inhibitor;
*investigational (Phase III) antiplatelet/
antithrombotic agent for unstable angina*
**intriptyline** INN *antidepressant* [also:
intriptyline HCl]
**intriptyline HCl** USAN *antidepressant*
[also: intriptyline]
**Introlan Half-Strength** liquid OTC
*enteral nutritional therapy* [lactose-free
formula]
**Introlite** liquid OTC *enteral nutritional
therapy* [lactose-free formula]

**Intron A** subcu or IM injection ℞ *antineoplastic for hairy cell leukemia and Kaposi sarcoma (orphan); antiviral for chronic hepatitis C* [interferon alfa-2b] 3, 5, 10, 18, 25, 50 million IU/vial

**Intropin** IV injection ℞ *vasopressor for cardiac, pulmonary, traumatic, septic, or renal shock* [dopamine HCl] 40, 80, 160 mg/mL ⧄ Ditropan; Isoptin

**inulin** USP *renal function test* 100 mg/mL injection ⧄ insulin

**invenol** [see: carbutamide]

**Inversine** tablets ℞ *antihypertensive* [mecamylamine HCl] 2.5 mg

**invert sugar** [see: sugar, invert]

**Invicorp** ℞ *investigational (NDA filed) treatment for organic-based erectile dysfunction*

**Invirase** capsules ℞ *antiviral protease inhibitor for HIV* [saquinavir mesylate] 200 mg

**iobenguane (¹³¹I)** INN

**iobenguane I 123** USP *radioactive agent*

**iobenguane sulfate I 123** USAN *radiopharmaceutical diagnostic aid for adrenomedullary disorders and neuroendocrine tumors*

**iobenguane sulfate I 131** *investigational (orphan) diagnostic aid for pheochromocytoma*

**iobenzamic acid** USAN, INN, BAN *cholecystographic radiopaque medium*

**Iobid DM** sustained-release tablets ℞ *antitussive; expectorant* [dextromethorphan hydrobromide; guaifenesin] 30•600 mg

**iobutoic acid** INN

**Iocare Balanced Salt** ophthalmic solution OTC *intraocular irrigating solution* [balanced saline solution]

**iocarmate meglumine** USAN *radiopaque medium* [also: meglumine iocarmate]

**iocarmic acid** USAN, INN, BAN *radiopaque medium*

**iocetamic acid** USAN, USP, INN, BAN *cholecystographic radiopaque medium*

**Iocon** shampoo OTC *antiseborrheic; antipsoriatic; antipruritic; antibacterial* [coal tar; alcohol]

**Iodal HD** liquid ℞ *narcotic antitussive; decongestant; antihistamine* [hydrocodone bitartrate; phenylephrine HCl; chlorpheniramine maleate] 1.67•5•2 mg/5 mL

**iodamide** USAN, INN, BAN *radiopaque medium*

**iodamide meglumine** USAN *radiopaque medium*

**iodecimol** INN

**iodecol** [see: iodecimol]

**iodetryl** INN

**Iodex; Iodex-P** ointment OTC *broad-spectrum antimicrobial* [povidone-iodine] 4.7%; 10%

**Iodex with Methyl Salicylate** salve OTC *counterirritant; topical anti-infective* [methyl salicylate; iodine; oil of wintergreen] ≟•4.7%•4.8%

**iodinated (¹²⁵I) human serum albumin** INN *radioactive agent; blood volume test* [also: albumin, iodinated I 125 serum]

**iodinated (¹³¹I) human serum albumin** INN, JAN *radioactive agent; intrathecal imaging agent; blood volume test* [also: albumin, iodinated I 131 serum]

**iodinated glycerol** [see: glycerol, iodinated]

**Iodinated Glycerol DM** liquid (discontinued 1993) ℞ *antitussive; expectorant* [iodinated glycerol; dextromethorphan hydrobromide]

**iodinated I 125 albumin** [see: albumin, iodinated I 125]

**iodinated I 131 aggregated albumin** [see: albumin, iodinated I 131 aggregated]

**iodinated I 131 albumin** [see: albumin, iodinated I 131]

**iodine** USP *broad-spectrum topical anti-infective; element (I)* 2% topical

**iodine I 123 murine MAb to alpha-fetoprotein (AFP)** *investigational (orphan) diagnostic aid for AFP-producing tumors, hepatocellular carcinoma, and hepatoblastoma*

**iodine I 123 murine MAb to human chorionic gonadotropin (hCG)** *investigational (orphan) diagnostic aid for hCG-producing tumors*

**iodine I 131 6B-iodomethyl-19-norcholesterol** *investigational (orphan) for adrenal cortical imaging*

**iodine I 131 Lym-1 MAb** *investigational (Phase III) treatment for non-Hodgkin's B-cell lymphoma; orphan status withdrawn 1994*

**iodine I 131 metaiodobenzylguanidine sulfate** [now: iobenguane sulfate I 131]

**iodine I 131 murine MAb IgG$_2$a to B cell** *investigational (orphan) for B-cell leukemia and lymphoma*

**iodine I 131 murine MAb to alpha-fetoprotein (AFP)** *investigational (orphan) treatment for AFP-producing tumors, hepatocellular carcinoma, and hepatoblastoma*

**iodine I 131 murine MAb to human chorionic gonadotropin (hCG)** *investigational (orphan) treatment for hCG-producing tumors*

**iodine I 131 radiolabeled B1 MAb** *investigational (orphan) for non-Hodgkin's B-cell lymphoma*

**iodipamide** USP, BAN [also: adipiodone]

**iodipamide meglumine** USP, BAN *radiopaque medium* [also: adipiodone meglumine]

**iodipamide methylglucamine** [see: iodipamide meglumine]

**iodipamide sodium** USP

**iodipamide sodium I 131** USAN *radioactive agent*

**iodisan** [see: prolonium iodide]

**iodixanol** USAN, INN, BAN *radiopaque medium*

**iodized oil** NF

**iodoalphionic acid** NF [also: pheniodol sodium]

**iodoantipyrine I 131** USAN *radioactive agent*

**iodobehenate calcium** NF

**iodobenzylguaninine sulfate I 123** [see: iobenguane sulfate I 123]

**iodocetylic acid ($^{123}$I)** INN *diagnostic aid* [also: iodocetylic acid I 123]

**iodocetylic acid I 123** USAN *diagnostic aid* [also: iodocetylic acid ($^{123}$I)]

**iodochlorhydroxyquin** [now: clioquinol]

**iodocholesterol ($^{131}$I)** INN *radioactive agent* [also: iodocholesterol I 131]

**iodocholesterol I 131** USAN *radioactive agent* [also: iodocholesterol ($^{131}$I)]

**iodoform** NF

**iodohippurate sodium I 123** USAN, USP *renal function test; radioactive agent*

**iodohippurate sodium I 125** USAN *radioactive agent*

**iodohippurate sodium I 131** USAN, USP *renal function test; radioactive agent* [also: sodium iodohippurate ($^{131}$I)]

**iodohydroxyquin** [see: clioquinol]

**iodol** USP

**iodomethamate sodium** NF

**Iodo-Niacin** controlled-action tablets (discontinued 1994) ℞ *expectorant* [potassium iodide; niacinamide hydroiodide] 135•25 mg

**Iodo-Pak** IV injection ℞ *intravenous nutritional therapy* [sodium iodide]

**iodopanoic acid** [see: iopanoic acid]

**Iodopen** IV injection ℞ *intravenous nutritional therapy* [sodium iodide] 118 μg/mL

**iodophthalein, soluble** [now: iodophthalein sodium]

**iodophthalein sodium** NF, INN

**iodopyracet** NF [also: diodone]

**iodopyracet I 125** USAN *radioactive agent*

**iodopyracet I 131** USAN *radioactive agent*

**iodoquinol** USAN, USP *amebicide; antimicrobial* [also: diiodohydroxyquinoline]

**Iodosorb** gel ℞ *investigational treatment of skin ulcers* [cadexomer iodine]

**iodothiouracil** INN, BAN

**iodothymol** [see: thymol iodide]

**Iodotope** capsules, oral solution ℞ *radioactive agent for hyperthyroidism and thyroid carcinoma* [sodium iodide I 131] 1–50 mCi; 7.05 mCi/mL

**iodoxamate meglumine** USAN, BAN *radiopaque medium*

**iodoxamic acid** USAN, INN, BAN *radiopaque medium*

**iodoxyl** [see: iodomethamate sodium]

**Iofed** extended-release capsules ℞ *decongestant; antihistamine* [pseudoephedrine HCl; brompheniramine maleate] 120•12 mg

**Iofed PD** extended-release capsules ℞ *pediatric decongestant and antihistamine* [pseudoephedrine HCl; brompheniramine maleate] 60•6 mg

**iofendylate** INN *radiopaque medium* [also: iophendylate]

**iofetamine ($^{123}$I)** INN *diagnostic aid; radioactive agent* [also: iofetamine HCl I 123]

**iofetamine HCl I 123** USAN *diagnostic aid; radioactive agent* [also: iofetamine ($^{123}$I)]

**Iofoam** (trademarked form) *foaming skin cleanser*

**ioglicic acid** USAN, INN, BAN *radiopaque medium*

**ioglucol** USAN, INN *radiopaque medium*

**ioglucomide** USAN, INN *radiopaque medium*

**ioglunide** INN

**ioglycamic acid** USAN, INN, BAN *cholecystographic radiopaque medium*

**iogulamide** USAN *radiopaque medium*

**iohexol** USAN, INN, BAN *radiopaque medium*

**Iohist D** elixir ℞ *decongestant; antihistamine* [phenylpropanolamine HCl; phenyltoloxamine citrate; pyrilamine maleate; pheniramine maleate] 12.5•4•4•4 mg/5 mL

**Iohist DM** syrup ℞ *antitussive; decongestant; antihistamine* [dextromethorphan hydrobromide; phenylpropanolamine HCl; brompheniramine maleate] 10•12.5•2 mg/5 mL

**iolidonic acid** INN

**iolixanic acid** INN

**iomeglamic acid** INN

**iomeprol** USAN, INN, BAN *radiopaque medium*

**iomethin I 125** USAN *neoplasm test; radioactive agent* [also: iometin ($^{125}$I)]

**iomethin I 131** USAN *neoplasm test; radioactive agent* [also: iometin ($^{131}$I)]

**iometin ($^{125}$I)** INN *neoplasm test; radioactive agent* [also: iomethin I 125]

**iometin ($^{131}$I)** INN *neoplasm test; radioactive agent* [also: iomethin I 131]

**iomorinic acid** INN

**Ionamin** capsules ℞ *anorexiant* [phentermine HCl resin complex] 15, 30 mg

**Ionax** foam OTC *topical cleanser for acne* [benzalkonium chloride]

**Ionax Astringent Skin Cleanser** liquid OTC *topical keratolytic cleanser for acne* [salicylic acid; isopropyl alcohol]

**Ionax Scrub** OTC *abrasive cleanser for acne* [benzalkonium chloride]

**Ionil** shampoo OTC *antiseborrheic; keratolytic; antiseptic* [salicylic acid; benzalkonium chloride]

**Ionil Plus** shampoo OTC *antiseborrheic; keratolytic* [salicylic acid] 2%

**Ionil T** shampoo OTC *antiseborrheic; antipsoriatic; keratolytic; antiseptic* [coal tar; salicylic acid; benzalkonium chloride]

**Ionil-T Plus** shampoo OTC *antiseborrheic; antipsoriatic; antipruritic; antibacterial* [coal tar] 2%

**ionphylline** [see: aminophylline]

**iopamidol** USAN, USP, INN, BAN *radiopaque medium*

**iopanoic acid** USP, INN, BAN *cholecystographic radiopaque medium*

**iopentol** USAN, INN, BAN *radiopaque medium*

**Iophen** tablets, elixir, drops ℞ *expectorant* [iodinated glycerol] 30 mg; 60 mg/5 mL; 50 mg/mL

**Iophen-C** liquid ℞ *narcotic antitussive; expectorant* [codeine phosphate; iodinated glycerol] 10•30 mg/5 mL

**Iophen-DM** liquid ℞ *antitussive; expectorant* [dextromethorphan hydrobromide; iodinated glycerol] 10•30 mg/5 mL

**iophendylate** USP, BAN *radiopaque medium* [also: iofendylate]

**iophenoic acid** INN [also: iophenoxic acid]

**iophenoxic acid** USP [also: iophenoic acid]

**Iophylline** elixir ℞ *antiasthmatic; bronchodilator; expectorant* [theophylline; iodinated glycerol] 120•30 mg/15 mL

**Iopidine** Drop-Tainer (eye drops) ℞ *topical antiglaucoma agent (sympathomimetic)* [apraclonidine HCl] 0.5%, 1%

**ioprocemic acid** USAN, INN *radiopaque medium*

**iopromide** USAN, INN, BAN *radiopaque imaging agent; source of iodine*

**iopronic acid** USAN, INN, BAN *cholecystographic radiopaque medium*

**iopydol** USAN, INN, BAN *bronchographic radiopaque medium*

**iopydone** USAN, INN, BAN *bronchographic radiopaque medium*

**Iosal II** extended-release tablets ℞ *decongestant; expectorant* [pseudoephedrine HCl; guaifenesin] 60•600 mg

**iosarcol** INN

**iosefamic acid** USAN, INN *radiopaque medium*

**ioseric acid** USAN, INN *radiopaque medium*

**iosimide** INN

**iosulamide** INN *radiopaque medium* [also: iosulamide meglumine]

**iosulamide meglumine** USAN *radiopaque medium* [also: iosulamide]

**iosulfan blue** *lymphography radiopaque medium*

**iosumetic acid** USAN, INN *radiopaque medium*

**iotalamic acid** INN *radiopaque medium* [also: iothalamic acid]

**iotasul** USAN, INN *radiopaque medium*

**iotetric acid** USAN, INN *radiopaque medium*

**iothalamate meglumine** USP *radiopaque medium* [also: meglumine iothalamate]

**iothalamate sodium** USP *radiopaque medium* [also: sodium iothalamate]

**iothalamate sodium I 125** USAN *radioactive agent* [also: sodium iotalamate ($^{125}$I)]

**iothalamate sodium I 131** USAN *radioactive agent* [also: sodium iotalamate ($^{131}$I)]

**iothalamic acid** USP, BAN *radiopaque medium* [also: iotalamic acid]

**iothiouracil sodium**

**iotranic acid** INN

**iotriside** INN

**iotrizoic acid** INN

**iotrol** [now: iotrolan]

**iotrolan** USAN, INN, BAN *radiopaque medium*

**iotroxic acid** USAN, INN, BAN *radiopaque medium*

**IoTuss** liquid (discontinued 1994) ℞ *narcotic antitussive; expectorant* [codeine phosphate; iodinated glycerol]

**IoTuss-DM** liquid (discontinued 1994) ℞ *antitussive; expectorant* [dextromethorphan hydrobromide; iodinated glycerol]

**Iotussin HC** syrup ℞ *narcotic antitussive; decongestant; antihistamine* [hydrocodone bitartrate; phenylephrine HCl; chlorpheniramine maleate] 2.5•5•2 mg/5 mL

**iotyrosine I 131** USAN *radioactive agent*

**ioversol** USAN, INN, BAN *radiopaque medium*

**ioxabrolic acid** INN

**ioxaglate meglumine** USAN *radiopaque medium* [also: meglumine ioxaglate]

**ioxaglate sodium** USAN *radiopaque medium* [also: sodium ioxaglate]

**ioxaglic acid** USAN, INN, BAN *radiopaque medium*

**ioxilan** USAN, INN *diagnostic aid*

**ioxitalamic acid** INN

**ioxotrizoic acid** USAN, INN *radiopaque medium*

**iozomic acid** INN

**IP 456** *investigational anxiolytic*

**ipazilide fumarate** USAN *antiarrhythmic*

**ipecac** USP *emetic* ②

**ipecac, powdered** USP

**ipexidine** INN *dental caries prophylactic* [also: ipexidine mesylate]

**ipexidine mesylate** USAN, INN *dental caries prophylactic* [also: ipexidine]

**ipodate calcium** USP *cholecystographic radiopaque medium*

**ipodate sodium** USAN, USP *cholecystographic radiopaque medium* [also: sodium ipodate; sodium iopodate]

**IPOL** subcu injection ℞ *poliomyelitis vaccine* [poliovirus vaccine, inactivated] 0.5 mL

***Ipomoea violacea* (morning glory) seeds** *contain lysergic acid amide, chemically similar to LSD, which produces hallucinations when ingested as a street drug* [see also: LSD]

**ipragratine** INN

**ipramidil** INN

**Ipran** tablets ℞ *antianginal; antihypertensive; antimigrainal* [propranolol HCl]

**ipratropium bromide** USAN, INN, BAN *bronchodilator; anticholinergic* 0.02% inhalation

**Ipravent** [see: Apo-Ipravent]

**iprazochrome** INN

**iprazone** [see: isoprazone]

**ipriflavone** INN

**iprindole** USAN, INN, BAN *antidepressant*

**iprocinodine HCl** USAN, BAN *veterinary antibacterial*

**iproclozide** INN, BAN

**iprocrolol** INN

**iprofenin** USAN *hepatic function test*

**iproheptine** INN

**iproniazid** INN, BAN

**ipronidazole** USAN, INN, BAN *antiprotozoal (Histomonas)*

**ipropethidine** [see: properidine]

**iproplatin** USAN, INN, BAN *antineoplastic*

**iprotiazem** INN

**iproxamine** INN *vasodilator* [also: iproxamine HCl]

**iproxamine HCl** USAN *vasodilator* [also: iproxamine]

**iprozilamine** INN

**ipsalazide** INN, BAN

**ipsapirone** INN, BAN *anxiolytic; investigational antidepressant* [also: ipsapirone HCl]

**ipsapirone HCl** USAN *anxiolytic; investigational antidepressant* [also: ipsapirone]

**Ipsatol Cough Formula for Children; Ipsatol Cough Formula for Adults** liquid OTC *antitussive; decongestant; expectorant* [dextromethorphan hydrobromide; phenylpropanolamine HCl; guaifenesin] 10•9•100 mg/5 mL

**IPTD (isopropyl-thiadiazol)** [see: glyprothiazol]

**IPV (inactivated poliomyelitis vaccine)** [see: poliovirus vaccine, inactivated]

**IPV (inactivated poliovaccine)** [see: poliovirus vaccine, inactivated]

**iquindamine** INN

**192Ir** [see: iridium Ir 192]

**irbesartan** USAN *antihypertensive; angiotensin II receptor antagonist*

**Ircon** tablets OTC *hematinic* [ferrous fumarate] 200 mg

**Ircon-FA** tablets OTC *hematinic* [ferrous fumarate; folic acid] 82•0.8 mg

**irgasan** [see: triclosan]

**iridium** *element (Ir)*

**iridium Ir 192** USAN *radioactive agent*

**irindalone** INN

**irinotecan** INN *antineoplastic for cervical, colon, and rectal cancers; topoisomerase I inhibitor* [also: irinotecan HCl]

**irinotecan HCl** USAN, JAN *antineoplastic for cervical, colon, and rectal cancers; topoisomerase I inhibitor* [also: irinotecan]

**irloxacin** INN

**irolapride** INN

**Iromin-G** tablets OTC *vitamin/iron supplement* [multiple vitamins; ferrous gluconate; folic acid] ±•30•0.8 mg

**iron** *element (Fe)*

**iron carbohydrate complex** [see: polyferose]

**iron dextran** USP *hematinic*

**iron heptonate** [see: gleptoferron]

**iron perchloride** [see: ferric chloride]

**iron polymalether** [see: ferropolimaler]

**iron sorbitex** USAN, USP *hematinic*

**Iron-Folic 500** timed-release tablets OTC *hematinic* [ferrous sulfate; multiple B vitamins; sodium ascorbate; folic acid] 105•±•500•0.8 mg

**Irospan** timed-release capsules, timed-release tablets OTC *hematinic* [ferrous sulfate; ascorbic acid] 60•150 mg

**Irrigate** eye wash OTC *extraocular irrigating solution* [sterile isotonic solution]

**irsogladine** INN

**irtemazole** USAN, INN, BAN *uricosuric*

**IS 5-MN (isosorbide 5-mononitrate)** [see: isorbide mononitrate]

**isaglidole** INN

**isamfazone** INN

**isamoltan** INN

**isamoxole** USAN, INN, BAN *antiasthmatic*

**isaxonine** INN

**isbogrel** INN

**iscador** *investigational (Phase I) antiviral for HIV and AIDS*

**I-Scrub** solution (name changed to Eye Scrub in 1996)

**Isda** *street drug slang* [see: heroin]

**Iselan** ℞ *investigational antianginal* [isosorbide mononitrate]

**Isepacin** injection ℞ *investigational aminoglycoside antibiotic for gram-positive and gram-negative infections* [isepamicin]

**isepamicin** USAN, INN, BAN *antibacterial; aminoglycoside*

**isethionate** USAN, BAN *combining name for radicals or groups* [also: isetionate]

**isetionate** INN *combining name for radicals or groups* [also: isethionate]

**ISG (immune serum globulin)** [see: globulin, immune]

**ISIS 2105** ℞ *investigational antiviral for genital warts*

**ISIS 2922** *investigational (Phase III) antiviral for AIDS-related cytomegalovirus retinitis*

**Ismelin** tablets ℞ *antihypertensive; investigational (orphan) for reflex sympathetic dystrophy and causalgia* [guanethidine monosulfate] 25 mg ⊘ Ritalin

**Ismelin Sulfate** tablets (name changed to Ismelin in 1993)

**Ismo** film-coated tablets ℞ *angina preventative* [isosorbide mononitrate] 20 mg

**Ismotic** solution ℞ *osmotic diuretic* [isosorbide] 45%

**iso-alcoholic elixir** NF

**isoaminile** INN, BAN

**isoamyl nitrate** [see: amyl nitrite]

**Iso-B** capsules OTC *vitamin supplement* [multiple B vitamins; folic acid; biotin] ±•200•100 μg

**Iso-Bid** sustained-release capsules (discontinued 1995) ℞ *antianginal* [isosorbide dinitrate] 40 mg

**isobromindione** INN

**isobucaine HCl** USP

**isobutamben** USAN, INN *topical anesthetic*

**isobutane** NF *aerosol propellant*

**isobutyl** *p*-aminobenzoate [see: isobutamben]

**isobutyl** α-phenylcyclohexaneglycolate [see: ibuverine]

**isobutyl 2-cyanoacrylate (IBC)** [see: bucrylate]

**isobutyl nitrite; butyl nitrite** *amyl nitrite substitutes, sold as euphoric*

street drugs, which produce a quick but short-lived "rush" [see also: amyl nitrite; volatile nitrites]

***p*-isobutylhydratropohydroxamic acid** [see: ibuproxam]

**isobutylhydrochlorothiazide** [see: buthiazide]

**isobutyramide** *investigational (orphan) for sickle cell disease, beta-thalassemia syndrome, and beta-hemoglobinopathies*

**isobuzole** BAN [also: glysobuzole]

**Isocaine HCl** injection ℞ *injectable local anesthetic* [mepivacaine HCl] 3%

**Isocaine HCl** injection ℞ *injectable local anesthetic* [mepivacaine HCl; levonordefrin] 2%•1:20 000

**Isocal** liquid OTC *enteral nutritional therapy* [lactose-free formula]

**Isocal HCN** ready-to-use liquid OTC *enteral nutritional therapy* [lactose-free formula]

**Isocal HN** liquid OTC *enteral nutritional therapy* [lactose-free formula]

**isocarboxazid** USP, INN, BAN *antidepressant; MAO inhibitor*

**Isocet** tablets ℞ *analgesic; anti-inflammatory; sedative* [acetaminophen; caffeine; butalbital] 325•40•50 mg

**Isoclor** Timesules (sustained-release capsules), tablets, liquid (discontinued 1995) OTC *decongestant; antihistamine* [pseudoephedrine HCl; chlorpheniramine maleate] 120•8 mg; 60•4 mg; 30•2 mg/5 mL

**Isoclor Expectorant** liquid ℞ *narcotic antitussive; decongestant; expectorant* [codeine phosphate; pseudoephedrine HCl; guaifenesin; alcohol 5%] 10•30•100 mg/5 mL

**Isocom** capsules ℞ *vasoconstrictor; sedative; analgesic (for migraine)* [isometheptene mucate; dichloralphenazone; acetaminophen] 65•100•325 mg

**isoconazole** USAN, INN, BAN *antibacterial; antifungal*

**isocromil** INN

**Isocult for Bacteriuria** culture paddles for professional use *in vitro diagnostic aid for nitrate, uropathogens, or bacteria in the urine*

**Isocult for Candida** culture paddles for professional use *in vitro diagnostic aid for Candida albicans in the vagina*

**Isocult for N gonorrhoeae and Candida** culture test for professional use OTC *in vitro diagnostic aid for gonorrhea and Candida in various specimens*

**Isocult for Neisseria gonorrhoeae** culture paddles for professional use *in vitro diagnostic aid for Neisseria gonorrhoeae*

**Isocult for Pseudomonas aeruginosa** culture test for professional use (discontinued 1995) *in vitro diagnostic aid for Pseudomonas aeruginosa in exudate or urine*

**Isocult for Staphylococcus aureus** culture paddles for professional use *in vitro diagnostic aid for Staphylococcus aureus in exudate*

**Isocult for Streptococcal pharyngitis** culture paddles for professional use *in vitro diagnostic test for streptococcal pharyngitis in throat swabs*

**Isocult for T vaginalis and Candida** culture test for professional use *in vitro diagnostic aid for Trichomonas and Candida in vaginal or urethral cultures*

**Isocult for Trichomonas vaginalis** culture test for professional use (discontinued 1995) *in vitro diagnostic aid for Trichomonas vaginalis in urethra or vagina*

**Isocult Throat Streptococci** test (name changed to Isocult for Streptococcal pharyngitis in 1995)

**isodapamide** [see: zidapamide]

*d*-**isoephedrine HCl** [see: pseudoephedrine HCl]

**isoetarine** INN *bronchodilator* [also: isoetharine]

**isoethadione** [see: paramethadione]

**isoetharine** USAN, BAN *bronchodilator* [also: isoetarine]

**isoetharine HCl** USP, BAN *bronchodilator* 0.08%, 0.1%, 0.125%, 0.167%, 0.17%, 0.2%, 0.25%, 1% inhalation

**isoetharine mesylate** USP, BAN *bronchodilator*

**isofezolac** INN

**isoflupredone** INN, BAN *anti-inflammatory* [also: isoflupredone acetate]

**isoflupredone acetate** USAN *anti-inflammatory* [also: isoflupredone]

**isoflurane** USAN, USP, INN, BAN *inhalation general anesthetic*

**isoflurophate** USP *antiglaucoma agent; irreversible cholinesterase inhibitor miotic* [also: dyflos]

**Isoject** (trademarked delivery system) *prefilled disposable syringe*

**Isolan** liquid OTC *enteral nutritional therapy* [lactose-free formula]

**isoleucine (L-isoleucine)** USAN, USP, INN, JAN *essential amino acid; symbols: Ile, I*

**isoleucine & leucine & valine** *investigational (orphan) for hyperphenylalaninemia*

**Isollyl Improved** tablets, capsules ℞ *analgesic; antipyretic; anti-inflammatory; sedative* [aspirin; caffeine; butalbital] 325•40•50 mg

**Isolyte E (G; H; M; P; R; S) with 5% Dextrose** IV infusion ℞ *intravenous nutritional/electrolyte therapy* [combined electrolyte solution; dextrose]

**Isolyte E; Isolyte S; Isolyte S pH 7.4** IV infusion ℞ *intravenous electrolyte therapy* [combined electrolyte solution]

**Isolyte S pH 7.4** IV infusion ℞ *intravenous electrolyte therapy* [combined electrolyte solution]

**isomazole** INN *cardiotonic* [also: isomazole HCl]

**isomazole HCl** USAN *cardiotonic* [also: isomazole]

**isomeprobamate** [see: carisoprodol]

**isomerol** USAN *antiseptic*

**isometamidium** BAN [also: isometamidium chloride]

**isometamidium chloride** INN [also: isometamidium]

**isomethadone** INN, BAN

**isomethepdrine chloride** [see: isomethepdrine]

**isometheptene** INN, BAN

**isometheptene HCl** [see: isometheptene]

**isometheptene mucate** USP *cerebral vasoconstrictor; "possibly effective" for migraine headaches*

**Isomil** liquid, powder OTC *hypoallergenic infant food* [soy protein formula] ☑ Esimil

**Isomil DF** ready-to-use liquid OTC *hypoallergenic infant food for management of diarrhea* [soy protein formula]

**Isomil SF** liquid OTC *hypoallergenic infant food* [soy protein formula, sucrose free]

**isomylamine HCl** USAN *smooth muscle relaxant*

**isoniazid** USP, INN, BAN *bactericidal; primary tuberculostatic* 50, 100, 300 mg oral; 50 mg/5 mL oral

**isonicophen** [see: aconiazide]

**isonicotinic acid hydrazide (INH)** [see: isoniazid]

**isonicotinic acid vanillylidenehydrazide** [see: ftivazide]

**1-isonicotinoyl-2-salicylidenehydrazine (INSH)** [see: salinazid]

**isonicotinylhydrazine** [see: isoniazid]

**isonixin** INN

**isooctadecanol** [see: isostearyl alcohol]

**isooctadecyl alcohol** [see: isostearyl alcohol]

**Isopan** liquid OTC *antacid* [magaldrate] 540 mg/5 mL

**Isopan Plus** liquid OTC *antacid; antiflatulent* [magaldrate; simethicone] 540•40 mg/5 mL

**Isopap** capsules ℞ *vasoconstrictor; sedative; analgesic (for migraine)* [isometheptene mucate; dichloralphenazone; acetaminophen] 65•100•325 mg

**isopentyl nitrite** [see: amyl nitrite]

**isophane insulin** BAN *antidiabetic* [also: insulin, isophane]

**isophenethanol** [see: nifenalol]

**isoprazone** INN, BAN

**isoprednidene** INN, BAN

**isopregnenone** [see: dydrogesterone]

**isoprenaline** INN, BAN *bronchodilator; vasopressor for shock* [also: isoproterenol HCl]

**L-isoprenaline** [see: levisoprenaline]

**isoprenaline HCl** [see: isoproterenol HCl]

**Isoprinosine** ℞ *investigational antiviral/immunomodulator for AIDS; investigational (orphan) for subacute sclerosing panencephalitis* [inosine pranobex]

**isoprofen** INN

**isopropamide iodide** USP, INN, BAN *peptic ulcer adjunct*

**isopropanol** [see: isopropyl alcohol]

**isopropicillin** INN

**isoproponum iodide** [see: isopropamide iodide]

**7-isopropoxyisoflavone** [see: ipriflavone]

**isopropyl alcohol** USP *topical anti-infective/antiseptic; solvent*

**isopropyl alcohol, rubbing** USP *rubefacient*

**N-isopropyl meprobamate** [see: carisoprodol]

**isopropyl myristate** NF *emollient*

**isopropyl palmitate** NF *oleaginous vehicle*

**isopropyl sebacate**

**isopropyl unoprostone** *investigational (Phase III) antiglaucoma agent*

**isopropylantipyrine** [see: propyphenazone]

**isopropylarterenol HCl** [see: isoproterenol HCl]

**isopropylarterenol sulfate** [see: isoproterenol sulfate]

**isoproterenol HCl** USP *bronchodilator; vasopressor for shock* [also: isoprenaline] 0.25%, 0.5%, 1% (1:400, 1:200, 1:100) inhalation; 0.25% aerosol; 0.2 mg/mL (1:5000) injection

**isoproterenol sulfate** USP *bronchodilator*

**Isoptin** film-coated tablets ℞ *antianginal; antiarrhythmic; antihypertensive; calcium channel blocker* [verapamil HCl] 40, 80, 120 mg ☑ Intropin

**Isoptin** IV injection ℞ *antitachyarrhythmic; calcium channel blocker* [verapamil HCl] 5 mg/2 mL

**Isoptin SR** film-coated sustained-release tablets ℞ *antihypertensive; calcium channel blocker* [verapamil HCl] 120, 180, 240 mg

**Isopto Alkaline** Drop-Tainers (eye drops) (discontinued 1995) OTC *ocular moisturizer/lubricant* [hydroxypropyl methylcellulose] 1%

**Isopto Atropine** Drop-Tainers (eye drops) ℞ *cycloplegic; mydriatic* [atropine sulfate] 0.5%, 1%

**Isopto Carbachol** Drop-Tainers (eye drops) ℞ *antiglaucoma agent; direct-acting miotic* [carbachol] 0.75%, 1.5%, 2.25%, 3%

**Isopto Carpine** Drop-Tainers (eye drops) ℞ *antiglaucoma agent; direct-acting miotic* [pilocarpine HCl] 0.25%, 0.5%, 1%, 2%, 3%, 4%, 5%, 6%, 8%, 10% ☑ Isopto Eserine

**Isopto Cetamide** Drop-Tainers (eye drops) ℞ *ophthalmic bacteriostatic* [sulfacetamide sodium] 15%

**Isopto Cetapred** eye drop suspension ℞ *ophthalmic topical corticosteroidal anti-inflammatory; bacteriostatic* [prednisolone acetate; sulfacetamide sodium] 0.25%•10%

**Isopto Eserine** eye drops (discontinued 1994) ℞ *antiglaucoma agent; reversible cholinesterase inhibitor miotic* [physostigmine salicylate] 0.25%, 0.5% ☑ Isopto Carpine

**Isopto Frin** eye drops (discontinued 1995) OTC *topical ocular decongestant* [phenylephrine HCl] 0.12%

**Isopto Homatropine** Drop-Tainers (eye drops) ℞ *cycloplegic; mydriatic* [homatropine hydrobromide] 2%, 5%

**Isopto Hyoscine** Drop-Tainers (eye drops) ℞ *cycloplegic; mydriatic* [scopolamine hydrobromide] 0.25%

**Isopto P-ES** Drop-Tainers (eye drops) (discontinued 1994) ℞ *antiglaucoma agent* [pilocarpine HCl; physostigmine salicylate] 2%•0.25%

**Isopto Plain; Isopto Tears** Drop-Tainers (eye drops) OTC *ocular moisturizer/lubricant* [hydroxypropyl methylcellulose] 0.5%

**Isordil** Titradose (tablets), Tembid (sustained-release capsules and tablets), sublingual ℞ *antianginal* [isosorbide dinitrate] 5, 10, 20, 30, 40 mg; 40 mg; 2.5, 5, 10 mg ☑ Isuprel

**isosorbide** USAN, USP, INN, BAN *osmotic diuretic*

**isosorbide dinitrate** USAN, USP, INN, BAN *coronary vasodilator; antianginal* 2.5, 5, 10, 20, 30, 40 mg oral

**isosorbide mononitrate** USAN, INN, BAN *coronary vasodilator*

**Isosource; Isosource HN** liquid OTC *enteral nutritional therapy* [lactose-free formula]

**isospaglumic acid** INN

**isospirilene** [see: spirilene]

**isostearyl alcohol** USAN *emollient; solvent*

**isosulfamerazine** [see: sulfaperin]

**isosulfan blue** USAN *lymphangiography aid* [also: sulphan blue]

**isosulpride** INN

**Isotein HN** powder OTC *enteral nutritional therapy* [lactose-free formula]

**3-isothiocyanato-1-propene** [see: allyl isothiocyanate]

**isothiocyanic acid, allyl ester** [see: allyl isothiocyanate]

**isothipendyl** INN, BAN

**isothipendyl HCl** [see: isothipendyl]

**isotiquimide** USAN, INN, BAN *antiulcerative*

**Isotrate** Timecelles (sustained-release capsules) (discontinued 1995) ℞ *antianginal* [isosorbide dinitrate] 40 mg

**isotretinoin** USAN, USP, INN, BAN *keratolytic for severe recalcitrant cystic acne*

**isotretinoin anisatil** USAN *keratolytic for acne vulgaris*

**Isotrex** ℞ *investigational keratolytic for acne* [isotretinoin]

**Isovex** capsules (discontinued 1996) ℞ *peripheral vasodilator* [ethaverine HCl] 100 mg

**Isovist** ℞ *investigational contrast medium for urography and angiography* [iotrolan]

**Isovorin** ℞ *investigational (orphan) antineoplastic and chemotherapy "rescue" agent* [L-leucovorin]

**Isovue-128; Isovue-200; Isovue-300; Isovue-370** injection ℞ *parenteral radiopaque agent* [iopamidol] 26%; 41%; 61%; 76%

**Isovue-M 200; Isovue-M 300** intrathecal injection ℞ *parenteral myelographic radiopaque agent* [iopamidol] 41%; 61%

**isoxaprolol** INN

**isoxepac** USAN, INN, BAN *anti-inflammatory*

**isoxicam** USAN, INN, BAN *nonsteroidal anti-inflammatory drug (NSAID); antiarthritic; analgesic; antipyretic*

**isoxsuprine** INN, BAN *peripheral vasodilator* [also: isoxsuprine HCl]

**isoxsuprine HCl** USP, JAN *peripheral vasodilator* [also: isoxsuprine] 10, 20 mg oral

**I-Soyalac** liquid OTC *hypoallergenic infant food* [soybean protein formula]

**isradipine** USAN, INN, BAN *antihypertensive; dihydropyridine calcium channel blocker*

**isrodipine** [see: isradipine]

**issues** *street drug slang* [see: cocaine, crack]

**Istin** (European name for U.S. product Norvasc)

**Isuprel** Glossets (sublingual tablets) (discontinued 1996) ℞ *bronchodilator for bronchial asthma and bronchospasm* [isoproterenol HCl] 10, 15 mg

**Isuprel** intracardiac, IV, IM, or subcu injection ℞ *vasopressor for cardiac, hypovolemic, or septic shock* [isoproterenol HCl] 1:5000 (0.2 mg/mL), 1:50 000 (0.02 mg/mL) ② Isordil

**Isuprel** Mistometer (metered-dose inhalation aerosol), solution for inhalation ℞ *bronchodilator for bronchial asthma and bronchospasm* [isoproterenol HCl] 131 μg/dose; 1:200 (0.5%)

**itanoxone** INN

**itasetron** USAN *anxiolytic; antidepressant; antiemetic; 5-HT$_3$ receptor antagonist*

**itazigrel** USAN, INN *platelet antiaggregatory agent*

**itazogrel** [see: itazigrel]

**Itch-X** spray, gel OTC *topical local anesthetic* [pramoxine HCl] 1%

**itobarbital** [see: butalbital]

**itraconazole** USAN, INN, BAN *systemic antifungal*

**itramin tosilate** INN [also: itramin tosylate]

**itramin tosylate** BAN [also: itramin tosilate]

**itrocainide** INN

**I-Valex-1** powder OTC *formula for infants with leucine catabolism disorder*

**I-Valex-2** powder OTC *enteral nutritional therapy for leucine catabolism disorder*

**Ivarest** cream, lotion OTC *topical poison ivy treatment* [calamine; benzocaine] 14%•5%

**ivarimod** INN

**Iveegam** freeze-dried powder for IV infusion ℞ *passive immunizing agent for HIV and Kawasaki syndrome; investigational (orphan) for acute myocarditis and juvenile rheumatoid arthritis* [immune globulin] 50 mg/mL

**ivermectin** USAN, INN, BAN *antiparasitic; anthelmintic for strongyloidiasis and onchocerciasis*

**ivermectin component B$_{1a}$**

**ivermectin component B$_{1b}$**

**IVIG (intravenous immunoglobulin)** [q.v.]

**Ivomec-SR** (name changed to Stromectol upon marketing release in 1997)

**ivoqualine** INN

**Ivy Shield** cream OTC *skin protectant*

**IvyBlock** OTC *topical poison ivy treatment* [bentoquatam] 5%

**Ivy-Chex** spray OTC *topical poison ivy treatment* [polyvinylpyrrolidone-vinylacetate copolymers; methyl salicylate; benzalkonium chloride]

**Ivy-Rid** spray OTC *topical poison ivy treatment* [polyvinylpyrrolidone-vinylacetate copolymers; benzalkonium chloride]

**jackpot** *street drug slang* [see: fentanyl]

**jam** *street drug slang* [see: amphetamine; cocaine]

**Jam Cecil** *street drug slang* [see: amphetamine]

**Jane** *street drug slang* [see: marijuana]

**Janimine** Filmtabs (film-coated tablets) (discontinued 1996) ℞ *tricyclic antidepressant; treatment for childhood enuresis* [imipramine HCl] 10, 25, 50 mg

**Japanese encephalitis (JE) virus vaccine** *active immunization vaccine*

**Jay; Jay smoke** *street drug slang for a marijuana cigarette* [see: marijuana]

**jee gee; jojee** *street drug slang* [see: heroin]

**Jeff** *street drug slang* [see: methcathinone]

**jellies** *street drug slang* [see: chloral hydrate]

**jelly** *street drug slang* [see: cocaine]

**jelly baby** *street drug slang* [see: amphetamines]

**jelly beans** *street drug slang* [see: amphetamines; chloral hydrate; cocaine, crack]

**Jenamicin** IV or IM injection ℞ *aminoglycoside-type antibiotic* [gentamicin sulfate] 40 mg/mL

**Jenest-28** tablets ℞ *biphasic oral contraceptive* [norethindrone; ethinyl estradiol] Phase 1: 0.5 mg•35 μg; Phase 2: 1 mg•35 μg

**jet** *street drug slang* [see: ketamine HCl]

**jet fuel** *street drug slang* [see: PCP]

**Jets** chewable tablets OTC *dietary supplement* [lysine; multiple vitamins] 300•± mg

**JE-VAX** powder for subcu injection ℞ *active immunizing agent* [Japanese encephalitis virus vaccine] 0.5 mL

**Jevity** liquid OTC *enteral nutritional therapy* [lactose-free formula]

**Jiffy Toothache Drops** (discontinued 1994) OTC *topical oral anesthetic; analgesic; antipruritic/counterirritant* [benzocaine; eugenol; menthol; alcohol 76%] 5%•9%•2%

**Jim Jones** *street drug slang for marijuana laced with cocaine and PCP* [see: marijuana; cocaine; PCP]

**jimsonweed** *the dried leaves or flowering tops of Datura stramonium, used as an antiasthmatic and abused as a street drug* [also known as: thorn apple; stramonium]

**jive** *street drug slang* [see: heroin; marijuana]

**jive doo jee** *street drug slang* [see: heroin]

**jive stick** *street drug slang for a marijuana cigarette* [see: marijuana]

**jodphthalein sodium** [see: iodophthalein sodium]

**Joe Friday** *street drug slang for Quaalude (methaqualone; disc. 1983), the tablet ID# matches Sgt. Friday's badge number on Dragnet* [see: methaqualone]

**jofendylate** [see: iophendylate]

**Johnson** *street drug slang* [see: cocaine, crack]

**Johnson grass** *street drug slang for low-potency Texas marijuana (President Lyndon Johnson was from Texas)* [see: marijuana]

**joint** *street drug slang for a marijuana cigarette* [see: marijuana]

**jojee; jee gee** *street drug slang* [see: heroin]

**jolly bean** *street drug slang* [see: amphetamines]

**jolly green** *street drug slang* [see: marijuana]

**Jones** *street drug slang* [see: heroin]

**jopanoic acid** [see: iopanoic acid]

**josamycin** USAN, INN *antibacterial*

**jotrizoic acid** [see: iotrizoic acid]

**joy flakes** *street drug slang* [see: heroin]

**joy juice** *street drug slang for chloral hydrate in an alcoholic beverage* [see: alcohol; chloral hydrate]

**joy plant** *street drug slang* [see: opium]

**joy powder** *street drug slang* [see: cocaine; heroin]

**joy smoke** *street drug slang* [see: marijuana]

**joy stick** *street drug slang for a marijuana cigarette* [see: marijuana]

**Juan Valdez** *street drug slang* [see: marijuana]

**Juanita** *street drug slang* [see: marijuana]

**Judas** *street drug slang, as in "the one who betrays" (a reference to Jesus' disciple)* [see: heroin]

**jugs** *street drug slang* [see: amphetamines]

**juice** *street drug slang for PCP or steroids* [see: PCP; anabolic steroids]

**juice joint** *street drug slang for a marijuana cigarette sprinkled with crack* [see: cocaine, crack; marijuana]

**ju-ju** *street drug slang for a marijuana cigarette* [see: marijuana]

**juniper tar** USP *antieczematic*

**junk** *street drug slang* [see: cocaine; heroin]

**Just Tears** eye drops OTC *ocular moisturizer/lubricant* [polyvinyl alcohol] 1.4%

**K+ 8; K+ 10** film-coated extended-release tablets ℞ *potassium supplement* [potassium chloride] 8 mEq (600 mg); 10 mEq (750 mg)

**K+ Care** powder ℞ *potassium supplement* [potassium chloride] 15, 20, 25 mEq/packet

**K+ Care ET** effervescent tablets ℞ *potassium supplement* [potassium bicarbonate] 20, 25 mEq

**⁴²K** [see: potassium chloride K 42]

**k82 ImmunoCap** test kit for professional use *in vitro diagnostic aid for specific latex allergies*

**Kabayo** *street drug slang* [see: heroin]

**Kabi 2234** *investigational treatment for urge incontinence*

**Kabikinase** powder for IV or intracoronary infusion ℞ *thrombolytic enzyme for lysis of thrombi and catheter clearance* [streptokinase] 250 000, 600 000, 750 000, 1 500 000 IU

**Kadian** polymer-coated sustained-release pellets in capsules ℞ *narcotic analgesic* [morphine sulfate] 20, 50, 100 mg

**Kainair** eye drops (discontinued 1994) ℞ *topical ophthalmic anesthetic* [proparacaine HCl]

**kainic acid** INN

**Kaksonjae** *street drug slang for smokable methamphetamine* [see: methamphetamine HCl]

**Kala** tablets OTC *dietary supplement; fever blister treatment; not generally regarded as safe and effective as an* *antidiarrheal* [Lactobacillus acidophilus (soy-based)] 200 million U

**kalafungin** USAN, INN *antifungal*

**Kali** *street drug slang* [see: marijuana]

**kallidinogenase** INN, BAN

**kalmopyrin** [see: calcium acetylsalicylate]

**kalsetal** [see: calcium acetylsalicylate]

**Kaltostat; Kaltostat Fortex** pads OTC *wound dressing* [calcium alginate fiber]

**kanamycin** INN, BAN *aminoglycoside bactericidal antibiotic; tuberculosis retreatment* [also: kanamycin sulfate] ⊘ Garamycin; gentamicin

**kanamycin B** [see: bekanamycin]

**kanamycin sulfate** USP *aminoglycoside bactericidal antibiotic; tuberculosis retreatment* [also: kanamycin] 75, 500, 1000 mg/vial injection

**kangaroo** *street drug slang* [see: cocaine, crack]

**Kank-a** liquid/film OTC *topical oral anesthetic* [benzocaine] 20%

**Kantrex** capsules, IV or IM injection, pediatric injection ℞ *aminoglycoside-type antibiotic* [kanamycin sulfate] 500 mg; 500, 1000 mg; 75 mg

**Kao Lectrolyte** powder for oral solution OTC *pediatric electrolyte replenisher*

**Kaochlor 10%; Kaochlor S-F** liquid ℞ *potassium supplement* [potassium chloride; alcohol 5%] 20 mEq/15 mL ⊘ K-Lor

**Kaodene Non-Narcotic** liquid OTC *antidiarrheal; GI adsorbent; antacid* [kaolin; pectin; bismuth subsalicylate] 3.9 g•194.4 mg• ⚤ per 30 mL ℞ codeine

**Kaodene Non-Narcotic** oral liquid OTC *antidiarrheal; GI adsorbent; antacid* [kaolin; pectin; bismuth subsalicylate] 130•6.48• ⚤ mg/mL

**kaolin** USP *GI adsorbent* ℞ Kaon

**Kaon** elixir ℞ *potassium supplement* [potassium gluconate] 20 mEq/15 mL ℞ kaolin

**Kaon-Cl; Kaon-Cl 10** extended-release tablets ℞ *potassium supplement* [potassium chloride] 500 mg (6.7 mEq); 750 mg (10 mEq)

**Kaon-Cl 20%** liquid ℞ *potassium supplement* [potassium chloride; alcohol 5%] 40 mEq/15 mL

**Kaopectate, Children's** chewable tablets (discontinued 1995) OTC *antidiarrheal; GI adsorbent* [attapulgite] 300 mg ℞ Kapectalin

**Kaopectate, Children's** liquid OTC *antidiarrheal; GI adsorbent* [attapulgite] 600 mg/15 mL ℞ Kapectalin

**Kaopectate II** caplets OTC *antidiarrheal* [loperamide HCl] 2 mg

**Kaopectate Advanced Formula** oral liquid OTC *antidiarrheal; GI adsorbent* [attapulgite] 750 mg/15 mL

**Kaopectate Maximum Strength** caplets OTC *antidiarrheal; GI adsorbent* [attapulgite] 750 mg

**Kao-Spen** oral suspension OTC *GI adsorbent; antidiarrheal* [kaolin; pectin] 5.2 g•260 mg per 30 mL

**Kapectolin** liquid OTC *GI adsorbent; antidiarrheal* [kaolin; pectin] 90•2 g/30 mL ℞ Kaopectate

**Kapectolin PG** liquid (discontinued 1994) ℞ *GI adsorbent; not generally regarded as safe and effective as an antidiarrheal* [opium; kaolin; pectin; hyoscyamine sulfate; atropine sulfate; scopolamine hydrobromide]

**kaps** *street drug slang* [see: PCP]

**Kapseal** (trademarked dosage form) *capsules sealed with a band*

**Karachi** *street drug slang (a reference to Karachi, Pakistan)* [see: heroin]

**Karidium** tablets, chewable tablets, drops ℞ *dental caries preventative*

[sodium fluoride] 2.2 mg; 2.2 mg; 0.275 mg/drop

**Karigel; Karigel-N** gel ℞ *topical dental caries preventative* [sodium fluoride] 1.1%

**kasal** USAN *food additive*

**Kasof** capsules OTC *stool softener* [docusate potassium] 240 mg

**kat; khat; q'at** *street drug slang for leaves of the Catha edulis plant* [see: Catha edulis, cathinone]

**Katadolon** ℞ *investigational narcotic analgesic and muscle relaxant* [flupirtine]

**Kato** powder (discontinued 1995) ℞ *potassium supplement* [potassium chloride] 20 mEq/packet

**Kay Ciel** liquid, powder ℞ *potassium supplement* [potassium chloride] 20 mEq/15 mL; 20 mEq/packet ℞ KCl

**kaya** *street drug slang* [see: marijuana]

**Kaybovite-1000** IM or subcu injection (discontinued 1994) ℞ *antianemic; vitamin $B_{12}$ supplement* [cyanocobalamin] 1000 µg/mL

**Kayexalate** powder ℞ *potassium-removing agent for hyperkalemia* [sodium polystyrene sulfonate]

**Kaylixir** liquid ℞ *potassium supplement* [potassium gluconate; alcohol 5%] 20 mEq/15 mL

**Kaysine** injection (discontinued 1995) ℞ *treatment for varicose veins with stasis dermatitis* [adenosine phosphate] 25 mg/mL

**K-blast** *street drug slang* [see: PCP]

**K-C** oral suspension OTC *antidiarrheal; GI adsorbent; antacid* [kaolin; pectin; bismuth subcarbonate] 5 g•260 mg• 260 mg per 30 mL

**KCl (potassium chloride)** [q.v.] ℞ Kay Ciel

**K-DEC** tablets (discontinued 1994) OTC *vitamin/mineral/iron supplement* [multiple vitamins & minerals; ferrous fumarate; folic acid; biotin] ≝ • 18 mg•0.4 mg•30 µg

**K-Dur 10; K-Dur 20** controlled-release tablets ℞ *potassium supplement* [potassium chloride] 750 mg (10 mEq); 1500 mg (20 mEq)

**kebuzone** INN

**Keflet** tablets (discontinued 1993) ℞ *cephalosporin-type antibiotic* [cephalexin monohydrate] 250, 500, 1000 mg ⍛ Keflex; Keflin

**Keflex** pediatric drops (discontinued 1995) ℞ *cephalosporin-type antibiotic* [cephalexin monohydrate] 100 mg/mL ⍛ Keflet; Keflin

**Keflex** Pulvules (capsules), oral suspension ℞ *cephalosporin-type antibiotic* [cephalexin monohydrate] 250, 500 mg; 125, 250 mg/5 mL ⍛ Keflet; Keflin

**Keflin, Neutral** powder for IV or IM injection (discontinued 1996) ℞ *cephalosporin-type antibiotic* [cephalothin sodium] 1, 2 g ⍛ Keflet; Keflex

**Keftab** tablets ℞ *cephalosporin-type antibiotic* [cephalexin HCl monohydrate] 500 mg

**Kefurox** powder for IV or IM injection ℞ *cephalosporin-type antibiotic* [cefuroxime sodium] 0.75, 1.5, 7.5 g

**Kefzol** powder for IV or IM injection ℞ *cephalosporin-type antibiotic* [cefazolin sodium] 0.25, 0.5, 1, 10, 20 g ⍛ Cefzil

**kellofylline** [see: visnafylline]

**Kemadrin** tablets ℞ *anticholinergic; antiparkinsonian agent* [procyclidine HCl] 5 mg ⍛ Coumadin

**Kemron** ℞ *investigational oral treatment for AIDS* [interferon alfa]

**Kemsol** ⓒⒶⓝ (U.S. product: Rimso-50) solution for bladder instillation ℞ *anti-inflammatory for symptomatic relief of interstitial cystitis* [dimethyl sulfoxide (DMSO)] 70%

**Kenacort** tablets, syrup ℞ *glucocorticoids* [triamcinolone] 4, 8 mg; 4 mg/5 mL

**Kenaject-40** IM, intra-articular, intrabursal, intradermal injection ℞ *glucocorticoids* [triamcinolone acetonide] 40 mg/mL

**Kenalog** ointment, cream, lotion, aerosol spray ℞ *topical corticosteroid* [triamcinolone acetonide] 0.025%, 0.1%, 0.5%; 0.025%, 0.1%, 0.5%; 0.025%, 0.1%; ⚕ ⍛ Ketalar

**Kenalog in Orabase** oral paste ℞ *topical corticosteroid* [triamcinolone acetonide] 0.1%

**Kenalog-10; Kenalog-40** IM, intra-articular, intrabursal, intradermal injection ℞ *glucocorticoids* [triamcinolone acetonide] 10 mg/mL; 40 mg/mL

**Kenalog-H** cream ℞ *topical corticosteroid* [triamcinolone acetonide] 0.1%

**Kendall's compound A** [see: dehydrocorticosterone]

**Kendall's compound B** [see: corticosterone]

**Kendall's compound E** [see: cortisone acetate]

**Kendall's compound F** [see: hydrocortisone]

**Kendall's desoxy compound B** [see: desoxycorticosterone acetate]

**Kenicef** ℞ *investigational cephalosporin antibiotic* [cefodizime]

**Kenonel** cream ℞ *topical corticosteroid* [triamcinolone acetonide] 1%

**Kentucky blue** *street drug slang* [see: marijuana]

**Kenwood Therapeutic** liquid OTC *vitamin/mineral supplement* [multiple vitamins & minerals] ⚕

**keoxifene HCl** [now: raloxifene HCl]

**keracyanin** INN

**Keralyte** gel (discontinued 1994) ℞ *topical keratolytic* [salicylic acid] 6%

**keratinocyte growth factor** *investigational GI protective agent*

**keratolytics** *a class of agents that cause sloughing of the horny layer of the epidermis and softening of the skin*

**Keri; Keri Light** lotion OTC *moisturizer; emollient*

**Keri Creme** OTC *moisturizer; emollient*

**Keri Facial Cleanser** liquid (discontinued 1994) OTC *soap-free therapeutic skin cleanser*

**KeriCort-10** cream OTC *topical corticosteroid* [hydrocortisone] 1%

**Kerledex** ℞ *investigational antihypertensive β-blocker and diuretic combination* [betaxolol HCl; chlorthalidone]

**Kerlone** tablets ℞ *antihypertensive; β-blocker* [betaxolol HCl] 10, 20 mg

**Kerodex #51** cream OTC *skin protectant for dry or oily work*

**Kerodex #71** cream OTC *water repellant skin protectant for wet work*

**Kestrone 5** IM injection ℞ *estrogen replacement therapy; antineoplastic for prostatic and breast cancer* [estrone] 5 mg/mL

**Ketalar** IV or IM injection ℞ *rapid-acting general anesthetic; sometimes abused as a street drug due to its "dissociative state" effects* [ketamine HCl] 10, 50, 100 mg/mL ⊠ Kenalog

**ketamine** INN, BAN *a rapid-acting general anesthetic; sometimes abused as a street drug due to its "dissociative state" effects* [also: ketamine HCl]

**ketamine HCl** USAN, USP, JAN *a rapid-acting general anesthetic; sometimes abused as a street drug due to its "dissociative state" effects* [also: ketamine]

**ketanserin** USAN, INN, BAN *serotonin antagonist*

**ketazocine** USAN, INN *analgesic*

**ketazolam** USAN, INN, BAN *minor tranquilizer*

**kethoxal** USAN *antiviral* [also: ketoxal]

**ketimipramine** INN *antidepressant* [also: ketipramine fumarate]

**ketimipramine fumarate** [see: ketipramine fumarate]

**ketipramine fumarate** USAN *antidepressant* [also: ketimipramine]

**ketobemidone** INN, BAN

**ketocaine** INN

**ketocainol** INN

**ketocholanic acid** [see: dehydrocholic acid]

**ketoconazole** USAN, USP, INN, BAN *broad-spectrum antifungal*

**ketoconazole & cyclosporine** orphan status withdrawn 1996

**Keto-Diastix** reagent strips *in vitro diagnostic aid for multiple urine products*

**ketohexazine** [see: cetohexazine]

**Ketonex-1** powder OTC *formula for infants with maple syrup urine disease*

**Ketonex-2** powder OTC *enteral nutritional therapy for maple syrup urine disease*

**ketoprofen** USAN, INN, BAN, JAN *antiarthritic; nonsteroidal anti-inflammatory drug (NSAID); analgesic* 25, 50, 75 mg oral

**ketorfanol** USAN, INN *analgesic*

**ketorolac** INN, BAN *analgesic; antipyretic; nonsteroidal anti-inflammatory drug (NSAID)* [also: ketorolac tromethamine]

**ketorolac tromethamine** USAN *analgesic; antipyretic; nonsteroidal anti-inflammatory drug (NSAID)* [also: ketorolac] 10 mg oral

**Ketostix** reagent strips for home use OTC *in vitro diagnostic aid for acetone (ketones) in the urine*

**ketotifen** INN, BAN *antiasthmatic* [also: ketotifen fumarate]

**ketotifen fumarate** USAN, JAN *antiasthmatic* [also: ketotifen]

**ketotrexate** INN

**ketoxal** INN *antiviral* [also: kethoxal]

**Kevadon** ℞ *investigational treatment for graft vs. host disease* [thalidomide]

**Key-Plex** injection ℞ *parenteral vitamin therapy* [multiple B vitamins; vitamin C] ± • 50 mg/mL

**Key-Pred 25; Key-Pred 50** IM injection ℞ *glucocorticoids* [prednisolone acetate] 25 mg/mL; 50 mg/mL

**Key-Pred-SP** IV or IM injection ℞ *glucocorticoids* [prednisolone sodium phosphate] 20 mg/mL

**keys to the kingdom** street drug slang [see: LSD]

**K-Flex** IV or IM injection (discontinued 1993) ℞ *skeletal muscle relaxant* [orphenadrine citrate]

**K-G Elixir** ℞ *potassium supplement* [potassium gluconate] 20 mEq/15 mL

**KGB** street drug slang for "killer green bud" [see: marijuana]

**khat; kat; q'at** street drug slang for leaves of the Catha edulis plant [see: Catha edulis, cathinone]

**khellin** INN

**khelloside** INN

**Kibbles and Bits** street drug slang for a combination of Talwin (pentazocine HCl) and Ritalin (methylphenidate HCl) or crumbs of crack [see: Talwin; pentazocine HCl; Ritalin; methylphenidate HCl; cocaine; crack]

**kick stick** street drug slang for a marijuana cigarette [see: marijuana]

**Kiddy Chews** chewable tablets (discontinued 1995) OTC *vitamin supple-*

*ment* [multiple vitamins; folic acid] ± •0.3 mg

**Kiddy Chews with Iron** chewable tablets (discontinued 1995) OTC *vitamin/iron supplement* [multiple vitamins; iron; folic acid] ± •15•0.3 mg

**KIE** syrup ℞ *decongestant; expectorant* [ephedrine HCl; potassium iodide] 8•150 mg/5 mL

**kif; kiff** *street drug slang for potent Moroccan marijuana or hashish* [see: hashish; marijuana]

**killer** *street drug slang* [see: marijuana; PCP]

**killer weed** *street drug slang for marijuana (1960s and 70s) or a combination of marijuana and PCP (1980s–)* [see: marijuana; PCP]

**kilter** *street drug slang* [see: marijuana]

**kind** *street drug slang* [see: marijuana]

**Kindercal** liquid OTC *enteral nutritional therapy* [lactose-free formula]

**Kinedak** ℞ *investigational treatment for diabetic neuropathy* [epalrestat]

**Kinesed** chewable tablets (discontinued 1995) ℞ *GI anticholinergic; sedative* [atropine sulfate; scopolamine hydrobromide; hyoscyamine hydrobromide; phenobarbital] 0.12•0.007•0.12•16 mg

**Kinevac** powder for IV injection ℞ *in vivo gallbladder function test* [sincalide] 1 μg/mL

**king ivory** *street drug slang* [see: fentanyl]

**King Kong pills** *street drug slang for barbiturate sleeping pills or other CNS depressants* [see: barbiturates]

**king's habit** *street drug slang* [see: cocaine]

**kitasamycin** USAN, INN, BAN, JAN *antibacterial* [also: acetylkitasamycin; kitasamycin tartrate]

**kitasamycin tartrate** JAN *antibacterial* [also: kitasamycin; acetylkitasamycin]

**KL4 surfactant** *investigational (orphan) for respiratory distress syndrome in adults and premature infants and meconium aspiration in newborn infants*

**Klaron** lotion ℞ *topical antibiotic acne treatment* [sodium sulfacetamide] 10%

**KLB6; Ultra KLB6** softgels OTC *dietary supplement* [vitamin B₆; multiple food supplements] 3.5• ± mg; 16.7• ± mg

**K-Lease** extended-release capsules ℞ *potassium supplement* [potassium chloride] 750 mg (10 mEq)

**Kleenex** *street drug slang* [see: MDMA]

**Klerist-D** tablets, sustained-release capsules ℞ *decongestant; antihistamine* [pseudoephedrine HCl; chlorpheniramine maleate] 60•4 mg; 120•8 mg

**Klonopin** tablets, Rx Pak (prescription package), Tel-E-Dose (unit dose package) ℞ *anticonvulsant; investigational (orphan) for hyperexplexia (startle disease)* [clonazepam] 0.5, 1, 2 mg ⍰ clonidine

**K-Lor** powder ℞ *potassium supplement* [potassium chloride] 15, 20 mEq/packet ⍰ Kaochlor

**Klor-Con; Klor-Con/25** powder ℞ *potassium supplement* [potassium chloride] 20 mEq/packet; 25 mEq/packet

**Klor-Con 8; Klor-Con 10** film-coated extended-release tablets ℞ *potassium supplement* [potassium chloride] 600 mg (8 mEq); 750 mg (10 mEq)

**Klor-Con/EF** effervescent tablets ℞ *potassium supplement* [potassium bicarbonate; potassium citrate] 25 mEq (K)

**Klorvess** liquid, effervescent granules, effervescent tablets ℞ *potassium supplement* [potassium chloride] 20 mEq/15 mL; 20 mEq/packet; 20 mEq

**Klotrix** film-coated controlled-release tablets ℞ *potassium supplement* [potassium chloride] 750 mg (10 mEq) ⍰ Liotrix

**K-Lyte; K-Lyte DS** effervescent tablets ℞ *potassium supplement* [potassium bicarbonate; potassium citrate] 25 mEq; 50 mEq (K)

**K-Lyte** ⍰ (U.S. product: Urocit-K) effervescent tablets ℞ *urinary alkalizer for hypocitruria* [potassium citrate] 2.5 g

**K-Lyte/Cl** powder ℞ *potassium supplement* [potassium chloride] 25 mEq/dose

**K-Lyte/Cl; K-Lyte/Cl 50** effervescent tablets Ŗ *potassium supplement* [potassium chloride] 25 mEq; 50 mEq

**KNI-272** *investigational (Phase I) antiviral for pediatric and adult HIV*

**knockout drops** *street drug slang for chloral hydrate mixed in an alcoholic beverage* [see: alcohol; chloral hydrate]

**K-Norm** controlled-release capsules Ŗ *potassium supplement* [potassium chloride] 750 mg (10 mEq)

**Koāte-HP** powder for IV injection Ŗ *antihemophilic to correct coagulation deficiency* [antihemophilic factor VIII] 250, 500, 1000, 1500 IU

**Koāte-HS** powder for IV injection (discontinued 1994) Ŗ *antihemophilic to correct coagulation deficiency* [antihemophilic factor VIII] ?

**Kof-Eze** lozenges OTC *topical antipruritic/counterirritant; mild local anesthetic* [menthol] 6 mg

**KoGENate** powder for IV injection Ŗ *antihemophilic for treatment of hemophilia A and presurgical prophylaxis of hemophiliacs (orphan)* [antihemophilic factor VIII, recombinant] ?

**KOH (potassium hydroxide)** [q.v.]

**Kokomo** *street drug slang* [see: cocaine, crack]

**Kolephrin** caplets OTC *decongestant; antihistamine; analgesic* [pseudoephedrine HCl; chlorpheniramine maleate; acetaminophen] 30•2•325 mg

**Kolephrin GG/DM** liquid OTC *antitussive; expectorant* [dextromethorphan hydrobromide; guaifenesin] 10•150 mg/5 mL

**Kolephrin/DM** caplets OTC *antitussive; decongestant; antihistamine; analgesic* [dextromethorphan hydrobromide; pseudoephedrine HCl; chlorpheniramine maleate; acetaminophen] 10•30•2•325 mg

**kolfocon A** USAN *hydrophobic contact lens material*

**kolfocon B** USAN *hydrophobic contact lens material*

**kolfocon C** USAN *hydrophobic contact lens material*

**kolfocon D** USAN *hydrophobic contact lens material*

**Kolyum** liquid Ŗ *potassium supplement* [potassium gluconate; potassium chloride] 20 mEq/15 mL (K)

**Kolyum** powder (discontinued 1993) Ŗ *potassium supplement* [potassium gluconate; potassium chloride] 20 mEq/packet (K)

**Komed** lotion (discontinued 1994) OTC *topical acne treatment* [salicylic acid; sodium thiosulfate; isopropyl alcohol] 2%•8%•25%

**Konakion** IM injection (discontinued 1997) Ŗ *coagulant; correct anticoagulant-induced prothrombin deficiency; vitamin K supplement* [phytonadione] 2 mg/mL

**Kondon's Nasal** jelly OTC *nasal decongestant* [ephedrine] 1%

**Kondremul Plain** emulsion OTC *emollient laxative* [mineral oil]

**Kondremul with Phenolphthalein** emulsion OTC *laxative* [mineral oil; phenolphthalein] 55%•150 mg/15 mL

**Konsyl** powder OTC *bulk laxative* [psyllium] 100%

**Konsyl Fiber** tablets OTC *bulk laxative; antidiarrheal* [calcium polycarbophil] 625 mg

**Konsyl-D; Konsyl Orange** powder OTC *bulk laxative* [psyllium hydrophilic mucilloid] 3.4 g/tbsp.

**Konyne 80** IV infusion Ŗ *antihemophilic to correct factor VIII (hemophilia A) and factor IX (hemophilia B; Christmas disease) deficiencies* [coagulation factors II, VII, IX, and X, heat treated] 20, 40 mL

**Kools** *street drug slang* [see: PCP]

**Kophane Cough & Cold Formula** liquid OTC *antitussive; decongestant; antihistamine* [dextromethorphan hydrobromide; phenylpropanolamine HCl; chlorpheniramine maleate] 10•12.5•2 mg/5 mL

**Korigesic** tablets (discontinued 1993) Ŗ *decongestant; antihistamine; analgesic* [phenylephrine HCl; chlorpheniramine maleate; acetaminophen; caffeine]

**Koromex** premedicated condom (discontinued 1995) OTC *spermicidal/barrier contraceptive* [nonoxynol 9] 5.6%

**Koromex** vaginal cream OTC *spermicidal contraceptive (for use with a diaphragm)* [octoxynol 9] 3%

**Koromex** vaginal foam, vaginal jelly OTC *spermicidal contraceptive* [nonoxynol 9] 12.5%; 3% 🔟 Komex

**Koromex Crystal Clear** vaginal gel OTC *spermicidal contraceptive (for use with a diaphragm)* [nonoxynol 9] 2%

**Kovitonic** liquid OTC *hematinic* [ferric pyrophosphate; multiple B vitamins; lysine; folic acid] 42•±•10•0.1 mg/15 mL

**K-Pek** oral suspension OTC *antidiarrheal; GI adsorbent* [attapulgite] 600 mg/15 mL

**K-Phen-50** injection ℞ *antihistamine; motion sickness; sleep aid; antiemetic; sedative* [promethazine HCl] 50 mg/mL

**K-Phos M.F.** tablets ℞ *urinary acidifier* [potassium acid phosphate; sodium acid phosphate] 155•350 mg (1.1 mEq potassium, 2.9 mEq sodium)

**K-Phos Neutral** film-coated tablets ℞ *urinary acidifier* [dibasic sodium phosphate; monobasic potassium phosphate; monobasic sodium phosphate] 852•155•130 mg (1.1 mEq potassium, 13.0 mEq sodium)

**K-Phos No. 2** tablets ℞ *urinary acidifier* [potassium acid phosphate; sodium acid phosphate] 305•700 mg (2.3 mEq potassium, 5.8 mEq sodium)

**K-Phos Original** tablets ℞ *urinary acidifier* [potassium acid phosphate] 500 mg (3.7 mEq potassium)

**K.P.N.** tablets OTC *vitamin/mineral/calcium/iron supplement* [multiple vitamins & minerals; calcium; iron; folic acid] ±•333•11•0.27 mg

**$^{81m}$Kr** [see: krypton Kr 81m]

**$^{85}$Kr** [see: krypton clathrate Kr 85]

**Kredex** (European name for U.S. product Coreg)

**Kronocap** (trademarked dosage form) *sustained-release capsule*

**Kronofed-A** sustained-release capsules ℞ *decongestant; antihistamine* [pseudoephedrine HCl; chlorpheniramine maleate] 120•8 mg

**Kronofed-A Jr.** Kronocaps (sustained-release capsules) ℞ *pediatric decongestant and antihistamine* [pseudoephedrine HCl; chlorpheniramine maleate] 60•4 mg

**Krypt Tonight** *street drug slang, a brand-name sound-alike to "kryptonite," the substance that makes Superman weak* [see: isobutyl nitrite]

**krypton** *element (Kr)*

**krypton clathrate Kr 85** USAN *radioactive agent*

**krypton Kr 81m** USAN, USP *radioactive agent*

**kryptonite** *street drug slang* [see: cocaine, crack]

**krystal; crystal; krystal joint; crystal joint** *street drug slang* [see: PCP]

**K-Tab** film-coated extended-release tablets ℞ *potassium supplement* [potassium chloride] 750 mg (10 mEq)

**Kudrox** oral suspension OTC *antacid* [aluminum hydroxide; magnesium hydroxide; simethicone] 500•450•40 mg/5 mL

**kumbo** *street drug slang* [see: marijuana]

**Kutapressin** subcu or IM injection ℞ *claimed to be an anti-inflammatory for multiple dermatoses* [liver derivative complex] 25.5 mg/mL

**Kutrase** capsules ℞ *digestive enzymes; antispasmodic; sedative* [amylase; protease; lipase; cellulase; hyoscyamine sulfate; phenyltoloxamine citrate] 30•6•75•2•0.0625•15 mg

**Ku-Zyme** capsules ℞ *digestive enzymes* [amylase; protease; lipase; cellulase] 30•6•75•2 mg

**Ku-Zyme HP** capsules ℞ *digestive enzymes* [lipase; protease; amylase] 8000•30 000•30 000 U

**Kwelcof** liquid ℞ *narcotic antitussive; expectorant* [hydrocodone bitartrate; guaifenesin] 5•100 mg/5 mL

**Kwell** cream, lotion, shampoo (discontinued 1996) ℞ *scabicide; pediculicide* [lindane] 1%

**Kwildane** lotion, shampoo ℞ *scabicide; pediculicide* [lindane]

**K-Y** vaginal jelly OTC *lubricant* [glycerin; hydroxyethyl cellulose]

**K-Y Plus** vaginal gel OTC *spermicidal contraceptive (for use with a diaphragm)* [nonoxynol 9] 2.2%

**kyamepromazin** [see: cyamemazine]

**Kybernin** ℞ *for thrombosis and pulmonary emboli of congenital AT-III deficiency (orphan)* [antithrombin III concentrate IV]

**Kynac** ℞ *investigational treatment for psoriasis and eczema*

**Kynacyte** ℞ *investigational cancer chemotherapy enhancer*

**Kytril** film-coated tablets, IV infusion ℞ *5-HT$_3$ antagonist; antiemetic/antinauseant for chemotherapy* [granisetron HCl] 1 mg; 1.12 mg/mL

**L-5 hydroxytryptophan (L-5HTP)** *investigational (orphan) for postanoxic intention myoclonus*

**L-696,229** [see: non-nucleoside reverse transcriptase inhibitor]

**L-697,661** *investigational non-nucleoside antiviral for AIDS (clinical trials discontinued 1994)*

**L.A.** *street drug slang for long-acting amphetamine* [see: amphetamines]

**L.A. glass; L.A. ice** *street drug slang for smokable methamphetamine* [see: methamphetamine HCl]

**L.A. turnarounds** *street drug slang, a reference to truckers' use of amphetamines for long-distance runs* [see: amphetamines]

**LA-12** IM injection ℞ *antianemic; vitamin B$_{12}$ supplement* [hydroxocobalamin] 1000 μg/mL

**LAAM (*l*-acetyl-α-methadol [or] *l*-alpha-acetyl-methadol)** [see: levomethadyl acetate]

**labetalol** INN, BAN *antihypertensive; antiadrenergic (α- and β-receptor)* [also: labetalol HCl]

**labetalol HCl** USAN, USP *antihypertensive; antiadrenergic (α- and β-receptor)* [also: labetalol]

**Labstix** reagent strips *in vitro diagnostic aid for multiple urine products*

**lace** *street drug slang for a combination of cocaine and marijuana* [see: cocaine; marijuana]

**Lac-Hydrin** cream, lotion ℞ *moisturizer; emollient* [ammonium lactate] 12%

**Lac-Hydrin Five** lotion OTC *moisturizer; emollient* [lactic acid]

**lacidipine** USAN, INN, BAN *antihypertensive; calcium channel blocker*

**Lacipil** (commercially available in Europe) ℞ *investigational antihypertensive; calcium channel blocker* [lacidipine]

**Lacril** eye drops OTC *ocular moisturizer/ lubricant* [hydroxypropyl methylcellulose] 0.5%

**Lacri-Lube NP; Lacri-Lube S.O.P.** ophthalmic ointment OTC *ocular moisturizer/lubricant* [white petrolatum; mineral oil; lanolin]

**Lacrisert** ophthalmic insert OTC *ocular moisturizer/lubricant* [hydroxypropyl cellulose] 5 mg

**LactAid** liquid, tablets OTC *digestive aid for lactose intolerance* [lactase enzyme] 250 U/drop; 3000 U

**lactalfate** INN

**lactase enzyme** *digestive enzyme for lactose intolerance*

**lactated potassic saline** [see: potassic saline, lactated]

**lactated Ringer's (LR) injection** [see: Ringer's injection, lactated]

**lactated Ringer's (LR) solution** [see: Ringer's injection, lactated]

**lactic acid** USP *pH adjusting agent*

**LactiCare** lotion OTC *emollient; moisturizer* [lactic acid]

**LactiCare-HC** lotion ℞ *topical corticosteroid* [hydrocortisone] 1%, 2.5%

**Lactinex** granules, chewable tablets OTC *dietary supplement; fever blister* treatment; *not generally regarded as safe and effective as an antidiarrheal* [Lactobacillus acidophilus; Lactobacillus bulgaricus]

**Lactinol** lotion ℞ *emollient; moisturizer* [lactic acid] 10%

**Lactinol-E** cream ℞ *emollient; moisturizer* [lactic acid; vitamin E] 10%•116.67 IU/g

**Lactisol; Lactisol-Forte** liquid (discontinued 1994) ℞ *topical keratolytic* [salicylic acid in a collodion base; lactic acid] 16.7%•16.7%; 20%•20%

**lactitol** INN, BAN

**Lactobacillus acidophilus** *dietary supplement; not generally regarded as safe and effective as an antidiarrheal*

**Lactobacillus bulgaricus** *dietary supplement; not generally regarded as safe and effective as an antidiarrheal*

**lactobin** *investigational (orphan) for AIDS-related diarrhea*

**lactobionic acid, calcium salt, dihydrate** [see: calcium lactobionate]

**Lactocal-F** film-coated tablets ℞ *vitamin/mineral/calcium/iron supplement* [multiple vitamins & minerals; calcium; iron; folic acid] ≟•200•65•1 mg

**lactoflavin** [see: riboflavin]

**Lactofree** liquid, powder OTC *hypoallergenic infant formula* [milk-based formula, lactose free]

**Lactogest** soft gel capsules (discontinued 1994) OTC *digestive aid for lactose intolerance* [lactase enzyme]

**β-lactone** [see: propiolactone]

**γ-lactone D-glucofuranuronic acid** see: glucurolactone

**lactose** NF *tablet and capsule diluent; dietary supplement*

**Lactrase** capsules OTC *digestive aid for lactose intolerance* [lactase enzyme] 250 mg

**lactulose** USAN, USP, INN, BAN *laxative*

**ladakamycin** [now: azacitidine]

**lady; lady caine; lady snow** *street drug slang* [see: cocaine]

**Lady Esther** cream OTC *moisturizer; emollient* [mineral oil] ≟

**laidlomycin** INN *veterinary growth stimulant* [also: laidlomycin propionate potassium]

**laidlomycin propionate potassium** USAN *veterinary growth stimulant* [also: laidlomycin]

**Lakbay diva** *street drug slang* [see: marijuana]

**Laki-Lorand factor** [see: factor XIII]

**Lambda** ℞ *investigational (Phase III) treatment for renal failure*

**lamb's bread** *street drug slang* [see: marijuana]

**Lamictal** tablets ℞ *phenyltriazine anticonvulsant; investigational (orphan) for Lennox-Gastaut syndrome* [lamotrigine] 25, 100, 150, 200 mg

**lamifiban** USAN, INN *GPIIb/IIIa receptor inhibitor; antiplatelet/antithrombotic agent for unstable angina*

**Lamisil** cream ℞ *topical allylamine antifungal* [terbinafine HCl] 1%

**Lamisil** tablets ℞ *systemic antifungal for onychomycosis* [terbinafine HCl] 250 mg

**lamivudine** USAN, INN, BAN *nucleoside reverse transcriptase inhibitor antiviral for HIV; investigational (Phase III) for hepatitis B*

**lamotrigine** USAN, INN, BAN *phenyltriazine anticonvulsant; investigational (orphan) for Lennox-Gastaut syndrome*

**Lampit** (available only from the Centers for Disease Control) ℞ *investigational anti-infective for Chagas disease* [nifurtimox]

**Lamprene** capsules ℞ *bactericidal; tuberculostatic; leprostatic (orphan)* [clofazimine] 50 mg

**lamtidine** INN, BAN

**Lanabiotic** ointment OTC *topical antibiotic; anesthetic* [polymyxin B sulfate; neomycin sulfate; bacitracin; lidocaine] 10 000 U•3.5 mg•500 U•40 mg per g

**Lanacaine** spray, cream OTC *topical local anesthetic; antiseptic* [benzocaine; benzethonium chloride] 20%•0.1%; 6%•0.1%

**Lanacaps** (dosage form) *timed-release capsules*

**Lanacort 5** cream, ointment OTC *topical corticosteroid* [hydrocortisone acetate] 0.5%

**Lanacort 10** cream OTC *topical corticosteroid* [hydrocortisone acetate] 1%

**Lanacort 10** ointment (discontinued 1997) OTC *topical corticosteroid* [hydrocortisone acetate] 1%

**Lanaphilic** cream OTC *moisturizer; emollient; keratolytic* [urea] 20%

**Lanaphilic** OTC *ointment base*

**Lanaphilic with Urea** OTC *ointment base* [urea] 10%

**Lanatabs** (dosage form) *sustained-release tablets*

**lanatoside** NF, INN, BAN

**Lanatuss Expectorant** liquid (discontinued 1994) OTC *decongestant; antihistamine; expectorant* [phenylpropanolamine HCl; chlorpheniramine maleate; guaifenesin]

**Lanazets Improved** lozenges (discontinued 1993) OTC *topical oral anesthetic; antiseptic* [benzocaine; cetylpyridinium chloride] 5•1 mg

**Laniazid** tablets, syrup R *tuberculostatic* [isoniazid] 50 mg; 50 mg/5 mL

**Laniazid C.T.** tablets R *tuberculostatic* [isoniazid] 300 mg

**lanolin** USP *ointment base; water-in-oil emulsion; emollient/protectant* ☑ Lanoline

**lanolin, anhydrous** USP *absorbent ointment base*

**lanolin alcohols** *ointment base ingredient*

**Lanolor** cream OTC *moisturizer; emollient*

**Lanophyllin** elixir R *bronchodilator* [theophylline] 80 mg/15 mL

**Lanophyllin-GG** capsules (discontinued 1993) R *antiasthmatic; expectorant* [theophylline; bronchodilator; guaifenesin]

**Lanoplex** elixir (discontinued 1993) OTC *vitamin supplement* [multiple B vitamins]

**Lanorinal** tablets, capsules R *analgesic; antipyretic; anti-inflammatory; sedative* [aspirin; caffeine; butalbital] 325•40•50 mg

**Lanoxicaps** capsules R *cardiac glycoside to increase cardiac output; antiarrhythmic* [digoxin] 0.05, 0.1, 0.2 mg

**Lanoxin** tablets, pediatric elixir, IV or IM injection R *cardiac glycoside to increase cardiac output; antiarrhythmic* [digoxin] 0.125, 0.25 mg; 0.05 mg/mL; 0.1, 0.25 mg/mL ☑ Levoxine

**lanreotide acetate** USAN *antineoplastic*

**lansoprazole** USAN, INN, BAN *antisecretory; proton pump inhibitor for duodenal ulcers, erosive esophagitis, and Zollinger-Ellison syndrome*

**lanthanum** *element (La)*

**Lanvisone** cream (discontinued 1993) R *topical corticosteroid; antifungal; antibacterial* [hydrocortisone; clioquinol]

**lapirium chloride** INN *surfactant* [also: lapyrium chloride]

**LAPOCA (L-asparaginase, Oncovin, cytarabine, Adriamycin)** *chemotherapy protocol*

**laprafylline** INN

**lapyrium chloride** USAN *surfactant* [also: lapirium chloride]

**laramycin** [see: zorbamycin]

**Largon** IV or IM injection R *sedative; analgesic adjunct* [propiomazine HCl] 20 mg/mL

**Lariam** tablets R *antimalarial for acute chloroquine-resistant malaria (orphan)* [mefloquine HCl] 250 mg

**Larobec** tablets (discontinued 1994) R *vitamin supplement* [multiple B vitamins; vitamin C; folic acid] ≛• 500•0.5 mg

**Larodopa** capsules R *antiparkinsonian* [levodopa] 100, 250, 500 mg

**Larodopa** tablets R *antiparkinsonian* [levodopa] 100, 250, 500 mg

**laroxyl** [see: amitriptyline]

**las mujercitas** (Spanish for "the little women") *street drug slang* [see: psilocybin]

**lasalocid** USAN, INN, BAN *coccidiostat for poultry*

**Lasan** cream, ointment R *topical antipsoriatic* [anthralin] 0.1%, 0.2%, 0.4%; 0.4%

**Lasan HP-1** cream R *topical antipsoriatic* [anthralin] 1%

**Lasix** tablets, oral solution, IM or IV injection R *loop diuretic* [furosemide] 20, 40, 80 mg; 10 mg/mL; 10 mg/mL ☑ Esidrix; Lidex

**lason sa daga** *street drug slang* [see: LSD]

**Lassar's paste** [betanaphthol (q.v.) + zinc oxide (q.v.)]

**latamoxef** INN, BAN *anti-infective* [also: moxalactam disodium]

**latamoxef disodium** [see: moxalactam disodium]

**latanoprost** USAN, INN *prostaglandin agonist for glaucoma and ocular hypertension*

**laudexium methylsulfate** [see: laudexium metilsulfate; laudexium methylsulphate]

**laudexium methylsulphate** BAN [also: laudexium metilsulfate]

**laudexium metilsulfate** INN [also: laudexium methylsulphate]

**laughing gas** *street drug slang* [see: nitrous oxide]

**laughing grass; laughing weed** *street drug slang* [see: marijuana]

**lauralkonium chloride** INN

**laureth 4** USAN *surfactant*

**laureth 9** USAN *spermaticide; surfactant*

**laureth 10S** USAN *spermaticide*

**lauril** INN *combining name for radicals or groups*

**laurilsulfate** INN *combining name for radicals or groups* [also: sodium lauryl sulfate]

**laurixamine** INN

**laurocapram** USAN, INN *excipient*

**lauroguadine** INN

**laurolinium acetate** INN, BAN

**lauromacrogol 400** INN

**lauryl isoquinolinium bromide** USAN *anti-infective*

**lavender oil** NF

**lavoltidine** INN *antiulcerative; histamine $H_2$-receptor blocker* [also: lavoltidine succinate; loxtidine]

**lavoltidine succinate** USAN *antiulcerative; histamine $H_2$-receptor blocker* [also: lavoltidine; loxtidine]

**Lavoptik Eye Wash** ophthalmic solution OTC *extraocular irrigating solution* [balanced saline solution]

**lawrencium** *element (Lr)*

**Lax Pills** tablets OTC *laxative* [yellow phenolphthalein] 90 mg

**Laxative Pills** tablets OTC *laxative* [yellow phenolphthalein] 90 mg

**lazabemide** USAN, INN *antiparkinsonian; investigational MAO B inhibitor for Alzheimer's disease*

**Lazer Creme** OTC *moisturizer; emollient* [vitamins A and E] 3333.3• 116.67 U/g

**Lazer Formalyde** solution ℞ *for hyperhidrosis and bromhidrosis* [formaldehyde] 10%

**LazerSporin-C** ear drops ℞ *topical corticosteroidal anti-inflammatory; antibiotic* [hydrocortisone; neomycin sulfate; polymyxin B sulfate] 1%•5 mg•10 000 U per mL

**LC-65** solution OTC *cleaning solution for hard, soft, or rigid gas permeable contact lenses*

**L-Caine** injection (discontinued 1995) ℞ *injectable local anesthetic* [lidocaine HCl] 1%

**LCD (liquor carbonis detergens)** [see: coal tar]

**LCR (leurocristine)** [see: vincristine]

**LCx Neisseria gonorrhoeae Assay** reagent kit for professional use *in vitro diagnostic aid for Neisseria gonorrhoeae*

**LDI-200** *investigational (Phase III) apoptosis inducer for myelodysplastic syndrome*

**lead** *element (Pb)*

**leaf** *street drug slang* [see: marijuana; cocaine]

**leaky bolla; leaky leak** *street drug slang* [see: PCP]

**leapers** *street drug slang* [see: amphetamines]

**Lebanese** *street drug slang for hashish from Lebanon* [see: hashish]

**lecimibide** USAN *hypocholesterolemic; antihyperlipidemic*

**lecithin** NF *emulsifying agent; dietary lipotropic supplement* 420, 1200 mg oral

**Ledercillin VK** tablets, powder for oral solution (discontinued 1997) ℞ *bactericidal antibiotic* [penicillin V potassium] 250, 500 mg; 250 mg/5 mL

**Lederject** (trademarked delivery system) *prefilled disposable syringe*

**Lederplex** capsules (discontinued 1995) OTC *vitamin supplement* [multiple B vitamins]

**lefetamine** INN

**leflunomide** INN *investigational (Phase II) antiarthritic; investigational (orphan) to prevent rejection of solid organ transplants*

**legal speed** *street drug slang for Mini Thin (ephedrine HCl), an over-the-counter asthma drug* [see: Mini Thin; ephedrine HCl]

**Legalon** Ŗ *orphan status withdrawn 1997* [disodium silibinin dihemisuccinate]

**Legatrin** tablets (discontinued 1995) OTC *prevention and treatment of nocturnal leg cramps* [quinine sulfate] 162.5 mg

**Legatrin PM** caplets OTC *prevention and treatment of nocturnal leg cramps* [diphenhydramine HCl; acetaminophen] 50•500 mg

**Legatrin Rub** gel (discontinued 1994) OTC *counterirritant; topical anesthetic* [menthol; benzocaine; alcohol 44%] 4%•2%

**leiopyrrole** INN

**lemidosul** INN

**Lemmon 714; Lemmons** *street drug slang for Quaalude (methaqualone; disc. 1983), refers to the manufacturer (Lemmon) and tablet ID# (714)* [see: methaqualone]

**lemon oil** NF

**lemonade** *street drug slang for heroin or poor-quality street drugs in general* [see: heroin]

**lenampicillin** INN

**Lenate** oral solution (discontinued 1993) OTC *expectorant; oral anti-infective; minor topical anesthetic* [menthol; guaifenesin; strong iodine tincture; phenol]

**leniquinsin** USAN, INN *antihypertensive*

**lenitzol** [see: amitriptyline]

**Lennons** *street drug slang for Quaalude (methaqualone; discontinued 1983), probably a reference to musician John Lennon* [see: methaqualone]

**lenograstim** USAN, INN *immunomodulator; investigational treatment for chemotherapy-induced neutropenia*

**Lenoxin** Ŗ *investigational topical ophthalmic corticosteroidal anti-inflammatory*

**lenperone** USAN, INN *antipsychotic*

**lens** *street drug slang* [see: LSD]

**Lens Clear** solution (discontinued 1995) OTC *surfactant cleaning solution for soft contact lenses*

**Lens Drops** solution OTC *rewetting solution for hard or soft contact lenses*

**Lens Fresh** solution (discontinued 1995) OTC *rewetting solution for hard or soft contact lenses*

**Lens Lubricant** solution OTC *rewetting solution for hard or soft contact lenses*

**Lens Plus Daily Cleaner** solution OTC *surfactant cleaning solution for soft contact lenses*

**Lens Plus Oxysept** products [see: Oxysept]

**Lens Plus Rewetting Drops** OTC *rewetting solution for soft contact lenses*

**Lens Plus Sterile Saline** aerosol solution OTC *rinsing/storage solution for soft contact lenses* [preservative-free saline solution]

**Lensept** solutions (discontinued 1995) OTC *two-step chemical disinfecting system for soft contact lenses* [hydrogen peroxide based] 3%

**Lens-Wet** solution (discontinued 1993) OTC *rewetting solution for soft or hard contact lenses*

**Lentaron** Ŗ *investigational aromatase inhibitor for the treatment of breast cancer*

**Lente Iletin I** subcu injection OTC *antidiabetic* [insulin zinc (beef-pork)] 100 U/mL

**Lente Iletin II (beef)** subcu injection (discontinued 1994) OTC *antidiabetic* [insulin zinc] 100 U/mL

**Lente Iletin II (pork)** subcu injection OTC *antidiabetic* [insulin zinc] 100 U/mL

**Lente Insulin** subcu injection (discontinued 1997) OTC *antidiabetic* [insulin zinc (beef)] 100 U/mL

**Lente L** subcu injection OTC *antidiabetic* [insulin zinc (pork)] 100 U/mL

**Lente Purified Pork Insulin** subcu injection (name changed to Lente L in 1994)

**lentin** [see: carbachol]

**lentinan** JAN *investigational (Phase II/III) immunomodulator for HIV and AIDS*

**lepirudin** *investigational (orphan) for heparin-associated thrombocytopenia type II*

**leprosatics** *a class of drugs effective against leprosy*

**leptacline** INN

**lergotrile** USAN, INN *prolactin enzyme inhibitor*

**lergotrile mesylate** USAN *prolactin enzyme inhibitor*

**Lescol** capsules ℞ *cholesterol-lowering antihyperlipidemic; HMG-CoA reductase inhibitor* [fluvastatin sodium] 20, 40 mg

**lesopitron** INN *investigational anxiolytic*

**lethal weapon** *street drug slang* [see: PCP]

**letimide** INN *analgesic* [also: letimide HCl]

**letimide HCl** USAN *analgesic* [also: letimide]

**letosteine** INN

**letrazuril** INN *investigational treatment for AIDS-related cryptosporidial diarrhea*

**letrozole** USAN, INN *hormonal antineoplastic/aromatase inhibitor for advanced breast cancer in postmenopausal women*

**leucarsone** [see: carbarsone]

**leucine (L-leucine)** USAN, USP, INN, JAN *essential amino acid; symbols: Leu, L*

**leucine & isoleucine & valine** *investigational (orphan) for hyperphenylalaninemia*

**leucinocaine** INN

**leucocianidol** INN

**Leucomax** (commercially available in 36 foreign countries) ℞ *investigational cytokine for AIDS; orphan status withdrawn 1996* [molgramostim]

**leucomycin** [see: kitasamycin; spiramycin]

**Leucotropin** ℞ *investigational (Phase III) antineoplastic* [granulocyte-macrophage colony-stimulating factor]

**L-leucovorin** *investigational (orphan) antineoplastic and chemotherapy "rescue" agent*

**leucovorin calcium** USP *antianemic; folate replenisher; antidote to folic acid antagonist; methotrexate "rescue" (orphan)* [also: calcium folinate] 5,

15, 25 mg oral; 3 mg/mL injection; 50, 100, 350 mg/vial injection

**leucovorin & fluorouracil** *investigational (orphan) for metastatic adenocarcinoma of colon and rectum*

**leukemia inhibitory factor (LIF)** *investigational multilineage cytokine for leukemia*

**Leukeran** tablets ℞ *nitrogen mustard-type alkylating antineoplastic for multiple leukemias, lymphomas, and neoplasms* [chlorambucil] 2 mg

**Leukine** powder for IV infusion ℞ *myeloid reconstitution after autologous bone marrow transplant (orphan); investigational (Phase III) for malignant melanoma; investigational for AIDS* [sargramostim] 250, 500 μg

**leukocyte interferon** [now: interferon alfa-n3]

**leukocyte protease inhibitor, secretory, recombinant** *investigational (orphan) for congenital alpha₁-antitrypsin deficiency, cystic fibrosis, and bronchopulmonary dysplasias*

**leukocyte typing serum** USP *in vitro blood test*

**leukopoietin** [see: sargramostim]

**LeukoScan** *investigational diagnostic aid for infectious lesions* [technetium Tc 99m sulesomab]

**leukotriene inhibitor** *investigational 5-lipoxygenase inhibitor for topical treatment of psoriasis*

**leukotriene receptor antagonists (LTRAs); leukotriene receptor inhibitors** *a class of antiasthmatics that inhibit bronchoconstriction when used prophylactically (will not reverse bronchospasm)*

**leupeptin** *investigational (orphan) aid to microsurgical peripheral nerve repair*

**leuprolide acetate** USAN *hormonal antineoplastic for various cancers; LHRH agonist for central precocious puberty (orphan)* [also: leuprorelin]

**leuprorelin** INN, BAN *antineoplastic; LHRH agonist* [also: leuprolide acetate]

**leurocristine (LCR)** [see: vincristine]

**leurocristine sulfate** [see: vincristine sulfate]

**Leustatin** IV infusion ℞ *antineoplastic for hairy-cell leukemia (orphan); investigational (orphan) for chronic lymphocytic leukemia and multiple sclerosis* [cladribine] 1 mg/mL

**Leutrol** (name changed to Zyflo upon marketing release in 1997)

**levacecarnine (acetyl L-carnitine)** *investigational treatment for Alzheimer's disease*

**levacetylmethadol** INN *narcotic analgesic* [also: levomethadyl acetate]

**levalbuterol** *investigational (Phase III) racemic albuterol bronchodilator for asthma and COPD*

**levallorphan** INN, BAN [also: levallorphan tartrate] 🔄 levorphanol

**levallorphan tartrate** USP [also: levallorphan]

**levamfetamine** INN *anorectic* [also: levamfetamine succinate; levamphetamine]

**levamfetamine succinate** USAN *anorectic* [also: levamfetamine; levamphetamine]

**levamisole** INN, BAN *antineoplastic; veterinary anthelmintic* [also: levamisole HCl]

**levamisole HCl** USAN *antineoplastic; veterinary anthelmintic; investigational immunomodulator for AIDS* [also: levamisole]

**levamphetamine** BAN *anorectic* [also: levamfetamine succinate; levamfetamine]

**Levaquin** tablets, IV infusion ℞ *fluoroquinolone antibiotic* [levofloxacin] 250, 500 mg

**levarterenol** [see: norepinephrine bitartrate]

**levarterenol bitartrate** [now: norepinephrine bitartrate]

**Levatol** tablets ℞ *antihypertensive; β-blocker* [penbutolol sulfate] 20 mg

**Levbid** extended-release tablets ℞ *GI anticholinergic; antispasmodic* [hyoscyamine sulfate] 0.375 mg

**levcromakalim** USAN, INN, BAN *antiasthmatic; antihypertensive*

**levcycloserine** USAN, INN *enzyme inhibitor; orphan status withdrawn 1994*

**levdobutamine** INN *cardiotonic* [also: levdobutamine lactobionate]

**levdobutamine lactobionate** USAN *cardiotonic* [also: levdobutamine]

**levdropizine** INN

**levemopamil** INN *investigational treatment for stroke*

**levisoprenaline** INN

**Levlen** tablets ℞ *monophasic oral contraceptive; emergency "morning after" contraceptive* [levonorgestrel; ethinyl estradiol] 0.15 mg•30 μg

**levlofexidine** INN

**levobetaxolol** INN *antiadrenergic (β-receptor)* [also: levobetaxolol HCl]

**levobetaxolol HCl** USAN *antiadrenergic (β-receptor)* [also: levobetaxolol]

**levobunolol** INN, BAN *antiadrenergic (β-receptor); topical antiglaucoma agent* [also: levobunolol HCl]

**levobunolol HCl** USAN, USP *antiadrenergic; topical antiglaucoma agent (β-blocker)* [also: levobunolol] 0.25%, 0.5% eye drops

**levocabastine** INN, BAN *antihistamine* [also: levocabastine HCl]

**levocabastine HCl** USAN *antihistamine; orphan status withdrawn 1994* [also: levocabastine]

**levocarbinoxamine tartrate** [see: rotoxamine tartrate]

**levocarnitine** USAN, USP, INN *dietary amino acid for genetic carnitine deficiency (orphan); investigational (orphan) for pediatric cardiomyopathy* 250 mg oral

**levodopa** USAN, USP, INN, BAN, JAN *antiparkinsonian* 🔄 methyldopa

**levodopa & carbidopa** *antiparkinsonian* 100•10, 100•25, 250•25 mg oral

**Levo-Dromoran** tablets, subcu or IV injection ℞ *narcotic analgesic; anxiolytic* [levorphanol tartrate] 2 mg; 2 mg/mL

**levofacetoperane** INN

**levofenfluramine** INN

**levofloxacin** USAN, INN, JAN *fluoroquinolone antibiotic*

**levofuraltadone** USAN, INN *antibacterial; antiprotozoal*

**levoglutamide** INN *nonessential amino acid*

**levoleucovorin calcium** USAN *antidote to folic acid antagonists*

**levomenol** INN

**levomepate** [see: atromepine]

**levomepromazine** INN *analgesic* [also: methotrimeprazine]

**levomethadone** INN

**levomethadyl acetate** USAN *narcotic analgesic* [also: levacetylmethadol]

**levomethadyl acetate HCl** USAN *narcotic analgesic; narcotic agonist for management of opiate dependence (orphan)*

**levomethorphan** INN, BAN

**levometiomeprazine** INN

**levomoprolol** INN

**levomoramide** INN, BAN

**levonantradol** INN, BAN *analgesic* [also: levonantradol HCl]

**levonantradol HCl** USAN *analgesic* [also: levonantradol]

**levonordefrin** USP *adrenergic; vasoconstrictor* [also: corbadrine]

**levonorgestrel** USAN, USP, INN, BAN *progestin; contraceptive implant*

**Levophed** IV infusion ℞ *vasopressor for acute hypotensive shock* [norepinephrine bitartrate] 1 mg/mL

**levophenacylmorphan** INN, BAN

**Levoprome** IM injection ℞ *central analgesic; CNS depressant* [methotrimeprazine HCl] 20 mg/mL

**levopropicillin** INN *antibacterial* [also: levopropylcillin potassium]

**levopropicillin potassium** [see: levopropylcillin potassium]

**levopropoxyphene** INN, BAN *antitussive* [also: levopropoxyphene napsylate]

**levopropoxyphene napsylate** USAN *antitussive* [also: levopropoxyphene]

**levopropylcillin potassium** USAN *antibacterial* [also: levopropicillin]

**levopropylhexedrine** INN

**levoprotiline** INN

**Levora** tablets (21 or 28) ℞ *monophasic oral contraceptive* [levonorgestrel; ethinyl estradiol] 0.15•0.03 mg

**levorin** INN

**levorphanol** INN, BAN *narcotic analgesic* [also: levorphanol tartrate] ⊡ levallorphan

**levorphanol tartrate** USP *narcotic analgesic* [also: levorphanol]

**Levo-T** tablets ℞ *thyroid hormone* [levothyroxine sodium] 25, 50, 75, 100, 125, 150, 200, 300 µg

**Levothroid** tablets, powder for injection ℞ *thyroid hormone* [levothyroxine sodium] 25, 50, 75, 88, 100, 112, 125, 137, 150, 175, 200, 300 µg; 200, 500 µg

**levothyroxine sodium (T₄)** USP, INN *thyroid hormone* [also: thyroxine] 0.1, 0.15, 0.2, 0.3 mg oral; 200, 500 µg/vial injection ⊡ liothyronine

**levothyroxine sodium & tiratricol** *investigational (orphan) to suppress thyroid-stimulating hormone (TSH) in thyroid cancer*

**Levovist** intracoronary injection ℞ *ultrasound contrast agent* [galactose]

**levoxadrol** INN *local anesthetic; smooth muscle relaxant* [also: levoxadrol HCl]

**levoxadrol HCl** USAN *local anesthetic; smooth muscle relaxant* [also: levoxadrol]

**Levoxine** powder for IV injection (discontinued 1994) ℞ *thyroid hormone* [levothyroxine sodium] 200, 500 µg ⊡ Lanoxin

**Levoxine** tablets (name changed to Levoxyl in 1994)

**Levoxyl** tablets ℞ *thyroid hormone* [levothyroxine sodium] 25, 50, 75, 88, 100, 112, 125, 137, 150, 175, 200, 300 µg

**Levsin** tablets, drops, IV, subcu or IM injection, elixir ℞ *GI anticholinergic; antispasmodic* [hyoscyamine sulfate] 0.125 mg; 0.125 mg/mL; 0.5 mg/mL; 0.125 mg/5 mL

**Levsin PB** drops ℞ *GI anticholinergic; sedative* [hyoscyamine sulfate; phenobarbital; alcohol 5%] 0.125•15 mg/mL

**Levsin with Phenobarbital** tablets ℞ *GI anticholinergic; sedative* [hyoscyamine sulfate; phenobarbital] 0.125•15 mg

**Levsinex** Timecaps (timed-release capsules) ℞ *GI anticholinergic; antispasmodic* [hyoscyamine sulfate] 0.375 mg

**Levsin-PB** drops ℞ *anticholinergic; sedative* [hyoscyamine sulfate; phenobarbital; alcohol 5%] 0.125•15 mg/mL

**Levsin/SL** sublingual tablets (also may be chewed or swallowed) ℞ *GI anticholinergic; antispasmodic* [hyoscyamine sulfate] 0.125 mg

**Levulan** ℞ *investigational (Phase III) photodynamic therapy for precancerous actinic keratoses of the skin* [5-aminolevulinic acid]

**levulose** BAN *nutrient; caloric replacement* [also: fructose]

**lexipafant** USAN *platelet activating factor (PAF) antagonist; investigational (Phase III) treatment for acute pancreatitis*

**lexithromycin** USAN, INN *antibacterial*

**lexofenac** INN

**Lexxel** film-coated combination-release tablets ℞ *antihypertensive; ACE inhibitor; calcium channel blocker* [enalapril maleate (immediate release); felodipine (extended release)] 5•5 mg

**LFA3TIP** *investigational anti-inflammatory*

**LHRF (luteinizing hormone-releasing factor) acetate hydrate** [see: gonadorelin acetate]

**LHRF diacetate tetrahydrate** [now: gonadorelin acetate]

**LHRF dihydrochloride** [now: gonadorelin HCl]

**LHRF HCl** [see: gonadorelin HCl]

**liarozole** INN, BAN *investigational antipsoriatic and antineoplastic for prostatic cancer*

**liarozole fumarate** USAN *antipsoriatic; aromatase inhibitor*

**liarozole HCl** USAN *antineoplastic; aromatase inhibitor*

**Lib** *street drug slang for Librium (chlordiazepoxide HCl)* [see: Librium; chlordiazepoxide HCl]

**libecillide** INN

**libenzapril** USAN, INN *angiotensin-converting enzyme (ACE) inhibitor*

**Librax** capsules ℞ *GI anticholinergic; anxiolytic* [clidinium bromide; chlordiazepoxide HCl] 2.5•5 mg

**Libritabs** film-coated tablets ℞ *anxiolytic* [chlordiazepoxide] 10, 25 mg

**Librium** capsules, powder for injection ℞ *anxiolytic; sometimes abused as a street drug* [chlordiazepoxide HCl] 5, 10, 25 mg; 100 mg

**Lice-Enz** foam shampoo OTC *pediculicide* [pyrethrins; piperonyl butoxide] 0.3%•3%

**Licetrol 400** liquid (discontinued 1993) OTC *pediculicide* [pyrethrins; piperonyl butoxide; petroleum distillate]

**Licoplex DS** IM injection (discontinued 1995) ℞ *hematinic* [ferrous gluconate; multiple B vitamins; procaine HCl] 3 mg/mL• ± •2%

**licryfilcon A** USAN *hydrophilic contact lens material*

**licryfilcon B** USAN *hydrophilic contact lens material*

**lid poppers; lip poppers** *street drug slang* [see: amphetamines]

**Lid Wipes-SPF** solution, pads OTC *eyelid cleansing wipes for blepharitis or contact lenses*

**Lidakol** ℞ *investigational (Phase III) topical antiviral treatment for herpes simplex* [aliphatic alcohol compound]

**Lida-Mantle-HC** cream ℞ *local anesthetic; topical corticosteroid* [lidocaine; hydrocortisone acetate] 3%•0.5%

**lidamidine** INN *antiperistaltic* [also: lidamidine HCl]

**lidamidine HCl** USAN *antiperistaltic* [also: lidamidine]

**Lidex** cream, gel, ointment, topical solution ℞ *topical corticosteroid* [fluocinonide] 0.05% ⃞ Lasix; Lidox; Wydase

**Lidex-E** cream ℞ *topical corticosteroid; emollient* [fluocinonide] 0.05%

**lidimycin** INN *antifungal* [also: lydimycin]

**lidocaine** USP, INN *topical local anesthetic; investigational (orphan) transdermal delivery for post-herpetic neuralgia* [also: lignocaine]

**lidocaine benzyl benzoate** [see: denatonium benzoate]

**lidocaine HCl** USP *topical/injectable local anesthetic; antiarrhythmic* [also: lignocaine HCl] 2%, 4%, 5% topical; 1%, 1.5%, 2% injection; 4%, 10%, 20% IV admixture

**Lidoderm** transdermal patch ℞ *investigational (orphan) for post-herpetic neuralgia* [lidocaine] 5%

**lidofenin** USAN, INN *hepatic function test*

**lidofilcon A** USAN *hydrophilic contact lens material*

**lidofilcon B** USAN *hydrophilic contact lens material*

**lidoflazine** USAN, INN, BAN *coronary vasodilator*

**Lidoject-1; Lidoject-2** injection ℞ *injectable local anesthetic* [lidocaine HCl] 1%; 2%

**LidoPen** auto-injector (automatic IM injection device) ℞ *emergency injection for cardiac arrhythmias* [lidocaine HCl] 10%

**Lidox** capsules (discontinued 1995) ℞ *GI anticholinergic; anxiolytic* [clidinium bromide; chlordiazepoxide HCl] 2.5•5 mg ⊠ Lidex

**Lids-N-Lashes** ℞ *investigational eyelid hygiene product*

**LIF (leukemia inhibitory factor)** [q.v.]

**lifarizine** USAN *platelet aggregation inhibitor; investigational neural cell protector in stroke*

**lifibrate** USAN, INN *antihyperlipoproteinemic*

**lifibrol** USAN, INN *antihyperlipidemic*

**Lifoject** IM injection (discontinued 1993) ℞ *antianemic; vitamin supplement* [liver extracts; vitamin $B_{12}$; folic acid]

**Lifolbex** IM injection (discontinued 1994) ℞ *hematinic; vitamin supplement* [liver extracts; folic acid; cyanocobalamin]

**Lifomin-R** IM injection (discontinued 1994) ℞ *antianemic; vitamin supplement* [liver extracts; vitamin $B_{12}$; folic acid]

**light mineral oil** [see: mineral oil, light]

**light stuff** *street drug slang* [see: marijuana]

**lightning** *street drug slang* [see: amphetamines]

**lignocaine** BAN *topical local anesthetic* [also: lidocaine]

**lignocaine HCl** BAN *local anesthetic; antiarrhythmic* [also: lidocaine HCl]

**lignosulfonic acid, sodium salt** [see: polignate sodium]

**lilopristone** INN

**Lima** *street drug slang* [see: marijuana]

**limaprost** INN

**limarsol** [see: acetarsone]

**Limbitrol DS 10-25** tablets ℞ *antidepressant; anxiolytic* [chlordiazepoxide; amitryptyline HCl] 10•25 mg

**limbo** *street drug slang* [see: marijuana]

**lime** USP *pharmaceutic necessity*

**lime, sulfurated (calcium polysulfide, calcium thiosulfate)** USP *wet dressing/soak for cystic acne and seborrhea*

**lime acid** *street drug slang* [see: LSD]

**linarotene** USAN, INN *antikeratinizing agent*

**Lincocin** capsules, pediatric capsules, IV or IM injection ℞ *antibiotic* [lincomycin HCl] 500 mg; 250 mg; 300 mg/mL ⊠ Cleocin; Indocin

**lincomycin** USAN, INN, BAN *bactericidal antibiotic*

**lincomycin HCl** USP *bactericidal antibiotic*

**Lincorex** IV or IM injection ℞ *antibiotic* [lincomycin HCl] 300 mg/mL

**lincosamides** *a class of antimicrobial antibiotics with potentially serious side effects, to which bacterial resistance has been shown*

**lindane** USAN, USP, INN, BAN *pediculicide; scabicide* 1% topical

**line** *street drug slang* [see: cocaine]

**Linguets** (trademarked form) *buccal tablets*

**linogliride** USAN, INN *antidiabetic*

**linogliride fumarate** USAN *antidiabetic*

**linolexamide** [see: clinolamide]

**Linomide** ℞ *investigational (Phase II) immunomodulator for HIV; investigational (orphan) for bone marrow transplant for leukemia; clinical trials for MS discontinued 1997* [roquinimex]

**linopiridine** USAN, INN *cognition enhancer for Alzheimer's disease*

**linsidomine** INN

**lintopride** INN

**Lioresal** intrathecal injection ℞ *skeletal muscle relaxant for intractable spasticity due to spinal cord injury or disease* *(orphan)* [baclofen] 10 mg/20 mL (500 µg/mL), 10 mg/5 mL (2000 µg/mL)

**Lioresal** tablets ℞ *skeletal muscle relaxant* [baclofen] 10, 20 mg

**liothyronine** INN, BAN *radioactive agent* [also: liothyronine I 125] 🔲 levothyroxine

**liothyronine I 125** USAN *radioactive agent* [also: liothyronine]

**liothyronine I 131** USAN *radioactive agent*

**liothyronine sodium (T₃)** USP, BAN *thyroid hormone; treatment of myxedema coma or precoma (orphan)* 25 µg oral

**liotrix** USAN, USP *thyroid hormone* 🔲 Klotrix

**Lip Medex** ointment OTC *topical antipruritic/counterirritant; mild local anesthetic* [camphor; phenol] 1%•0.54%

**lipancreatin** [see: pancrelipase]

**lipase of pancreas** [see: pancrelipase]

**lipase triacylglycerol** [see: pancrelipase]

**Lipidil** capsules (discontinued 1994) ℞ *triglyceride-lowering agent* [fenofibrate]

**Lipidox** ℞ *investigational antineoplastic for breast cancer* [liposomal doxorubicin]

**Lipisorb** powder OTC *enteral nutritional therapy* [lactose-free formula]

**Lipitor** film-coated tablets ℞ *cholesterol-lowering antihyperlipidemic; HMG-CoA reductase inhibitor* [atorvastatin calcium] 10, 20, 40 mg

**Liple** (commercially available in Japan) ℞ *investigational agent for peripheral arterial occlusive disease and diabetic peripheral neuropathy* [liposomal PGE₁]

**Lipoflavonoid** capsules OTC *dietary lipotropic with vitamin supplementation* [choline; inositol; multiple B vitamins; vitamin C; lemon bioflavonoids] 111.3•111.3•≚•100•100 mg

**Lipogen** capsules, caplets OTC *dietary lipotropic with vitamin supplementation* [choline; inositol; multiple vitamins] 111•111•≚ mg

**Lipomul** liquid OTC *dietary fat supplement* [corn oil] 10 g/15 mL

**Lipo-Nicin/100** tablets (discontinued 1996) ℞ *peripheral vasodilator* [niacin; niacinamide; multiple vitamins] 100•75•≚ mg

**Lipo-Nicin/250** tablets (discontinued 1994) ℞ *peripheral vasodilator* [niacin; niacinamide; multiple vitamins] 250•75•≚ mg

**Lipo-Nicin/300** timed-release capsules (discontinued 1996) ℞ *peripheral vasodilator* [niacin; multiple vitamins] 300•≚ mg

**Liponol** capsules OTC *dietary lipotropic with vitamin supplementation* [choline; inositol; methionine; multiple B vitamins] 115•83•110•≚ mg

**liposomal gentamicin** [see: gentamicin liposome]

**liposome-encapsulated recombinant interleukin-2** [see: interleukin-2, liposome-encapsulated recombinant]

**liposome-encapsulated T4 endonuclease V** [see: T4 endonuclease V, liposome encapsulated]

**Liposyn II 10%; Liposyn III 10%** IV infusion (discontinued 1996) ℞ *nutritional therapy* [intravenous fat emulsion]

**Liposyn II 20%; Liposyn III 20%** IV infusion ℞ *nutritional therapy* [intravenous fat emulsion]

**Lipo-Tears** eye drops (discontinued 1993) OTC *ocular moisturizer/lubricant*

**Lipotriad** caplets OTC *dietary lipotropic with vitamin supplementation* [choline; inositol; multiple vitamins] 111•≚•≚ mg

**Lipotriad** liquid (discontinued 1994) OTC *dietary lipotropic with vitamin supplementation* [choline; inositol; multiple B vitamins] 334•≚•≚ mg/5 mL

**lipotropics** *a class of oral nutritional supplements*

**Lipovite** capsules (discontinued 1995) OTC *vitamin supplement* [multiple B vitamins] ≚

**Liquaemin Sodium** IV or deep subcu injection (discontinued 1997) ℞ *anticoagulant* [heparin sodium] 1000, 5000, 10 000, 20 000, 40 000 U/mL

**liquefied phenol** [see: phenol, liquefied]

**Liquibid** sustained-release tablet ℞ *expectorant* [guaifenesin] 600 mg

**Liquibid-D** sustained-release tablets ℞ *decongestant; expectorant* [phenylephrine HCl; guaifenesin] 40•600 mg

**Liqui-Char** oral liquid OTC *adsorbent antidote for poisoning* [activated charcoal] 12.5 g/60 mL, 15 g/75 mL, 25 g/120 mL, 30 g/120 mL, 50 g/240 mL

**Liquid Caps** (dosage form) *soft liquid-filled capsules*

**liquid ecstasy; liquid E; liquid ex; liquid X** *street drug slang* [see: GHB]

**liquid glucose** [see: glucose, liquid]

**Liquid Lather** body wash (discontinued 1995) OTC *bath emollient*

**liquid petrolatum** [see: mineral oil]

**Liquid Pred** syrup ℞ *glucocorticoids* [prednisone; alcohol 5%] 5 mg/5 mL

**Liquid Tabs** (dosage form) *liquid-filled tablets*

**Liqui-Doss** emulsion OTC *emollient laxative* [mineral oil]

**Liquifilm Tears; Liquifilm Forte** eye drops OTC *ocular moisturizer/lubricant* [polyvinyl alcohol] 1.4%; 3%

**Liquifilm Wetting** solution OTC *wetting solution for hard contact lenses*

**Liqui-Histine DM** syrup ℞ *antitussive; decongestant; antihistamine* [dextromethorphan hydrobromide; phenylpropanolamine HCl; brompheniramine maleate] 10•12.5•2 mg/5 mL

**Liqui-Histine-D** elixir ℞ *decongestant; antihistamine* [phenylpropanolamine HCl; phenyltoloxamine citrate; pyrilamine maleate; pheniramine maleate] 12.5•4•4•4 mg/5 mL

**Liquimat** lotion OTC *antibacterial and exfoliant for acne* [sulfur] 4%

**Liquipake** suspension ℞ *GI contrast radiopaque agent* [barium sulfate] 100%

**Liquiprin** elixir (discontinued 1997) OTC *analgesic; antipyretic* [acetaminophen] 160 mg/5 mL

**Liquiprin Drops for Children** OTC *analgesic; antipyretic* [acetaminophen] 80 mg/1.66 mL

**Liquitab** (trademarked dosage form) *chewable tablet*

**LiquiVent** ℞ *investigational (Phase III) treatment for pediatric acute respiratory distress syndrome (ARDS)*

**liquor carbonis detergens (LCD)** [see: coal tar]

**liroldine** INN

**lisadimate** USAN, INN *sunscreen*

**lisinopril** USAN, INN, BAN *antihypertensive; angiotensin-converting enzyme (ACE) inhibitor for CHF and acute MI*

**lisofylline (LSF)** USAN *investigational (Phase III) immunomodulator and cytokine inhibitor for RBC replenishment following bone marrow transplants*

**Listerex Scrub** lotion (discontinued 1995) OTC *topical keratolytic for acne* [salicylic acid] 2%

**Listerine; Cool-Mint Listerine; FreshBurst Listerine** mouthwash/gargle OTC *oral antiseptic* [thymol; eucalyptol; methyl salicylate; menthol; alcohol 22%–26%] 0.06%•0.09%•0.06%•0.04%

**Listerine Throat; Listerine Antiseptic** lozenges (discontinued 1994) OTC *oral antiseptic* [hexylresorcinol] 2.4 mg; 4 mg

**Listermint Arctic Mint** mouthwash/gargle OTC

**Listermint with Fluoride** oral rinse (discontinued 1995) OTC *topical dental caries preventative* [sodium fluoride] 0.02%

**lisuride** INN [also: lysuride]

**Lithane** tablets ℞ *antipsychotic* [lithium carbonate] 300 mg

**lithium** *element (Li)*

**lithium benzoate** NF

**lithium carbonate** USAN, USP *antimanic; immunity booster in chemotherapy and AIDS* 150, 300, 600 mg oral

**lithium citrate** USP *antimanic; immunity booster in chemotherapy and AIDS* 300 mg/5 mL oral

**lithium hydroxide** USP *antimanic*

**lithium hydroxide monohydrate** [see: lithium hydroxide]

**lithium salicylate** NF

**Lithobid** slow-release tablets ℞ *antipsychotic* [lithium carbonate] 300 mg

**Lithonate** capsules ℞ *antipsychotic* [lithium carbonate] 300 mg

**Lithostat** tablets ℞ *adjunctive therapy in chronic urea-splitting urinary tract infections* [acetohydroxamic acid] 250 mg

**Lithotabs** film-coated tablets ℞ *antipsychotic* [lithium carbonate] 300 mg

**litracen** INN

**little bomb** *street drug slang* [see: amphetamines; heroin]

**little ones** *street drug slang* [see: PCP]

**little smoke** *street drug slang* [see: marijuana; psilocybin; psilocin]

**live ones** *street drug slang* [see: PCP]

**Liver Combo No. 5** IM injection ℞ *antianemic; vitamin supplement* [liver extracts; vitamin $B_{12}$; folic acid] 10 μg•100 μg•0.4 mg per mL

**liver derivative complex** *claimed to be an anti-inflammatory for various dermatological conditions*

**liver extracts** *source of vitamin* $B_{12}$

**Livial** (commercially available in Europe, Asia, and South America) ℞ *investigational agent for hormone replacement therapy*

**lividomycin** INN

**Livifol** IM injection (discontinued 1994) ℞ *antianemic; vitamin supplement* [liver extracts; vitamin $B_{12}$; folic acid]

**Livitamin** capsules (discontinued 1995) OTC *hematinic* [ferrous fumarate; desiccated liver; multiple vitamins] 33•150•± mg

**Livitamin** chewable tablets (discontinued 1995) OTC *hematinic* [ferrous fumarate; multiple B vitamins; vitamin C] 16.4•±•100 mg

**Livitamin** liquid (discontinued 1995) OTC *hematinic* [peptonized iron; liver fraction 1; multiple B vitamins] 35.5•500•± mg/15 mL

**Livitamin with Intrinsic Factor** capsules (discontinued 1995) ℞ *hematinic* [ferrous fumarate; multiple B vitamins; ascorbic acid; desiccated liver; intrinsic factor concentrate] 33 mg•±•100 mg•150 mg•0.33 U

**Livitrinsic-f** capsules ℞ *hematinic* [ferrous fumarate; cyanocobalamin; ascorbic acid; intrinsic factor concentrate; folic acid] 110 mg•15 μg•75 mg•240 mg•0.5 mg

**Livostin** eye drop suspension ℞ *topical antihistamine for allergic conjunctivitis* [levocarbastine HCl] 0.05%

**Livostin** nasal spray ℞ *investigational treatment for seasonal allergic rhinitis* [levocarbastine HCl]

**Livroben** IM injection (discontinued 1993) ℞ *antianemic; vitamin supplement* [liver extracts; vitamin $B_{12}$; folic acid]

**lixazinone sulfate** USAN *cardiotonic; phosphodiesterase inhibitor*

**LKV Infant Drops** powder + liquid OTC *vitamin supplement* [multiple vitamins; biotin] ±•75 μg/0.6 mL

**LLD factor** [see: cyanocobalamin]

**Llesca** *street drug slang* [see: marijuana]

**10% LMD** IV injection ℞ *plasma volume expander for shock due to hemorrhage, burns, or surgery* [dextran 40] 10%

**LMD (low molecular weight dextran)** [see: dextran 40]

**LMF (Leukeran, methotrexate, fluorouracil)** *chemotherapy protocol*

**LMWD (low molecular weight dextran)** [see: dextran 40]

**loads** *street drug slang for a combination of Doriden (glutethimide; discontinued 1990) and codeine* [see: glutethimide; codeine]

**loaf** *street drug slang* [see: marijuana]

**Lobac** capsules ℞ *skeletal muscle relaxant; analgesic* [salicylamide; phenyltoloxamine; acetaminophen] 200•20•300 mg

**Lobana Body** lotion OTC *moisturizer; emollient*

**Lobana Body Shampoo; Lobana Liquid Lather** liquid OTC *soap-free therapeutic skin cleanser* [chloroxylenol]

**Lobana Derm-Ade** cream OTC *moisturizer; emollient* [vitamins A, D, and E]

**Lobana Peri-Garde** ointment OTC *moisturizer; emollient; antiseptic* [vitamins A, D, and E; chloroxylenol]

**lobeline** INN *nicotine withdrawal aid* [also: lobeline HCl]

**lobeline HCl** JAN *nicotine withdrawal aid* [also: lobeline]

**lobeline sulfate** *investigational (Phase III) nicotine withdrawal aid; clinical trials discontinued 1997*

**lobendazole** USAN, INN *veterinary anthelmintic*

**lobenzarit** INN *antirheumatic* [also: lobenzarit sodium]

**lobenzarit sodium** USAN *antirheumatic* [also: lobenzarit]

**lobo** (Spanish for "wolf") *street drug slang* [see: marijuana]

**lobucavir** USAN *antiviral; investigational (Phase I) for AIDS-related asymptomatic cytomegalovirus*

**lobuprofen** INN

**Loceryl** cream, nail lacquer (commercially available in Europe) ℞ *investigational antifungal* [amorolfine]

**locicortolone dicibate** INN

**locicortone** [see: locicortolone dicibate]

**locker room** *street drug slang* [see: isobutyl nitrite]

**loco** (Spanish for "crazy" or "insane") *street drug slang* [see: marijuana]

**Locoid** cream, ointment, solution ℞ *topical corticosteroid* [hydrocortisone butyrate] 0.1%

**locoweed** *street drug slang* [see: marijuana; jimsonweed]

**lodaxaprine** INN

**lodazecar** INN

**lodelaben** USAN, INN *antiarthritic; emphysema therapy adjunct*

**Lodine** film-coated tablets, capsules ℞ *nonsteroidal anti-inflammatory drug (NSAID); analgesic; antiarthritic* [etodolac] 200, 300, 400, 500 mg

**Lodine XL** extended-release film-coated tablets ℞ *once-daily nonsteroidal anti-inflammatory drug (NSAID); analgesic; antiarthritic* [etodolac] 400, 600 mg

**lodinixil** INN

**lodiperone** INN

**Lodosyn** tablets ℞ *antiparkinsonian agent when used with levodopa (no effect when given alone)* [carbidopa] 25 mg

**lodoxamide** INN, BAN *antiallergic; antiasthmatic* [also: lodoxamide ethyl]

**lodoxamide ethyl** USAN *antiallergic; antiasthmatic* [also: lodoxamide]

**lodoxamide trometamol** BAN *antiallergic; antiasthmatic* [also: lodoxamide tromethamine]

**lodoxamide tromethamine** USAN *antiasthmatic; antiallergic for vernal keratoconjunctivitis (orphan)* [also: lodoxamide trometamol]

**Lodrane LD** sustained-release capsules ℞ *decongestant; antihistamine* [pseudoephedrine HCl; brompheniramine maleate] 60•6 mg

**Loestrin 21 1/20; Loestrin 21 1.5/30** tablets ℞ *monophasic oral contraceptive* [norethindrone acetate; ethinyl estradiol] 1 mg•20 μg; 1.5 mg•30 μg

**Loestrin Fe 1/20; Loestrin Fe 1.5/30** tablets ℞ *monophasic oral contraceptive; iron supplement* [norethindrone acetate; ethinyl estradiol; ferrous fumarate] 1 mg•20 μg•75 mg; 1.5 mg•30 μg•75 mg

**lofemizole** INN *anti-inflammatory; analgesic; antipyretic* [also: lofemizole HCl]

**lofemizole HCl** USAN *anti-inflammatory; analgesic; antipyretic* [also: lofemizole]

**Lofenalac** powder OTC *special diet for infants with phenylketonuria*

**lofendazam** INN, BAN

**Lofene** tablets (discontinued 1993) ℞ *antidiarrheal* [diphenoxylate HCl; atropine sulfate]

**lofentanil** INN, BAN *narcotic analgesic* [also: lofentanil oxalate]

**lofentanil oxalate** USAN *narcotic analgesic* [also: lofentanil]

**lofepramine** INN, BAN *antidepressant* [also: lofepramine HCl]

**lofepramine HCl** USAN *antidepressant* [also: lofepramine]

**lofexidine** INN, BAN *antihypertensive* [also: lofexidine HCl]

**lofexidine HCl** USAN *antihypertensive* [also: lofexidine]

**loflucarban** INN

**LoFrin** ℞ *5-lipoxygenase inhibitor* [fenleuton]

**log** *street drug slang for a marijuana cigarette or PCP* [see: marijuana; PCP]

**Logen** tablets ℞ *antidiarrheal* [diphenoxylate HCl; atropine sulfate] 2.5•0.025 mg

**Logiparin** ℞ *investigational antithrombotic for deep vein thrombosis* [low molecular weight heparin]

**logor** *street drug slang* [see: LSD]

**LOMAC (leucovorin, Oncovin, methotrexate, Adriamycin, cyclophosphamide)** *chemotherapy protocol*

**Lomanate** liquid ℞ *antidiarrheal* [diphenoxylate HCl; atropine sulfate] 2.5•0.025 mg/5 mL

**lombazole** INN, BAN

**lomefloxacin** USAN, INN, BAN *antibacterial*

**lomefloxacin HCl** USAN *broad-spectrum fluoroquinolone bactericidal antibiotic*

**lomefloxacin mesylate** USAN *antibacterial*

**lometraline** INN *antipsychotic; antiparkinsonian* [also: lometraline HCl]

**lometraline HCl** USAN *antipsychotic; antiparkinsonian* [also: lometraline]

**lometrexol** INN *antineoplastic* [also: lometrexol sodium]

**lometrexol sodium** USAN *antineoplastic* [also: lometrexol]

**lomevactone** INN

**lomifylline** INN

**Lomodix** tablets (discontinued 1993) ℞ *antidiarrheal* [diphenoxylate HCl; atropine sulfate]

**lomofungin** USAN *antifungal*

**Lomotil** tablets, liquid ℞ *antidiarrheal* [diphenoxylate HCl; atropine sulfate] 2.5•0.025 mg; 2.5•0.025 mg/5 mL

**lomustine** USAN, INN, BAN *nitrosourea-type alkylating antineoplastic for brain tumors and Hodgkin's disease*

**Lonalac** powder OTC *enteral nutritional therapy* [milk-based formula]

**lonapalene** USAN *antipsoriatic*

**lonaprofen** INN

**lonazolac** INN

**lonidamine** INN

**Loniten** tablets ℞ *antihypertensive; vasodilator* [minoxidil] 2.5, 10 mg ⑨ clonidine

**Lonox** tablets ℞ *antidiarrheal* [diphenoxylate HCl; atropine sulfate] 2.5•0.025 mg

**loop diuretics** *a class of diuretic agents that inhibit the reabsorption of sodium and chloride*

**Lo/Ovral** tablets ℞ *monophasic oral contraceptive; emergency "morning after" contraceptive* [norgestrel; ethinyl estradiol] 0.3 mg•30 µg

**loperamide** INN, BAN *antiperistaltic; antidiarrheal* [also: loperamide HCl]

**loperamide HCl** USAN, USP, JAN *antiperistaltic; antidiarrheal* [also: loperamide] 2 mg oral; 1 mg/5 mL oral

**loperamide oxide** INN, BAN *investigational antiperistaltic*

**Lophophora williamsii** *a flowering Mexican cactus whose heads (mescal buttons) are used to produce mescaline, a hallucinogenic street drug*

**Lopid** film-coated tablets ℞ *antihyperlipidemic for hypertriglyceridemia and coronary heart disease* [gemfibrozil] 600 mg (300 mg capsules available in Canada)

**Lopid-SR** ℞ *investigational cholesterol-lowering agent* [gemfibrozil]

**lopirazepam** INN

**loprazolam** INN, BAN

**lopremone** [now: protirelin]

**Lopressor** tablets, IV injection ℞ *antianginal; antihypertensive; β-blocker* [metoprolol tartrate] 50, 100 mg; 1 mg/mL

**Lopressor HCT 50/25; Lopressor HCT 100/25; Lopressor HCT 100/50** tablets ℞ *antihypertensive* [metoprolol tartrate; hydrochlorothiazide] 50•25 mg; 100•25 mg; 100•50 mg

**loprodiol** INN

**Loprox** cream, lotion ℞ *topical antifungal* [ciclopirox olamine] 1%

**Lorabid** Pulvules (capsules), powder for oral suspension ℞ *carbacephem-type antibiotic* [loracarbef] 200, 400, 500 mg; 100, 200 mg/5 mL

**loracarbef** USAN, INN *antibacterial*

**lorajmine** INN *antiarrhythmic* [also: lorajmine HCl]

**lorajmine HCl** USAN *antiarrhythmic* [also: lorajmine]

**lorapride** INN

**loratadine** USAN, INN, BAN *antihistamine*

**lorazepam** USAN, USP, INN, BAN *anxiolytic; minor tranquilizer* 0.5, 1, 2 mg oral; 2 mg/mL oral; 2, 4 mg/mL injection

**lorbamate** USAN, INN *muscle relaxant*

**lorcainide** INN, BAN *antiarrhythmic* [also: lorcainide HCl]

**lorcainide HCl** USAN *antiarrhythmic* [also: lorcainide]

**Lorcet; Lorcet Plus; Lorcet 10/650** tablets ℞ *narcotic analgesic* [hydrocodone bitartrate; acetaminophen] 5•500 mg; 7.5•650 mg; 10•650 mg

**Lorcet-HD** capsules ℞ *narcotic analgesic* [hydrocodone bitartrate; acetaminophen] 5•500 mg ⊡ Fioricet

**lorcinadol** USAN, INN, BAN *analgesic*

**loreclezole** USAN, INN, BAN *antiepileptic*

**Lorelco** tablets (discontinued 1996) ℞ *serum cholesterol reduction* [probucol] 250, 500 mg

**lorglumide** INN

**lormetazepam** USAN, INN, BAN *sedative; hypnotic*

**lornoxicam** USAN, INN, BAN *analgesic; anti-inflammatory*

**Lorothidol** (available only from the Centers for Disease Control) ℞ *investigational anti-infective for paragonimiasis and fascioliasis* [bithionol]

**Loroxide** lotion OTC *topical keratolytic for acne* [benzoyl peroxide] 5.5%

**lorpiprazole** INN

**Lortab** elixir ℞ *narcotic analgesic* [hydrocodone bitartrate; acetaminophen] 2.5•167 mg/5 mL

**Lortab 2.5/500; Lortab 5/500; Lortab 7.5/500; Lortab 10/500** tablets ℞ *narcotic analgesic* [hydrocodone bitartrate; acetaminophen] 2.5•500 mg; 5•500 mg; 7.5•500 mg; 10•500 mg

**Lortab ASA** tablets ℞ *narcotic analgesic* [hydrocodone bitartrate; aspirin] 5•500 mg

**lortalamine** USAN, INN *antidepressant*

**lorzafone** USAN, INN *minor tranquilizer*

**losartan** INN *antihypertensive; angiotensin II antagonist* [also: losartan potassium]

**losartan potassium** USAN *antihypertensive; angiotensin II receptor antagonist* [also: losartan]

**Losec** (foreign name for U.S. product Prilosec)

**losigamone** INN

**losindole** INN

**losmiprofen** INN

**Losotron Plus** liquid (discontinued 1994) OTC *antacid; antiflatulent* [magaldrate; simethicone] 108•4 mg/mL

**losoxantrone** INN *antineoplastic* [also: losoxantrone HCl]

**losoxantrone HCl** USAN *antineoplastic* [also: losoxantrone]

**losulazine** INN *antihypertensive* [also: losulazine HCl]

**losulazine HCl** USAN *antihypertensive* [also: losulazine]

**Lotema** eye drop suspension ℞ *investigational (Phase III) ophthalmic anti-inflammatory* [loteprednol etabonate] 0.5%

**Lotensin** tablets ℞ *antihypertensive; angiotensin-converting enzyme (ACE) inhibitor* [benazepril HCl] 5, 10, 20, 40 mg

**Lotensin HCT 5/6.25; Lotensin HCT 10/12.5; Lotensin HCT 20/12.5; Lotensin HCT 20/25** tablets ℞ *antihypertensive* [benazepril; hydrochlorothiazide] 5•6.25 mg; 10•12.5 mg; 20•12.5 mg; 20•25 mg

**loteprednol** INN *topical anti-inflammatory* [also: loteprednol etabonate]

**loteprednol etabonate** USAN *topical anti-inflammatory; investigational (NDA filed) ophthalmic antiallergy suspension* [also: loteprednol]

**lotifazole** INN

**Lotrel** capsules ℞ *antihypertensive* [amlodipine besylate; benazepril HCl] 2.5•10, 5•10, 5•20 mg

**lotrifen** INN

**Lotrimin** cream, solution, lotion ℞ *topical antifungal* [clotrimazole] 1% ⊡ Otrivin

**Lotrimin AF** cream, solution, lotion OTC *topical antifungal* [clotrimazole] 1%

**Lotrimin AF** powder, spray powder, spray liquid OTC *topical antifungal* [miconazole nitrate] 2%

**Lotrisone** cream ℞ *topical corticosteroid; antifungal* [betamethasone dipropionate; clotrimazole] 0.05%•1%

**lotucaine** INN

**Lovan** ℞ *investigational obesity and bulimia treatment* [fluoxetine]

**lovastatin** USAN, INN, BAN *antihyperlipidemic; HMG-CoA reductase inhibitor*

**love** *street drug slang* [see: cocaine, crack]

**love affair** *street drug slang* [see: cocaine]

**love boat** *street drug slang for PCP or marijuana dipped in formaldehyde* [see: marijuana; PCP]

**love drug** *street drug slang for Quaalude (methaqualone; discontinued 1983)* [see: methaqualone]

**love drug of the '80s and '90s** *street drug slang* [see: MDMA]

**love pearls; love pills** *street drug slang* [see: alpha-ethyltryptamine]

**love trip** *street drug slang for a combination of mescaline and MDMA* [see: mescaline; MDMA]

**love weed** *street drug slang* [see: marijuana]

**lovelies** *street drug slang for marijuana laced with PCP* [see: marijuana; PCP]

**lovely** *street drug slang* [see: PCP]

**Lovenox** subcu injection ℞ *anticoagulant/antithrombotic for prevention of deep vein thrombosis (DVT) following knee, hip, or abdominal surgery* [enoxaparin sodium (low molecular weight heparin)] 30 mg/0.3 mL

**lovers** *street drug slang for Quaalude (methaqualone; discontinued 1983)* [see: methaqualone]

**loviride** INN *investigational treatment for AIDS*

**low molecular weight dextran (LMD; LMWD)** [see: dextran 40]

**low molecular weight heparins** *a class of anticoagulants*

**Lowila Cake** bar OTC *soap-free therapeutic skin cleanser*

**Low-Quel** tablets (discontinued 1993) ℞ *antidiarrheal* [diphenoxylate HCl; atropine sulfate]

**Lowsium** chewable tablets, oral suspension (tablets discontinued and suspension renamed Lowsium Plus in 1994)

**Lowsium Plus** oral suspension OTC *antacid; antiflatulent* [magaldrate; simethicone] 540•40 mg/5 mL

**loxanast** INN

**loxapine** USAN, INN, BAN *minor tranquilizer; antipsychotic*

**loxapine HCl** *minor tranquilizer; antipsychotic*

**loxapine succinate** USAN *minor tranquilizer; antipsychotic* 5, 10, 25, 50 mg oral

**loxiglumide** INN

**Loxitane** capsules ℞ *antipsychotic* [loxapine succinate] 5, 10, 25, 50 mg

**Loxitane C** oral concentrate ℞ *antipsychotic* [loxapine HCl] 25 mg/mL

**Loxitane IM** injection ℞ *antipsychotic* [loxapine HCl] 50 mg/mL

**loxoprofen** INN

**loxoribine** USAN, INN *immunostimulant; vaccine adjuvant; orphan status withdrawn 1996*

**loxotidine** [now: lavoltidine succinate]

**loxtidine** BAN *antiulcerative; histamine $H_2$-receptor blocker* [also: lavoltidine succinate; lavoltidine]

**lozilurea** INN

**Lozi-Tabs** (trademarked form) *lozenges*

**Lozol** film-coated tablets ℞ *antihypertensive; diuretic* [indapamide] 1.25, 2.5 mg

**L-PAM (L-phenylalanine mustard)** [see: melphalan]

**LR (lactated Ringer's) solution** [see: Ringer's injection, lactated]

**LSD (lysergic acid diethylamide)** *hallucinogenic street drug associated with disorders of sensory and temporal perception, depersonalization, and ataxia* [medically known as lysergide]

**LSF (lisofylline)** [q.v.]

**LTRAs (leukotriene receptor antagonists)** *a class of antiasthmatics*

**lubage** *street drug slang* [see: marijuana]

**lubeluzole** INN *investigational therapy for ischemic stroke*

**LubraSol Bath Oil** OTC *bath emollient*

**Lubricating Gel** OTC *vaginal antimicrobial and lubricant* [chlorhexidine gluconate; glycerin]

**Lubricating Jelly** OTC *vaginal lubricant* [glycerin; propylene glycol]

**Lubriderm** cream, lotion OTC *moisturizer; emollient*

**Lubriderm Bath Oil** OTC *bath emollient*

**Lubrin** vaginal inserts OTC *lubricant for sexual intercourse* [glycerin; caprylic triglyceride] ⚠

**LubriTears** eye drops OTC *ocular moisturizer/lubricant* [hydroxypropyl methylcellulose] 0.3%

**LubriTears** ophthalmic ointment OTC *ocular moisturizer/lubricant* [white petrolatum; mineral oil; lanolin]

**lucanthone** INN, BAN *antischistosomal* [also: lucanthone HCl]

**lucanthone HCl** USAN, USP *antischistosomal* [also: lucanthone]

**lucartamide** INN

**Lucas** *street drug slang* [see: marijuana]

**lucensomycin** [see: lucimycin]

**lucimycin** INN

**Lucy; Lucy in the sky with diamonds** *street drug slang* [see: LSD]

**'ludes** *street drug slang for Quaalude (methaqualone; discontinued 1983)* [see: methaqualone]

**Ludiomil** coated tablets ℞ *tetracyclic antidepressant* [maprotiline HCl] 25, 50, 75 mg

**lufironil** USAN, INN *collagen inhibitor*

**lufuradom** INN

**Lufyllin** tablets, elixir, IM injection ℞ *bronchodilator* [dyphylline] 200 mg; 100 mg/15 mL; 250 mg/mL

**Lufyllin 400** tablets ℞ *bronchodilator* [dyphylline] 400 mg

**Lufyllin-EPG** tablets, elixir ℞ *antiasthmatic; bronchodilator; decongestant; expectorant; sedative* [dyphylline; ephedrine HCl; guaifenesin; phenobarbital] 100•16•200•16 mg; 150•24•300•24 mg/15 mL

**Lufyllin-GG** tablets, elixir ℞ *antiasthmatic; bronchodilator; expectorant* [dyphylline; guaifenesin] 200•200 mg; 100•100 mg/15 mL

**Lugol** solution ℞ *thyroid-blocking therapy; topical antimicrobial* [iodine; potassium iodide] 5%•10%

**lumber** *street drug slang for marijuana stems and waste* [see: marijuana]

**LumenHance** ℞ *investigational GI contrast agent for MRI* [manganese chloride]

**Luminal Sodium** IV or IM injection ℞ *long-acting barbiturate sedative, hypnotic, and anticonvulsant; also abused as a street drug* [phenobarbital sodium] 130 mg/mL ⚠ Tuinal

**Lumirem** (European name for U.S. product Gastromark)

**Lung Check** sputum test for professional use (discontinued 1993) *in vitro diagnostic aid for precancerous lung cells*

**lung surfactant, synthetic** [see: colfosceril palmitate]

**2,6-lupetidine** [see: nanofin]

**lupitidine** INN *veterinary antagonist to histamine $H_2$ receptors* [also: lupitidine HCl]

**lupitidine HCl** USAN *veterinary antagonist to histamine $H_2$ receptors* [also: lupitidine]

**Lupron; Lupron Pediatric** subcu injection (daily) ℞ *hormonal chemotherapy for prostatic cancer and central precocious puberty (orphan)* [leuprolide acetate] 5 mg/mL

**Lupron Depot** microspheres for IM injection (monthly) ℞ *hormonal chemotherapy for prostatic cancer, endometriosis, and uterine fibroids* [leuprolide acetate] 3.75, 7.5 mg

**Lupron Depot–3 month; Lupron Depot–4 month** microspheres for IM injection ℞ *hormonal chemotherapy for prostatic cancer* [leuprolide acetate] 11.5, 22.5 mg; 30 mg

**Lupron Depot-Ped** microspheres for IM injection (monthly) ℞ *hormonal chemotherapy for prostatic cancer, endometriosis, uterine fibroids, and central precocious puberty (CPP)* [leuprolide acetate] 7.5, 11.25, 15 mg

**luprostiol** INN, BAN

**Luramide** tablets (discontinued 1993) ℞ *loop diuretic* [furosemide]

**Luride** Lozi-Tabs (chewable tablets), drops, gel ℞ *dental caries preventative* [sodium fluoride] 0.25, 1.1, 2.2 mg; 1.1 mg/mL; 1.2%

**Luride SF** Lozi-Tabs (lozenges) ℞ *dental caries preventative* [sodium fluoride] 2.2 mg

**Lurline PMS** tablets OTC *analgesic; antipyretic; diuretic; vitamin* [acetaminophen; pamabrom; pyridoxine] 500•25•50 mg

**lurosetron mesylate** USAN *antiemetic*

**lurtotecan dihydrochloride** USAN *antineoplastic; topoisomerase I inhibitor*

**luteinizing hormone-releasing factor acetate hydrate** [see: gonadorelin acetate]

**luteinizing hormone-releasing factor diacetate tetrahydrate** [now: gonadorelin acetate]

**luteinizing hormone-releasing factor dihydrochloride** [now: gonadorelin HCl]

**luteinizing hormone-releasing factor HCl** [see: gonadorelin HCl]

**lutetium** *element (Lu)*

**lutrelin** INN *luteinizing hormone-releasing hormone (LHRH) agonist* [also: lutrelin acetate]

**lutrelin acetate** USAN *luteinizing hormone-releasing hormone (LHRH) agonist* [also: lutrelin]

**Lutrepulse** powder for continuous ambulatory infusion R *gonadotropin-releasing hormone for hypothalamic amenorrhea (orphan)* [gonadorelin acetate] 0.8, 3.2 mg

**LuVax** R *investigational treatment for small cell lung cancer* [anti-idiotypic antiboby vaccine] 🔄 Luvox

**Luvox** film-coated tablets R *selective serotonin reuptake inhibitor (SSRI) for depression and obsessive-compulsive disorder; investigational (Phase III) for panic disorder* [fluvoxamine maleate] 50, 100 mg 🔄 LuVax

**luxabendazole** INN, BAN

**L-VAM (leuprolide acetate, vinblastine, Adriamycin, mitomycin)** *chemotherapy protocol*

**LY 293111** *investigational antiasthmatic*

**lyapolate sodium** USAN *anticoagulant* [also: sodium apolate]

**lycetamine** USAN *topical antimicrobial*

**lycine HCl** [see: betaine HCl]

**Lycolan** elixir (discontinued 1993) OTC *oral amino acid supplement* [L-lysine]

**lydimycin** USAN *antifungal* [also: lidimycin]

**Lyme borreliosis vaccine** *investigational (NDA filed) inactivated subunit vaccine for Lyme disease (caused by the spirochete Borrelia burgdorferi)*

**lymecycline** INN, BAN

**Lymphazurin 1%** injection R *adjunct radiopaque agent for lymphography* [isosulfan blue] 1%

**LymphoCide** R *investigational* [humanized lymphoma antibody]

**lymphocyte immune globulin, antithymocyte** *passive immunizing agent; investigational (orphan) to prevent allograft rejection in organ and bone marrow transplants*

**lymphogranuloma venereum antigen** USP

**lymphoma antibody, humanized** *investigational*

**LymphoScan** R *investigational (Phase III, orphan) for diagnostic aid for B-cell leukemias and non-Hodgkin's lymphomas* [technetium Tc 99m bectumomab]

**lynestrenol** USAN, INN *progestin* [also: lynoestrenol]

**lynoestrenol** BAN *progestin* [also: lynestrenol]

**Lyo-Ject** (trademarked delivery system) *prefilled dual-chambered syringe with lyophilized powder and diluent*

**Lyphazome** R *investigational treatment for burns* [liposomal silver sulfadiazine]

**Lyphocin** powder for IV or IM injection R *glycopeptide-type antibiotic* [vancomycin HCl] 0.5, 1, 5 g

**Lypholized Vitamin B Complex & Vitamin C with B$_{12}$** injection R *parenteral vitamin therapy* [multiple B vitamins; vitamin C] ≛•50 mg/mL

**Lypholyte; Lypholyte II** IV admixture R *intravenous electrolyte therapy* [combined electrolyte solution]

**lypressin** USAN, USP, INN, BAN *posterior pituitary hormone; antidiuretic; vasoconstrictor*

**lysergic acid diethylamide (LSD)** *street drug* [see: LSD; lysergide]

**lysergide** INN, BAN, DCF

**lysine (L-lysine)** USAN, INN *essential amino acid; symbols: Lys, K* 312, 500, 1000 mg oral

**lysine acetate** USP *amino acid*

326   DL-lysine acetylsalicylate

**DL-lysine acetylsalicylate** *orphan status withdrawn 1993* [see: aspirin DL-lysine]
**lysine HCl** USAN, USP *amino acid*
**L-lysine monoacetate** [see: lysine acetate]
**L-lysine monohydrochloride** [see: lysine HCl]
**8-L-lysine vasopressin** [see: lypressin]
**Lysodase** *investigational (orphan) for chronic enzyme replacement in Gaucher's disease* [PEG-glucocerebrosidase]

**Lysodren** tablets ℞ *antisteroidal antineoplastic for inoperable adrenal cortical carcinoma and Cushing syndrome* [mitotane] 500 mg
**lysostaphin** USAN *antibacterial enzyme*
**LysPro** [see: Humalog]
**lysuride** BAN [also: lisuride]

**M-2 protocol (vincristine, carmustine, cyclophosphamide, melphalan, prednisone)** *chemotherapy protocol*
**MAA (macroaggregated albumin)** [see: albumin, aggregated]
**Maalox** chewable tablets, oral suspension OTC *antacid* [aluminum hydroxide; magnesium hydroxide] 200•200, 350•350 mg; 225•200 mg/5 mL ⑨ Marax
**Maalox, Extra Strength** oral suspension OTC *antacid; antiflatulent* [aluminum hydroxide; magnesium hydroxide; simethicone] 500•450•40 mg/5 mL
**Maalox Antacid** caplets OTC *antacid* [calcium carbonate] 1 g
**Maalox Anti-Diarrheal** caplets OTC *antidiarrheal* [loperamide HCl] 2 mg
**Maalox Anti-Gas** chewable tablets OTC *antiflatulent* [simethicone] 80 mg
**Maalox Daily Fiber Therapy** powder OTC *bulk laxative* [psyllium hydrophilic mucilloid] 3.4 g/dose
**Maalox HRF (Heartburn Relief Formula)** liquid OTC *antacid* [aluminum hydroxide; magnesium carbonate] 140•175 mg/5 mL
**Maalox Plus** chewable tablets, oral suspension OTC *antacid; antiflatulent* [aluminum hydroxide; magnesium hydroxide; simethicone] 200•200•25 mg; 500•450•40 mg/5 mL

**Maalox TC** chewable tablets, oral suspension (tablets discontinued 1994; suspension renamed Maalox Therapeutic Concentrate)
**Maalox Therapeutic Concentrate** oral suspension OTC *antacid* [aluminum hydroxide; magnesium hydroxide] 600•300 mg/5 mL
**MAb; MAB (monoclonal antibody)**
**MABOP (Mustargen, Adriamycin, bleomycin, Oncovin, prednisone)** *chemotherapy protocol*
**mabuterol** INN
**MAC (methotrexate, actinomycin D, chlorambucil)** *chemotherapy protocol*
**MAC; MAC III (methotrexate, actinomycin D, cyclophosphamide)** *chemotherapy protocol*
**MAC (mitomycin, Adriamycin, cyclophosphamide)** *chemotherapy protocol*
**MACC (methotrexate, Adriamycin, cyclophosphamide, CCNU)** *chemotherapy protocol*
**machinery** *street drug slang* [see: marijuana]
**MACHO (methotrexate, asparaginase, cyclophosphamide, hydroxydaunomycin, Oncovin)** *chemotherapy protocol*
**Macon** *street drug slang* [see: marijuana]
**MACOP-B (methotrexate, Adriamycin, cyclophosphamide,**

Oncovin, prednisone, bleomycin) *chemotherapy protocol*

**Macritonin** ℞ *investigational (Phase II/III) oral treatment for osteoporosis* [calcitonin (salmon)]

**macroaggregated albumin (MAA)** [see: albumin, aggregated]

**macroaggregated iodinated ($^{131}$I) human albumin** [see: macrosalb ($^{131}$I)]

**Macrobid** capsules ℞ *urinary bacteriostatic* [nitrofurantoin (macrocrystals); nitrofurantoin monohydrate] 25•75 mg

**Macrodantin** capsules ℞ *urinary bacteriostatic* [nitrofurantoin (macrocrystals)] 25, 50, 100 mg

**Macrodantin** MACPAC (box of 7 cards of 4 capsules each) (discontinued 1993) ℞ *urinary antibacterial* [nitrofurantoin (macrocrystals)]

**Macrodex** IV infusion ℞ *plasma volume expander for shock due to hemorrhage, burns, or surgery* [dextran 70] 6%

**macrogol 4000** INN, BAN [also: polyethylene glycol 4000]

**macrogol ester 2000** INN *surfactant* [also: polyoxyl 40 stearate]

**macrogol ester 400** INN *surfactant* [also: polyoxyl 8 stearate]

**macrolides** *a class of antibiotics that are bacteriostatic or bactericidal, depending on such factors as drug concentration*

**Macrolin** ℞ *investigational agent for fungal disease and advanced cancer* [macrophage colony-stimulating factor (CSF)]

**macrophage colony-stimulating factor (M-CSF)** *investigational antiviral for AIDS and various forms of cancer*

**macrophage-targeted β-glucocerebrosidase** now: alglucerase

**macrosalb ($^{131}$I)** INN, BAN

**macrosalb ($^{99m}$Tc)** INN, BAN [also: technetium ($^{99m}$Tc) labeled macroaggregated human ...]

**Macroscint** ℞ *investigational inflammation and infection imaging aid* [indium In 111 IGIV pentetate]

**Macrulin** ℞ *investigational (Phase I) oral insulin formulation*

**Macstim** ℞ *investigational antineoplastic for various cancers; investigational antihyperlipidemic* [macrophage colony-stimulating factor]

**MAD (MeCCNU, Adriamycin)** *chemotherapy protocol*

**mad dog** *street drug slang for PCP or Mogen David 20/20 fortified wine* [see: PCP; alcohol]

**MADDOC (mechlorethamine, Adriamycin, dacarbazine, DDP, Oncovin, cyclophosphamide)** *chemotherapy protocol*

**madman** *street drug slang* [see: PCP]

**maduramicin** USAN, INN *anticoccidal*

**mafenide** USAN, INN, BAN *bacteriostatic; adjunct to burn therapy*

**mafenide acetate** USP *bacteriostatic; investigational (orphan) to prevent meshed autograft loss on burn wounds*

**mafenide HCl**

**mafilcon A** USAN *hydrophilic contact lens material*

**mafoprazine** INN

**mafosfamide** INN

**Mag-200** tablets OTC *magnesium supplement* [magnesium oxide] 400 mg

**magaldrate** USAN, USP, INN *antacid* 540 mg/5 mL oral

**Magaldrate Plus** oral suspension OTC *antacid; antiflatulent* [magaldrate; simethicone] 540•40 mg/5 mL

**Magalox Plus** chewable tablets OTC *antacid; antiflatulent* [aluminum hydroxide; magnesium hydroxide; simethicone] 200•200•25 mg

**Magan** tablets ℞ *analgesic; antirheumatic* [magnesium salicylate] 545 mg

**Mag-Cal** tablets OTC *dietary supplement* [calcium carbonate; vitamin D; multiple minerals] 416.7 mg•66.7 IU• ≛

**Mag-Cal Mega** tablets OTC *mineral supplement* [magnesium; calcium] 800•400 mg

**magic; magic dust** *street drug slang* [see: PCP]

**magic mushroom** *street drug slang* [see: psilocybin; psilocin]

**magic smoke** *street drug slang* [see: marijuana]

**Magnacal** ready-to-use liquid OTC *enteral nutritional therapy* [lactose-free formula]

**Magnagel** chewable tablets (discontinued 1994) OTC *antacid* [aluminum hydroxide; magnesium carbonate]

**Magnalox** liquid OTC *antacid* [aluminum hydroxide; magnesium hydroxide] 225•220 mg/5 mL

**Magnaprin; Magnaprin Arthritis Strength Captabs** film-coated tablets OTC *analgesic; antipyretic; antiinflammatory; antirheumatic* [aspirin (buffered with aluminum hydroxide, magnesium hydroxide, and calcium carbonate)] 325 mg

**Magnatril** chewable tablets (discontinued 1994) OTC *antacid* [aluminum hydroxide; magnesium hydroxide; magnesium trisilicate]

**Magnatril** oral suspension (discontinued 1994) OTC *antacid* [aluminum hydroxide; calcium carbonate; magnesium trisilicate] 30•16•80 mg/mL

**magnesia, milk of** USP *antacid; laxative* [also: magnesium hydroxide] 400 mg/5 mL oral

**magnesia magma** [now: magnesia, milk of]

**magnesium** *element (Mg)*

**magnesium aluminosilicate hydrate** [see: almasilate]

**magnesium aluminum silicate** NF *suspending agent*

**magnesium amino acid chelate** *dietary magnesium supplement*

**magnesium aspartate** [see: potassium aspartate & magnesium aspartate]

**magnesium carbonate** USP *antacid; dietary magnesium supplement*

**magnesium carbonate hydrate** [see: magnesium carbonate]

**magnesium chloride** USP *electrolyte replenisher* 1.97 mEq/mL (20%) injection

**magnesium chloride hexahydrate** [see: magnesium chloride]

**magnesium citrate** USP *saline laxative*

**magnesium clofibrate** INN

**magnesium D-gluconate dihydrate** [see: magnesium gluconate]

**magnesium D-gluconate hydrate** [see: magnesium gluconate]

**magnesium gluconate** USP *magnesium replenisher*

**magnesium glycinate** USAN

**magnesium hydroxide** USP *antacid; saline laxative* [also: magnesia, milk of]

**magnesium oxide** USP *antacid; sorbent* 500 mg oral

**magnesium phosphate** USP *antacid*

**magnesium phosphate pentahydrate** [see: magnesium phosphate]

**magnesium salicylate** USP *analgesic; antipyretic; anti-inflammatory; antirheumatic*

**magnesium salicylate tetrahydrate** [see: magnesium salicylate]

**magnesium silicate** NF *tablet excipient*

**magnesium silicate hydrate** [see: magnesium trisilicate]

**magnesium stearate** NF *tablet and capsule lubricant*

**magnesium sulfate** USP, JAN *anticonvulsant; saline laxative; electrolyte replenisher* 0.8, 1, 4 mEq/mL (10%, 12.5%, 50%) injection

**magnesium sulfate heptahydrate** [see: magnesium sulfate]

**magnesium trisilicate** USP *antacid*

**Magnevist** injection R *parenteral radioopaque agent for magnetic imaging of the brain and spine* [gadopentetate dimeglumine] 46.9%

**Magnox** oral suspension OTC *antacid* [aluminum hydroxide; magnesium hydroxide] 225•200 mg/5 mL

**Magonate** tablets, liquid OTC *magnesium supplement* [magnesium gluconate] 500 mg; 54 mg/5 mL

**Mag-Ox 400** tablets OTC *antacid; magnesium supplement* [magnesium oxide] 400 mg

**Magsal** tablets R *analgesic; antipyretic; anti-inflammatory; antihistamine* [magnesium salicylate; phenyltoloxamine citrate] 600•25 mg

**Mag-Tab SR** sustained-release caplets OTC *magnesium supplement* [magnesium lactate] 7 mEq (84 mg)

**Magtrate** tablets OTC *magnesium supplement* [magnesium gluconate] 500 mg

**MAID (mesna [rescue], Adriamycin, ifosfamide, dacarbazine)** *chemotherapy protocol*

**MainStream** R̲ *investigational IV system*

**maitansine** INN *antineoplastic* [also: maytansine]

**Maitec** injection R̲ *investigational (orphan) for disseminated Mycobacterium avium-intracellulare infection* [gentamicin liposome]

**Major-Con** chewable tablets OTC *antiflatulent* [simethicone] 80 mg

**Major-gesic** tablets OTC *antihistamine; analgesic* [phenyltoloxamine citrate; acetaminophen] 30•325 mg

**MAK 195 F** *investigational therapy for graft vs. host disease* [monoclonal antibodies]

**Malatal** tablets R̲ *GI anticholinergic; sedative* [atropine sulfate; scopolamine hydrobromide; hyoscyamine hydrobromide; phenobarbital] 0.0194•0.0065•0.1037•16.2 mg

**malathion** USP, BAN *pediculicide*

**maletamer** INN *antiperistaltic* [also: malethamer]

**malethamer** USAN *antiperistaltic* [also: maletamer]

**maleylsulfathiazole** INN

**malic acid** NF *acidifying agent*

**malidone** [see: aloxidone]

**Mallamint** chewable tablets OTC *antacid* [calcium carbonate] 420 mg

**Mallazine** eye drops OTC *topical ocular decongestant/vasoconstrictor* [tetrahydrozoline HCl] 0.05%

**Mallergan VC Cough** syrup (discontinued 1994) R̲ *narcotic antitussive; decongestant; antihistamine* [codeine phosphate; phenylephrine HCl; promethazine HCl; alcohol]

**Mallisol** ointment OTC *broad-spectrum antimicrobial* [povidone-iodine]

**malonal** [see: barbital]

**malotilate** USAN, INN *liver disorder treatment*

**Maltsupex** liquid OTC *bulk laxative* [nondiastatic barley malt extract] 16 g/tbsp.

**Maltsupex** powder OTC *bulk laxative* [nondiastatic barley malt extract] 8 g/tbsp.

**Maltsupex** tablets OTC *bulk laxative* [nondiastatic barley malt extract] 750 mg

**Mama Coca** *street drug slang* [see: cocaine]

**Mammol** ointment OTC *emollient for nipples of nursing mothers* [bismuth subnitrate] 40%

***m*-AMSA (acridinylamine methanesulphon anisidide)** [see: amsacrine]

**man** *street drug slang* [see: heroin]

**Mandameth** enteric-coated tablets R̲ *urinary bactericidal* [methenamine mandelate] 0.5, 1 g

**Mandelamine** film-coated tablets (discontinued 1995) R̲ *urinary bactericidal* [methenamine mandelate] 0.5, 1 g

**Mandelamine** oral suspension, suspension forte, granules (discontinued 1993) R̲ *urinary bactericidal* [methenamine mandelate] 50 mg/mL; 100 mg/mL; 1 g/dose

**mandelic acid** NF

**Mandol** powder for IV or IM injection R̲ *cephalosporin-type antibiotic* [cefamandole nafate] 1, 2 g ⑨ nadolol

**Manerex** ⑭ tablets R̲ *antidepressant* [moclobemide] 100, 150 mg

**manganese** *element* (Mn)

**manganese chloride** USP *dietary manganese supplement; investigational GI contrast agent for MRI* 0.1 mg/mL injection

**manganese chloride tetrahydrate** [see: manganese chloride]

**manganese gluconate (manganese D-gluconate)** USP *dietary manganese supplement*

**manganese glycerophosphate** NF

**manganese hypophosphite** NF

**manganese phosphinate** [see: manganese hypophosphite]

**manganese sulfate** USP *dietary manganese supplement* 0.1 mg/mL injection

**manganese sulfate monohydrate** [see: manganese sulfate]

**Manhattan silver** *street drug slang* [see: marijuana]

**manidipine 6300** INN

**manna sugar** [see: mannitol]

**mannite** [see: mannitol]

**mannitol (D-mannitol)** USP *renal function test aid; osmotic diuretic; urologic irrigant* 10%, 15%, 20%, 25% injection

**mannitol hexanitrate** INN

**mannityl nitrate** [see: mannitol hexanitrate]

**mannomustine** INN, BAN

**mannosulfan** INN

**Manoplax** film-coated tablets (discontinued 1993) ℞ *vasodilator for congestive heart failure* [flosequinan]

**manozodil** INN

**Mantadil** cream ℞ *topical corticosteroid; antihistamine* [hydrocortisone acetate; chlorcyclizine HCl] 0.5%•2%

**Mantoux test** [see: tuberculin]

**MAOIs (monoamine oxidase inhibitors)** *a class of antidepressants that increase CNS monoamine neurotransmitters (epinephrine, norepinephrine, and serotonin)*

**Maolate** tablets ℞ *skeletal muscle relaxant* [chlorphenesin carbamate] 400 mg

**Maox** tablets (name changed to Maox 420 in 1995)

**Maox 420** tablets OTC *antacid* [magnesium oxide] 420 mg

**MAP (mitomycin, Adriamycin, Platinol)** *chemotherapy protocol*

**Mapap** tablets OTC *analgesic; antipyretic* [acetaminophen] 325, 500 mg

**Mapap, Children's** liquid OTC *analgesic; antipyretic* [acetaminophen] 160 mg/5 mL

**Mapap Cold Formula** tablets OTC *antitussive; decongestant; antihistamine; analgesic* [dextromethorphan hydrobromide; pseudoephedrine HCl; chlorpheniramine maleate; acetaminophen] 15•30•2•325 mg

**Mapap Infant Drops** OTC *analgesic; antipyretic* [acetaminophen] 100 mg/mL

**maprotiline** USAN, INN *tetracyclic antidepressant*

**maprotiline HCl** USP *tetracyclic antidepressant* 25, 50, 75 mg oral

**Maranox** tablets OTC *analgesic; antipyretic* [acetaminophen] 325 mg

**marathons** *street drug slang* [see: amphetamines]

**Marax** tablets ℞ *antiasthmatic; bronchodilator; decongestant* [theophylline; ephedrine sulfate] 130•25 mg ⓭ Atarax; Maalox

**Marax-DF** pediatric syrup ℞ *antiasthmatic; bronchodilator; decongestant; anxiolytic* [theophylline; ephedrine sulfate; hydroxyzine HCl] 97.5•18.75•7.5 mg/15 mL

**Marbaxin 750** tablets (discontinued 1993) ℞ *skeletal muscle relaxant* [methocarbamol]

**Marbec** tablets (discontinued 1995) OTC *dietary supplement* [multiple B vitamins; vitamin C; brewer's yeast] ±•300•120 mg

**Marblen** tablets, liquid OTC *antacid* [calcium carbonate; magnesium carbonate] 520•400 mg; 540•400 mg/5 mL

**Marcaine HCl** injection ℞ *injectable local anesthetic* [bupivacaine HCl] 0.25%, 0.5%, 0.75%

**Marcaine HCl** injection ℞ *injectable local anesthetic* [bupivacaine HCl; epinephrine bitartrate] 0.25%•1:200 000, 0.5%•1:200 000, 0.75%•1:200 000 ⓭ Narcan

**Marcaine Spinal** injection ℞ *injectable local anesthetic* [bupivacaine HCl] 0.75%

**Marcaine with Epinephrine** injection (discontinued 1996) ℞ *injectable local anesthetic* [bupivacaine HCl; epinephrine] 0.5%•1:200 000

**Marcillin** capsules, powder for oral suspension ℞ *penicillin-type antibiotic* [ampicillin trihydrate] 500 mg; 250 mg/100 mL

**Marcof Expectorant** syrup ℞ *narcotic antitussive; expectorant* [hydrocodone bitartrate; potassium guaiacolsulfonate] 5•300 mg/5 mL

**Marezine** IM injection (discontinued 1993) ℞ *antiemetic; anticholinergic; antihistamine; motion sickness preventative* [cyclizine lactate] 50 mg/mL

**Marezine** tablets OTC *antiemetic; anticholinergic; antihistamine; motion sickness preventative* [cyclizine HCl] 50 mg

**Marflex** tablets (discontinued 1993) ℞ *skeletal muscle relaxant* [orphenadrine citrate]

**Margesic** capsules ℞ *analgesic; anti-inflammatory; sedative* [acetaminophen; caffeine; butalbital] 325•40•50 mg

**Margesic H** capsules ℞ *narcotic analgesic* [hydrocodone bitartrate; acetaminophen] 5•500 mg

**Margesic No. 3** tablets (discontinued 1996) ℞ *narcotic analgesic* [codeine phosphate; acetaminophen] 30•650 mg

**maridomycin** INN

**marijuana; marihuana** *euphoric/hallucinogenic street drug made from the dried leaves and flowering tops of the cannabis plant* [see also: cannabis]

**marimastat** USAN *investigational (Phase III) antineoplastic; matrix metalloproteinase (MMP) inhibitor*

**Marine Lipid Concentrate** softgels OTC *dietary supplement* [omega-3 fatty acids] 1200 mg

**Marinol** soft gelatin capsules ℞ *antiemetic for chemotherapy; appetite stimulant for AIDS patients (orphan)* [dronabinol] 2.5, 5, 10 mg

**mariptiline** INN

**Marley** *street drug slang* [see: marijuana]

**Marlin Salt System** tablets OTC *rinsing/storage solution for soft contact lenses* [sodium chloride for normal saline solution] 250 mg

**Marlin Salt System II** tablets OTC *rinsing/storage solution for soft contact lenses* [sodium chloride for normal saline solution] 250 mg

**Marlipids III** capsules (discontinued 1993) OTC *dietary supplement* [omega-3 fatty acids] 1000 mg

**Marmine** IV or IM injection ℞ *antinauseant; antiemetic; antivertigo; motion sickness preventative* [dimenhydrinate] 50 mg/mL

**Marmine** tablets OTC *antinauseant; antiemetic; antivertigo; motion sickness preventative* [dimenhydrinate] 50 mg

**Marnal** tablets, capsules ℞ *analgesic; antipyretic; anti-inflammatory; sedative* [aspirin; caffeine; butalbital] 325•40•50 mg

**Marnatal-F** film-coated tablets ℞ *vitamin/mineral/calcium/iron supplement* [multiple vitamins & minerals; calcium; iron; folic acid] ≚•250•60•1 mg

**Marogen** ℞ *investigational substitute for blood transfusion; investigational (orphan) for anemia of end-stage renal disease* [epoetin beta]

**maroxepin** INN

**Marplan** tablets (discontinued 1994) ℞ *antidepressant; monoamine oxidase (MAO) inhibitor* [isocarboxazid] 10 mg

**Marpres** tablets ℞ *antihypertensive* [hydrochlorothiazide; reserpine; hydralazine HCl] 15•0.1•25 mg

**MART-1 adenoviral gene therapy** *investigational (orphan) for metastatic malignant melanoma*

**Marthritic** tablets ℞ *analgesic; antipyretic; anti-inflammatory; antirheumatic* [salsalate] 750 mg

**Mary; Mari** *street drug slang* [see: marijuana]

**Mary and Johnny** *street drug slang* [see: marijuana]

**Mary Ann; Mary Jane; Mary Warner** *street drug slang* [see: marijuana]

**masoprocol** USAN, INN *antineoplastic for actinic keratoses (AK)*

**Massé Breast** cream OTC *moisturizer and emollient for nipples of nursing women*

**Massengill Baking Soda Freshness** solution OTC *vaginal cleanser and deodorizer; acidity modifier* [sodium bicarbonate]

**Massengill Disposable Douche** solution OTC *antiseptic/germicidal; vaginal cleanser and deodorizer; acidity modifier* [cetylpyridinium chloride; lactic acid; sodium lactate]

**Massengill Disposable Douche; Massengill Vinegar & Water Extra Mild** solution OTC *vaginal cleanser and deodorizer; acidity modifier* [vinegar (acetic acid)]

**Massengill Douche** powder OTC *astringent; antipruritic/counterirritant; vaginal cleanser and deodorizer* [ammonium alum; phenol; methyl salicylate; menthol; thymol]

**Massengill Douche** solution concentrate OTC *vaginal cleanser and deodorizer; acidity modifier* [lactic acid; sodium lactate; sodium bicarbonate]

**Massengill Feminine Cleansing Wash** liquid OTC *for external perivaginal cleansing*

**Massengill Medicated** towelettes OTC *topical corticosteroidal anti-inflammatory* [hydrocortisone] 0.5%

**Massengill Medicated Douche with Cepticin; Massengill Medicated Disposable Douche with Cepticin** solution OTC *antiseptic/germicidal; vaginal cleanser and deodorizer* [povidone-iodine] 12%; 10%

**Massengill Unscented** solution (discontinued 1995) OTC *vaginal cleanser and deodorizer; acidity modifier* [lactic acid]

**Massengill Vinegar & Water Extra Cleansing with Puraclean** solution OTC *antiseptic/germicidal; vaginal cleanser and deodorizer; acidity modifier* [cetylpyridinium chloride; vinegar (acetic acid)]

**Materna** tablets (discontinued 1997) ℞ *vitamin/mineral/calcium/iron supplement* [multiple vitamins & minerals; calcium; iron; folic acid; biotin] ± • 250•60•1•0.03 mg

**matrix metalloproteinase (MMP) inhibitors** *a class of investigational (Phase III) antineoplastics and investigational (orphan) agents to treat corneal ulcers*

**Matsakow** *street drug slang* [see: heroin]

**Matulane** capsules ℞ *antibiotic antineoplastic for Hodgkin's disease; investigational for lymphoma, brain and lung cancer* [procarbazine HCl] 50 mg

**Maui wowie; Maui waui** *street drug slang for marijuana from Hawaii* [see: marijuana]

**Mavik** tablets ℞ *antihypertensive; angiotensin converting enzyme (ACE) inhibitor* [trandolapril] 1, 2, 4 mg

**Max** *street drug slang for GHB dissolved in water and mixed with amphetamine* [see: GHB; amphetamines]

**Maxair** Autohaler (breath-activated metered-dose inhaler) ℞ *bronchodilator for bronchospasm* [pirbuterol acetate] 0.2 mg/dose

**Maxalt** ℞ *investigational (Phase III) antimigraine agent* [rizatriptan benzoate]

**Maxamine** ℞ *investigational (Phase III) treatment for malignant melanoma*

**Maxaquin** film-coated tablets ℞ *broad-spectrum fluoroquinolone antibiotic* [lomefloxacin HCl] 400 mg

**Max-Caro** capsules (discontinued 1996) OTC *to reduce photosensitivity reaction* [beta-carotene] 15 mg

**MaxEPA** soft capsules OTC *dietary supplement* [omega-3 fatty acids; multiple vitamins & minerals] 1000• ± mg

**Maxibolin** *an anabolic steroid abused as a street drug* [see: ethylestrenol]

**Maxicam** ℞ *investigational nonsteroidal anti-inflammatory drug (NSAID); antiarthritic; analgesic; antipyretic* [isoxicam]

**Maxidex** Drop-Tainers (eye drop suspension), ophthalmic ointment ℞ *ophthalmic topical corticosteroidal anti-inflammatory* [dexamethasone] 0.1%; 0.05%

**Maxiflor** cream, ointment ℞ *topical corticosteroidal anti-inflammatory* [diflorasone diacetate] 0.05%

**Maxilube Personal Lubricant** jelly OTC *vaginal lubricant*

**Maximum Blue Label; Maximum Green Label** tablets OTC *vitamin/mineral supplement* [multiple vitamins & minerals; folic acid; biotin] ± •130•50 µg

**Maximum Red Label** tablets OTC *vitamin/mineral/iron supplement* [multiple vitamins & minerals; iron; folic acid; biotin] ± •3.3 mg•0.13 mg•50 µg

**"Maximum Strength"** products [see under product name]

**Maxipime** powder for IV or IM injection ℞ *broad-spectrum cephalosporin antibiotic* [cefepime HCl] 0.5, 1, 2 g

**Maxitrol** eye drop suspension, ophthalmic ointment ℞ *topical ophthalmic corticosteroidal anti-inflammatory; antibiotic* [dexamethasone; neomycin sulfate; polymyxin B sulfate] 0.1%•0.35%•10 000 U/mL; 0.1%•0.35%•10 000 U/g

**Maxivate** ointment, cream, lotion ℞ *topical corticosteroid* [betamethasone diproprionate] 0.05%

**Maxivent** ℞ *investigational antiasthmatic* [doxofylline]

**Maxi-Vite** tablets OTC *vitamin/mineral/calcium/iron supplement* [multiple vitamins & minerals; calcium; iron; folic acid; biotin] ±•53.5•1.5•0.4•0.001 mg

**Maxolon** tablets ℞ *antidopaminergic; antiemetic for chemotherapy; peristaltic* [metoclopramide monohydrochloride monohydrate] 10 mg

**Maxovite** sustained-release tablets OTC *vitamin/mineral supplement* [multiple vitamins & minerals; folic acid; biotin] ±•330•11.7 μg

**Maxzide** tablets ℞ *diuretic; antihypertensive* [triamterene; hydrochlorothiazide] 37.5•25, 75•50 mg

**Mayo** *street drug slang* [see: cocaine; heroin]

**maytansine** USAN *antineoplastic* [also: maitansine]

**May-Vita** elixir ℞ *vitamin supplement* [multiple B vitamins; folic acid] ±•0.1 mg

**Mazanor** tablets ℞ *anorexiant* [mazindol] 1 mg

**mazapertine succinate** USAN *antipsychotic; dopamine receptor antagonist*

**mazaticol** INN

**MAZE (*m*-AMSA, azacitidine, etoposide)** *chemotherapy protocol*

**Mazicon** IV injection (name changed to Romazicon in 1993)

**mazindol** USAN, USP, INN, BAN *anorexiant; investigational (orphan) treatment for Duchenne muscular dystrophy* ② mebendazole

**mazipredone** INN

**MB (methylene blue)** [q.v.]

**m-BACOD; M-BACOD (methotrexate, bleomycin, Adriamycin, cyclophosphamide, Oncovin, dexamethasone)** *chemotherapy protocol* "m" is 200 mg/m$^2$; "M" is 3 g/m$^2$

**M-BACOS (methotrexate, bleomycin, Adriamycin, cyclophosphamide, Oncovin, Solu-Medrol)** *chemotherapy protocol*

**MBC (methotrexate, bleomycin, cisplatin)** *chemotherapy protocol*

**MBD (methotrexate, bleomycin, DDP)** *chemotherapy protocol*

**MBR (methylene blue, reduced)** [see: methylene blue]

**MC (mitoxantrone, cytarabine)** *chemotherapy protocol*

**M-Caps** capsules ℞ *urinary acidifier to control ammonia production* [racemethionine] 200 mg

**MCBP (melphalan, cyclophosphamide, BCNU, prednisone)** *chemotherapy protocol*

**MCH (microfibrillar collagen hemostat)** [q.v.]

**MCP (melphalan, cyclophosphamide, prednisone)** *chemotherapy protocol*

**M-CSF (macrophage colony-stimulating factor)** [q.v.]

**MCT** oil OTC *dietary fat supplement* [medium chain triglycerides from coconut oil]

**MCT (medium chain triglycerides)** [q.v.]

**MCV (methotrexate, cisplatin, vinblastine)** *chemotherapy protocol*

**MD-60; MD-76** injection ℞ *parenteral radiopaque agent* [diatrizoate meglumine; diatrizoate sodium] 52%•8%; 66%•10%

**MDA (methylenedioxyamphetamine)** [see: MDMA, MDEA]

**MDEA (3,4-methylenedioxyethamphetamine)** *a hallucinogenic amphetamine derivative closely related to MDMA, abused as a street drug, which causes dependence* [also see: amphetamines; MDMA]

**MD-Gastroview** solution ℞ *GI contrast radiopaque agent* [diatrizoate meglumine; diatrizoate sodium] 66%•10%

**MDL 27,192** *investigational anticonvulsant*

**MDL 28,314** *investigational antineoplastic for leukemia and solid tumors*

**MDL 28,574** *investigational (Phase II) antiviral glucosidase inhibitor for HIV*

**MDL 100,240** *investigational treatment for hypertension and congestive heart failure*

**MDL 201,404** *investigational agent for adult respiratory disorders*

**MDMA (3,4-methylenedioxymethamphetamine)** *widely abused hallucinogenic street drug that is chemically related to amphetamines and mescaline and causes dependence* [see also: amphetamines; mescaline; MDEA]

**MDP (methylene diphosphonate)** [now: medronate disodium]

**MEA (mercaptoethylamine)** [see: mercaptamine]

**mean green** *street drug slang* [see: PCP]

**measles, mumps & rubella virus vaccine, live** USP *active immunizing agent for measles (rubeola), mumps and rubella*

**measles immune globulin** USP

**measles & rubella virus vaccine, live** USP *active immunizing agent for measles (rubeola) and rubella*

**measles virus vaccine, live** USP *active immunizing agent for measles (rubeola)*

**Mebadin** (available only from the Centers for Disease Control) Ŗ *investigational anti-infective for amebiasis and amebic dysentery* [dehydroemetine]

**meballymal** [see: secobarbital]

**mebamoxine** [see: benmoxin]

**mebanazine** INN, BAN

**Mebaral** tablets Ŗ *long-acting barbiturate sedative, hypnotic and anticonvulsant* [mephobarbital] 32, 50, 100 mg ⊘ Medrol; Mellaril

**mebendazole** USAN, USP, INN *anthelmintic for trichuriasis, enterobiasis, ascariasis, and uncinariasis* 100 mg oral ⊘ mazindol

**mebenoside** INN

**mebeverine** INN *smooth muscle relaxant* [also: mebeverine HCl]

**mebeverine HCl** USAN *smooth muscle relaxant* [also: mebeverine]

**mebezonium iodide** INN, BAN

**mebhydrolin** INN, BAN

**mebiquine** INN

**mebolazine** INN

**mebrofenin** USAN, INN *hepatobiliary function test*

**mebrophenhydramine HCl** [see: embramine HCl]

**mebubarbital** [see: pentobarbital]

**mebumal** [see: pentobarbital]

**mebutamate** USAN, INN *antihypertensive*

**mebutizide** INN

**mecamylamine** INN *antihypertensive* [also: mecamylamine HCl]

**mecamylamine HCl** USP *antihypertensive* [also: mecamylamine]

**mecamylamine HCl & nicotine** *investigational (Phase III) transdermal patch for smoking cessation*

**mecarbinate** INN

**mecarbine** [see: mecarbinate]

**mecasermin** INN, BAN *investigational (NDA filed, orphan) for amyotrophic lateral sclerosis, growth hormone insufficiency, and post-poliomyelitis syndrome* [previously known as insulin-like growth factor 1]

**MeCCNU (methyl chloroethylcyclohexyl-nitrosourea)** [see: semustine]

**mecetronium ethylsulfate** USAN *antiseptic* [also: mecetronium etilsulfate]

**mecetronium etilsulfate** INN *antiseptic* [also: mecetronium ethylsulfate]

**mechlorethamine HCl** USP *nitrogen mustard-type alkylating antineoplastic* [also: chlormethine; mustine; nitrogen mustard N-oxide HCl]

**Mechol** tablets (discontinued 1994) OTC *dietary supplement* [multiple B vitamins; vitamin C] ≛•75 mg

**meciadanol** INN

**mecillinam** INN, BAN *antibacterial* [also: amdinocillin]

**mecinarone** INN

**Meclan** cream Ŗ *topical antibiotic for acne* [meclocycline sulfosalicylate] 1% ⊘ Meclomen; Mezlin

**meclizine HCl** USP *antiemetic; antihistamine; anticholinergic; motion sickness relief* [also: meclozine] 12.5, 25, 50 mg oral ⊘ mescaline

**meclocycline** USAN, INN, BAN *antibacterial*

**meclocycline sulfosalicylate** USAN, USP *antibacterial antibiotic*

**meclofenamate sodium** USAN, USP *analgesic; antiarthritic; nonsteroidal anti-inflammatory drug (NSAID)* 50, 100 mg oral

**meclofenamic acid** USAN, INN *nonsteroidal anti-inflammatory drug (NSAID)*

**meclofenoxate** INN, BAN

**Meclomen** capsules (discontinued 1996) ℞ *nonsteroidal anti-inflammatory drug (NSAID); antiarthritic; analgesic* [meclofenamate sodium] 50, 100 mg ② Meclan

**meclonazepam** INN

**mecloqualone** USAN, INN *sedative; hypnotic*

**mecloralurea** INN

**meclorisone** INN, BAN *topical anti-inflammatory* [also: meclorisone dibutyrate]

**meclorisone dibutyrate** USAN *topical anti-inflammatory* [also: meclorisone]

**mecloxamine** INN

**meclozine** INN, BAN *antiemetic; antihistamine; anticholinergic; motion sickness relief* [also: meclizine HCl] ② mescaline

**mecobalamin** USAN, INN *vitamin; hematopoietic*

**mecrilate** INN *tissue adhesive* [also: mecrylate]

**mecrylate** USAN *tissue adhesive* [also: mecrilate]

**Mectizan** ℞ *investigational antiparasitic*

**MECY (methotrexate, cyclophosphamide)** *chemotherapy protocol*

**mecysteine** INN

**Med Timolol** ⓒᴬᴺ (U.S. product: Timoptic) eye drops ℞ *antiglaucoma agent (β-blocker)* [timolol maleate] 0.25%, 0.5%

**Meda Cap** capsules OTC *analgesic; antipyretic* [acetaminophen] 500 mg

**Meda Tab** tablets OTC *analgesic; antipyretic* [acetaminophen] 325 mg

**Medacote** lotion OTC *topical antihistamine; astringent; antipruritic* [pyrilamine maleate; zinc oxide] 1%•²

**Medadyne** liquid OTC *topical oral anesthetic; antiseptic; astringent* [benzocaine; methylbenzethonium chloride; tannic acid; camphor; menthol]

**Medadyne** throat spray OTC *topical anesthetic; oral antiseptic* [lidocaine; cetalkonium chloride]

**Medalone 40; Medalone 80** [see: depMedalone 40; depMedalone 80]

**Medamint** throat lozenges OTC *topical oral anesthetic* [benzocaine]

**Medatussin** syrup, pediatric syrup (discontinued 1994) OTC *antitussive; expectorant; demulcent* [dextromethorphan hydrobromide; guaifenesin; potassium citrate; citric acid]

**Medatussin Plus** syrup (discontinued 1994) ℞ *decongestant; antihistamine; antitussive; expectorant* [phenylpropanolamine HCl; chlorpheniramine maleate; phenyltoloxamine citrate; dextromethorphan hydrobromide; guaifenesin]

**medazepam** INN *minor tranquilizer* [also: medazepam HCl]

**medazepam HCl** USAN *minor tranquilizer* [also: medazepam]

**medazomide** INN

**medazonamide** [see: medazomide]

**medetomidine** INN, BAN *veterinary analgesic; veterinary sedative* [also: medetomidine HCl]

**medetomidine HCl** USAN *veterinary analgesic; veterinary sedative* [also: medetomidine]

**MEDI 488** *investigational HIV vaccine*

**MEDI 493** *investigational (Phase III) monoclonal antibody for prophylaxis of respiratory syncytial virus (RSV) in infants*

**Mediatric** capsules (discontinued 1993) ℞ *geriatric dietary supplement with hormones* [multiple B vitamins; iron; methyltestosterone; conjugated estrogens; methamphetamine HCl]

**medibazine** INN

**medical air** [see: air, medical]

**Medicated Acne Cleanser** OTC *topical acne treatment* [colloidal sulfur; resorcinol] 4%•2%

**medicinal zinc peroxide** [see: zinc peroxide, medicinal]

**Medicone** anorectal ointment OTC *topical local anesthetic* [benzocaine] 20%

**Medicone** rectal suppositories OTC *topical vasoconstrictor* [phenylephrine HCl] 0.25%

**Medi-Flu** caplets, liquid (discontinued 1995) OTC *antitussive; decongestant; antihistamine; analgesic* [dextromethorphan hydrobromide; pseudoephedrine HCl; chlorpheniramine maleate; acetaminophen] 15•30•2•500 mg; 5•10•0.67•167 mg/5 mL

**medifoxamine** INN

**Medigesic** capsules ℞ *analgesic; antipyretic; sedative* [acetaminophen; caffeine; butalbital] 325•40•50 mg

**Medihaler-Epi** inhalation aerosol (discontinued 1996) OTC *bronchodilator for bronchial asthma* [epinephrine bitartrate] 0.3 mg/dose

**Medihaler-Iso** inhalation aerosol ℞ *bronchodilator* [isoproterenol sulfate] 0.2% (80 μg/dose)

**Medilax** chewable tablets OTC *laxative* [phenolphthalein] 120 mg

**medinal** [see: barbital sodium]

**Medipain 5** capsules ℞ *narcotic analgesic* [hydrocodone bitartrate; acetaminophen] 5•500 mg

**Mediplast** plaster OTC *topical keratolytic* [salicylic acid] 40%

**Mediplex** Tabules (tablets) OTC *vitamin/mineral supplement* [multiple vitamins & minerals] ±

**Medipren** tablets, caplets (discontinued 1996) OTC *nonsteroidal antiinflammatory drug (NSAID); antiarthritic; analgesic* [ibuprofen] 200 mg

**Medi-Quik** aerosol (discontinued 1995) OTC *topical local anesthetic; antiseptic* [lidocaine HCl; benzalkonium chloride]

**Medi-Quik** ointment OTC *topical antibiotic* [polymyxin B sulfate; neomycin; bacitracin] 5000 U•3.5 mg•400 U per g

**Medi-Quik** spray OTC *topical local anesthetic; antiseptic* [lidocaine; benzalkonium chloride] 2%•0.13%

**medium chain triglycerides (MCT)** *dietary lipid supplement*

**medorinone** USAN, INN *cardiotonic*

**medorubicin** INN

**Medotar** ointment OTC *topical antipsoriatic; antiseborrheic; astringent; antiseptic* [coal tar; zinc oxide] 1%• ±

**MEDR-640** *investigational agent to prevent reperfusion injury following a heart attack*

**Medralone 40; Medralone 80** intralesional, soft tissue, and IM injection ℞ *glucocorticoid; anti-inflammatory; immunosuppressant* [methylprednisolone acetate] 40 mg/mL; 80 mg/mL

**medrogestone** USAN, INN, BAN *progestin*

**Medrol** tablets, Dosepak (unit of use package) ℞ *glucocorticoid; anti-inflammatory; immunosuppressant* [methylprednisolone] 2, 4, 8, 16, 24, 32 mg ② Mebaral

**Medrol Acetate Topical** ointment (discontinued 1993) ℞ *topical corticosteroid* [methylprednisolone acetate] 0.25%, 1%

**medronate disodium** USAN *pharmaceutic aid*

**medronic acid** USAN, INN, BAN *pharmaceutic aid*

**medroxalol** USAN, INN, BAN *antihypertensive*

**medroxalol HCl** USAN *antihypertensive*

**medroxiprogesterone acetate** [see: medroxyprogesterone acetate]

**medroxyprogesterone** INN, BAN *progestin; antineoplastic* [also: medroxyprogesterone acetate]

**medroxyprogesterone acetate** USP *progestin for secondary amenorrhea or abnormal uterine bleeding; antineoplastic* [also: medroxyprogesterone] 10 mg oral

**MED-Rx** controlled-release tablets (14-day, 56-tablet regimen) ℞ *decongestant; expectorant* [pseudoephedrine HCl + guaifenesin (blue tablets); guaifenesin (white tablets)] 60•600 mg; 600 mg

**MED-Rx DM** controlled-release tablets (14-day, 56-tablet regimen) ℞ *decongestant; expectorant; antitussive* [pseudoephedrine HCl + guaifenesin (blue tablets); dextromethorphan hydrobromide + guaifenesin (green tablets)] 60•600 mg; 30•600 mg

**medrylamine** INN

**medrysone** USAN, USP, INN *glucocorticoid; ophthalmic anti-inflammatory*

**mefeclorazine** INN

**mefenamic acid** USAN, USP, INN, BAN *analgesic; nonsteroidal anti-inflammatory drug (NSAID)*

**mefenidil** USAN, INN *cerebral vasodilator*

**mefenidil fumarate** USAN *cerebral vasodilator*

**mefenidramium metilsulfate** INN

**mefenorex** INN *anorectic* [also: mefenorex HCl]

**mefenorex HCl** USAN *anorectic* [also: mefenorex]

**mefeserpine** INN

**mefexamide** USAN, INN *CNS stimulant*

**mefloquine** USAN, INN, BAN *antimalarial schizonticide*

**mefloquine HCl** USAN *antimalarial schizonticide (orphan)*

**Mefoxin** powder for IV or IM injection ℞ *cephalosporin-type antibiotic* [cefoxitin sodium] 1, 2, 10 g

**mefruside** USAN, INN *diuretic*

**Meg; Megg; Meggie** *street drug slang* [see: marijuana]

**Mega B with C** tablets (discontinued 1995) OTC *vitamin supplement* [multiple B vitamins; vitamin C; folic acid; biotin] ± •500 mg•400 μg•100 μg

**Mega VM-80** tablets OTC *geriatric vitamin/mineral supplement* [multiple vitamins & minerals; folic acid; biotin] ± •400•80 μg

**Mega-B** tablets OTC *vitamin supplement* [multiple B vitamins; folic acid; biotin] ± •100•100 μg

**Megace** oral suspension ℞ *antineoplastic for breast or endometrial cancer; treatment for AIDS-related anorexia and cachexia (orphan)* [megestrol acetate] 40 mg/mL

**Megace** tablets ℞ *antineoplastic for advanced carcinoma of the breast or endometrium* [megestrol acetate] 20, 40 mg

**Megadose** tablets (discontinued 1995) OTC *geriatric vitamin/mineral supplement* [multiple vitamins & minerals; folic acid; biotin] ± •400•80 μg

**megallate** INN *combining name for radicals or groups*

**megalomicin** INN *antibacterial* [also: megalomicin potassium phosphate]

**megalomicin potassium phosphate** USAN *antibacterial* [also: megalomicin]

**Megalone** ℞ *investigational quinolone antibiotic* [fleroxacin]

**Megaton** elixir ℞ *vitamin/mineral supplement* [multiple B vitamins & minerals; folic acid] ± •0.1 mg

**megestrol** INN, BAN *antineoplastic* [also: megestrol acetate]

**megestrol acetate** USAN, USP *antineoplastic for breast or endometrial cancer; therapy for AIDS-related anorexia and cachexia (orphan)* [also: megestrol] 20, 40 mg oral

**meglitinide** INN

**meglucycline** INN

**meglumine** USP, INN *radiopaque medium*

**meglumine diatrizoate** BAN *radiopaque medium* [also: diatrizoate meglumine]

**meglumine iocarmate** BAN *radiopaque medium* [also: iocarmate meglumine]

**meglumine iothalamate** BAN *radiopaque medium* [also: iothalamate meglumine]

**meglumine ioxaglate** BAN *radiopaque medium* [also: ioxaglate meglumine]

**meglutol** USAN, INN *antihyperlipoproteinemic*

**mel B** [see: melarsoprol]

**mel W** [see: melarsonyl potassium]

**Melacine** ℞ *investigational (NDA filed, orphan) theraccine for invasive stage III-IV melanoma; investigational (Phase III) for early-stage melanoma* [melanoma vaccine]

**meladrazine** INN, BAN

**melafocon A** USAN *hydrophobic contact lens material*

**Melaine** ℞ *investigational oral contraceptive and for use in hormone replacement therapy* [ethinyl estradiol; gestodene]

**Melanex** solution ℞ *hyperpigmentation bleaching agent* [hydroquinone] 3%

**melanoma vaccine** *investigational (NDA filed, orphan) therapeutic vaccine for invasive stage III-IV melanoma; investigational (Phase III) for early-stage melanoma*

**melarsonyl potassium** INN, BAN

**melarsoprol** INN, BAN, DCF *investigational anti-infective for trypanosomiasis*

**melatonin** *sleep aid; investigational (orphan) for circadian rhythm sleep disorders in blind people with no light perception*

**melengestrol** INN *antineoplastic; progestin* [also: melengestrol acetate]

**melengestrol acetate** USAN *antineoplastic; progestin* [also: melengestrol]

**meletimide** INN

**melfalan** [see: melphalan]

**Melfiat-105** Unicelles (sustained-release capsules) ℞ *anorexiant* [phendimetrazine tartrate] 105 mg

**Melimmune** *investigational (orphan) for non-Hodgkin's B-cell lymphoma* [indium In 111 murine MAb (2B8-MXDTPA); Y-90 murine MAB (2B8-MXDTPA)]

**melinamide** INN

**melitracen** INN *antidepressant* [also: melitracen HCl]

**melitracen HCl** USAN *antidepressant* [also: melitracen]

**melizame** USAN, INN *sweetener*

**Mellaril** tablets, oral concentrate ℞ *antipsychotic* [thioridazine HCl] 10, 15, 25, 50, 100, 150, 200 mg; 30, 100 mg/mL ② Elavil; Mebaral; Moderil

**Mellaril-S** oral suspension ℞ *antipsychotic* [thioridazine HCl] 25, 100 mg/5 mL

**mellow drug of America** *street drug slang, for MDA (methylenedioxyamphetamine), now called MDMA (methylenedioxymethamphetamine)* [see: MDMA]

**mellow yellow** *street drug slang for LSD or banana peels used for smoking* [see: LSD]

**meloxicam** INN

**Melpaque HP** cream ℞ *hyperpigmentation bleaching agent; sunscreen* [hydroquinone in a sunblock base] 4%

**melperone** INN, BAN

**melphalan (MPL)** USAN, USP, INN, BAN, JAN *nitrogen mustard-type alkylating antineoplastic for multiple myeloma and ovarian cancer; investigational (orphan) for metastatic melanoma*

**Melquin HP** cream ℞ *hyperpigmentation bleaching agent* [hydroquinone] 4%

**MelVax** ℞ *investigational treatment for malignant melanoma* [melanoma vaccine]

**memantine** INN

**Memorette** (trademarked packaging form) *patient compliance package*

**memotine** INN *antiviral* [also: memotine HCl]

**memotine HCl** USAN *antiviral* [also: memotine]

**menabitan** INN *analgesic* [also: menabitan HCl]

**menabitan HCl** USAN *analgesic* [also: menabitan]

**menadiol** BAN *vitamin $K_4$; prothrombogenic* [also: menadiol sodium diphosphate]

**menadiol sodium diphosphate** USP *vitamin $K_4$; prothrombogenic* [also: menadiol]

**menadiol sodium sulfate** INN

**menadione** USP *vitamin $K_3$; prothrombogenic*

**menadione sodium bisulfite** USP, INN

**Menadol** tablets OTC *nonsteroidal anti-inflammatory drug (NSAID); antiarthritic; analgesic* [ibuprofen] 200 mg

**menaphthene** [see: menadione]

**menaphthone** [see: menadione]

**menaphthone sodium bisulfite** [see: menadione sodium bisulfite]

**menaquinone** *vitamin $K_2$; prothrombogenic*

**menatetrenone** INN

**menbutone** INN, BAN

**mendelevium** *element (Md)*

**Menest** film-coated tablets ℞ *estrogen replacement therapy; hypogonadism; inoperable prostatic and breast cancer* [esterified estrogens] 0.3, 0.625, 1.25, 2.5 mg

**menfegol** INN

**menglytate** INN

**menichlopholan** [see: niclofolan]

**Meni-D** capsules ℞ *anticholinergic; antivertigo agent; motion sickness preventative* [meclizine HCl] 25 mg

**meningococcal polysaccharide vaccine, group A** USP *active bacterin for meningitis (Neisseria meningitidis)*

**meningococcal polysaccharide vaccine, group C** USP *active bacterin for meningitis (Neisseria meningitidis)*

**meningococcal polysaccharide vaccine, group W-135** *active bacterin for meningitis (Neisseria meningitidis)*

**meningococcal polysaccharide vaccine, group Y** *active bacterin for meningitis (Neisseria meningitidis)*

**menitrazepam** INN

**menoctone** USAN, INN *antimalarial*

**menogaril** USAN, INN *antibiotic antineoplastic*

**Menogen; Menogen H.S.** tablets ℞ *estrogen/androgen for menopausal vasomotor symptoms* [esterified estrogens; methyltestosterone] 1.25•2.5 mg; 0.625•1.25 mg

**Menomune-A/C/Y/W-135** powder for subcu injection ℞ *meningitis vaccine* [meningococcal polysaccharide vaccine, groups A, C, Y, and W-135] 200 μg/0.5 mL

**Menoplex** tablets OTC *analgesic; antipyretic; antihistamine* [acetaminophen; phenyltoloxamine citrate] 325•30 mg

**Menorest** transdermal patch ℞ *investigational estrogen replacement therapy for postmenopausal disorders* [estradiol]

**menotropins** USAN, USP *gonad-stimulating principle; gonadotropin*

**menotropins & human luteinizing hormone (hLH), recombinant** *investigational (orphan) for chronic anovulation due to hypogonadotropic hypogonadism*

**Menrium 5-2; Menrium 5-4; Menrium 10-4** tablets ℞ *estrogen replacement therapy for postmenopausal disorders* [chlordiazepoxide; esterified estrogens] 5•0.2 mg; 5•0.4 mg; 10•0.4 mg

**Mentane** ℞ *investigational cholinesterase inhibitor for Alzheimer's disease* [velnacrine]

**Mentax** cream ℞ *topical benzylamine antifungal* [butenafine HCl] 1%

**menthol** USP *topical antipruritic/antiseptic; mild local anesthetic*

**MenthoRub** vaporizing ointment OTC *counterirritant* [menthol; camphor; eucalyptus oil; oil of turpentine] 2.6%•4.73%•♯•♯

**meobentine** INN *antiarrhythmic* [also: meobentine sulfate]

**meobentine sulfate** USAN *antiarrhythmic* [also: meobentine]

**mepacrine** INN *anthelmintic; antimalarial* [also: quinacrine HCl]

**mepacrine HCl** [see: quinacrine HCl]

**meparfynol** [see: methylpentynol]

**mepartricin** USAN, INN *antifungal; antiprotozoal*

**mepazine acetate** [see: pecazine]

**mepenzolate bromide** USP, INN *peptic ulcer adjunct*

**mepenzolate methylbromide** [see: mepenzolate bromide]

**mepenzolone bromide** [see: mepenzolate bromide]

**Mepergan** injection ℞ *narcotic analgesic; sedative* [meperidine HCl; promethazine HCl] 25•25 mg/mL

**Mepergan Fortis** capsules ℞ *narcotic analgesic; sedative* [meperidine HCl; promethazine HCl] 50•25 mg

**meperidine HCl** USP *narcotic analgesic; also abused as a street drug* [also: pethidine] 50, 100 mg oral; 50 mg/5 mL oral; 10, 25, 50, 75, 100 mg/mL injection ▨ meprobamate

**Mephaquin** ℞ *antimalarial for acute chloroquine-resistant malaria (orphan)* [mefloquine HCl]

**mephenesin** NF, INN

**mephenhydramine** [see: moxastine]

**mephenoxalone** INN

**mephentermine** INN *adrenergic; vasoconstrictor; vasopressor for hypotensive shock* [also: mephentermine sulfate]

**mephentermine sulfate** USP *adrenergic; vasoconstrictor; vasopressor for hypotensive shock* [also: mephentermine]

**mephenytoin** USAN, USP, INN *hydantoin-type anticonvulsant* [also: methoin] ▨ Mephyton; Mesantoin

**mephobarbital** USP, JAN *anticonvulsant; sedative* [also: methylphenobarbital; methylphenobarbitone]

**Mephyton** tablets ℞ *coagulant; correct anticoagulant-induced prothrombin deficiency; vitamin K supplement* [phytonadione] 5 mg ▨ mephenytoin; methadone

**mepicycline** [see: pipacycline]

**MEPIG (mucoid exopolysaccharide *Pseudomonas* [hyper]-immune globulin)** [q.v.]

**mepindolol** INN, BAN

**mepiperphenidol bromide**
**mepiprazole** INN, BAN
**mepirizole** [see: epirizole]
**mepiroxol** INN
**mepitiostane** INN
**mepivacaine** INN *local anesthetic* [also: mepivacaine HCl]
**mepivacaine HCl** USP *local anesthetic* [also: mepivacaine] 1%, 2% injection
**mepixanox** INN
**mepramidil** INN
**meprednisone** USAN, USP, INN
**meprobamate** USP, INN, BAN, JAN *sedative; hypnotic; anxiolytic; minor tranquilizer; also abused as a street drug* 200, 400 mg oral ⊘ meperidine
**Meprogesic Q** tablets (discontinued 1995) ℞ *analgesic; antipyretic; antiinflammatory; anxiolytic* [aspirin; meprobamate] 325•200 mg
**Mepron** film-coated tablets (discontinued 1995) ℞ *antiprotozoal for AIDS-related Pneumocystis carinii pneumonia (PCP)* [atovaquone] 250 mg
**Mepron** oral suspension ℞ *antipneumocystic for Pneumocystis carinii pneumonia (orphan); investigational (orphan) antiprotozoal for Toxoplasma gondii encephalitis* [atovaquone] 750 mg/5 mL
**meproscillarin** INN, BAN
**Meprospan** sustained-release capsules (discontinued 1997) ℞ *anxiolytic* [meprobamate] 200, 400 mg ⊘ Naprosyn
**meprothixol** BAN [also: meprotixol]
**meprotixol** INN [also: meprothixol]
**meprylcaine** INN *local anesthetic* [also: meprylcaine HCl]
**meprylcaine HCl** USP *local anesthetic* [also: meprylcaine]
**meptazinol** INN, BAN *analgesic* [also: meptazinol HCl]
**meptazinol HCl** USAN *analgesic* [also: meptazinol]
**mepyramine** INN, BAN *antihistamine* [also: pyrilamine maleate]
**mepyramine maleate** [see: pyrilamine maleate]
**mepyrium** [see: amprolium]
**mepyrrotazine** [see: dimelazine]
**mequidox** USAN, INN *antibacterial*
**mequinol** INN

**mequitamium iodide** INN
**mequitazine** INN, BAN
**mequitazium iodide** [see: mequitamium iodide]
**meragidone sodium**
**meralein sodium** USAN, INN *topical anti-infective*
**meralluride** NF, INN
**merbaphen** USP
**merbromin** NF, INN *general antiseptic*
**mercaptamine** INN *antiurolithic* [also: cysteamine]
**mercaptoarsenical** [see: arsthinol]
**mercaptoarsenol** [see: arsthinol]
**mercaptoethylamine (MEA)** [see: mercaptamine]
**mercaptomerin (MT6)** INN [also: mercaptomerin sodium]
**mercaptomerin sodium** USP [also: mercaptomerin]
**mercaptopurine (6-MP)** USP, INN *antimetabolic antineoplastic*
**Merck** *street drug slang for pharmaceutical cocaine, a reference to the manufacturer* [see: cocaine]
**mercuderamide** INN
**mercufenol chloride** USAN *topical anti-infective*
**mercumatilin sodium** INN
**mercuric oxide, yellow** NF *ophthalmic antiseptic (FDA ruled it "not safe and effective" in 1992)*
**mercuric salicylate** NF
**mercuric succinimide** NF
**mercurobutol** INN
**Mercurochrome** solution OTC *antiseptic* [merbromin] 2%
**mercurophylline** NF, INN
**mercurous chloride** [see: calomel]
**mercury** *element (Hg)*
**mercury, ammoniated** USP *topical anti-infective; antipsoriatic*
**mercury amide chloride** [see: mercury, ammoniated]
**mercury oleate** NF
**merethoxylline procaine**
**mergocriptine** INN
**Meridia** ℞ *investigational anorexiant and antidepressant* [sibutramine HCl]
**merisoprol acetate Hg 197** USAN *radioactive agent*

**merisoprol acetate Hg 203** USAN radioactive agent

**merisoprol Hg 197** USAN renal function test; radioactive agent

**Meritene** powder OTC enteral nutritional therapy [milk-based formula]

**Meritene** ready-to-use liquid (discontinued 1994) OTC enteral nutritional therapy [milk-based formula] 250 mL

**meropenem** USAN, INN, BAN broad-spectrum carbapenem antibiotic for intra-abdominal infections and bacterial meningitis

**Merrem** powder for IV infusion ℞ broad-spectrum carbapenem antibiotic for intra-abdominal infections and bacterial meningitis [meropenem] 500, 1000 mg

**mersalyl** INN

**mersalyl sodium** [see: mersalyl]

**Mersol** solution, tincture OTC antiseptic; antibacterial; antifungal [thimerosal] 1:1000

**mertiatide** INN

**Meruvax II** powder for subcu injection ℞ rubella vaccine [rubella virus vaccine, live] 0.5 mL

**mesabolone** INN

**mesalamine** USAN anti-inflammatory; treatment of ulcerative colitis and proctitis [also: mesalazine]

**mesalazine** INN, BAN anti-inflammatory; treatment of ulcerative colitis and proctitis [also: mesalamine]

**Mesantoin** tablets ℞ hydantoin-type anticonvulsant [mephenytoin] 100 mg ⧉ mephenytoin; Mestinon; Metatensin

**mesc'; mez** street drug slang [see: mescaline]

**mescal** street drug slang for mescaline or an intoxicating distilled beverage from the same plant [see: mescaline]

**mescaline** hallucinogenic street drug derived from the flowering heads (mescal buttons) of a Mexican cactus ⧉ meclizine

**Mescolor** film-coated, sustained-release tablets ℞ decongestant; antihistamine; anticholinergic [pseudoephedrine HCl; chlorpheniramine maleate; methscopolamine nitrate] 120•8•2.5 mg

**meseclazone** USAN, INN anti-inflammatory

**meserole** street drug slang for a marijuana cigarette [see: marijuana]

**mesifilcon A** USAN hydrophilic contact lens material

**mesilate** INN combining name for radicals or groups [also: mesylate]

**M-Eslon** ⒸⒶⓃ (U.S. product: Capros)

**mesna** USAN, INN, BAN urotoxic antidote for hemorrhagic cystitis (orphan); investigational (orphan) for cyclophosphamide-induced urotoxicity

**Mesnex** IV injection ℞ urotoxic antidote for hemorrhagic cystitis (orphan); investigational (orphan) for cyclophosphamide-induced urotoxicity [mesna] 100 mg/mL

**mesocarb** INN

**meso-inositol** [see: inositol]

**meso-NDGA (nordihydroguaiaretic acid)** [see: masoprocol]

**meso-nordihydroguaiaretic acid (NDGA)** [see: masoprocol]

**mesoridazine** USAN, INN antipsychotic

**mesoridazine besylate** USP antipsychotic

**mespirenone** INN

**mestanolone** INN, BAN

**mestenediol** [see: methandriol]

**mesterolone** USAN, INN, BAN androgen; also abused as a street drug

**Mestinon** tablets, Timespan (sustained-release tablets), syrup, IM or IV injection ℞ anticholinesterase muscle stimulant; muscle relaxant reversal [pyridostigmine bromide] 60 mg; 180 mg; 60 mg/5 mL; 5 mg/mL ⧉ Mesantoin; Metatensin

**mestranol** USAN, USP, INN estrogen

**mesudipine** INN

**mesulergine** INN

**mesulfamide** INN

**mesulfen** INN [also: mesulphen]

**mesulphen** BAN [also: mesulfen]

**mesuprine** INN vasodilator; smooth muscle relaxant [also: mesuprine HCl]

**mesuprine HCl** USAN vasodilator; smooth muscle relaxant [also: mesuprine]

**mesuximide** INN anticonvulsant [also: methsuximide]

**mesylate** USAN, USP, BAN *combining name for radicals or groups* [also: mesilate]

**metabromsalan** USAN, INN *disinfectant*

**metabutethamine HCl** NF

**metabutoxycaine HCl** NF

**metacetamol** INN, BAN

**metaclazepam** INN

**metacycline** INN *antibacterial* [also: methacycline]

**metaglycodol** INN

**metahexamide** INN

**metahexanamide** [see: metahexamide]

**Metahydrin** tablets ℞ *diuretic; antihypertensive* [trichlormethiazide] 4 mg ⧖ Metandren

**metalkonium chloride** INN

**metallibure** INN *anterior pituitary activator for swine* [also: methallibure]

**metalol HCl** USAN *antiadrenergic (β-receptor)*

**metamelfalan** INN

**metamfazone** INN [also: methamphazone]

**metamfepramone** INN [also: dimepropion]

**metamfetamine** INN *CNS stimulant; widely abused as a street drug* [also: methamphetamine HCl]

**metamizole sodium** INN *analgesic; antipyretic* [also: dipyrone]

**metampicillin** INN

**Metamucil** effervescent powder OTC *bulk laxative; antacid* [psyllium hydrophilic mucilloid; sodium bicarbonate; potassium bicarbonate] 3.4•⧖•⧖ g/packet

**Metamucil** powder, wafers OTC *bulk laxative* [psyllium hydrophilic mucilloid] 3.4 g/tsp.; 1.7 g

**metandienone** INN [also: methandrostenolone; methandienone]

**metanixin** INN

**metaoxedrine chloride** [see: phenylephrine HCl]

**metaphosphoric acid, potassium salt** [see: potassium metaphosphate]

**metaphosphoric acid, trisodium salt** [see: sodium trimetaphosphate]

**metaphyllin** [see: aminophylline]

**metapramine** INN

**Metaprel** syrup ℞ *bronchodilator* [metaproterenol sulfate] 10 mg/5 mL

**Metaprel** tablets, inhalation aerosol powder, solution for inhalation (discontinued 1996) ℞ *bronchodilator* [metaproterenol sulfate] 10, 20 mg; 0.65 mg/dose; 0.4%, 0.6%, 5%

**metaproterenol polistirex** USAN *bronchodilator* [also: orciprenaline] ⧖ metoprolol

**metaproterenol sulfate** USAN, USP *bronchodilator* 10, 20 mg oral; 10 mg/5 mL oral; 0.4%, 0.6%, 5% inhalation

**metaradrine bitartrate** [see: metaraminol bitartrate]

**metaraminol** INN *adrenergic; vasopressor for acute hypotensive shock, anaphylaxis, or traumatic shock* [also: metaraminol bitartrate]

**metaraminol bitartrate** USP *adrenergic; vasopressor for acute hypotensive shock, anaphylaxis, or traumatic shock* [also: metaraminol]

**Metasome** ℞ *investigational antiasthmatic* [liposomal metaproterenol]

**Metastron** IV injection ℞ *analgesic for metastatic bone pain* [strontium chloride Sr 89] 10.9–22.6 mg/mL (4 mCi)

**Metatensin #2; Metatensin #4** tablets ℞ *antihypertensive* [trichlormethiazide; reserpine] 2•0.1 mg; 4•0.1 mg ⧖ Mesantoin; Mestinon

**metaterol** INN

**metaxalone** USAN, INN, BAN *skeletal muscle relaxant* ⧖ metolazone

**metazamide** INN

**metazepium iodide** [see: buzepide metiodide]

**metazide** INN

**metazocine** INN, BAN

**metbufen** INN

**metcaraphen HCl**

**metembonate** INN *combining name for radicals or groups*

**meteneprost** USAN, INN *oxytocic; prostaglandin*

**metenolone** INN *anabolic steroid; also abused as a street drug* [also: methenolone acetate; methenolone; metenolone acetate]

**metenolone acetate** JAN *anabolic steroid; also abused as a street drug* [also:

methenolone acetate; metenolone; methenolone]

**metenolone enanthate** JAN *anabolic steroid; also abused as a street drug* [also: methenolone enanthate]

**metergoline** INN, BAN

**metergotamine** INN

**metescufylline** INN

**metesculetol** INN

**metesind glucuronate** USAN *specific thymidylate synthase (TS) inhibitor antineoplastic* ⊡ *medicine*

**metethoheptazine** INN

**metetoin** INN *anticonvulsant* [also: methetoin]

**metformin** USAN, INN, BAN *biguanide-type antidiabetic* [also: metformin HCl]

**metformin HCl** USAN, JAN *biguanide antidiabetic* [also: metformin]

**meth** *street drug slang* [see: methamphetamine HCl]

**methacholine bromide** NF

**methacholine chloride** USP, INN *cholinergic; bronchoconstrictor for pulmonary challenge tests*

**methacrylic acid copolymer** NF *tablet-coating agent*

**methacycline** USAN *antibacterial* [also: metacycline]

**methacycline HCl** USP *gram-negative and gram-positive bacteriostatic; antirickettsial*

**methadol** [see: dimepheptanol]

**methadone** INN *narcotic analgesic; often abused as a street drug* [also: methadone HCl] ⊡ Mephyton

**methadone HCl** USP *narcotic analgesic; often abused as a street drug* [also: methadone] 5, 10, 40 mg oral; 5, 10 mg/5 mL oral; 10 mg/mL oral

**methadonium chloride** [see: methadone HCl]

**Methadose** tablets ℞ *narcotic analgesic; narcotic addiction detoxicant; often abused as a street drug* [methadone HCl] 5, 10 mg

**methadyl acetate** USAN *narcotic analgesic* [also: acetylmethadol]

**methafilcon B** USAN *hydrophilic contact lens material*

**Methagual** OTC *counterirritant* [methyl salicylate; guaiacol] 8%•2%

**Methalgen** cream OTC *counterirritant* [methyl salicylate; menthol; camphor; mustard oil]

**methallenestril** INN

**methallenestrol** [see: methallenestril]

**methallibure** USAN *anterior pituitary activator for swine* [also: metallibure]

**methalthiazide** USAN *diuretic; antihypertensive*

**methamoctol**

**methamphazone** BAN [also: metamfazone]

**methamphetamine HCl** USP *CNS stimulant; widely abused as a street drug* [also: metamfetamine]

**methampyrone** [now: dipyrone]

**methanabol** [see: methandriol]

**methandienone** BAN [also: methandrostenolone; metandienone]

**methandriol**

**methandrostenolone** USP *steroid; discontinued for human use, but the veterinary product is still available and sometimes abused as a street drug* [also: metandienone; methandienone]

**methaniazide** INN

**methanol** [see: methyl alcohol]

**methantheline bromide** USP *peptic ulcer adjunct* [also: methanthelinium bromide]

**methanthelinium bromide** INN, BAN *anticholinergic* [also: methantheline bromide]

**methaphenilene** INN, BAN [also: methaphenilene HCl]

**methaphenilene HCl** NF [also: methaphenilene]

**methapyrilene** INN [also: methapyrilene fumarate]

**methapyrilene fumarate** USP [also: methapyrilene]

**methapyrilene HCl** USP

**methaqualone** USAN, USP, INN, BAN *hypnotic; sedative; widely abused as a street drug, which leads to dependence*

**methaqualone HCl** USP

**metharbital** USP, INN, JAN *anticonvulsant* [also: metharbitone]

**metharbitone** BAN *anticonvulsant* [also: metharbital]

**MethaSite** ℞ *investigational ophthalmic steroidal anti-inflammatory* [fluorometholone]

**methastyridone** INN

**Methatropic** capsules OTC *dietary lipotropic with vitamin supplementation* [choline; inositol; methionine; multiple B vitamins] 115•83•110• ± mg

**methazolamide** USP, INN *carbonic anhydrase inhibitor* 25, 50 mg oral

**Methblue 65** tablets ℞ *urinary anti-infective/antiseptic; antidote to cyanide poisoning* [methylene blue] 65 mg

**methcathinone** *a highly addictive manufactured street drug similar to cathinone, with amphetamine-like effects* [see also: cathinone; *Catha edulis*]

**methdilazine** USP, INN *antipruritic*

**methdilazine HCl** USP *antipruritic; antihistamine*

**methenamine** USP, INN *urinary bactericidal* ⑨ methionine

**methenamine hippurate** USAN, USP *urinary bactericidal* [also: hexamine hippurate]

**methenamine mandelate** USP *urinary bactericidal* 0.5, 1 g oral; 0.5 g/5 mL oral

**methenolone** BAN *anabolic steroid; also abused as a street drug* [also: methenolone acetate; metenolone; metenolone acetate]

**methenolone acetate** USAN *anabolic steroid; also abused as a street drug* [also: metenolone; methenolone; metenolone acetate]

**methenolone enanthate** USAN *anabolic steroid; also abused as a street drug* [also: metenolone enanthate]

**metheptazine** INN

**Methergine** coated tablets, IV or IM injection ℞ *control postpartum uterine atony; postpartum hemorrhage* [methylergonovine maleate] 0.2 mg; 0.2 mg/mL

**methestrol** INN

**methetharimide** [see: bemegride]

**methetoin** USAN *anticonvulsant* [also: metetoin]

**methicillin sodium** USAN, USP *bactericidal antibiotic* [also: meticillin]

**methimazole** USP *thyroid inhibitor* [also: thiamazole]

**methindizate** BAN [also: metindizate]

**methiodal sodium** USP, INN

**methiomeprazine** INN

**methiomeprazine HCl** [see: methiomeprazine]

**methionine (DL-methionine)** NF, JAN *urinary acidifier* [also: racemethionine] 500 mg oral

**methionine (L-methionine)** USAN, USP, INN, JAN *essential amino acid; investigational (orphan) for AIDS myelopathy; symbols: Met, M* ⑨ methenamine

**methionine-enkephalin** *investigational (Phase I) immunomodulator for AIDS*

**methionyl granulocyte CSF, recombinant** *orphan status withdrawn 1994*

**methionyl human granulocyte CSF, recombinant** *orphan status withdrawn 1994*

**methionyl neurotropic factor, brain-derived, recombinant** *investigational (orphan) for amyotrophic lateral sclerosis*

**methionyl stem cell factor, recombinant human** *investigational (orphan) for progressive bone marrow failure*

**methionyl stem cell factor, recombinant human & filgrastim** *investigational (orphan) adjunct to myelosuppressive or myeloablative therapy*

**methiothepin** [see: metitepine]

**methisazone** USAN *antiviral* [also: metisazone]

**methisoprinol** [now: inosine pranobex]

**methitural** INN

**methixene HCl** USAN *smooth muscle relaxant* [also: metixene] ⑨ methoxsalen

**methocamphone methylsulfate** [see: trimethidinium methosulfate]

**methocarbamol** USP, INN, BAN, JAN *skeletal muscle relaxant* 500, 750 mg oral; 100 mg/mL injection

**methocidin** INN

**methohexital** USP, INN *barbiturate general anesthetic* [also: methohexitone]

**methohexital sodium** USP *barbiturate general anesthetic*

**methohexitone** BAN *barbiturate general anesthetic* [also: methohexital]

**methoin** BAN *anticonvulsant* [also: mephenytoin]

**methonaphthone** [see: menbutone]

**methophedrine** [see: methoxyphedrine]

**methophenazine** [see: metofenazate]

**methopholine** USAN *analgesic* [also: metofoline]

**methoprene** INN

**methopromazine** INN

**methopromazine maleate** [see: methopromazine]

**methopyrimazole** [see: epirizole]

*d*-**methorphan** [see: dextromethorphan]

*d*-**methorphan hydrobromide** [see: dextromethorphan hydrobromide]

**methoserpidine** INN, BAN

**methotrexate (MTX)** USAN, USP, INN, BAN, JAN *antimetabolic antineoplastic; antirheumatic; systemic antipsoriatic; investigational (orphan) for juvenile rheumatoid arthritis* 2.5 mg oral; 1 g injection

**methotrexate & laurocapram** *investigational (orphan) for topical treatment of Mycosis fungoides*

**Methotrexate LPF Sodium** *preservative-free injection (discontinued 1994)* ℞ *antineoplastic for leukemia, psoriasis and rheumatoid arthritis* [methotrexate sodium] 1 g

**methotrexate sodium** USP *antirheumatic; antimetabolic antineoplastic for osteogenic sarcoma (orphan)* 2.5 mg oral; 20, 1000 mg/vial injection; 2.5, 25 mg/mL injection

**methotrimeprazine** USAN, USP *central analgesic; CNS depressant* [also: levomepromazine]

**methoxamine** INN *adrenergic; vasoconstrictor; vasopressor for hypotensive shock during surgery* [also: methoxamine HCl]

**methoxamine HCl** USP *adrenergic; vasoconstrictor; vasopressor for hypotensive shock during surgery* [also: methoxamine]

**methoxiflurane** [see: methoxyflurane]

**methoxsalen** USP *pigmentation agent for vitiligo; antipsoriatic; investigational*

*(orphan) for diffuse systemic sclerosis and cardiac allografts* ⑫ methixene

**methoxy polyethylene glycol** [see: polyethylene glycol monomethyl ether]

**8-methoxycarbonyloctyl oligosaccharides** *investigational (Phase III) E. coli neutralizer for traveler's diarrhea and hemolytic uremic syndrome (HUS)*

**methoxyfenoserpin** [see: mefeserpine]

**methoxyflurane** USAN, USP, INN, BAN *inhalation general anesthetic*

**methoxyphedrine** INN

*p*-**methoxyphenacyl** [see: anisatil]

**methoxyphenamine** INN [also: methoxyphenamine HCl]

**methoxyphenamine HCl** USP [also: methoxyphenamine]

**4-methoxyphenol** [see: mequinol]

*o*-**methoxyphenyl salicylate acetate** [see: guacetisal]

**methoxypromazine maleate** [see: methopromazine]

**8-methoxypsoralen (8-MOP)** [see: methoxsalen]

**5-methoxyresorcinol** [see: flamenol]

**methphenoxydiol** [see: guaifenesin]

**methscopolamine bromide** USP *peptic ulcer adjunct* [also: hyoscine methobromide]

**methsuximide** USP, BAN *anticonvulsant* [also: mesuximide]

**methyclothiazide** USAN, USP, INN *diuretic; antihypertensive* 2.5, 5 mg oral

**methydromorphine** [see: methyldihydromorphine]

**methyl alcohol** NF *solvent*

**methyl benzoquate** BAN *coccidiostat for poultry* [also: nequinate]

**methyl cresol** [see: cresol]

**methyl cysteine** [see: mecysteine]

**methyl *p*-hydroxybenzoate** [see: methylparaben]

**methyl isobutyl ketone** NF *alcohol denaturant*

**methyl nicotinate** USAN

**methyl palmoxirate** USAN *antidiabetic*

**methyl phthalate** [see: dimethyl phthalate]

**methyl salicylate** NF *flavoring agent; counterirritant; topical anesthetic*

**methyl sulfoxide** [see: dimethyl sulfoxide]

**methyl violet** [see: gentian violet]

*l***-methylaminoethanolcatechol** [see: epinephrine]

**methylaminopterin** [see: methotrexate]

**methylandrostenediol** [see: methandriol]

**methylatropine nitrate** USAN *anticholinergic* [also: atropine methonitrate]

**methylbenactyzium bromide** INN

**methylbenzethonium chloride** USP, INN *topical anti-infective/antiseptic*

**α-methylbenzylhydrazine** [see: mebanazine]

**methylcarbamate of salicylanilide** [see: anilamate]

**methyl-CCNU (chloroethyl-cyclohexyl-nitrosourea)** [see: semustine]

**methylcellulose** USP, INN *suspending and viscosity-increasing agent*

**methylcellulose, propylene glycol ether of** [see: hydroxypropyl methylcellulose]

**methylchromone** INN, BAN

**methyldesorphine** INN, BAN

**methyldigoxin** [see: metildigoxin]

**methyldihydromorphine** INN

**methyldihydromorphinone HCl** [see: metopon]

**methyldinitrobenzamide** [see: dinitolmide]

**methyldioxatrine** [see: meletimide]

**N-methyldiphenethylamine** [see: demelverine]

**α-methyl-DL-thyroxine ethyl ester** see: etiroxate

**methyldopa** USAN, USP, INN, BAN, JAN *centrally acting antiadrenergic antihypertensive* 125, 250, 500 mg oral ☒ levodopa

**α-methyldopa** [now: methyldopa]

**methyldopate** BAN *centrally acting antiadrenergic antihypertensive* [also: methyldopate HCl]

**methyldopate HCl** USAN, USP *centrally acting antiadrenergic antihypertensive* [also: methyldopate] 50 mg/mL injection

**6-methylenandrosta-1,4-diene-3,17-dione** *orphan status withdrawn 1996*

**methylene blue (MB)** USP *antimethemoglobinemic; GU antiseptic; antidote to cyanide poisoning* [also: methylthioninium chloride] 65 mg oral; 10 mg/mL injection

**methylene chloride** NF *solvent*

**methylene diphosphonate (MDP)** [now: medronate disodium]

**methylenedioxyamphetamine (MDA)** [see: MDMA, MDEA]

**3,4-methylenedioxyethamphetamine (MDEA)** [q.v.]

**3,4-methylenedioxymethamphetamine (MDMA)** [q.v.]

**6-methyleneoxytetracycline (MOTC)** [see: methacycline]

**methylenprednisolone** [see: prednylidene]

**methylergometrine** INN *oxytocic* [also: methylergonovine maleate]

**methylergometrine maleate** [see: methylergonovine maleate]

**methylergonovine maleate** USP *oxytocic* [also: methylergometrine]

**methylergonovinium bimaleate** [see: methylergonovine maleate]

**methylergotamine** [see: metergotamine]

**methylestrenolone** [see: normethandrone]

**methyl-GAG (methylglyoxal-*bis*-guanylhydrazone)** [see: mitoguazone]

**methylglyoxal-*bis*-guanylhydrazone (methyl-GAG; MGBG)** [see: mitoguazone]

**1-methylhexylamine** [see: tuaminoheptane]

**1-methylhexylamine sulfate** [see: tuaminoheptane sulfate]

**N-methylhydrazine** [see: procarbazine]

**methylmorphine** [see: codeine]

**methylnaltrexone** *investigational (orphan) treatment for chronic opioid-induced constipation*

**methyl-nitro-imidazole** [see: carnidazole]

**methylnortestosterone** [see: normethandrone]

**methylparaben** USAN, NF *antifungal agent; preservative*

**methylparaben sodium** USAN, NF *antimicrobial preservative*

**methylparafynol** [see: meparfynol]

**methylpentynol** INN, BAN

**methylperidol** [see: moperone]

**(+)-methylphenethylamine** [see: dextroamphetamine]

**(–)-methylphenethylamine** [see: lev-amphetamine]

**methylphenethylamine HCl** [see: amphetamine HCl]

**methylphenethylamine phosphate** [see: amphetamine phosphate]

**(–)-methylphenethylamine succi-nate** [see: levamfetamine succinate]

**methylphenethylamine sulfate** [see: amphetamine sulfate]

**(+)-methylphenethylamine sulfate** [see: dextroamphetamine sulfate]

**methylphenidate** INN, BAN *CNS stimulant for attention deficit hyperactivity disorder (ADHD) and narcolepsy; also abused as a street drug* [also: methylphenidate HCl]

**methylphenidate HCl** USP, JAN *CNS stimulant for attention deficit hyperactivity disorder (ADHD) and narcolepsy; also abused as a street drug* [also: methylphenidate] 5, 10, 20 mg oral

**methylphenobarbital** INN *anticonvulsant; sedative* [also: mephobarbital; methylphenobarbitone]

**methylphenobarbitone** BAN *anticonvulsant; sedative* [also: mephobarbital; methylphenobarbital]

**d-methylphenylamine sulfate** [see: dextroamphetamine sulfate]

**methylphytyl napthoquinone** [see: phytonadione]

**methylprednisolone** USP, INN, BAN, JAN *corticosteroid; anti-inflammatory; immunosuppressant* 4, 16 mg oral

**methylprednisolone aceponate** INN

**methylprednisolone acetate** USP, JAN *corticosteroid; anti-inflammatory; immunosuppressant* 20, 40, 80 mg/mL injection

**methylprednisolone hemisuccinate** USP *corticosteroid*

**methylprednisolone sodium phosphate** USAN *corticosteroid* 40, 125, 500, 1000 mg/vial injection

**methylprednisolone sodium succinate** USP, JAN *corticosteroid; anti-inflammatory; immunosuppressant*

**methylprednisolone suleptanate** USAN, INN *anti-inflammatory*

**methylpromazine**

**4-methylpyrazole (4-MP)** [see: fomepizole]

**methylrosaniline chloride** [now: gentian violet]

**methylrosanilinium chloride** INN *topical anti-infective* [also: gentian violet]

**methylscopolazole bromide** [see: methscopolamine bromide]

**methylsulfate** USP *combining name for radicals or groups* [also: metilsulfate]

**methyltestosterone** USP, INN, BAN *oral androgen; also abused as a street drug* 10, 25 mg oral

**methyltheobromine** [see: caffeine]

**methylthionine chloride** [see: methylene blue]

**methylthionine HCl** [see: methylene blue]

**methylthioninium chloride** INN *antimethemoglobinemic; antidote to cyanide poisoning* [also: methylene blue]

**methylthiouracil** USP, INN

**methyltrienolone** [see: metribolone]

**methynodiol diacetate** USAN *progestin* [also: metynodiol]

**methyprylon** USP, INN *sedative; hypnotic* [also: methprylone]

**methyprylone** BAN *sedative* [also: methyprylon]

**methyridene** BAN [also: metyridine]

**methysergide** USAN, INN, BAN *migraine-specific vasoconstrictor*

**methysergide maleate** USP *migraine-specific vasoconstrictor*

**metiamide** USAN, INN *antagonist to histamine $H_2$ receptors*

**metiapine** USAN, INN *antipsychotic*

**metiazinic acid** INN

**metibride** INN

**meticillin** INN *antibacterial* [also: methicillin sodium]

**meticillin sodium** [see: methicillin sodium]

**Meticorten** tablets ℞ *glucocorticoid; anti-inflammatory; immunosuppressant* [prednisone] 1 mg

**meticrane** INN

**metildigoxin** INN

**metilsulfate** INN *combining name for radicals or groups* [also: methylsulfate]

**Metimyd** eye drop suspension, ophthalmic ointment ℞ *ophthalmic topical corticosteroidal anti-inflammatory; bacteriostatic* [prednisolone acetate; sulfacetamide sodium] 0.5%•10%

**metindizate** INN [also: methindizate]

**metioprim** USAN, INN, BAN *antibacterial*

**metioxate** INN

**metipirox** INN

**metipranolol** USAN, INN, BAN *ophthalmic antihypertensive (β-blocker)*

**metipranolol HCl** *topical antiglaucoma agent (β-blocker)*

**metiprenaline** INN

**metirosine** INN *antihypertensive* [also: metyrosine]

**metisazone** INN *antiviral* [also: methisazone]

**metitepine** INN

**metixene** INN *smooth muscle relaxant* [also: methixene HCl]

**metixene HCl** [see: methixene HCl]

**metizoline** INN *adrenergic; vasoconstrictor* [also: metizoline HCl]

**metizoline HCl** USAN *adrenergic; vasoconstrictor* [also: metizoline]

**metkefamide** INN *analgesic* [also: metkephamid acetate]

**metkefamide acetate** [see: metkephamid acetate]

**metkephamid acetate** USAN *analgesic* [also: metkefamide]

**metochalcone** INN

**metocinium iodide** INN

**metoclopramide** INN *antiemetic for chemotherapy; GI stimulant; antidopaminergic* [also: metoclopramide HCl]

**metoclopramide HCl** USAN, USP *antiemetic for chemotherapy; GI stimulant; antidopaminergic* [also: metoclopramide] 5, 10 mg oral; 5, 10 mg/5 mL oral; 10 mg/mL oral; 5 mg/mL injection

**metoclopramide monohydrochloride monohydrate** *antiemetic for chemotherapy; GI stimulant; antidopaminergic* 5, 10 mg oral; 5, 10 mg/5 mL oral; 5 mg/mL injection

**metocurine iodide** USAN, USP *neuromuscular blocker; muscle relaxant* 2 mg/mL injection

**metofenazate** INN

**metofoline** INN *analgesic* [also: methopholine]

**metogest** USAN, INN *hormone*

**metolazone** USAN, INN *diuretic; antihypertensive* ② metaxalone

**metomidate** INN, BAN

**metopimazine** USAN, INN *antiemetic*

**Metopirone** softgels ℞ *pituitary function test* [metyrapone] 250 mg ② metyrapone

**Metopirone** tablets (discontinued 1994) ℞ *pituitary function test* [metyrapone] 250 mg ② metyrapone

**metopon** INN

**metopon HCl** [see: metopon]

**metoprine** USAN *antineoplastic*

**metoprolol** USAN, INN, BAN *antiadrenergic (β-receptor)* ② metaproterenol

**metoprolol fumarate** USAN *antihypertensive*

**metoprolol succinate** USAN *antianginal; antihypertensive*

**metoprolol tartrate** USAN, USP *antiadrenergic (β-receptor)* 50, 100 mg oral; 1 mg/mL injection

**metoquizine** USAN, INN *anticholinergic*

**metoserpate** INN *veterinary sedative* [also: metoserpate HCl]

**metoserpate HCl** USAN *veterinary sedative* [also: metoserpate]

**metostilenol** INN

**metoxepin** INN

**metoxiestrol** [see: moxestrol]

**Metra** tablets (discontinued 1994) ℞ *anorexiant* [phendimetrazine tartrate] 35 mg

**metrafazoline** INN

**metralindole** INN

**metrazifone** INN

**metrenperone** USAN, INN, BAN *veterinary myopathic*

**Metreton Ophthalmic** eye drops (discontinued 1993) ℞ *ophthalmic topical corticosteroidal anti-inflammatory* [prednisolone sodium phosphate]

**metribolone** INN

**Metric 21** tablets (discontinued 1995) ℞ *antibiotic; antiprotozoal; amebicide* [metronidazole]

**metrifonate** INN *investigational treatment for Alzheimer's disease* [also: metriphonate]

**metrifudil** INN

**metriphonate** BAN *investigational treatment for Alzheimer's disease* [also: metrifonate]

**metrizamide** USAN, INN *radiopaque medium*

**metrizoate sodium** USAN *radiopaque medium* [also: sodium metrizoate]

**Metro I.V.** ready-to-use injection ℞ *antibiotic; antiprotozoal; amebicide* [metronidazole] 500 mg/100 mL

**MetroCream** ℞ *topical antibiotic, antiprotozoal, and amebicide for rosacea* [metronidazole] 0.75%

**Metrodin** powder for IM injection ℞ *ovulation stimulant in polycystic ovarian disease (orphan)* [urofollitropin] 0.83, 1.66 mg/ampule

**Metrodin HP** ℞ *investigational infertility treatment* [urofollitropin]

**MetroGel** ℞ *antibacterial; antiprotozoal; acne rosacea treatment (orphan); investigational (orphan) for decubitus ulcers and perioral dermatitis* [metronidazole] 0.75%

**MetroGel Vaginal** gel ℞ *antibacterial; antiprotozoal* [metronidazole] 0.75%

**metronidazole** USAN, USP, INN, BAN *antibiotic; antiprotozoal/amebicide; acne rosacea treatment (orphan); investigational (orphan) for decubitus ulcers and perioral dermatitis* 250, 500 mg oral; 500 mg/100 mL injection

**metronidazole benzoate** *antiprotozoal (Trichomonas)*

**metronidazole HCl** USAN *antibiotic; antiprotozoal; amebicide*

**metronidazole phosphate** USAN *antibacterial; antiprotozoal*

**Metubine Iodide** IV injection ℞ *anesthesia adjunct* [metocurine iodide] 2 mg/mL

**metuclazepam** [see: metaclazepam]

**meturedepa** USAN, INN *antineoplastic*

**metynodiol** INN *progestin* [also: methynodiol diacetate]

**metynodiol diacetate** [see: methynodiol diacetate]

**metyrapone** USAN, USP, INN *pituitary function test* ⚗ Metopirone; metyrosine

**metyrapone tartrate** USAN *pituitary function test*

**metyridine** INN [also: methyridene]

**metyrosine** USAN, USP *antihypertensive; pheochromocytomic agent* ⚗ metyrapone

**Mevacor** tablets ℞ *cholesterol-lowering antihyperlipidemic; HMG-CoA reductase inhibitor; antiatherosclerotic* [lovastatin] 10, 20, 40 mg

**mevastatin** INN

**mevinolin** [now: lovastatin]

**mexafylline** INN

**mexazolam** INN

**mexenone** INN, BAN

**Mexican brown** *street drug slang* [see: heroin; marijuana]

**Mexican horse; Mexican mud** *street drug slang* [see: heroin]

**Mexican mushrooms** *street drug slang* [see: psilocybin; psilocin]

**Mexican red** *street drug slang* [see: marijuana]

**Mexican Valium** *street drug slang* [see: Rohypnol; flunitrazepam]

**mexiletine** INN, BAN *antiarrhythmic* [also: mexiletine HCl]

**mexiletine HCl** USAN, USP *antiarrhythmic* [also: mexiletine] 150, 200, 250 mg oral

**mexiprostil** INN

**Mexitil** capsules ℞ *antiarrhythmic* [mexiletine HCl] 150, 200, 250 mg

**mexoprofen** INN

**mexrenoate potassium** USAN, INN *aldosterone antagonist*

**Mexsana Medicated** powder OTC *topical diaper rash treatment* [kaolin; zinc oxide; eucalyptus oil; camphor; corn starch]

**mez; mesc'** *street drug slang* [see: mescaline]

**mezacopride** INN

**mezepine** INN

**mezilamine** INN

**Mezlin** powder for IV or IM injection ℞ *extended-spectrum penicillin-type antibiotic* [mezlocillin sodium] 1, 2, 3, 4, 20 g ⑨ Meclan

**mezlocillin** USAN, INN *antibacterial*

**mezlocillin sodium** USP *bactericidal antibiotic*

**MF (methotrexate [with leucovorin rescue], fluorouracil)** *chemotherapy protocol*

**MF (mitomycin, fluorouracil)** *chemotherapy protocol*

**MFP (melphalan, fluorouracil, medroxyprogesterone acetate)** *chemotherapy protocol*

**MG Cold Sore Formula** solution OTC *topical oral anesthetic; antipruritic/counterirritant* [lidocaine; menthol] ≟•1%

**MG217 Dual Treatment** lotion OTC *topical antipsoriatic; antiseborrheic* [coal tar solution] 5%

**MG217 Medicated** conditioner OTC *topical antipsoriatic; antiseborrheic* [coal tar solution] 2%

**MG217 Medicated** ointment, shampoo OTC *topical antipsoriatic; antiseborrheic; antifungal; keratolytic* [coal tar solution; colloidal sulfur; salicylic acid] 2%•1.1%•1.5%; 5%•1.5%•2%

**MG400** shampoo OTC *antiseborrheic; keratolytic* [salicylic acid; sulfur] 3%•5%

**MGA (melengestrol acetate)** [q.v.]

**MGBG (methylglyoxal-*bis*-guanylhydrazone)** [see: mitoguazone]

**MGW (magnesium sulfate + glycerin + water)** enema [q.v.]

**Miacalcin** nasal spray ℞ *calcium regulator for postmenopausal osteoporosis (only)* [calcitonin (salmon)] 200 IU/0.09 mL dose

**Miacalcin** subcu or IM injection ℞ *calcium regulator for hypercalcemia, Paget's disease, and postmenopausal osteoporosis* [calcitonin (salmon)] 200 IU/mL

**Mi-Acid** gelcaps OTC *antacid* [calcium carbonate; magnesium carbonate] 311•232 mg

**Mi-Acid; Mi-Acid II** liquid OTC *antacid; antiflatulent* [aluminum hydroxide; magnesium hydroxide; simethicone] 200•200•20 mg/5 mL; 400•400•40 mg/5 mL

**mianserin** INN *serotonin inhibitor; antihistamine; investigational antidepressant* [also: mianserin HCl]

**mianserin HCl** USAN *serotonin inhibitor; antihistamine; investigational antidepressant* [also: mianserin]

**mibefradil** INN *vasodilator and calcium channel blocker for hypertension and chronic stable angina* [also: mibefradil dihydrochloride]

**mibefradil dihydrochloride** USAN *vasodilator and calcium channel blocker for hypertension and chronic stable angina* [also: mibefradil]

**MIBG-I-123** [see: iobenguane sulfate I 123]

**mibolerone** USAN, INN *anabolic; androgen*

**Micanol** cream ℞ *topical antipsoriatic* [anthralin] 1%

**Micatin** cream, powder, aerosol powder, liquid spray OTC *topical antifungal* [miconazole nitrate] 2%

**MICE (mesna [rescue], ifosfamide, carboplatin, etoposide)** *chemotherapy protocol* [also: ICE]

**Mi-Cebrin; Mi-Cebrin T** tablets (discontinued 1993) OTC *vitamin/mineral/iron supplement* [multiple vitamins & minerals; iron]

**micinicate** INN

**Mickey Finn** *street drug slang for chloral hydrate mixed in an alcoholic beverage* [see: chloral hydrate; alcohol]

**miconazole** USP, INN, BAN, JAN *fungicidal*

**miconazole nitrate** USAN, USP, JAN *antifungal* 2% topical

**Micrainin** tablets ℞ *analgesic; antipyretic; anti-inflammatory; anxiolytic* [aspirin; meprobamate] 325•200 mg

**MICRhoGAM** IM injection ℞ *obstetric Rh factor immunity suppressant* [$Rh_0(D)$ immune globulin] 50 μg ⑨ microgram

**microbubble contrast agent** *investigational (orphan) neurosonographic diagnostic aid for intracranial tumors*

**microcrystalline cellulose** [see: cellulose, microcrystalline]

**microcrystalline wax** [see: wax, microcrystalline]

**microdot** *street drug slang* [see: LSD]

**microfibrillar collagen hemostat (MCH)** *topical local hemostatic*

**Micro-K; Micro-K 10** Extencaps (controlled-release capsules) ℞ *potassium supplement* [potassium chloride] 600 mg (8 mEq); 750 mg (10 mEq)

**Micro-K LS** extended-release powder ℞ *potassium supplement* [potassium chloride] 20 mEq/packet

**Microlipid** emulsion OTC *dietary fat supplement* [safflower oil] 50%

**Micronase** tablets ℞ *sulfonylurea antidiabetic* [glyburide] 1.25, 2.5, 5 mg

**microNefrin** solution for inhalation OTC *bronchodilator for bronchial asthma and COPD* [racepinephrine] 2.25%

**micronized aluminum** *astringent*

**Micronized Glyburide** tablets ℞ *sulfonylurea antidiabetic* [glyburide] 1.5, 3 mg

**micronomicin** INN

**Micronor** tablets ℞ *oral contraceptive (progestin only)* [norethindrone] 0.35 mg

**Microstix-3** reagent strips for professional use *in vitro diagnostic aid for nitrate, uropathogens, or bacteria in the urine*

**MicroTrak Chlamydia trachomatis** slide test for professional use *in vitro diagnostic aid for Chlamydia trachomatis*

**MicroTrak HSV 1/HSV 2 Culture Identification/Typing Test** culture test for professional use *in vitro diagnostic aid for herpes simplex virus in tissue cultures*

**MicroTrak HSV 1/HSV 2 Direct Specimen Identification/Typing Test** slide test for professional use *in vitro diagnostic aid for herpes simplex virus in external lesions*

**MicroTrak Neisseria gonorrhoeae Culture Confirmation Test** reagent kit for professional use *in vitro diagnostic aid for Neisseria gonorrhoeae*

**Microzide** capsules ℞ *once-daily antihypertensive; thiazide diuretic* [hydrochlorothiazide] 12.5 mg

**mic's; mikes** *street drug slang for microdots of LSD* [see: LSD]

**mictine** [see: aminometradine]

**Micturin** ℞ *investigational agent for urinary incontinence (clinical trials discontinued in 1994)* [terodiline HCl]

**midaflur** USAN, INN *sedative*

**midaglizole** INN

**midalcipran** [see: milnacipran]

**midamaline** INN

**Midamine** ℞ *investigational (orphan) vasopressor for idiopathic orthostatic hypotension (OH)* [midodrine HCl]

**Midamor** tablets ℞ *potassium-sparing diuretic* [amiloride HCl] 5 mg

**midazogrel** INN

**midazolam** INN, BAN, JAN *short-acting benzodiazepine general anesthetic* [also: midazolam HCl]

**midazolam HCl** USAN *short-acting benzodiazepine general anesthetic* [also: midazolam]

**midazolam maleate** USAN *intravenous anesthetic*

**Midchlor** capsules ℞ *vasoconstrictor; sedative; analgesic (for migraine)* [isometheptene mucate; dichloralphenazone; acetaminophen] 65•100•325 mg

**midecamycin** INN

**midkine factor** *investigational protectant for nerve cells*

**midnight oil** *street drug slang* [see: opium]

**midodrine** INN, BAN *antihypotensive; vasoconstrictor; vasopressor for orthostatic hypotension (OH)* [also: midodrine HCl]

**midodrine HCl** USAN, JAN *antihypotensive; vasoconstrictor; vasopressor for orthostatic hypotension (orphan)* [also: midodrine]

**Midol; Midol for Cramps** caplets (discontinued 1995) OTC *analgesic; antipyretic; anti-inflammatory; muscle relaxant* [aspirin; caffeine; cinnamedrine HCl] 545•32.4•14.9 mg; 500•32.4•14.9 mg

**Midol, Teen** caplets OTC *analgesic; anti-inflammatory; diuretic* [acetaminophen; pamabrom] 400•25 mg

**Midol 200** tablets (discontinued 1996) OTC *nonsteroidal anti-inflamma-*

*tory drug (NSAID); antiarthritic; analgesic* [ibuprofen] 200 mg

**Midol IB** tablets OTC *nonsteroidal anti-inflammatory drug (NSAID); antiarthritic; analgesic* [ibuprofen] 200 mg

**Midol Multi-Symptom Formula** caplets OTC *analgesic; anti-inflammatory; antihistaminic sleep aid* [acetaminophen; pyrilamine maleate] 325•12.5 mg

**Midol Multi-Symptom Menstrual** caplets OTC *analgesic; anti-inflammatory; antihistaminic sleep aid* [acetaminophen; caffeine; pyrilamine maleate] 500•60•15 mg

**Midol PM** caplets OTC *analgesic; antipyretic; antihistaminic sleep aid* [acetaminophen; diphenhydramine] 500•25 mg

**Midol PMS** caplets, gelcaps OTC *analgesic; anti-inflammatory; diuretic; antihistaminic sleep aid* [acetaminophen; pamabrom; pyrilamine maleate] 500•25•15 mg

**Midon** ℞ *investigational treatment for orthostatic hypotension* [midodrine]

**Midrin** capsules ℞ *vasoconstrictor; sedative; analgesic (for migraine)* [isometheptene mucate; dichloralphenazone; acetaminophen] 65•100•325 mg ⊡ Mydfrin

**Midstream Pregnancy Test** kit for home use OTC *in vitro diagnostic aid for urine pregnancy test*

**MIFA (mitomycin, fluorouracil, Adriamycin)** *chemotherapy protocol*

**mifarmonab** [see: imciromab pentetate]

**Mifegyne** (available in France, Sweden, and the U.K.) ℞ *abortifacient; investigational glucocorticosteroid antagonist for Cushing syndrome* [mifepristone]

**mifentidine** INN

**mifepristone** INN, BAN *progesterone antagonist; abortifacient; investigational (Phase III) for unresectable meningioma*

**mifobate** USAN, INN *antiatherosclerotic*

**mighty mezz** *street drug slang for a marijuana cigarette* [see: marijuana]

**Mighty Quinn** *street drug slang* [see: LSD]

**miglitol** USAN, INN, BAN *antidiabetic agent for type 2 diabetes; α-glucosidase inhibitor that delays the digestion of dietary carbohydrates*

**Migranol** nasal spray ℞ *investigational (NDA filed) rapid-acting antimigraine agent* [dihydroergotamine mesylate]

**Migrastat** intranasal ℞ *investigational antimigraine agent* [propranolol HCl]

**Migratine** capsules ℞ *vasoconstrictor; sedative; analgesic (for migraine)* [isometheptene mucate; dichloralphenazone; acetaminophen] 65•100•325 mg

**mikamycin** INN, BAN

**mikes; mic's** *street drug slang for microdots of LSD* [see: LSD]

**milacemide** INN *anticonvulsant; antidepressant* [also: milacemide HCl]

**milacemide HCl** USAN *anticonvulsant; antidepressant* [also: milacemide]

**milameline HCl** USAN *partial muscarinic agonist for Alzheimer's disease*

**mild silver protein** [see: silver protein, mild]

**milenperone** USAN, INN, BAN *antipsychotic*

**Miles Nervine** caplets OTC *antihistaminic sleep aid* [diphenhydramine HCl] 25 mg

**milipertine** USAN, INN *antipsychotic*

**milk of bismuth** [see: bismuth, milk of]

**milk of magnesia** [see: magnesia, milk of]

**Milk of Magnesia-Cascara, Concentrated** oral suspension OTC *antacid; laxative* [milk of magnesia; aromatic cascara fluidextract; alcohol 7%] 30•5 mL/15 mL

**Milkinol** emulsion OTC *emollient laxative* [mineral oil]

**milnacipran** INN *investigational antidepressant*

**milodistim** USAN *antineutropenic; hematopoietic stimulant; granulocyte macrophage colony-stimulating factor (GM-CSF) + interleukin 3*

**Milontin** Kapseals (capsules) ℞ *anticonvulsant* [phensuximide] 500 mg ⊡ Miltown; Mylanta

**Milophene** tablets ℞ *ovulation stimulant* [clomiphene citrate] 50 mg

**miloxacin** INN

**milrinone** USAN, INN, BAN *cardiotonic*

**milrinone lactate** *vasodilator for congestive heart failure*

**miltefosine** INN

**Miltown; Miltown-600** tablets ℞ *anxiolytic; also abused as a street drug* [meprobamate] 200, 400 mg; 600 mg ⊚ Milontin

**milverine** INN

**mimbane** INN *analgesic* [also: mimbane HCl]

**mimbane HCl** USAN *analgesic* [also: mimbane]

**minalrestat** USAN *aldose reductase inhibitor for diabetic neuropathy and other long-term diabetic complications*

**minaprine** USAN, INN, BAN *psychotropic*

**minaprine HCl** USAN *antidepressant*

**minaxolone** USAN, INN *anesthetic*

**mind detergent** *street drug slang* [see: LSD]

**mindodilol** INN

**mindolic acid** [see: clometacin]

**mindoperone** INN

**MINE (mesna [rescue], ifosfamide, Novantrone, etoposide)** *chemotherapy protocol*

**MINE-ESHAP (alternating cycles of MINE and ESHAP)** *chemotherapy protocol*

**minepentate** INN, BAN

**Mineral Ice** [see: Therapeutic Mineral Ice]

**mineral oil** USP *emollient/protectant; laxative; solvent*

**mineral oil, light** NF *tablet and capsule lubricant; vehicle*

**mineralocorticoids** *a class of adrenal cortical steroids that are used for partial replacement therapy in adrenocortical insufficiency*

**Mini Thin Asthma Relief** tablets OTC *decongestant; expectorant* [ephedrine HCl; guaifenesin] 25•100, 25•200 mg

**Mini Thin Pseudo** tablets OTC *nasal decongestant* [pseudoephedrine HCl] 60 mg

**mini-BEAM (BCNU, etoposide, ara-C, melphalan)** *chemotherapy protocol*

**minibennie** *street drug slang* [see: amphetamines]

**mini-COAP (cyclophosphamide, Oncovin, ara-C, prednisone)** *chemotherapy protocol*

**Minidyne** solution OTC *broad-spectrum antimicrobial* [povidone-iodine] 10%

**Mini-Gamulin Rh** IM injection ℞ *obstetric Rh factor immunity suppressant* [Rh₀(D) immune globulin] 50 μg

**Miniguard** disposable pads *adhesive foam pad to seal urethral opening for stress urinary incontinence in women*

**Min-I-Mix** (delivery system) *dual-chambered prefilled syringe*

**Minipress** capsules ℞ *antihypertensive; antiadrenergic* [prazosin HCl] 1, 2, 5 mg

**Minipress XL** extended-release tablets ℞ *antihypertensive* [prazosin HCl]

**Minitran** transdermal patch ℞ *antianginal* [nitroglycerin] 9, 18, 36, 54 mg

**Minit-Rub** OTC *counterirritant* [methyl salicylate; menthol; camphor] 15%•3.5%•2.3%

**Minizide 1; Minizide 2; Minizide 5** capsules ℞ *antihypertensive* [prazosin HCl; polythiazide] 1•0.5 mg; 2•0.5 mg; 5•0.5 mg

**Minocin** pellet-filled capsules, oral suspension, powder for IV injection ℞ *tetracycline-type antibiotic; orphan status withdrawn 1996* [minocycline HCl] 50, 100 mg; 50 mg/5 mL; 100 mg ⊚ Indocin; Mithracin; niacin

**minocromil** USAN, INN, BAN *prophylactic antiallergic*

**minocycline** USAN, INN, BAN *gram-negative and gram-positive bacteriostatic; antirickettsial*

**minocycline HCl** USP *antibacterial; orphan status withdrawn 1996* 50, 100 mg oral

**Minodyl** tablets (discontinued 1993) ℞ *antihypertensive; vasodilator* [minoxidil]

**minoxidil** USAN, USP, INN, BAN *antihypertensive; peripheral vasodilator; hair growth stimulant* 2.5, 10 mg oral

**Minoxidil for Men** topical solution OTC *hair growth stimulant* [minoxidil; alcohol 60%] 2%

**mint leaf; mint weed** *street drug slang* [see: PCP]

**Mintezol** chewable tablets, oral suspension ℞ *anthelmintic for strongyloidiasis (threadworm), larva migrans, and trichinosis* [thiabendazole] 500 mg; 500 mg/5 mL

**Mintox** chewable tablets, oral suspension OTC *antacid* [aluminum hydroxide; magnesium hydroxide] 200•200 mg; 225•200 mg/5 mL

**Mintox Plus** liquid OTC *antacid; antiflatulent* [aluminum hydroxide; magnesium hydroxide; simethicone] 500•450•40 mg/5 mL

**Minulet** ℞ *investigational monophasic oral contraceptive* [gestodene]

**45-minute psychosis** *street drug slang* [see: dimethyltryptamine]

**Minute-Gel** ℞ *topical dental caries preventative* [acidulated phosphate fluoride] 1.23%

**Miochol** solution (discontinued 1996) ℞ *direct-acting miotic for ophthalmic surgery* [acetylcholine chloride] 1:100

**Miochol-E** solution ℞ *direct-acting miotic for ophthalmic surgery* [acetylcholine chloride] 1:100

**mioflazine** INN, BAN *coronary vasodilator* [also: mioflazine HCl]

**mioflazine HCl** USAN *coronary vasodilator* [also: mioflazine]

**Miostat** solution ℞ *direct-acting miotic for ophthalmic surgery* [carbachol] 0.01%

**miotics** *a class of drugs that cause the pupil of the eye to contract*

**MIP-1 alpha** *investigational antineoplastic*

**mipafilcon A** USAN *hydrophilic contact lens material*

**mipimazole** INN

**mira** (Spanish for "look" or "watch") *street drug slang* [see: opium]

**Mirac** [see: Tilarin]

**Miradon** tablets ℞ *indandione-derivative anticoagulant* [anisindione] 50 mg

**MiraFlow** solution OTC *cleaning solution for hard or soft contact lenses*

**Mirapex** tablets ℞ *dopamine agonist for Parkinson's disease* [pramipexole] 0.125, 0.25, 1, 1.5 mg

**MiraSept System** solutions OTC *two-step chemical disinfecting system for soft contact lenses* [hydrogen peroxide based] 3%

**mirfentanil** INN *analgesic* [also: mirfentanil HCl]

**mirfentanil HCl** USAN *analgesic* [also: mirfentanil]

**mirincamycin** INN *antibacterial; antimalarial* [also: mirincamycin HCl]

**mirincamycin HCl** USAN *antibacterial; antimalarial* [also: mirincamycin]

**mirisetron maleate** USAN *anxiolytic*

**miristalkonium chloride** INN

**miroprofen** INN

**mirosamicin** INN

**mirtazapine** USAN, INN *tetracyclic antidepressant; 5-HT$_{1A}$ agonist*

**misonidazole** USAN, INN *antiprotozoal (Trichomonas)*

**misoprostol** USAN, INN, BAN *prevention of NSAID-induced gastric ulcers*

**Miss Emma** *street drug slang* [see: morphine]

**missile basing** *street drug slang for a combination of crack liquid and PCP* [see: cocaine, crack; PCP]

**Mission Prenatal; Mission Prenatal F.A.; Mission Prenatal H.P.** tablets OTC *vitamin/iron supplement* [multiple vitamins; ferrous gluconate; folic acid] ≛•30•0.4 mg; ≛•30•0.8 mg; ≛•30•0.8 mg

**Mission Prenatal Rx** tablets ℞ *vitamin/calcium/iron supplement* [multiple vitamins; calcium; iron; folic acid] ≛•175•29.5•1 mg

**Mission Surgical Supplement** tablets OTC *vitamin/iron supplement* [multiple vitamins; ferrous gluconate] ≛•27 mg

**mist** *street drug slang for crack smoke or PCP* [see: cocaine, crack; PCP]

**Mister Blue** *street drug slang* [see: morphine]

**Mister Brownstone** *street drug slang for hashish or brown heroin* [see: hashish; heroin]

**Mister Natural** *street drug slang* [see: LSD]

**Mistometer** (trademarked form) *metered-dose inhalation aerosol*

**Mithracin** powder for IV infusion ℞ *antineoplastic for testicular cancer* [plicamycin] 2.5 mg ⑨ Minocin

**mithramycin** [now: plicamycin] ⊠ mitomycin

**mitindomide** USAN, INN *antineoplastic*

**mitobronitol** INN, BAN

**mitocarcin** USAN, INN *antineoplastic*

**mitoclomine** INN, BAN

**mitocromin** USAN *antineoplastic*

**mitoflaxone** INN

**mitogillin** USAN, INN *antineoplastic*

**mitoguazone** INN *investigational antineoplastic for multiple myeloma and head, esophagus, and prostate cancer; investigational (orphan) for non-Hodgkin's lymphoma*

**mitolactol** INN *investigational (orphan) antineoplastic for brain tumors and recurrent or metastatic cervical squamous cell carcinoma*

**mitomalcin** USAN, INN *antineoplastic*

**mitomycin** USAN, USP, INN, BAN *antibiotic antineoplastic; investigational (orphan) for refractory glaucoma and glaucoma surgery* ⊠ mithramycin; Mutamycin

**mitomycin C (MTC)** [see: mitomycin]

**mitonafide** INN

**mitopodozide** INN, BAN

**mitoquidone** INN, BAN

**mitosper** USAN, INN *antineoplastic*

**mitotane** USAN, USP, INN *antineoplastic; adrenal cytotoxic agent*

**mitotenamine** INN, BAN

**mitotic inhibitors** *a class of antineoplastics that inhibit cell division (mitosis)*

**mitoxantrone** INN *antibiotic antineoplastic* [also: mitoxantrone HCl; mitozantrone]

**mitoxantrone HCl** USAN *antibiotic antineoplastic for prostate cancer and acute myelogenous (nonlymphocytic) leukemia (orphan)* [also: mitoxantrone; mitozantrone]

**mitozantrone** BAN *antineoplastic* [also: mitoxantrone HCl; mitoxantrone]

**mitozolomide** INN, BAN

**Mitran** capsules ℞ *anxiolytic* [chlordiazepoxide HCl] 10 mg

**Mitrolan** chewable tablets OTC *bulk laxative; antidiarrheal* [calcium polycarbophil] 500 mg

**mitronal** [see: cinnarizine]

**MIV (mitoxantrone, ifosfamide, VePesid)** *chemotherapy protocol*

**Mivacron** IV infusion ℞ *muscle relaxant; adjunct to anesthesia* [mivacurium chloride] 0.5, 2 mg/mL

**mivacurium chloride** USAN, INN, BAN *neuromuscular blocking agent*

**mixed respiratory vaccine (MRV)** *active bacterin for respiratory tract infections*

**mixed tocopherols** [see: vitamin E]

**mixidine** USAN, INN *coronary vasodilator*

**Mix-O-Vial** (trademarked packaging form) *two-compartment vial*

**Mixtard 70/30** subcu injection (discontinued 1994) OTC *antidiabetic* [isophane insulin (pork); insulin (pork)]

**Mixtard Human 70/30** subcu injection (discontinued 1994) OTC *antidiabetic* [isophane insulin (human semisynthetic); human insulin (semisynthetic)]

**mizoribine** INN

**MK-383** *investigational fibrinogen receptor antagonist for cardiac platelet aggregation disorders*

**MK-462** *investigational serotonin reuptake receptor inhibitor for migraine*

**MK-499** *investigational calcium channel blocker for atrial and ventricular arrhythmias*

**MK-966** *investigational (Phase III) COX-2 inhibitor for pain, inflammation, and fever*

**M-KYA** capsules (discontinued 1996) OTC *prevention and treatment of nocturnal leg cramps* [quinine sulfate] 64.8 mg

**MM (mercaptopurine, methotrexate)** *chemotherapy protocol*

**MMOPP (methotrexate, mechlorethamine, Oncovin, procarbazine, prednisone)** *chemotherapy protocol*

**MMP (matrix metalloproteinase) inhibitors** [q.v.]

**MMR (measles, mumps & rubella vaccines)** [q.v.]

**M-M-R II** powder for subcu injection ℞ *measles, mumps and rubella vaccine* [measles, mumps & rubella virus vaccine, live] 0.5 mL

**M.O.; M.U.** *street drug slang* [see: marijuana]

**MOB (mechlorethamine, Oncovin, bleomycin)** *chemotherapy protocol*

**MOB-III (mitomycin, Oncovin, bleomycin, cisplatin)** *chemotherapy protocol*

**Moban** tablets, oral concentrate ℞ *antipsychotic* [molindone HCl] 5, 10, 25, 50, 100 mg; 20 mg/mL ☒ Mobidin; Modane

**mobecarb** INN

**mobenzoxamine** INN

**Mobidin** tablets ℞ *analgesic; antipyretic; anti-inflammatory; antirheumatic* [magnesium salicylate] 600 mg ☒ Moban

**Mobigesic** tablets OTC *analgesic; antipyretic; anti-inflammatory; antihistamine* [magnesium salicylate; phenyltoloxamine citrate] 325•30 mg

**Mobisyl Creme** OTC *topical analgesic* [trolamine salicylate] 10%

**moccasin snake antivenin** [see: antivenin (Crotalidae) polyvalent]

**mocimycin** INN

**mociprazine** INN

**moclobemide** USAN, INN, BAN *antidepressant; investigational treatment for panic disorder and social phobia*

**moctamide** INN

**Moctanin** biliary infusion ℞ *anticholelithogenic for dissolution of cholesterol gallstones (orphan)* [monoctanoin]

**modafinil** USAN, INN *analeptic; investigational (orphan) for excessive daytime sleepiness of narcolepsy*

**modaline** INN *antidepressant* [also: modaline sulfate]

**modaline sulfate** USAN *antidepressant* [also: modaline]

**modams** *street drug slang* [see: marijuana]

**Modane** tablets OTC *laxative* [white phenolphthalein] 130 mg ☒ Moban; Mudrane

**Modane Bulk** liquid OTC *bulk laxative* [psyllium hydrophilic mucilloid] 50%

**Modane Plus** tablets OTC *laxative; stool softener* [white phenolphthalein; docusate sodium] 65•100 mg

**Modane Soft** capsules OTC *stool softener* [docusate sodium] 100 mg

**modecainide** USAN, INN *antiarrhythmic*

**Moderil** tablets (discontinued 1995) ℞ *antihypertensive* [rescinnamine] 0.25, 0.5 mg ☒ Mellaril

**Modicon** tablets ℞ *monophasic oral contraceptive* [norethindrone; ethinyl estradiol] 0.5 mg•35 μg ☒ Mylicon

**modified bovine lung surfactant extract** [see: beractant]

**modified Burow solution** [see: aluminum acetate solution]

**modified cellulose gum** [now: croscarmellose sodium]

**modified Shohl solution (sodium citrate & citric acid)** *urinary alkalinizer; compounding agent*

**Modiodal** (commercially available in France) ℞ *investigational analeptic for narcolepsy and hypersomnia* [modafinil]

**Modivid** ℞ *investigational cephalosporin antibiotic* [cefodizime]

**Modrastane** capsules (discontinued 1995) ℞ *adrenal steroid inhibitor; antisteroidal antineoplastic for Cushing syndrome* [trilostane] 30, 60 mg

**Moducal** powder OTC *carbohydrate caloric supplement* [glucose polymers]

**Moduretic** tablets ℞ *diuretic; antihypertensive* [amiloride HCl; hydrochlorothiazide] 5•50 mg

**moexipril** INN, BAN *antihypertensive*

**moexipril HCl** USAN *antihypertensive; angiotensin-converting enzyme (ACE) inhibitor*

**moexiprilat** INN

**MOF (MeCCNU, Oncovin, fluorouracil)** *chemotherapy protocol*

**mofebutazone** INN

**mofedione** [see: oxazidione]

**mofegiline** INN *antiparkinsonian; investigational Alzheimer's treatment; investigational antiasthmatic* [also: mofegiline HCl]

**mofegiline HCl** USAN *antiparkinsonian; investigational Alzheimer's treatment; investigational antiasthmatic* [also: mofegiline]

**mofetil** USAN, INN *combining name for radicals or groups*

**mofloverine** INN

**mofoxime** INN

**MOF-STREP; MOF-Strep (MeCCNU, Oncovin, fluoroura-**

**cil, streptozocin)** *chemotherapy protocol*

**Mogadon** ℞ *investigational benzodiazepine-type tranquilizer; anxiolytic; anticonvulsant; hypnotic* [nitrazepam]

**moguisteine** INN

**Mohasky** *street drug slang* [see: marijuana]

**Moist Again** vaginal gel OTC *lubricant* [glycerin; aloe vera]

**Moi-Stir** oral spray, Swabsticks OTC *saliva substitute* ⑫ moisture

**Moi-Stir 10** oral spray (name changed to Entertainer's Secret Throat Relief in 1994)

**Moisture Drops** eye drops OTC *ocular moisturizer/lubricant* [hydroxypropyl methylcellulose] 0.5%

**Moisturel** lotion (discontinued 1997) OTC *moisturizer; emollient* [dimethicone] 3%

**mojo** *street drug slang* [see: cocaine; heroin; morphine]

**molecusol & carbamazepine** *orphan status withdrawn 1996*

**molfarnate** INN

**molgramostim** USAN, INN, BAN *antineutropenic; hematopoietic stimulant; investigational cytokine to AIDS; orphan status withdrawn 1996*

**molinazone** USAN, INN *analgesic*

**molindone** INN *antipsychotic* [also: molindone HCl]

**molindone HCl** USAN *antipsychotic* [also: molindone]

**Mol-Iron** tablets OTC *hematinic* [ferrous sulfate] 195 mg

**Mol-Iron with Vitamin C** tablets OTC *hematinic* [ferrous sulfate; ascorbic acid] 39•75 mg

**Mollifene Ear Wax Removing Formula** drops OTC *agent to emulsify and disperse ear wax* [carbamide peroxide] 6.5%

**molracetam** INN

**molsidomine** USAN, INN *antianginal; coronary vasodilator*

**molybdenum** *element (Mo)*

**Molypen** IV injection ℞ *intravenous nutritional therapy* [ammonium molybdate tetrahydrate] 25 μg/mL

**Momentum** caplets OTC *analgesic; antipyretic; anti-inflammatory; antihistamine* [aspirin; phenyltoloxamine citrate] 500•15 mg

**Momentum Muscular Backache Formula** caplets OTC *analgesic; antipyretic; anti-inflammatory* [magnesium salicylate] 580 mg

**mometasone** INN, BAN *topical corticosteroid* [also: mometasone furoate]

**mometasone furoate** USAN *topical corticosteroid; investigational agent for allergic rhinitis in nasal spray form* [also: mometasone]

**MOMP (mechlorethamine, Oncovin, methotrexate, prednisone)** *chemotherapy protocol*

**Monafed** sustained-release tablets ℞ *expectorant* [guaifenesin] 600 mg

**Monafed DM** tablets ℞ *antitussive; expectorant* [dextromethorphan hydrobromide; guaifenesin] 30•600 mg

**monalazone disodium** INN

**monalium hydrate** [see: magaldrate]

**monatepil** INN *antianginal; antihypertensive* [also: monatepil maleate]

**monatepil maleate** USAN *antianginal; antihypertensive* [also: monatepil]

**monensin** USAN, INN *antiprotozoal; antibacterial; antifungal*

**Monistat 3** vaginal suppositories + cream OTC *antifungal* [miconazole nitrate] 200 mg; 2%

**Monistat 5** tampons (discontinued 1994; previously available only in California) ℞ *antifungal* [miconazole nitrate] 100 mg

**Monistat 7** vaginal suppositories, vaginal cream OTC *antifungal* [miconazole nitrate] 100 mg; 2%

**Monistat 7 Combination Pack** vaginal suppositories + cream OTC *antifungal* [miconazole nitrate] 100 mg; 2%

**Monistat Dual-Pak** vaginal suppositories + cream ℞ *antifungal* [miconazole nitrate] 200 mg; 2%

**Monistat i.v.** intrathecal or IV injection ℞ *systemic antifungal* [miconazole] 10 mg/mL

**Monistat-Derm** cream ℞ *topical antifungal* [miconazole nitrate] 2%

**monkey** *street drug slang for a cigarette made from cocaine paste and tobacco* [see: cocaine; tobacco]

**monkey dust; monkey tranquilizer** *street drug slang* [see: PCP]

**mono- & di-acetylated monoglycerides** NF *plasticizer*

**mono- & di-glycerides** NF *emulsifying agent*

**monoamine oxidase inhibitors (MAOIs)** *a class of antidepressants that increase CNS monoamine neurotransmitters (epinephrine, norepinephrine, and serotonin)*

**monobactams** *a class of antibiotics*

**monobasic potassium phosphate** [see: potassium phosphate, monobasic]

**monobasic sodium phosphate** [see: sodium phosphate, monobasic]

**monobenzone** USP, INN *depigmenting agent for vitiligo*

**monobenzyl ether of hydroquinone** [see: monobenzone]

**monobromated camphor** [see: camphor, monobromated]

**monocalcium phosphate** [see: calcium phosphate, dibasic] 🔲 ]

**Monocaps** tablets OTC *vitamin/mineral/iron supplement* [multiple vitamins & minerals; ferrous fumerate; folic acid; biotin] ±•14 mg•0.1 mg•15 μg

**Monocete** liquid (discontinued 1995) ℞ *cauterant; keratolytic* [monochloroacetic acid] 80% 🔲 Monoket

**Mono-Chlor** liquid ℞ *cauterant; keratolytic* [monochloroacetic acid] 80% 🔲 Monocor

**monochloroacetic acid** *strong keratolytic/cauterant*

**monochlorothymol** [see: chlorothymol]

**monochlorphenamide** [see: clofenamide]

**Monocid** powder for IV or IM injection ℞ *cephalosporin-type antibiotic* [cefonicid sodium] 0.5, 1, 10 g

**Monoclate** powder for IV injection (discontinued 1996) ℞ *antihemophilic to correct coagulation deficiency* [antihemophilic factor VIII:C, heat treated] ≟

**Monoclate P** powder for IV injection ℞ *antihemophilic to correct coagulation deficiency* [antihemophilic factor VIII:C] ≟

**monoclonal antibody 17-1A** *orphan status withdrawn 1997* [now: edrecolomab]

**monoclonal antibody 7E3** [see: abciximab]

**monoclonal antibody anti-idiotype melanoma assorted antigen, murine** *orphan status withdrawn 1997*

**monoclonal antibody B43.13** *investigational (orphan) for epithelial ovarian cancer*

**monoclonal antibody E5** [now: edobacomab]

**monoclonal antibody IgG** *investigational treatment for multiple sclerosis*

**monoclonal antibody PM-81** *investigational (orphan) for acute myelogenous leukemia*

**monoclonal antibody PM-81 & AML-2-23** *investigational (orphan) for bone marrow transplant for acute myelogenous leukemia*

**monoclonal antibody r24** *investigational treatment for Hodgkin's disease*

**monoclonal antibody to B-cell lymphoma, murine or human** *orphan status withdrawn 1996*

**monoclonal antibody to CD4** [see: 5A8 MAb to CD4]

**monoclonal antibody to cytomegalovirus, human** *investigational (orphan) prophylaxis for CMV retinitis and CMV disease in solid organ transplants*

**monoclonal antibody to hepatitis B virus, human** *investigational (orphan) hepatitis B prophylaxis for liver transplant*

**monoclonal antibody to lupus nephritis** *investigational (orphan) for immunization against lupus nephritis*

**monoclonal antiendotoxin antibody XMMEN-OE5** *orphan status withdrawn 1994; clinical trials discontinued 1997* [now: edobacomab]

**monoclonal factor IX** [see: factor IX complex]

**monoctanoin** USAN, BAN *antichole-lithogenic for dissolution of cholesterol gallstones (orphan)*

**monoctanoin component A**
**monoctanoin component B**
**monoctanoin component C**
**monoctanoin component D**

**Mono-Diff** reagent kit for professional use *in vitro diagnostic aid for mononucleosis*

**Monodox** capsules ℞ *antibiotic* [doxycycline monohydrate] 50, 100 mg

**Mono-Drop** (trademarked delivery system) *prefilled eye drop dispenser*

**monoethanolamine** NF *surfactant*

**monoethanolamine oleate** INN *sclerosing agent* [also: ethanolamine oleate]

**Monogen** ℞ *investigational treatment for T-cell leukemia* [monoclonal antibodies]

**Mono-Gesic** film-coated tablets ℞ *analgesic; antipyretic; anti-inflammatory; antirheumatic* [salsalate] 750 mg

**Mono-IX** ℞ *investigational treatment for hemophilia B* [factor IX complex]

**Monoket** tablets ℞ *angina preventative* [isosorbide mononitrate] 10, 20 mg ⊇ Monocete

**Mono-Latex** reagent kit for professional use *in vitro diagnostic aid for mononucleosis*

**monolaurin** *investigational (orphan) for congenital primary ichthyosis*

**monometacrine** INN

**N-monomethyl arginine (NMA)** *investigational treatment for septic shock and hypotension following chemotherapy*

**Mononine** powder for IV infusion ℞ *antihemophilic for factor IX deficiency (hemophilia B; Christmas disease) (orphan)* [factor IX complex] 100 IU/mL

**monooctanoin** [see: monoctanoin]

**monophenylbutazone** [see: mofebutazone]

**monophosphoryl lipid A (MPL-A)** *investigational (Phase I) vaccine for AIDS; investigational for septic shock in surgical patients*

**monophosphoryl lipid C (MPL-C)** *investigational agent to prevent cardiac reperfusion injury*

**monophosphoryl lipid S (MPL-S)** *investigational immunostimulant for sepsis*

**monophosphothiamine** INN

**Mono-Plus** reagent kit for professional use *in vitro diagnostic aid for mononucleosis*

**monopotassium 4-aminosalicylate** [see: aminosalicylate potassium]

**monopotassium carbonate** [see: potassium bicarbonate]

**monopotassium D-gluconate** [see: potassium gluconate]

**monopotassium monosodium tartrate tetrahydrate** [see: potassium sodium tartrate]

**monopotassium phosphate** [see: potassium phosphate, monobasic]

**Monopril** tablets ℞ *antihypertensive; angiotensin-converting enzyme (ACE) inhibitor* [fosinopril sodium] 10, 20, 40 mg

**monos** *street drug slang for cigarettes made from cocaine paste and tobacco* [see: cocaine; tobacco]

**monosodium p-aminohippurate** [see: aminohippurate sodium]

**monosodium 4-aminosalicylate dihydrate** [see: aminosalicylate sodium]

**monosodium carbonate** [see: sodium bicarbonate]

**monosodium D-gluconate** [see: sodium gluconate]

**monosodium D-thyroxine hydrate** [see: dextrothyroxine sodium]

**monosodium glutamate** NF *flavoring agent; perfume*

**monosodium L-ascorbate** [see: sodium ascorbate]

**monosodium L-thyroxine hydrate** [see: levothyroxine sodium]

**monosodium phosphate dihydrate** [see: sodium phosphate, monobasic]

**monosodium phosphate monohydrate** [see: sodium phosphate, monobasic]

**monosodium salicylate** [see: sodium salicylate]

**monosodium sulfite** [see: sodium bisulfite]

**Monospot** slide test for professional use *in vitro diagnostic aid for mononucleosis*

**monostearin** [see: glyceryl monostearate]

**Monosticon Dri-Dot** slide test for professional use *in vitro diagnostic aid for mononucleosis*

**monosulfiram** BAN [also: sulfiram]

**Mono-Sure** slide test for professional use *in vitro diagnostic aid for mononucleosis*

**Mono-Test** slide test for professional use *in vitro diagnostic aid for mononucleosis*

**Mono-Test (FTB)** test kit for professional use (discontinued 1994) *in vitro diagnostic aid for mononucleosis*

**monothioglycerol** NF *preservative*

**Mono-Vacc Test (O.T.)** single-use intradermal puncture test device ℞ *tuberculosis skin test* [old tuberculin] 5 U

**monoxerutin** INN

**monte** (Spanish for "mountain") *street drug slang for marijuana from South America* [see: marijuana]

**montelukast sodium** USAN *antiasthmatic; leukotriene $D_4$ antagonist*

**monteplase** INN

**montirelin** INN

**Monuril** (foreign name for U.S. product Monurol)

**Monurol** granules for oral solution ℞ *broad-spectrum bactericidal antibiotic for urinary tract infections* [fosfomycin tromethamine] 3 g per packet

**mooca; moocah** *street drug slang* [see: marijuana]

**moon** *street drug slang* [see: mescaline]

**moonrock** *street drug slang for a combination of crack and heroin* [see: cocaine, crack; heroin]

**mooster** *street drug slang* [see: marijuana]

**moota; mooters; mootie; mootos; muta; mutah** *street drug slang for a marijuana cigarette* [see: marijuana]

**8-MOP** capsules ℞ *to increase tolerance to sunlight and enhance pigmentation* [methoxsalen] 10 mg

**MOP (mechlorethamine, Oncovin, prednisone)** *chemotherapy protocol*

**MOP (mechlorethamine, Oncovin, procarbazine)** *chemotherapy protocol*

**8-MOP (8-methoxypsoralen)** [see: methoxsalen]

**MOP-BAP (mechlorethamine, Oncovin, procarbazine, bleomycin, Adriamycin, prednisone)** *chemotherapy protocol*

**moperone** INN

**mopidamol** INN

**mopidralazine** INN

**MOPP (mechlorethamine, Oncovin, procarbazine, prednisone)** *chemotherapy protocol*

**MOPP (mustine HCl, Oncovin, procarbazine, prednisone)** *chemotherapy protocol*

**MOPP/ABV (mechlorethamine, Oncovin, procarbazine, prednisone, Adriamycin, bleomycin, vinblastine)** *chemotherapy protocol*

**MOPP/ABVD (alternating cycles of MOPP and ABVD)** *chemotherapy protocol*

**MOPP-BLEO; MOPP-Bleo (mechlorethamine, Oncovin, procarbazine, prednisone, bleomycin)** *chemotherapy protocol*

**MOPPHDB (mechlorethamine, Oncovin, procarbazine, prednisone, high-dose bleomycin)** *chemotherapy protocol*

**MOPPLDB (mechlorethamine, Oncovin, procarbazine, prednisone, low-dose bleomycin)** *chemotherapy protocol*

**MOPr (mechlorethamine, Oncovin, procarbazine)** *chemotherapy protocol*

**moprolol** INN

**moquizone** INN

**mor a grifa** *street drug slang* [see: marijuana]

**moracizine** INN, BAN *antiarrhythmic* [also: moricizine]

**morantel** INN *anthelmintic* [also: morantel tartrate]

**morantel tartrate** USAN *anthelmintic* [also: morantel]

**Moranyl** (available only from the Centers for Disease Control) ℞ *investigational anti-infective for trypanosomiasis and onchocerciasis* [suramin sodium]

**morazone** INN, BAN

**morclofone** INN

**more** *street drug slang* [see: PCP]

**More-Dophilus** powder OTC *dietary supplement; fever blister treatment; not generally regarded as safe and effective as an antidiarrheal* [Lactobacillus acidophilus] 4 billion U/g

**morfina** (Spanish for "morphine") *street drug* [see: morphine]

**morforex** INN

**moricizine** USAN *antiarrhythmic* [also: moracizine]

**moricizine HCl** *antiarrhythmic*

**morinamide** INN

**morniflumate** USAN, INN *anti-inflammatory*

**morning glory (Ipomoea violacea) seeds** *contain lysergic acid amide, chemically similar to LSD, which produce hallucinations when ingested as a street drug* [see also: LSD]

**morocromen** INN

**morotgara** *street drug slang* [see: heroin]

**moroxydine** INN, BAN

**morph'** *street drug slang* [see: morphine]

**morphazinamide** [see: morinamide]

**morpheridine** INN, BAN

**morphine** BAN *narcotic analgesic; widely abused as a street drug, which leads to dependence* [also: morphine sulfate]

**morphine dinicotinate ester** [see: nicomorphine]

**morphine HCl** USP *narcotic analgesic preferred in Germany and Great Britain; widely abused as a street drug, which leads to dependence*

**morphine sulfate (MS)0** USP *narcotic analgesic preferred in the U.S.; intraspinal microinfusion for intractable chronic pain (orphan)* [also: morphine] 25, 50 mg/mL injection

**4-morpholinecarboximidoylguanidine** [see: moroxydine]

**2-morpholinoethylrutin** [see: ethoxazorutoside]

**3-morpholinosydnoneimine** [see: linsidomine]

**morpholinyl succinimide** [see: morsuximide]

**morpholinylethyl morphine** [see: pholcodine]

**morphy** *street drug slang* [see: morphine]

**morrhuate sodium** USP *sclerosing agent* [also: sodium morrhuate] 50 mg/mL injection

**morsuximide** INN

**morsydomine** [see: molsidomine]

**mortal combat** *street drug slang for high-potency heroin* [see: heroin]

**Morton Salt Substitute; Morton Seasoned Salt Substitute** OTC *salt substitute* [potassium chloride] 64 mEq/5 g; 56 mEq/5 g

**Mosco** liquid OTC *topical keratolytic* [salicylic acid in flexible collodion] 17.6%

**mosquitos** *street drug slang* [see: cocaine]

**Mostarinia** ℞ *investigational antineoplastic for leukemia, lymphoma, ovarian, breast, and prostatic cancers* [prednimustine]

**mota; moto** (Spanish for "speck") *street drug slang* [see: marijuana]

**motapizone** INN

**MOTC (methyleneoxytetracycline)** [see: methacycline]

**mother** *street drug slang* [see: marijuana]

**mother's little helper** *street drug slang* [see: Valium; diazepam]

**Motilium** ℞ *investigational antiemetic for diabetic gastroparesis* [domperidone]

**Motofen** tablets ℞ *antidiarrheal* [difenoxin HCl; atropine sulfate] 1•0.025 mg

**motrazepam** INN

**motretinide** USAN, INN *keratolytic*

**Motrin** tablets, chewable tablets, oral suspension ℞ *nonsteroidal anti-inflammatory drug (NSAID); antiarthritic; analgesic* [ibuprofen] 300, 400, 600, 800 mg; 50, 100 mg; 100 mg/5 mL

**Motrin, Children's** drops OTC *nonsteroidal anti-inflammatory drug (NSAID); analgesic; antipyretic* [ibuprofen] 40 mg/mL

**Motrin, Children's** oral suspension OTC *nonsteroidal anti-inflammatory drug (NSAID); analgesic; antipyretic* [ibuprofen] 100 mg/5 mL

**Motrin, Junior** film-coated caplets, chewable tablets OTC *nonsteroidal*

*anti-inflammatory drug (NSAID); anti-arthritic; analgesic* [ibuprofen] 100 mg

**Motrin IB** caplets, tablets, gelcaps OTC *nonsteroidal anti-inflammatory drug (NSAID); antiarthritic; analgesic* [ibuprofen] 200 mg

**Motrin IB Sinus** caplets OTC *decongestant; analgesic* [pseudoephedrine HCl; ibuprofen] 30•200 mg

**MouthKote** oral spray OTC *saliva substitute*

**MouthKote F/R** oral rinse OTC *topical dental caries preventative* [sodium fluoride] 0.04%

**MouthKote O/R** mouthwash OTC *anesthetic and antimicrobial throat irrigation* [benzyl alcohol; menthol]

**MouthKote O/R** oral solution OTC *topical antihistamine* [diphenhydramine] 1.25%

**MouthKote P/R** oral solution, ointment OTC *topical antihistamine* [diphenhydramine HCl] 1.25%; 25%

**moveltipril** INN

**movie star drug** *street drug slang* [see: cocaine]

**moxadolen** INN

**moxalactam disodium** USAN, USP *bactericidal antibiotic* [also: latamoxef]

**moxantrazole** [now: teloxantrone HCl]

**moxaprindine** INN

**moxastine** INN

**moxaverine** INN, BAN

**moxazocine** USAN, INN *analgesic; antitussive*

**moxestrol** INN

**moxicoumone** INN

**moxidectin** USAN, INN *veterinary antiparasitic*

**moxipraquine** INN, BAN

**moxiraprine** INN

**moxisylyte** INN [also: thymoxamine]

**moxnidazole** USAN, INN *antiprotozoal (Trichomonas)*

**moxonidine** INN *investigational antihypertensive*

**Moxy Compound** tablets (discontinued 1993) ℞ *antiasthmatic; bronchodilator; decongestant; anxiolytic* [theophylline; ephedrine sulfate; hydroxyzine HCl]

**MP (melphalan, prednisone)** *chemotherapy protocol*

**4-MP (4-methylpyrazole)** [see: fomepizole]

**6-MP (6-mercaptopurine)** [see: mercaptopurine]

**MPF** [see: Mucoprotective Factor]

**m-PFL (methotrexate, Platinol, fluorouracil, leucovorin [rescue])** *chemotherapy protocol*

**MPL (melphalan)** [q.v.]

**MPL + PRED (melphalan, prednisone)** *chemotherapy protocol*

**MPL-A (monophosphoryl lipid A)** [q.v.]

**MPL-C (monophosphoryl lipid C)** [q.v.]

**MPL-S (monophosphoryl lipid S)** [q.v.]

**M-Prednisol-40; M-Prednisol-80** intralesional, soft tissue, and IM injection ℞ *glucocorticoid; anti-inflammatory; immunosuppressant* [methylprednisolone acetate] 40 mg/mL; 80 mg/mL

**MRV** subcu injection ℞ *active respiratory bacteria immunizing agent* [mixed respiratory vaccine]

**MRV (mixed respiratory vaccine)** [q.v.]

**M-R-Vax II** powder for subcu injection ℞ *measles and rubella vaccine* [measles & rubella virus vaccine, live] 0.5 mL

**MS (magnesium salicylate)** [q.v.]

**MS (morphine sulfate)** [q.v.]

**MS Contin** controlled-release tablets ℞ *narcotic analgesic; preoperative sedative and anxiolytic* [morphine sulfate] 15, 100, 200 mg

**MSI-78** *investigational (Phase III) broad-spectrum antibacterial for impetigo and diabetic foot ulcers*

**MSIR** immediate-release tablets, capsules, oral solution, oral concentrate ℞ *narcotic analgesic; preoperative sedative and anxiolytic* [morphine sulfate] 15, 30 mg; 15, 30 mg; 10, 20 mg/5 mL; 20 mg/mL

**MS/L; MS/L Concentrate** oral liquid ℞ *narcotic analgesic; preoperative sedative and anxiolytic; also abused as a*

*street drug* [morphine sulfate] 10 mg/5 mL; 100 mg/5 mL

**MS/S** suppositories ℞ *narcotic analgesic; preoperative sedative and anxiolytic* [morphine sulfate] 5, 10, 20, 30 mg

**MSTA (Mumps Skin Test Antigen)** intradermal injection ℞ *diagnostic aid to assess immune system competency (not effective in testing immunity to mumps virus)* [mumps skin test antigen] 0.1 mL (4 U/0.1 mL)

**MT6 (mercaptomerin)** [q.v.]

**MTC (mitomycin C)** [see: mitomycin]

**M.T.E.-4; M.T.E.-5; M.T.E.-6; M.T.E.-7; M.T.E.-4 Concentrated; M.T.E.-5 Concentrated; M.T.E.-6 Concentrated** IV injection ℞ *intravenous nutritional therapy* [multiple trace elements (metals)]

**mTHPC** [see: temoporfin]

**MTX (methotrexate)** [q.v.]

**MTX + MP (methotrexate, mercaptopurine)** *chemotherapy protocol*

**MTX + MP + CTX (methotrexate, mercaptopurine, cyclophosphamide)** *chemotherapy protocol*

**MTXCP-PDAdr (methotrexate [with leucovorin rescue], cisplatin, doxorubicin)** *chemotherapy protocol*

**M.U.; M.O.** *street drug slang* [see: marijuana]

**Muco-Fen-DM** timed-release tablets ℞ *antitussive; expectorant* [dextromethorphan hydrobromide; guaifenesin] 30•600 mg

**Muco-Fen-LA** timed-release tablets ℞ *expectorant* [guaifenesin] 600 mg

**mucoid exopolysaccharide *Pseudomonas* hyperimmune globulin (MEPIG)** *investigational (orphan) for pulmonary infections of cystic fibrosis*

**mucolytics** *a class of respiratory inhalant drugs that destroy or inhibit mucin*

**Mucomyst** solution for nebulization or intratracheal instillation ℞ *mucolytic; investigational (orphan) for severe acetaminophen overdose* [acetylcysteine sodium] 10%, 20%

**Mucomyst 10** IV ℞ *investigational (orphan) for moderate to severe acetaminophen overdose* [acetylcysteine]

**Mucoplex** tablets (discontinued 1995) OTC *dietary supplement* [vitamins $B_2$ and $B_{12}$; liver fraction] 1.5 mg•5 µg•750 mg

**Mucoprotective Factor (MPF)** (trademarked ingredient) *aromatic flavored syrup* [eriodictyon]

**Mucosil-10; Mucosil-20** solution for nebulization or intratracheal instillation ℞ *mucolytic* [acetylcysteine sodium] 10%; 20%

**mud** *street drug slang* [see: heroin; morphine; opium]

**Mudrane** tablets ℞ *antiasthmatic; bronchodilator; decongestant; expectorant; sedative* [aminophylline; ephedrine HCl; potassium iodide; phenobarbital] 111•16•195•8 mg ⌯ Modane

**Mudrane GG** elixir (discontinued 1995) ℞ *antiasthmatic; decongestant; expectorant; sedative* [theophylline; ephedrine HCl; guaifenesin; phenobarbital] 4•0.8•5.2•0.5 mg/mL

**Mudrane GG** tablets ℞ *antiasthmatic; decongestant; expectorant; sedative* [theophylline; ephedrine HCl; guaifenesin; phenobarbital] 111•16•100•8 mg

**Mudrane GG-2** tablets ℞ *antiasthmatic; bronchodilator; expectorant* [theophylline; guaifenesin] 111•100 mg

**Mudrane-2** tablets (discontinued 1995) ℞ *antiasthmatic; expectorant* [aminophylline; potassium iodide] 111•195 mg

**muggie; muggies; muggles** *street drug slang for a marijuana cigarette* [see: marijuana]

**mujer** (Spanish for "woman" or "wife") *street drug slang* [see: cocaine]

**mulka** *street drug slang* [see: methcathinone]

**MulTE-Pak-4; MulTE-Pak-5** IV injection ℞ *intravenous nutritional therapy* [multiple trace elements (metals)] ≛

**Multi 75** timed-release tablets OTC *vitamin/mineral supplement* [multiple vitamins & minerals; folic acid; biotin] ± •0.4• ≟ mg

**Multi Vit** drops (discontinued 1993) OTC *vitamin supplement* [multiple vitamins]

**Multi Vit with Iron** drops OTC *vitamin/iron supplement* [multiple vitamins; iron] ± •10 mg/mL

**Multi Vitamin Concentrate** injection ℞ *parenteral vitamin supplement* [multiple vitamins] ±

**Multibret-500 Hematinic** timed-release tablets (discontinued 1995) ℞ *hematinic* [ferrous sulfate; multiple B vitamins; sodium ascorbate] 105• ± •500 mg

**Multibret-Folic-500** timed-release tablets (discontinued 1995) ℞ *hematinic* [ferrous sulfate; multiple B vitamins; sodium ascorbate; folic acid] 105• ± •500•0.8 mg

**Multi-Day** tablets OTC *vitamin supplement* [multiple vitamins; folic acid] ± •0.4 mg

**Multi-Day Plus Iron** tablets OTC *vitamin/iron supplement* [multiple vitamins; iron; folic acid] ± •18•0.4 mg

**Multi-Day Plus Minerals** tablets OTC *vitamin/mineral/iron supplement* [multiple vitamins & minerals; iron; folic acid; biotin] ± •18 mg•0.4 mg•30 μg

**Multi-Day with Calcium and Extra Iron** tablets OTC *vitamin/calcium/iron supplement* [multiple vitamins; calcium; iron; folic acid] ± • ≟ •27•0.4 mg

**Multilex; Multilex-T & M** tablets OTC *vitamin/mineral/iron supplement* [multiple vitamins & minerals; iron] ± •15 mg

**Multilyte** effervescent tablets (discontinued 1993) OTC *vitamin/mineral supplement* [multiple vitamins & minerals; folic acid; biotin; phenylalanine]

**Multilyte-20; Multilyte-40** IV admixture ℞ *intravenous electrolyte therapy* [combined electrolyte solution]

**Multi-Mineral** tablets OTC *mineral supplement* [multiple minerals]

**Multiple Trace Element; Multiple Trace Element Concentrated; Multiple Trace Element Neona-** **tal; Multiple Trace Element Pediatric** IV injection ℞ *intravenous nutritional therapy* [multiple trace elements (metals)]

**Multiple Trace Element with Selenium; Multiple Trace Element with Selenium Concentrated** IV injection ℞ *intravenous nutritional therapy* [multiple trace elements (metals)]

**Multistix; Multistix 2; Multistix 7; Multistix 8 SG; Multistix 9; Multistix 9 SG; Multistix 10 SG; Multistix SG** reagent strips *in vitro diagnostic aid for multiple urine products*

**Multitest CMI** single-use intradermal skin test device ℞ *skin test for multiple allergen sensitivity* [skin test antigens (seven different); glycerin (one for test control)]

**Multitrace-5 Concentrate** IV injection ℞ *intravenous nutritional therapy* [multiple trace elements (metals)] ±

**Multi-Vita-Drops** (discontinued 1993) OTC *vitamin supplement* [multiple vitamins]

**Multi-Vita-Drops with Fluoride** (discontinued 1993) ℞ *pediatric vitamin supplement and dental caries preventative* [multiple vitamins; fluoride]

**Multi-Vita-Drops with Iron** (discontinued 1993) OTC *vitamin/iron supplement* [multiple vitamins; iron]

**multivitamin infusion, neonatal formula** *investigational (orphan) total parenteral nutrition for very low birthweight infants*

**Multi-Vitamin Mineral with Beta-Carotene** tablets OTC *vitamin/mineral/iron supplement* [multiple vitamins & minerals; ferrous fumarate; folic acid; biotin] ± •27•0.4•0.45 mg

**Multivitamin with Fluoride** drops ℞ *pediatric vitamin supplement and dental caries preventative* [multiple vitamins; fluoride] ± •0.25, ± •0.5 mg/mL

**Multivitamins** capsules OTC *vitamin supplement* [multiple vitamins] ±

**Mulvidren-F** Softabs (chewable tablets) ℞ *pediatric vitamin supplement and dental caries preventative* [multiple vitamins; fluoride] ± •1 mg

**Mumps Skin Test Antigen** [see: MSTA]

**mumps skin test antigen (MSTA)** USP *diagnostic aid to assess immune system competency*

**mumps vaccine** [see: mumps virus vaccine, inactivated]

**mumps virus vaccine, inactivated** NF

**mumps virus vaccine, live** USP *active immunizing agent for mumps*

**Mumpsvax** powder for subcu injection R *mumps vaccine* [mumps virus vaccine, live] 0.5 mL

**mupirocin** USAN, INN, BAN *topical antibacterial antibiotic*

**mupirocin calcium** USAN *topical antibacterial antibiotic*

**muplestim** USAN *progenitor cell stimulator for neutropenia and thrombocytopenia*

**murabutide** INN

**muramyl-tripeptide** *investigational immunomodulator for AIDS (clinical trials discontinued 1994)*

**murder 8** *street drug slang* [see: fentanyl]

**murder one** *street drug slang for combination of heroin and cocaine* [see: cocaine; heroin]

**Murine** eye drops OTC *ocular moisturizer/lubricant* [polyvinyl alcohol] 0.5%

**Murine Ear Drops** OTC *agent to emulsify and disperse ear wax* [carbamide peroxide; alcohol] 6.5%•6.3%

**murine MAb** [see: muromonab-CD3]

**Murine Plus** eye drops OTC *topical ocular decongestant/vasoconstrictor* [tetrahydrozoline HCl] 0.05%

**Murine Regular Formula** ophthalmic solution (discontinued 1993) OTC *extraocular irrigating solution* [balanced saline solution]

**Muro 128** eye drops, ophthalmic ointment OTC *corneal edema-reducing agent* [hypertonic saline solution] 2%, 5%; 5%

**Muro Tears** eye drops (discontinued 1993) OTC *ocular moisturizer/lubricant*

**murocainide** INN

**Murocel** eye drops OTC *ocular moisturizer/lubricant* [methylcellulose] 1%

**Murocoll-2** eye drops R *cycloplegic; mydriatic* [scopolamine hydrobromide; phenylephrine HCl] 0.3%•10%

**murodermin** INN

**muromonab-CD3** USAN, INN *monoclonal antibody immunosuppressive for renal, hepatic, and cardiac transplants*

**Muroptic-5** eye drops OTC *corneal edema-reducing agent* [hypertonic saline solution] 5%

**Muro's Opcon** eye drops (discontinued 1995) R *topical ocular decongestant/vasoconstrictor* [naphazoline HCl] 0.1%

**Murphy** *street drug slang* [see: morphine]

**muscarinic agonists** *investigational analgesic*

**MuscleRub** ointment OTC *counterirritant* [methyl salicylate; menthol] 15%•10%

**Muse** single-use intraurethral suppository R *vasodilator for erectile dysfunction* [alprostadil] 125, 150, 500, 1000 μg

**mushrooms** *street drug slang* [see: psilocybin; psilocin]

**musk** *street drug slang* [see: psilocybin; psilocin]

**Mus-Lax** capsules (discontinued 1996) R *skeletal muscle relaxant; analgesic* [chlorzoxazone; acetaminophen] 250•300 mg

**mustaral oil** [see: allyl isothiocyanate]

**mustard oil** [see: allyl isothiocyanate]

**Mustargen** powder for IV or intracavitary injection R *alkylating antineoplastic for multiple myelomas, lymphomas and leukemias, and breast, lung, and ovarian cancers* [mechlorethamine HCl] 10 mg

**Musterole Deep Strength Rub** OTC *counterirritant* [methyl salicylate; methyl nicotinate; menthol] 30%•0.5%•3%

**Musterole Extra Strength** OTC *counterirritant* [camphor; menthol] 5%•3%

**mustine** BAN *nitrogen mustard-type alkylating antineoplastic* [also: mechlorethamine HCl; chlormethine; nitrogen mustard N-oxide HCl]

**mustine HCl** [see: mechlorethamine HCl]

**muta; mutah; moota; mooters; mootie; mootos** *street drug slang for a marijuana cigarette* [see: marijuana]

**Mutamycin** powder for IV injection ℞ *antibiotic antineoplastic for stomach, pancreatic, breast, colon, head, neck, and lung cancers* [mitomycin] 5, 20, 40 mg ⊡ mitomycin

**muzolimine** USAN, INN *diuretic; antihypertensive*

**muzzle** *street drug slang* [see: heroin]

**MV (mitomycin, vinblastine)** *chemotherapy protocol*

**MV (mitoxantrone, VePesid)** *chemotherapy protocol*

**MVAC; M-VAC (methotrexate, vinblastine, Adriamycin, cisplatin)** *chemotherapy protocol*

**M.V.C. 9+3** injection (discontinued 1995) ℞ *parenteral vitamin supplement* [multiple vitamins; folic acid; biotin] ±•0.4 mg•60 μg per 5 mL

**M.V.C. 9+4 Pediatric** powder for injection ℞ *vitamin therapy* [multiple vitamins; folic acid; biotin]

**MVF (mitoxantrone, vincristine, fluorouracil)** *chemotherapy protocol*

**M.V.I. Neonatal** IV infusion ℞ *investigational (orphan) total parenteral nutrition for very low birthweight infants* [multiple vitamin infusion, neonatal formula]

**M.V.I. Pediatric** injection ℞ *parenteral vitamin supplement* [multiple vitamins; folic acid; biotin] ±•140•20 μg/5 mL

**M.V.I.-12** injection ℞ *parenteral vitamin supplement* [multiple vitamins; folic acid; biotin] ±•400•60 μg/5 mL

**M.V.M.** capsules OTC *vitamin/mineral/iron supplement* [multiple vitamins & minerals; iron; folic acid; biotin] ±•3.6 mg•0.08 mg•160 μg

**MVP (mitomycin, vinblastine, Platinol)** *chemotherapy protocol*

**MVPP (mechlorethamine, vinblastine, procarbazine, prednisone)** *chemotherapy protocol*

**MVT (mitoxantrone, VePesid, thiotepa)** *chemotherapy protocol*

**MVVPP (mechlorethamine, vincristine, vinblastine, procarbazine, prednisone)** *chemotherapy protocol*

**Myadec** tablets OTC *vitamin/mineral/iron supplement* [multiple vitamins & minerals; iron; folic acid; biotin] ±•18 mg•0.4 mg•30 μg

**Myambutol** film-coated tablets ℞ *tuberculostatic* [ethambutol HCl] 100, 400 mg ⊡ Nembutal

**Myapap** drops (discontinued 1997) ℞ *analgesic; antipyretic* [acetaminophen] 100 mg/mL

**Mycelex** cream, solution ℞ *topical antifungal* [clotrimazole] 1%

**Mycelex** troches ℞ *antifungal; oral candidiasis prophylaxis or treatment* [clotrimazole] 10 mg

**Mycelex OTC** cream, solution OTC *topical antifungal* [clotrimazole] 1%

**Mycelex Twin Pack** vaginal tablets + cream ℞ *antifungal* [clotrimazole] 500 mg; 1%

**Mycelex-7** vaginal cream, vaginal tablets, combination pack (cream + vaginal suppositories) OTC *antifungal* [clotrimazole] 1%; 100 mg

**Mycelex-G** vaginal cream (discontinued 1994) ℞ *antifungal* [clotrimazole] 500 mg

**Mycelex-G** vaginal tablets ℞ *antifungal* [clotrimazole] 500 mg

**Mycifradin Sulfate** oral solution ℞ *aminoglycoside-type antibiotic* [neomycin sulfate] 125 mg/5 mL

**Myciguent** ointment, cream OTC *topical antibiotic* [neomycin sulfate] 3.5 mg/g

**Mycinette** throat spray OTC *topical anesthetic; oral antiseptic; astringent* [phenol; alum] 1.4%•0.3%

**Mycinettes** lozenges OTC *topical oral anesthetic* [benzocaine] 15 mg

**Myci-Spray** nasal spray OTC *nasal decongestant; antihistamine* [phenylephrine HCl; pyrilamine maleate] 0.25%•0.15%

**Mycitracin Plus** ointment OTC *topical antibiotic; local anesthetic* [polymyxin B sulfate; neomycin sulfate; bacitracin; lidocaine] 5000 U•3.5 mg•500 U•40 mg per g

**Mycitracin Triple Antibiotic** ointment OTC *topical antibiotic* [polymyxin B sulfate; neomycin sulfate; bacitracin] 5000 U•3.5 mg•500 U per g

*Mycobacterium avium* **sensitin RS-10** *investigational (orphan) diagnostic aid for Mycobacterium avium infection in immunocompromised patients*

**Mycobax** ℞ *investigational immunizing agent for high-risk tuberculosis populations* [BCG vaccine]

**Myco-Biotic II** cream ℞ *topical corticosteroid; antifungal* [triamcinolone acetonide; neomycin sulfate; nystatin] 0.1%•0.5%•100 000 U per g

**Mycobutin** capsules ℞ *antiviral/antibacterial for prevention of Mycobacterium avium complex (MAC) in advanced HIV patients (orphan)* [rifabutin] 150 mg

**Mycocide NS** solution OTC *topical antiseptic* [benzalkonium chloride] ≗

**Mycogen II** cream, ointment ℞ *topical corticosteroid; antifungal* [triamcinolone acetonide; nystatin] 0.1%•100 000 U per g

**Mycolog-II** cream, ointment ℞ *topical corticosteroid; antifungal* [triamcinolone acetonide; nystatin] 0.1%•100 000 U per g

**Myconel** cream ℞ *topical corticosteroid; antifungal* [triamcinolone acetonide; nystatin] 0.1%•100 000 U per g

**mycophenolate mofetil** USAN *immunomodulator; purine biosynthesis inhibitor; kidney transplant rejection preventative*

**mycophenolic acid** USAN, INN *antineoplastic*

**Mycostatin** cream, ointment, powder, vaginal tablets ℞ *topical antifungal* [nystatin] 100 000 U/g; 100 000 U/g; 100 000 U/g; 100 000 U

**Mycostatin** film-coated tablets ℞ *systemic antifungal* [nystatin] 500 000 U

**Mycostatin** oral suspension, Pastilles (troches) ℞ *antifungal; oral candidiasis treatment* [nystatin] 100 000 U/mL; 200 000 U

**Myco-Triacet II** cream, ointment ℞ *topical corticosteroid; antifungal* [triamcinolone acetonide; nystatin] 0.1%•100 000 U per g

**mydeton** [see: tolperisone]

**Mydfrin 2.5%** eye drops ℞ *ophthalmic decongestant/vasoconstrictor; mydriatic* [phenylephrine HCl] 2.5% ℞ Midrin; Myfedrine

**Mydrapred** Drop-Tainers (eye drop suspension) (discontinued 1994) ℞ *ophthalmic topical corticosteroidal anti-inflammatory; cycloplegic; mydriatic* [prednisolone acetate; atropine sulfate] 0.25%•1%

**Mydriacyl** Drop-Tainers (eye drops) ℞ *cycloplegic; mydriatic* [tropicamide] 0.5%, 1%

**mydriatics** *a class of drugs that cause the pupil of the eye to dilate*

**myelin** *investigational (orphan) for multiple sclerosis*

**myelosan** [see: busulfan]

**myfadol** INN

**Myfedrine** liquid (discontinued 1993) OTC *nasal decongestant* [pseudoephedrine HCl] ℞ Mydfrin

**Myfedrine Plus** liquid (discontinued 1993) OTC *decongestant; antihistamine* [pseudoephedrine HCl; chlorpheniramine maleate]

**Mygel; Mygel II** oral suspension OTC *antacid; antiflatulent* [aluminum hydroxide; magnesium hydroxide; simethicone] 200•200•20 mg/5 mL; 400•400•40 mg/5 mL

**Myidyl** syrup ℞ *antihistamine* [triprolidine HCl] 1.25 mg/5 mL

**Mykinac** cream ℞ *topical antifungal* [nystatin]

**Mykrox** tablets ℞ *diuretic; antihypertensive* [metolazone] 0.5 mg

**Mylagen** gelcaps OTC *antacid* [calcium carbonate; magnesium carbonate] 311•232 mg

**Mylagen; Mylagen II** liquid OTC *antacid; antiflatulent* [aluminum hydroxide; magnesium hydroxide; simethicone] 200•200•20 mg/5 mL; 400•400•40 mg/5 mL

**Mylanta** chewable tablets, liquid OTC *antacid; antiflatulent* [aluminum hydroxide; magnesium hydroxide; simethicone] 200•200•20, 400•400•40 mg; 200•200•20, 400•400•40 mg/5 mL ℞ Milontin

**Mylanta** gelcaps OTC *antacid* [calcium carbonate; magnesium carbonate] 311•232 mg

**Mylanta** lozenges OTC *antacid* [calcium carbonate] 600 mg

**Mylanta, Children's** oral liquid, chewable tablets OTC *antacid* [calcium carbonate] 400 mg/5 mL; 400 mg

**Mylanta AR** tablets OTC *"acid reducer" for heartburn and acid indigestion* [famotidine] 10 mg

**Mylanta Gas** chewable tablets OTC *antiflatulent* [simethicone] 40, 80, 125 mg

**Mylanta Natural Fiber Supplement** powder OTC *laxative* [psyllium hydrophilic mucilloid] 3.4 g/tsp.

**Myleran** tablets ℞ *alkylating antineoplastic for chronic myelogenous leukemia (CML)* [busulfan] 2 mg ⑨ Mylicon

**Mylicon** drops OTC *antiflatulent* [simethicone] 40 mg/0.6 mL ⑨ Modicon; Myleran

**Myloral** ℞ *investigational (Phase III) oral treatment for multiple sclerosis* [bovine myelin]

**Myminic** syrup (discontinued 1993) OTC *antihistamine; decongestant* [phenylpropanolamine HCl; chlorpheniramine maleate]

**Myminic Expectorant** liquid OTC *decongestant; expectorant* [phenylpropanolamine HCl; guaifenesin; alcohol 5%] 12.5•100 mg/5 mL

**Myminicol** liquid OTC *antitussive; decongestant; antihistamine* [dextromethorphan hydrobromide; phenylpropanolamine HCl; chlorpheniramine maleate] 10•12.5•2 mg/5 mL

**Mynatal** capsules ℞ *vitamin/mineral/calcium/iron supplement* [multiple vitamins & minerals; calcium; iron; folic acid; biotin] ≟•300•65•1•0.03 mg

**Mynatal FC** caplets ℞ *vitamin/mineral/calcium/iron supplement* [multiple vitamins & minerals; calcium; iron; folic acid; biotin] ≟•250•60•1•0.03 mg

**Mynatal P.N.** captabs ℞ *vitamin/calcium/iron supplement* [multiple vitamins; calcium; iron; folic acid] ≟• 125•60•1 mg

**Mynatal P.N. Forte** caplets ℞ *vitamin/mineral/calcium/iron supplement* [multiple vitamins & minerals; calcium; iron; folic acid] ≟•250•60•1 mg

**Mynatal Rx** caplets ℞ *vitamin/mineral/calcium/iron supplement* [multiple vitamins & minerals; calcium; iron; folic acid; biotin] ≟•200•60•1•0.03 mg

**Mynate 90 Plus** delayed-release caplets ℞ *vitamin/calcium/iron supplement* [multiple vitamins; calcium; iron; folic acid] ≟•250•90•1 mg

**Myochrysine** IM injection (discontinued 1996) ℞ *antirheumatic* [gold sodium thiomalate] 25, 50 mg/mL

**Myocide NS** solution OTC *topical antiseptic* [benzalkonium chloride] ≟

**Myoflex Creme** OTC *topical analgesic* [trolamine salicylate] 10%

**Myolin** IV or IM injection ℞ *skeletal muscle relaxant* [orphenadrine citrate] 30 mg/mL

**Myoscint** (commercially available in Europe) ℞ *investigational (orphan) imaging agent for cardiac necrosis and myocarditis* [imciromab pentetate]

**Myotonachol** tablets ℞ *cholinergic urinary stimulant for postsurgical and postpartum urinary retention* [bethanechol chloride] 10, 25 mg

**Myotrophin** injection ℞ *investigational adjunct to chemotherapy; investigational (NDA filed, orphan) for amyotrophic lateral sclerosis* [mecasermin]

**Myoview** ℞ *investigational cardiovascular imaging aid* [technetium Tc 99m tetrofosmin]

**Myphetane DC Cough** syrup ℞ *narcotic antitussive; decongestant; antihistamine* [codeine phosphate; phenylpropanolamine HCl; brompheniramine maleate; alcohol 1.2%] 10•12.5•2 mg/5 mL

**Myphetane DX Cough** syrup ℞ *antitussive; decongestant; antihistamine* [dextromethorphan hydrobromide; pseudoephedrine HCl; brompheniramine maleate; alcohol 1%] 10•30• 2 mg/5 mL

**Myphetapp** elixir (discontinued 1993) OTC *decongestant; antihistamine* [phenylpropanolamine HCl; brompheniramine maleate]

**myralact** INN, BAN

**myricodine** [see: myrophine]

**myristica oil** [see: nutmeg oil]

**myristyl alcohol** NF *stiffening agent*

**myristyltrimethylammonium bromide** *antiseborrheic*

**myrophine** INN, BAN

**myrtecaine** INN

**Mysoline** tablets, oral suspension ℞ *anticonvulsant for grand mal, psychomotor, or focal epileptic seizures* [primidone] 50, 250 mg; 250 mg/5 mL

**myspamol** [see: proquamezine]

**Mytelase** caplets ℞ *anticholinesterase muscle stimulant; myasthenia gravis treatment* [ambenonium chloride] 10 mg

**Mytrex** cream, ointment ℞ *topical corticosteroid; antifungal* [triamcinolone acetonide; nystatin] 0.1%•100 000 U/g

**Mytussin** syrup OTC *expectorant* [guaifenesin; alcohol 3.5%] 100 mg/5 mL

**Mytussin AC Cough** syrup ℞ *narcotic antitussive; expectorant* [codeine phosphate; guaifenesin; alcohol 3.5%] 10•100 mg/5 mL

**Mytussin DAC** syrup ℞ *narcotic antitussive; decongestant; expectorant* [codeine phosphate; pseudoephedrine HCl; guaifenesin; alcohol 1.7%] 10•30•100 mg/5 mL

**Mytussin DM** liquid OTC *antitussive; expectorant* [dextromethorphan hydrobromide; guaifenesin; alcohol 1.6%] 10•100 mg/5 mL

**myuizone** [see: thioacetazone; thiacetazone]

**My-Vitalife** capsules OTC *vitamin/mineral/calcium/iron supplement* [multiple vitamins & minerals; calcium; iron; folic acid; biotin] ±•130•27•0.4•0.03 mg

**MZM** tablets ℞ *carbonic anhydrase inhibitor; diuretic* [methazolamide] 25, 50 mg

**MZM (methazolamide)** [q.v.]

**N₂ (nitrogen)** [q.v.]

**N-3 polyunsaturated fatty acids** [see: doconexent; icosapent; omega-3 marine triglycerides]

**N901-blocked ricin** *investigational antineoplastic for small cell lung cancer*

**²²Na** [see: sodium chloride Na 22]

**nabazenil** USAN, INN *anticonvulsant*

**nabilone** USAN, INN, BAN *minor tranquilizer*

**nabitan** INN *analgesic* [also: nabitan HCl]

**nabitan HCl** USAN *analgesic* [also: nabitan]

**naboctate** INN *antiglaucoma agent; antinauseant* [also: naboctate HCl]

**naboctate HCl** USAN *antiglaucoma agent; antinauseant* [also: naboctate]

**nabumetone** USAN, INN, BAN *nonsteroidal anti-inflammatory drug; antiarthritic*

**nabutan HCl** [now: nabitan HCl]

**NAC (nitrogen mustard, Adriamycin, CCNU)** *chemotherapy protocol*

**nacartocin** INN

**NaCl (sodium chloride)** [q.v.]

**NAD (nicotinamide-adenine dinucleotide)** [see: nadide]

**nadide** USAN, INN *antagonist to alcohol and narcotics*

**nadisan** [see: carbutamide]

**nadolol** USAN, USP, INN, BAN *antianginal; antihypertensive; antiadrenergic (β-receptor)* 20, 40, 80, 120, 160 mg oral ⊘ Nandol

**nadoxolol** INN

**naepaine HCl** NF

**nafamostat** INN *anticoagulant; antifibrinolytic* [also: nafamostat mesylate; nafamostat mesilate]

**nafamostat mesilate** JAN *anticoagulant; antifibrinolytic* [also: nafamostat mesylate; nafamostat]

**nafamostat mesylate** USAN *anticoagulant; antifibrinolytic* [also: nafamostat; nafamostat mesilate]

**nafarelin** INN, BAN *luteinizing hormone-releasing hormone (LHRH) agonist* [also: nafarelin acetate]

**nafarelin acetate** USAN *luteinizing hormone-releasing hormone (LHRH) agonist for central precocious puberty (orphan) and endometriosis* [also: nafarelin]

**Nafazair** eye drops ℞ *topical ocular decongestant/vasoconstrictor* [naphazoline HCl] 0.1%

**Nafazair A** eye drops (discontinued 1995) ℞ *topical ocular decongestant and antihistamine* [naphazoline HCl; pheniramine maleate] 0.025%•0.3%

**nafazatrom** INN, BAN

**nafcaproic acid** INN

**Nafcil** powder for IV or IM injection ℞ *bactericidal antibiotic (penicillinase-resistant penicillin)* [nafcillin sodium] 0.5, 1, 2, 10 g

**nafcillin** INN *antibacterial* [also: nafcillin sodium]

**nafcillin sodium** USAN, USP *bactericidal antibiotic* [also: nafcillin] 0.5, 1, 2, 10 g/vial injection

**nafenodone** INN

**nafenopin** USAN, INN *antihyperlipoproteinemic*

**nafetolol** INN

**nafimidone** INN *anticonvulsant* [also: nafimidone HCl]

**nafimidone HCl** USAN *anticonvulsant* [also: nafimidone]

**nafiverine** INN

**naflocort** USAN, INN *topical adrenocortical steroid*

**nafomine** INN *muscle relaxant* [also: nafomine malate]

**nafomine malate** USAN *muscle relaxant* [also: nafomine]

**nafoxadol** INN

**nafoxidine HCl** USAN, INN *antiestrogen*

**nafronyl oxalate** USAN *vasodilator* [also: naftidrofuryl]

**naftalofos** USAN, INN *veterinary anthelmintic*

**naftazone** INN, BAN

**naftidrofuryl** INN *vasodilator* [also: nafronyl oxalate]

**naftifine** INN, BAN *broad-spectrum antifungal* [also: naftifine HCl]

**naftifine HCl** USAN *broad-spectrum antifungal* [also: naftifine]

**Naftin** cream, gel ℞ *topical antifungal* [naftifine HCl] 1%

**naftopidil** INN

**naftoxate** INN

**naftypramide** INN *antibacterial*

**Naganol** (available only from the Centers for Disease Control) ℞ *investigational anti-infective for trypanosomiasis and onchocerciasis* [suramin sodium]

**naganol** [see: suramin sodium]

**nail** *street drug slang for a marijuana cigarette* [see: marijuana]

**nalazosulfamide** [see: salazosulfamide]

**nalbuphine** INN, BAN *narcotic agonist-antagonist analgesic; narcotic antagonist* [also: nalbuphine HCl]

**nalbuphine HCl** USAN *narcotic agonist-antagonist analgesic; narcotic antagonist* [also: nalbuphine] 10, 20 mg/mL injection

**Naldec Pediatric** syrup ℞ *decongestant; antihistamine* [phenylpropanolamine HCl; phenylephrine HCl; phenyltoloxamine citrate; chlorpheniramine maleate]

**Naldecon** sustained-release tablets, syrup, pediatric syrup, pediatric drops ℞ *decongestant; antihistamine* [phenylpropanolamine HCl; phenylephrine HCl; chlorpheniramine maleate; phenyltoloxamine citrate] 40•10•5•15 mg; 20•5•2.5•7.5 mg/5 mL; 5•1.25•0.5•2 mg/5 mL; 5•1.25•0.5•2 mg/mL ⊡ Nalfon

**Naldecon CX Adult** liquid ℞ *narcotic antitussive; decongestant; expectorant* [codeine phosphate; phenylpropanolamine HCl; guaifenesin] 10•12.5•200 mg/5 mL

**Naldecon DX** children's syrup, pediatric drops OTC *pediatric antitussive, decongestant, and expectorant* [dextromethorphan hydrobromide; phenylpropanolamine HCl; guaifenesin] 5•6.25•100 mg/5 mL; 5•6.25•50 mg/mL

**Naldecon DX Adult** liquid OTC *antitussive; decongestant; expectorant* [dextromethorphan hydrobromide;

phenylpropanolamine HCl; guaifenesin] 10•12.5•200 mg/5 mL

**Naldecon EX** children's syrup, pediatric drops OTC *pediatric decongestant and expectorant* [phenylpropanolamine HCl; guaifenesin] 6.25•100 mg/5 mL; 6.25•50 mg/5 mL

**Naldecon Senior DX** liquid OTC *antitussive; expectorant* [dextromethorphan hydrobromide; guaifenesin] 10•200 mg/5 mL

**Naldecon Senior EX** liquid OTC *expectorant* [guaifenesin] 200 mg/5 mL

**Naldegesic** tablets OTC *decongestant; analgesic* [pseudoephedrine HCl; acetaminophen]

**Naldelate** syrup, pediatric syrup ℞ *decongestant; antihistamine* [phenylpropanolamine HCl; phenylephrine HCl; chlorpheniramine maleate; phenyltoloxamine citrate] 20•5•2.5•7.5 mg/5 mL; 5•1.25•0.5•2 mg/5 mL

**Naldelate DX Adult** liquid OTC *antitussive; decongestant; expectorant* [dextromethorphan hydrobromide; phenylpropanolamine HCl; guaifenesin] 10•12.5•200 mg/5 mL

**Nalfon** Pulvules (capsules) ℞ *nonsteroidal anti-inflammatory drug (NSAID); antiarthritic; analgesic* [fenoprofen calcium] 200, 300 mg ⑨ Naldecon

**Nalfon** tablets (discontinued 1994) ℞ *nonsteroidal anti-inflammatory drug (NSAID); antiarthritic; analgesic* [fenoprofen calcium] 600 mg

**Nalgest** sustained-release tablets, syrup, pediatric syrup, pediatric drops ℞ *decongestant; antihistamine* [phenylpropanolamine HCl; phenylephrine HCl; chlorpheniramine maleate; phenyltoloxamine citrate] 40•10•5•15 mg; 20•5•2.5•7.5 mg/5 mL; 5•1.25•0.5•2 mg/5 mL; 5•1.25•0.5•2 mg/mL

**nalidixane** [see: nalidixic acid]

**nalidixate sodium** USAN *antibacterial*

**nalidixic acid** USAN, USP, INN *urinary bactericidal*

**Nallpen** IV or IM injection ℞ *bactericidal antibiotic (penicillinase-resistant penicillin)* [nafcillin sodium] 0.5, 1, 2, 10 g

**nalmefene** USAN, INN, BAN *narcotic antagonist; investigational treatment for stroke, interstitial cystitis, and pruritus*

**nalmefene HCl** *narcotic antagonist*

**nalmetrene** [now: nalmefene]

**nalmexone** INN *analgesic; narcotic antagonist* [also: nalmexone HCl]

**nalmexone HCl** USAN *analgesic; narcotic antagonist* [also: nalmexone]

**nalorphine** INN [also: nalorphine HCl]

**nalorphine HCl** USP [also: nalorphine]

**naloxiphane tartrate** [see: levallorphan tartrate]

**naloxone** INN *narcotic antagonist; investigational treatment for constipation* [also: naloxone HCl]

**naloxone HCl** USAN, USP *narcotic antagonist; investigational treatment for constipation* [also: naloxone] 0.02, 0.4 mg/mL injection

**naloxone HCl & pentazocine** *narcotic agonist-antagonist analgesic* 0.5•50 mg oral

**Nalspan** syrup (discontinued 1993) ℞ *decongestant; antihistamine* [phenylpropanolamine HCL; phenylephrine HCl; chlorpheniramine maleate; phenyltoloxamine citrate]

**naltrexone** USAN, INN, BAN *narcotic antagonist*

**naltrexone HCl** *opiate blockage and maintenance in formerly opiate-dependent individuals (orphan)*

**naminterol** INN

**[¹³N]ammonia** [see: ammonia N 13]

**namoxyrate** USAN, INN *analgesic*

**namuron** [see: cyclobarbitone]

**nanafrocin** INN

**Nandrobolic** IM injection (discontinued 1994) ℞ *anabolic steroid for metastatic breast cancer in women* [nandrolone phenpropionate] 25 mg/mL

**nandrolone** BAN *anabolic* [also: nandrolone cyclotate]

**nandrolone cyclotate** USAN *anabolic* [also: nandrolone]

**nandrolone decanoate** USAN, USP *androgen; anabolic steroid; sometimes abused as a street drug* 50, 100, 200 mg/mL injection (in oil)

**nandrolone phenpropionate** USP *androgen; anabolic steroid; sometimes* *abused as a street drug* 25, 50 mg/mL injection (in oil)

**naniopine** [see: nanofin]

**nanofin** INN

**Nanoo** *street drug slang* [see: heroin]

**nanterinone** INN, BAN

**nantradol** INN *analgesic* [also: nantradol HCl]

**nantradol HCl** USAN *analgesic* [also: nantradol]

**Napa** Ṛ *investigational antiarrhythmic* [acecainide HCl]

**NAPA (N-acetyl-*p*-aminophenol)** [see: acetaminophen]

**NAPA (N-acetylprocainamide)** [q.v.]

**napactadine** INN *antidepressant* [also: napactadine HCl]

**napactadine HCl** USAN *antidepressant* [also: napactadine]

**napadisilate** INN *combining name for radicals or groups* [also: napadisylate]

**napadisylate** BAN *combining name for radicals or groups* [also: napadisilate]

**napamezole** INN *antidepressant* [also: napamezole HCl]

**napamezole HCl** USAN *antidepressant* [also: napamezole]

**Napamide** capsules Ṛ *antiarrhythmic* [disopyramide phosphate]

**Naphazole-A** eye drops (discontinued 1995) Ṛ *topical ocular decongestant and antihistamine* [naphazoline HCl; pheniramine maleate] 0.025%•0.3%

**naphazoline** INN, BAN *topical ocular vasoconstrictor; nasal decongestant* [also: naphazoline HCl; naphazoline nitrate]

**naphazoline HCl** USP *topical ocular vasoconstrictor; nasal decongestant* [also: naphazoline; naphazoline nitrate] 0.1% eye drops

**naphazoline HCl & antazoline phosphate** *topical ocular decongestant and antihistamine* 0.05%•0.5%

**naphazoline HCl & pheniramine maleate** *topical ocular decongestant and antihistamine* 0.025%•0.3% eye drops

**naphazoline nitrate** JAN *topical ocular vasoconstrictor; nasal decongestant* [also: naphazoline HCl; naphazoline]

**Naphazoline Plus** eye drops OTC *topical ocular decongestant and antihista-*

*mine* [naphazoline HCl; pheniramine maleate] 0.025%•0.3%

**Naphazoline-A** eye drops (name changed to Naphazoline Plus in 1993)

**Naphcon** eye drops OTC *topical ocular decongestant/vasoconstrictor* [naphazoline HCl] 0.012%

**Naphcon Forte** Drop-Tainers (eye drops) Ṛ *topical ocular decongestant/ vasoconstrictor* [naphazoline HCl] 0.1%

**Naphcon-A** Drop-Tainers (eye drops) OTC *topical ocular decongestant and antihistamine* [naphazoline HCl; pheniramine maleate] 0.025%•0.3%

**Naphoptic-A** eye drops Ṛ *topical ocular decongestant and antihistamine* [naphazoline HCl; pheniramine maleate] 0.025%•0.3%

**2-naphthol** [see: betanaphthol]

**naphthonone** INN

**naphthypramide** [see: naftypramide]

**Naphuride** (available only from the Centers for Disease Control) Ṛ *investigational anti-infective for trypanosomiasis and onchocerciasis* [suramin sodium]

**napirimus** INN

**napitane mesylate** USAN *antidepressant; α-adrenergic blocker; norepinephrine uptake antagonist*

**Naprelan** controlled-release tablets Ṛ *once-daily nonsteroidal anti-inflammatory drug (NSAID); antiarthritic; analgesic* [naproxen (from naproxen sodium)] 375 (412.5), 500 (550) mg

**Napril** tablets (discontinued 1994) OTC *decongestant; antihistamine* [pseudoephedrine HCl; chlorpheniramine maleate] 60•4 mg

**naprodoxime** INN

**Napron X** tablets Ṛ *nonsteroidal anti-inflammatory drug (NSAID); antiarthritic; analgesic* [naproxen] 500 mg

**Naprosyn** tablets, oral suspension Ṛ *nonsteroidal anti-inflammatory drug (NSAID); antiarthritic; analgesic* [naproxen] 250, 375, 500 mg; 125 mg/5 mL ⊡ Meprospan; naproxen; Natacyn

**Naprosyn EC** [see: EC-Naprosyn]

**Naprosyn SR** Ṛ *investigational nonsteroidal anti-inflammatory drug*

*(NSAID); antiarthritic; analgesic* [naproxen]

**naproxen** USAN, USP, INN, BAN, JAN *analgesic; antiarthritic; nonsteroidal anti-inflammatory drug (NSAID); antipyretic* 250, 375, 500 mg oral; 125 mg/5 mL oral ☒ Naprosyn

**naproxen sodium** USAN, USP *analgesic; antiarthritic; nonsteroidal anti-inflammatory drug (NSAID); antipyretic* 220, 250, 500 mg oral

**naproxol** USAN, INN *anti-inflammatory; analgesic; antipyretic*

**napsagatran** USAN, INN *antithrombotic*

**napsilate** INN *combining name for radicals or groups* [also: napsylate]

**napsylate** USAN, BAN *combining name for radicals or groups* [also: napsilate]

**Naqua** tablets ℞ *diuretic; antihypertensive* [trichlormethiazide] 2, 4 mg

**naranol** INN *antipsychotic* [also: naranol HCl]

**naranol HCl** USAN *antipsychotic* [also: naranol]

**narasin** USAN, INN, BAN *coccidiostat; veterinary growth stimulant*

**naratriptan** INN, BAN *antimigraine agent* [also: naratriptan HCl]

**naratriptan HCl** USAN *antimigraine agent* [also: naratriptan]

**Narcan** IV, IM, or subcu injection, neonatal injection ℞ *narcotic antagonist for opiate dependence or overdose; hypotension treatment* [naloxone HCl] 0.4, 1 mg/mL; 0.02 mg/mL ☒ Marcaine

**narcotic agonist-antagonists** *a class of opioid or morphine-like analgesics with lower abuse potential than pure narcotic agonist analgesics*

**narcotic agonists** *a class of opioid analgesics*

**narcotine** [see: noscapine]

**narcotine HCl** [see: noscapine HCl]

**Nardil** sugar-coated tablets ℞ *antipsychotic; monoamine oxidase inhibitor (MAOI) for treatment-resistant atypical depression* [phenelzine sulfate] 15 mg ☒ Norinyl

**Naropin** injection ℞ *long-acting local anesthetic* [ropivacaine HCl] 2, 5, 7.5, 10 mg/mL

**Nasabid** prolonged-action capsules ℞ *decongestant; expectorant* [pseudoephedrine HCl; guaifenesin] 90•250 mg

**Nasacort** nasal spray ℞ *intranasal steroidal anti-inflammatory* [triamcinolone acetonide] 55 µg/spray

**Nasacort AQ** metered-dose aerosol ℞ *once-daily aqueous intranasal corticosteroidal anti-inflammatory* [triamcinolone acetonide] 55 µg/spray

**Nasahist** sustained-release capsules (discontinued 1993) ℞ *decongestant; antihistamine* [phenylpropanolamine HCl; phenylephrine HCl; chlorpheniramine maleate]

**Nasahist B** subcu or IM injection ℞ *antihistamine; anaphylaxis* [brompheniramine maleate] 10 mg/mL

**NāSal** nasal spray, nose drops OTC *nasal moisturizer* [sodium chloride (saline)] 0.65%

**Nasal Decongestant** spray OTC *nasal decongestant* [oxymetazoline HCl] 0.05%

**Nasal Moist** nasal spray OTC *nasal moisturizer* [sodium chloride (saline)] 0.65%

**Nasal Relief** nasal spray OTC *nasal decongestant* [oxymetazoline HCl] 0.05%

**Nasalcrom** nasal spray OTC *bronchodilator for bronchial asthma and bronchospasm* [cromolyn sodium] 4% (5.2 mg/dose)

**Nasalide** nasal spray ℞ *intranasal steroidal anti-inflammatory* [flunisolide] 25 µg/dose

**Nasarel** metered dose nasal spray ℞ *intranasal steroidal anti-inflammatory* [flunisolide] 0.025% (25 µg/dose)

**Nasatab LA** long-acting film-coated tablets ℞ *decongestant; expectorant* [pseudoephedrine HCl; guaifenesin] 120•500 mg

**Nashville rabbit antithymocyte serum** [see: lymphocyte immune globulin, antithymocyte]

**Natabec Rx** Kapseals (capsules) (discontinued 1995) ℞ *vitamin/calcium/iron supplement* [multiple vitamins;

calcium; iron; folic acid] ± • 240 • 30 • 1 mg

**Natacomp-FA** film-coated tablets (discontinued 1993) ℞ *vitamin/mineral/iron supplement* [multiple vitamins & minerals; iron; folic acid]

**Natacyn** eye drop suspension ℞ *ophthalmic antifungal agent* [natamycin] 5% ⌧ Naprosyn

**Natafort** Filmseal (film-coated tablets) (discontinued 1995) ℞ *vitamin/calcium/iron supplement* [multiple vitamins; calcium; iron; folic acid] ± • 350 • 65 • 1 mg

**Natalins** tablets OTC *vitamin/calcium/iron supplement* [multiple vitamins; calcium; iron; folic acid] ± • 200 • 30 • 0.5 mg

**Natalins Rx** tablets ℞ *vitamin/calcium/iron supplement* [multiple vitamins; calcium; iron; folic acid; biotin] ± • 200 • 60 • 1 • 0.03 mg

**natamycin** USAN, USP, INN, BAN *ophthalmic fungicidal antibiotic* [also: pimaricin]

**Natarex Prenatal** tablets ℞ *vitamin/calcium/iron supplement* [multiple vitamins; calcium; iron; folic acid; biotin] ± • 200 • 60 • 1 • 0.03 mg

**natural killer cell stimulatory factor** [see: interleukin-12]

· **Natural Vegetable** powder OTC *bulk laxative* [psyllium hydrophilic mucilloid] 3.4 g/tsp.

**Naturalyte** oral solution OTC *electrolyte replacement* [sodium, potassium, and chloride electrolytes] 240 mL, 1 L

**Nature's Bounty 1** timed-release tablets (discontinued 1995) OTC *vitamin/mineral/calcium/iron supplement* [multiple vitamins & minerals; calcium; iron; folic acid; biotin] ± • 50 • 10 • 0.4 • 0.05 mg

**Nature's Remedy** tablets OTC *laxative* [cascara sagrada] 150 mg

**Nature's Tears** eye drops OTC *ocular moisturizer/lubricant* [hydroxypropyl methylcellulose] 0.4%

**Naturetin** tablets ℞ *diuretic; antihypertensive* [bendroflumethiazide] 5, 10 mg

**Naus-A-Way** solution (discontinued 1997) OTC *antinauseant; antiemetic*

[phosphorated carbohydrate solution (fructose, dextrose, and orthophosphoric acid)]

**Nausea Relief** solution OTC *antinauseant; antiemetic* [phosphorated carbohydrate solution (dextrose, levulose, and phosphoric acid)]

**Nausetrol** solution OTC *antinauseant; antiemetic* [phosphorated carbohydrate solution (fructose, dextrose, and orthophosphoric acid)]

**Navane** capsules ℞ *antipsychotic* [thiothixene] 1, 2, 5, 10, 20 mg

**Navane** oral concentrate, IM solution (discontinued 1997) ℞ *antipsychotic* [thiothixene HCl] 5 mg/mL; 2 mg/mL

**Navane** powder for IM injection ℞ *antipsychotic* [thiothixene HCl] 5 mg/mL

**Navelbine** IV injection ℞ *antineoplastic for Hodgkin's disease and lung, breast and ovarian cancer* [vinorelbine tartrate] 10 mg/mL

**Navoban** ℞ *investigational treatment for nausea and vomiting related to chemotherapy* [tropisetron]

**naxagolide** INN *antiparkinsonian; dopamine agonist* [also: naxagolide HCl]

**naxagolide HCl** USAN *antiparkinsonian; dopamine agonist* [also: naxagolide]

**naxaprostene** INN

**N-B-P** ointment (discontinued 1994) OTC *topical antibiotic* [polymyxin B sulfate; neomycin sulfate; bacitracin] 5000 U • 3.5 mg • 400 U per g

**9-NC (9-nitro-20-(S)-camptothecin)** [q.v.]

**ND Clear** sustained-release capsules ℞ *decongestant; antihistamine* [pseudoephedrine HCl; chlorpheniramine maleate] 120 • 8 mg

**ND Stat** subcu or IM injection ℞ *antihistamine; anaphylaxis* [brompheniramine maleate] 10 mg/mL

**ND-Gesic** tablets OTC *decongestant; antihistamine; analgesic* [phenylephrine HCl; chlorpheniramine maleate; pyrilamine maleate; acetaminophen] 5 • 2 • 12.5 • 300 mg

**nealbarbital** INN [also: nealbarbitone]

**nealbarbitone** BAN [also: nealbarbital]

**nebacumab** USAN, INN, BAN *antiendotoxin monoclonal antibody; investigational (orphan) for gram-negative bacteremia in endotoxin shock*

**nebbies** *street drug slang* [see: Nembutal Sodium; pentobarbital sodium]

**Nebcin** IV or IM injection, pediatric injection, powder for injection ℞ *aminoglycoside-type antibiotic* [tobramycin sulfate] 10, 40 mg/mL; 10 mg/mL; 30 mg/mL

**nebidrazine** INN

**nebivolol** USAN, INN *antihypertensive (β-blocker)*

**nebracetam** INN

**nebramycin** USAN, INN *antibacterial*

**nebramycin factor 6** [see: tobramycin]

**NebuPent** inhalation aerosol ℞ *antiprotozoal; treatment and prophylaxis of Pneumocystis carinii pneumonia (orphan)* [pentamidine isethionate] 300 mg

**nedocromil** USAN, INN, BAN *prophylactic antiallergic*

**nedocromil calcium** USAN *prophylactic antiallergic*

**nedocromil sodium** USAN *prophylactic antiallergic; antiasthmatic*

**N.E.E. 1/35** tablets ℞ *monophasic oral contraceptive* [norethindrone; ethinyl estradiol] 1 mg•35 μg

**nefazodone** INN *antidepressant* [also: nefazodone HCl]

**nefazodone HCl** USAN *antidepressant* [also: nefazodone]

**neflumozide** INN *antipsychotic* [also: neflumozide HCl]

**neflumozide HCl** USAN *antipsychotic* [also: neflumozide]

**nefocon A** USAN *hydrophobic contact lens material*

**nefopam** INN *analgesic* [also: nefopam HCl]

**nefopam HCl** USAN *analgesic* [also: nefopam]

**nefrolan** [see: clorexolone]

**NegGram** caplets, oral suspension ℞ *urinary bactericidal* [nalidixic acid] 250, 500, 1000 mg; 250 mg/5 mL

**neldazosin** INN

**nelezaprine** INN *muscle relaxant* [also: nelezaprine maleate]

**nelezaprine maleate** USAN *muscle relaxant* [also: nelezaprine]

**nelfilcon A** USAN *hydrophilic contact lens material*

**nelfinavir mesylate** USAN *antiretroviral HIV-1 protease inhibitor*

**Nelova 1/35E; Nelova 0.5/35E** tablets ℞ *monophasic oral contraceptive* [norethindrone; ethinyl estradiol] 1 mg•35 μg; 0.5 mg•35 μg

**Nelova 1/50M** tablets ℞ *monophasic oral contraceptive* [norethindrone; mestranol] 1 mg•50 μg

**Nelova 10/11** tablets ℞ *biphasic oral contraceptive* [norethindrone; ethinyl estradiol] Phase 1: 0.5 mg•35 μg; Phase 2: 1 mg•35 μg

**Nelulen 1/35E; Nelulen 1/50E** tablets (discontinued 1994) ℞ *oral contraceptive* [ethynodiol diacetate; ethinyl estradiol] 1 mg•35 μg; 1 mg•50 μg

**nemadectin** USAN, INN *veterinary antiparasitic*

**nemazoline** INN *nasal decongestant* [also: nemazoline HCl]

**nemazoline HCl** USAN *nasal decongestant* [also: nemazoline]

**Nembutal** elixir (discontinued 1993) ℞ *sedative; hypnotic* [pentobarbital] Ⓓ Myambutal

**Nembutal Sodium** capsules, IV or IM injection, suppositories ℞ *sedative; hypnotic; also abused as a street drug* [pentobarbital sodium] 50, 100 mg; 50 mg/mL; 30, 60, 120, 200 mg

**nemish** *street drug slang* [see: Nembutal Sodium; pentobarbital sodium]

**neoarsphenamine** NF, INN

**Neocaf** ℞ *investigational (orphan) for apnea of prematurity* [caffeine]

**Neo-Calglucon** syrup OTC *calcium supplement* [calcium glubionate] 1.8 g/5 mL

**neocarzinostatin** [now: zinostatin]

**Neo-Castaderm** liquid (discontinued 1995) OTC *topical antifungal; astringent; antiseptic* [resorcinol; boric acid; acetone; sodium bisulfite; phenol; alcohol]

**Neocate One +** ready-to-use liquid OTC *pediatric enteral nutritional therapy* [lactose-free formula] 237 mL

**Neocera** (trademarked ingredient) *suppository base* [PEG 400, 1450, 8000; polysorbate 60]

**neocid** [see: chlorophenothane]

**Neocidin** eye drops (discontinued 1993) ℞ *ophthalmic antibiotic* [polymyxin B sulfate; neomycin sulfate; gramicidin]

**neocinchophen** NF, INN

**NeoCitran DM Coughs & Colds** (CAN) powder for oral solution OTC *antitussive; decongestant; antihistamine* [dextromethorphan hydrobromide; phenylephrine HCl; pheniramine maleate] 30•10•20 mg/dose

**Neo-Cortef** cream (discontinued 1993) ℞ *topical corticosteroid; antibiotic* [hydrocortisone; neomycin sulfate] 1%•0.5%

**Neo-Cortef** ointment (discontinued 1997) ℞ *topical corticosteroid; antibiotic* [hydrocortisone; neomycin sulfate] 0.5%•0.5%, 1%•0.5%

**Neo-Cultol** jelly OTC *emollient laxative* [mineral oil]

**Neocyten** IV or IM injection (discontinued 1993) ℞ *skeletal muscle relaxant* [orphenadrine citrate]

**NeoDecadron** cream ℞ *topical corticosteroid; antibiotic* [dexamethasone phosphate; neomycin sulfate] 0.1%•0.5%

**NeoDecadron** Ocumeter (eye drops), ophthalmic ointment ℞ *topical ophthalmic corticosteroidal anti-inflammatory; antibiotic* [dexamethasone sodium phosphate; neomycin sulfate] 0.1%•0.35%; 0.05%•0.35%

**Neo-Dexair** eye drops ℞ *topical ophthalmic corticosteroidal anti-inflammatory; antibiotic* [dexamethasone sodium phosphate; neomycin sulfate] 0.1%•0.35%

**Neo-Dexameth** eye drops ℞ *topical ophthalmic corticosteroidal anti-inflammatory; antibiotic* [dexamethasone sodium phosphate; neomycin sulfate] 0.1%•0.35%

**Neo-Diaral** capsules OTC *antidiarrheal* [loperamide] 2 mg

**Neo-Durabolic** IM injection ℞ *anabolic steroid for anemia of renal insufficiency* [nandrolone decanoate] 50, 200 mg/mL

**neodymium** *element (Nd)*

**Neo-fradin** oral solution ℞ *aminoglycoside-type antibiotic* [neomycin sulfate] 125 mg/5 mL

**Neoloid** oil OTC *stimulant laxative* [castor oil] 36.4%

**Neomac** ointment OTC *topical antibiotic* [polymyxin B sulfate; neomycin sulfate; bacitracin]

**Neo-Medrol Acetate** liquid (discontinued 1993) ℞ *topical corticosteroid; antibiotic* [methylprednisolone acetate; neomycin sulfate] 0.25%•0.5%, 1%•0.5%

**neo-mercazole** [see: carbimazole]

**Neomixin** ointment OTC *topical antibiotic* [polymyxin B sulfate; neomycin sulfate; bacitracin zinc] 5000 U•3.5 mg•400 U per g ② neomycin

**neomycin** INN, BAN *antibacterial* [also: neomycin palmitate] ② Neomixin

**neomycin B** [see: framycetin]

**neomycin palmitate** USAN *antibacterial* [also: neomycin]

**neomycin sulfate** USP *aminoglycoside antibacterial antibiotic* 500 mg oral; 3.5 mg/g topical

**neomycin undecenoate** [see: neomycin undecylenate]

**neomycin undecylenate** USAN *antibacterial; antifungal*

**neon** *element (Ne)*

**Neopap** suppositories OTC *analgesic; antipyretic* [acetaminophen] 125 mg

**neopenyl** [see: clemizole penicillin]

**neoquate** [see: nequinate]

**Neoquess** IM injection (discontinued 1994) ℞ *gastrointestinal antispasmodic* [dicyclomine HCl] 10 mg/mL

**Neoquess** tablets (discontinued 1994) ℞ *gastrointestinal antispasmodic* [hyoscyamine sulfate] 0.125 mg

**Neoral** soft gelatin capsules for microemulsion, oral solution for microemulsion ℞ *immunosuppressant for allogenic*

kidney, liver, and heart transplants [cyclosporine] 25, 100 mg; 100 mg/mL

**NeoRespin** timed-release capsules OTC *bronchodilator for bronchial asthma and bronchospasm* [ephedrine HCl]

**Neosar** powder for IV injection ℞ *nitrogen mustard-type alkylating antineoplastic for multiple leukemias, lymphomas, blastomas, sarcomas and organ cancers* [cyclophosphamide] 100 mg

**Neosporin** cream OTC *topical antibiotic* [polymyxin B sulfate; neomycin sulfate] 10 000 U•3.5 mg per g

**Neosporin** Drop Dose (eye drops) ℞ *ophthalmic antibiotic* [polymyxin B sulfate; neomycin sulfate; gramicidin] 10 000 U•1.75 mg•0.025 mg per mL

**Neosporin** ointment OTC *topical antibiotic* [polymyxin B sulfate; neomycin sulfate; bacitracin] 5000 U•3.5 mg•400 U, 10 000 U•3.5 mg•500 U per g

**Neosporin** ophthalmic ointment ℞ *ophthalmic antibiotic* [polymyxin B sulfate; neomycin sulfate; bacitracin zinc] 10 000 U•3.5 mg•400 U per g

**Neosporin G.U. Irrigant** solution ℞ *bactericidal* [neomycin sulfate; polymyxin B sulfate] 40 mg•200 000 U per mL

**Neosporin Plus** cream OTC *topical antibiotic; anesthetic* [polymyxin B sulfate; neomycin; lidocaine] 10 000 U•3.5 mg•40 mg per g

**Neosporin Plus** ointment OTC *topical antibiotic; anesthetic* [polymyxin B sulfate; bacitracin zinc; neomycin; lidocaine] 10 000 U•500 U•3.5 mg•40 mg per g

**neostigmine** BAN *cholinergic muscle stimulant* [also: neostigmine bromide]

**neostigmine bromide** USP, INN, BAN *cholinergic muscle stimulant* [also: neostigmine] 15 mg oral

**neostigmine methylsulfate** USP *anticholinesterase muscle stimulant; cholinergic urinary stimulant* 1:1000 (1 mg/mL), 1:2000 (0.5 mg/mL) injection

**Neostrata AHA for Age Spots and Skin Lightening** gel OTC *hyperpigmentation bleaching agent; sunscreen* [hydroquinone; glycolic acid] 2%• ±

**Neo-Synalar** cream (discontinued 1995) ℞ *topical corticosteroid; antibacterial* [fluocinolone acetonide; neomycin sulfate] 0.025%•0.5%

**Neo-Synephrine** eye drops, viscous solution ℞ *ophthalmic decongestant/ vasoconstrictor; mydriatic* [phenylephrine HCl] 2.5%, 10%; 10%

**Neo-Synephrine** nasal spray, nose drops OTC *nasal decongestant* [phenylephrine HCl] 0.25%, 0.5%, 1%; 0.125%, 0.25%, 0.5%, 1%

**Neo-Synephrine 12 Hour** nasal spray OTC *nasal decongestant* [oxymetazoline HCl] 0.05%

**Neo-Synephrine** IV, IM, or subcu injection ℞ *vasopressor for hypotensive or cardiac shock* [phenylephrine HCl] 1% (10 mg/mL)

**Neo-Tabs** tablets ℞ *aminoglycoside-type antibiotic* [neomycin sulfate] 500 mg

**Neotal** ophthalmic ointment (discontinued 1995) ℞ *ophthalmic antibiotic* [polymyxin B sulfate; neomycin sulfate; bacitracin zinc] 5000 U•5 mg•400 U per g

**Neothylline** tablets (discontinued 1996) ℞ *bronchodilator* [dyphylline] 200, 400 mg

**Neothylline-GG** tablets (discontinued 1995) ℞ *antiasthmatic; bronchodilator; expectorant* [dyphylline; guaifenesin] 200•200 mg

**Neotrace-4** IV injection ℞ *intravenous nutritional therapy* [multiple trace elements (metals)]

**Neotricin HC** ophthalmic ointment ℞ *ophthalmic topical corticosteroidal anti-inflammatory; antibiotic* [hydrocortisone acetate; neomycin sulfate; bacitracin zinc; polymyxin B sulfate] 1%•3.5%•400 U/g•10 000 U/g

**Neovastat** ℞ *investigational (Phase III) antineoplastic/angiogenesis inhibitor for lung, prostate, and breast cancers*

**Nephplex Rx** tablets ℞ *vitamin supplement* [multiple B vitamins; ascorbic acid; folic acid; biotin] ±•60• 1•0.3 mg

**NephrAmine 5.4%** IV infusion ℞ *nutritional therapy for renal failure*

[multiple essential amino acids; electrolytes]

**Nephrobiss** ℞ *investigational atrial natriuretic peptide to prevent renal failure after heart transplant* [urodilatin]

**Nephro-Calci** tablets OTC *calcium supplement* [calcium carbonate] 1.5 g

**Nephrocaps** capsules ℞ *vitamin supplement* [multiple B vitamins; vitamin C; folic acid; biotin] ± • 100 mg • 1 mg • 150 μg

**Nephro-Derm** cream (discontinued 1996) OTC *moisturizer; emollient; antipruritic; counterirritant* [camphor; menthol]

**Nephro-Fer** tablets OTC *hematinic* [ferrous fumarate] 350 mg

**Nephro-Fer Rx** film-coated tablets ℞ *hematinic* [ferrous fumarate; folic acid] 106.9 • 1 mg

**Nephron** solution for inhalation OTC *bronchodilator for bronchial asthma* [racepinephrine] 2.25%

**Nephron FA** tablets (name changed to Nephplex Rx in 1995; reintroduced with a different formulation in 1996—see below)

**Nephron FA** tablets ℞ *hematinic* [ferrous fumarate; multiple B vitamins; ascorbic acid; folic acid; biotin; docusate sodium] 66.6 • ± • 40 • 1 • 0.3 • 75 mg

**Nephro-Vite Rx** film-coated tablets ℞ *vitamin supplement* [multiple B vitamins; vitamin C; folic acid; biotin] ± • 60 mg • 1 mg • 300 μg

**Nephro-Vite Rx + Fe** film-coated tablets ℞ *hematinic* [ferrous fumarate; multiple B vitamins; ascorbic acid; folic acid; biotin] 100 • ± • 60 • 1 • 0.3 mg

**Nephro-Vite Vitamin B Complex and C Supplement** tablets OTC *vitamin supplement* [multiple B vitamins; vitamin C; folic acid; biotin] ± • 60 • 0.8 • 0.3 mg

**Nephrox** oral suspension OTC *antacid; laxative* [aluminum hydroxide; mineral oil 10%] 320 mg/5 mL

**Nepro** oral liquid OTC *enteral nutritional therapy for acute or chronic renal failure* [lactose-free formula] 240 mL

**neptamustine** INN *antineoplastic* [also: pentamustine]

**Neptazane** tablets ℞ *carbonic anhydrase inhibitor; diuretic* [methazolamide] 25, 50 mg

**neptunium** *element (Np)*

**nequinate** USAN, INN *coccidiostat for poultry* [also: methyl benzoquate]

**neraminol** INN

**nerbacadol** INN

**nerelimomab** USAN *monoclonal antibody; investigational (Phase III) cytokine modulator for septic shock*

**neridronic acid** INN

**nerve growth factor (NGF)** *investigational agent for chemotherapy-induced peripheral neuropathy*

**nerve growth factor receptor antagonist** *investigational treatment for degenerative CNS disorders*

**Nervine Nighttime Sleep-Aid** tablets (name changed to Miles Nervine in 1993)

**Nervocaine 1%** injection ℞ *injectable local anesthetic* [lidocaine HCl] 1%

**Nervocaine 2%** injection (discontinued 1995) ℞ *injectable local anesthetic* [lidocaine HCl] 2%

**Nesacaine; Nesacaine MPF** injection ℞ *injectable local anesthetic* [chloroprocaine HCl] 1%, 2%; 2%, 3%

**nesapidil** INN

**nesosteine** INN

**Nestabs** tablets OTC *vitamin/calcium/iron supplement* [multiple vitamins; calcium; ferrous fumarate; folic acid] ± • 200 • 36 • 0.8 mg

**Nestabs FA** tablets ℞ *vitamin/calcium/iron supplement* [multiple vitamins; calcium; ferrous fumarate; folic acid] ± • 200 • 36 • 1 mg

**Nestrex** tablets OTC *vitamin supplement* [pyridoxine HCl] 25 mg

**nethalide** [see: pronetalol]

**netilmicin** INN, BAN *aminoglycoside bactericidal antibiotic* [also: netilmicin sulfate]

**netilmicin sulfate** USAN, USP *aminoglycoside bactericidal antibiotic* [also: netilmicin]

**netobimin** USAN, INN, BAN *veterinary anthelmintic*

**netrafilcon A** USAN *hydrophilic contact lens material*

**Netromicina** (Mexican name for U.S. product Netromycin)

**Netromycin** IV or IM injection ℞ *aminoglycoside-type antibiotic* [netilmicin sulfate] 100 mg/mL

**NEU differentiation factor** *investigational treatment for breast cancer*

**Neucef** ℞ *investigational cephalosporin antibiotic* [cefodizime]

**Neumega** ℞ *investigational (orphan) prophylaxis for thrombocytopenia related to chemotherapy or radiation* [oprelvekin]

**Neupogen** IV or subcu injection ℞ *investigational (orphan) for severe chronic neutropenia and myelodysplastic syndrome; investigational (Phase III, orphan) cytokine for CMV retinitis of AIDS* [filgrastim] 300 μg/mL

**Neuprex** ℞ *investigational (Phase III) agent for sepsis, hemorrhagic shock, and meningococcemia* [rBPI-21]

**Neuralgon** (name changed to Lioresal upon marketing release in 1996)

**Neuramate** tablets ℞ *anxiolytic* [meprobamate] 400 mg

**NeuRecover-DA; NeuRecover-LT; NeuRecover-SA** capsules OTC *dietary supplement* [multiple vitamins, minerals, and amino acids; folic acid] ≛•0.067 mg; ≛•0.03 mg; ≛•0.067 mg

**Neurelan** *investigational (orphan) for multiple sclerosis* [fampridine]

**NeuroCRIB** ℞ *investigational treatment for Alzheimer's and Parkinson's diseases* [cellular implants]

**Neurodep** injection OTC *parenteral vitamin therapy* [multiple B vitamins; vitamin C] ≛•50 mg/mL

**Neurodep-Caps** capsules OTC *vitamin supplement* [vitamins B$_1$, B$_6$, and B$_{12}$] 125•125•1 mg

**Neurogard** ℞ *investigational stroke treatment* [dizocilpine]

**Neurolite** injection ℞ *imaging aid for SPECT brain scans* [technetium Tc 99m bicisate]

**Neuromax** ℞ *investigational muscle relaxant* [doxacurium]

**Neurontin** capsules ℞ *anticonvulsant; investigational (orphan) for amyotrophic lateral sclerosis* [gabapentin] 100, 300, 400 mg

**neurosin** [see: calcium glycerophosphate]

**NeuroSlim** capsules OTC *dietary supplement* [multiple vitamins, minerals, and amino acids; folic acid; biotin] ≛•0.066•0.05 mg

**neurotrophic growth factor** [see: methionyl neurotrophic factor]

**neurotrophin-1** *investigational (orphan) for motor neuron disease and amyotrophic lateral sclerosis*

**neurotrophin-2** *investigational treatment for amyotrophic lateral sclerosis*

**neurotrophin-3** *investigational agent for treating peripheral neuropathies*

**neustab** [see: thioacetazone; thiacetazone]

**Neut** IV or subcu injection ℞ *pH buffer for metabolic acidosis; urinary alkalinizer* [sodium bicarbonate] 4% (0.48 mEq/mL)

**neutral acriflavine** [see: acriflavine]

**neutral insulin** INN, BAN *antidiabetic* [also: insulin, neutral]

**neutramycin** USAN, INN *antibacterial*

**Neutra-Phos** capsules (discontinued 1994) OTC *phosphorus supplement* [monobasic sodium phosphate; monobasic potassium phosphate; dibasic sodium phosphate; dibasic potassium phosphate] 250 mg (P)

**Neutra-Phos** powder OTC *phosphorus supplement* [monobasic sodium phosphate; monobasic potassium phosphate; dibasic sodium phosphate; dibasic potassium phosphate] 250 mg/packet (P)

**Neutra-Phos-K** capsules (discontinued 1994) OTC *phosphorus supplement* [monobasic potassium phosphate; dibasic potassium phosphate] 250 mg (P)

**Neutra-Phos-K** powder OTC *phosphorus supplement* [monobasic potassium phosphate; dibasic potassium phosphate] 250 mg/packet (P)

**NeuTrexin** powder for IV injection ℞ *antineoplastic for AIDS-related Pneu-*

*mocystis carinii pneumonia (orphan); investigational (orphan) for multiple other cancers* [trimetrexate glucuronate] 25 mg

**neutroflavine** [see: acriflavine]

**Neutrogena Acne Mask** OTC *topical keratolytic cleansing mask for acne* [benzoyl peroxide] 5%

**Neutrogena Antiseptic Cleanser for Acne-Prone Skin** liquid OTC *topical cleanser for acne* [benzethonium chloride]

**Neutrogena Body** lotion, oil OTC *moisturizer; emollient*

**Neutrogena Drying** gel OTC *topical astringent and antiseptic for acne* [hamamelis water; isopropyl alcohol]

**Neutrogena Moisture** lotion OTC *moisturizer; emollient*

**Neutrogena Non-Drying Cleansing** lotion OTC *soap-free therapeutic skin cleanser*

**Neutrogena Norwegian Formula Hand** cream OTC *moisturizer; emollient*

**Neutrogena Oil-Free Acne Wash** liquid OTC *topical keratolytic cleanser for acne* [salicylic acid] 2%

**Neutrogena Soap; Neutrogena Cleansing for Acne-Prone Skin; Neutrogena Baby Cleansing Formula Soap; Neutrogena Dry Skin Soap; Neutrogena Oily Skin Soap** bar OTC *therapeutic skin cleanser*

**Neutrogena T/Derm** oil OTC *topical antipsoriatic; antiseborrheic* [coal tar] 5%

**Neutrogena T/Gel** shampoo, conditioner OTC *antiseborrheic; antipsoriatic; antipruritic; antibacterial* [coal tar] 2%; 1.5%

**Neutrogena T/Sal** shampoo OTC *antiseborrheic; antipsoriatic; antipruritic; antibacterial* [salicylic acid; coal tar] 2%•2%

**nevirapine** USAN, INN *antiviral; nonnucleoside reverse transcriptase inhibitor (NNRTI) for HIV-1*

**new acid** *street drug slang* [see: PCP]

**New Decongest** syrup (discontinued 1993) R *decongestant; antihistamine* [phenylpropanolamine HCl; phenyl-

ephrine HCl; chlorpheniramine maleate; phenyltoloxamine citrate]

**New Decongest Pediatric** syrup, drops (name changed to Tri-Phen-Mine in 1995)

**New Decongestant** sustained-release tablets (discontinued 1993) R *decongestant; antihistamine* [phenylpropanolamine HCl; phenylephrine HCl; chlorpheniramine maleate; phenyltoloxamine citrate]

**New Jack Swing** *street drug slang for a combination of heroin and morphine* [see: heroin; morphine]

**new magic** *street drug slang* [see: PCP]

**new-estranol 1** [see: diethylstilbestrol]

**new-oestranol 1** [see: diethylstilbestrol]

**new-oestranol 11** [see: diethylstilbestrol dipropionate]

**NewPaks** (trademarked delivery form) *ready-to-use closed system containers*

**New-Skin** liquid, spray OTC *skin protectant; antiseptic* [hydroxyquinoline]

**nexeridine** INN *analgesic* [also: nexeridine HCl]

**nexeridine HCl** USAN *analgesic* [also: nexeridine]

**NFL (Novantrone, fluorouracil, leucovorin [rescue])** *chemotherapy protocol*

**NG-29** *investigational (orphan) diagnostic aid for pituitary release of growth hormone*

**NGD 91-1** *investigational anxiolytic*

**NGF (nerve growth factor)** [q.v.]

**N.G.T.** cream R *topical corticosteroid; antifungal* [triamcinolone acetonide; nystatin] 0.1%•100 000 U per g

**Nia-Bid** sustained-action capsules OTC *vitamin supplement* [niacin] 400 mg

**Niac** timed-release capsules (discontinued 1994) OTC *vitamin supplement* [niacin] 300 mg

**Niacels** timed-release capsules (discontinued 1997) OTC *vitamin supplement* [niacin] 400 mg

**niacin** USP *vitamin $B_3$; vasodilator; antihyperlipidemic* [also: nicotinic acid] 25, 50, 100, 125, 250, 500 mg oral; 100 mg/mL injection ② Minocin

**niacinamide** USP *vitamin B₃; enzyme cofactor* [also: nicotinamide] 50, 100, 125, 250, 500 mg oral

**niacinamide hydroiodide** *expectorant*

**Niacor** immediate-release tablets ℞ *antihyperlipidemic* [niacin] 500 mg

**nialamide** NF, INN

**niaprazine** INN

**Niaspan** extended-release tablets ℞ *vasodilator; antihyperlipidemic; vitamin B₃* [niacin] 375, 500, 750, 1000 mg

**Niazide** tablets (discontinued 1993) ℞ *diuretic; antihypertensive* [trichlormethiazide]

**nibroxane** USAN, INN *topical antimicrobial*

**Nicabate** (European name for U.S. product Nicoderm)

**nicafenine** INN

**nicainoprol** INN

**nicametate** INN, BAN

**nicaraven** INN

**nicarbazin** BAN

**nicardipine** INN, BAN *vasodilator; calcium channel blocker* [also: nicardipine HCl]

**nicardipine HCl** USAN *vasodilator; calcium channel blocker* [also: nicardipine] 20, 30 mg oral

**NicCheck I** reagent strips *in vitro diagnostic aid for urine nicotine, used to determine the smoking status of the subject*

**NicCheck II** reagent strips *investigational in vitro diagnostic aid for urine nicotine, used to determine exposure to passive cigarette smoke*

**N'Ice** throat spray OTC *topical antipruritic/counterirritant; mild local anesthetic* [menthol] 0.12%

**N'Ice; N'Ice 'n Clear** lozenges OTC *topical antipruritic/counterirritant; mild local anesthetic* [menthol] 5 mg

**nice and easy** *street drug slang* [see: heroin]

**N'Ice Vitamin C Drops** (lozenges) OTC *vitamin supplement* [ascorbic acid; menthol; sorbitol] 60 mg

**NicErase-SL** ℞ *investigational (Phase III) treatment for nicotine withdrawal; clinical trials discontinued 1997* [lobeline sulfate]

**nicergoline** USAN, INN *vasodilator*

**niceritrol** INN, BAN

**nicethamide** BAN [also: nikethamide]

**niceverine** INN

**nickel** *element (Ni)*

**nickel desk** *street drug slang* [see: heroin]

**Niclocide** chewable tablets (discontinued 1995) ℞ *anthelmintic for cestodiasis (tapeworm)* [niclosamide] 500 mg

**niclofolan** INN, BAN

**niclosamide** USAN, INN *anthelmintic for cestodiasis (tapeworm)*

**Nico-400** timed-release capsules OTC *vitamin supplement* [niacin] 400 mg

**Nicobid** Tempules (timed-release capsules) OTC *niacin therapy* [niacin] 125, 250, 500 mg ⊡ Nitro-Bid

**nicoboxil** INN

**nicoclonate** INN

**nicocodine** INN, BAN

**nicocortonide** INN

**Nicoderm** transdermal patch ℞ *smoking deterrent; nicotine withdrawal aid* [nicotine] 36, 78, 114 mg

**Nicoderm CQ** transdermal patch OTC *smoking deterrent; nicotine withdrawal aid* [nicotine] 7, 14, 21 mg/day

**Nicoderm HP** transdermal patch ℞ *investigational high-potency form* [nicotine]

**nicodicodine** INN, BAN

**nicoduozide (isoniazid + nicothiazone)**

**nicofibrate** INN

**nicofuranose** INN

**nicofurate** INN

**nicogrelate** INN

**Nicolar** tablets ℞ *niacin therapy; antihyperlipidemic* [niacin] 500 mg

**nicomol** INN

**nicomorphine** INN, BAN

**nicopholine** INN

**nicorandil** USAN, INN *coronary vasodilator*

**Nicorette** chewing pieces OTC *smoking deterrent; nicotine withdrawal aid* [nicotine polacrilex] 2 mg

**Nicorette** nasal spray, inhaler, throat pastilles *investigational delivery forms* [nicotine]

**Nicorette DS** chewing pieces ℞ *smoking deterrent; nicotine withdrawal aid* [nicotine polacrilex] 4 mg

**nicothiazone** INN

**nicotinaldehyde thiosemicarbazone** [see: nicothiazone]

**nicotinamide** INN, BAN, JAN *vitamin B₃; enzyme cofactor* [also: niacinamide]

**nicotinamide-adenine dinucleotide (NAD)** [now: nadide]

**nicotine** *a very poisonous alkaloid used as an insecticide and external parasiticide; the principal drug in tobacco* [also see: tobacco]

**nicotine & mecamylamine HCl** *investigational (Phase III) transdermal patch for smoking cessation*

**nicotine OT** *investigational (Phase II) oral transmucosal form for smoking cessation*

**nicotine polacrilex** USAN *smoking deterrent; nicotine withdrawal aid*

**nicotine resin complex** [see: nicotine polacrilex]

**Nicotinex** elixir OTC *vitamin supplement* [niacin] 50 mg/5 mL

**nicotinic acid** INN, BAN, JAN *vitamin B₃; vasodilator; antihyperlipidemic* [also: niacin]

**nicotinic acid amide** [see: niacinamide]

**nicotinic acid 1-oxide** [see: oxiniacic acid]

**nicotinohydroxamic acid** [see: nicoxamat]

**6-nicotinoyl dihydrocodeine** [see: nicodicodine]

**6-nicotinoylcodeine** [see: nicocodine]

**4-nicotinoylmorpholine** [see: nicopholine]

**nicotinyl alcohol** USAN, BAN *peripheral vasodilator*

**nicotinyl tartrate**

**Nicotrol** transdermal patch OTC *smoking deterrent; nicotine withdrawal aid* [nicotine] 15 mg

**Nicotrol** transdermal patch ℞ *smoking deterrent; nicotine withdrawal aid; investigational treatment for ulcerative colitis* [nicotine] 8.3, 16.6, 24.9 mg

**Nicotrol NS** nasal spray, oral inhaler ℞ *smoking deterrent; nicotine withdrawal aid* [nicotine] 0.5 mg/spray

**nicotylamide** [see: niacinamide]

**nicoumalone** BAN [also: acenocoumarol]

**Nico-Vert** capsules (discontinued 1995) ℞ *anticholinergic; antiemetic; antivertigo agent; motion sickness preventative* [meclizine] 30, 50 mg

**nicoxamat** INN

**nictiazem** INN

**nictindole** INN

**nidroxyzone** INN

**Nidryl** elixir (discontinued 1996) OTC *antihistamine; antitussive* [diphenhydramine HCl] 12.5 mg/5 mL

**nie; nigh** *street drug slang* [see: nitrous oxide]

**niebla** (Spanish for "fog" or "haze") *street drug slang* [see: PCP]

**nifedipine** USAN, USP, INN, BAN *coronary vasodilator; calcium channel blocker; investigational (orphan) for interstitial cystitis* 10, 20 mg oral

**nifenalol** INN

**nifenazone** INN, BAN

**Niferex** film-coated tablets, elixir OTC *hematinic* [polysaccharide-iron complex] 50 mg; 100 mg/5 mL

**Niferex Forte** elixir (discontinued 1996) ℞ *hematinic* [polysaccharide-iron complex; cyanocobalamin; folic acid] 300 mg•75 μg•3 mg per 15 mL

**Niferex with Vitamin C** chewable tablets OTC *hematinic* [polysaccharide-iron complex; ascorbic acid; sodium ascorbate] 50•100•169 mg

**Niferex-150** capsules OTC *hematinic* [polysaccharide-iron complex] 150 mg

**Niferex-150 Forte** capsules ℞ *hematinic* [polysaccharide-iron complex; cyanocobalamin; folic acid] 150 mg•25 μg•1 mg

**Niferex-PN** film-coated tablets ℞ *prenatal vitamin/iron supplement* [polysaccharide-iron complex; multiple vitamins and minerals; folic acid] 60• ± •1 mg

**Niferex-PN Forte** film-coated tablets ℞ *prenatal vitamin/mineral/calcium/ iron supplement* [multiple vitamins & minerals; calcium; polysaccharide-iron complex; folic acid] ± •250• 60•1 mg

**niflumic acid** INN
**nifluridide** USAN *ectoparasiticide*
**nifungin** USAN, INN
**nifuradene** USAN, INN *antibacterial*
**nifuralazine** [see: furalazine]
**nifuraldezone** USAN, INN *antibacterial*
**nifuralide** INN
**nifuramizone** [see: nifurethazone]
**nifuratel** USAN, INN *antibacterial; antifungal; antiprotozoal (Trichomonas)*
**nifuratrone** USAN, INN *antibacterial*
**nifurazolidone** [see: furazolidone]
**nifurdazil** USAN, INN *antibacterial*
**nifurethazone** INN
**nifurfoline** INN
**nifurhydrazone** [see: nihydrazone]
**nifurimide** USAN, INN *antibacterial*
**nifurizone** INN
**nifurmazole** INN
**nifurmerone** USAN, INN *antifungal*
**nifuroquine** INN
**nifuroxazide** INN
**nifuroxime** NF, INN
**nifurpipone (NP)** INN
**nifurpirinol** USAN, INN *antibacterial*
**nifurprazine** INN
**nifurquinazol** USAN, INN *antibacterial*
**nifursemizone** USAN, INN *antiprotozoal for poultry (Histomonas)*
**nifursol** USAN, INN *antiprotozoal for poultry (Histomonas)*
**nifurthiazole** USAN, INN *antibacterial*
**nifurthiline** [see: thiofuradene]
**nifurtimox** INN, BAN *investigational anti-infective for Chagas disease (available only from Centers for Disease Control and Prevention)*
**nifurtoinol** INN
**nifurvidine** INN
**nifurzide** INN
**Night-Time Effervescent Cold** tablets for oral solution OTC *decongestant; antihistamine; analgesic; antipyretic* [phenylpropanolamine HCl; diphenhydramine citrate; aspirin] 15•38.33•325 mg
**niguldipine** INN
**nihydrazone** INN
**nikethamide** NF, INN [also: nicethamide]
**Nilandron** tablets ℞ *antiandrogen antineoplastic adjunct to surgical or chemical castration for metastatic prostate cancer* [nilutamide] 50 mg
**nileprost** INN
**nilestriol** INN *estrogen* [also: nylestriol]
**nilprazole** INN
**Nilstat** cream, ointment ℞ *topical antifungal* [nystatin] 100 000 U/g ☒ Nitrostat; nystatin
**Nilstat** film-coated tablets ℞ *systemic antifungal* [nystatin] 500 000 U
**Nilstat** oral suspension, powder for oral suspension ℞ *antifungal; oral candidiasis treatment* [nystatin] 100 000 U/mL; 150 million, 500 million, 1 billion, 2 billion U
**Nilstat** vaginal tablets (discontinued 1993) ℞ *topical antifungal* [nystatin]
**niludipine** INN
**nilutamide** USAN, INN, BAN *antiandrogen antineoplastic adjunct to surgical or chemical castration for metastatic prostate cancer*
**nilvadipine** USAN, INN, JAN *calcium channel antagonist*
**nimazone** USAN, INN *anti-inflammatory*
**Nimbex** IV infusion ℞ *nondepolarizing neuromuscular blocking agent for anesthesia* [cisatracurium besylate] 2, 10 mg/mL
**nimbies** *street drug slang* [see: Nembutal Sodium; pentobarbital sodium]
**Nimbus; Nimbus Quick Strip** test kit for home use OTC *in vitro diagnostic aid for urine pregnancy test* [monoclonal antibody-based enzyme immunoassay]
**Nimbus Plus** test kit for professional use *in vitro diagnostic aid for urine pregnancy test*
**nimesulide** INN, BAN
**nimetazepam** INN
**nimidane** USAN, INN *veterinary acaricide*
**nimodipine** USAN, INN, BAN *vasodilator; calcium channel blocker; investigational Alzheimer's treatment*
**nimorazole** INN, BAN
**Nimotop** soft liquid-filled capsules ℞ *calcium channel blocker for subarachnoid hemorrhage; investigational Alzheimer's treatment* [nimodipine] 30 mg
**nimustine** INN
**niobium** *element (Nb)*

**niometacin** INN

**Nion B Plus C** caplets OTC *vitamin supplement* [multiple B vitamins; vitamin C] ± • 300 mg

**Nipent** powder for IV injection R *antibiotic antineoplastic for hairy cell and chronic lymphocytic leukemias (orphan)* [pentostatin] 10 mg

**niperotidine** INN

**nipradilol** INN

**niprofazone** INN

**niridazole** USAN, INN *antischistosomal*

**nisbuterol** INN *bronchodilator* [also: nisbuterol mesylate]

**nisbuterol mesylate** USAN *bronchodilator* [also: nisbuterol]

**nisobamate** USAN, INN *minor tranquilizer*

**nisoldipine** USAN, INN, BAN, JAN *coronary vasodilator; calcium channel blocker for hypertension*

**nisoxetine** USAN, INN *antidepressant*

**nisterime** INN *androgen* [also: nisterime acetate]

**nisterime acetate** USAN *androgen* [also: nisterime]

**nitarsone** USAN, INN *antiprotozoal (Histomonas)*

**nitazoxanide (NTZ)** INN *investigational (Phase II, orphan) anti-infective for AIDS-related cryptosporidiosis*

**Nite Time Cold Formula** liquid OTC *antitussive; decongestant; antihistamine; analgesic* [dextromethorphan hydrobromide; pseudoephedrine HCl; doxylamine succinate; acetaminophen; alcohol 25%] 5 • 10 • 1.25 • 167 mg/5 mL

**NiteLite** OTC *investigational cough/cold medication*

**nithiamide** USAN *veterinary antibacterial* [also: aminitrozole; acinitrazole]

**nitracrine** INN

**nitrafudam** INN *antidepressant* [also: nitrafudam HCl]

**nitrafudam HCl** USAN *antidepressant* [also: nitrafudam]

**nitralamine HCl** USAN *antifungal*

**nitramisole** INN *anthelmintic* [also: nitramisole HCl]

**nitramisole HCl** USAN *anthelmintic* [also: nitramisole]

**nitraquazone** INN

**nitrates** *a class of antianginal agents that cause the relaxation of vascular smooth muscles*

**nitratophenylmercury** [see: phenylmercuric nitrate]

**nitrazepam** USAN, INN, BAN, JAN *anticonvulsant; hypnotic*

**Nitrazine** paper for professional use *in vitro diagnostic aid for urine pH determination*

**nitre, sweet spirit of** [see: ethyl nitrite]

**nitrefazole** INN, BAN

**Nitrek** transdermal patch R *antianginal* [nitroglycerin] 22.4, 44.8, 67.2 mg

**nitrendipine** USAN, INN, BAN, JAN *antihypertensive; calcium channel blocker*

**nitric acid** NF *acidifying agent*

**nitric oxide** *investigational (orphan) for neonatal persistent pulmonary hypertension and adult acute respiratory distress syndrome*

**nitricholine perchlorate** INN

**nitro; nitrogen** *street drug slang* [see: nitrous oxide]

**9-nitro-20-(S)-camptothecin (9-NC)** *investigational (orphan) for pancreatic cancer*

***p*-nitrobenzenearsonic acid** [see: nitarsone]

**Nitro-Bid** ointment R *antianginal* [nitroglycerin] 2% (15 mg/inch) ☑ Nicobid

**Nitro-Bid** Plateau Caps (controlled-release capsules) (discontinued 1996) R *antianginal* [nitroglycerin] 2.5, 6.5, 9 mg ☑ Nicobid

**Nitro-Bid IV** infusion R *antianginal; perioperative antihypertensive; for congestive heart failure with myocardial infarction* [nitroglycerin] 5 mg/mL

**Nitrocine** Timecaps (timed-release capsules) (discontinued 1996) R *antianginal* [nitroglycerin] 2.5, 6.5, 9 mg

**Nitrocine** transdermal patch (discontinued 1995) R *antianginal* [nitroglycerin] 187.5 mg

**nitroclofene** INN

**nitrocycline** USAN, INN *antibacterial*

**nitrodan** USAN, INN *anthelmintic*

**Nitro-Derm** transdermal patch R *antianginal* [nitroglycerin] 160 mg

**Nitrodisc** transdermal patch ℞ *antianginal* [nitroglycerin] 16, 24, 32 mg

**Nitro-Dur** transdermal patch ℞ *antianginal* [nitroglycerin] 20, 40, 60, 80, 120, 160 mg

**nitroethanolamine** [see: aminoethyl nitrate]

**Nitrofan** capsules ℞ *urinary bacteriostatic* [nitrofurantoin] 50, 100 mg

**nitrofuradoxadone** [see: furmethoxadone]

**nitrofural** INN *broad-spectrum bactericidal; adjunct to burn treatment* [also: nitrofurazone]

**nitrofurantoin** USP, INN *urinary bacteriostatic* 50, 100 mg oral

**nitrofurantoin sodium**

**nitrofurazone** USP, BAN *broad-spectrum bactericidal; adjunct to burn treatment* [also: nitrofural] 0.2% topical

**nitrofurmethone** [see: furaltadone]

**nitrofuroxizone** [see: nidroxyzone]

**Nitrogard** transmucosal extended-release tablets *antianginal* [nitroglycerin] 1, 2, 3 mg

**nitrogen (N$_2$)** NF *air displacement agent; element (N)*

**nitrogen monoxide** [see: nitrous oxide]

**nitrogen mustard N-oxide HCl** JAN *alkylating antineoplastic* [also: mechlorethamine HCl; chlormethine; mustine]

**nitrogen mustards** *a class of alkylating antineoplastics*

**nitrogen oxide (N$_2$O)** [see: nitrous oxide]

**nitroglycerin** USP *coronary vasodilator; antianginal* [also: glyceryl trinitrate] 2.5, 6.5, 9 mg oral; 5 mg/mL injection; 16–187.5 mg transdermal; 2% topical ② Nitroglyn

**Nitroglyn** extended-release capsules ℞ *antianginal* [nitroglycerin] 2.5, 6.5, 9, 13 mg ② nitroglycerin

**nitrohydroxyquinoline** [see: nitroxoline]

**Nitrol** ointment, Appli-Kit (ointment & adhesive dosage covers) ℞ *antianginal* [nitroglycerin] 2% (15 mg/inch)

**Nitrolan** liquid OTC *enteral nutritional therapy* [lactose-free formula]

**Nitrolingual Spray** lingual aerosol ℞ *antianginal* [nitroglycerin] 0.4 mg/spray

**nitromannitol** [see: mannitol hexanitrate]

**nitromersol** USP *topical anti-infective*

**nitromide** USAN *coccidiostat for poultry; antibacterial*

**nitromifene** INN

**nitromifene citrate** USAN *antiestrogen*

**Nitrong** sustained-release tablets ℞ *antianginal* [nitroglycerin] 2.6, 6.5, 9 mg

**Nitropress** powder for IV injection, flip-top vials ℞ *emergency antihypertensive* [sodium nitroprusside] 50 mg/dose

**nitroprusside sodium** [see: sodium nitroprusside]

**nitroscanate** USAN, INN *veterinary anthelmintic*

**nitrosoureas** *a class of alkylating antineoplastics*

**Nitrostat** sublingual tablets ℞ *antianginal* [nitroglycerin] 0.3, 0.4, 0.6 mg

**nitrosulfathiazole** INN [also: paranitrosulfathiazole]

**Nitro-Time** extended-release capsules ℞ *antianginal* [nitroglycerin] 2.5, 6.5, 9 mg

**nitrous acid, sodium salt** [see: sodium nitrite]

**nitrous oxide (N$_2$O)** USP *a weak inhalation general anesthetic; sometimes abused as a street drug to create a dreamy or floating sensation*

**nitroxinil** INN

**nitroxoline** INN, BAN

**nivacortol** INN *glucocorticoid* [also: nivazol]

**nivadipine** [see: nilvadipine]

**nivaquine** [see: chloroquine phosphate]

**nivazol** USAN *glucocorticoid* [also: nivacortol]

**Nivea After Tan; Nivea Moisturizing; Nivea Moisturizing Extra Enriched** lotion OTC *moisturizer; emollient*

**Nivea Moisturizing; Nivea Skin** oil OTC *moisturizer; emollient*

**Nivea Moisturizing Creme Soap** bar OTC *therapeutic skin cleanser*

**Nivea Ultra Moisturizing Creme** OTC *moisturizer; emollient*

**nivimedone sodium** USAN *antiallergic*

**Nix** creme rinse (discontinued 1993) OTC *pediculicide; scabicide* [permethrin; alcohol 20%] 1%

**Nixon** *street drug slang for low-potency heroin* [see: heroin]

**nixylic acid** INN

**nizatidine** USAN, USP, INN, BAN, JAN *treatment of gastric and duodenal ulcers; histamine $H_2$ antagonist*

**nizofenone** INN

**Nizoral** cream, shampoo ℞ *topical antifungal* [ketoconazole] 2%

**Nizoral** tablets ℞ *systemic antifungal; orphan status withdrawn 1996* [ketoconazole] 200 mg

**NMA (N-monomethyl arginine)** [q.v.]

**N-Multistix; N-Multistix SG** reagent strips *in vitro diagnostic aid for multiple urine products*

**NNRTIs (non-nucleoside reverse transcriptase inhibitors)** [q.v.]

**no more burn; no more ouchies** spray (discontinued 1995) OTC *topical local anesthetic; antiseptic* [lidocaine HCl; benzethonium chloride] 2.3%•0.13%

**no more germies** soap (discontinued 1995) OTC *antiseptic; disinfectant* [triclosan] 0.25%

**no more germies** towelettes (discontinued 1995) OTC *antiseptic wipes* [benzalkonium chloride]

**no more itchies** spray (discontinued 1995) OTC *topical corticosteroid* [hydrocortisone] 1%

**No Pain-HP** roll-on OTC *topical analgesic* [capsaicin] 0.075%

**nobelium** *element (No)*

**noberastine** USAN, INN, BAN *antihistamine*

**nocloprost** INN

**nocodazole** USAN, INN *antineoplastic*

**NōDōz** chewable tablets OTC *CNS stimulant; analeptic* [caffeine] 100 mg

**nofecainide** INN

**nofetumomab merpentan** *monoclonal antibody imaging agent for small cell lung cancer*

**nogalamycin** USAN, INN *antineoplastic*

**noggin** *investigational neurotrophic factor for neurologic diseases*

**No-Hist** capsules ℞ *nasal decongestant* [phenylephrine HCl; phenylpropanolamine HCl; pseudoephedrine HCl] 5•40•40 mg

**noise** *street drug slang* [see: heroin]

**Nolahist** tablets OTC *antihistamine* [phenindamine tartrate] 25 mg

**Nolamine** timed-release tablets ℞ *decongestant; antihistamine* [phenylpropanolamine HCl; chlorpheniramine maleate; phenindamine tartrate] 50•4•24 mg

**Nolex LA** long-acting tablets (name changed to Exgest LA in 1994)

**nolinium bromide** USAN, INN *antisecretory; antiulcerative*

**Noludar 300** capsules (discontinued 1993) ℞ *sedative; hypnotic* [methyprylon] 300 mg

**Nolvadex** tablets ℞ *antiestrogen antineoplastic for advanced postmenopausal breast cancer* [tamoxifen citrate] 10, 20 mg

**nomegestrol** INN

**nomelidine** INN

**nomifensine** INN *antidepressant* [also: nomifensine maleate]

**nomifensine maleate** USAN *antidepressant* [also: nomifensine]

**nonabine** INN, BAN

**nonabsorbable surgical suture** [see: suture, nonabsorbable surgical]

**nonachlazine** [now: azaclorzine HCl]

**nonanedioic acid** [see: azelaic acid]

**nonaperone** INN

**nonapyrimine** INN

**nonathymulin** INN

**nondestearinated cod liver oil** [see: cod liver oil, nondestearinated]

**nonivamide** INN

**non-nucleoside reverse transcriptase inhibitors (NNRTIs)** *a class of antivirals that inhibit HIV replication* [reverse transcriptase is also known as DNA polymerase]

**nonoxinol 4** INN *surfactant* [also: nonoxynol 4]

**nonoxinol 9** INN *wetting and solubilizing agent; spermaticide* [also: nonoxynol 9]

**nonoxinol 15** INN *surfactant* [also: nonoxynol 15]

**nonoxinol 30** INN *surfactant* [also: nonoxynol 30]

**nonoxynol 4** USAN *surfactant* [also: nonoxinol 4]

**nonoxynol 9** USAN, USP *wetting and solubilizing agent; spermicide* [also: nonoxinol 9]

**nonoxynol 10** NF *surfactant*

**nonoxynol 15** USAN *surfactant* [also: nonoxinol 15]

**nonoxynol 30** USAN *surfactant* [also: nonoxinol 30]

**nonsteroidal anti-inflammatory drugs (NSAIDs)** *a class of anti-inflammatory drugs that have analgesic and antipyretic effects*

**nonylphenoxypolyethoxyethanol** [see: nonoxynol 4, 9, 15, & 30]

**Nootropic** ℞ *investigational treatment for Alzheimer's disease* [oxiracetam]

**Nootropil** ℞ *cognition adjuvant; investigational (orphan) for myoclonus* [piracetam]

**noracymethadol** INN *analgesic* [also: noracymethadol HCl]

**noracymethadol HCl** USAN *analgesic* [also: noracymethadol]

**Noradex** tablets (discontinued 1993) ℞ *skeletal muscle relaxant* [orphenadrine citrate]

**noradrenaline bitartrate** [see: norepinephrine bitartrate]

**Noralac** chewable tablets OTC *antacid* [calcium carbonate; magnesium carbonate; bismuth subnitrate]

**noramidopyrine methanesulfonate sodium** [see: dipyrone]

**norandrostenolone phenylpropionate** [see: nandrolone phenpropionate]

**norastemizole** *investigational antihistamine for allergy*

**norbolethone** USAN *anabolic* [also: norboletone]

**norboletone** INN *anabolic* [also: norbolethone]

**norbudrine** INN [also: norbutrine]

**norbutrine** BAN [also: norbudrine]

**Norcept-E 1/35** tablets (discontinued 1994) ℞ *monophasic oral contraceptive* [norethindrone; ethinyl estradiol] 1 mg•35 μg

**Norcet** capsules (discontinued 1995) ℞ *narcotic analgesic* [hydrocodone bitartrate; acetaminophen] 5•500 mg

**norclostebol** INN

**Norco** tablets ℞ *narcotic analgesic* [hydrocodone bitartrate; acetaminophen] 10•325 mg

**norcodeine** INN, BAN

**Norcuron** powder for IV injection ℞ *nondepolarizing neuromuscular blocker; adjunct to anesthesia* [vecuronium bromide] 10, 20 mg/vial

**norcycline** [see: sancycline]

**nordazepam** INN

**nordefrin HCl** NF

**Nordette** tablets ℞ *monophasic oral contraceptive; emergency "morning after" contraceptive* [levonorgestrel; ethinyl estradiol] 0.15 mg•30 μg

**Nordiate** ℞ *investigational treatment for hemophilia* [antihemophilic factor]

**Nordimmun** ℞ *investigational antibody replacement therapy for immunologic thrombocytic disorders* [immunoglobulin]

**nordinone** INN

**Norditropin** powder for subcu injection ℞ *growth hormone for congenital or renal-induced growth failure (orphan); investigational (orphan) for severe burns* [somatropin] 4, 8 mg (12, 24 IU) per vial

**Norel** capsules ℞ *decongestant; expectorant* [phenylephrine HCl; phenylpropanolamine HCl; guaifenesin] 5•45•200 mg

**Norel Plus** capsules ℞ *decongestant; antihistamine; analgesic* [phenylpropanolamine HCl; chlorpheniramine maleate; phenyltoloxamine dihydrogen citrate; acetaminophen] 25•4•25•325 mg

**norephedrine HCl** [see: phenylpropanolamine HCl]

**norepinephrine** INN *adrenergic; vasoconstrictor; vasopressor for shock* [also: norepinephrine bitartrate]

**norepinephrine bitartrate** USAN, USP *adrenergic; vasoconstrictor; vasopressor for acute hypotensive shock* [also: norepinephrine]

**norethandrolone** NF, INN

**Norethin 1/35E** tablets ℞ *monophasic oral contraceptive* [norethindrone; ethinyl estradiol] 1 mg•35 μg

**Norethin 1/50M** tablets ℞ *monophasic oral contraceptive* [norethindrone; mestranol] 1 mg•50 μg

**norethindrone** USP *progestin for amenorrhea, abnormal uterine bleeding, and endometriosis* [also: norethisterone]

**norethindrone acetate** USP *progestin for amenorrhea, abnormal uterine bleeding, and endometriosis*

**norethisterone** INN, BAN, JAN *progestin* [also: norethindrone]

**norethynodrel** USAN, USP *progestin* [also: noretynodrel]

**noretynodrel** INN *progestin* [also: norethynodrel]

**noreximide** INN

**norfenefrine** INN

**Norflex** sustained-release tablets, IV or IM injection ℞ *skeletal muscle relaxant* [orphenadrine citrate] 100 mg; 30 mg/mL

**norfloxacin** USAN, USP, INN, BAN, JAN *broad-spectrum bactericidal antibiotic*

**norfloxacin succinil** INN

**norflurane** USAN, INN *inhalation anesthetic*

**Norforms** powder OTC *absorbs vaginal moisture; astringent* [cornstarch; zinc oxide]

**Norforms** vaginal suppositories OTC *feminine deodorant*

**Norgesic; Norgesic Forte** tablets ℞ *skeletal muscle relaxant; analgesic* [orphenadrine citrate; aspirin; caffeine] 25•385•30 mg; 50•770•60 mg

**norgesterone** INN

**norgestimate** USAN, INN, BAN *progestin*

**Norgestimate/EE** ℞ *investigational cyclophasic oral contraceptive*

**norgestomet** USAN, INN *progestin*

**norgestrel** USAN, USP, INN *progestin*

**d-norgestrel** *(incorrect enantiomer designation)* [now: levonorgestrel]

**D-norgestrel** [see: levonorgestrel]

**norgestrienone** INN

**Norinyl 1 + 35** tablets ℞ *monophasic oral contraceptive* [norethindrone; ethinyl estradiol] 1 mg•35 μg ⊡ Nardil

**Norinyl 1 + 50** tablets ℞ *monophasic oral contraceptive* [norethindrone; mestranol] 1 mg•50 μg

**Norisodrine** Aerotrol (inhalation aerosol) ℞ *bronchodilator* [isoproterenol HCl]

**Norisodrine with Calcium Iodide** syrup ℞ *bronchodilator; expectorant* [isoproterenol sulfate; calcium iodide; alcohol 6%] 3•150 mg

**Norlac Rx** tablets (discontinued 1995) ℞ *vitamin/mineral/calcium/iron supplement* [multiple vitamins & minerals; calcium; iron; folic acid] ± •200•60•1 mg

**Norlestrin 1/50** tablets (discontinued 1993) ℞ *monophasic oral contraceptive* [norethindrone acetate; ethinyl estradiol] 1 mg•50 μg

**Norlestrin 21 2.5/50** tablets (discontinued 1994) ℞ *monophasic oral contraceptive* [norethindrone acetate; ethinyl estradiol] 2.5 mg•50 μg

**Norlestrin Fe 1/50; Norlestrin Fe 2.5/50** tablets (discontinued 1994) ℞ *monophasic oral contraceptive* [norethindrone acetate; ethinyl estradiol; ferrous fumarate] 1 mg•50 μg•75 mg

**norletimol** INN

**norleusactide** INN [also: pentacosactride]

**norlevorphanol** INN, BAN

**norlupinanes** *a class of antibiotics* [also called: quinolizidines]

**Norlutate** tablets (discontinued 1995) ℞ *progestin for amenorrhea, abnormal uterine bleeding, or endometriosis* [norethindrone acetate] 5 mg ⊡ Norlutin

**Norlutin** tablets (discontinued 1995) ℞ *progestin for amenorrhea, abnormal uterine bleeding, or endometriosis* [norethindrone] 5 mg ⊡ Norlutate

**½ normal saline (½ NS; 0.45% sodium chloride)** *electrolyte replacement*

**normal saline (NS; 0.9% sodium chloride)** *electrolyte replacement* [also: saline solution]

**normal serum albumin** [see: albumin, human]

**normethadone** INN, BAN

**normethandrolone** [see: normethandrone]

**normethandrone**

**normethisterone** [see: normethandrone]

**Normiflo** deep subcu injection ℞ *low molecular weight heparin-type anticoagulant for prevention of deep vein thrombosis (DVT) following knee surgery* [ardeparin sodium] 5000, 10 000 anti-Xa U/0.5 mL

**Normodyne** film-coated tablets, IV infusion ℞ *antihypertensive; alpha- and beta-adrenergic blocking agent* [labetalol HCl] 100, 200, 300 mg; 5 mg/mL

**normorphine** INN, BAN

**Normosang** ℞ *investigational (orphan) for acute symptomatic porphyria and myelodysplastic syndrome* [heme arginate]

**Normosol-M and 5% Dextrose; Normosol-R and 5% Dextrose** IV infusion ℞ *intravenous nutritional/ electrolyte therapy* [combined electrolyte solution; dextrose]

**Normosol-R; Normosol-R pH 7.4** IV infusion ℞ *intravenous electrolyte therapy* [combined electrolyte solution]

**Normozide** film-coated tablets (discontinued 1994) ℞ *antihypertensive* [labetalol HCl; hydrochlorothiazide] 100•25, 200•25, 300•25 mg

**Normylin** ℞ *investigational antidiabetic* [AC 137 (code name—generic name not yet approved)]

**Noroxin** film-coated tablets ℞ *broad-spectrum fluoroquinolone-type antibiotic* [norfloxacin] 400 mg

**Norpace** capsules ℞ *antiarrhythmic* [disopyramide phosphate] 100, 150 mg

**Norpace CR** controlled-release capsules ℞ *antiarrhythmic* [disopyramide phosphate] 100, 500 mg

**norpipanone** INN, BAN

**Norplant** implantable Silastic capsules ℞ *implant contraceptive system* [levonorgestrel] 36 mg

**Norplant II** ℞ *investigational implant contraceptive system* [levonorgestrel]

**Norpramin** film-coated tablets ℞ *tricyclic antidepressant* [desipramine HCl] 10, 25, 50, 75, 100, 150 mg ☒ imipramine

**norpseudoephedrine** [see: cathine]

**Nor-Q.D.** tablets ℞ *oral contraceptive (progestin only)* [norethindrone] 0.35 mg

**nortestosterone phenylpropionate** [see: nandrolone phenpropionate]

**Nor-Tet** capsules ℞ *broad-spectrum antibiotic* [tetracycline HCl] 250, 500 mg

**nortetrazepam** INN

**nortriptyline HCl** USAN, USP, INN *tricyclic antidepressant* [10, 25, 50, 75 mg oral] ☒ amitriptyline

**Norvasc** tablets ℞ *antianginal; antihypertensive; calcium channel blocker* [amlodipine] 2.5, 5, 10 mg

**norvinisterone** INN

**norvinodrel** [see: norgesterone]

**Norvir** capsules, oral solution ℞ *antiviral protease inhibitor for HIV* [ritonavir] 100 mg; 80 mg/mL

**Norwich** tablets OTC *analgesic; antipyretic; anti-inflammatory; antirheumatic* [aspirin] 325, 500 mg

**Norzine** IM injection, suppositories, tablets ℞ *antiemetic* [thiethylperazine maleate] 5 mg/mL; 10 mg; 10 mg

**NoSalt; NoSalt Seasoned** (discontinued 1997) OTC *salt substitute* [potassium chloride] 64 mEq/5 g; 34 mEq/5 g

**nosantine** INN, BAN

**noscapine** USP, INN *antitussive*

**noscapine HCl** NF

**nose** *street drug slang* [see: heroin]

**nose candy; nose powder; nose stuff** *street drug slang* [see: cocaine]

**nose drops** *street drug slang for liquefied heroin* [see: heroin]

**nosiheptide** USAN, INN *veterinary growth stimulant*

**Nōstril; Children's Nōstril** nasal spray OTC *nasal decongestant* [phenylephrine HCl] 0.5%; 0.25%

**Nōstrilla** nasal spray OTC *nasal decongestant* [oxymetazoline HCl] 0.05%

**notensil maleate** [see: acepromazine]

**Novacet** lotion ℞ *topical acne treat-ment* [sodium sulfacetamide; sulfur] 10%•5%

**Nova-Dec** tablets OTC *vitamin/mineral/iron supplement* [multiple vitamins & minerals; iron; folic acid; biotin] ± • 30 mg•0.4 mg•30 μg

**Novafed** timed-release capsules (dis-continued 1996) ℞ *nasal decongestant* [pseudoephedrine HCl] 120 mg

**Novafed A** sustained-release capsules ℞ *decongestant; antihistamine* [pseu-doephedrine HCl; chlorpheniramine maleate] 120•8 mg

**Novagest Expectorant with Codeine** liquid ℞ *narcotic antitussive; decongestant; expectorant* [codeine phosphate; pseudoephed-rine HCl; guaifenesin; alcohol 1.4%] 10•30•100 mg/5 mL

**Novahistine** elixir (discontinued 1997) OTC *decongestant; antihistamine* [phenylephrine HCl; chlorphenir-amine maleate] 5•2 mg/5 mL

**Novahistine DH** liquid (discontinued 1997) ℞ *narcotic antitussive; decongestant; antihistamine* [codeine phos-phate; pseudoephedrine HCl; chlor-pheniramine maleate; alcohol 5%] 10•30•2 mg/5 mL

**Novahistine DMX** liquid (discontin-ued 1997) OTC *antitussive; decongestant; expectorant* [dextromethorphan hydrobromide; pseudoephedrine HCl; guaifenesin; alcohol 10%] 10• 30•100 mg/5 mL

**Novahistine Expectorant** liquid (dis-continued 1997) ℞ *narcotic antitussive; decongestant; expectorant* [codeine phosphate; pseudoephed-rine HCl; guaifenesin; alcohol 7.5%] 10•30•100 mg/5 mL

**novamidon** [see: aminopyrine]

**Novamine; Novamine 15%** IV infu-sion ℞ *total parenteral nutrition; periph-eral parenteral nutrition* [multiple essen-tial and nonessential amino acids]

**Novantrone** IV injection ℞ *antibiotic antineoplastic for prostate cancer or acute myelogenous (nonlymphocytic) leukemia (orphan)* [mitoxantrone HCl] 2 mg/mL

**Novapren** ℞ *investigational (Phase I) antiviral for HIV*

**Novastan** injection ℞ *investigational (Phase III) thrombin inhibitor for hepa-rin-induced thrombocytopenia (HIT) and thrombosis; investigational (Phase II) for myocardial infarction* [argatroban]

**novel plasminogen activator (NPA)** *investigational treatment for heart attack and blood clotting disor-ders; modified tPA*

**novobiocin** INN, BAN *bacteriostatic antibiotic* [also: novobiocin calcium]

**novobiocin calcium** USP *bacteriostatic antibiotic* [also: novobiocin]

**novobiocin sodium** USP *bacteriostatic antibiotic*

**Novocain** injection ℞ *injectable local anesthetic* [procaine HCl] 1%, 2%, 10%

**Novo-Gemfibrozil** ⒸⒶⓃ (U.S. product: Lopid) tablets ℞ *antihyperlipidemic for hypertriglyceridemia and coronary heart disease* [gemfibrozil] 600 mg

**Novolin 70/30** subcu injection OTC *antidiabetic* [isophane human insulin (rDNA); human insulin (rDNA)] 100 U/mL

**Novolin 70/30 PenFill** NovoPen car-tridge OTC *antidiabetic* [isophane human insulin (rDNA); human insulin (rDNA)] 150 U/1.5 mL

**Novolin 70/30 Prefilled** syringes OTC *antidiabetic* [isophane human insulin (rDNA); human insulin (rDNA)] 150 U/1.5 mL

**Novolin ge 30/70** ⒸⒶⓃ (U.S. product: Novolin 70/30) vials for subcu injec-tion, prefilled cartridges OTC *antidia-betic* [insulin; isophane insulin] 100 U/mL; 1.5, 3 mL

**Novolin ge 50/50** ⒸⒶⓃ (U.S. product: Novolin 50/50) prefilled cartridges OTC *antidiabetic* [insulin; isophane insulin] 300 U/3 mL

**Novolin ge Lente** ⒸⒶⓃ (U.S. product: Novolin L) vials for subcu injection, prefilled cartridges OTC *antidiabetic* [insulin zinc] 100 U/mL; 3 mL

**Novolin ge NPH** ⒸⒶⓃ (U.S. product: Novolin N) vials for subcu injec-tion, prefilled cartridges OTC *antidia-*

*betic* [isophane insulin] 100 U/mL; 1.5, 3 mL

**Novolin ge Toronto** Ⓒ (U.S. product: Novolin R) vials for subcu injection, prefilled cartridges OTC *antidiabetic* [insulin] 100 U/mL; 1.5, 3 mL

**Novolin ge Ultralente** Ⓒ (U.S. product: Humulin U Ultralente) vials for subcu injection, prefilled cartridges OTC *antidiabetic* [insulin zinc] 100 U/mL; 1.5 mL

**Novolin L** subcu injection OTC *antidiabetic* [human insulin zinc (rDNA)] 100 U/mL

**Novolin N** subcu injection OTC *antidiabetic* [isophane human insulin (rDNA)] 100 U/mL

**Novolin N PenFill** NovoPen cartridge OTC *antidiabetic* [isophane human insulin (rDNA)] 150 U/1.5 mL

**Novolin N Prefilled** syringes OTC *antidiabetic* [isophane human insulin (rDNA)] 150 U/1.5 mL

**Novolin R** subcu injection OTC *antidiabetic* [human insulin (rDNA)] 100 U/mL

**Novolin R PenFill** NovoPen cartridges OTC *antidiabetic* [human insulin (rDNA)] 150 U/1.5 mL

**Novolin R Prefilled** syringes OTC *antidiabetic* [human insulin (rDNA)] 150 U/1.5 mL

**NovoNorm** ℞ *investigational antidiabetic agent; stimulates pancreatic insulin production*

**NovoPen 1.5** prefilled reusable syringe *uses Novolin PenFill cartridges and NovoFine 30-gauge disposable needles* [insulin (several types available)] 1–40 U/injection

**NovoSeven** ℞ *investigational antihemophilic* [recombinant factor VIIa]

**Novo-Timol** Ⓒ (U.S. product: Timoptic) eye drops ℞ *antiglaucoma agent (β-blocker)* [timolol maleate] 0.25%, 0.5%

**NOVP (Novantrone, Oncovin, vinblastine, prednisone)** *chemotherapy protocol*

**noxiptiline** INN [also: noxiptyline]
**noxiptyline** BAN [also: noxiptiline]
**noxythiolin** BAN [also: noxytiolin]
**noxytiolin** INN [also: noxythiolin]

**NP (nifurpipone)** [q.v.]

**NP-27** solution, powder, spray powder, cream OTC *topical antifungal* [tolnaftate] 1%

**NPA (novel plasminogen activator)** [q.v.]

**NPH (neutral protamine Hagedorn) insulin** [see: insulin, isophane]

**NPH Iletin I** subcu injection OTC *antidiabetic* [isophane insulin (beef-pork)] 100 U/mL

**NPH Iletin I (beef)** subcu injection (discontinued 1994) OTC *antidiabetic* [isophane insulin]

**NPH Iletin I (pork)** subcu injection (discontinued 1994) OTC *antidiabetic* [isophane insulin]

**NPH Iletin II (beef)** subcu injection (discontinued 1994) OTC *antidiabetic* [isophane insulin]

**NPH Iletin II (pork)** subcu injection OTC *antidiabetic* [isophane insulin] 100 U/mL

**NPH Insulin** subcu injection (discontinued 1997) OTC *antidiabetic* [isophane insulin (beef)] 100 U/mL

**NPH Purified Pork Isophane Insulin** subcu injection (name changed to NPH-N in 1994)

**NPH-N** subcu injection OTC *antidiabetic* [isophane insulin (pork)] 100 U/mL

**NR-LU-10-PE** *investigational diagnostic aid for small cell lung cancer*

**NS (normal saline)** [q.v.]

**NSAIDs (nonsteroidal anti-inflammatory drugs)** [q.v.]

**NTBC** *investigational (orphan) for tyrosinemia type I*

**NTS** transdermal patches ℞ *antianginal* [nitroglycerin]

**NTZ (nitazoxanide)** [q.v.]

**NTZ Long Acting** nasal spray, nose drops OTC *nasal decongestant* [oxymetazoline HCl] 0.05%

**Nubain** IV, subcu or IM injection ℞ *narcotic agonist-antagonist analgesic* [nalbuphine HCl] 10, 20 mg/mL

**nubs** *street drug slang* [see: mescaline]
**nuclomedone** INN
**nuclotixene** INN
**Nucofed** capsules, syrup ℞ *narcotic antitussive; decongestant* [codeine

phosphate; pseudoephedrine HCl] 20•60 mg; 20•60 mg/5 mL

**Nucofed Expectorant; Nucofed Pediatric Expectorant** syrup R *narcotic antitussive; decongestant; expectorant* [codeine phosphate; pseudoephedrine HCl; guaifenesin; alcohol 12.5%•6%] 20•60•200 mg/5 mL; 10•30•100 mg/5 mL

**Nucotuss Expectorant; Nucotuss Pediatric Expectorant** liquid *narcotic antitussive; decongestant; expectorant* [codeine phosphate; pseudoephedrine HCl; guaifenesin; alcohol 12.5%•6%] 20•60•200 mg/5 mL; 10•30•100 mg/5 mL

**nufenoxole** USAN, INN *antiperistaltic*

**nuggets** *street drug slang* [see: amphetamines; cocaine, crack]

**Nu-Iron** elixir OTC *hematinic* [polysaccharide-iron complex] 100 mg/5 mL

**Nu-Iron 150** capsules OTC *hematinic* [polysaccharide-iron complex] 150 mg

**Nu-Iron Plus** elixir R *hematinic* [polysaccharide iron complex; cyanocobalamin; folic acid] 300 mg•75 μg• 3 mg per 15 mL

**Nu-Iron V** film-coated tablets R *vitamin/iron supplement* [polysaccharide iron complex; multiple vitamins; folic acid] 60• ± •1 mg

**Nu-knit** (trademarked form) *oxidized cellulose hemostatic pad*

**Nulicaine** injection (discontinued 1995) R *injectable local anesthetic* [lidocaine HCl] 1%, 2%

**Nullo** tablets (discontinued 1996) OTC *vulnerary; fecal and urinary odor control* [chlorophyllin copper complex] 33.3 mg

**NuLytely** powder for oral solution R *pre-procedure bowel cleansing* [polyethylene glycol-electrolyte solution (plus electrolytes)] 105 g/L

**number** *street drug slang for a marijuana cigarette* [see: marijuana]

**number 3** *street drug slang* [see: cocaine; heroin]

**number 4; number 8** *street drug slang* [see: heroin]

**Numorphan** IV, IM, or subcu injection, suppositories R *narcotic analgesic; preoperative support of anesthesia; investigational (orphan) for intractable pain in narcotic-tolerant patients* [oxymorphone HCl] 1, 1.5 mg/mL; 5 mg

**Numzident** gel OTC *topical oral anesthetic* [benzocaine] 10%

**Numzit Teething** gel OTC *topical oral anesthetic* [benzocaine] 7.5%

**Numzit Teething** lotion OTC *topical oral anesthetic* [benzocaine; alcohol 12.1%] 0.2%

**Nupercainal** ointment, cream OTC *topical local anesthetic* [dibucaine] 1%; 0.5%

**Nupercainal** rectal suppositories OTC *emollient; astringent* [cocoa butter; zinc oxide] 2.1•0.25 g

**Nuprin** tablets, caplets OTC *nonsteroidal anti-inflammatory drug (NSAID); antiarthritic; analgesic* [ibuprofen] 200 mg

**Nuquin HP** cream, gel R *hyperpigmentation bleaching agent; sunscreen* [hydroquinone; dioxybenzone] 4%•30 mg

**Nuromax** IV injection R *nondepolarizing neuromuscular blocker; adjunct to anesthesia* [doxacurium chloride] 1 mg/mL

**Nursette** (trademarked form) *prefilled disposable bottle*

**Nursoy** liquid, powder (discontinued 1996) OTC *hypoallergenic infant food* [soy protein formula]

**Nu-Salt** OTC *salt substitute* [potassium chloride] 68 mEq/5 g

**Nu-Tears** eye drops OTC *ocular moisturizer/lubricant* [polyvinyl alcohol] 1.4%

**Nu-Tears II** eye drops OTC *ocular moisturizer/lubricant* [polyvinyl alcohol; polyethylene glycol 400] 1%•1%

**Nu-Timolol** ⓒ (U.S. product: Timoptic) eye drops R *antiglaucoma agent (β-blocker)* [timolol maleate] 0.25%, 0.5%

**nutmeg oil** NF

**Nutracort** cream R *topical corticosteroid* [hydrocortisone] 1%

**Nutracort** lotion (discontinued 1997) R *topical corticosteroid* [hydrocortisone] 1%

**Nutraderm** cream, lotion OTC *moisturizer; emollient*

**Nutraderm** OTC *lotion base*

**Nutraderm Bath Oil** OTC *bath emollient*

**Nutraloric** powder OTC *enteral nutritional therapy* [milk-based formula]

**Nutramigen** liquid, powder OTC *hypoallergenic infant food* [enzymatically hydrolyzed protein formula]

**Nutra-Plex** liquid (discontinued 1995) OTC *vitamin/mineral supplement* [multiple B vitamins & minerals; alcohol 13.5%]

**Nutraplus** cream, lotion OTC *moisturizer; emollient; keratolytic* [urea] 10%

**Nutra-Soothe** bath oil OTC *bath emollient* [colloidal oatmeal; light mineral oil]

**NutraTear** eye drops (discontinued 1994) OTC *ocular moisturizer/lubricant*

**Nutren 1.0** liquid OTC *enteral nutritional therapy* [lactose-free formula]

**Nutren 1.5** liquid OTC *enteral nutritional therapy* [lactose-free formula]

**Nutren 2.0** ready-to-use liquid OTC *enteral nutritional therapy* [lactose-free formula]

**Nutricon** tablets OTC *vitamin/mineral/calcium/iron supplement* [multiple vitamins & minerals; calcium; iron; folic acid; biotin] ≗•200•20•0.4•0.15 mg

**Nutrilan** ready-to-use liquid OTC *enteral nutritional therapy* [lactose-free formula]

**Nutrilyte; Nutrilyte II** IV admixture ℞ *intravenous electrolyte therapy* [combined electrolyte solution]

**Nutrineal Peritoneal Dialysis Solution with 1.1% Amino Acid** ℞ *investigational (orphan) nutritional supplement for continuous ambulatory peritoneal dialysis patients*

**Nutropin** powder for subcu injection ℞ *growth hormone for congenital or renal-induced growth failure and Turner syndrome (orphan); investigational (orphan) for severe burns* [somatropin] 5, 10 mg (13, 26 IU) per vial

**Nutropin AQ** subcu injection ℞ *growth hormone for congenital or renal-induced growth failure and Turner syndrome (orphan); investigational (orphan) for severe burns* [somatropin] 10 mg (30 IU) per vial

**Nutrox** capsules OTC *dietary supplement* [multiple vitamins, minerals, and amino acids] ≗

**nuvenzepine** INN

**nyctal** [see: carbromal]

**nydrane** [see: benzchlorpropamid]

**Nydrazid** IM injection ℞ *tuberculostatic* [isoniazid] 100 mg/mL

**nylestriol** USAN *estrogen* [also: nilestriol]

**nylidrin HCl** USP *peripheral vasodilator* [also: buphenine]

**Nyotran** ℞ *investigational (NDA filed) empiric systemic therapy for fungal infections* [nystatin liposomal]

**NyQuil Allergy/Head Cold, Children's** liquid (discontinued 1995) OTC *pediatric decongestant and antihistamine* [pseudoephedrine HCl; chlorpheniramine maleate] 10•0.67 mg/5 mL

**NyQuil Hot Therapy** powder for oral solution OTC *antitussive; decongestant; antihistamine; analgesic* [dextromethorphan hydrobromide; pseudoephedrine HCl; doxylamine succinate; acetaminophen] 30•60•12.5•1000 mg/packet

**NyQuil LiquiCaps** (liquid-filled capsules) OTC *antitussive; decongestant; antihistamine; analgesic* [dextromethorphan hydrobromide; pseudoephedrine HCl; doxylamine succinate; acetaminophen] 10•30•6.25•250 mg

**NyQuil Multisymptom Cold Flu Relief; NyQuilNighttime Cold/Flu Medicine** liquid OTC *antitussive; decongestant; antihistamine; analgesic* [dextromethorphan hydrobromide; pseudoephedrine HCl; doxylamine succinate; acetaminophen; alcohol 10%•25%] 5•10•2.1•167 mg/5 mL; 5•10•1.25•167 mg/5 mL

**NyQuil Nighttime Cough/Cold, Children's** liquid OTC *pediatric antitussive, decongestant, and antihistamine* [dextromethorphan hydrobromide; pseudoephedrine HCl; chlorpheniramine maleate] 5•10•0.67 mg/5 mL

**nystatin** USP, INN, BAN, JAN *polyene antifungal* 100 000, 500 000 U/mL oral; 100 000 mg vaginal; 100 000 U/g topical ② Nilstat; Nitrostat

**nystatin liposomal** *investigational (NDA filed) empiric systemic therapy for fungal infections*

**Nystatin-LF** (liposomal formulation) IV injection ℞ *investigational (Phase II) antiviral for HIV* [AR-121 (code name—generic name not yet approved)]

**Nystex** cream, ointment ℞ *topical antifungal* [nystatin] 100 000 U/g

**Nystex** oral suspension ℞ *antifungal; oral candidiasis treatment* [nystatin] 100 000 U/mL

**Nytcold Medicine** liquid OTC *antitussive; decongestant; antihistamine; analgesic* [dextromethorphan hydrobromide; pseudoephedrine HCl; doxylamine succinate; acetaminophen; alcohol 25%] 5•10•1.25• 167 mg/5 mL

**Nytol** tablets OTC *antihistaminic sleep aid* [diphenhydramine HCl] 25, 50 mg

**O; O.P.** *street drug slang* [see: opium]

**O₂ (oxygen)** [q.v.]

**OAP (Oncovin, ara-C, prednisone)** *chemotherapy protocol*

**oatmeal, colloidal** *demulcent*

**Obalan** tablets (discontinued 1996) ℞ *anorexiant* [phendimetrazine tartrate] 35 mg

**obecalp** *placebo (spelled backward)*

**Obe-nix** capsules ℞ *appetite suppressant* [phentermine HCl] 37.5 mg

**Obephen** capsules ℞ *anorexiant* [phentermine HCl] 30 mg

**Obetrol** tablets (name changed to Adderall in 1994)

**obidoxime chloride** USAN, INN *cholinesterase reactivator*

**Oby-Cap** capsules ℞ *anorexiant* [phentermine HCl] 30 mg

**O-Cal f.a.** tablets ℞ *vitamin/mineral/calcium/iron supplement and dental caries preventative* [multiple vitamins & minerals; calcium; iron; folic acid; sodium fluoride] ± •200•66•1•1.1 mg

**ocaperidone** USAN, INN, BAN *antipsychotic*

**Occlusal** liquid (discontinued 1994) OTC *topical keratolytic* [salicylic acid in polyacrylic vehicle] 17%

**Occlusal-HP** liquid OTC *topical keratolytic* [salicylic acid in polyacrylic vehicle] 17%

**Occucoat** ophthalmic solution ℞ *ophthalmic surgical aid* [hydroxypropyl methylcellulose] 2%

**Ocean Mist** nasal spray OTC *nasal moisturizer* [sodium chloride (saline)] 0.65%

**ocfentanil** INN *narcotic analgesic* [also: ocfentanil HCl]

**ocfentanil HCl** USAN *narcotic analgesic* [also: ocfentanil]

**ociltide** INN

**ocinaplon** USAN *anxiolytic*

**OCL** oral solution ℞ *pre-procedure bowel evacuant* [polyethylene glycol-electrolyte solution]

**ocrase** INN

**ocrilate** INN *tissue adhesive* [also: ocrylate]

**ocrylate** USAN *tissue adhesive* [also: ocrilate]

**octabenzone** USAN, INN *ultraviolet screen*

**octacaine** INN

**octacosactrin** BAN [also: tosactide]

**octadecafluorodecehydronaphthalene** [see: perflunafene]

**octadecanoic acid, calcium salt** [see: calcium stearate]

**octadecanoic acid, sodium salt** [see: sodium stearate]

**octadecanoic acid, zinc salt** [see: zinc stearate]

**1-octadecanol** [see: stearyl alcohol]
**9-octadecenylamine hydrofluoride** [see: dectaflur]
**octafonium chloride** INN
**Octamide PFS** IV or IM injection ℞ *antiemetic for chemotherapy; GI stimulant; peristaltic* [metoclopramide monohydrochloride monohydrate] 5 mg/mL
**octamoxin** INN
**octamylamine** INN
**octane** *street drug slang for PCP laced with gasoline* [see: PCP; petroleum distillate inhalants]
**octanoic acid** USAN, INN *antifungal*
**octapinol** INN
**octastine** INN
**octatropine methylbromide** INN, BAN *anticholinergic; peptic ulcer adjunct* [also: anisotropine methylbromide]
**octatropone bromide** [see: anisotropine methylbromide]
**octaverine** INN, BAN
**octazamide** USAN, INN *analgesic*
**octenidine** INN, BAN *topical anti-infective* [also: octenidine HCl]
**octenidine HCl** USAN *topical anti-infective* [also: octenidine]
**octenidine saccharin** USAN *dental plaque inhibitor*
**Octicare** ear drops, ear drop suspension ℞ *topical corticosteroidal anti-inflammatory; antibiotic* [hydrocortisone; neomycin sulfate; polymyxin B sulfate] 1%•5 mg•10 000 U per mL
**octicizer** USAN *plasticizer*
**octil** INN *combining name for radicals or groups*
**octimibate** INN
**octisamyl** [see: octamylamine]
**Octocaine HCl** injection ℞ *injectable local anesthetic* [lidocaine HCl; epinephrine] 2%•1:50 000, 2%• 1:100 000
**octoclothepine** [see: clorotepine]
**octocrilene** INN *ultraviolet screen* [also: octocrylene]
**octocrylene** USAN *ultraviolet screen* [also: octocrilene]
**octodecactide** [see: codactide]
**octodrine** USAN, INN *adrenergic; vasoconstrictor; local anesthetic*
**octopamine** INN

**octotiamine** INN
**octoxinol** INN *surfactant/wetting agent* [also: octoxynol 9]
**octoxynol 9** USAN, NF *surfactant/wetting agent; spermicide* [also: octoxinol]
**OctreoScan** powder for injection ℞ *parenteral radiopaque agent* [oxidronate sodium] 2 mg
**OctreoScan 111** ℞ *investigational tumor imaging agent for SPECT scans* [indium In 111 pentetreotide]
**octreotide** USAN, INN, BAN *gastric antisecretory*
**octreotide acetate** USAN *gastric antisecretory*
**octriptyline** INN *antidepressant* [also: octriptyline phosphate]
**octriptyline phosphate** USAN *antidepressant* [also: octriptyline]
**octrizole** USAN, INN *ultraviolet screen*
**S-octyl thiobenzoate** [see: tioctilate]
**octyl-2-cyanoacrylate** [see: ocrylate]
**octyldodecanol** NF *oleaginous vehicle*
**OcuCaps** caplets OTC *vitamin/mineral supplement* [vitamins A, C, and E; multiple minerals] 5000 IU•400 mg•182 mg• ≛
**Ocu-Carpine** eye drops (discontinued 1995) ℞ *antiglaucoma agent; direct-acting miotic* [pilocarpine HCl] 0.5%, 1%, 2%, 3%, 4%, 6%
**OcuClear** eye drops OTC *topical ocular decongestant/vasoconstrictor* [oxymetazoline HCl] 0.025%
**OcuClenz** solution, pads (discontinued 1996) OTC *eyelid cleanser for blepharitis or contact lenses*
**OcuCoat** prefilled syringe OTC *ophthalmic surgical aid* [hydroxypropyl methylcellulose] 2%
**OcuCoat; OcuCoat PF** eye drops OTC *ocular moisturizer/lubricant* [hydroxypropyl methylcellulose] 0.8%
**Ocudose** (trademarked delivery device) *single-use eye drop dispenser*
**Ocufen** eye drops ℞ *ocular nonsteroidal anti-inflammatory drug (NSAID); intraoperative miosis inhibitor* [flurbiprofen sodium] 0.03%
**ocufilcon A** USAN *hydrophilic contact lens material*

**ocufilcon B** USAN *hydrophilic contact lens material*

**ocufilcon C** USAN *hydrophilic contact lens material*

**ocufilcon D** USAN *hydrophilic contact lens material*

**Ocuflox** eye drops ℞ *ophthalmic quinolone-type antibiotic for corneal ulcers (orphan)* [ofloxacin] 3 mg/mL

**Oculinum** powder (name changed to Botox in 1993)

**Ocumeter** (trademarked delivery device) *prefilled eye drop dispenser*

**Ocupress** eye drops ℞ *topical antiglaucoma agent (β-blocker)* [carteolol HCl] 1%

**Ocusert Pilo-20; Ocusert Pilo-40** continuous-release ocular wafer ℞ *antiglaucoma agent; direct-acting miotic* [pilocarpine] 20 μg/hour; 40 μg/hour

**OCuSOFT** solution, pads OTC *eyelid cleanser for blepharitis or contact lenses*

**OCuSoft VMS** film-coated tablets OTC *vitamin/mineral supplement* [vitamins A, C, and E; multiple minerals] 5000 IU•60 mg•30 mg• ±

**Ocusulf-10** eye drops ℞ *ophthalmic bacteriostatic* [sulfacetamide sodium] 10%

**Ocutears** ⒸⒶⓃ eye drops OTC *ocular moisturizer/lubricant* [hydroxypropyl methylcellulose] 0.5%

**Ocutricin** eye drops (discontinued 1995) ℞ *ophthalmic antibiotic* [polymyxin B sulfate; neomycin sulfate; gramicidin] 10 000 U•1.75 mg•0.025 mg per mL

**Ocutricin** ophthalmic ointment ℞ *ophthalmic antibiotic* [polymyxin B sulfate; neomycin sulfate; bacitracin zinc] 10 000 U•3.5 mg•400 U per g

**Ocuvite** film-coated tablets OTC *vitamin/mineral supplement* [vitamins A, C, and E; multiple minerals] 5000 IU•60 mg•30 IU• ±

**Ocuvite Extra** tablets OTC *vitamin/mineral supplement* [vitamins A, C, and E; multiple minerals] 6000 IU•200 mg•50 IU• ±

**OCuZIN** tablets OTC *vitamin/mineral supplement* [vitamins A, C, and E; zinc; copper; selenium]

**Odor Free ArthriCare** [see: ArthriCare, Odor Free]

**Oesto-Mins** powder OTC *vitamin/mineral supplement* [vitamins C and D; calcium; magnesium; potassium] 500 mg•100 IU•250 mg•250 mg•45 mg per 4.5 g

**oestradiol** BAN *estrogen* [also: estradiol]

**oestradiol benzoate** BAN [also: estradiol benzoate]

**oestradiol valerate** BAN *estrogen* [also: estradiol valerate]

**Oestring** (Swedish name for U.S. product Estring)

**oestriol succinate** BAN *estrogen* [also: estriol; estriol succinate]

**oestrogenine** [see: diethylstilbestrol]

**oestromenin** [see: diethylstilbestrol]

**oestrone** BAN *estrogen* [also: estrone]

**Off-Ezy Corn & Callus Remover** kit (liquid + cushion pads) OTC *topical keratolytic* [salicylic acid in a collodion-like vehicle] 17%

**Off-Ezy Wart Remover** liquid OTC *topical keratolytic* [salicylic acid in a collodion-like vehicle] 17%

**O-Flex** IV or IM injection (discontinued 1993) ℞ *skeletal muscle relaxant* [orphenadrine citrate]

**ofloxacin** USAN, INN, BAN, JAN *broad-spectrum quinolone-type bactericidal antibiotic; topical corneal ulcer treatment (orphan)*

**ofornine** USAN, INN *antihypertensive*

**oftasceine** INN

**Ogen** tablets ℞ *hormone replacement therapy for postmenopausal disorders* [estrogen (from estropipate)] 0.625 (0.75), 1.25 (1.5), 2.5 (3) mg

**Ogen** vaginal cream ℞ *topical estrogen replacement for postmenopausal disorders* [estropipate] 1.5 mg/g

**ogoy** street drug slang [see: heroin]

**oidiomycin** *diagnostic aid for cell-mediated immunity; extract of the Oidiomycetes fungus family*

**oil** street drug slang for hashish oil, heroin, or PCP [see: hashish; heroin; PCP]

**oil of mustard** [see: allyl isothiocyanate]

**Oil of Olay Foaming Face Wash** liquid OTC *topical cleanser for acne*

**oil ricini** [see: castor oil]

**Oilatum Soap** bar OTC *therapeutic skin cleanser*

**ointment, hydrophilic** USP *ointment base; oil-in-water emulsion*

**ointment, white** USP *oleaginous ointment base*

**ointment, yellow** USP *ointment base*

**O.J.** *street drug slang* [see: marijuana]

**OK-B7** *investigational monoclonal antibody used for the treatment of lymphoma*

**olaflur** USAN, INN, BAN *dental caries prophylactic*

**olamine** USAN, INN *combining name for radicals or groups*

**olanzapine** USAN, INN *thienobenzodiazepine antipsychotic for schizophrenia and other psychotic disorders*

**olaquindox** INN, BAN

**Old Steve** *street drug slang* [see: heroin]

**old tuberculin (OT)** [see: tuberculin]

**oleandomycin** INN [also: oleandomycin phosphate]

**oleandomycin, triacetate ester** [see: troleandomycin]

**oleandomycin phosphate** NF [also: oleandomycin]

**oleic acid** NF *emulsion adjunct*

**oleic acid I 125** USAN *radioactive agent*

**oleic acid I 131** USAN *radioactive agent*

**oleovitamin A** [now: vitamin A]

**oleovitamin A & D** USP *source of vitamins A and D*

**oleovitamin D, synthetic** [now: ergocalciferol]

**olethytan 20** [see: polysorbate 80]

**oletimol** INN

**oleum caryophylii** [see: clove oil]

**oleum gossypii seminis** [see: cottonseed oil]

**oleum maydis** [see: corn oil]

**oleum ricini** [see: castor oil]

**oleyl alcohol** NF *emulsifying agent; emollient*

**oligomycin D** [see: rutamycin]

**olive oil** NF *pharmaceutic aid*

**olivomycin** INN

**olmidine** INN

**olopatadine** INN *antiallergic; antiasthmatic*

**olopatadine HCl** USAN *antiallergic; antiasthmatic; ophthalmic antihistamine*

**olpimedone** INN

**olsalazine** INN, BAN *GI anti-inflammatory* [also: olsalazine sodium]

**olsalazine sodium** USAN *GI anti-inflammatory; treatment of ulcerative colitis* [also: olsalazine]

**oltipraz** INN

**olvanil** USAN, INN *analgesic*

**OLX-102** *investigational adjuvant to chemotherapy in small-cell lung cancer*

**OM 401** *investigational (orphan) for sickle cell disease*

**OMAD (Oncovin, methotrexate/ citrovorum factor, Adriamycin, dactinomycin)** *chemotherapy protocol*

**omega-3 fatty acids** [see: doconexent; icosapent; omega-3 marine triglycerides]

**omega-3 fatty acids with all double bonds in the *cis* configuration** *investigational (orphan) preventative for organ graft rejection*

**omega-3 marine triglycerides** BAN [12% doconexent (q.v.) + 18% icosapent (q.v.)]

**omeprazole** USAN, INN, BAN, JAN *gastric acid antisecretory; proton pump inhibitor*

**omeprazole sodium** USAN *gastric antisecretory*

**omidoline** INN

**Omnicef** ℞ *investigational broad-spectrum cephalosporin antibiotic* [cefdinir]

**OmniHIB** powder for IM injection, prefilled syringes ℞ *Haemophilus influenzae type b (HIB) vaccine* [Hemophilus b conjugate vaccine; tetanus toxoid] 10•24 μg/0.5 mL

**OMNIhist L.A.** long-acting tablets ℞ *decongestant; antihistamine; anticholinergic* [phenylephrine HCl; chlorpheniramine maleate; methscopolamine nitrate] 20•8•2.5 mg

**Omnipaque** injection ℞ *parenteral radiopaque agent* [iohexol] 140, 180, 210, 240, 300, 350 mg/mL

**Omnipen** capsules ℞ *penicillin-type antibiotic* [ampicillin, anhydrous] 250, 500 mg ⚇ Unipen

**Omnipen** powder for oral suspension ℞ *penicillin-type antibiotic* [ampicillin trihydrate] 125, 250 mg/5 mL

**Omnipen-N** powder for IV or IM injection ℞ *penicillin-type antibiotic* [ampicillin sodium] 0.125, 0.25, 0.5, 1, 2, 10 g

**Omniscan** IV injection ℞ *magnetic resonance imaging agent for the central nervous system* [gadodiamide] 287 mg/mL

**omoconazole** INN *antifungal*

**omoconazole nitrate** USAN *antifungal*

**omonasteine** INN

**OMS Concentrate** drops ℞ *narcotic analgesic* [morphine sulfate] 20 mg/mL

**onapristone** INN *investigational antineoplastic for hormone-dependent cancers*

**Oncaspar** IV or IM injection ℞ *antineoplastic for acute lymphocytic leukemia (orphan) and acute lymphoblastic leukemia* [pegaspargase] 750 IU/mL

**Oncet** capsules ℞ *narcotic antitussive; analgesic* [hydrocodone bitartrate; acetaminophen] 5•500 mg

**Oncoject** ℞ *investigational antineoplastic*

**Oncolym** ℞ *investigational (Phase III) treatment for non-Hodgkin's B-cell lymphoma* [iodine I 131 Lym-1 MAb]

**Oncolysin B** ℞ *investigational (Phase III) antineoplastic for B-cell lymphoma, leukemia, AIDS lymphoma, and myeloma; clinical trials discontinued 1997* [anti-B4-blocked ricin MAb]

**Oncolysin CD6** ℞ *investigational treatment for cutaneous T-cell lymphoma* [CD6-blocked ricin]

**Oncolysin M** ℞ *investigational treatment for myeloid leukemias* [anti-My9-blocked ricin]

**Oncolysin S** ℞ *investigational antineoplastic for small cell lung cancer* [N901-blocked ricin]

**Onconase** ℞ *investigational (Phase III) treatment for pancreatic, breast, colorectal, prostate, and small cell lung cancers* [p30 protein]

**OncoPurge** ℞ *investigational antineoplastic for breast cancer* [*Pseudomonas* exotoxin monoclonal antibody]

**OncoRad GI103** ℞ *investigational antineoplastic for gastrointestinal cancer* [CYT-103-Y-90 (code name—generic name not yet approved)]

**OncoRad OV103** ℞ *investigational antineoplastic for colorectal cancer; investigational (orphan) for ovarian cancer* [CYT-103-Y-90 (code name—generic name not yet approved)]

**OncoRad-Prostate** ℞ *investigational antineoplastic for prostatic cancer* [CYT-356-Y-90 (code name—generic name not yet approved)]

**OncoScint CR372** ℞ *investigational imaging aid for colorectal cancer detection and staging* [CYT-372-In-111 (code name—generic name not yet approved)]

**OncoScint CR/OV** ℞ *investigational imaging aid for colorectal cancer; imaging aid for ovarian cancer (orphan)* [indium In 111 satumomab pendetide]

**OncoScint OV103** ℞ *orphan status withdrawn 1994* [indium In 111 murine MAb B72.3]

**OncoScint PR356** ℞ *investigational imaging aid for prostatic cancer detection and staging* [CYT-356-In-111 (code name—generic name not yet approved)]

**OncoScint-Breast** ℞ *investigational imaging aid for breast cancer detection and staging* [TC-CYT-380 (code name—generic name not yet approved)]

**OncoScint-NSC Lung** ℞ *investigational imaging aid for non-small cell lung cancer detection and staging* [TC-CYT-380 fragment (code name—generic name not yet approved)]

**OncoSpect** ℞ *investigational imaging aid for colon cancer* [monoclonal antibodies]

**Oncostate** ℞ *investigational (orphan) for renal cell carcinoma* [coumarin]

**OncoTher 130** ℞ *investigational treatment for breast and ovarian cancer* [aminopterin sodium]

**OncoTICE** (foreign name for U.S. product Tice BCG)

**OncoTrac** imaging kit ℞ *investigational (orphan) for diagnostic imaging agent for metastasis of malignant melanoma* [technetium Tc 99m antimelanoma murine MAb]

**OncoVax-P** ℞ *investigational (Phase I/II) antineoplastic for prostate cancer*

**Oncovin** IV injection, Hyporets (pre-filled syringes) ℞ *antineoplastic for lung and breast cancers, various leukemias, lymphomas, and sarcomas* [vincristine sulfate] 1 mg/mL ② Ancobon

**Oncovite** tablets OTC *vitamin supplement* [multiple vitamins] ±

**Oncozole** ℞ *investigational antineoplastic* [3-deazaguanine]

**ondansetron** INN, BAN 5-$HT_3$ *antiemetic for chemotherapy; antischizophrenic; anxiolytic; investigational Alzheimer's treatment* [also: ondansetron HCl]

**ondansetron HCl** USAN 5-$HT_3$ *antiemetic for chemotherapy; antischizophrenic; anxiolytic; investigational Alzheimer's treatment* [also: ondansetron]

**Ondrox** sustained-release tablets OTC *vitamin/mineral/calcium/iron supplement* [multiple vitamins, minerals and amino acids; calcium; iron; folic acid; biotin] ±•25•3•0.67•0.005 mg

**1 + 1-F Creme** ℞ *topical corticosteroid; antifungal; antibacterial; local anesthetic* [hydrocortisone; clioquinol; pramoxine] 1%•3%•1%

**1% HC** ointment ℞ *topical corticosteroid* [hydrocortisone] 1%

**One Step Midstream Pregnancy Test** stick for home use OTC *in vitro diagnostic aid for urine pregnancy test*

**One Touch** reagent strips for home use OTC *in vitro diagnostic aid for blood glucose*

**one way** *street drug slang* [see: LSD]

**1069C** *investigational antineoplastic*

**1370U** *investigational antidepressant*

**141W94** *investigational (Phase III) antiviral protease inhibitor for HIV and AIDS* [also: VX-478]

**142780** *investigational antiestrogen steroid for advanced breast cancer*

**One-A-Day 55 Plus** tablets OTC *geriatric vitamin/mineral supplement* [multiple vitamins and minerals; folic acid; biotin] ±•400•30 μg

**One-A-Day Essential** tablets OTC *vitamin supplement* [multiple vitamins; folic acid] ±•0.4 mg

**One-A-Day Extras Antioxidant** softgel capsules OTC *vitamin/mineral supplement* [vitamins A, C, and E;

multiple minerals] 5000 IU•250 mg•200 IU• ±

**One-A-Day Extras Vitamin C** tablets OTC *vitamin supplement* [vitamin C] 500 mg

**One-A-Day Extras Vitamin E** soft gel capsules OTC *vitamin supplement* [vitamin E] 400 IU

**One-A-Day Maximum Formula** tablets OTC *vitamin/mineral/iron supplement* [multiple vitamins & minerals; iron; folic acid; biotin] ±•18 mg•0.4 mg•30 μg

**One-A-Day Men's Vitamins** tablets OTC *vitamin supplement* [multiple vitamins; folic acid] ±•0.4 mg

**One-A-Day Plus Extra C** tablets (discontinued 1994) OTC *vitamin supplement* [multiple vitamins; folic acid] ±•0.4 mg

**One-A-Day Stressgard** tablets (discontinued 1994) OTC *vitamin/mineral/iron supplement* [multiple vitamins & minerals; iron; folic acid] ±•18•0.4 mg

**One-A-Day Within** (name changed to One-A-Day Women's Formula in 1993)

**One-A-Day Women's Formula** tablets OTC *vitamin/calcium/iron supplement* [multiple vitamins; calcium; iron; folic acid] ±•450•27•0.4 mg

**one-fifty-one; fifty-one** *street drug slang* [see: cocaine, crack]

**One-Tablet-Daily** OTC *vitamin supplement* [multiple vitamins; folic acid] ±•0.4 mg

**One-Tablet-Daily with Iron** OTC *vitamin/iron supplement* [multiple vitamins; iron; folic acid] ±•18•0.4 mg

**One-Tablet-Daily with Minerals** OTC *vitamin/mineral/iron supplement* [multiple vitamins & minerals; iron; folic acid; biotin] ±•18 mg•0.4 mg•30 μg

**ONO-1078** *investigational leukotriene antagonist for asthma*

**ontazolast** USAN *antiasthmatic; leukotriene biosynthesis inhibitor*

**ontianil** INN

**Ontosein** ℞ *investigational treatment for osteoarthritis* [orgotein]

**Ony-Clear** solution ℞ *topical antifungal* [miconazole nitrate] 2%

**Ony-Clear Nail** (name changed to Ony-Clear in 1996)

**OPA (Oncovin, prednisone, Adriamycin)** *chemotherapy protocol*

**OPAL (Oncovin, prednisone, L-asparaginase)** *chemotherapy protocol*

**OPC-14117** *investigational vitamin E-like antioxidant for cognitive impairment and HIV-related nerve damage*

**Opcon** eye drops (name changed to Muro's Opcon in 1993)

**Opcon-A** eye drops OTC *topical ocular decongestant, antihistamine, and lubricant* [naphazoline HCl; pheniramine maleate; hydroxypropyl methylcellulose] 0.027%•0.315%•0.5%

**ope** *street drug slang* [see: opium]

**OPEN (Oncovin, prednisone, etoposide, Novantrone)** *chemotherapy protocol*

**Operand** solution, prep pads, swab sticks, surgical scrub, perineal wash concentrate, aerosol, Iofoam skin cleanser, ointment OTC *broad-spectrum antimicrobial* [povidone-iodine] 1%; 1%; 1%; 7.5%; 1%; 0.5%; 1%; 1%

**Operand Douche** concentrate OTC *antiseptic/germicidal; vaginal cleanser and deodorizer* [povidone-iodine]

**Ophthacet** eye drops (discontinued 1993) ℞ *ophthalmic bacteriostatic* [sodium sulfacetamide]

**Ophthaine** eye drops (discontinued 1997) ℞ *topical ophthalmic anesthetic* [proparacaine HCl] 0.5%

**Ophthalgan** eye drops ℞ *corneal edema-reducing and clearing agent* [glycerin]

**Ophthetic** eye drops ℞ *topical ophthalmic anesthetic* [proparacaine HCl] 0.5%

**Ophthifluor** IV injection ℞ *corneal disclosing agent* [fluorescein sodium] 10%

**Ophthocort** ophthalmic ointment (discontinued 1996) ℞ *ophthalmic topical corticosteroidal anti-inflammatory; antibiotic* [hydrocortisone acetate; chloramphenicol; polymyxin B sulfate] 0.5%•1%•10 000 U/g ⌧ Ophthochlor

**opiniazide** INN

**opipramol** INN *antidepressant; antipsychotic* [also: opipramol HCl]

**opipramol HCl** USAN *antidepressant; antipsychotic* [also: opipramol]

**opium** USP *narcotic analgesic; widely abused as a street drug, which is highly addictive* 10% oral

**opium, powdered** USP *narcotic analgesic*

**OPOL** ℞ *investigational oral polio vaccine*

**O.P.P.** *street drug slang* [see: PCP]

**OPP (Oncovin, procarbazine, prednisone)** *chemotherapy protocol*

**OPPA (Oncovin, prednisone, procarbazine, Adriamycin)** *chemotherapy protocol*

**oprelvekin** USAN *hematopoietic cytokine for thrombocytopenia of chemotherapy or radiation*

**optical illusions** *street drug slang* [see: LSD]

**Opticare PMS** tablets OTC *vitamin/mineral supplement; digestive enzymes* [multiple vitamins & minerals; iron; folic acid; biotin; amylase; protease; lipase] ≛•2.5 mg•0.033 mg•10.4 μg•2500 U•2500 U•200 U

**Opti-Clean** solution OTC *cleaning solution for hard, soft, or rigid gas permeable contact lenses*

**Opti-Clean II** solution OTC *cleaning solution for hard or soft contact lenses*

**Opti-Clean II Especially for Sensitive Eyes** solution OTC *cleaning solution for rigid gas permeable contact lenses*

**Opticrom 4%** eye drops (discontinued 1993) ℞ *ocular antiallergic for vernal keratoconjunctivitis (orphan)* [cromolyn sodium]

**Opticyl** eye drops ℞ *cycloplegic; mydriatic* [tropicamide] 0.5%, 1%

**Opti-Free** solution OTC *chemical disinfecting solution for soft contact lenses* [note: one of four different products with the same name]

**Opti-Free** solution OTC *rewetting solution for soft contact lenses* [note: one of four different products with the same name]

**Opti-Free** solution OTC *surfactant cleaning solution for soft contact lenses* [note: one of four different products with the same name]

**Opti-Free** tablets OTC *enzymatic cleaner for soft contact lenses* [pork pancreatin; note: one of four different products with the same name]

**Optigene** ophthalmic solution OTC *extraocular irrigating solution* [sterile isotonic solution]

**Optigene 3** eye drops OTC *topical ocular decongestant/vasoconstrictor* [tetrahydrozoline HCl] 0.05%

**Optilets-500** Filmtabs (film-coated tablets) OTC *vitamin supplement* [multiple vitamins] ±

**Optilets-M-500** Filmtabs (film-coated tablets) OTC *vitamin/mineral/iron supplement* [multiple vitamins & minerals; iron] ± • 20 mg

**Optimine** tablets ℞ *antihistamine* [azatadine maleate] 1 mg

**Optimmune** ℞ *investigational (orphan) for severe keratoconjunctivitis sicca in Sjögren syndrome* [cyclosporine]

**Optimoist** oral spray OTC *saliva substitute*

**Optimox Prenatal** tablets OTC *vitamin/mineral/calcium/iron supplement* [multiple vitamins & minerals; calcium; iron; folic acid] ± • 100 • 5 • 0.133 mg

**Optimyd** eye drops (discontinued 1995) ℞ *topical ophthalmic corticosteroidal anti-inflammatory; bacteriostatic* [prednisolone sodium phosphate; sulfacetamide sodium] 0.5% • 10%

**Opti-One** solution OTC *rewetting solution for soft contact lenses*

**Opti-One Multi-Purpose** solution OTC *chemical disinfecting solution for soft contact lenses*

**OptiPranolol** eye drops ℞ *topical antiglaucoma agent (β-blocker)* [metipranolol HCl] 0.3%

**Opti-Pure** aerosol solution (discontinued 1993) OTC *rinsing/storage solution for soft contact lenses*

**Optiray 160; Optiray 240; Optiray 320; Optiray 350** injection ℞ *parenteral radiopaque agent* [ioversol (source of iodine)] 34% (16%); 51% (24%); 68% (32%); 74% (35%)

**Optised** eye drops (discontinued 1993) OTC *topical ocular decongestant; astringent; antiseptic* [phenylephrine HCl; zinc sulfate]

**Opti-Soft Especially for Sensitive Eyes** solution OTC *rinsing/storage solution for soft contact lenses* [preserved saline solution]

**Opti-Tears** solution OTC *rewetting solution for hard or soft contact lenses*

**Optivite P.M.T.** tablets OTC *geriatric vitamin/mineral supplement* [multiple vitamins & minerals; folic acid; biotin] ± • 30 • ² μg

**Opti-Zyme Enzymatic Cleaner Especially for Sensitive Eyes** tablets OTC *enzymatic cleaner for soft or rigid gas permeable contact lenses* [pork pancreatin]

**OPV (oral poliovirus vaccine)** [see: poliovirus vaccine, live oral]

**ORA5** liquid OTC *oral anti-infective* [copper sulfate; iodine; potassium iodide] ² • ² • ²

**Orabase** gel OTC *mucous membrane anesthetic* [benzocaine] 15%

**Orabase Baby** gel OTC *topical oral anesthetic* [benzocaine] 7.5%

**Orabase HCA** oral paste ℞ *topical corticosteroid* [hydrocortisone acetate] 0.5%

**Orabase Lip Healer** cream OTC *topical oral anesthetic; antipruritic/counterirritant; vulnerary* [benzocaine; menthol; allantoin] 5% • 0.5% • 1.5%

**Orabase-B** oral paste OTC *topical oral anesthetic* [benzocaine] 20% ▢ Orinase

**Orabase-O** orthodontic gel (discontinued 1994) OTC *topical oral anesthetic* [benzocaine] 20%

**Orabase-Plain** oral paste OTC *relief from minor oral irritations* [plasticized hydrocarbon gel]

**Oracin** lozenges (discontinued 1994) OTC *topical oral anesthetic; antipruritic/counterirritant* [benzocaine; menthol] 6.25 mg • 0.1% ▢ orarsan; Orasone

**Oracit** solution ℞ *urinary alkalinizing agent* [sodium citrate; citric acid] 490 • 640 mg/5 mL

**Oradex-C** lozenges (discontinued 1995) OTC *topical anesthetic; counterirritant* [dyclonine HCl] 3 mg

**Oradex-C** troches (discontinued 1994) OTC *topical oral anesthetic; anti-*

*septic* [benzocaine; cetylpyridinium chloride] 10•2.5 mg

**Ora-Fresh** mouthwash (discontinued 1994) OTC *oral antiseptic/antifungal* [methylparaben; zinc chloride]

**Oragest SR** sustained-release capsules (discontinued 1993) ℞ *decongestant; antihistamine* [phenylpropanolamine HCl; chlorpheniramine maleate]

**Oragrafin Calcium** granules for oral suspension ℞ *oral cholecystographic radiopaque agent* [ipodate calcium] 3 g/packet

**Oragrafin Sodium** capsules ℞ *oral cholecystographic radiopaque agent* [ipodate sodium] 500 mg

**Orajel** liquid OTC *topical oral anesthetic* [benzocaine; alcohol 44.2%] 20%

**Orajel; Orajel Brace-aid; Orajel/d; Denture Orajel; Baby Orajel; Baby Orajel Nighttime Formula** gel OTC *topical oral anesthetic* [benzocaine] 20%; 20%; 10%; 10%; 7.5%; 10%

**Orajel Brace-aid** rinse (discontinued 1993) OTC *topical oral anti-inflammatory/anti-infective for braces* [carbamide peroxide] 10%

**Orajel Mouth-Aid** liquid, gel OTC *mucous membrane anesthetic* [benzocaine] 20%

**Orajel Perioseptic** liquid OTC *topical oral anti-inflammatory/anti-infective for braces* [carbamide peroxide] 15%

**Orajel Tooth & Gum Cleanser, Baby** gel OTC *removes plaque-like film* [poloxamer 407; simethicone] 2%•0.12%

**Oralease** ℞ *investigational (Phase III) analgesic for pain due to oral ulcers*

**Oralet** (trademarked dosage form) *oral lozenge/lollipop*

**Oralone Dental** paste ℞ *topical corticosteroid* [triamcinolone acetonide] 0.1%

**Oramide** tablets ℞ *antidiabetic* [tolbutamide]

**Oraminic II** subcu or IM injection ℞ *antihistamine; anaphylaxis* [brompheniramine maleate] 10 mg/mL

**Oramorph SR** sustained-release tablets ℞ *narcotic analgesic* [morphine sulfate] 15, 30, 60, 100 mg

**orange** *street drug slang for Desoxyn (methamphetamine HCl), a reference to the capsule color* [see: Desoxyn; methamphetamine HCl]

**orange barrels; orange cubes; orange haze; orange micro; orange wedges** *street drug slang* [see: LSD]

**orange crystal** *street drug slang* [see: PCP]

**orange cupcakes** *street drug slang for a combination of LSD, methamphetamine, strychnine, and STP* [see: LSD; methamphetamine HCl; strychnine; STP]

**orange flower oil** NF *flavoring agent; perfume*

**orange flower water** NF

**orange oil** NF

**orange peel tincture, sweet** NF

**orange spirit, compound** NF

**orange syrup** NF

**oranges** *street drug slang* [see: amphetamines]

**Orap** tablets ℞ *antipsychotic* [pimozide] 2 mg

**Oraphen-PD** elixir OTC *analgesic; antipyretic* [acetaminophen] 120 mg/5 mL

**orarsan** [see: acetarsone] ② Oracin; Orasone

**OraScan** ℞ *investigational diagnostic aid for oral cancers*

**Orasept** liquid OTC *oral astringent; antiseptic* [tannic acid; methylbenzethonium chloride; alcohol 53.31%] 12.16%•1.53%

**Orasept** throat spray OTC *topical oral anesthetic; antiseptic* [benzocaine; methylbenzethonium chloride] 0.996%•1.037%

**Orasol** liquid OTC *topical oral anesthetic; antipruritic/counterirritant; antiseptic* [benzocaine; phenol; alcohol 70%] 6.3%•0.5%

**Orasone** tablets ℞ *glucocorticoid; anti-inflammatory; immunosuppressant* [prednisone] 1, 5, 10, 20, 50 mg ② Oracin; orarsan

**OraSure** reagent kit for home use OTC *in vitro diagnostic aid for HIV antibodies*

**OraSure HIV-1** reagent kit for professional use ℞ *in vitro diagnostic aid for HIV antibodies using oral mucosal*

*transudate* [single-sample, three-test kit: two ELISA assays plus Western Blot assay]

**Oratect** gel (discontinued 1995) OTC *topical oral anesthetic* [benzocaine; alcohol 65.8%] 15%

**orazamide** INN

**Orazinc** capsules, tablets OTC *zinc supplement* [zinc sulfate] 220 mg; 110 mg

**orbofiban acetate** USAN *platelet aggregation inhibitor; fibrinogen receptor antagonist*

**orbutopril** INN

**orciprenaline** INN, BAN *bronchodilator* [also: metaproterenol polistirex]

**orciprenaline polistirex** [see: metaproterenol polistirex]

**orconazole** INN *antifungal* [also: orconazole nitrate]

**orconazole nitrate** USAN *antifungal* [also: orconazole]

**Ordrine AT** extended-release capsules ℞ *antitussive; decongestant* [caramiphen edisylate; phenylpropanolamine HCl] 40•75 mg

**Ordrine S.R.** sustained-release capsules ℞ *decongestant; antihistamine* [phenylpropanolamine HCl; chlorpheniramine maleate]

**orestrate** INN

**orestrol** [see: diethylstilbestrol dipropionate]

**Oretic** tablets ℞ *diuretic; antihypertensive* [hydrochlorothiazide] 25, 50 mg ☒ Oreton

**Oreticyl 25; Oreticyl 50; Oreticyl Forte** tablets (discontinued 1994) ℞ *antihypertensive* [hydrochlorothiazide; deserpidine] 25•0.125 mg; 50•0.125 mg; 25•0.25 mg

**Oreton Methyl** tablets, buccal tablets ℞ *androgen for male hypogonadism, impotence and breast cancer* [methyltestosterone] 10 mg ☒ Oretic

**Orex** oral solution (discontinued 1994) OTC *saliva substitute* ☒ Ornex

**Orexin** chewable tablets OTC *vitamin supplement* [vitamins $B_1$, $B_6$, and $B_{12}$] 8.1 mg•4.1 mg•25 μg

**Org 32489** *investigational recombinant follicle-stimulating hormone for infertility*

**organic Quaalude** *street drug slang* [see: GHB]

**Organidin** tablets, elixir, drops (discontinued 1993; Organidin NR ["Newly Reformulated"] replaced it in 1994) ℞ *expectorant* [iodinated glycerol] 30 mg; 60 mg/5 mL; 50 mg/mL

**Organidin NR** tablets, oral liquid ℞ *expectorant* [guaifenesin] 200 mg; 100 mg/5 mL

**organoclay** [see: bentoquatam]

**Orgaran** subcu injection ℞ *anticoagulant/antithrombotic for prevention of deep vein thrombosis (DVT) following hip replacement surgery* [danaproid sodium] 750 anti-Xa IU/0.6 mL

**orgotein** USAN, INN, BAN *anti-inflammatory; antirheumatic; investigational (orphan) for amyotrophic lateral sclerosis and to prevent donor organ reperfusion injury* [previously known as superoxide dismutase (SOD)]

**orgotein, recombinant human** *investigational (orphan) for bronchopulmonary dysplasia of premature neonates*

**orienticine A; orienticine D** [see: orientiparcin]

**orientiparcin** INN [a mixture of orienticine A and orienticine D]

**Orimune** oral suspension ℞ *poliomyelitis vaccine* [poliovirus vaccine, live oral trivalent] 0.5 mL

**Orinase** tablets ℞ *sulfonylurea-type antidiabetic* [tolbutamide] 500 mg ☒ Orabase; Ornade; Ornex; Tolinase

**Orinase Diagnostic** powder for IV injection ℞ *in vivo pancreas function test* [tolbutamide sodium] 1 g

**Orlaam** IV injection ℞ *narcotic agonist for management of opiate dependence (orphan)* [levomethadyl acetate HCl] 10 mg/mL

**orlipastat** [see: orlistat]

**orlistat** USAN, INN *pancreatic lipase inhibitor; investigational adjunct to weight loss*

**ormaplatin** USAN *antineoplastic*

**Ormazine** IV or IM injection ℞ *antipsychotic* [chlorpromazine HCl] 25 mg/mL

**ormetroprim** USAN, INN *antibacterial*

**Ornade** Spansules (sustained-release capsules) ℞ *decongestant; antihistamine* [phenylpropanolamine HCl; chlorpheniramine maleate] 75•12 mg ☐ Orinase; Ornex

**Ornex** caplets (name changed to Ornex No Drowsiness in 1995) ☐ Orex; Orinase; Ornade

**Ornex No Drowsiness** caplets OTC *decongestant; analgesic; antipyretic* [pseudoephedrine HCl; acetaminophen] 30•325 mg

**Ornex Severe Cold No Drowsiness** caplets (discontinued 1995) OTC *antitussive; decongestant; analgesic* [dextromethorphan hydrobromide; pseudoephedrine HCl; acetaminophen] 15•30•500 mg

**ornidazole** USAN, INN *anti-infective*

**Ornidyl** IV injection concentrate ℞ *antiprotozoal for Trypanosoma brucei gambiense infection (orphan)* [eflornithine HCl] 200 mg/mL

**ornipressin** INN

**ornithine (L-ornithine)** INN

**ornithine vasopressin** [see: ornipressin]

**ornoprostil** INN

**orotic acid** INN

**orotirelin** INN

**orpanoxin** USAN, INN *anti-inflammatory*

**orphenadrine citrate** [see: orphenadrine citrate]

**orphenadrine** INN, BAN *skeletal muscle relaxant; antihistamine* [also: orphenadrine citrate]

**orphenadrine citrate** USP *skeletal muscle relaxant; antihistamine* [also: orphenadrine] 100 mg oral; 30 mg/mL injection

**Orphenate** IV or IM injection (discontinued 1993) ℞ *skeletal muscle relaxant* [orphenadrine citrate]

**Orphengesic; Orphengesic Forte** tablets (discontinued 1996) ℞ *skeletal muscle relaxant; analgesic; CNS stimulant* [orphenadrine citrate; aspirin; caffeine] 25•385•30 mg; 50•770•60 mg

**orpressin** [see: ornipressin]

**ortetamine** INN

**orthesin** [see: benzocaine]

**Ortho Dienestrol** vaginal cream ℞ *estrogen replacement for postmenopausal disorders* [dienestrol] 0.01%

**Ortho Drops** eye drop suspension (discontinued 1993) ℞ *topical ophthalmic corticosteroidal anti-inflammatory; antibiotic* [hydrocortisone acetate; neomycin sulfate]

**Ortho Tri-Cept** ℞ *investigational triphasic oral contraceptive* [ethinyl estradiol; desogestrel]

**Ortho Tri-Cyclen** tablets ℞ *triphasic oral contraceptive; treatment for acne vulgaris in females* [norgestimate; ethinyl estradiol] Phase 1: 0.18 mg•35 μg; Phase 2: 0.215 mg•35 μg; Phase 3: 0.25 mg•35 μg

**Ortho-Cept** tablets ℞ *monophasic oral contraceptive* [desogestrel; ethinyl estradiol] 0.15 mg•30 μg

**Orthoclone OKT3** IV injection ℞ *immunosuppressant for renal, cardiac, and hepatic transplants* [muromonab-CD3] 5 mg/5 mL ☐ Ortho-Creme

**Orthoclone OKT4A** ℞ *investigational immunosuppressant for cardiac and hepatic transplantation* ☐ Ortho-Creme

**Ortho-Creme** vaginal cream (discontinued 1994) OTC *spermicidal contraceptive* [nonoxynol 9] 2% ☐ Orthoclone

**orthocresol** NF

**Ortho-Cyclen** tablets ℞ *monophasic oral contraceptive* [norgestimate; ethinyl estradiol] 0.25 mg•35 μg

**Ortho-Est** tablets ℞ *hormone replacement therapy for postmenopausal disorders* [estropipate] 0.75, 1.5 mg

**Ortho-Est Plus** ℞ *investigational hormone for menopause*

**Ortho-Gynol** vaginal gel OTC *spermicidal contraceptive (for use with a diaphragm)* [octoxynol 9] 1%

**Ortholinum** ℞ *investigational (orphan) for spasmodic torticollis* [botulinum toxin, type F]

**Ortho-Novum 1/35** tablets ℞ *monophasic oral contraceptive* [norethindrone; ethinyl estradiol] 1 mg•35 μg

**Ortho-Novum 1/50** tablets ℞ *monophasic oral contraceptive* [norethindrone; mestranol] 1 mg•50 μg

**Ortho-Novum 7/7/7** tablets ℞ *triphasic oral contraceptive* [norethindrone; ethinyl estradiol] Phase 1: 0.5 mg•35 μg; Phase 2: 0.75 mg•35 μg; Phase 3: 1 mg•35 μg

**Ortho-Novum 10/11** tablets ℞ *biphasic oral contraceptive* [norethindrone; ethinyl estradiol] Phase 1: 0.5 mg•35 μg; Phase 2: 1 mg•35 μg

**orthotolidine**

**Orthovisc** (available in the European Community countries) ℞ *investigational (Phase III) treatment for osteoarthritis and temporomandibular joint syndrome* [hyaluronate sodium]

**Orthoxicol Cough** syrup OTC *antitussive; decongestant; antihistamine* [dextromethorphan hydrobromide; phenylpropanolamine HCl; chlorpheniramine maleate; alcohol 8%] 6.7•8.3•1.3 mg/5 mL

**Orthozyme-CD5+** ℞ *investigational graft vs. host disease preventative* [zolimomab aritox]

**Orudis** capsules ℞ *nonsteroidal anti-inflammatory drug (NSAID); antiarthritic; analgesic* [ketoprofen] 25, 50, 75 mg

**Orudis KT** tablets OTC *nonsteroidal anti-inflammatory drug (NSAID); analgesic; antiarthritic* [ketoprofen] 12.5 mg

**Orudis SR** ℞ *investigational once-daily anti-inflammatory* [ketoprofen]

**Oruvail** sustained-release pellets in capsules ℞ *once-daily nonsteroidal anti-inflammatory drug (NSAID); antiarthritic; analgesic* [ketoprofen] 100, 150, 200 mg

**osalmid** INN

**osarsal** [see: acetarsone]

**Os-Cal 250+D; Os-Cal 500+D** film-coated tablets OTC *dietary supplement* [calcium carbonate; vitamin D] 250 mg•125 IU; 500 mg•125 IU

**Os-Cal 500** tablets, chewable tablets OTC *calcium supplement* [calcium carbonate] 1.25 g

**Os-Cal Fortified** tablets OTC *vitamin/calcium/iron supplement* [multiple vitamins; calcium carbonate; iron] ≐•250•5 mg

**Os-Cal Fortified Multivitamin & Minerals** tablets OTC *vitamin/mineral/calcium/iron supplement* [multiple vitamins & minerals; calcium carbonate; iron] ≐•250•5 mg

**Os-Cal Plus** tablets (discontinued 1995) OTC *vitamin/calcium/iron supplement* [multiple vitamins; calcium carbonate; iron] ≐•250•16.6 mg

**osmadizone** INN

**Osmitrol** IV infusion ℞ *osmotic diuretic* [mannitol] 5%, 10%, 15%, 20%

**osmium** *element* (Os)

**Osmoglyn** solution ℞ *osmotic diuretic* [glycerin] 50%

**Osmolite; Osmolite HN** liquid OTC *enteral nutritional therapy* [lactose-free formula]

**osmotic diuretics** *a class of diuretics that increase excretion of sodium and chloride and decrease tubular absorption of water*

**Osmovist** injection ℞ *parenteral radiopaque agent* [iotrolan]

**Ossirene** ℞ *investigational bone marrow protectant for chemotherapy*

**Osteocalcin** subcu or IM injection ℞ *calcium regulator for hypercalcemia, Paget's disease, and postmenopausal osteoporosis* [calcitonin (salmon)] 200 IU/mL

**Osteo-D** ℞ *calcium regulator; investigational (orphan) for familial hypophosphatemic rickets* [secalciferol]

**Osteo-F** slow-release tablets ℞ *investigational treatment for postmenopausal osteoporosis* [sodium fluoride]

**Osteomark** ℞ *investigational enzyme-linked immunoassay for monitoring breakdown of bone mass* [monoclonal antibodies]

**Osteo-Mins** powder OTC *dietary supplement* [multiple minerals; vitamins C and D] ≐•500 mg•100 IU

**Ostiderm** lotion OTC *for hyperhidrosis and bromhidrosis* [aluminum sulfate; zinc oxide] 14.5•≐ mg/g

**Ostiderm** roll-on OTC *for hyperhidrosis and bromhidrosis* [aluminum chlorohydrate; camphor; alcohol] ≐•≐•≐

**ostreogrycin** INN, BAN

**osvarsan** [see: acetarsone]

**OT (old tuberculin)** [see: tuberculin]

**Otic Domeboro** ear drops ℞ *antibac-terial/antifungal* [acetic acid; aluminum acetate] 2%• ?

**Otic Tridesilon** ear drops (discontinued 1995) ℞ *topical corticosteroidal anti-inflammatory; antibacterial/antifungal* [desonide; acetic acid] 0.05%•2%

**Otic-Care** ear drops, otic suspension ℞ *topical corticosteroidal anti-inflammatory; antibiotic* [hydrocortisone; neomycin sulfate; polymyxin B sulfate] 1%•5 mg•10 000 U per mL

**otilonium bromide** INN, BAN

**Oti-Med** ear drops ℞ *topical corticosteroidal anti-inflammatory; antibacterial; topical local anesthetic* [hydrocortisone; chloroxylenol; pramoxine HCl] 10•1•10 mg/mL

**otimerate sodium** INN

**OtiTricin** otic suspension ℞ *topical corticosteroidal anti-inflammatory; antibiotic* [hydrocortisone; neomycin sulfate; polymyxin B sulfate] 1%•5 mg•10 000 U per mL

**Otobiotic Otic** ear drops ℞ *topical corticosteroidal anti-inflammatory; antibiotic* [hydrocortisone; polymyxin B sulfate] 0.5%•10 000 U per mL ⅁ Urobiotic

**Otocain** ear drops ℞ *topical local anesthetic* [benzocaine] 20%

**Otocalm** ear drops ℞ *topical local anesthetic; analgesic* [benzocaine; antipyrine] 1.4%•5.4%

**Otocort** ear drops, otic suspension ℞ *topical corticosteroidal anti-inflammatory; antibiotic* [hydrocortisone; neomycin sulfate; polymyxin B sulfate] 1%•5 mg•10 000 U per mL

**Otomycet-HC** ear drops ℞ *topical corticosteroidal anti-inflammatory; antibacterial/antifungal* [hydrocortisone; acetic acid] 1%•2%

**Otomycin-HPN Otic** ear drops ℞ *topical corticosteroidal anti-inflammatory; antibiotic* [hydrocortisone; neomycin sulfate; polymyxin B sulfate] 1%•5 mg•10 000 U per mL

**Otosporin** ear drops ℞ *topical corticosteroidal anti-inflammatory; antibiotic*

[hydrocortisone; neomycin sulfate; polymyxin B sulfate] 1%•5 mg•10 000 U per mL

**Otrivin** nasal spray, nose drops, pediatric drops OTC *nasal decongestant* [xylometazoline HCl] 0.1%; 0.1%; 0.05% ⅁ Lotrimin

**ouabain** USP

**outer limits** *street drug slang for a combination of crack and LSD* [see: cocaine, crack; LSD]

**Outgro** solution OTC *pain relief for ingrown toenails* [tannic acid; chlorobutanol; isopropyl alcohol 83%] 25%•5%

**ovandrotone albumin** INN, BAN

**Ovarex** *investigational (orphan) for epithelial ovarian cancer* [monoclonal antibody B43.13]

**Ovastat** ℞ *investigational (orphan) for ovarian cancer* [treosulfan]

**Ovcon-35; Ovcon-50** tablets ℞ *monophasic oral contraceptive* [norethindrone; ethinyl estradiol] 1 mg•35 μg; 1 mg•50 μg

**Ovide** lotion ℞ *pediculicide* [malathion; isopropyl alcohol 78%] 0.5%

**ovine corticotropin-releasing hormone** [see: corticorelin ovine triflutate]

**Ovoid** (trademarked dosage form) *sugar-coated tablet*

**Ovral** tablets ℞ *monophasic oral contraceptive; emergency "morning after" contraceptive* [norgestrel; ethinyl estradiol] 0.5 mg•50 μg

**Ovrette** tablets ℞ *oral contraceptive (progestin only)* [norgestrel] 0.075 mg

**OvuGen** test kit OTC *in vitro diagnostic aid to predict ovulation time*

**OvuKIT Self-Test** kit for home use OTC *in vitro diagnostic aid to predict ovulation time*

**OvuQuick Self-Test** kit for home use OTC *in vitro diagnostic aid to predict ovulation time*

**[¹⁵O]water** [see: water O 15]

**Owsley; Owsley's acid; white Owsley** *street drug slang* [see: LSD]

**ox bile extract** [see: bile salts]

**oxabolone cipionate** INN

**oxabrexine** INN

**oxaceprol** INN
**oxacillin** INN *antibacterial* [also: oxacillin sodium]
**oxacillin sodium** USAN, USP *bactericidal antibiotic* [also: oxacillin] 250, 500 mg oral; 0.25, 0.5, 1, 2, 4, 10 g/ vial injection
**oxadimedine** INN
**oxadimedine HCl** [see: oxadimedine]
**oxaflozane** INN
**oxaflumazine** INN
**oxafuradene** [see: nifuradene]
**oxagrelate** USAN, INN *platelet antiaggregatory agent*
**oxalinast** INN
**oxaliplatin** INN *investigational (orphan) for ovarian cancer*
**oxamarin** INN *hemostatic* [also: oxamarin HCl]
**oxamarin HCl** USAN *hemostatic* [also: oxamarin]
**oxametacin** INN
**oxamisole** INN *immunoregulator* [also: oxamisole HCl]
**oxamisole HCl** USAN *immunoregulator* [also: oxamisole]
**oxamniquine** USAN, USP, INN *antischistosomal; anthelmintic for schistosomiasis (flukes)*
**oxamphetamine hydrobromide** [see: hydroxyamphetamine hydrobromide]
**oxamycin** [see: cycloserine]
**oxanamide** INN
**Oxandrin** tablets ℞ *anabolic steroid for weight gain; investigational (orphan) for Turner syndrome, growth and puberty delay, AIDS; abused as a street drug* [oxandrolone] 2.5 mg
**oxandrolone** USAN, USP, INN, BAN, JAN *androgen/anabolic steroid; investigational (orphan) for Turner syndrome, growth and puberty delay, AIDS, and hepatitis; abused as a street drug*
**oxantel** INN *anthelmintic* [also: oxantel pamoate]
**oxantel pamoate** USAN *anthelmintic* [also: oxantel]
**oxantrazole HCl** [see: piroxantrone HCl]
**oxapadol** INN
**oxapium iodide** INN
**oxaprazine**

**oxapropanium iodide** INN
**oxaprotiline** INN *antidepressant* [also: oxaprotiline HCl]
**oxaprotiline HCl** USAN *antidepressant* [also: oxaprotiline]
**oxaprozin** USAN, INN, BAN *nonsteroidal anti-inflammatory drug (NSAID) for rheumatoid arthritis and osteoarthritis*
**oxarbazole** USAN, INN *antiasthmatic*
**oxarutine** [see: ethoxazorutoside]
**oxatomide** USAN, INN *antiallergic; antiasthmatic*
**oxazafone** INN
**oxazepam** USAN, USP, INN *anxiolytic; minor tranquilizer; alcohol withdrawal therapy* 10, 15, 30 mg oral
**oxazidione** INN
**oxazolam** INN
**oxazolidin** [see: oxyphenbutazone]
**oxazolidinediones** *a class of anticonvulsants*
**oxazorone** INN
**oxcarbazepine** INN *antiepileptic*
**oxdralazine** INN
**oxeladin** INN, BAN
**oxendolone** USAN, INN *antiandrogen for benign prostatic hypertrophy*
**oxepinac** INN
**oxerutins** BAN
**oxetacaine** INN *topical anesthetic* [also: oxethazaine]
**oxetacillin** INN
**2-oxetanone** [see: propiolactone]
**oxethazaine** USAN, BAN *topical anesthetic* [also: oxetacaine]
**oxetorone** INN *migraine-specific analgesic* [also: oxetorone fumarate]
**oxetorone fumarate** USAN *migraine-specific analgesic* [also: oxetorone]
**oxfenamide** [see: oxiramide]
**oxfendazole** USAN, INN *anthelmintic*
**oxfenicine** USAN, INN, BAN *vasodilator*
**oxibendazole** USAN, INN *anthelmintic*
**oxibetaine** INN
**oxibuprocaine chloride** [see: benoxinate HCl]
**oxichlorochine sulfate** [see: hydroxychloroquine sulfate]
**oxicinchophen** [see: oxycinchophen]
**oxiconazole** INN, BAN *antifungal* [also: oxiconazole nitrate]

**oxiconazole nitrate** USAN *antifungal* [also: oxiconazole]

**oxicone** [see: oxycodone]

**oxidized cellulose** [see: cellulose, oxidized]

**oxidized cholic acid** [see: dehydrocholic acid]

**oxidized regenerated cellulose** [see: cellulose, oxidized regenerated]

**oxidopamine** USAN, INN *ophthalmic adrenergic*

**oxidronic acid** USAN, INN, BAN *calcium regulator*

**oxifenamate** [see: hydroxyphenamate]

**oxifentorex** INN

**Oxi-Freeda** tablets OTC *dietary supplement* [multiple vitamins, minerals, and amino acids] ±

**oxifungin** INN *antifungal* [also: oxifungin HCl]

**oxifungin HCl** USAN *antifungal* [also: oxifungin]

**oxilorphan** USAN, INN *narcotic antagonist*

**oximetazoline HCl** [see: oxymetazoline HCl]

**oximetholone** [see: oxymetholone]

**oximonam** USAN, INN *antibacterial*

**oximonam sodium** USAN *antibacterial*

**oxindanac** INN

**oxiniacic acid** INN

**oxiperomide** USAN, INN *antipsychotic*

**oxipertine** [see: oxypertine]

**oxipethidine** [see: hydroxypethidine]

**oxiphenbutazone** [see: oxyphenbutazone]

**oxiphencyclimine chloride** [see: oxyphencyclimine HCl]

**Oxipor VHC** lotion OTC *topical antipsoriatic; antiseborrheic; keratolytic* [coal tar solution; alcohol 79%] 25%

**oxiprocaine** [see: hydroxyprocaine]

**oxiprogesterone caproate** [see: hydroxyprogesterone caproate]

**oxipurinol** INN *xanthine oxidase inhibitor* [also: oxypurinol]

**oxiracetam** INN, BAN *investigational treatment for Alzheimer's disease*

**oxiramide** USAN, INN *antiarrhythmic*

**oxisopred** INN

**Oxistat** cream, lotion ℞ *topical antifungal* [oxiconazole nitrate] 1%

**oxistilbamidine isethionate** [see: hydroxystilbamidine isethionate]

**oxisuran** USAN, INN *antineoplastic*

**oxitefonium bromide** INN

**oxitetracaine** [see: hydroxytetracaine]

**oxitetracycline** [see: oxytetracycline]

**oxitriptan** INN

**oxitriptyline** INN

**oxitropium bromide** INN, BAN

**oxmetidine** INN, BAN *antagonist to histamine $H_2$ receptors* [also: oxmetidine HCl]

**oxmetidine HCl** USAN *antagonist to histamine $H_2$ receptors* [also: oxmetidine]

**oxmetidine mesylate** USAN *antagonist to histamine $H_2$ receptors*

**oxodipine** INN

**oxogestone** INN *progestin* [also: oxogestone phenpropionate]

**oxogestone phenpropionate** USAN *progestin* [also: oxogestone]

**oxoglurate** INN *combining name for radicals or groups*

**oxolamine** INN

**oxolinic acid** USAN, INN *antibacterial*

**oxomemazine** INN

**oxonazine** INN

**4-oxopentanoic acid, calcium salt** [see: calcium levulinate]

**oxophenarsine** INN [also: oxophenarsine HCl]

**oxophenarsine HCl** USP [also: oxophenarsine]

**5-oxoproline** [see: pidolic acid]

**oxoprostol** INN, BAN

**oxothiazolidine carboxylate (L-2-oxothiazolidine-4-carboxylic acid)** *investigational (Phase II) immunomodulator for AIDS; investigational (orphan) for adult respiratory distress syndrome and amyotrophic lateral sclerosis*

**oxozepam** [see: oxazepam]

**oxpentifylline** BAN *vasodilator; hemorheologic agent* [also: pentoxifylline]

**oxpheneridine** INN

**oxprenoate potassium** INN

**oxprenolol** INN *coronary vasodilator* [also: oxprenolol HCl]

**oxprenolol HCl** USAN, USP *coronary vasodilator* [also: oxprenolol]

**OxSODrol** ℞ *investigational (Phase III) anti-inflammatory and antirheumatic* [orgotein (previously known as superoxide dismutase, or SOD)]

**Oxsoralen** capsules (discontinued 1993) R̲ *antipsoriatic* [methoxsalen] 10 mg

**Oxsoralen** lotion R̲ *repigmenting adjunct with ultraviolet A for vitiligo; investigational treatment for scleroderma* [methoxsalen] 1%

**Oxsoralen-Ultra** capsules R̲ *antipsoriatic* [methoxsalen] 10 mg

**oxtriphylline** USP *bronchodilator* [also: choline theophyllinate] 100, 200 mg oral; 50, 100 mg/5 mL oral

**Oxy 5** lotion (discontinued 1994) OTC *topical keratolytic for acne* [benzoyl peroxide] 5%

**Oxy 5 Advanced Formula for Sensitive Skin** gel (name changed to Advanced Formula Oxy 5 for Sensitive Skin in 1995)

**Oxy 5 for Sensitive Skin, Advanced Formula; Oxy for Sensitive Skin, Advanced Formula** gel OTC *topical keratolytic for acne* [benzoyl peroxide] 5%; 2.5%

**Oxy 5 Tinted** lotion OTC *topical keratolytic for acne* [benzoyl peroxide] 5%

**Oxy 10** lotion, cover cream (discontinued 1994) OTC *topical keratolytic for acne* [benzoyl peroxide] 10%

**Oxy 10 Advanced Formula** gel OTC *topical keratolytic for acne* [benzoyl peroxide] 10%

**Oxy 10 Wash** liquid OTC *topical keratolytic for acne* [benzoyl peroxide] 10%

**Oxy Clean Lathering Facial** scrub (discontinued 1994) OTC *abrasive cleanser for acne* [sodium tetraborate decahydrate dissolving particles]

**Oxy Clean Soap** bar (discontinued 1994) OTC *medicated cleanser for acne* [salicylic acid] 3.5%

**Oxy Medicated Cleanser & Pads** OTC *topical keratolytic cleanser for acne* [salicylic acid; alcohol] 0.5%•22%, 0.5%•40%, 2%•50%

**Oxy Medicated Soap** bar OTC *medicated cleanser for acne* [triclosan] 1%

**Oxy Night Watch; Oxy Night Watch for Sensitive Skin** lotion OTC *topical keratolytic for acne* [salicylic acid] 2%; 1%

**Oxy ResiDon't Medicated Face Wash** liquid OTC *topical cleanser for acne* [triclosan] 0.6%

**oxybenzone** USAN, USP, INN *ultraviolet screen*

**oxybuprocaine** INN, BAN *topical anesthetic* [also: benoxinate HCl; oxybuprocaine HCl]

**oxybuprocaine HCl** JAN *topical anesthetic* [also: benoxinate HCl; oxybuprocaine]

**oxybutynin** INN, BAN *anticholinergic; urinary antispasmodic* [also: oxybutynin chloride]

**oxybutynin chloride** USAN, USP *anticholinergic; urinary antispasmodic* [also: oxybutynin] 5 mg oral

**Oxycel** pads, pledgets, strips R̲ *topical local hemostat for surgery* [oxidized cellulose]

**oxychlorosene** USAN *topical anti-infective*

**oxychlorosene sodium** USAN *topical anti-infective*

**oxycinchophen** INN, BAN

**oxyclipine** INN *anticholinergic* [also: propenzolate HCl]

**oxyclipine HCl** [see: propenzolate HCl]

**oxyclozanide** INN, BAN

**oxycodone** USAN, INN, BAN *narcotic analgesic; also abused as a street drug*

**oxycodone HCl** USAN, USP *narcotic analgesic; also abused as a street drug*

**oxycodone terephthalate** USP *narcotic analgesic; also abused as a street drug*

**OxyContin** controlled-release tablets R̲ *narcotic analgesic* [oxycodone HCl] 10, 20, 40, 80 mg

**Oxydess II** tablets R̲ *CNS stimulant; amphetamine* [dextroamphetamine sulfate] 10 mg

**oxydimethylquinazine** [see: antipyrine]

**oxydipentonium chloride** INN

**oxyethyltheophylline** [see: etofylline]

**oxyfedrine** INN, BAN

**oxyfenamate** INN *minor tranquilizer* [also: hydroxyphenamate]

**oxyfilcon A** USAN *hydrophilic contact lens material*

**oxygen ($O_2$)** USP *medicinal gas; element (O)*

**oxygen, polymeric** *investigational (orphan) for sickle cell anemia*

**oxygen 93 percent** USP *medicinal gas*

**Oxygent** ℞ *investigational blood substitute* [perflubron]

**OxyIR** immediate-release capsules ℞ *narcotic analgesic* [oxycodone HCl] 5 mg

**oxymesterone** INN, BAN

**oxymetazoline** INN, BAN *topical ocular vasoconstrictor; nasal decongestant* [also: oxymetazoline HCl] ⧉ oxymetholone

**oxymetazoline HCl** USAN, USP *topical ocular vasoconstrictor; nasal decongestant* [also: oxymetazoline] 0.05% nose drops or spray

**oxymetholone** USAN, USP, INN, BAN *androgen; anabolic steroid; also abused as a street drug* ⧉ oxymetazoline; oxymorphone

**oxymethylene urea** [see: polynoxylin]

**oxymorphone** INN, BAN *narcotic analgesic* [also: oxymorphone HCl] ⧉ oxymetholone

**oxymorphone HCl** USP *narcotic analgesic; investigational (orphan) for intractable pain in narcotic-tolerant patients* [also: oxymorphone]

**oxypendyl** INN

**oxypertine** USAN, INN *antidepressant*

**oxyphenbutazone** USP, INN *antiinflammatory; antirheumatic; antipyretic; analgesic*

**oxyphencyclimine** INN *anticholinergic* [also: oxyphencyclimine HCl]

**oxyphencyclimine HCl** USP *peptic ulcer adjunct* [also: oxyphencyclimine]

**oxyphenhydrazine** [see: carsalam]

**oxyphenisatin** BAN *laxative* [also: oxyphenisatin acetate; oxyphenisatine]

**oxyphenisatin acetate** USAN *laxative* [also: oxyphenisatine; oxyphenisatin]

**oxyphenisatine** INN *laxative* [also: oxyphenisatin acetate; oxyphenisatin]

**oxyphenonium bromide**

**oxyphylline** [see: etofylline]

**oxypurinol** USAN *xanthine oxidase inhibitor* [also: oxipurinol]

**oxypyrronium bromide** INN

**oxyquinoline** USAN *disinfectant/antiseptic*

**oxyquinoline benzoate** [see: benzoxiquine]

**oxyquinoline sulfate** USAN, NF *complexing agent*

**oxyridazine** INN

**Oxysept** solution + tablets OTC *two-step chemical disinfecting system for soft contact lenses* [hydrogen peroxide-based] 3%

**Oxysept 2** solution OTC *rinsing/storage solution for soft contact lenses* [preservative-free saline solution]

**oxysonium iodide** INN

**oxytetracycline** USP, INN *bacteriostatic antibiotic; antirickettsial*

**oxytetracycline calcium** USP *antibacterial*

**oxytetracycline HCl** USP *bacteriostatic antibiotic; antirickettsial* 250 mg oral

**oxytocics** *a class of posterior pituitary hormones that stimulate contraction of the myometrium (uterine muscle)*

**oxytocin** USP, INN *oxytocic; posterior pituitary hormone* 10 U/mL injection

**Oxyzal Wet Dressing** liquid OTC *antiseptic dressing for minor infections* [oxyquinoline sulfate; benzalkonium chloride]

**Oysco 500** chewable tablets OTC *calcium supplement* [calcium carbonate] 1.25 g

**Oysco D** tablets (discontinued 1993) OTC *dietary supplement* [calcium carbonate; vitamin D] 250 mg•125 IU

**Oyst-Cal 500** film-coated tablets OTC *calcium supplement* [calcium carbonate] 1.25 g

**Oyst-Cal-D** film-coated tablets OTC *dietary supplement* [calcium carbonate; vitamin D] 250 mg•125 IU

**Oyster Calcium** tablets OTC *dietary supplement* [calcium carbonate; vitamins A and D] 375 mg•800 IU•200 IU

**Oyster Calcium 500 + D** tablets OTC *dietary supplement* [calcium carbonate; vitamin D] 500 mg•125 IU

**Oyster Calcium with Vitamin D** tablets OTC *dietary supplement* [calcium carbonate; vitamin D] 250 mg•125 IU

**Oyster Shell Calcium with Vitamin D** tablets OTC *calcium supplement* [calcium carbonate; vitamin D] 250 mg•125 IU

**Oyster Shell Calcium-500** tablets OTC *calcium supplement* [calcium carbonate] 1.25 g

**Oystercal 500** tablets OTC *calcium supplement* [calcium carbonate] 1.25 g

**Oystercal-D 250** tablets OTC *dietary supplement* [calcium carbonate; vitamin D] 250 mg•125 IU

**ozagrel** INN *investigational antiasthmatic*

**ozolinone** USAN, INN *diuretic*

**ozone** *street drug slang* [see: PCP]

**Ozzie's stuff** *street drug slang, probably a reference to Ozzie Osborne* [see: LSD]

**P & S** liquid OTC *antimicrobial hair dressing* [phenol]

**P & S** shampoo OTC *antiseborrheic; keratolytic* [salicylic acid] 2%

**P & S Plus** gel OTC *topical antipsoriatic; antiseborrheic; keratolytic* [coal tar solution; salicylic acid] 8%•2%

**$P_1E_1$; $P_2E_1$; $P_3E_1$; $P_4E_1$; $P_6E_1$** Drop-Tainers (eye drops) ℞ *antiglaucoma agent* [pilocarpine HCl; epinephrine bitartrate] 1%•1%; 2%•1%; 3%•1%; 4%•1%; 6%•1%

**P-280** *investigational (Phase III) diagnostic imaging agent for deep vein thrombosis (DVT)*

**p30 protein** *investigational (Phase III) adjunct to chemotherapy for pancreatic, breast, colorectal, prostate, and small cell lung cancers*

**$^{32}$P** [see: chromic phosphate P 32]

**$^{32}$P** [see: polymetaphosphate P 32]

**$^{32}$P** [see: sodium phosphate P 32]

**P829 Techtide** *investigational (Phase III) radiopharmaceutical imaging agent for lung cancer, malignant melanoma, and neuroendocrine tumors*

**PAB (para-aminobenzoate)** [see: aminobenzoic acid]

**PABA (para-aminobenzoic acid)** [now: aminobenzoic acid]

**PABA sodium** [see: aminobenzoate sodium]

**Pabalate** enteric-coated tablets OTC *analgesic; antipyretic; anti-inflammatory* [sodium salicylate; aminobenzoate sodium] 300•300 mg

**Pabalate-SF** enteric-coated tablets (discontinued 1995) ℞ *analgesic; antipyretic; anti-inflammatory* [potassium salicylate; potassium aminobenzoate] 300•300 mg

**PAB-Esc-C (Platinol, Adriamycin, bleomycin, escalating doses of cyclophosphamide)** *chemotherapy protocol*

**pabestrol D** [see: diethylstilbestrol dipropionate]

**P-A-C** tablets (discontinued 1995) OTC *analgesic; antipyretic; anti-inflammatory* [aspirin; caffeine] 400•32 mg

**PAC; PAC-I (Platinol, Adriamycin, cyclophosphamide)** *chemotherapy protocol*

**paca lolo; pakalolo** *street drug slang (a Hawaiian term)* [see: marijuana]

**PACE (Platinol, Adriamycin, cyclophosphamide, etoposide)** *chemotherapy protocol*

**PACIS** ⓒ injection ℞ *immunizing agent* [BCG vaccine, Montreal strain] 2–10 × 10⁶ CFU (colony-forming units)

**pack** *street drug slang* [see: heroin; marijuana]

**pack of rocks** *street drug slang for a marijuana cigarette* [see: marijuana]

**Packer's Pine Tar** shampoo, soap OTC *antiseborrheic; antipsoriatic; antipruritic; antibacterial* [pine tar]

**paclitaxel** USAN, INN, BAN *antineoplastic; investigational (orphan) for AIDS-related Kaposi sarcoma*

**pacrinolol** INN

**padimate** INN *ultraviolet screen* [also: padimate A]

**padimate A** USAN *ultraviolet screen* [also: padimate]

**padimate O** USAN *ultraviolet screen*

**pafenolol** INN

**pagoclone** USAN *anxiolytic*

**PAH (para-aminohippurate)** [see: aminohippuric acid]

**PAHA (para-aminohippuric acid)** [see: aminohippuric acid]

**Pain Bust-R II** cream OTC *topical local anesthetic; counterirritant* [methyl salicylate; menthol] 17%•12%

**Pain Doctor** cream OTC *topical analgesic; topical anesthetic; antipruritic* [capsaicin; methyl salicylate; menthol] 0.025%•25%•10%

**Pain Gel Plus** OTC *counterirritant* [menthol] 4%

**Pain Reliever** tablets OTC *analgesic; antipyretic; anti-inflammatory* [acetaminophen; aspirin; caffeine] 250•250•65 mg

**Pain-X** gel OTC *topical analgesic; counterirritant* [capsaicin; menthol; camphor] 0.05%•5%•4%

**Pakistani black** *street drug slang* [see: marijuana]

**PALA disodium** [see: sparfosate sodium]

**palatrigine** INN, BAN

**paldimycin** USAN, INN *antibacterial*

**paldimycin A** [see: paldimycin]

**paldimycin B** [see: paldimycin]

**palestrol** [see: diethylstilbestrol]

**palinavir** USAN *antiviral; HIV-1 protease inhibitor*

**palinum** [see: cyclobarbitone]

**palladium** *element (Pd)*

**palmidrol** INN

**Palmitate-A 5000** tablets OTC *vitamin supplement* [vitamin A] 5000 IU

**palmoxirate sodium** USAN *antidiabetic* [also: palmoxiric acid]

**palmoxiric acid** INN *antidiabetic* [also: palmoxirate sodium]

**palonosetron HCl** USAN *antiemetic; antinauseant; 5-HT$_3$ antagonist*

**PALS** coated tablets OTC *systemic deodorant for ostomy, breath, and body odors* [chlorophyllin copper complex] 100 mg

**PAM; L-PAM (phenylalanine mustard)** [see: melphalan]

**2-PAM (2-pyridine aldoxime methylchloride)** [see: pralidoxime chloride]

**pamabrom** USAN *nonprescription diuretic*

**pamaqueside** USAN *hypocholesterolemic; cholesterol absorption inhibitor; antiatherosclerotic*

**pamaquine naphthoate** NF

**pamatolol** INN *antiadrenergic (β-receptor)* [also: pamatolol sulfate]

**pamatolol sulfate** USAN *antiadrenergic (β-receptor)* [also: pamatolol]

**Pamelor** capsules, oral solution R *tricyclic antidepressant* [nortriptyline HCl] 10, 25, 50, 75 mg; 10 mg/5 mL ⊅ Dymelor

**pamidronate disodium** USAN *bisphosphonate bone resorption suppressant for Paget's disease, hypercalcemia of malignancy, and multiple myeloma*

**pamidronic acid** INN, BAN

**Pamine** tablets R *anticholinergic; peptic ulcer treatment* [methscopolamine bromide] 2.5 mg

**Pamisyl** R *investigational (orphan) for ulcerative colitis* [aminosalicylic acid]

**pamoate** USAN, USP *combining name for radicals or groups* [also: embonate]

**Pamprin** caplets (name changed to Multi-Symptom Pamprin in 1994)

**Pamprin, Multi-Symptom** caplets, tablets OTC *analgesic; antipyretic; diuretic; antihistaminic sleep aid* [acetaminophen; pamabrom; pyrilamine maleate] 500•25•15 mg

**Pamprin, Nighttime** powder OTC *antihistaminic sleep aid; analgesic* [diphenhydramine HCl; acetaminophen] 50•650 mg

**Pamprin Maximum Cramp Relief** caplets (name changed to Multi-Symptom Pamprin in 1994)

**Pamprin Maximum Pain Relief** caplets OTC *analgesic; antipyretic; diuretic* [acetaminophen; magnesium salicylate; pamabrom] 250•250•25 mg

**Pamprin-IB** coated tablets (discontinued 1993) OTC *nonsteroidal antiinflammatory drug (NSAID); antiarthritic; analgesic* [ibuprofen] 200 mg

**Pan C-500** tablets OTC *dietary supplement* [vitamin C; citrus bioflavonoids & hesperidin] 1000•250 mg

**Panacet 5/500** tablets ℞ *narcotic analgesic* [hydrocodone bitartrate; acetaminophen] 5•500 mg

**panadiplon** USAN, INN *anxiolytic*

**Panadol** tablets, caplets OTC *analgesic; antipyretic* [acetaminophen] 500 mg

**Panadol, Children's** chewable tablets, liquid OTC *analgesic; antipyretic* [acetaminophen] 80 mg; 160 mg/5 mL

**Panadol, Infants'** drops OTC *analgesic; antipyretic* [acetaminophen] 100 mg/mL

**Panadol, Junior** caplets OTC *analgesic; antipyretic* [acetaminophen] 160 mg

**Panadyl Forte** sustained-release tablets (discontinued 1993) ℞ *decongestant; antihistamine* [phenylpropanolamine HCl; phenylephrine HCl; chlorpheniramine maleate]

**Panafil** ointment ℞ *topical enzyme for wound debridement; vulnerary; wound deodorant* [papain; urea; chlorophyllin copper complex] 10%•10%•0.5%

**Panafil White** ointment ℞ *topical enzyme for wound debridement; vulnerary* [papain; urea] 10%•10%

**Panalgesic** cream OTC *counterirritant* [methyl salicylate; menthol] 35%•4%

**Panalgesic Gold** liniment OTC *counterirritant; topical antiseptic* [methyl salicylate; camphor; menthol; alcohol 22%] 55%•3.1%•1.25%

**Panama cut; Panama gold; Panama red** *street drug slang* [see: marijuana]

**Panasal 5/500** tablets ℞ *narcotic analgesic* [hydrocodone bitartrate; aspirin] 5•500 mg

**Panasol-S** tablets ℞ *glucocorticoid; anti-inflammatory; immunosuppressant* [prednisone] 1 mg ⌧ Pranscol

**panatella** *street drug slang for a large cigar-shaped marijuana cigarette* [see: marijuana]

**pancakes and syrup** *street drug slang for a combination of glutethimide and codeine cough syrup* [see: glutethimide; codeine]

**pancopride** USAN, INN *antiemetic; anxiolytic; peristaltic stimulant*

**Pancrease; Pancrease MT 4; Pancrease MT 10; Pancrease MT 16; Pancrease MT 20** capsules containing enteric-coated microtablets ℞ *digestive enzymes* [lipase; protease; amylase] 4.5•25•20; 4.5•12•12; 10•30•30; 16•48•48; 20•44•56 thousand USP units

**Pancrease MT 25; Pancrease MT 32** capsules containing enteric-coated microtablets (discontinued 1994) ℞ *digestive enzymes* [lipase; protease; amylase] 25 000•70 000•55 000 U; 32 000•90 000•70 000 U

**pancreatin** USP *digestive enzyme*

**Pancreatin, 4X; Pancreatin, 8X** tablets OTC *digestive enzymes* [pancreatin; lipase; protease; amylase] 2400 mg•12 000 U•60 000 U•60 000 U; 7200 mg•22 500 U•180 000 U•180 000 U

**pancrelipase** USAN, USP *digestive enzyme*

**Pancrezyme 4X** tablets OTC *digestive enzymes* [pancreatin; lipase; protease; amylase] 2400 mg•12 000 U•60 000 U•60 000 U

**pancuronium bromide** USAN, INN *nondepolarizing neuromuscular blocker; muscle relaxant; adjunct to anesthesia* 1, 2 mg/mL injection

**Pandel** cream ℞ *topical corticosteroid* [hydrocortisone buteprate] 0.1%

**pane** *street drug slang, a short form of "window pane," a reference to the glassine packaging* [see: LSD]

**Panex; Panex 500** tablets (discontinued 1997) OTC *analgesic; antipyretic* [acetaminophen] 325 mg; 500 mg

**pangonadalot** *street drug slang* [see: heroin]

**Panhematin** powder for IV injection ℞ *enzyme inhibitor for acute intermittent porphyria (AIP), porphyria variegata, and hereditary coproporphyria (orphan)* [hemin] 7 mg/mL

**panidazole** INN, BAN

**Panmycin** capsules ℞ *broad-spectrum antibiotic* [tetracycline HCl] 250 mg

**panomifene** INN

**Panorex** ℞ *orphan status withdrawn 1997* [edrecolomab] ⊡ Panarex

**Panoxyl** cleansing bar ℞ *topical keratolytic for acne* [benzoyl peroxide] 5%, 10% ⊡ Benoxyl

**Panoxyl AQ 2½; Panoxyl 5; Panoxyl AQ 5; Panoxyl 10; Panoxyl AQ 10** gel ℞ *topical keratolytic for acne* [benzoyl peroxide] 2.5%; 5%; 5%; 10%; 10%

**Panretin** capsules ℞ *investigational (Phase III) treatment for Kaposi sarcoma, psoriasis, myelodysplastic syndrome (MDS), and acute promyelocytic leukemia (APL)* [9-cis-retinoic acid]

**Panretin** gel ℞ *investigational (Phase III) topical delivery form for AIDS-related Kaposi sarcoma* [9-cis-retinoic acid]

**Panscol** lotion, ointment OTC *topical keratolytic* [salicylic acid] 3% ⊡ Panasol

**pantenicate** INN

**panthenol** USAN, USP, INN *B complex vitamin*

**D-panthenol** [see: dexpanthenol]

**Panthoderm** cream OTC *antipruritic; vulnerary; emollient* [dexpanthenol] 2%

**Pantopon** injection (discontinued 1993) ℞ *narcotic analgesic; sedative; hypnotic* [opium alkaloids HCl] 20 mg/mL ⊡ Parafon

**pantoprazole** USAN, INN, BAN *antiulcerative*

**pantothenic acid** BAN *vitamin $B_5$; enzyme cofactor* [also: calcium pantothenate]

**DL-pantothenic acid** [see: calcium pantothenate, racemic]

**pantothenol** [see: dexpanthenol]

**pantothenyl alcohol** [see: panthenol]

**D-pantothenyl alcohol** [see: dexpanthenol]

**panuramine** INN, BAN

**Panwarfin** tablets (discontinued 1993) ℞ *anticoagulant* [warfarin sodium] 2, 2.5, 5, 7.5, 10 mg

**Papadeine #3** tablets ℞ *narcotic analgesic* [codeine phosphate; acetaminophen]

**papain** USP *topical proteolytic enzyme for necrotic tissue debridement*

**papaverine** BAN *peripheral vasodilator; smooth muscle relaxant; orphan status withdrawn 1996* [also: papaverine HCl]

**papaverine HCl** USP *peripheral vasodilator; smooth muscle relaxant for cerebral, myocardial, and peripheral ischemias* [also: papaverine] 150 mg oral

**papaveroline** INN, BAN

**Papaya Enzyme** chewable tablets OTC *digestive enzymes* [papain; amylase] 60•60 mg

**paper acid** *street drug slang* [see: LSD]

**paper blunts** *street drug slang for a marijuana cigarette rolled in cigarette paper rather than a tobacco leaf casing* [see: marijuana]

**Paplex** solution (discontinued 1994) ℞ *topical keratolytic* [salicylic acid in flexible collodion; lactic acid] 17%•17%

**Paplex Ultra** solution ℞ *topical keratolytic* [salicylic acid in flexible collodion] 26%

**Par Decon** sustained-action tablets (discontinued 1993) ℞ *decongestant; antihistamine* [phenylpropanolamine HCl; phenylephrine HCl; phenyltoloxamine citrate; chlorpheniramine maleate]

**Par Glycerol** elixir ℞ *expectorant* [iodinated glycerol] 60 mg/5 mL

**Par Glycerol C** liquid (discontinued 1993) ℞ *narcotic antitussive; expectorant* [codeine phosphate; iodinated glycerol]

**Par Glycerol DM** liquid (discontinued 1993) ℞ *expectorant; antitussive* [iodinated glycerol; dextromethorphan hydrobromide]

**para-aminobenzoate (PAB)** [see: aminobenzoic acid]

**Para-Aminobenzoic Acid** tablets, powder OTC *"possibly effective" for scleroderma and other skin diseases, and Peyronie's disease* [aminobenzoic acid] 100, 500 mg; 120 g

**para-aminobenzoic acid (PABA)** [now: aminobenzoic acid]

**para-aminohippurate (PAH)** [see: aminohippuric acid]

**para-aminohippurate sodium** [see: aminohippurate sodium]

**para-aminohippuric acid (PAHA)** [see: aminohippuric acid]

**para-aminosalicylate (PAS)** [see: aminosalicylic acid]

**para-aminosalicylic acid (PASA)** [see: aminosalicylic acid]

**Parabolan** *brand name for trenbolone hexahydrobenzylcarbonate, a European veterinary anabolic steroid abused as a street drug*

**parabromdylamine maleate** [see: brompheniramine maleate]

**paracetaldehyde** [see: paraldehyde]

**paracetamol** INN, BAN *analgesic; antipyretic* [also: acetaminophen]

**parachlorometaxylenol (PCMX)** *topical antiseptic; broad-spectrum antibacterial*

**parachlorophenol (PCP)** USP *topical antibacterial*

**parachlorophenol, camphorated** USP *topical dental anti-infective*

**parachute** *street drug slang for heroin or crack and PCP smoked together* [see: cocaine, crack; PCP; heroin]

**paracodin** [see: dihydrocodeine]

**Paradione** *capsules, oral solution (discontinued 1994)* ℞ *anticonvulsant* [paramethadione] 150, 300 mg

**paradise; paradise white** *street drug slang* [see: cocaine]

**paraffin** NF *stiffening agent*

**paraffin, liquid** [see: mineral oil]

**paraffin, synthetic** NF *stiffening agent*

**Paraflex** *caplets* ℞ *skeletal muscle relaxant* [chlorzoxazone] 250 mg

**paraflutizide** INN

**Parafon Forte DSC** *caplets* ℞ *skeletal muscle relaxant* [chlorzoxazone] 500 mg ② Pantopon

**paraformaldehyde** USP

**Para-Hist AT** *syrup (discontinued 1994)* ℞ *narcotic antitussive; decongestant; antihistamine* [codeine phosphate; phenylephrine HCl; promethazine HCl; alcohol] 10•5•6.25 mg/5 mL

**Para-Hist HD** *liquid* ℞ *narcotic antitussive; decongestant; antihistamine* [hydrocodone bitartrate; phenyleph-rine HCl; chlorpheniramine maleate] 1.67•5•2 mg/5 mL

**parahydrecin** [now: isomerol]

**Paral** *oral liquid, rectal liquid* ℞ *sedative; hypnotic* [paraldehyde]

**paraldehyde** USP *hypnotic; sedative; anticonvulsant* 1 g/mL oral or rectal

**paramethadione** USP, INN, BAN *anticonvulsant* ② paramethasone

**paramethasone** INN *glucocorticoid* [also: paramethasone acetate] ② paramethadione

**paramethasone acetate** USAN, USP *glucocorticoid* [also: paramethasone]

**para-nitrosulfathiazole** NF [also: nitrosulfathiazole]

**paranyline HCl** USAN *anti-inflammatory* [also: renytoline]

**parapenzolate bromide** USAN, INN *anticholinergic*

**Paraplatin** *powder for IV injection* ℞ *alkylating antineoplastic for ovarian and other cancers* [carboplatin] 50, 150, 450 mg

**parapropamol** INN

**pararosaniline embonate** INN *antischistosomal* [also: pararosaniline pamoate]

**pararosaniline pamoate** USAN *antischistosomal* [also: pararosaniline embonate]

**parasympathomimetics** *a class of agents that produce effects similar to those of the parasympathetic nervous system* [also called: cholinergic agonists]

**Parathar** *powder for IV injection* ℞ *in vivo diagnostic aid for parathyroid-induced hypocalcemia (orphan)* [teriparatide acetate] 200 U

**parathesin** [see: benzocaine]

**parathiazine** INN

**parathyroid** USP *hormone*

**parathyroid hormone (1-34), biosynthetic human** [see: teriparatide]

**paraxazone** INN

**parbendazole** USAN, INN *anthelmintic*

**parconazole** INN *antifungal* [also: parconazole HCl]

**parconazole HCl** USAN *antifungal* [also: parconazole]

**Par-Drix** sustained-release tablets (discontinued 1994) ℞ *decongestant; antihistamine* [pseudoephedrine sulfate; dexbrompheniramine maleate] 120•6 mg

**Paredrine** eye drops ℞ *mydriatic* [hydroxyamphetamine hydrobromide] 1%

**paregoric (PG) (a preparation of opium, anise oil, benzoic acid, camphor, alcohol, and glycerin)** USP *antiperistaltic; narcotic analgesic; sometimes abused as a street drug* 2 mg/5 mL oral

**Paremyd** eye drops ℞ *mydriatic; weak cycloplegic* [hydroxyamphetamine hydrobromide; tropicamide] 1%• 0.25%

**parenabol** [see: boldenone undecylenate]

**Parepectolin** concentrated liquid OTC *GI adsorbent; antidiarrheal* [attapulgite] 600 mg/15 mL

**pareptide** INN *antiparkinsonian* [also: pareptide sulfate]

**pareptide sulfate** USAN *antiparkinsonian* [also: pareptide]

**parethoxycaine** INN

**parethoxycaine HCl** [see: parethoxycaine]

**Par-F** tablets ℞ *vitamin/mineral/calcium/iron supplement* [multiple vitamins & minerals; calcium; iron; folic acid] ≐•250•60•1 mg

**pargeverine** INN

**pargolol** INN

**pargyline** INN *antihypertensive* [also: pargyline HCl]

**pargyline HCl** USAN, USP *antihypertensive* [also: pargyline]

**Parhist SR** sustained-release capsules (discontinued 1995) ℞ *decongestant; antihistamine* [phenylpropanolamine HCl; chlorpheniramine maleate] 75•12 mg

**paridocaine** INN

**parlay** *street drug slang* [see: cocaine, crack]

**Parlodel** SnapTabs (scored tablets), capsules ℞ *antiparkinsonian; lactation preventative; treats acromegaly, infer-* tility, and hypogonadism [bromocriptine mesylate] 2.5 mg; 5 mg

**Par-Natal Plus 1 Improved** tablets ℞ *vitamin/calcium/iron supplement* [multiple vitamins; calcium; iron; folic acid] ≐•200•65•1 mg

**Parnate** film-coated tablets ℞ *monoamine oxidase inhibitor (MAOI) for reactive depression (a major depressive episode without melancholia)* [tranylcypromine sulfate] 10 mg

**parodilol** INN

**parodyne** [see: antipyrine]

**paroleine** [see: mineral oil]

**paromomycin** INN, BAN *aminoglycoside bactericidal antibiotic; amebicide* [also: paromomycin sulfate]

**Paromomycin** ℞ *investigational (orphan) for tuberculosis, Mycobacterium avium complex, and visceral leishmaniasis* [aminosidine]

**paromomycin sulfate** USP *aminoglycoside bactericidal antibiotic; amebicide* [also: paromomycin]

**paroxetine** USAN, INN, BAN *selective serotonin reuptake inhibitor (SSRI) for depression, obsessive-compulsive disorder, and panic disorder*

**paroxetine HCl** *selective serotonin reuptake inhibitor (SSRI) for depression, obsessive-compulsive disorder, and panic disorder*

**paroxyl** [see: acetarsone]

**paroxypropione** INN

**parpanit HCl** [see: caramiphen HCl]

**parsalmide** INN

**Parsidol** tablets (discontinued 1997) ℞ *anticholinergic; antiparkinsonian* [ethopropazine HCl] 10, 50 mg

**parsley** *street drug slang* [see: marijuana; PCP]

**Partapp** elixir (discontinued 1994) OTC *decongestant; antihistamine* [phenylpropanolamine HCl; brompheniramine maleate] 12.5•2 mg/5 mL

**Partapp TD** timed-release tablets (discontinued 1995) ℞ *decongestant; antihistamine* [phenylpropanolamine HCl; phenylephrine HCl; brompheniramine maleate] 15•15•12 mg

**partricin** USAN, INN *antifungal; antiprotozoal*

**Partuss LA** long-acting tablets ℞ *decongestant; expectorant* [phenylpropanolamine HCl; guaifenesin] 75•400 mg

**parvaquone** INN, BAN

**Parvlex** tablets OTC *hematinic* [ferrous fumarate; multiple B vitamins and minerals; vitamin C; folic acid] 100• ± •50•0.1 mg

**PAS (para-aminosalicylate)** [see: aminosalicylic acid]

**PASA (para-aminosalicylic acid)** [see: aminosalicylic acid]

**Paser** granules ℞ *tuberculostatic (orphan)* [aminosalicylic acid] 4 g/packet

**pasiniazid** INN

**PassHIV** ℞ *investigational immunotherapy for HIV and AIDS*

**paste** *street drug slang* [see: cocaine, crack]

**Pastilles** (dosage form) *troches*

**Pat** *street drug slang* [see: marijuana]

**Patanol** Drop-Tainer (eye drops) ℞ *ophthalmic antihistamine for allergic conjunctivitis* [olopatadine HCl] 0.1%

**PATCO (prednisone, ara-C, thioguanine, cyclophosphamide, Oncovin)** *chemotherapy protocol*

**Pathilon** film-coated tablets ℞ *peptic ulcer treatment adjunct* [tridihexethyl chloride] 25 mg ② Pathocil

**Pathocil** capsules, powder for oral suspension ℞ *bactericidal antibiotic (penicillinase-resistant penicillin)* [dicloxacillin sodium monohydrate] 250, 500 mg; 62.5 mg/5 mL ② Bactocill; Pathilon; Placidyl

**'patico** *street drug slang, from the Spanish "simpático," meaning "nice" or "pleasant"* [see: cocaine, crack]

**paulomycin** USAN, INN *antibacterial*

**Pavabid** Plateau Caps (controlled-release capsules) ℞ *peripheral vasodilator; smooth muscle relaxant for cerebral, myocardial, and peripheral ischemias* [papaverine HCl] 150 mg ② Pavased

**Pavabid HP** capsulets (tablets) (discontinued 1995) ℞ *peripheral vasodilator; smooth muscle relaxant for cerebral, myocardial, and peripheral ischemias* [papaverine HCl] 300 mg

**Pavagen TD** timed-release capsules ℞ *peripheral vasodilator; smooth muscle relaxant for cerebral, myocardial, and peripheral ischemias* [papaverine HCl] 150 mg

**Pavarine** Spancaps (timed-release capsules) (discontinued 1997) ℞ *peripheral vasodilator; smooth muscle relaxant for cerebral, myocardial, and peripheral ischemias* [papaverine HCl] 150 mg

**Pavased** timed-release capsules (discontinued 1996) ℞ *peripheral vasodilator; smooth muscle relaxant for cerebral, myocardial, and peripheral ischemias* [papaverine HCl] 150 mg

**Pavatine** timed-release capsules (discontinued 1997) ℞ *peripheral vasodilator; smooth muscle relaxant for cerebral, myocardial, and peripheral ischemias* [papaverine HCl] 150 mg ② Pavatym

**PAVe (procarbazine, Alkeran, Velban)** *chemotherapy protocol*

**Paverolan** Lanacaps (timed-release capsules) (discontinued 1997) ℞ *peripheral vasodilator; smooth muscle relaxant for cerebral, myocardial, and peripheral ischemias* [papaverine HCl] 150 mg ② Pavulon

**Pavulon** IM injection ℞ *nondepolarizing neuromuscular blocker; adjunct to anesthesia* [pancuronium bromide] 1, 2 mg/mL ② Paverolan

**paxamate** INN

**Paxarel** tablets ℞ *anxiolytic; sedative* [acetylcarbromal] 250 mg

**Paxil** film-coated tablets ℞ *selective serotonin reuptake inhibitor (SSRI) for depression, obsessive-compulsive disorder, and panic disorder* [paroxetine HCl] 10, 20, 30, 40 mg

**Paxipam** tablets (discontinued 1995) ℞ *anxiolytic* [halazepam] 20, 40 mg

**paz** *street drug slang* [see: PCP]

**pazelliptine** INN

**pazinaclone** USAN *anxiolytic*

**Pazo Hemorrhoid** ointment OTC *temporary relief of hemorrhoidal symptoms; topical vasoconstrictor; counter-irritant; astringent* [ephedrine sulfate; camphor; zinc oxide] 0.2%•2%•5%

**Pazo Hemorrhoid** suppositories OTC *temporary relief of hemorrhoidal symptoms; topical vasoconstrictor; astringent* [ephedrine sulfate; zinc oxide] 3.8•96.5 mg

**pazoxide** USAN, INN *antihypertensive*

**PBV (Platinol, bleomycin, vinblastine)** *chemotherapy protocol*

**PBZ** elixir (discontinued 1997) ℞ *antihistamine* [tripelennamine HCl] 37.5 mg/5 mL

**PBZ** tablets ℞ *antihistamine* [tripelennamine HCl] 25, 50 mg

**PBZ (pyribenzamine)** [see: tripelennamine]

**PBZ-SR** sustained-release tablets ℞ *antihistamine* [tripelennamine HCl] 100 mg

**PC (paclitaxel, carboplatin)** *chemotherapy protocol*

**PC (phosphatidylcholine)** [see: lecithin]

**PCE** Dispertabs (delayed-release tablets) ℞ *macrolide antibiotic* [erythromycin] 333, 500 mg

**PCE (Platinol, cyclophosphamide, etoposide)** *chemotherapy protocol*

**PCE (polymer-coated erythromycin)** [see: erythromycin]

**PCMX (parachlorometaxylenol)** [q.v.]

**PCP (parachlorophenol)** [q.v.]

**PCP (phenylcyclohexyl piperidine)** *a powerful veterinary analgesic/anesthetic widely abused as a hallucinogenic street drug* [medically known as phencyclidine HCl]

**PCPA** *street drug slang* [see: PCP]

**PCV (procarbazine, CCNU, vincristine)** *chemotherapy protocol*

**PDA-641** *investigational anti-inflammatory and bronchodilator for asthma*

**PDGA (pteroyldiglutamic acid)**

**PDLA (phosphinicodilactic acid)** [see: foscolic acid]

**P-dope** *street drug slang for 20-30% pure heroin* [see: heroin]

**PDP Liquid Protein** OTC *dietary supplement* [hydrolyzed protein; L-tryptophan] 15• 2/30 mL

**PE (phenylephrine)** [q.v.]

**PE (polyethylene)** [q.v.]

**peace** *street drug slang* [see: LSD; PCP]

**peace pill** *street drug slang* [see: PCP]

**peace tablets** *street drug slang* [see: LSD]

**peace weed** *street drug slang for PCP or a combination of marijuana and PCP* [see: marijuana; PCP]

**peaches** *street drug slang for Benzedrine (amphetamine sulfate; discontinued 1982)* [see: amphetamine sulfate]

**peanut butter** *street drug slang for PCP mixed with peanut butter* [see: PCP]

**peanut oil** NF *solvent*

**peanuts** *street drug slang for barbiturate sleeping pills* [see: barbiturates]

**pearl** *street drug slang* [see: cocaine]

**pearls** *street drug slang* [see: amyl nitrite]

**pearly gates** *street drug slang for LSD or a variety of psychedelic morning glory seeds* [see: LSD; morning glory seeds]

**PEB (Platinol, etoposide, bleomycin)** *chemotherapy protocol*

**pebbles** *street drug slang* [see: cocaine, crack]

**pecazine** INN, BAN

**pecazine acetate** [see: pecazine]

**pecilocin** INN, BAN

**pecocycline** INN

**pectin** USP *suspending agent; protectant; GI adsorbent*

**Pedameth** capsules, liquid ℞ *urinary acidifier to control ammonia production* [racemethionine] 200 mg; 75 mg/5 mL

**PediaCare Allergy Formula** liquid OTC *antihistamine* [chlorpheniramine maleate] 1 mg/5 mL

**PediaCare Cold-Allergy** chewable tablets OTC *pediatric decongestant and antihistamine* [pseudoephedrine HCl; chlorpheniramine maleate] 15•1 mg

**PediaCare Cough-Cold Formula** chewable tablets, liquid OTC *pediatric antitussive, decongestant, and antihistamine* [dextromethorphan hydrobromide; pseudoephedrine HCl; chlorpheniramine maleate] 5•15•1 mg; 5•15•1 mg/5 mL

**PediaCare Infant's Decongestant** drops OTC *nasal decongestant* [pseudoephedrine HCl] 7.5 mg/0.8 mL

**PediaCare NightRest Cough-Cold** liquid OTC *pediatric antitussive, decon-*

**gestant, and antihistamine** [dextromethorphan hydrobromide; pseudoephedrine HCl; chlorpheniramine maleate] 7.5•15•1 mg/5 mL

**Pediacof** syrup ℞ *pediatric narcotic antitussive, decongestant, antihistamine, and expectorant* [codeine phosphate; phenylephrine HCl; chlorpheniramine maleate; potassium iodide; alcohol 5%] 5•2.5•0.75•75 mg/5 mL

**Pediacon DX** children's syrup, pediatric drops OTC *pediatric antitussive, decongestant, and expectorant* [dextromethorphan hydrobromide; phenylpropanolamine HCl; guaifenesin] 5•6.25•100 mg/5 mL; 5•6.25•50 mg/mL

**Pediacon EX** pediatric drops OTC *pediatric decongestant and expectorant* [phenylpropanolamine HCl; guaifenesin] 6.25•50 mg/mL

**Pediaflor** drops ℞ *dental caries preventative* [sodium fluoride] 1.1 mg/mL

**Pedialyte** oral solution, freezer pops OTC *electrolyte replacement* [sodium, potassium, and chloride electrolytes]

**PediaPatch** transdermal patch (name changed to Trans-Ver-Sal Pedia-Patch in 1995)

**Pediapred** oral liquid ℞ *glucocorticoids* [prednisolone sodium phosphate] 5 mg/5 mL

**PediaProfen** oral suspension (name changed to Children's Motrin in 1993)

**PediaSure** ready-to-use liquid OTC *total or supplementary infant feeding*

**Pediatric Electrolyte** oral solution OTC *electrolyte replacement* [dextrose; multiple electrolytes] 1 L

**Pediazole** oral suspension ℞ *antibiotic* [erythromycin ethylsuccinate; sulfisoxazole acetyl] 200•600 mg/5 mL

**Pedi-Bath Salts** OTC *bath emollient*

**Pedi-Boro Soak Paks** powder packets OTC *astringent wet dressing (modified Burow solution)* [aluminum sulfate; calcium acetate]

**Pedi-Cort V Creme** ℞ *topical corticosteroid; antifungal; antibacterial* [hydrocortisone; clioquinol] 1%•3%

**pediculocides** *a class of agents effective against head and pubic lice*

**Pedi-Dri** powder ℞ *topical antifungal* [nystatin] 100 000 U/g

**Pediotic** ear drop suspension ℞ *topical corticosteroidal anti-inflammatory; antibiotic* [hydrocortisone; neomycin sulfate; polymyxin B sulfate] 1%•5 mg•10 000 U per mL

**Pedi-Pro** foot powder OTC *topical antifungal; anhidrotic* [zinc undecylenate; aluminum chlorhydroxide; menthol; chloroxylenol]

**Pedituss Cough** syrup ℞ *pediatric narcotic antitussive, decongestant, antihistamine, and expectorant* [codeine phosphate; phenylephrine HCl; chlorpheniramine maleate; potassium iodide] 5•2.5•0.75•75 mg/5 mL

**Pedi-Vit-A Creme** OTC *moisturizer; emollient* [vitamin A] 100 000 U/30 g

**Pedotic** otic suspension ℞ *topical corticosteroidal anti-inflammatory; antibiotic* [hydrocortisone; neomycin sulfate; polymyxin B sulfate] 1%•5 mg•10 000 U per mL

**PedTE-Pak-4** IV injection ℞ *intravenous nutritional therapy* [multiple trace elements (metals)] ±

**Pedtrace-4** IV injection ℞ *intravenous nutritional therapy* [multiple trace elements (metals)]

**PedvaxHIB** powder for IM injection ℞ *Haemophilus influenzae type b (HIB) vaccine* [Hemophilus b conjugate vaccine]

**Pee Wee** *street drug slang* [see: cocaine, crack]

**peep** *street drug slang* [see: PCP]

**PeeWee's Children's Vitamins** chewable tablets (discontinued 1995) OTC *vitamin/iron supplement* [multiple vitamins; iron; folic acid] ±•15•0.3 mg

**pefloxacin** USAN, INN, BAN *antibacterial*

**pefloxacin mesylate** USAN *antibacterial*

**Peg** *street drug slang* [see: heroin]

**PEG (polyethylene glycol)** [q.v.]

**PEG-ADA (polyethylene glycol-adenosine deaminase)** [see: pegademase bovine]

**pegademase** INN *adenosine deaminase (ADA) replacement* [also: pegademase bovine]

**pegademase bovine** USAN *adenosine deaminase (ADA) replacement for severe combined immunodeficiency disease (orphan)* [also: pegademase]

**PEG-adenosine deaminase (PEG-ADA)** [see: pegademase bovine]

**Peganone** tablets ℞ *hydantoin-type anticonvulsant* [ethotoin] 250, 500 mg

**pegaspargase (PEG-L-asparaginase)** USAN, INN *antineoplastic for acute lymphocytic leukemia (orphan) and acute lymphoblastic leukemia*

**PEG-ES (polyethylene glycol-electrolyte solution)** [q.v.]

**PEG-glucocerebrosidase (polyethylene glycol-glucocerebrosidase)** *investigational (orphan) for chronic enzyme replacement in Gaucher's disease*

**PEG-hemoglobin (polyethylene glycol-hemoglobin)** *investigational blood replacement*

**PEG-interleukin-2 (polyethylene glycol-interleukin-2)** *investigational (Phase II) cytokine for AIDS; investigational (orphan) for primary immunodeficiencies associated with T-cell defects*

**PEG-intron A (polyethylene glycol-intron A)** *investigational (Phase III) for hepatitis C*

**PEG-L-asparaginase** [see: pegaspargase]

**peglicol 5 oleate** USAN *emulsifying agent*

**pegorgotein** USAN *investigational free-radical scavenger to prevent irreversible brain damage after head trauma*

**pegoterate** USAN, INN *suspending agent*

**pegoxol 7 stearate** USAN *emulsifying agent*

**PEG-SOD (polyethylene glycol-superoxide dismutase)** [see: pegorgotein]

**Pelamine** tablets ℞ *antihistamine* [tripelennamine HCl] 50 mg

**pelanserin** INN *antihypertensive; vasodilator; serotonin adrenergic blocker* [also: pelanserin HCl]

**pelanserin HCl** USAN *antihypertensive; vasodilator; serotonin adrenergic blocker* [also: pelanserin]

**peldesine** USAN *purine nucleoside phosphorylase inhibitor for cutaneous T-cell lymphoma and psoriasis*

**peliomycin** USAN, INN *antineoplastic*

**pellets** *street drug slang* [see: LSD]

**pelretin** USAN, INN *antikeratinizing agent*

**pelrinone** INN *cardiotonic* [also: pelrinone HCl]

**pelrinone HCl** USAN *cardiotonic* [also: pelrinone]

**PEM-420** *investigational oral analgesic*

**pemedolac** USAN, INN *analgesic*

**pemerid** INN *antitussive* [also: pemerid nitrate]

**pemerid nitrate** USAN *antitussive* [also: pemerid]

**pemirolast** INN *antiallergic; mediator release inhibitor* [also: pemirolast potassium]

**pemirolast potassium** USAN *antiallergic; mediator release inhibitor* [also: pemirolast]

**pemoline** USAN, INN, BAN, JAN *CNS stimulant for attention deficit hyperactivity disorders (ADHD) and narcolepsy*

**pempidine** INN, BAN

**pen yan** *street drug slang* [see: opium]

**penamecillin** USAN, INN, BAN *antibacterial*

**penbutolol** INN, BAN *antiadrenergic (β-receptor)* [also: penbutolol sulfate]

**penbutolol sulfate** USAN *antiadrenergic (β-receptor)* [also: penbutolol]

**penciclovir** USAN, INN, BAN *topical antiviral for herpes*

**pendecamaine** INN, BAN

**pendiomide** [see: azamethonium bromide]

**Penecare** cream, lotion OTC *moisturizer; emollient*

**Penecort** cream, solution ℞ *topical corticosteroid* [hydrocortisone] 1%

**penems** *a class of broad-spectrum antibiotics*

**Penetrex** film-coated tablets ℞ *broad-spectrum fluoroquinolone-type antibiotic* [enoxacin] 200, 400 mg

**PenFill** (trademarked form) *insulin injector refill cartridge*

**penfluridol** USAN, INN *antipsychotic*

**penflutizide** INN

**pengitoxin** INN

**penicillamine** USAN, USP, INN *metal chelating agent; antirheumatic* ⟦?⟧ penicillin

**penicillin aluminum**

penicillin benzathine phenoxy-methyl [now: penicillin V benzathine]

penicillin calcium USP

penicillin G benzathine USP *bactericidal antibiotic* [also: benzathine benzylpenicillin; benzathine penicillin; benzylpenicillin benzathine]

penicillin G hydrabamine

penicillin G potassium USP *bactericidal antibiotic* [also: benzylpenicillin potassium] 200, 250, 400, 500 thousand U oral; 1, 2, 3, 5, 10, 20 million U/vial injection

penicillin G procaine USP *bactericidal antibiotic* [also: procaine penicillin]

penicillin G redox [see: redox-penicillin G]

penicillin G sodium USP *bactericidal antibiotic* [also: benzylpenicillin sodium]

penicillin hydrabamine phenoxy-methyl [now: penicillin V hydrabamine]

penicillin N [see: adicillin]

penicillin O [see: almecillin]

penicillin O chloroprocaine

penicillin O potassium

penicillin O sodium

penicillin phenoxymethyl [now: penicillin V]

penicillin potassium G [see: penicillin G potassium]

penicillin potassium phenoxymethyl [now: penicillin V potassium]

penicillin V USAN, USP *bactericidal antibiotic* [also: phenoxymethylpenicillin]

penicillin V benzathine USAN, USP *antibacterial*

penicillin V hydrabamine USAN, USP *antibacterial*

penicillin V potassium USAN, USP *bactericidal antibiotic*

penicillin-152 potassium [see: phenethicillin potassium] ⏃ penicillamine; Polycillin

penicillinase INN, BAN

penicillinase-resistant penicillins *a class of bactericidal antibiotics*

penicillinphenyrazine [see: phenyracillin]

penicillins *a class of bactericidal antibiotics*

**Penicillin-VK** tablets, oral solution ℞ *bactericidal antibiotic* [penicillin V potassium] 250, 500 mg; 125, 250 mg/5 mL

penidural [see: benzathine penicillin]

penimepicycline INN

penimocycline INN

penirolol INN

**Pen-Kera** cream OTC *moisturizer; emollient*

penmesterol INN

**Pennsaid** ℞ *investigational (NDA filed) therapy for rheumatoid arthritis*

penoctonium bromide INN

penprostene INN

pentabamate USAN, INN *minor tranquilizer*

**Pentacarinat** IV or IM injection ℞ *antiprotozoal; treatment and prophylaxis of Pneumocystis carinii pneumonia (orphan)* [pentamidine isethionate] 300 mg

**Pentacef** powder for IV or IM injection ℞ *cephalosporin-type antibiotic* [ceftazidime]

pentacosactride BAN [also: norleusactide]

pentacynium chloride INN

pentacyone chloride [see: pentacynium chloride]

pentaerithritol tetranicotinate [see: niceritrol]

pentaerithrityl tetranitrate INN *vasodilator* [also: pentaerythritol tetranitrate]

pentaerythritol tetranitrate (PETN) USP *vasodilator; "possibly effective" antianginal* [also: pentaerithrityl tetranitrate]

pentaerythritol trinitrate [see: pentrinitrol]

pentafilcon A USAN *hydrophilic contact lens material*

pentafluranol INN

pentagastrin USAN, INN *gastric secretion indicator*

pentagestrone INN

pentalamide INN, BAN

pentalyte USAN, USP, NF *electrolyte combination*

**Pentam 300** IV or IM injection ℞ *antiprotozoal; treatment and prophylaxis of Pneumocystis carinii pneumo-*

nia *(orphan)* [pentamidine isethionate] 300 mg

**pentamethazene** [see: azamethonium bromide]

**pentamethonium bromide** INN, BAN

**pentamethylenetetrazol** [see: pentylenetetrazol]

**pentamidine** INN, BAN

**pentamidine isethionate** *antiprotozoal; treatment and prophylaxis of Pneumocystis carinii pneumonia (orphan)* 300 mg injection

**pentamin** [see: azamethonium bromide]

**pentamorphone** USAN, INN *narcotic analgesic*

**pentamoxane** INN

**pentamoxane HCl** [see: pentamoxane]

**pentamustine** USAN *antineoplastic* [also: neptamustine]

**pentanedial** [see: glutaral]

**pentanitrol** [see: pentaerythritol tetranitrate]

**pentaphonate**

**pentapiperide** INN

**pentapiperium methylsulfate** USAN *anticholinergic* [also: pentapiperium metilsulfate]

**pentapiperium metilsulfate** INN *anticholinergic* [also: pentapiperium methylsulfate]

**pentaquine** INN [also: pentaquine phosphate]

**pentaquine phosphate** USP [also: pentaquine]

**Pentasa** controlled-release capsules ℞ *for ulcerative colitis, proctosigmoiditis, and proctitis; investigational for Crohn's disease* [mesalamine] 250 mg

**pentasodium colistinmethanesulfonate** [see: colistimethate sodium]

**Pentaspan** ℞ *leukapheresis adjunct to improve leukocyte yield (orphan)* [pentastarch]

**pentastarch** USAN, BAN *leukapheresis adjunct; red cell sedimenting agent; centrifugal leukocyte harvesting aid (orphan)*

**pentavalent gas gangrene antitoxin**

**Pentazine** injection ℞ *antihistamine; motion sickness; sleep aid; antiemetic; sedative* [promethazine HCl] 50 mg/mL ⓩ Phenazine

**Pentazine VC with Codeine** liquid ℞ *narcotic antitussive; antihistamine* [codeine phosphate; promethazine HCl] 10•6.25 mg/5 mL

**pentazocine** USAN, USP, INN, BAN *narcotic agonist-antagonist analgesic; also abused as a street drug*

**pentazocine HCl** USAN, USP *narcotic agonist-antagonist analgesic; also abused as a street drug*

**pentazocine lactate** USAN, USP *analgesic*

**pentazocine & naloxone HCl** *narcotic agonist-antagonist analgesic; also abused as a street drug* 50•0.5 mg oral

**pentetate calcium trisodium** USAN *plutonium chelating agent* [also: calcium trisodium pentetate]

**pentetate calcium trisodium Yb 169** USAN *radioactive agent*

**pentetate disodium** [see: pentetic acid, sodium salts]

**pentetate indium disodium In 111** USAN *diagnostic aid; radioactive agent*

**pentetate monosodium** [see: pentetic acid, sodium salts]

**pentetate pentasodium** [see: pentetic acid, sodium salts]

**pentetate tetrasodium** [see: pentetic acid, sodium salts]

**pentetate trisodium** [see: pentetic acid, sodium salts]

**pentetate trisodium calcium** [see: pentetate calcium trisodium]

**pentethylcyclanone** [see: cyclexanone]

**pentetic acid** USAN, BAN *diagnostic aid*

**pentetic acid, sodium salts** *diagnostic aid*

**pentetrazol** INN [also: pentylenetetrazol]

**penthanil diethylenetriamine pentaacetic acid (DTPA)** [see: pentetic acid]

**penthienate bromide** NF

**Penthrane** liquid for vaporization ℞ *inhalation general anesthetic* [methoxyflurane]

**penthrichloral** INN, BAN

**pentiapine** INN *antipsychotic* [also: pentiapine maleate]

**pentiapine maleate** USAN *antipsychotic* [also: pentiapine]

**penticide** [see: chlorophenothane]

**Pentids '400'; Pentids '800'** tablets (discontinued 1993) ℞ *bactericidal antibiotic* [penicillin G potassium] 400 000 U; 800 000 U

**Pentids '400' for Syrup** powder for oral solution (discontinued 1993) ℞ *bactericidal antibiotic* [penicillin G potassium] 400 000 U/5 mL

**pentifylline** INN, BAN

**pentigetide** USAN, INN *antiallergic*

**pentisomicin** USAN, INN *anti-infective*

**pentisomide** INN

**pentizidone** INN *antibacterial* [also: pentizidone sodium]

**pentizidone sodium** USAN *antibacterial* [also: pentizidone]

**pentobarbital** USP, INN *sedative; hypnotic; also abused as a street drug* [also: pentobarbitone; pentobarbital calcium] ⊡ phenobarbital

**pentobarbital calcium** JAN *sedative; hypnotic; also abused as a street drug* [also: pentobarbital; pentobarbitone]

**pentobarbital sodium** USP, JAN *sedative; hypnotic; also abused as a street drug* [also: pentobarbitone sodium] 100 mg oral; 50 mg/mL injection

**pentobarbitone** BAN *sedative; hypnotic; also abused as a street drug* [also: pentobarbital]

**pentobarbitone sodium** BAN *sedative; hypnotic; also abused as a street drug* [also: pentobarbital sodium]

**Pentolair** eye drops ℞ *mydriatic; cycloplegic* [cyclopentolate HCl] 1%

**pentolinium tartrate** NF [also: pentolonium tartrate]

**pentolonium tartrate** INN [also: pentolinium tartrate]

**pentolonum bitartrate** [see: pentolinium tartrate]

**pentomone** USAN, INN *prostate growth inhibitor*

**pentopril** USAN, INN *angiotensin-converting enzyme (ACE) inhibitor*

**pentorex** INN

**pentosalen** BAN

**pentosan polysulfate sodium** USAN, INN *urinary tract anti-inflammatory and analgesic for interstitial cystitis (orphan)* [also: pentosan polysulphate sodium]

**pentosan polysulphate sodium** BAN *urinary tract anti-inflammatory and analgesic* [also: pentosan polysulfate sodium]

**Pentostam** (available only from the Centers for Disease Control) ℞ *investigational anti-infective for leishmaniasis* [sodium stibogluconate]

**pentostatin** USAN, INN *potentiator; antibiotic antineoplastic for hairy cell and chronic lymphocytic leukemias (orphan)*

**Pentothal** powder for IV injection ℞ *barbiturate general anesthetic* [thiopental sodium] 2%, 2.5% (20, 25 mg/mL) ⊡ pentrinitrol

**Pentothal** rectal suspension (discontinued 1997) ℞ *barbiturate general anesthetic* [thiopental sodium] 400 mg/g ⊡ pentrinitrol;

**pentoxifylline** USAN, INN *vasodilator; hemorheologic agent* [also: oxpentifylline] 400 mg oral

**pentoxiverine citrate** [see: carbetapentane citrate]

**pentoxyverine** INN [also: carbetapentane citrate]

**pentoxyverine citrate** [see: carbetapentane citrate]

**Pentrax; Pentrax Gold** shampoo OTC *antiseborrheic; antipsoriatic; antipruritic; antibacterial* [coal tar] 4.3%; 4%

**pentrinitrol** USAN, INN *coronary vasodilator* ⊡ Pentothal

***tert*-pentyl alcohol** [see: amylene hydrate]

**Pentylan** tablets (discontinued 1995) ℞ *antianginal* [pentaerythritol tetranitrate] 10, 20 mg

**6-pentyl-*m*-cresol** [see: amylmetacresol]

**pentylenetetrazol** NF [also: pentetrazol]

**pentymal** [see: amobarbital]

**Pen-V** tablets ℞ *bactericidal antibiotic* [penicillin V potassium] 250, 500 mg

**Pen-Vee K** tablets, powder for oral solution ℞ *bactericidal antibiotic* [penicillin V potassium] 250, 500 mg; 125, 250 mg/5 mL

**pep pills** *street drug slang* [see: amphetamines]

**Pepcid** film-coated tablets, powder for oral suspension, IV injection, preloaded syringes for IV ℞ *gastric and duodenal ulcer treatment; histamine H₂ antagonist* [famotidine] 20, 40 mg; 40 mg/5 mL; 10 mg/mL; 20 mg

**Pepcid AC** tablets OTC *"acid controller" for heartburn and acid indigestion* [famotidine] 10 mg

**pepleomycin** [see: peplomycin sulfate]

**peplomycin** INN *antineoplastic* [also: peplomycin sulfate]

**peplomycin sulfate** USAN *antineoplastic* [also: peplomycin]

**peppermint** NF *flavoring agent; perfume*

**peppermint oil** NF *flavoring agent*

**peppermint spirit** USP *flavoring agent; perfume*

**peppermint water** NF *flavored vehicle*

**pepsin** *digestive aid*

**pepstatin** USAN, INN *pepsin enzyme inhibitor*

**Peptamen** ready-to-use liquid OTC *enteral nutritional therapy for GI impairment*

**Peptavlon** subcu injection ℞ *in vivo gastrointestinal function test* [pentagastrin] 250 μg/mL

**peptide copper compound** *investigational treatment for peptic ulcers, surgical wound repair, and bone healing*

**peptide metal compound** *investigational hair growth enhancer*

**peptide T** *investigational antiviral for AIDS (clinical trials discontinued 1994)*

**Pepto Diarrhea Control** oral solution OTC *antidiarrheal* [loperamide HCl] 1 mg/5 mL

**Pepto-Bismol** chewable tablets, caplets, liquid OTC *antidiarrheal; antinauseant* [bismuth subsalicylate] 262 mg; 262 mg; 262, 524 mg/15 mL

**peraclopone** INN

**peradoxime** INN

**perafensine** INN

**peralopride** INN

**peraquinsin** INN

**perastine** INN

**peratizole** INN, BAN

**perbufylline** INN

**Perchloracap** capsules ℞ *pertechnetate Tc 99m accumulation blocker; for hyperthyroidism* [potassium perchlorate] 200 mg

**Percocet** tablets ℞ *narcotic analgesic* [oxycodone HCl; acetaminophen] 5•325 mg

**Percodan; Percodan-Demi** tablets ℞ *narcotic analgesic; also abused as a street drug* [oxycodone HCl; oxycodone terephthalate; aspirin] 4.5• 0.38•325 mg; 2.25•0.19•325 mg ⊡ Decadron

**Percogesic** tablets OTC *antihistamine; analgesic* [phenyltoloxamine citrate; acetaminophen] 30•325 mg

**perc's; perks** *street drug slang* [see: Percodan; oxycodone HCl]

**Perdiem** granules OTC *laxative* [psyllium husks; senna extract] 3.25•0.74 g/tsp. ⊡ Pyridium

**Perdiem Fiber** granules OTC *laxative* [psyllium] 4.03 g/tsp.

**perfect high** *street drug slang* [see: heroin]

**Perfectoderm** gel OTC *topical keratolytic for acne* [benzoyl peroxide] 5%

**perfilcon A** USAN *hydrophilic contact lens material*

**perflenapent** USAN *ultrasound contrast agent*

**perflisopent** USAN *ultrasound contrast agent*

**perfluamine** INN, BAN

**perflubron** USAN, INN *blood substitute; MRI imaging agent*

**perflunafene** INN, BAN

**perfluorochemical (PFC) emulsion** (discontinued 1995) *synthetic blood oxygen carrier for PTCA*

**perfomedil** INN

**perfosfamide** USAN *antineoplastic; orphan status withdrawn 1996*

**Pergamid** ℞ *investigational antineoplastic; orphan status withdrawn 1996* [perfosfamide]

**pergolide** INN, BAN *dopamine agonist; antiparkinsonian* [also: pergolide mesylate]

**pergolide mesylate** USAN *dopamine agonist; antiparkinsonian* [also: pergolide]

**Pergonal** powder for IM injection ℞ *ovulation stimulant for women; spermatogenesis stimulant for men* [menotropins] 75, 150 IU/ampule

**perhexiline** INN *coronary vasodilator* [also: perhexiline maleate]

**perhexiline maleate** USAN *coronary vasodilator* [also: perhexiline]

**Periactin** tablets, syrup ℞ *antihistamine; cold urticaria; anticholinergic* [cyproheptadine HCl] 4 mg; 2 mg/5 mL ② Taractan

**periciazine** INN [also: pericyazine]

**perico** (Spanish for "parakeet") *street drug slang* [see: cocaine]

**Peri-Colace** capsules, syrup OTC *laxative; stool softener* [casanthranol; docusate sodium] 30•100 mg; 30•60 mg/15 mL

**pericyazine** BAN [also: periciazine]

**Peridex** mouth rinse ℞ *antimicrobial; gingivitis treatment; investigational (orphan) for oral mucositis in bone marrow transplant patients* [chlorhexidine gluconate; alcohol 11.6%] 0.12%

**Peridin-C** tablets OTC *vitamin supplement* [ascorbic acid; hesperidin complex; hesperidin methyl chalcone bioflavonoids] 200•150•50 mg

**Peri-Dos** softgels OTC *laxative; stool softener* [casanthranol; docusate sodium] 30•100 mg

**Perimed** oral rinse (discontinued 1994) OTC *oral antibacterial* [hydrogen peroxide; povidone-iodine] 1.5%•5%

**perimetazine** INN

**perindopril** USAN, INN, BAN *angiotensin-converting enzyme (ACE) inhibitor*

**perindopril erbumine** USAN *antihypertensive*

**perindoprilat** INN, BAN

**PerioGard** mouth rinse ℞ *antimicrobial; gingivitis treatment* [chlorhexidine gluconate; alcohol 11.6%] 0.12%

**Periostat** ℞ *investigational (NDA filed) collagenase inhibitor* [doxycycline]

**peripheral vasodilators** *a class of cardiovascular drugs that cause dilation of the blood vessels*

**perisoxal** INN

**Peritrate** tablets (discontinued 1995) ℞ *antianginal* [pentaerythritol tetranitrate] 10, 20, 40 mg

**Peritrate SA** sustained-action tablets (discontinued 1995) ℞ *antianginal* [pentaerythritol tetranitrate] 80 mg

**perlapine** USAN, INN *hypnotic*

**Perle** (dosage form) *soft gelatin capsule*

**permanganic acid, potassium salt** [see: potassium permanganate]

**Permapen** Isoject (unit dose syringe) ℞ *bactericidal antibiotic* [penicillin G benzathine] 1 200 000 U

**Permax** tablets ℞ *antiparkinsonian agent* [pergolide mesylate] 0.05, 0.25, 1 mg

**permethrin** USAN, INN, BAN *ectoparasiticide*

**Permitil** tablets, oral concentrate ℞ *antipsychotic* [fluphenazine HCl] 2.5, 5, 10 mg; 5 mg/mL

**Pernox Scrub; Pernox Lathering Lotion** OTC *abrasive cleanser for acne* [sulfur; salicylic acid]

**peroxide, dibenzoyl** [see: benzoyl peroxide]

**Peroxin A 5; Peroxin A 10** gel ℞ *topical keratolytic for acne* [benzoyl peroxide] 5%; 10%

**Peroxyl** mouth rinse, oral gel OTC *cleansing of oral wounds* [hydrogen peroxide] 1.5%

**perp** *street drug slang for fake crack made of candle wax and baking soda (to "perpetrate" a fraud)*

**perphenazine** USP, INN *antipsychotic; antiemetic; antidopaminergic; intractable hiccough relief* 2, 4, 8, 16 mg oral

**Persa-Gel; Persa-Gel W 5%; Persa-Gel W 10%** gel ℞ *topical keratolytic for acne* [benzoyl peroxide] 5%, 10%; 5%; 10%

**Persantine** sugar-coated tablets ℞ *antiplatelet agent* [dipyridamole] 25, 50, 75 mg ② Pertofrane

**Persantine IV** injection ℞ *in vivo coronary artery function test* [dipyridamole] 10 mg

**persic oil** NF *vehicle*

**persilic acid** INN

**Pertofrane** capsules (discontinued 1996) ℞ *tricyclic antidepressant* [desipramine HCl] 25, 50 mg ② Persantine

**Pertropin** capsules OTC *dietary lipo-tropic agent* [linolenic acid; multiple essential fatty acids] 7 mins.

**Pertussin All-Night PM** liquid (discontinued 1994) OTC *decongestant; antihistamine; antitussive; analgesic* [pseudoephedrine HCl; doxylamine succinate; dextromethorphan hydrobromide; acetaminophen; alcohol 25%] 2•0.25•1•33.4 mg/mL

**Pertussin AM** liquid (discontinued 1994) OTC *decongestant; antitussive; expectorant* [pseudoephedrine HCl; dextromethorphan hydrobromide; guaifenesin; alcohol]

**Pertussin CS; Pertussin ES** syrup OTC *antitussive* [dextromethorphan hydrobromide] 3.5 mg/5 mL; 15 mg/5 mL

**Pertussin PM** liquid (discontinued 1994) OTC *decongestant; antihistamine; antitussive; analgesic* [pseudoephedrine HCl; doxylamine succinate; dextromethorphan hydrobromide; acetaminophen; alcohol]

**pertussis immune globulin** USP *passive immunizing agent*

**pertussis immune human globulin** [now: pertussis immune globulin]

**pertussis vaccine** USP *active immunizing agent*

**pertussis vaccine adsorbed** USP *active immunizing agent*

**Peruvian; Peruvian flake; Peruvian lady** *street drug slang* [see: cocaine]

**Peruvian balsam** NF *topical local protectant; rubefacient*

**Peter** *street drug slang* [see: chloral hydrate]

**Peter Pan** *street drug slang* [see: PCP]

**peth** *street drug slang, from "pethidine," the official British and International name for meperidine HCl* [see: Demerol HCl; meperidine HCl]

**pethidine** INN, BAN *narcotic analgesic; also abused as a street drug* [also: meperidine HCl]

**pethidine HCl** [see: meperidine HCl]

**PETN (pentaerythritol tetranitrate)** [q.v.]

**petrichloral** INN

**petrol** *street drug slang (and a British term) for gasoline* [see: petroleum distillate inhalants]

**petrolatum** USP *ointment base; emollient/protectant* [also: yellow petrolatum]

**petrolatum, hydrophilic** USP *absorbent ointment base; topical protectant*

**petrolatum, liquid** [see: mineral oil]

**petrolatum, liquid emulsion** [see: mineral oil emulsion]

**petrolatum, white** USP, JAN *oleaginous ointment base; topical protectant*

**petrolatum gauze** [see: gauze, petrolatum]

**petroleum benzin** [see: benzin, petroleum]

**petroleum distillate inhalants** *vapors from butane, toluene, acetone, benzene, gasoline, etc., which produce psychoactive effects, abused as street drugs* [see also: nitrous oxide; volatile nitrites]

**petroleum jelly** [see: petrolatum]

**pexantel** INN

**peyote** *street drug slang* [see: mescaline]

**PFA (phosphonoformic acid)** [see: foscarnet sodium]

**PFC (perfluorochemical) emulsion** [q.v.]

**Pfeiffer's Allergy** tablets OTC *antihistamine* [chlorpheniramine maleate] 4 mg

**Pfeiffer's Cold Sore** lotion OTC *topical oral anesthetic; antipruritic/counterirritant* [gum benzoin; camphor; menthol; eucalyptol; alcohol 85%] 7%•<u>?</u>•<u>?</u>•<u>?</u>

**Pfizerpen** powder for injection ℞ *bactericidal antibiotic* [penicillin G potassium] 5, 20 million units

**Pfizerpen-AS** IM injection (discontinued 1997) ℞ *bactericidal antibiotic* [penicillin G procaine] 300 000 U/mL

**PFL (Platinol, fluorouracil, leucovorin [rescue])** *chemotherapy protocol*

**PFT (L-phenylalanine mustard, fluorouracil, tamoxifen)** *chemotherapy protocol*

**P-funk** *street drug slang for heroin or a combination of crack and PCP* [see: heroin; cocaine, crack; PCP]

**PG (paregoric)** [q.v.]

**PG (prostaglandin)** [q.v.]

**PGA (pteroylglutamic acid)** [see: folic acid]

**PGE₁ (prostaglandin E₁)** [now: alprostadil]

**PGE₂ (prostaglandin E₂)** [now: dinoprostone]

**PGF₂α (prostaglandin F₂α)** [see: dinoprost]

**PGF₂α (prostaglandin F₂α) THAM** [see: dinoprost tromethamine]

**PGI₂ (prostaglandin I₂)** [now: epoprostenol]

**PGX (prostaglandin X)** [now: epoprostenol]

**Phacotron Gold** ℞ *investigational phacoemulsification system for cataract surgery*

**Phanacōl Cough** syrup (discontinued 1995) OTC *decongestant; antitussive; expectorant; analgesic; antipyretic* [phenylpropanolamine HCl; dextromethorphan hydrobromide; guaifenesin; acetaminophen] 25•10•100• 325 mg/5 mL

**Phanadex Cough** syrup OTC *antitussive; decongestant; antihistamine; expectorant* [dextromethorphan hydrobromide; phenylpropanolamine HCl; pyrilamine maleate; guaifenesin] 15•25•40•100 mg/5 mL

**Phanatuss Cough** syrup OTC *antitussive; expectorant* [dextromethorphan hydrobromide; guaifenesin] 10•85 mg/5 mL

**phanchinone** [see: phanquinone; phanquone]

**phanquinone** INN [also: phanquone]

**phanquone** BAN [also: phanquinone]

**pharmaceutical glaze** [see: glaze, pharmaceutical]

**Pharmaflur; Pharmaflur df; Pharmaflur 1.1** chewable tablets ℞ *dental caries preventative* [sodium fluoride] 2.2 mg; 2.2 mg; 1.1 mg

**Pharmalgen** subcu or IM injection ℞ *venom sensitivity testing (subcu); venom desensitization therapy (IM)* [extracts of honeybee, yellow jacket, yellow hornet, white-faced hornet, mixed vespid, and wasp venom]

**Pharmorubicin PFS; Pharmorubicin RDF** ⒶⓃ injection ℞ *antibiotic*

*antineoplastic* [epirubicin HCl] 2 mg/mL; 10, 20, 50, 150 mg

**Phazyme** tablets, drops OTC *antiflatulent* [simethicone] 60 mg; 40 mg/0.6 mL ☒ Pherazine

**Phazyme 95** tablets OTC *antiflatulent* [simethicone] 95 mg

**Phazyme 125** softgels OTC *antiflatulent* [simethicone] 125 mg

**phebutazine** [see: febuverine]

**phebutyrazine** [see: febuverine]

**phemfilcon A** USAN *hydrophilic contact lens material*

**phenacaine** INN [also: phenacaine HCl]

**phenacaine HCl** USP [also: phenacaine]

**PhenaCal** capsules (discontinued 1993) OTC *dietary supplement* [multiple amino acids, vitamins, and minerals]

**phenacemide** USP, INN, BAN *anticonvulsant*

**phenacetin** USP, INN *(withdrawn from market)* ☒ phenazocine

**phenacon** [see: fenaclon]

**phenactropinium chloride** INN, BAN

**phenacyl 4-morpholineacetate** [see: mobecarb]

**N-phenacylhomatropinium chloride** [see: phenactropinium chloride]

**phenacylpivalate** [see: pibecarb]

**Phenadex Children's Cough/Cold** syrup OTC *pediatric antitussive, decongestant, and expectorant* [dextromethorphan hydrobromide; phenylpropanolamine HCl; guaifenesin; alcohol 5%] 5•6.25•100 mg/5 mL

**Phenadex Pediatric Cough/Cold** drops OTC *pediatric antitussive, decongestant, and expectorant* [dextromethorphan hydrobromide; phenylpropanolamine HCl; guaifenesin] 5•6.25• 50 mg/mL

**Phenadex Senior** liquid OTC *antitussive; expectorant* [dextromethorphan hydrobromide; guaifenesin] 10•200 mg/5 mL

**phenadoxone** INN, BAN

**phenaglycodol** INN

**Phenahist-TR** sustained-release tablets ℞ *decongestant; antihistamine; anticholinergic* [phenylpropanolamine HCl; phenylephrine HCl; chlorpheniramine maleate; hyoscyamine sulfate; atropine sulfate; scopolamine hydrobromide] 50•25•8•0.19• 0.04•0.01 mg

**phenamazoline** INN

**phenamazoline HCl** [see: phenamazoline]

**Phenameth** tablets ℞ *antihistamine; motion sickness; sleep aid; antiemetic; sedative* [promethazine HCl] 25 mg

**Phenameth DM** syrup ℞ *antitussive; antihistamine* [dextromethorphan hydrobromide; promethazine HCl; alcohol] 15•6.25 mg/5 mL

**phenampromide** INN

**Phenapap Sinus Headache & Congestion** tablets OTC *decongestant; antihistamine; analgesic* [pseudoephedrine HCl; chlorpheniramine maleate; acetaminophen] 30•2•325 mg

**Phenaphen** caplets (discontinued 1993) OTC *analgesic; antipyretic* [acetaminophen] 325 mg ② Betapen; Phenergan

**Phenaphen with Codeine No. 2** capsules (discontinued 1993) ℞ *narcotic analgesic* [codeine phosphate; acetaminophen] 15•325 mg

**Phenaphen with Codeine No. 3 & No. 4** capsules ℞ *narcotic analgesic* [codeine phosphate; acetaminophen] 30•325 mg; 60•325 mg

**Phenaphen-650 with Codeine** tablets (discontinued 1995) ℞ *narcotic analgesic* [codeine phosphate; acetaminophen] 30•650 mg

**phenaphthazine**

**phenarbutal** [see: phetharbital]

**phenarsone sulfoxylate** INN

**Phenaseptic** mouthwash/gargle (discontinued 1995) OTC *topical antipruritic/counterirritant; mild local anesthetic* [phenol] 1.4%

**Phenate** timed-release tablets ℞ *decongestant; antihistamine; analgesic* [phenylpropanolamine HCl; chlorpheniramine maleate; acetaminophen] 40•4•325 mg

**Phenazine 25** injection (discontinued 1996) ℞ *antihistamine; motion sickness; sleep aid; antiemetic; sedative* [promethazine HCl] 25 mg/mL ②

Pentazine; phenelzine; Phenoxine; Pherazine

**Phenazine 50** injection ℞ *antihistamine; motion sickness; sleep aid; antiemetic; sedative* [promethazine HCl] 50 mg/mL ② Pentazine; phenelzine; Phenoxine; Pherazine

**Phenazo** Ⓒ (U.S. product: Pyridium) tablets ℞ *urinary analgesic* [phenazopyridine HCl] 100, 200 mg

**phenazocine** INN ② phenacetin

**phenazocine hydrobromide** [see: phenazocine]

**Phenazodine** tablets (discontinued 1996) ℞ *urinary analgesic* [phenazopyridine HCl] 100, 200 mg

**phenazone** INN, BAN *analgesic* [also: antipyrine]

**phenazopyridine** INN, BAN *urinary tract analgesic* [also: phenazopyridine HCl]

**phenazopyridine HCl** USAN, USP *urinary tract analgesic* [also: phenazopyridine] 100, 200 mg oral

**phenbenicillin** BAN [also: fenbenicillin]

**phenbutazone sodium glycerate** USAN *anti-inflammatory*

**phenbutrazate** BAN [also: fenbutrazate]

**phencarbamide** USAN *anticholinergic* [also: fencarbamide]

**Phencen-50** injection (discontinued 1994) ℞ *sedative; antihistamine* [promethazine HCl] 50 mg/mL

**Phenchlor S.H.A.** sustained-release tablets ℞ *decongestant; antihistamine; anticholinergic* [phenylpropanolamine HCl; phenylephrine HCl; chlorpheniramine maleate; hyoscyamine sulfate; atropine sulfate; scopolamine hydrobromide] 50•25•8•0.19• 0.04•0.01 mg

**phencyclidine** INN *anesthetic* [also: phencyclidine HCl]

**phencyclidine HCl** USAN *anesthetic* [also: phencyclidine]

**phendimetrazine** INN *anorexiant* [also: phendimetrazine tartrate] 35 mg oral

**phendimetrazine tartrate** USP *anorexiant; CNS stimulant* [also: phendimetrazine] 35, 105 mg oral

**Phendry; Phendry Children's Allergy Medicine** elixir OTC *anti-*

*histamine* [diphenhydramine HCl] 12.5 mg/5 mL

**phenelzine** INN, BAN *antidepressant; MAO inhibitor* [also: phenelzine sulfate] ⊉ Phenazine; Phenylzin

**phenelzine sulfate** USP *antidepressant; MAO inhibitor* [also: phenelzine]

**phenemal** [see: phenobarbital]

**Phenerbel-S** tablets ℞ *GI anticholinergic; sedative; analgesic* [belladonna alkaloids; phenobarbital; ergotamine tartrate] 0.2•40•0.6 mg

**Phenergan** tablets, suppositories, injection ℞ *antihistamine; motion sickness; sleep aid; antiemetic; sedative* [promethazine HCl] 12.5, 25 mg; 12.5, 25, 50 mg; 25, 50 mg/mL ⊉ Phenaphen; Theragran

**Phenergan Fortis** syrup ℞ *antihistamine; motion sickness; sleep aid; antiemetic; sedative* [promethazine HCl; alcohol 1.5%] 25 mg/5 mL

**Phenergan Plain** syrup ℞ *antihistamine; motion sickness; sleep aid; antiemetic; sedative* [promethazine HCl] 6.25 mg/5 mL

**Phenergan VC** syrup ℞ *decongestant; antihistamine* [phenylephrine HCl; promethazine HCl; alcohol 7%] 5•6.25 mg/5 mL

**Phenergan VC with Codeine** syrup ℞ *narcotic antitussive; decongestant; antihistamine* [codeine phosphate; phenylephrine HCl; promethazine HCl; alcohol 7%] 10•5•6.25 mg/5 mL

**Phenergan with Codeine** syrup ℞ *narcotic antitussive; antihistamine* [codeine phosphate; promethazine HCl; alcohol 7%] 10•6.25 mg/5 mL

**Phenergan with Dextromethorphan** syrup ℞ *antitussive; antihistamine* [dextromethorphan hydrobromide; promethazine HCl; alcohol 7%] 15•6.25 mg/5 mL

**pheneridine** INN

**phenethanol** [see: phenylethyl alcohol]

**phenethazine** [see: fenethazine]

**phenethicillin potassium** USP [also: pheneticillin]

**phenethyl alcohol** BAN *antimicrobial agent* [also: phenylethyl alcohol]

**N-phenethylanthranilic acid** [see: enfenamic acid]

**phenethylazocine bromide** [see: phenazocine hydrobromide]

**phenethylhydrazine sulfate** [see: phenelzine sulfate]

**pheneticillin** INN [also: phenethicillin potassium]

**pheneticillin potassium** [see: phenethicillin potassium]

**Phenetron** tablets, syrup (discontinued 1997) ℞ *antihistamine; antitussive* [chlorpheniramine maleate] 4 mg; 2 mg/5 mL

**Phenetron Compound** sugar-coated tablets (discontinued 1993) OTC *antihistamine; analgesic* [chlorpheniramine maleate; aspirin; caffeine]

**phenetsal** [see: acetaminosalol]

**pheneturide** INN, BAN [also: acetylpheneturide]

**Phenex-1** powder OTC *formula for infants with phenylketonuria*

**Phenex-2** powder OTC *enteral nutritional therapy for phenylketonuria*

**phenformin** INN, BAN *biguanide hypoglycemic agent* [also: phenformin HCl]

**phenformin HCl** USP *hypoglycemic agent (removed from market by FDA in 1977, now available as an investigational drug)* [also: phenformin]

**phenglutarimide** INN, BAN

**Phenhist DH with Codeine** liquid ℞ *narcotic antitussive; decongestant; antihistamine* [codeine phosphate; pseudoephedrine HCl; chlorpheniramine maleate; alcohol 5%] 10•30•2 mg/5 mL

**Phenhist Expectorant** liquid ℞ *narcotic antitussive; decongestant; expectorant* [codeine phosphate; pseudoephedrine HCl; guaifenesin; alcohol 7.5%] 10•30•100 mg/5 mL

**phenicarbazide** INN

**phenidiemal** [see: phetharbital]

**phenindamine** INN *antihistamine* [also: phenindamine tartrate]

**phenindamine tartrate** USAN *antihistamine* [also: phenindamine]

**phenindione** USP, INN *anticoagulant*

**pheniodol sodium** INN [also: iodoalphionic acid]

**pheniprazine** INN, BAN
**pheniprazine HCl** [see: pheniprazine]
**pheniramine** INN [also: pheniramine maleate]
**pheniramine maleate** USAN [also: pheniramine]
**pheniramine maleate & naphazoline HCl** *topical ocular antihistamine and decongestant* 0.3%•0.025% eye drops
**phenisonone hydrobromide**
**Phenistix** reagent strips for professional use (discontinued 1994) *in vitro diagnostic aid for phenylketonuria*
**phenmetraline HCl** [see: phenmetrazine HCl]
**phenmetrazine** INN, BAN *anorexiant; CNS stimulant; also abused as a street drug* [also: phenmetrazine HCl]
**phenmetrazine HCl** USP *anorexiant; CNS stimulant; also abused as a street drug* [also: phenmetrazine]
**phennies; fennies** *street drug slang* [see: phenobarbital]
**phenobamate** [see: febarbamate]
**phenobarbital** USP, INN, JAN *anticonvulsant; hypnotic; sedative; also abused as a street drug* [also: phenobarbitone] 15, 30, 60, 100 mg oral; 15, 20 mg/5 mL oral ⚕ pentobarbital
**phenobarbital sodium** USP, INN, JAN *anticonvulsant; hypnotic; sedative; also abused as a street drug* 30, 60, 65, 130 mg/mL injection
**phenobarbitone** BAN *anticonvulsant; hypnotic; sedative; also abused as a street drug* [also: phenobarbital]
**phenobutiodil** INN
**phenododecinium bromide** [see: domiphen bromide]
**Phenoject-50** injection ℞ *antihistamine; motion sickness; sleep aid; antiemetic; sedative* [promethazine HCl] 50 mg/mL
**phenol** USP *topical antiseptic/antipruritic; local anesthetic; preservative*
**phenol, liquefied** USP *topical antipruritic*
**phenol, sodium salt** [see: phenolate sodium]
**phenol red** [see: phenolsulfonphthalein]
**phenolate sodium** USAN *disinfectant*

**Phenolated Calamine** lotion OTC *topical poison ivy treatment* [calamine; zinc oxide; phenol] 8%•8%•1%
**Phenolax** wafers OTC *laxative* [phenolphthalein] 64.8 mg
**phenolphthalein** USP, INN *stimulant laxative*
**phenolphthalein, white** [see: phenolphthalein]
**phenolphthalein, yellow** USP *stimulant laxative*
**phenolsulfonphthalein** USP
**phenolsulphonate sodium** USP
**phenomorphan** INN, BAN
**phenomycilline** [see: penicillin V]
**phenoperidine** INN, BAN
**phenopryldiasulfone sodium** [see: solasulfone]
**Phenoptic** eye drops ℞ *ophthalmic decongestant/vasoconstrictor; mydriatic* [phenylephrine HCl] 2.5%
**pheno's; feno's** *street drug slang* [see: phenobarbital]
**phenosulfophthalein** [see: phenolsulfonphthalein]
**phenothiazine** NF, INN *antipsychotic*
**phenothiazines** *a class of drugs with antipsychotic, hypotensive, antiemetic, antispasmodic, and antihistaminic activity*
**phenothrin** INN, BAN
**phenoxazoline HCl** [see: fenoxazoline HCl]
**Phenoxine** tablets OTC *diet aid* [phenylpropanolamine HCl] 25 mg ⚕ Phenazine
**phenoxybenzamine** INN *antihypertensive* [also: phenoxybenzamine HCl]
**phenoxybenzamine HCl** USP *antihypertensive; pheochromocytomic agent* [also: phenoxybenzamine]
**phenoxymethylpenicillin** INN *bactericidal antibiotic* [also: penicillin V]
**phenoxypropazine** BAN [also: fenoxypropazine]
**phenoxypropylpenicillin** [see: propicillin]
**phenozolone** [see: fenozolone]
**phenprobamate** INN, BAN
**phenprocoumon** USAN, USP, INN *anticoagulant*

**phenprocumone** [see: phenpro-
coumon]

**phenpromethadrine** [see: phenpro-
methamine]

**phenpromethamine** INN

**phenpropamine citrate** [see: alverine
citrate]

**phensuximide** USP, INN, BAN *anticonvulsant*

**phentermine** USAN, INN *anorexiant;
an adrenergic isomeric of amphetamine*
🔄 phentolamine

**phentermine HCl** USP *anorexiant;
CNS stimulant; the water-soluble form
of phentermine for oral administration*
8, 15, 18.75, 30, 37.5 mg oral

**phenthiazine** [see: phenothiazine]

**phentolamine** INN, BAN *antihypertensive; pheochromocytomic agent* [also:
phentolamine HCl] 🔄 phentermine;
Ventolin

**phentolamine HCl** USP *antihypertensive; pheochromocytomic agent* [also:
phentolamine]

**phentolamine mesilate** INN, JAN *antiadrenergic; antihypertensive; pheochromocytomic agent* [also: phentolamine
mesylate]

**phentolamine mesylate** USP *antiadrenergic; antihypertensive; pheochromocytomic agent; investigational (Phase
III) oral treatment for erectile dysfunction* [also: phentolamine mesilate]

**phentolamine methanesulfonate**
[now: phentolamine mesylate]

**Phentrol** tablets (discontinued 1996) ℞
*anorexiant* [phentermine HCl] 8 mg

**Phentrol 2; Phentrol 4; Phentrol 5**
capsules ℞ *anorexiant* [phentermine
HCl] 30 mg

**phentydrone**

**Phenurone** tablets (discontinued
1997) ℞ *anticonvulsant* [phenace-
mide] 500 mg

**phenyl aminosalicylate** USAN, BAN
*antibacterial; tuberculostatic* [also:
fenamisal]

**phenyl salicylate** NF *analgesic; not
generally regarded as safe and effective
as an antidiarrheal*

**phenylalanine (L-phenylalanine)**
USAN, USP, INN *essential amino acid;
symbols: Phe, F*

**phenylalanine ammonia-lyase** *investigational (orphan) for hyperphenylalaninemia*

**phenylalanine mustard (PAM)** [see:
melphalan]

**L-phenylalanine mustard (L-PAM)**
[see: melphalan]

**Phenylase** *investigational (orphan) for
hyperphenylalaninemia* [phenylalanine
ammonia-lyase]

**phenylazo diamino pyridine HCl**
[see: phenazopyridine HCl]

**phenylbenzyl atropine** [see: xenytropium bromide]

**phenylbutazone** USP, INN *antirheumatic; anti-inflammatory; antipyretic;
analgesic*

**phenylbutyrate sodium** [see: sodium
phenylbutyrate]

**2-phenylbutyrylurea** [see: pheneturide; acetylpheneturide]

**phenylcarbinol** [see: benzyl alcohol]

**phenylcinchoninic acid** [now: cin-
chophen]

**α-phenyl-*p*-cresol carbamate** [see:
diphenan]

**phenylcyclohexyl piperidine (PCP)**
[see: PCP; phencyclidine HCl]

**2-phenylcyclopentylamine HCl**
[see: cypenamine HCl]

**phenyldimazone** [see: normethadone]

**Phenyldrine** timed-release tablets
OTC *diet aid* [phenylpropanolamine
HCl] 75 mg

**phenylephrine (PE)** INN, BAN *nasal
decongestant; ocular vasoconstrictor;
vasopressor for hypotensive or cardiac
shock* [also: phenylephrine HCl]

**phenylephrine bitartrate** *bronchodilator; vasoconstrictor*

**phenylephrine HCl** USP *nasal decongestant; ocular vasoconstrictor; vasopressor for hypotensive or cardiac shock*
[also: phenylephrine] 0.25%, 0.5%,
1% nose drops or spray; 2.5%, 10%
eye drops; 1% injection

**phenylephrine tannate, chlorphen-
iramine tannate, and pyrilamine**

**tannate** *decongestant; antihistamine* 25•8•25 mg oral

**phenylethanol** [see: phenylethyl alcohol]

**phenylethyl alcohol** USP *antimicrobial agent; preservative* [also: phenethyl alcohol]

**phenylethylmalonylurea** [see: phenobarbital]

**Phenylfenesin L.A.** extended-action tablets R *decongestant; expectorant* [phenylpropanolamine HCl; guaifenesin] 75•400 mg

**Phenylfenesin L.A.** long-acting tablets R *decongestant; expectorant* [phenylpropanolamine HCl; guaifenesin] 75•400 mg

**Phenyl-Free** liquid OTC *special diet for infants with phenylketonuria (PKU)*

**Phenylgesic** tablets OTC *antihistamine; analgesic* [phenyltoloxamine citrate; acetaminophen] 30•325 mg

**phenylindanedione** [see: phenindione]

**phenylmercuric acetate** NF *antimicrobial agent; preservative*

**phenylmercuric borate** INN

**phenylmercuric chloride** NF

**phenylmercuric nitrate** NF *antimicrobial agent; preservative; topical antiseptic*

**phenylone** [see: antipyrine]

**phenylpropanolamine (PPA)** INN, BAN *vasoconstrictor; nasal decongestant; nonprescription diet aid* [also: phenylpropanolamine HCl]

**phenylpropanolamine HCl** USP *vasoconstrictor; nasal decongestant; nonprescription diet aid* [also: phenylpropanolamine] 25, 50, 75 mg oral

**phenylpropanolamine polistirex** USAN *adrenergic; vasoconstrictor*

**1-phenylsemicarbazide** [see: phenicarbazide]

**phenylthilone** [see: phenythilone]

**phenyltoloxamine** INN

**phenyltoloxamine citrate** *antihistamine*

**phenyltriazines** *a class of anticonvulsants*

**Phenylzin** eye drops (discontinued 1993) OTC *topical ocular decongestant; astringent; antiseptic* [phenylephrine HCl; zinc sulfate] ☑ phenelzine

**phenyracillin** INN

**phenyramidol HCl** USAN *analgesic; skeletal muscle relaxant* [also: fenyramidol]

**phenythilone** INN

**phenytoin** USAN, USP, INN, BAN *hydantoin-type anticonvulsant*

**phenytoin redox** [see: redox-phenytoin]

**phenytoin sodium** USP *hydantoin-type anticonvulsant* 100 mg oral; 50 mg/mL injection

**Pherazine DM** syrup R *antitussive; antihistamine* [dextromethorphan hydrobromide; promethazine HCl; alcohol 7%] 15•6.25 mg/5 mL

**Pherazine VC** syrup (name changed to Promethazine VC Plain in 1995)

**Pherazine VC with Codeine** syrup R *narcotic antitussive; decongestant; antihistamine* [codeine phosphate; phenylephrine HCl; promethazine HCl; alcohol 7%] 10•5•6.25 mg/5 mL

**Pherazine with Codeine** syrup R *narcotic antitussive; antihistamine* [codeine phosphate; promethazine HCl; alcohol 7%] 10•6.25 mg/5 mL

**phetharbital** INN

**phezathion** [see: fezatione]

**Phicon** cream OTC *topical anesthetic; emollient* [pramoxine HCl; vitamins A and E] 0.5%•7500 IU•2000 IU

**Phicon F** cream OTC *topical anesthetic; antifungal* [pramoxine HCl; undecylenic acid] 0.05%•8%

**Phillies blunt** *street drug slang for a cigar hollowed out and filled with marijuana* [see: marijuana]

**Phillips' Chewable** tablets OTC *antacid* [magnesium hydroxide] 311 mg

**Phillips' Laxative** gelcaps OTC *laxative; stool softener* [phenolphthalein; docusate sodium] 90•83 mg

**Phillips' LaxCaps** capsules OTC *laxative; stool softener* [phenolphthalein; docusate sodium] 90•83 mg

**Phillips' Milk of Magnesia; Concentrated Phillips' Milk of Magnesia** liquid OTC *antacid; laxative* [magnesium hydroxide] 400 mg/5 mL; 800 mg/5 mL

**pHisoDerm; pHisoDerm for Baby** liquid OTC *soap-free therapeutic skin cleanser*

**pHisoDerm Cleansing Bar** OTC *therapeutic skin cleanser*

**pHisoHex** liquid ℞ *bacteriostatic skin cleanser* [hexachlorophene] 3% ☒ Fostex

**phloropropiophenone** [see: flopropione]

**pholcodine** INN

**pholedrine** INN, BAN

**pholescutol** [see: folescutol]

**PhosChol** softgels, liquid concentrate OTC *neurotransmitter; lipotropic* [phosphatidylcholine] 565, 900 mg; 3 g/5 mL

**phoscolic acid** [see: foscolic acid]

**Phos-Ex 62.5 Mini-Tabs; Phos-Ex 167; Phos-Ex 250** tablets (discontinued 1994) OTC *calcium supplement* [calcium acetate] 250 mg; 668 mg; 1000 mg

**Phos-Ex 125** capsules (discontinued 1994) OTC *calcium supplement* [calcium acetate] 500 mg

**Phos-Flur** oral rinse ℞ *dental caries preventative* [acidulated phosphate fluoride] 0.44 mg/mL

**PhosLo** tablets ℞ *buffering agent for hyperphosphatemia in end-stage renal disease (orphan)* [calcium acetate] 667 mg

**pHos-pHaid E.C.** enteric-coated tablets (discontinued 1993) ℞ *urinary acidifier* [ammonium biphosphate; sodium biphosphate; sodium acid pyrophosphate] 95•100•55, 190•200•110 mg

**Phosphaljel** oral suspension (discontinued 1994) OTC *no longer labeled for use as an antacid* [aluminum phosphate gel] 44.6 mg/mL

**phosphate salt of tricyclic nucleoside** [now: triciribine phosphate]

**phosphatidylcholine (PC)** [see: lecithin]

**phosphinic acid** [see: hypophosphorous acid]

**2,2′-phosphinicodilactic acid (PDLA)** [see: foscolic acid]

**Phosphocol P 32** suspension for intracavitary instillation, interstitial injection ℞ *radiopharmaceutical antineoplastic* [chromic phosphate P 32] 10, 15 mCi

**phosphocysteamine** *investigational (orphan) for cystinosis*

**Phospholine Iodide** powder for eye drops ℞ *antiglaucoma agent; irreversible cholinesterase inhibitor miotic* [echothiophate iodide] 0.03%, 0.06%, 0.125%, 0.25%

**phosphonoformic acid (PFA)** [see: foscarnet sodium]

**phosphorated carbohydrate solution (hyperosmolar solution with phosphoric acid)** *antinauseant; antiemetic*

**phosphoric acid** NF *solvent; acidifying agent*

**phosphoric acid, aluminum salt** [see: aluminum phosphate gel]

**phosphoric acid, calcium salt** [see: calcium phosphate, dibasic]

**phosphoric acid, chromium salt** [see: chromic phosphate Cr 51 & P 32]

**phosphoric acid, diammonium salt** [see: ammonium phosphate]

**phosphoric acid, dipotassium salt** [see: potassium phosphate, dibasic]

**phosphoric acid, disodium salt heptahydrate** [see: sodium phosphate, dibasic]

**phosphoric acid, disodium salt hydrate** [see: sodium phosphate, dibasic]

**phosphoric acid, magnesium salt** [see: magnesium phosphate]

**phosphoric acid, monopotassium salt** [see: potassium phosphate, monobasic]

**phosphoric acid, monosodium salt dihydrate** [see: sodium phosphate, monobasic]

**phosphoric acid, monosodium salt monohydrate** [see: sodium phosphate, monobasic]

**phosphorofluoridic acid, disodium salt** [see: sodium monofluorophosphate]

**phosphorus** *element (P)*

**Phospho-Soda** [see: Fleet Phospho-Soda]

**phosphothiamine** [see: monophosphothiamine]

**Photofrin** powder for IV injection *laser light-activated antineoplastic for photodynamic therapy of esophageal cancer (orphan); investigational (orphan) for bladder cancer* [porfimer sodium] 75 mg

**phoxim** INN, BAN

**Phrenilin** tablets ℞ *analgesic; antipyretic; sedative* [acetaminophen; butalbital] 325•50

**Phrenilin Forte** capsules ℞ *analgesic; antipyretic; sedative* [acetaminophen; butalbital] 650•50 mg

**PHRT (procarbazine, hydroxyurea, radiotherapy)** *chemotherapy protocol*

**phthalofyne** USAN *veterinary anthelmintic* [also: ftalofyne]

**phthalylsulfacetamide** NF

**phthalylsulfamethizole** INN

**phthalylsulfathiazole** USP, INN

**phylcardin** [see: aminophylline]

**phyllindon** [see: aminophylline]

**Phyllocontin** controlled-release tablets ℞ *bronchodilator* [aminophylline] 225 mg

**phylloquinone** [see: phytonadione]

**Phylorinol** liquid OTC *topical antipruritic/counterirritant; mild local anesthetic; antiseptic; astringent; oral deodorant* [phenol; boric acid; strong iodine solution; chlorophyllin copper complex] 0.6%•⁇•⁇•⁇

**Phylorinol** mouthwash/gargle OTC *topical antipruritic/counterirritant; mild local anesthetic* [phenol] 0.6%

**physiological irrigating solution** *for general irrigating, washing and rinsing; not for injection*

**Physiolyte** liquid ℞ *sterile irrigant* [physiological irrigating solution]

**PhysioSol** liquid ℞ *sterile irrigant* [physiological irrigating solution]

**Physiotens** ℞ *investigational antihypertensive* [monoxidine]

**physostigmine** USP, BAN *investigational (Phase III) reversible cholinesterase inhibitor miotic for glaucoma* ⑨ pyridostigmine; Prostigmin

**physostigmine salicylate** USP *cholinergic to reverse anticholinergic overdose; investigational (orphan) for Friedreich's and other inherited ataxias*

**physostigmine sulfate** USP *ophthalmic cholinergic*

**phytate persodium** USAN *pharmaceutic aid*

**phytate sodium** USAN *calcium-chelating agent*

**phytic acid** [see: fytic acid]

**phytomenadione** INN, BAN *vitamin K₁; prothrombogenic* [also: phytonadione]

**phytonadiol sodium diphosphate** INN

**phytonadione** USP, JAN *vitamin K₁; prothrombogenic* [also: phytomenadione] 2 mg/mL injection

**PIA (Platinol, ifosfamide, Adriamycin)** *chemotherapy protocol*

**pibecarb** INN

**piberaline** INN

**picafibrate** INN

**picartamide** INN

**picenadol** INN *analgesic* [also: picenadol HCl]

**picenadol HCl** USAN *analgesic* [also: picenadol]

**picilorex** INN

**piclamilast** USAN *phosphodiesterase type IV inhibitor for asthma*

**piclonidine** INN

**piclopastine** INN

**picloxydine** INN, BAN

**picobenzide** INN

**picodralazine** INN

**picolamine** INN

**piconol** INN

**picoperine** INN

**picoprazole** INN

**picotrin** INN *keratolytic* [also: picotrin diolamine]

**picotrin diolamine** USAN *keratolytic* [also: picotrin]

**picric acid** [see: trinitrophenol]

**picrotoxin** NF

**picumast** INN, BAN

**picumeterol** INN, BAN *bronchodilator* [also: picumeterol fumarate]

**picumeterol fumarate** USAN *bronchodilator* [also: picumeterol]

**pidolacetamol** INN

**pidolic acid** INN

**piece** *street drug slang* [see: cocaine; cocaine, crack]

**piedras** (Spanish for "stones") *street drug slang* [see: cocaine, crack]

**pifarnine** USAN, INN *gastric antiulcerative*

**pifenate** INN, BAN

**pifexole** INN

**piflutixol** INN

**pifoxime** INN

**pig killer** *street drug slang* [see: PCP]

**piketoprofen** INN

**Pilagan** eye drops ℞ *antiglaucoma agent; direct-acting miotic* [pilocarpine nitrate] 1%, 2%, 4%

**pildralazine** INN

**piles** *street drug slang* [see: cocaine, crack]

**Pilocar** eye drops ℞ *antiglaucoma agent; direct-acting miotic* [pilocarpine HCl] 0.5%, 1%, 2%, 3%, 4%, 6%

**pilocarpine** USP, BAN *antiglaucoma agent; ophthalmic cholinergic*

**pilocarpine HCl** USP *ophthalmic cholinergic; antiglaucoma miotic; for radiation xerostomia (orphan); investigational (orphan) for keratoconjunctivitis sicca* 0.5%, 1%, 2%, 4%, 6%, 8% eye drops

**pilocarpine nitrate** USP *ophthalmic cholinergic; antiglaucoma agent; miotic*

**Pilocarpine SME** ℞ *investigational glaucoma treatment* [pilocarpine]

**Pilopine HS** ophthalmic gel ℞ *antiglaucoma agent; direct-acting miotic* [pilocarpine HCl] 4%

**Piloptic-½; Piloptic-1; Piloptic-2; Piloptic-3; Piloptic-4; Piloptic-6** eye drops ℞ *antiglaucoma agent; direct-acting miotic* [pilocarpine HCl] 0.5%; 1%; 2%; 3%; 4%; 6%

**Pilopto-Carpine** eye drops ℞ *antiglaucoma agent; direct-acting miotic* [pilocarpine HCl] 4%

**Pilostat** eye drops ℞ *antiglaucoma agent; direct-acting miotic* [pilocarpine HCl] 0.5%, 1%, 2%, 3%, 4%, 6%

**Pilpak** (trademarked packaging form) *patient compliance package*

**Pima** syrup ℞ *expectorant* [potassium iodide] 325 mg/5 mL

**pimagedine HCl** USAN *advanced glycosylation inhibitor for type 1 diabetes;* *investigational (Phase III) for diabetics in end-stage renal disease*

**pimaricin** JAN *ophthalmic antibacterial/ antifungal antibiotic* [also: natamycin]

**pimeclone** INN

**pimefylline** INN

**pimelautide** INN

**pimetacin** INN

**pimethixene** INN

**pimetine** INN *antihyperlipoproteinemic* [also: pimetine HCl]

**pimetine HCl** USAN *antihyperlipoproteinemic* [also: pimetine]

**pimetixene** [see: pimethixene]

**pimetremide** INN

**pimeverine** [see: pimetremide]

**piminodine** INN [also: piminodine esylate]

**piminodine esylate** NF [also: piminodine]

**piminodine ethanesulfonate** [see: piminodine esylate]

**pimobendan** USAN, INN *cardiotonic*

**pimonidazole** INN, BAN

**pimozide** USAN, USP, INN, BAN, JAN *antipsychotic; neuroleptic; suppresses symptoms of Tourette syndrome*

**pimp** *street drug slang* [see: cocaine]

**pin; pinhead** *street drug slang for a thinly rolled marijuana cigarette* [see: marijuana]

**pin gun; pin yen** *street drug slang* [see: opium]

**pinacidil** USAN, INN *antihypertensive*

**pinadoline** USAN, INN *analgesic*

**pinafide** INN

**pinaverium bromide** INN

**pinazepam** INN

**pincainide** INN

**Pindac** ℞ *investigational antihypertensive* [pinacidil]

**pindolol** USAN, USP, INN, BAN *vasodilator; antiadrenergic (β-receptor)* 5, 10 mg oral

**pine needle oil** NF

**pine tar** USP

**pineapple** *street drug slang for a combination of heroin and Ritalin (methylphenidate HCl) or amphetamine* [see: heroin; Ritalin; methylphenidate HCl; amphetamines]

**Pink Bismuth** liquid OTC *antidiarrheal; antinauseant* [bismuth subsalicylate] 130, 262 mg/15 mL

**pink blotters** *street drug slang* [see: LSD]

**pink hearts** *street drug slang* [see: amphetamines]

**Pink Panther; pink robots; pink wedge; pink witches** *street drug slang* [see: LSD]

**pink spoons** *street drug slang* [see: Percodan; oxycodone HCl]

**pinks** *street drug slang* [see: Seconal Sodium; secobarbital sodium]

**pinolcaine** INN

**pinoxepin** INN *antipsychotic* [also: pinoxepin HCl]

**pinoxepin HCl** USAN *antipsychotic* [also: pinoxepin]

**Pin-Rid** soft gel capsules, liquid OTC *anthelmintic for ascariasis (roundworm) and enterobiasis (pinworm)* [pyrantel pamoate] 180 mg; 50 mg/mL

**Pin-X** liquid OTC *anthelmintic for ascariasis (roundworm) and enterobiasis (pinworm)* [pyrantel pamoate] 50 mg/mL

**pioglitazone** INN *antidiabetic* [also: pioglitazone HCl]

**pioglitazone HCl** USAN *antidiabetic* [also: pioglitazone]

**pipacycline** INN

**pipamazine** INN

**pipamperone** USAN, INN *antipsychotic*

**pipaneperone** [see: pipamperone]

**pipazetate** INN *antitussive* [also: pipazethate]

**pipazethate** USAN *antitussive* [also: pipazetate]

**pipebuzone** INN

**pipecuronium bromide** USAN, INN, BAN *muscle relaxant; nondepolarizing neuromuscular blocker; adjunct to anesthesia*

**pipemidic acid** INN

**pipenzolate bromide** INN

**pipenzolate methylbromide** [see: pipenzolate bromide]

**pipenzolone bromide** [see: pipenzolate bromide]

**pipequaline** INN

**piperacetazine** USAN, USP, INN *antipsychotic* ☐ piperazine

**piperacillin** INN, BAN *penicillin-type bactericidal antibiotic* [also: piperacillin sodium]

**piperacillin sodium** USAN, USP, JAN *penicillin-type bactericidal antibiotic* [also: piperacillin]

**piperamide** INN *anthelmintic* [also: piperamide maleate]

**piperamide maleate** USAN *anthelmintic* [also: piperamide]

**piperamine** [see: bamipine]

**piperazine** USP *anthelmintic for enterobiasis (pinworm) and ascariasis (roundworm)* ☐ piperacetazine

**piperazine calcium edetate** INN *anthelmintic* [also: piperazine edetate calcium]

**piperazine citrate** USP *anthelmintic* 250 mg oral; 500 mg/mL oral

**piperazine citrate hydrate** [see: piperazine citrate]

**piperazine edetate calcium** USAN *anthelmintic* [also: piperazine calcium edetate]

**piperazine estrone sulfate** [now: estropipate]

**piperazine hexahydrate** [see: piperazine citrate]

**piperazine phosphate**

**piperazine phosphate monohydrate** [see: piperazine phosphate]

**piperazine theophylline ethanoate** [see: acefylline piperazine]

**piperidine phosphate**

**piperidines** *a class of antihistamines*

**piperidolate** INN [also: piperidolate HCl]

**piperidolate HCl** USP [also: piperidolate]

**piperilate** [see: pipethanate]

**piperine** USP

**piperocaine** INN [also: piperocaine HCl]

**piperocaine HCl** USP [also: piperocaine]

**piperonyl butoxide** *pediculicide*

**piperoxan** INN

**piperphenidol HCl**

**piperylone** INN

**pipethanate** INN

**pipobroman** USAN, USP, INN *alkylating antineoplastic*

**pipoctanone** INN

**pipofezine** INN

piposulfan USAN, INN *antineoplastic*
pipotiazine INN *antipsychotic* [also: pipotiazine palmitate]
pipotiazine palmitate USAN *antipsychotic* [also: pipotiazine]
pipoxizine INN
pipoxolan INN *muscle relaxant* [also: pipoxolan HCl]
pipoxolan HCl USAN *muscle relaxant* [also: pipoxolan]
**Pipracil** powder for IV or IM injection ℞ *extended-spectrum penicillin-type antibiotic* [piperacillin sodium] 2, 3, 4, 20 g
pipradimadol INN
pipradrol INN [also: pipradrol HCl]
pipradrol HCl NF [also: pipradrol]
pipramadol INN
pipratecol INN
piprinhydrinate INN, BAN
piprocurarium iodide INN
piprofurol INN
piprozolin USAN, INN *choleretic*
piquindone INN *antipsychotic* [also: piquindone HCl]
piquindone HCl USAN *antipsychotic* [also: piquindone]
piquizil INN *bronchodilator* [also: piquizil HCl]
piquizil HCl USAN *bronchodilator* [also: piquizil]
piracetam USAN, INN, BAN *cognition adjuvant; investigational (orphan) for myoclonus* ⊘ piroxicam
pirandamine INN *antidepressant* [also: pirandamine HCl]
pirandamine HCl USAN *antidepressant* [also: pirandamine]
pirarubicin INN
piraxelate INN
pirazmonam INN *antimicrobial* [also: pirazmonam sodium]
pirazmonam sodium USAN *antimicrobial* [also: pirazmonam]
pirazofurin INN *antineoplastic* [also: pyrazofurin]
pirazolac USAN, INN, BAN *antirheumatic*
pirbenicillin INN *antibacterial* [also: pirbenicillin sodium]
pirbenicillin sodium USAN *antibacterial* [also: pirbenicillin]
pirbuterol INN *bronchodilator* [also: pirbuterol acetate]

pirbuterol acetate USAN *bronchodilator* [also: pirbuterol]
pirbuterol HCl USAN *bronchodilator*
pirdonium bromide INN
pirenoxine INN
pirenperone USAN, INN, BAN *tranquilizer*
pirenzepine INN, BAN *antiulcerative* [also: pirenzepine HCl]
pirenzepine HCl USAN, JAN *antiulcerative* [also: pirenzepine]
pirepolol INN
piretanide USAN, INN *diuretic*
pirfenidone USAN, INN *analgesic; anti-inflammatory; antipyretic*
piribedil INN
piribenzyl methylsulfate [see: bevonium metilsulfate]
piridicillin INN *antibacterial* [also: piridicillin sodium]
piridicillin sodium USAN *antibacterial* [also: piridicillin]
piridocaine INN
piridocaine HCl [see: piridocaine]
piridoxilate INN, BAN
piridronate sodium USAN *calcium regulator*
piridronic acid INN
pirifibrate INN
pirinidazole INN
pirinitramide [see: piritramide]
pirinixic acid INN
pirinixil INN
piriprost USAN *antiasthmatic*
piriprost potassium USAN *antiasthmatic*
piriqualone INN
pirisudanol INN
piritramide INN, BAN
piritrexim INN *antiproliferative agent* [also: piritrexim isethionate]
piritrexim isethionate USAN *antiproliferative; orphan status withdrawn 1996* [also: piritrexim]
pirlimycin HCl USAN *antibacterial*
pirlindole INN
pirmagrel USAN, INN *thromboxane synthetase inhibitor*
pirmenol INN *antiarrhythmic* [also: pirmenol HCl]
pirmenol HCl USAN *antiarrhythmic* [also: pirmenol]
pirnabin INN *antiglaucoma agent* [also: pirnabine]

**pirnabine** USAN *antiglaucoma agent*
[also: pirnabin]
**piroctone** USAN, INN *antiseborrheic*
**piroctone olamine** USAN *antiseborrheic*
**pirodavir** USAN, INN, BAN *antiviral*
**pirogliride** INN *antidiabetic* [also:
pirogliride tartrate]
**pirogliride tartrate** USAN *antidiabetic*
[also: pirogliride]
**piroheptine** INN
**pirolate** USAN, INN *antiasthmatic*
**pirolazamide** USAN, INN *antiarrhythmic*
**piromidic acid** INN
**piroxantrone** INN *antineoplastic* [also:
piroxantrone HCl]
**piroxantrone HCl** USAN *antineoplastic*
[also: piroxantrone]
**piroxicam** USAN, USP, INN, BAN, JAN
*antiarthritic; nonsteroidal anti-inflam-
matory drug (NSAID); analgesic; antiarthritic* 10, 20 mg oral ⍰ piracetam
**piroxicam betadex** USAN *analgesic;
anti-inflammatory; antirheumatic*
**piroxicam cinnamate** USAN *anti-
inflammatory*
**piroxicam olamine** USAN *analgesic;
anti-inflammatory*
**piroxicillin** INN
**piroximone** USAN, INN, BAN *cardiotonic*
**pirozadil** INN
**pirprofen** USAN, INN, BAN *anti-inflammatory*
**pirquinozol** USAN, INN *antiallergic*
**pirralkonium bromide** INN
**pirroksan** [now: proroxan HCl]
**pirsidomine** USAN, INN *vasodilator*
**pirtenidine** INN
**pit** *street drug slang* [see: PCP]
**pitenodil** INN
**Pitocin** IV, IM injection ℞ *induction of
labor; postpartum bleeding; incomplete
abortion* [oxytocin] 10 U/mL ⍰
Pitressin
**pitofenone** INN
**Pitressin Synthetic** IM or subcu
injection ℞ *pituitary antidiuretic hormone for diabetes insipidus or prevention of abdominal distention* [vaso-
pressin] 20 U/mL ⍰ Pitocin
**pituitary, anterior**
**pituitary, posterior** USP *antidiuretic
hormone*

**pituxate** INN
**pivalate** USAN, INN, BAN *combining
name for radicals or groups*
**pivampicillin** INN *antibacterial* [also:
pivampicillin HCl]
**pivampicillin HCl** USAN *antibacterial*
[also: pivampicillin]
**pivampicillin pamoate** USAN *antibacterial*
**pivampicillin probenate** USAN *antibacterial*
**pivenfrine** INN
**pivmecillinam** INN, BAN *antibacterial*
[also: amdinocillin pivoxil; pivmecillinam HCl]
**pivmecillinam HCl** JAN *antibacterial*
[also: amdinocillin pivoxil; pivmecil-
linam]
**pivopril** USAN *antihypertensive*
**pivoxazepam** INN
**pivoxetil** USAN, INN *combining name
for radicals or groups*
**pivoxil** USAN, INN *combining name for
radicals or groups*
**pivsulbactam** BAN *β-lactamase inhibitor; penicillin/cephalosporin synergist*
[also: sulbactam pivoxil]
**pix pini** [see: pine tar]
**pixies** *street drug slang* [see: amphet-
amines]
**Pixykine** ℞ *investigational second-generation colony stimulating factor for
neutropenia and thrombocytopenia*
[milodistim]
**pizotifen** INN, BAN *anabolic; antidepressant; serotonin inhibitor (migraine specific)* [also: pizotyline]
**pizotyline** USAN *anabolic; antidepressant; serotonin inhibitor (migraine specific)* [also: pizotifen]
**placebo** *no medicinal value* [also: obecalp]
**Placidyl** capsules ℞ *hypnotic* [eth-
chlorvynol] 200, 500, 750 mg ⍰
Pathocil
**plafibride** INN
**plague vaccine** USP *active bacterin for
plague (Yersinia pestis)* $1.8–2.2 \times 10^8$
bacilli/mL IM injection
**planadalin** [see: carbromal]
**plantago seed** USP *laxative*
**plantain seed** [see: plantago seed]

**Plaquase** powder for injection ℞ *investigational (orphan) for Peyronie's disease* [collagenase]

**Plaquenil Sulfate** tablets ℞ *antimalarial; antirheumatic* [hydroxychloroquine sulfate] 200 mg

**Plasbumin-5; Plasbumin-25** IV infusion ℞ *blood volume expander for shock, burns, and hypoproteinemia* [human albumin] 5%; 25%

**plasma, antihemophilic human** USP

**plasma concentrate factor IX** [see: factor IX complex]

**plasma expanders** *a class of therapeutic blood modifiers used to increase the volume of circulating blood*

**plasma protein fraction** USP *blood volume supporter*

**plasma protein fraction, human** [now: plasma protein fraction]

**plasma protein fractions** *a class of therapeutic blood modifiers used to regulate the volume of circulating blood*

**plasma thromboplastin component (PTC)** [see: factor IX]

**Plasma-Lyte A pH 7.4; Plasma-Lyte R; Plasma-Lyte 56; Plasma-Lyte 148** IV infusion ℞ *intravenous electrolyte therapy* [combined electrolyte solution]

**Plasma-Lyte M (R; 56; 148) and 5% Dextrose** IV infusion ℞ *intravenous nutritional/electrolyte therapy* [combined electrolyte solution; dextrose]

**Plasmanate** IV infusion ℞ *blood volume expander for shock due to burns, trauma and surgery* [plasma protein fraction] 5%

**Plasma-Plex** IV infusion ℞ *blood volume expander for shock due to burns, trauma and surgery* [plasma protein fraction] 5%

**Plasmatein** IV infusion ℞ *blood volume expander for shock due to burns, trauma and surgery* [plasma protein fraction] 5%

**plasmin** BAN [also: fibrinolysin, human]

**Plateau Cap** (trademarked dosage form) *controlled-release capsule*

**platelet cofactor II** [see: factor IX]

**platelet concentrate** USP *platelet replensher*

**platelet factor 4, recombinant (rPF4)** *investigational antineoplastic for various cancers and heparin neutralizer*

**platelet-derived growth factor** *investigational treatment for diabetic skin ulcers and pressure ulcers*

**Platinol** powder for IV injection (discontinued 1997) ℞ *alkylating antineoplastic for testicular, ovarian, bladder, lung, head, neck, and esophageal cancers* [cisplatin] 10, 50 mg

**Platinol-AQ** IV injection ℞ *alkylating antineoplastic for metastatic testicular tumors, metastatic ovarian tumors, and advanced bladder cancer* [cisplatin] 1 mg/mL

**platinum** *element (Pt)*

**cis-platinum** [now: cisplatin]

**cis-platinum II** [now: cisplatin]

**platinum diamminodichloride** [see: cisplatin]

**platters** *street drug slang* [see: hashish]

**plaunotol** INN

**plauracin** USAN, INN *veterinary growth stimulant*

**Plax, Advanced Formula** mouthwash/gargle OTC [sodium pyrophosphate]

**Plegine** tablets ℞ *anorexiant* [phendimetrazine tartrate] 35 mg

**Plegisol** solution ℞ *cardioplegic solution* [calcium chloride; magnesium chloride; potassium chloride; sodium chloride] 17.6•325.3•119.3•643 mg/100 mL

**Plendil** extended-release tablets ℞ *antihypertensive; investigational antianginal* [felodipine] 2.5, 5, 10 mg

**pleuromulin** INN

**Pliagel** solution OTC *surfactant cleaning solution for soft contact lenses*

**plicamycin** USAN, USP, INN *antibiotic antineoplastic*

**plomestane** USAN *antineoplastic; aromatase inhibitor*

**plutonium** *element (Pu)*

**PMB 200; PMB 400** tablets ℞ *estrogen replacement therapy for postmenopausal disorders* [conjugated estrogens; meprobamate] 0.45•200 mg; 0.45•400 mg

**PMEA** *investigational (Phase I/II) antiviral nucleoside analog for HIV and various herpesvirus types* [GS 393]

**PMMA (polymethylmethacrylate)** [q.v.]

**PMS-Bethanechol Chloride** Ⓒ (U.S. product: Duvoid) tablets ℞ *cholinergic urinary stimulant for postsurgical and postpartum urinary retention* [bethanechol chloride] 10, 25, 50 mg

**PMS-Dicitrate** Ⓒ (U.S. product: Bicitra) oral solution ℞ *urinary alkalinizing agent* [sodium citrate; citric acid] 500•334 mg/5 mL

**P-MVAC (Platinol, methotrexate, vinblastine, Adriamycin, carboplatin)** *chemotherapy protocol*

**pneumococcal vaccine, polyvalent** *active bacterin for pneumococcal pneumonia (23 types)*

**Pneumomist** sustained-release tablets ℞ *expectorant* [guaifenesin] 600 mg

**Pneumopent** for inhalation ℞ *investigational (orphan) prophylaxis of Pneumocystis carinii pneumonia* [pentamidine isethionate]

**Pneumotussin HC** syrup ℞ *narcotic antitussive; expectorant* [hydrocodone bitartrate; guaifenesin] 5•100 mg/5 mL

**Pneumovax 23** subcu or IM injection ℞ *pneumonia vaccine* [pneumococcal vaccine, polyvalent] 0.5 mL

**Pnu-Imune 23** subcu or IM injection ℞ *pneumonia vaccine* [pneumococcal vaccine, polyvalent] 0.5 mL

**pobilukast edamine** USAN *antiasthmatic*

**POC (procarbazine, Oncovin, CCNU)** *chemotherapy protocol*

**POCA (prednisone, Oncovin, cytarabine, Adriamycin)** *chemotherapy protocol*

**POCC (procarbazine, Oncovin, cyclophosphamide, CCNU)** *chemotherapy protocol*

**pocket rocket** *street drug slang* [see: marijuana]

**Pockethaler** (trademarked delivery device) *nasal inhalation aerosol*

**pod** *street drug slang* [see: marijuana]

**Pod-Ben-25** liquid (discontinued 1994) ℞ *topical keratolytic* [podophyllum resin] 25%

**podilfen** INN

**Podocon-25** liquid ℞ *topical keratolytic for genital warts* [podophyllum resin] 25%

**podofilox** USAN *topical antimitotic* [also: podophyllotoxin]

**Podofin** liquid ℞ *topical keratolytic for genital warts* [podophyllum resin] 25% ② podophyllin

**podophyllin** [see: podophyllum resin] ② Podofin

**podophyllotoxin** BAN *topical antimitotic* [also: podofilox]

**podophyllotoxins** *a class of mitotic-inhibiting antineoplastics derived from podophyllotoxin*

**podophyllum** USP *pharmaceutic necessity*

**podophyllum resin** USP *caustic; cytotoxic agent for genital warts*

**Point-Two** oral rinse ℞ *topical dental caries preventative* [sodium fluoride; alcohol 6%] 0.2%

**poison** *street drug slang* [see: heroin; fentanyl]

**Poison Antidote Kit** OTC *emergency treatment for various poisons* [syrup of ipecac; charcoal suspension] 30•60 mL

**poison ivy extract, alum precipitated** USAN *ivy poisoning counteractant*

**poison oak extract** USAN *antiallergic*

**Poison Oak-N-Ivy Armor** lotion OTC *topical poison ivy protectant*

**poke** *street drug slang* [see: marijuana]

**polacrilin** USAN, INN *pharmaceutic aid*

**polacrilin potassium** USAN, NF *tablet disintegrant*

**Poladex** timed-release tablets ℞ *antihistamine* [dexchlorpheniramine maleate] 4, 6 mg

**Polaramine** tablets, Repetabs (repeat-action tablets), syrup ℞ *antihistamine* [dexchlorpheniramine maleate] 2 mg; 6 mg; 2 mg/5 mL

**Polaramine Expectorant** liquid ℞ *decongestant; antihistamine; expectorant* [pseudoephedrine sulfate; dexchlorpheniramine maleate; guaifenesin; alcohol 7.2%] 20•2•100 mg/5 mL

**poldine methylsulfate** USAN, USP *anticholinergic* [also: poldine metilsulfate]

**poldine metilsulfate** INN *anticholinergic* [also: poldine methylsulfate]

**policapram** USAN, INN *tablet binder*

**policresulen** INN

**polidexide sulfate** INN

**polidocanol**

**polifeprosan** INN *pharmaceutic aid; implantable, biodegradable drug carrier* [also: polifeprosan 20]

**polifeprosan 20** USAN *pharmaceutic aid; implantable, biodegradable drug carrier* [also: polifeprosan]

**poligeenan** USAN, INN *dispersing agent*

**poliglecaprone 25** USAN *absorbable surgical suture material*

**poliglecaprone 90** USAN *absorbable surgical suture coating*

**poliglusam** USAN *antihemorrhagic*

**polignate sodium** USAN *pepsin enzyme inhibitor*

**polihexanide** INN [also: polyhexanide]

**poliomyelitis vaccine** [now: poliovirus vaccine, inactivated]

**Poliovax** subcu injection (discontinued 1993) ℞ *poliomyelitis vaccine* [poliovirus vaccine, inactivated] 0.5 mL

**poliovirus vaccine, enhanced inactivated (eIPV)** *active immunizing agent for poliomyelitis*

**poliovirus vaccine, inactivated (IPV)** USP *active immunizing agent for poliomyelitis*

**poliovirus vaccine, live oral (OPV)** USP *active immunizing agent for poliomyelitis*

**polipropene 25** USAN *tablet excipient*

**polisaponin** INN

**politef** INN *prosthetic aid* [also: polytef]

**polixetonium chloride** USAN, INN *preservative*

**Polocaine** injection ℞ *injectable local anesthetic* [mepivacaine HCl] 1%, 2%, 3%

**Polocaine** injection ℞ *injectable local anesthetic* [mepivacaine HCl; levonordefrin] 2%•1:20 000

**Polocaine MPF** injection ℞ *injectable local anesthetic* [mepivacaine HCl] 1%, 1.5%, 2%

**polonium** *element (Po)*

**Poloris Dental Poultice** (discontinued 1994) OTC *topical oral anesthetic; antipruritic/counterirritant* [benzocaine; capsicum] 7.5•4.6 mg

**poloxalene** USAN, INN, BAN *surfactant*

**poloxamer** USAN, NF, INN, BAN *ointment and suppository base; tablet binder*

**poloxamer 124** USAN *surfactant; emulsifier; solubilizer; stabilizer*

**poloxamer 188** USAN *surfactant; emulsifier; solubilizer; investigational (orphan) for sickle cell crisis and severe burns*

**poloxamer 237** USAN *surfactant; emulsifier; solubilizer; stabilizer*

**poloxamer 331** *investigational (orphan) for toxoplasmosis of AIDS*

**poloxamer 338** USAN *surfactant; emulsifier; solubilizer; stabilizer*

**poloxamer 407** USAN *surfactant; emulsifier; solubilizer; stabilizer*

**polvo** (Spanish for "powder" or "dust") *street drug slang* [see: heroin; PCP]

**polvo blanco** (Spanish for "white powder") *street drug slang* [see: cocaine]

**polvo de angel; polvo de estrellas** (Spanish for "angel dust"; "star dust") *street drug slang* [see: PCP]

**poly I: poly C12U** *investigational (Phase III, orphan) antiviral/immunomodulator for AIDS, renal cell carcinoma, metastatic melanoma, and chronic fatigue syndrome*

**polyamine resin** [see: polyamine-methylene resin]

**polyamine-methylene resin**

**polyanhydroglucose** [see: dextran]

**polyanhydroglucuronic acid** [see: dextran]

**polybenzarsol** INN

**polybutester** USAN *surgical suture material*

**polybutilate** USAN *surgical suture coating*

**polycarbokane** [see: polycarbophil]

**polycarbophil** USP, INN, BAN *bulk laxative*

**Polycillin** capsules, powder for oral suspension, pediatric drops ℞ *penicillin-type antibiotic* [ampicillin trihydrate] 250, 500 mg; 125, 250, 500 mg/5 mL; 100 mg/mL ② penicillin

**Polycillin-N** powder for IV or IM injection ℞ *penicillin-type antibiotic* [ampicillin sodium] 0.125, 0.25, 0.5, 1, 2, 10 g

**Polycillin-PRB** powder for oral suspension ℞ *antibiotic for Neisseria gonorrhoeae* [ampicillin trihydrate; probenecid] 3.5•1 g

**Polycitra** syrup ℞ *urinary alkalinizing agent* [potassium citrate; sodium citrate; citric acid] 550•500•334 mg/5 mL

**Polycitra-K** oral solution, crystals for oral solution ℞ *urinary alkalizing agent; orphan status withdrawn 1994* [potassium citrate; citric acid] 1100•334 mg/5 mL; 3300•1002 mg/packet

**Polycitra-LC** solution ℞ *urinary alkalizing agent; orphan status withdrawn 1994* [potassium citrate; sodium citrate; citric acid] 550•500•334 mg/5 mL

**Polycose** liquid, powder OTC *carbohydrate caloric supplement* [glucose polymers]

**polydextrose** USAN *food additive*

**polydimethylsiloxane** *surgical aid (retinal tamponade) for retinal detachment*

**Polydine** ointment, scrub, solution OTC *broad-spectrum antimicrobial* [povidone-iodine]

**polydioxanone** USAN *absorbable surgical suture material*

**polyelectrolyte 211** [see: sodium alginate]

**polyenes** *a class of antifungals produced by a species of Streptomyces that damage fungal cell membranes*

**polyestradiol phosphate** INN, BAN *antineoplastic; estrogen*

**polyetadene** INN *antacid* [also: polyethadene]

**polyethadene** USAN *antacid* [also: polyetadene]

**polyethylene excipient** NF *stiffening agent*

**polyethylene glycol (PEG)** NF *ointment and suppository base; solvent*

**polyethylene glycol** *n* [*n* refers to the molecular weight: 300, 400, 1000, etc.]

**polyethylene glycol** *n* **dioleate** [*n* refers to the molecular weight: 300, 400, 1000, etc.]

**polyethylene glycol 8 monostearate** [see: polyoxyl 8 stearate]

**polyethylene glycol 1000 monocetyl ether** [see: cetomacrogol 1000]

**polyethylene glycol 1540** NF

**polyethylene glycol 4000** USP [also: macrogol 4000]

**polyethylene glycol 6000** USP

**polyethylene glycol monoleyl ether** [see: polyoxyl 10 oleyl ether]

**polyethylene glycol monomethyl ether** NF *excipient*

**polyethylene glycol monostearate** [see: polyoxyl 40 & 50 stearate]

**polyethylene glycol-electrolyte solution (PEG-ES)** *pre-procedure bowel evacuant* [contains PEG 3350]

**polyethylene glycol-superoxide dismutase (PEG-SOD)** [see: pegorgotein]

**polyethylene oxide** NF *suspending and viscosity agent; tablet binder*

**polyferose** USAN *hematinic*

**Polygam** powder for IV infusion ℞ *passive immunizing agent for HIV* [immune globulin] 50 mg/mL

**Polygam S/D** freeze-dried powder for IV infusion ℞ *passive immunizing agent for HIV, idiopathic thrombocytopenic purpura (ITP), and B-cell chronic lymphocytic leukemia* [immune globulin, solvent/detergent treated] 50 mg/mL

**polygeline** INN, BAN

**polyglactin 370** USAN *absorbable surgical suture coating*

**polyglactin 910** USAN *absorbable surgical suture material*

**polyglycolic acid** USAN, INN *surgical suture material*

**polyglyconate** USAN, BAN *absorbable surgical suture material*

**PolyHeme** ℞ *investigational (Phase III) blood substitute* [human hemoglobin cross-linked with glutaral]

**polyhexanide** BAN [also: polihexanide]

**Poly-Histine** elixir ℞ *antihistamine* [pheniramine maleate; pyrilamine maleate; phenyltoloxamine citrate] 4•4•4 mg/5 mL

**Poly-Histine CS** syrup ℞ *narcotic antitussive; decongestant; antihistamine* [codeine phosphate; phenylpropanolamine HCl; brompheniramine maleate] 10•12.5•2 mg/5 mL

**Poly-Histine DM** syrup ℞ *antitussive; decongestant; antihistamine* [dextromethorphan hydrobromide; phenylpropanolamine HCl; brompheniramine maleate] 10•12.5•2 mg/5 mL

**Poly-Histine-D** sustained-release capsules, elixir ℞ *decongestant; antihistamine* [phenylpropanolamine HCl; phenyltoloxamine citrate; pyrilamine maleate; pheniramine maleate] 50•16•16•16 mg; 12.5•4•4•4 mg/5 mL

**Poly-Histine-D Ped Caps** sustained-release capsules ℞ *pediatric decongestant and antihistamine* [phenylpropanolamine HCl; phenyltoloxamine citrate; pyrilamine maleate; pheniramine maleate] 25•8•8•8 mg

**poly-ICLC** *investigational (orphan) for primary brain tumors*

**polyloxyl 8 stearate** USAN *surfactant*

**polymacon** USAN *hydrophilic contact lens material*

**polymanoacetate** [now: acemannan]

**polymeric oxygen** [see: oxygen, polymeric]

**polymetaphosphate P 32** USAN *radioactive agent*

**polymethyl methacrylate (PMMA)** *rigid hydrophobic polymer used for hard contact lenses*

**polymixin E** [see: colistin sulfate]

**polymonine**

**Polymox** capsules, powder for oral suspension, pediatric drops ℞ *penicillin-type antibiotic* [amoxicillin trihydrate] 250, 500 mg; 125, 250 mg/5 mL; 50 mg/mL

**polymyxin** BAN *bactericidal antibiotic* [also: polymyxin B sulfate; polymyxin B]

**polymyxin B** INN *bactericidal antibiotic* [also: polymyxin B sulfate; polymyxin]

**polymyxin B sulfate** USP *bactericidal antibiotic* [also: polymyxin B; polymyxin] 500 000 U/vial eye drops or injection

**polymyxin B₁** [see: polymyxin B]
**polymyxin B₂** [see: polymyxin B]
**polymyxin B₃** [see: polymyxin B]
**polymyxin E** [see: colistin sulfate]

**polynoxylin** INN, BAN

**polyoxyethylene 20 sorbitan monolaurate** [see: polysorbate 20]

**polyoxyethylene 20 sorbitan monooleate** [see: polysorbate 80]

**polyoxyethylene 20 sorbitan monopalmitate** [see: polysorbate 40]

**polyoxyethylene 20 sorbitan monostearate** [see: polysorbate 60]

**polyoxyethylene 20 sorbitan trioleate** [see: polysorbate 85]

**polyoxyethylene 20 sorbitan tristearate** [see: polysorbate 65]

**polyoxyethylene 50 stearate** [now: polyoxyl 50 stearate]

**polyoxyethylene glycol 1000 monocetyl ether** [see: cetomacrogol 1000]

**polyoxyethylene nonyl phenol** *surfactant/wetting agent*

**polyoxyl 10 oleyl ether** NF *surfactant*

**polyoxyl 20 cetostearyl ether** NF *surfactant*

**polyoxyl 35 castor oil** NF *emulsifying agent; surfactant*

**polyoxyl 40 hydrogenated castor oil** NF *emulsifying agent; surfactant*

**polyoxyl 40 stearate** USAN, NF *surfactant*

**polyoxyl 50 stearate** NF *surfactant; emulsifying agent*

**polyoxypropylene 15 stearyl ether** USAN *solvent*

**polyphosphoric acid, sodium salt** [see: sodium polyphosphate]

**Poly-Pred** eye drop suspension ℞ *topical ophthalmic corticosteroidal antiinflammatory; antibiotic* [prednisolone acetate; neomycin sulfate; polymyxin B sulfate] 0.5%•0.35%•10 000 U per mL

**polypropylene glycol** NF

**polyribonucleotide** [see: poly I: poly C12U]

**polysaccharide-iron complex** *hematinic* 150 mg oral

**Polysorb Hydrate** cream OTC *moisturizer; emollient*

**polysorbate 20** USAN, NF, INN *surfactant/wetting agent*

**polysorbate 40** USAN, NF, INN *surfactant*

**polysorbate 60** USAN, NF, INN *surfactant*

**polysorbate 65** USAN, INN *surfactant*

**polysorbate 80** USAN, NF, INN *surfactant/wetting agent; viscosity-increasing agent*

**polysorbate 85** USAN, INN *surfactant*

**Polysporin** aerosol spray (discontinued 1993) OTC *topical/ophthalmic antibiotic* [polymyxin B sulfate; bacitracin zinc] 2222•111 U/mL

**Polysporin** ointment, powder OTC *topical antibiotic* [polymyxin B sulfate; bacitracin zinc] 10 000•500 U/g

**Polysporin** ophthalmic ointment OTC *ophthalmic antibiotic* [polymyxin B sulfate; bacitracin zinc] 10 000•500 U/g

**Polytabs-F** chewable tablets ℞ *pediatric vitamin supplement and dental caries preventative* [multiple vitamins; fluoride; folic acid] ±•1•0.3 mg

**Polytar** shampoo, soap OTC *antiseborrheic; antipsoriatic; antipruritic; antibacterial* [coal tar, pine tar, and juniper tar solution] 2.5%; 1%

**Polytar Bath** oil OTC *antipsoriatic; antiseborrheic; antipruritic; emollient* [coal tar, pine tar, and juniper tar solution] 25%

**polytef** USAN *prosthetic aid* [also: politef]

**polytetrafluoroethylene (PTFE)** [see: polytef]

**polythiazide** USAN, USP, INN *diuretic; antihypertensive*

**Polytrim** eye drops ℞ *ophthalmic antibiotic* [polymyxin B sulfate; trimethoprim] 10 000 U•1 mg per mL

**polyurethane foam** USAN *internal bone splint*

**polyvalent Crotaline antivenin** [see: antivenin (Crotalidae) polyvalent]

**polyvalent gas gangrene antitoxin** [see: gas gangrene antitoxin, pentavalent]

**polyvidone** INN *dispersing, suspending and viscosity-increasing agent* [also: povidone]

**Poly-Vi-Flor** chewable tablets ℞ *pediatric vitamin supplement and dental caries preventative* [multiple vitamins; sodium fluoride; folic acid] ±•0.25•0.3, ±•0.5•0.3, ±•1•0.3 mg

**Poly-Vi-Flor** drops ℞ *pediatric vitamin supplement and dental caries preventative* [multiple vitamins; sodium fluoride] ±•0.25, ±•0.5 mg/mL

**Poly-Vi-Flor with Iron** chewable tablets ℞ *pediatric vitamin/iron supplement and dental caries preventative* [multiple vitamins & minerals; sodium fluoride; iron; folic acid] ±•0.25•12•0.3, ±•0.5•12•0.3, ±•1•12•0.3 mg

**Poly-Vi-Flor with Iron** drops ℞ *pediatric vitamin/iron supplement and dental caries preventative* [multiple vitamins & minerals; sodium fluoride; iron] ±•0.25•10, ±•0.5•10 mg/mL

**polyvinyl acetate phthalate** NF *coating agent*

**polyvinyl alcohol (PVA)** USP *viscosity-increasing agent* ·

**polyvinylpyrrolidone** [now: povidone]

**Poly-Vi-Sol** chewable tablets OTC *vitamin supplement* [multiple vitamins; folic acid] ±•0.3 mg

**Poly-Vi-Sol** drops OTC *vitamin supplement* [multiple vitamins] ±

**Poly-Vi-Sol with Iron** chewable tablets OTC *vitamin/iron supplement* [multiple vitamins; iron; folic acid] ±•12•0.3 mg

**Poly-Vi-Sol with Iron** drops OTC *vitamin/iron supplement* [multiple vitamins; iron] ±•10 mg/mL

**Poly-Vitamin** drops OTC *vitamin supplement* [multiple vitamins] ±

**Polyvitamin Fluoride** chewable tablets ℞ *pediatric vitamin supplement and dental caries preventative* [multiple vitamins; fluoride; folic acid] ±•0.5•0.3, ±•1•0.3 mg

**Polyvitamin Fluoride** drops ℞ *pediatric vitamin supplement and dental caries preventative* [multiple vitamins; fluoride] ±•0.25, ±•0.5 mg/mL

**Polyvitamin Fluoride with Iron** chewable tablets ℞ *pediatric vitamin/iron supplement and dental caries pre-*

*ventative* [multiple vitamins & minerals; fluoride; iron; folic acid] ≛•1•12•0.3 mg

**Poly-Vitamin with Iron** drops OTC *vitamin/iron supplement* [multiple vitamins; iron] ≛•10 mg/mL

**Polyvitamin with Iron and Fluoride** drops ℞ *pediatric vitamin/iron supplement and dental caries preventative* [multiple vitamins; iron; fluoride] ≛•10•0.25 mg/mL

**Polyvitamins with Fluoride and Iron** chewable tablets ℞ *pediatric vitamin/iron supplement and dental caries preventative* [multiple vitamins; fluoride; iron; folic acid] ≛•0.5•12•0.3 mg

**Polyvite with Fluoride** drops (discontinued 1993) ℞ *pediatric vitamin deficiency and dental caries prevention* [multiple vitamins; fluoride]

**POMP (prednisone, Oncovin, methotrexate, Purinethol)** *chemotherapy protocol*

**ponalrestat** USAN, INN, BAN *aldose reductase inhibitor*

**Pondimin** tablets ℞ *anorexiant; CNS depressant* [fenfluramine HCl] 20 mg

**ponfibrate** INN

**Ponstel** capsules ℞ *nonsteroidal antiinflammatory drug (NSAID); analgesic; for primary dysmenorrhea* [mefenamic acid] 250 mg ⌦ Pronestyl

**Pontocaine** cream OTC *topical local anesthetic* [tetracaine HCl] 1%

**Pontocaine** ointment OTC *topical local anesthetic* [tetracaine; menthol] 0.5%•0.5%

**Pontocaine HCl** Mono-Drop (eye drops) ℞ *topical ophthalmic anesthetic* [tetracaine HCl] 0.5%

**Pontocaine HCl** ophthalmic ointment (discontinued 1995) ℞ *topical ophthalmic anesthetic* [tetracaine HCl] 0.5%

**Pontocaine HCl** solution ℞ *nose/throat anesthetic to abolish laryngeal and esophageal reflex* [tetracaine HCl; chlorobutanol] 2%•0.4%

**Pontocaine HCl** spinal injection, powder for reconstitution ℞ *injectable local anesthetic* [tetracaine HCl] 0.2%, 0.3%, 1%

**pony** *street drug slang* [see: cocaine, crack]

**poor man's speedball** *street drug slang for a combination of heroin and methamphetamine* [see: heroin; methamphetamine HCl]

**Po-Pon-S** sugar-coated tablets OTC *vitamin/mineral supplement* [multiple vitamins & minerals] ≛

**poppers** *street drug slang* [see: isobutyl nitrite; amyl nitrite]

**poppy** *street drug slang* [see: heroin]

**poractant alfa** BAN *porcine lung extract containing 90% phospholipids*

**Porcelana** cream OTC *hyperpigmentation bleaching agent* [hydroquinone] 2%

**Porcelana with Sunscreen** cream OTC *hyperpigmentation bleaching agent; sunscreen* [hydroquinone; padimate O] 2%•2.5%

**porcine fetal neural dopaminergic cells (or precursors)** *investigational (orphan) intracerebral implant for stage 4 and 5 Parkinson's disease*

**porcine fetal neural gabaergic cells (or precursors)** *investigational (orphan) intracerebral implant for Huntington's disease*

**porcine islet preparation, encapsulated** *investigational (orphan) antidiabetic for type 1 patients on immunosuppression*

**porfimer sodium** USAN, INN *light-activated antineoplastic for photodynamic therapy (PDT) of esophageal cancer (orphan); investigational (orphan) for bladder cancer*

**porfiromycin** USAN, INN, BAN *antibacterial; investigational (Phase III, orphan) antineoplastic for head, neck, and cervical cancers*

**porofocon A** USAN *hydrophobic contact lens material*

**porofocon B** USAN *hydrophobic contact lens material*

**Portagen** powder OTC *enteral nutritional therapy* [lactose-free formula]

**porton asparaginase** [see: Erwinia L-asparaginase]

**posatirelin** INN

**posedrine** [see: benzchlorpropamid]

**Posicor** tablets ℞ *vasodilator and calcium channel blocker for hypertension and chronic stable angina* [mibefradil dihydrochloride] 50, 100 mg

**poskine** INN, BAN

**posterior pituitary** [see: pituitary, posterior]

**Posture** tablets OTC *calcium supplement* [calcium phosphate, tribasic] 1565.2 mg

**Posture-D** film-coated tablets OTC *dietary supplement* [calcium phosphate, tribasic; vitamin D] 600 mg•125 IU

**pot** *street drug slang* [see: marijuana]

**pot liquor; pot likker** *street drug slang for a tea brewed from marijuana waste* [see: marijuana]

**Potaba** tablets, capsules, Envules (powder for reconstitution), powder ℞ *"possibly effective" for scleroderma and other skin diseases, and Peyronie's disease* [aminobenzoate potassium] 500 mg; 500 mg; 2 g; 100 g, 1 lb.

**Potable Aqua** tablets OTC *emergency disinfectant for drinking water* [tetraglycine hydroperiodide (source of iodine)] 16.7% (6.68%)

**Potasalan** liquid ℞ *potassium supplement* [potassium chloride; alcohol 4%] 20 mEq/15 mL

**potash, sulfurated** USP *source of sulfides*

**potassic saline, lactated** NF

**potassium** *element (K)*

**potassium acid phosphate** *urinary acidifier*

**potassium alpha-phenoxyethyl penicillin** [see: phenethicillin potassium]

**potassium alum** [see: alum, potassium]

**potassium aspartate** [see: L-aspartate potassium]

**potassium aspartate & magnesium aspartate** USAN *nutrient*

**potassium benzoate** NF *preservative*

**potassium benzyl penicillin** [see: penicillin G potassium]

**potassium bicarbonate** USP *pH buffer; electrolyte replacement*

**potassium bitartrate** USAN

**potassium borate** *pH buffer*

**potassium canrenoate** JAN *aldosterone antagonist* [also: canrenoate potassium; canrenoic acid]

**potassium carbonate** USP *alkalizing agent*

**potassium chloride (KCl)** USP *electrolyte replenisher* 600, 750 mg oral; 20, 40 mEq/15 mL oral; 20 mEq/pkt oral; 2, 10, 20, 30, 40, 60, 90 mEq/mL injection

**potassium chloride K 42** USAN *radioactive agent*

**potassium citrate** USP *urinary alkalizer; electrolyte replacement; nephrolithiasis and hypocitruria prevention (orphan)*

**potassium citrate & citric acid** *orphan status withdrawn 1994*

**potassium clavulanate & amoxicillin** [see: amoxicillin]

**potassium clavulanate & ticarcillin** [see: ticarcillin disodium]

**potassium dichloroisocyanurate** [see: troclosene potassium]

**potassium glucaldrate** USAN, INN *antacid*

**potassium gluconate** USP *electrolyte replenisher* 500, 595 mg oral; 20 mEq/15 mL oral

**potassium guaiacolsulfonate** USP *expectorant* [also: sulfogaiacol]

**potassium hydroxide (KOH)** NF *alkalizing agent*

**potassium hydroxymethoxybenzenesulfonate hemihydrate** [see: potassium guaiacolsulfonate]

**potassium iodide** USP *antifungal; expectorant; iodine supplement* 1 g/mL oral

**potassium mercuric iodide** NF

**potassium metabisulfite** NF *antioxidant*

**potassium metaphosphate** NF *buffering agent*

**potassium nitrate** *tooth desensitizer*

**potassium nitrazepate** INN

**potassium para-aminobenzoate (PAB)** [see: aminobenzoate potassium]

**potassium penicillin G** [see: penicillin G potassium]

**potassium perchlorate** *adjunct in radioimaging*

**potassium permanganate** USP *topical anti-infective*

**potassium phosphate, dibasic** USP *calcium regulator; phosphorus replacement; pH buffer*

**potassium phosphate, monobasic** NF *pH buffer; phosphorus replacement*

**potassium sodium tartrate** USP *laxative*

**potassium sorbate** NF *antimicrobial agent*

**potassium tetraborate** *pH buffer*

**potassium thiocyanate** NF

**potassium-sparing diuretics** *a class of diuretic agents that interfere with sodium reabsorption thus decreasing potassium secretion*

**potato** *street drug slang* [see: LSD]

**potato chips** *street drug slang for crack cut with benzocaine* [see: cocaine, crack]

**potten bush** *street drug slang* [see: marijuana]

**Povidine** ointment, scrub, solution OTC *broad-spectrum antimicrobial* [povidone-iodine] 10%, 5%, 10%

**povidone** USAN, USP *dispersing, suspending and viscosity-increasing agent* [also: polyvidone]

**povidone I 125** USAN *radioactive agent*

**povidone I 131** USAN *radioactive agent*

**povidone-iodine** USP, BAN *broad-spectrum antimicrobial* 10% topical

**powder** *street drug slang* [see: heroin; amphetamines]

**powder diamonds** *street drug slang* [see: cocaine]

**powdered cellulose** [see: cellulose, powdered]

**powdered ipecac** [see: ipecac, powdered]

**powdered opium** [see: opium, powdered]

**PowerMate** tablets OTC *vitamin/mineral supplement* [multiple vitamins & minerals] ≚

**PowerVites** tablets OTC *vitamin/mineral supplement* [multiple vitamins and minerals; folic acid; biotin] ≚•150•25 μg

**pox** *street drug slang* [see: opium]

**PPA (phenylpropanolamine)** [q.v.]

**PPD (purified protein derivative [of tuberculin])** [see: tuberculin]

**PPG-15 stearyl ether** [now: polyoxypropylene 15 stearyl ether]

**PPI-002** *orphan status withdrawn 1996*

**P.R. (Panama Red)** *street drug slang* [see: marijuana]

**PR-122 (redox-phenytoin)** *orphan status withdrawn 1996*

**PR-225 (redox-acyclovir)** *orphan status withdrawn 1996*

**PR-239 (redox penicillin G)** *orphan status withdrawn 1996*

**PR-320 (molecusol & carbamazepine)** *orphan status withdrawn 1996*

**practolol** USAN, INN *antiadrenergic (β-receptor)*

**prajmalium bitartrate** INN, BAN

**pralidoxime chloride** USAN, USP *cholinesterase reactivator for organophosphate poisoning and anticholinesterase overdose* 600 mg injection ⧆ pyridoxine; pramoxine

**pralidoxime iodide** USAN, INN *cholinesterase reactivator* ⧆ pyridoxine; pramoxine

**pralidoxime mesylate** USAN *cholinesterase reactivator* ⧆ pyridoxine; pramoxine

**PrameGel** gel OTC *topical local anesthetic* [pramoxine HCl; menthol] 1%•0.5%

**Pramet FA** controlled-release Filmtabs (film-coated tablets) (discontinued 1995) ℞ *prenatal vitamin/calcium/iron supplement* [multiple vitamins; calcium; iron; folic acid] ≚•250•60•1 mg

**Pramilet FA** Filmtabs (film-coated tablets) ℞ *prenatal vitamin/mineral/calcium/iron supplement* [multiple vitamins & minerals; calcium; iron; folic acid] ≚•250•40•1 mg

**pramipexole** USAN, INN *dopamine agonist for Parkinson's disease; investigational for depression and schizophrenia*

**pramiracetam** INN *cognition adjuvant* [also: pramiracetam HCl]

**pramiracetam HCl** USAN *cognition adjuvant* [also: pramiracetam]

**pramiracetam sulfate** USAN *cognition adjuvant; orphan status withdrawn 1996*

**pramiverine** INN, BAN

**pramlintide** USAN *investigational (Phase III) antidiabetic for type 1 and type 2 diabetes mellitus*

**pramocaine** INN *topical anesthetic* [also: pramoxine HCl; pramoxine]

**pramocaine HCl** [see: pramoxine HCl]

**Pramosone** cream, lotion, ointment ℞ *topical corticosteroid; local anesthetic* [hydrocortisone acetate; pramoxine] 1%•1%, 2.5%•1%; 2.5%•1%; 2.5%•1% ② pramoxine

**pramoxine** BAN *topical local anesthetic* [also: pramoxine HCl; pramocaine] ② pralidoxime; Pramosone

**Pramoxine HC** anorectal aerosol foam ℞ *topical corticosteroidal anti-inflammatory; local anesthetic* [hydrocortisone acetate; pramoxine HCl] 1%•1%

**pramoxine HCl** USP *topical local anesthetic* [also: pramocaine; pramoxine]

**prampine** INN, BAN

**Prandase** ⓒⒶⓃ (U.S. product: Precose) tablets ℞ *alpha-glucosidase inhibitor for type 2 diabetes mellitus* [acarbose] 50, 100 mg

**pranidipine** INN

**pranlukast** INN *investigational treatment for asthma*

**pranolium chloride** USAN, INN *antiarrhythmic*

**pranoprofen** INN

**pranosal** INN

**praseodymium** *element (Pr)*

**prasterone** INN

**Pravachol** tablets ℞ *cholesterol-lowering antihyperlipidemic; HMG-CoA reductase inhibitor; antiatherosclerotic; reduces CHD mortality* [pravastatin sodium] 10, 20, 40 mg ② Primacor

**pravadoline** INN *analgesic* [also: pravadoline maleate]

**pravadoline maleate** USAN *analgesic* [also: pravadoline]

**pravastatin** INN, BAN *antihyperlipidemic; HMG-CoA reductase inhibitor* [also: pravastatin sodium]

**pravastatin sodium** USAN, JAN *antihyperlipidemic; HMG-CoA reductase inhibitor* [also: pravastatin]

**Prax** lotion, cream OTC *topical local anesthetic* [pramoxine HCl] 1%

**praxadine** INN

**prazepam** USAN, USP, INN *sedative* 5 mg oral ② prazepine; prazosin

**prazepine** INN ② prazepam

**praziquantel** USAN, USP, INN, BAN *anthelmintic for schistosomiasis (flukes); orphan status withdrawn 1994*

**prazitone** INN, BAN

**prazocillin** INN

**prazosin** INN, BAN *antihypertensive; $\alpha_1$-adrenergic blocker* [also: prazosin HCl] 1, 2, 5 mg oral ② prazepam

**prazosin HCl** USAN, USP, JAN *antihypertensive; $\alpha_1$-adrenergic blocker* [also: prazosin]

**Pre-Attain** liquid OTC *enteral nutritional therapy* [lactose-free formula]

**Precef** powder for IV or IM injection, StrapKap vials (discontinued 1993) ℞ *cephalosporin-type antibiotic* [ceforanide]

**precipitated calcium carbonate** JAN *antacid; calcium replenisher* [also: calcium carbonate]

**precipitated chalk** [see: calcium carbonate]

**precipitated sulfur** [see: sulfur, precipitated]

**Precision High Nitrogen Diet** powder OTC *enteral nutritional therapy* [lactose-free formula]

**Precision Isotonic Diet** powder (discontinued 1994) OTC *oral nutritional supplement* 58.4 g/packet

**Precision LR Diet** powder OTC *enteral nutritional therapy* [lactose-free formula]

**preclamol** INN

**Precose** tablets ℞ *alpha-glucosidase inhibitor for type 2 diabetes mellitus* [acarbose] 50, 100 mg

**Pred Mild; Pred Forte** eye drop suspension ℞ *ophthalmic topical corticosteroidal anti-inflammatory* [prednisolone acetate] 0.12%; 1%

**Predaject-50** IM injection (discontinued 1996) ℞ *glucocorticoid* [prednisolone acetate] 50 mg/mL

**Predalone 50** IM injection ℞ *glucocorticoids* [prednisolone acetate] 50 mg/mL

**Predalone T.B.A.** intra-articular, intralesional, or soft tissue injection (discontinued 1994) ℞ *glucocorticoids* [prednisolone tebutate] 20 mg/mL

**Predcor-25** IM injection (discontinued 1994) ℞ *glucocorticoids* [prednisolone acetate] 25 mg/mL

**Predcor-50** IM injection ℞ *glucocorticoids* [prednisolone acetate] 50 mg/mL

**Pred-G** eye drop suspension ℞ *topical ophthalmic corticosteroidal anti-inflammatory; antibiotic* [prednisolone acetate; gentamicin sulfate] 1%•0.3%

**Pred-G S.O.P.** ophthalmic ointment ℞ *ophthalmic topical corticosteroidal anti-inflammatory; antibiotic* [prednisolone acetate; gentamicin sulfate; chlorobutanol] 0.6%•0.3%•0.5%

**prednazate** USAN, INN *anti-inflammatory*

**prednazoline** INN

**prednicarbate** USAN, INN *glucocorticoid*

**Prednicen-M** tablets ℞ *glucocorticoid; anti-inflammatory; immunosuppressant* [prednisone] 5 mg

**prednimustine** USAN, INN *antineoplastic; investigational (orphan) for malignant non-Hodgkin's lymphomas*

**Prednisol TBA** intra-articular, intralesional, or soft tissue injection ℞ *glucocorticoids* [prednisolone tebutate] 20 mg/mL

**prednisolamate** INN, BAN

**prednisolone** USP, INN *glucocorticoid* 5 mg oral ⚕ prednisone

**prednisolone acetate** USP, BAN *glucocorticoid; ophthalmic anti-inflammatory* 1% eye drops; 25, 50 mg/mL injection

**prednisolone hemisuccinate** USP *glucocorticoid*

**prednisolone sodium phosphate** USP *glucocorticoid; ophthalmic anti-inflammatory* 0.125%, 1% eye drops

**prednisolone sodium succinate** USP *glucocorticoid*

**prednisolone steaglate** INN, BAN

**prednisolone tebutate** USP *glucocorticoid* 20 mg/mL injection

**prednisone** USP, INN *glucocorticoid; anti-inflammatory; immunosuppressant* 1, 5, 20 mg oral ⚕ prednisolone

**prednival** USAN *glucocorticoid*

**prednylidene** INN, BAN

**Predsulfair** eye drop suspension, ophthalmic ointment (discontinued 1993) ℞ *topical ophthalmic corticosteroidal anti-inflammatory; bacteriostatic* [prednisolone acetate; sulfacetamide sodium]

**prefenamate** INN

**Prefill** (dosage form) *prefilled applicator*

**Preflex Daily Cleaner Especially for Sensitive Eyes** solution OTC *surfactant cleaning solution for soft contact lenses*

**Prefrin Liquifilm** eye drops OTC *topical ocular decongestant* [phenylephrine HCl] 0.12%

**Prefrin-A** eye drops (discontinued 1993) ℞ *topical ocular decongestant and antihistamine; local anesthetic* [phenylephrine HCl; pyrilamine maleate; antipyrine]

**pregelatinized starch** [see: starch, pregelatinized]

**Pregestimil** powder OTC *hypoallergenic infant food for severe malabsorption disorders* [enzymatically hydrolyzed protein formula]

**pregnandiol** JAN

**pregneninolone** [see: ethisterone]

**pregnenolone** INN *non-hormonal sterol derivative* [also: pregnenolone succinate]

**pregnenolone succinate** USAN *non-hormonal sterol derivative* [also: pregnenolone]

**Pregnosis** slide test for home use OTC *in vitro diagnostic aid for urine pregnancy test* [latex agglutination test]

**Pregnyl** powder for IM injection ℞ *hormone for prepubertal cryptorchidism and hypogonadism; ovulation stimulant* [chorionic gonadotropin] 1000 U/mL

**Pre-H Cal** tablets (discontinued 1995) ℞ *vitamin/calcium/iron supplement* [multiple vitamins; calcium; iron; folic acid] ≐•47.5•51.7•0.5 mg

**Prehist** sustained-release capsules ℞ *decongestant; antihistamine* [phenylephrine HCl; chlorpheniramine maleate] 20•8 mg

**Prehist D** sustained-release tablets, sustained-release capsules ℞ *decongestant; antihistamine; anticholinergic* [phenylephrine HCl; chlorpheniramine maleate; methscopolamine nitrate] 20•8•2.5 mg

**Prelone** syrup ℞ *glucocorticoids* [prednisolone; alcohol 5%] 15 mg/5 mL

**Prelu-2** timed-release capsules ℞ *anorexiant* [phendimetrazine tartrate] 105 mg

**preludes** *street drug slang for Preludin (phenmetrazine HCl; discontinued 1992)* [see: phenmetrazine HCl]

**premafloxacin** USAN, INN *veterinary antibacterial*

**Premarin** tablets ℞ *estrogen replacement therapy; palliative therapy for prostatic and breast cancer* [conjugated estrogens] 0.3, 0.625, 0.9, 1.25, 2.5 mg

**Premarin** vaginal cream ℞ *estrogen replacement therapy for postmenopausal disorders* [conjugated estrogens] 0.625 mg/g

**Premarin Intravenous** IV or IM injection ℞ *treatment of abnormal uterine bleeding due to hormonal imbalance* [conjugated estrogens] 25 mg

**Premarin MPA** ℞ *investigational osteoporosis treatment* [conjugated estrogens; medroxyprogesterone acetate]

**Premarin with Methyltestosterone** tablets ℞ *estrogen/androgen for menopausal vasomotor symptoms* [conjugated estrogens; methyltestosterone] 0.625•5, 1.25•10 mg

**premazepam** INN, BAN

**Premphase** tablets (28 per package, 14 of each phase) ℞ *treatment of menopausal symptoms including osteoporosis* [Phase 1: conjugated estrogens; Phase 2: medroxyprogesterone acetate] 0.625 mg; 5 mg

**Prempro** tablets (the single-phase product replaced the two-phase product in 1996) [Phase 1: conjugated estrogens; Phase 2: medroxyprogesterone acetate] 0.625 mg; 2.5 mg

**Prempro** tablets ℞ *treatment of menopausal symptoms including osteoporosis* [conjugated estrogens; medroxyprogesterone acetate] 0.625•2.5 mg

**Prēmsyn PMS** caplets OTC *analgesic; antipyretic; diuretic; antihistaminic sleep aid* [acetaminophen; pamabrom; pyrilamine maleate] 500•25•15 mg

**prenalterol** INN, BAN *adrenergic* [also: prenalterol HCl]

**prenalterol HCl** USAN *adrenergic* [also: prenalterol]

**Prenatal Maternal** tablets ℞ *vitamin/mineral/calcium/iron supplement* [multiple vitamins & minerals; calcium; iron; folic acid; biotin] ±•250•60•1•0.03 mg

**Prenatal MR 90** film-coated delayed-release tablets ℞ *vitamin/calcium/iron supplement* [multiple vitamins; calcium; iron; folic acid] ±•250•90•1 mg

**Prenatal One** film-coated tablets (discontinued 1995) ℞ *vitamin/calcium/iron supplement* [multiple vitamins; calcium; iron; folic acid] ±•200•65•1 mg

**Prenatal Plus** tablets ℞ *vitamin/calcium/iron supplement* [multiple vitamins; calcium; iron; folic acid] ±•200•65•1 mg

**Prenatal Plus Improved** tablets ℞ *vitamin/calcium/iron supplement* [multiple vitamins; calcium; iron; folic acid] ±•200•65•1 mg

**Prenatal Plus with Betacarotene** tablets ℞ *vitamin/calcium/iron supplement* [multiple vitamins; calcium; iron; folic acid] ±•200•65•1 mg

**Prenatal Rx** tablets (name changed to Prenatal Rx with Betacarotene in 1995)

**Prenatal Rx with Betacarotene** tablets ℞ *vitamin/calcium/iron supplement* [multiple vitamins; calcium; iron; folic acid; biotin] ±•200•60•1•0.03 mg

**Prenatal with Folic Acid** tablets OTC *vitamin/calcium/iron supplement* [multiple vitamins; calcium; iron; folic acid] ±•200•60•0.8 mg

**Prenatal Z** film-coated delayed-release tablets ℞ *vitamin/calcium/iron supplement* [multiple vitamins; calcium; iron; folic acid] ±•300•65•1 mg

**Prenatal-1 + Iron** tablets ℞ *vitamin/calcium/iron supplement* [multiple vitamins; calcium; iron; folic acid] ±•200•65•1 mg

**Prenatal-S** tablets OTC *vitamin/calcium/ iron supplement* [multiple vitamins; calcium; iron; folic acid] ≚•200• 60•0.8 mg

**Prenate 90; Prenate Ultra** film-coated delayed-release tablets ℞ *vitamin/calcium/iron supplement* [multiple vitamins; calcium; iron; folic acid] ≚•250•90•1 mg; ≚•200• 90•1 mg

**Prenavite** tablets OTC *vitamin/calcium/ iron supplement* [multiple vitamins; calcium; iron; folic acid] ≚•200• 60•0.8 mg

**prenisteine** INN

**prenoverine** INN

**prenoxdiazine** INN

**prenylamine** USAN, INN *coronary vasodilator*

**Preparation H** anorectal cream, anorectal ointment OTC *temporary relief of hemorrhoidal symptoms* [shark liver oil; phenylephrine HCl] 3%•0.25%

**Preparation H** cleansing tissues OTC *moisturizer and cleanser for external rectal/vaginal areas* [propylene glycol]

**Preparation H** rectal suppositories OTC *temporary relief of hemorrhoidal symptoms* [shark liver oil] 3%

**prepared chalk** [see: calcium carbonate]

**Prepcat** suspension ℞ *GI contrast radiopaque agent* [barium sulfate] 1.5%

**Pre-Pen** solution for dermal scratch test ℞ *penicillin hypersensitivity assessment* [benzylpenicilloyl polylysine] 0.25 mL

**Pre-Pen/MDM** solution for dermal scratch test ℞ *investigational (orphan) for penicillin hypersensitivity assessment* [benzylpenicillin]

**Prepidil** gel ℞ *prostaglandin for cervical ripening at term* [dinoprostone] 0.5 mg

**Prepulsid** ⓒ (U.S. product: Propulsid) tablets ℞ *treatment for nocturnal heartburn due to gastroesophageal reflux disease (GERD)* [cisapride] 10, 20 mg

**Presalin** tablets (discontinued 1995) OTC *analgesic; antipyretic; anti-inflammatory; antacid* [acetaminophen; aspirin; salicylamide; aluminum hydroxide] 120•260•120•100 mg

**Presaril** (name changed to Demadex in 1993)

**prescription** *street drug slang for a marijuana cigarette* [see: marijuana]

**press** *street drug slang* [see: cocaine; cocaine, crack]

**pretamazium iodide** INN, BAN

**pretendica; pretendo** (Spanish for "pretender") *street drug slang* [see: marijuana]

**prethcamide**

**prethrombin** [see: prothrombin complex, activated]

**pretiadil** INN

**Pretts Diet-Aid** chewable tablets OTC *diet aid* [sodium carboxymethylcellulose; alginic acid; sodium bicarbonate] 100•200•70 mg

**Pretty Feet & Hands** cream OTC *moisturizer; emollient*

**Pretz** solution OTC *nasal moisturizer* [sodium chloride (saline)] 0.6%

**Pretz Irrigating** solution OTC *for postoperative irrigation* [sodium chloride (saline); glycerin; eriodictyon] 0.75%

**Pretz Moisturizing** nose drops OTC *nasal moisturizer* [sodium chloride (saline); glycerin; eriodictyon] 0.75%

**Pretz-D** nasal spray OTC *nasal decongestant and moisturizer* [ephedrine sulfate] 0.25%

**PretzPak** ointment OTC *antimicrobial postoperative nasal pack* [benzyl alcohol; PEG; carboxymethylcellulose; urea; allantoin]

**Prevacid** enteric-coated granules in delayed-release capsules ℞ *antisecretory; proton pump inhibitor for duodenal ulcers, erosive esophagitis, and Zollinger-Ellison syndrome* [lansoprazole] 15, 30 mg

**Prevalite** powder for oral suspension ℞ *cholesterol-lowering antihyperlipidemic; also used for biliary obstruction* [cholestyramine resin] 4 g/dose

**PreviDent** topical gel (for self-application) ℞ *dental caries preventative* [sodium fluoride] 1.1%

**PreviDent Rinse** oral solution ℞ *dental caries preventative* [sodium fluoride] 0.2%

**prezatide copper acetate** USAN, INN *immunomodulator*

**pribecaine** INN

**pridefine** INN *antidepressant* [also: pridefine HCl]

**pridefine HCl** USAN *antidepressant* [also: pridefine]

**prideperone** INN ·

**pridinol** INN

**prifelone** USAN, INN *dermatologic antiinflammatory*

**prifinium bromide** INN

**prifuroline** INN

**priliximab** USAN *monoclonal antibody to treat autoimmune lymphoproliferative diseases and in organ transplants*

**prilocaine** INN *local anesthetic* [also: prilocaine HCl]

**prilocaine HCl** USAN, USP *local anesthetic* [also: prilocaine]

**Prilosec** delayed-release capsules ℞ *proton pump inhibitor for gastric and duodenal ulcers and gastroesophageal reflux disease* [omeprazole] 10, 20 mg

**primachine phosphate** [see: primaquine phosphate]

**Primacor** IV infusion ℞ *vasodilator for congestive heart failure* [milrinone lactate] 0.2, 1 mg/mL ② Pravachol

**Primacor in 5% Dextrose** IV infusion ℞ *vasodilator for congestive heart failure* [milrinone lactate; dextrose] 200 μg/mL; 5% ② Pravachol

**Primaderm-B** anorectal ointment (discontinued 1995) OTC *topical anesthetic; astringent* [benzocaine; zinc oxide; cod liver oil]

**primaperone** INN

**primaquine** INN *antimalarial* [also: primaquine phosphate]

**primaquine phosphate** USP *cure for malaria; prevention of malarial relapse* [also: primaquine] 26.3 mg oral

**primaquine phosphate & clindamycin HCl** *investigational (orphan) for AIDS-associated Pneumocystis carinii pneumonia*

**Primatene** tablets OTC *antiasthmatic; bronchodilator; decongestant; sedative* [theophylline; ephedrine HCl; phenobarbital] 130•24•7.5 mg

**Primatene Dual Action** tablets OTC *antiasthmatic; bronchodilator; decongestant; expectorant* [theophylline; ephedrine HCl; guaifenesin] 60•12.5•100 mg

**Primatene Mist** inhalation aerosol OTC *bronchodilator for bronchial asthma* [epinephrine] 0.2 mg/dose

**Primatene Mist Suspension** inhalation aerosol OTC *bronchodilator for bronchial asthma* [epinephrine bitartrate] 0.3 mg/dose

**Primatuss Cough Mixture 4** liquid OTC *antitussive; antihistamine* [dextromethorphan hydrobromide; chlorpheniramine maleate; alcohol 10%] 15•2 mg/5 mL

**Primatuss Cough Mixture 4D** liquid OTC *antitussive; decongestant; expectorant* [dextromethorphan hydrobromide; pseudoephedrine HCl; guaifenesin; alcohol 10%] 10•20•67 mg/5 mL

**Primaxin I.M.** powder for injection ℞ *thienamycin-type bactericidal antibiotic* [imipenem; cilastatin sodium] 500•500, 750•750 mg

**Primaxin I.V.** powder for injection ℞ *thienamycin-type bactericidal antibiotic* [imipenem; cilastatin sodium] 250•250, 500•500 mg

**primidolol** USAN, INN *antihypertensive; antianginal; antiarrhythmic*

**primidone** USP, INN, BAN *anticonvulsant for grand mal, psychomotor, or focal epileptic seizures* 250 mg oral

**primo** (Spanish for "priority") *street drug slang for crack, marijuana and crack, or cigarettes with cocaine and heroin* [see: cocaine, crack; marijuana; cocaine; heroin]

**Primobolan** *brand name for methenolone acetate, a European anabolic steroid abused as a street drug*

**Primobolan Depot** *brand name for methenolone enanthate, a European anabolic steroid abused as a street drug*

**primycin** INN

**Principen** capsules, powder for oral suspension ℞ *penicillin-type antibiotic* [ampicillin trihydrate] 250, 500 mg; 125, 250 mg/5 mL

**Principen with Probenecid** capsules ℞ *antibiotic for Neisseria gonorrhoeae* [ampicillin trihydrate; probenecid]

**Prinivil** tablets ℞ *antihypertensive; angiotensin-converting enzyme (ACE) inhibitor for CHF and acute MI* [lisinopril] 2.5, 5, 10, 20, 40 mg

**prinodolol** [see: pindolol]

**prinomide** INN *antirheumatic* [also: prinomide tromethamine]

**prinomide tromethamine** USAN *antirheumatic* [also: prinomide]

**prinoxodan** USAN, INN *cardiotonic*

**Prinzide** tablets ℞ *antihypertensive* [hydrochlorothiazide; lisinopril] 12.5•10 mg

**Prinzide 12.5; Prinzide 25** tablets ℞ *antihypertensive* [hydrochlorothiazide; lisinopril] 12.5•20 mg; 25•20 mg

**Priscoline HCl** IV injection ℞ *antihypertensive* [tolazoline HCl] 25 mg/mL ⊡ Apresoline

**pristinamycin** INN, BAN

**Privine** nasal spray, nose drops OTC *nasal decongestant* [naphazoline HCl] 0.05%

**prizidilol** INN, BAN *antihypertensive* [also: prizidilol HCl]

**prizidilol HCl** USAN *antihypertensive* [also: prizidilol]

**Pro Skin** capsules OTC *vitamin/zinc supplement* [vitamins A, B₅, C, and E; zinc] 6250 IU•10 mg•100 mg•100 IU•10 mg

**Pro-50** injection ℞ *antihistamine; motion sickness; sleep aid; antiemetic; sedative* [promethazine HCl] 50 mg/mL

**proadifen** INN *non-specific synergist* [also: proadifen HCl]

**proadifen HCl** USAN *non-specific synergist* [also: proadifen]

**Pro-Air** ℞ *investigational antiasthmatic* [procaterol]

**ProAmatine** tablets ℞ *vasopressor for orthostatic hypotension (OH)* [midodrine HCl] 2.5, 5 mg

**Probalan** tablets (discontinued 1997) ℞ *uricosuric for gout* [probenecid] 500 mg

**Probampacin** powder for oral suspension ℞ *antibiotic for Neisseria gonorrhoeae* [ampicillin trihydrate; probenecid] 3.5•1 g

**Pro-Banthīne** tablets ℞ *peptic ulcer treatment adjunct; antispasmodic; antisecretory* [propantheline bromide] 7.5, 15 mg

**probarbital sodium** NF, INN

**Probax** gel OTC *relief from minor oral irritations* [propolis] 2%

**Probec-T** tablets OTC *vitamin supplement* [multiple B vitamins; vitamin C] ≛•600 mg

**Proben-C** tablets (discontinued 1997) ℞ *treatment for frequent, recurrent attacks of gouty arthritis* [probenecid; colchicine] 500•0.5 mg

**probenecid** USP, INN, BAN *uricosuric for gout* 500 mg oral

**probenecid & colchicine** *treatment for frequent, recurrent attacks of gouty arthritis* 500•0.5 mg oral

**Probeta** ℞ *investigational antihypertensive (β-blocker)* [bisoprolol]

**probicromil calcium** USAN *prophylactic antiallergic* [also: ambicromil]

**Pro-Bionate** capsules, powder OTC *dietary supplement; fever blister treatment; not generally regarded as safe and effective as an antidiarrheal* [Lactobacillus acidophilus] 2 billion U; 2 billion U/g

**probucol** USAN, USP, INN *antihyperlipoproteinemic*

**procainamide** INN *antiarrhythmic* [also: procainamide HCl]

**procainamide HCl** USP *antiarrhythmic* [also: procainamide] 250, 375, 500, 750 mg oral; 100, 500 mg/mL injection

**procaine** INN *local anesthetic* [also: procaine borate] ⊡ Procan

**procaine borate** NF *local anesthetic* [also: procaine] ⊡ Procan

**procaine HCl** USP *injectable local anesthetic* 1%, 2% ⊡ Procan

**procaine penicillin** BAN *bactericidal antibiotic* [also: penicillin G procaine] ⊡ Procan

**ProcalAmine** IV infusion ℞ *peripheral parenteral nutrition* [multiple essential and nonessential amino acids; electrolytes]

**Pro-Cal-Sof** capsules OTC *stool softener* [docusate calcium] 240 mg

**Procan SR** sustained-release tablets (replaced by Procanbid in 1996) ℞ antiarrhythmic [procainamide HCl] 250, 500, 750, 1000 mg ⑨ procaine

**Procanbid** extended-release film-coated tablets ℞ twice-daily antiarrhythmic [procainamide HCl] 500, 1000 mg

**procarbazine** INN antibiotic antineoplastic [also: procarbazine HCl] ⑨ dacarbazine

**procarbazine HCl** USAN, USP antibiotic antineoplastic for Hodgkin's disease [also: procarbazine]

**Procardia** capsules ℞ antianginal [nifedipine] 10, 20 mg

**Procardia XL** film-coated sustained-release tablets ℞ antianginal; antihypertensive [nifedipine] 30, 60, 90 mg

**procaterol** INN, BAN bronchodilator [also: procaterol HCl]

**procaterol HCl** USAN bronchodilator [also: procaterol]

**prochlorperazine** USP, INN antiemetic; antipsychotic; antidopaminergic 25 mg suppositories

**prochlorperazine edisylate** USP antiemetic; antipsychotic 5 mg/mL injection

**prochlorperazine ethanedisulfonate** [see: prochlorperazine edisylate]

**prochlorperazine maleate** USP antiemetic; antipsychotic 5, 10, 25 mg oral

**procinolol** INN

**procinonide** USAN, INN adrenocortical steroid

**proclonol** USAN, INN anthelmintic; antifungal

**procodazole** INN

**proconvertin** [see: factor VII]

**Procort** cream, spray OTC topical corticosteroid [hydrocortisone] 1%

**Procrit** IV or subcu injection ℞ stimulates RBC production; for anemia of chronic renal failure, HIV, or chemotherapy (orphan) [epoetin alfa] 2000, 3000, 4000, 10 000, 20 000 U/mL

**Proctocort** anorectal cream ℞ topical corticosteroidal anti-inflammatory [hydrocortisone] 1%

**ProctoCream-HC** anorectal cream ℞ topical corticosteroidal anti-inflammatory [hydrocortisone acetate] 2.5%

**ProctoCream-HC** anorectal cream ℞ topical corticosteroidal anti-inflammatory; local anesthetic [hydrocortisone acetate; pramoxine HCl] 1%•1%

**ProctoFoam NS** anorectal aerosol foam OTC topical local anesthetic [pramoxine HCl] 1%

**Proctofoam-HC** anorectal aerosol foam ℞ topical corticosteroidal anti-inflammatory; local anesthetic [hydrocortisone acetate; pramoxine HCl] 1%•1%

**Pro-Cute** lotion OTC moisturizer; emollient

**ProCycle Gold** tablets OTC vitamin/mineral/iron supplement [multiple vitamins & minerals; iron; folic acid; biotin] ±•3•0.067• ≟ mg

**procyclidine** INN antiparkinsonian; skeletal muscle relaxant; anticholinergic [also: procyclidine HCl]

**procyclidine HCl** USP antiparkinsonian; skeletal muscle relaxant; anticholinergic [also: procyclidine]

**procymate** INN

**Procysteine** ℞ investigational (Phase II) immunomodulator for AIDS; investigational (orphan) for adult respiratory distress syndrome and amyotrophic lateral sclerosis [oxothiazolidine carboxylate]

**prodeconium bromide** INN

**Pro-Depo** IM injection (discontinued 1993) ℞ progestin for amenorrhea and dysfunctional uterine bleeding [hydroxyprogesterone caproate in oil]

**Proderm Topical** dressing OTC dressing for decubitus ulcers [castor oil; balsam Peru] 650•72.5 mg/0.82 mL

**prodilidine** INN analgesic [also: prodilidine HCl]

**prodilidine HCl** USAN analgesic [also: prodilidine]

**prodipine** INN

**Prodium** tablets OTC urinary analgesic [phenazopyridine HCl] 95 mg

**prodolic acid** USAN, INN anti-inflammatory

**pro-drugs** a class of agents which metabolize into a therapeutic or more potent form in the body

**profadol** INN analgesic [also: profadol HCl]

**profadol HCl** USAN *analgesic* [also: profadol]

**Profasi** powder for IM injection ℞ *hormone for prepubertal cryptorchidism and hypogonadism; ovulation stimulant* [chorionic gonadotropin] 500, 1000 U/mL

**Profasi HP** powder for IM injection (name changed to Profasi in 1994)

**Profen II; Profen LA** timed-release tablets ℞ *decongestant; expectorant* [phenylpropanolamine HCl; guaifenesin] 37.5•600 mg; 75•600 mg

**Profen II DM** timed-release tablets ℞ *decongestant; expectorant; antitussive* [phenylpropanolamine HCl; guaifenesin; dextromethorphan hydrobromide] 37.5•600•30 mg

**Profenal** Drop-Tainers (eye drops) ℞ *ocular nonsteroidal anti-inflammatory drug (NSAID); intraoperative miosis inhibitor* [suprofen] 1%

**profenamine** INN *antiparkinsonian* [also: ethopropazine HCl; ethopropazine]

**profenamine HCl** [see: ethopropazine HCl]

**profexalone** INN

**Profiber** liquid OTC *enteral nutritional therapy* [lactose-free formula]

**Profilate HP** IV injection ℞ *antihemophilic to correct coagulation deficiency* [antihemophilic factor VIII:C in heptane] ≟

**Profilate OSD** IV injection (discontinued 1996) ℞ *antihemophilic to correct coagulation deficiency* [antihemophilic factor VIII:C] ≟

**Profilnine Heat-Treated** IV suspension (discontinued 1995) ℞ *anticoagulant to correct factor IX deficiency (hemophilia B; Christmas disease)* [factor IX complex, heat treated] ≟

**Profilnine SD** powder for IV injection ℞ *anticoagulant to correct factor IX deficiency (hemophilia B; Christmas disease)* [coagulation factors II, VII, IX, and X, solvent/detergent treated]

**proflavine** INN [also: proflavine dihydrochloride]

**proflavine dihydrochloride** NF [also: proflavine]

**proflavine sulfate** NF

**proflazepam** INN

**ProFree/GP Weekly Enzymatic Cleaner** tablets OTC *enzymatic cleaner for rigid gas permeable contact lenses* [papain]

**progabide** USAN, INN *anticonvulsant; muscle relaxant*

**Pro-gesic** liquid (discontinued 1995) OTC *topical analgesic* [trolamine salicylate] 10%

**Progestasert** IUD ℞ *intrauterine contraceptive* [progesterone] 38 mg

**progesterone** USP, INN *progestin; intrauterine contraceptive; investigational (orphan) for in vitro fertilization and embryo transfer* 50 mg/mL IM injection (in oil); also available as powder for compounding

**progestins** *a class of sex hormones that cause a sloughing of the endometrial lining, also used as a hormonal antineoplastic*

**proglumetacin** INN

**proglumide** USAN, INN *anticholinergic; investigational antiulcerative*

**Proglycem** capsules, oral suspension ℞ *glucose-elevating agent* [diazoxide] 50 mg; 50 mg/mL

**Prograf** capsules ℞ *liver and kidney transplant rejection preventative; investigational preventative for other transplant rejection* [tacrolimus] 1, 5 mg

**Prograf** IV infusion ℞ *liver transplant rejection preventative* [tacrolimus] 5 mg/mL

**proguanil** INN, BAN [also: chloroguanide HCl]

**proguanil HCl** [see: chloroguanide HCl]

**ProHance** injection ℞ *contrast media for magnetic imaging of the brain and spine* [gadoteridol] 279.3 mg/mL

**proheptazine** INN

**ProHIBiT** IM injection ℞ *Haemophilus influenzae type b (HIB) vaccine* [Hemophilus b conjugate vaccine] 0.5 mL

**proinsulin human** USAN *antidiabetic*

**Prokine** powder for IV infusion (discontinued 1993) ℞ *myeloid reconstitution after autologous bone marrow transplant* [sargramostim] 250, 500 μg

**prolactin** *investigational immune stimulator for burns and chemotherapy*

**Prolastin** IV injection ℞ *replacement therapy for alpha₁-proteinase inhibitor deficiency (orphan)* [alpha₁-proteinase inhibitor] 20 mg/mL

**Proleukin** powder for IV infusion ℞ *antineoplastic for metastatic renal cell carcinoma (orphan); investigational (orphan) for immunodeficiency diseases* [aldesleukin] 18 million IU/mL

**Proleukin-PEG** ℞ *investigational immune enhancer for AIDS and human papillomavirus* [aldesleukin; polyethylene glycol]

**proligestone** INN

**proline (L-proline)** USAN, USP, INN *nonessential amino acid; symbols: Pro, P* ⧉ Prolene

**prolintane** INN *antidepressant* [also: prolintane HCl]

**prolintane HCl** USAN *antidepressant* [also: prolintane]

**Prolixin** tablets, elixir, oral concentrate, IM injection ℞ *antipsychotic* [fluphenazine HCl] 1, 2.5, 5, 10 mg; 2.5 mg/5 mL; 5 mg/mL; 2.5 mg/mL

**Prolixin Decanoate** subcu or IM injection, Unimatic (prefilled) syringe ℞ *antipsychotic* [fluphenazine decanoate] 25 mg/mL

**Prolixin Enanthate** subcu or IM injection ℞ *antipsychotic* [fluphenazine enanthate] 25 mg/mL

**prolonium iodide** INN

**Proloprim** tablets ℞ *anti-infective; antibacterial* [trimethoprim] 100, 200 mg

**ProMACE (prednisone, methotrexate [with leucovorin rescue], Adriamycin, cyclophosphamide, etoposide)** *chemotherapy protocol*

**ProMACE/cytaBOM (ProMACE [above], cytarabine, bleomycin, Oncovin, mitoxantrone)** *chemotherapy protocol*

**ProMACE/MOPP (full course of ProMACE, followed by MOPP)** *chemotherapy protocol*

**promazine** INN *antipsychotic* [also: promazine HCl] ⧉ Promethazine

**promazine HCl** USP *antipsychotic* [also: promazine] 25, 50 mg/mL injection

**Promedrol** ℞ *investigational treatment for asthma, shock, and kidney transplant rejection* [methylprednisolone suleptanate]

**Promega** Pearls (softgels) OTC *dietary supplement* [omega-3 fatty acids; multiple vitamins & minerals] 600•≛, 1000•≛ mg

**promegestone** INN

**promelase** INN

**promestriene** INN

**Prometa** syrup (discontinued 1995) ℞ *bronchodilator* [metaproterenol sulfate] 10 mg/5 mL

**Prometh** syrup (discontinued 1996) ℞ *antihistamine* [promethazine HCl; alcohol]

**Prometh VC Plain** liquid ℞ *decongestant; antihistamine* [phenylephrine HCl; promethazine HCl] 5•6.25 mg/5 mL

**Prometh VC with Codeine** syrup ℞ *narcotic antitussive; decongestant; antihistamine* [codeine phosphate; phenylephrine HCl; promethazine HCl; alcohol] 10•5•6.25 mg/5 mL

**Prometh with Codeine** syrup ℞ *narcotic antitussive; antihistamine* [codeine phosphate; promethazine HCl] 10•6.25 mg/5 mL

**Prometh with Dextromethorphan** syrup ℞ *antitussive; antihistamine* [dextromethorphan hydrobromide; promethazine HCl; alcohol 7%] 15•6.25 mg/5 mL

**Prometh-50** injection ℞ *antihistamine; motion sickness; sleep aid; antiemetic; sedative* [promethazine HCl] 50 mg/mL

**promethazine** INN *antiemetic; antihistamine; antidopaminergic; motion sickness relief* [also: promethazine HCl]

**Promethazine DC Plain** syrup (discontinued 1993) ℞ *decongestant; antihistamine* [promethazine HCl; phenylephrine HCl; alcohol] ⧉ promazine

**Promethazine DM** syrup ℞ *antitussive; antihistamine* [dextr+methorphan hydrobromide; promethazine HCl; alcohol] 15•6.25 mg/5 mL

**promethazine HCl** USP *antiemetic; antihistamine; antidopaminergic* [also: promethazine] 12.5, 25, 50 mg oral; 6.25, 25 mg/5 mL oral; 50 mg suppositories; 25, 50 mg/mL injection

**promethazine teoclate** INN

**Promethazine VC** syrup ℞ *decongestant; antihistamine* [phenylephrine HCl; promethazine HCl] 5•6.25 mg/5 mL

**Promethazine VC Plain** syrup ℞ *decongestant; antihistamine* [phenylephrine HCl; promethazine HCl; alcohol 7%] 5•6.25 mg/5 mL

**Promethazine VC with Codeine** syrup ℞ *narcotic antitussive; decongestant; antihistamine* [codeine phosphate; phenylephrine HCl; promethazine HCl; alcohol] 10•5•6.25 mg/5 mL

**promethestrol** [see: methestrol]

**Promethist with Codeine** syrup ℞ *narcotic antitussive; decongestant; antihistamine* [codeine phosphate; phenylephrine HCl; promethazine HCl; alcohol] 10•5•6.25 mg/5 mL

**promethium** *element (Pm)*

**Prometrium** ℞ *investigational oral progesterone for secondary amenorrhea and abnormal uterine bleeding*

**Promine** capsules ℞ *antiarrhythmic* [procainamide HCl]

**Prominol** tablets ℞ *analgesic; antipyretic; sedative* [acetaminophen; butalbital] 650•50 mg

**Promise with Fluoride** toothpaste (discontinued 1994) OTC *tooth desensitizer; dental caries preventative* [potassium nitrate; sodium monofluorophosphate]

**Promit** IV injection ℞ *monovalent hapten for prophylaxis of dextran-induced anaphylactic reactions* [dextran 1] 150 mg/mL

**ProMod** powder OTC *oral protein supplement* [D-whey protein concentrate; soy lecithin]

**promolate** INN

**promoxolane** INN

**prompt insulin zinc** [see: insulin zinc, prompt]

**Promycin** *investigational (Phase III, orphan) antineoplastic for head, neck, and cervical cancers* [porfiromycin]

**Pronemia Hematinic** capsules ℞ *hematinic* [ferrous fumarate; cyanocobalamin; ascorbic acid; intrinsic factor concentrate; folic acid] 115 mg•15 μg•150 mg•75 mg•1 mg

**Pronestyl** capsules, tablets, IV or IM injection ℞ *antiarrhythmic* [procainamide HCl] 250, 375, 500 mg; 250, 375, 500 mg; 100, 500 mg/mL ☒ Ponstel

**Pronestyl-SR** sustained-release tablets ℞ *antiarrhythmic* [procainamide HCl] 500 mg

**pronetalol** INN [also: pronethalol]

**pronethalol** BAN [also: pronetalol]

**Pronto** shampoo + creme rinse OTC *pediculicide* [pyrethrins; piperonyl butoxide] 0.33%•4%

**Propa P.H. with Aloe** cleansing pads (discontinued 1994) OTC *topical acne treatment* [salicylic acid; alcohol] 0.5%•25%

**Propa P.H. with Aloe** cream (discontinued 1993) OTC *topical acne treatment* [salicylic acid] 2%

**Propac** powder OTC *oral protein supplement* [whey protein; lactose]

**Propacet 100** film-coated tablets ℞ *narcotic analgesic* [propoxyphene napsylate; acetaminophen] 100•650 mg

**propacetamol** INN

**propafenone** INN, BAN *antiarrhythmic* [also: propafenone HCl]

**propafenone HCl** USAN *antiarrhythmic* [also: propafenone]

**Propagest** tablets OTC *nasal decongestant; diet aid* [phenylpropanolamine HCl] 25 mg

**propamidine** INN, BAN, DCF

**propamidine isethionate** *orphan status withdrawn 1996*

**propaminodiphen** [see: pramiverine]

**propane** NF *aerosol propellant*

**1,2-propanediol** [see: propylene glycol]

**propanidid** USAN, INN *intravenous anesthetic*

**propanocaine** INN

**propanoic acid, sodium salt hydrate** [see: sodium propionate]

**2-propanol** [see: isopropyl alcohol]

**2-propanone** [see: acetone]

**propantheline bromide** USP, INN *peptic ulcer adjunct* 15 mg oral

**PROPApH Acne** cream OTC *topical keratolytic for acne* [salicylic acid] 2%

**PROPApH Cleansing; PROPApH Cleansing for Sensitive Skin; PROPApH Cleansing Maximum Strength** pads OTC *topical keratolytic for acne* [salicylic acid] 0.5%; 0.5%; 2%

**PROPApH Cleansing for Normal/ Combination Skin; PROPApH Cleansing for Oily Skin** lotion OTC *topical keratolytic for acne* [salicylic acid] 0.5%

**PROPApH Foaming Face Wash** liquid Rx *topical keratolytic cleanser for acne* [salicylic acid] 2%

**PROPApH Peel-Off Acne Mask** OTC *topical keratolytic for acne* [salicylic acid] 2%

**proparacaine HCl** USP *topical ophthalmic anesthetic* [also: proxymetacaine] 0.5% eye drops

**proparacaine HCl & fluorescein sodium** *topical ophthalmic anesthetic; corneal disclosing agent* 0.5%•0.25%

**propatyl nitrate** USAN *coronary vasodilator* [also: propatylnitrate]

**propatylnitrate** INN *coronary vasodilator* [also: propatyl nitrate]

**propazolamide** INN

**Propecia** Rx *investigational (Phase III) oral treatment for androgenic alopecia* [finasteride]

**1-propene homopolymer** [see: polipropene 25]

**propenidazole** INN

**propentofylline** INN

*p*-**propenylanisole** [see: anethole]

**propenzolate HCl** USAN *anticholinergic* [also: oxyclipine]

**propericiazine** [see: periciazine]

**properidine** INN, BAN

**propetamide** INN

**propetandrol** INN

**prophenamine HCl** [see: ethopropazine HCl]

**Pro-Phree** powder OTC *supplement to breast milk* [protein-free formula with vitamins & minerals]

**Prophyllin** ointment OTC *topical antifungal; vulnerary; wound deodorant* [sodium propionate; chlorophyll derivatives] 5%•0.0125%

**Prophyllin** powder (discontinued 1994) OTC *topical antifungal; vulnerary; wound deodorant* [sodium propionate; chlorophyll derivatives] 1%•0.0025%

**propicillin** INN, BAN

**propikacin** USAN, INN *antibacterial*

**Propimex-1** powder OTC *formula for infants with propionic or methylmalonicacidemia*

**Propimex-2** powder OTC *enteral nutritional therapy for propionic or methylmalonicacidemia*

**Propine** eye drops Rx *antiglaucoma agent* [dipivefrin HCl] 0.1%

**propinetidine** INN

**propiodal** [see: prolonium iodide]

**propiolactone (β-propiolactone)** USAN, INN *disinfectant*

**propiomazine** USAN, INN *preanesthetic sedative*

**propiomazine HCl** USP *sedative; analgesic adjunct*

**propionic acid** NF *antimicrobial; acidifying agent*

**propionyl erythromycin lauryl sulfate** [see: erythromycin estolate]

**propipocaine** INN

**propiram** INN *narcotic analgesic* [also: propiram fumarate]

**propiram fumarate** USAN *narcotic analgesic* [also: propiram]

**propisergide** INN

**propitocaine HCl** [now: prilocaine HCl]

**propiverine** INN

**propizepine** INN

**Proplex T** IV infusion Rx *antihemophilic to correct factor VII, VIII (hemophilia A), and IX (hemophilia B; Christmas disease) deficiencies* [coagulation factors II, VII, IX, and X, heat treated] 30 mL

**propofol** USAN, INN, BAN *rapid-acting general anesthetic*

**propoxate** INN

**propoxycaine** INN *local anesthetic* [also: propoxycaine HCl]

**propoxycaine HCl** USP *local anesthetic* [also: propoxycaine]

**propoxyphene HCl** USAN, USP *narcotic analgesic* [also: dextro-propoxyphene HCl] 65 mg oral

**propoxyphene napsylate** USAN, USP *narcotic analgesic*

**propranolol** INN, BAN *antiarrhythmic; migraine preventative; antiadrenergic (β-receptor)* [also: propranolol HCl]

**propranolol HCl** USAN, USP *antiarrhythmic; migraine preventative; antiadrenergic (β-receptor)* [also: propranolol] 10, 20, 40, 60, 80, 90, 120, 160 mg oral; 4, 8, 80 mg/mL oral; 1 mg/mL injection

**Propulsid** tablets, oral suspension ℞ *treatment for nocturnal heartburn due to gastroesophageal reflux disease (GERD)* [cisapride] 10, 20 mg; 1 mg/mL

**propyl *p*-aminobenzoate** [see: risocaine]

**propyl docetrizoate** INN, BAN

**propyl gallate** NF *antioxidant*

**propyl *p*-hydroxybenzoate** [see: propylparaben]

**propyl *p*-hydroxybenzoate, sodium salt** [see: propylparaben sodium]

**N-propylajmalinium tartrate** [see: prajmalinum bitartrate]

**propylene carbonate** NF *gelling agent*

**propylene glycol** USP *humectant; solvent; suspending and viscosity-increasing agent*

**propylene glycol alginate** NF *suspending agent; viscosity-increasing agent*

**propylene glycol diacetate** NF *solvent*

**propylene glycol ether of methylcellulose** [see: hydroxypropyl methylcellulose]

**propylene glycol monostearate** NF *emulsifying agent*

**propylhexedrine** USP, INN, BAN *vasoconstrictor; nasal decongestant*

**propyliodone** USP, INN *radiopaque medium*

**propylorvinol** [see: etorphine]

**propylparaben** USAN, NF *antifungal agent; preservative*

**propylparaben sodium** USAN, NF *antimicrobial preservative*

**2-propylpentanoic acid** [see: valproic acid]

**propylthiouracil (PTU)** USP, INN *thyroid inhibitor*

**2-propylvaleramide** [see: valpromide]

**propylvaleric acid** [see: valproic acid]

**5-propynylarabinofuranosyluracil** *investigational treatment for varicella-zoster virus*

**propyperone** INN

**propyphenazone** INN, BAN

**propyromazine bromide** INN

**proquamezine** BAN [also: aminopromazine]

**proquazone** USAN, INN *anti-inflammatory*

**proquinolate** USAN, INN *coccidiostat for poultry*

**prorenoate potassium** USAN, INN *aldosterone antagonist*

**Prorex-25; Prorex-50** injection ℞ *antihistamine; motion sickness; sleep aid; antiemetic; sedative* [promethazine HCl] 25 mg/mL; 50 mg/mL

**proroxan** INN *antiadrenergic (α-receptor)* [also: proroxan HCl]

**proroxan HCl** USAN *antiadrenergic (α-receptor)* [also: proroxan]

**Proscar** film-coated tablets ℞ *androgen hormone inhibitor for benign prostatic hyperplasia (BPH)* [finasteride] 5 mg

**proscillaridin** USAN, INN *cardiotonic*

**proscillaridin A** [see: proscillaridin]

**Prosed/DS** sugar-coated tablets ℞ *urinary anti-infective; antiseptic; analgesic; antispasmodic* [methenamine; phenyl salicylate; methylene blue; benzoic acid; atropine sulfate; hyoscyamine sulfate] 81.6•36.2•10.8•9•0.06•0.06 mg

**ProSobee** liquid, powder OTC *hypoallergenic infant food* [soy protein formula]

**Pro-Sof Plus** capsules OTC *laxative; stool softener* [casanthranol; docusate sodium] 30•100 mg

**ProSom** tablets ℞ *sedative; hypnotic* [estazolam] 1, 2 mg

**Prosorba** ℞ *investigational treatment for rheumatoid arthritis*

**prospidium chloride** INN

**prostacyclin** [now: epoprostenol]

**prostaglandin E₁ (PGE₁)** [now: alprostadil]

**prostaglandin E₁ alphacyclodextrin** *orphan status withdrawn 1996*

**prostaglandin E₂ (PGE₂)** [see: dinoprostone]

**prostaglandin F₂ₐ (PGF₂ₐ)** [see: dinoprost]

**prostaglandin I₂ (PGI₂)** [now: epoprostenol]

**prostaglandin X (PGX)** [now: epoprostenol]

**prostaglandins** *a class of agents that stimulate uterine contractions, used for abortions, cervical ripening, and postpartum hemorrhage*

**prostalene** USAN, INN *prostaglandin*

**Prostaphlin** capsules, powder for oral solution, powder for IV or IM injection ℞ *bactericidal antibiotic (penicillinase-resistant penicillin)* [oxacillin sodium] 250, 500 mg; 250 mg/5 mL; 0.5, 1, 2, 4, 10 g

**ProstaScint** ℞ *imaging agent for prostate cancer and its metastases* [capromab pendetide]

**ProStep** transdermal patch ℞ *smoking deterrent; nicotine withdrawal aid* [nicotine] 15, 30 mg

**Prostigmin** subcu or IM injection ℞ *cholinergic urinary stimulant for postsurgical urinary retention* [neostigmine methylsulfate] 1:1000 (1 mg/mL), 1:2000 (0.5 mg/mL), 1:4000 (0.25 mg/mL) (1:400 [2.5 mg/mL] available in Canada) ⊡ *physostigmine*

**Prostigmin** tablets ℞ *myasthenia gravis treatment; antidote for neuromuscular blockers* [neostigmine bromide] 15 mg

**Prostin E2** vaginal suppository ℞ *prostaglandin-type abortifacient* [dinoprostone] 20 mg

**Prostin VR Pediatric** IV injection ℞ *vasodilator; platelet aggregation inhibitor* [alprostadil] 500 μg/mL

**prosulpride** INN

**prosultiamine** INN

**Protac** troches (discontinued 1994) OTC *topical oral anesthetic; antiseptic* [benzocaine; cetylpyridinium chloride] 10•2.5 mg

**protactinium** *element (Pa)*

**protamine sulfate** USP, INN *antidote to heparin overdose* [also: protamine sulphate] 10 mg/mL injection

**protamine sulphate** BAN *antidote to heparin overdose* [also: protamine sulfate]

**protamine zinc insulin (PZI)** INN *antidiabetic* [also: insulin, protamine zinc]

**Protar Protein** shampoo OTC *antiseborrheic; antipsoriatic; antipruritic; antibacterial* [coal tar] 5%

**protargin, mild** [see: silver protein, mild]

**protease inhibitors** *a class of antivirals that block HIV replication*

**ProTec** ℞ *investigational immunomodulator* [lisofylline]

**ProTech First Aid Stick** liquid OTC *topical antiseptic; analgesic* [lidocaine; povidone-iodine] 2.5%•10%

**Protectol Medicated** powder OTC *topical antifungal* [calcium undecylenate] 15%

**Protegra** softgels OTC *vitamin/mineral supplement* [multiple vitamins & minerals] ≝

**protein C concentrate** *investigational (orphan) anticoagulant for protein C deficiency*

**protein hydrolysate** USP *fluid and nutrient replenisher*

**α₁-proteinase inhibitor** [see: alpha₁-proteinase inhibitor]

**Protenate** IV infusion ℞ *blood volume expander for shock due to burns, trauma and surgery* [plasma protein fraction] 5%

**proterguride** INN

**Prothazine** subcu or IM injection ℞ *antihistamine; motion sickness; sleep aid; antiemetic; sedative* [promethazine HCl] 25, 50 mg/mL

**Prothazine Plain** syrup ℞ *antihistamine; motion sickness; sleep aid; antiemetic; sedative* [promethazine HCl] 6.25 mg/5 mL

**protheobromine** INN

**Prothera** liquid (discontinued 1995) OTC *soap-free therapeutic skin cleanser*

**Prothiaden** ℞ *investigational tricyclic antidepressant* [dothiepin HCl]

**prothionamide** BAN [also: protionamide]

**prothipendyl** INN

**prothipendyl HCl** [see: prothipendyl]

**prothixene** INN

**prothrombin complex, activated** BAN

**Protilase** capsules containing enteric-coated spheres ℞ *digestive enzymes* [lipase; protease; amylase] 4000•25 000•20 000 U

**ProTime** test kit for home use OTC *in vitro diagnostic aid for the management of anticoagulation therapy*

**protiofate** INN

**protionamide** INN [also: prothionamide]

**protirelin** USAN, INN, BAN *prothyrotropin; investigational (orphan) for infant respiratory distress syndrome of prematurity*

**protizinic acid** INN

**protokylol HCl**

**proton pump inhibitor** [see: reversible proton pump inhibitor]

**proton pump inhibitors** *a class of gastric antisecretory agents that inhibit the ATPase "proton pump" within the cell* [also called: ATPase inhibitors; substituted benzimidazoles]

**Protopam Chloride** IV injection ℞ *antidote for organophosphate poisoning and anticholinesterase overdose* [pralidoxime chloride] 1 g ☒ Protamine

**Protopam Chloride** tablets (discontinued 1995) ℞ *antidote for organophosphate and anticholinesterase chemicals* [pralidoxime chloride] 500 mg ☒ Protamine

**Protostat** tablets ℞ *antibiotic; antiprotozoal; amebicide* [metronidazole] 250, 500 mg

**protoveratrine A**

**Protovir** ℞ *investigational antiviral for cytomegalovirus* [sevirumab]

**Protox** ℞ *investigational (orphan) for toxoplasmosis of AIDS* [poloxamer 331]

**protriptyline** INN *tricyclic antidepressant* [also: protriptyline HCl]

**protriptyline HCl** USAN, USP *tricyclic antidepressant* [also: protriptyline] 5, 10 mg oral

**Protropin** powder for IM or subcu injection ℞ *growth hormone for congenital growth failure (orphan) or due to chronic renal insufficiency; investigational (orphan) for Turner syndrome* [somatrem] 5, 10 mg (13, 26 IU) per vial

**Protropin II** ℞ *growth hormone for congenital or renal-induced growth failure (orphan); investigational (orphan) for Turner syndrome, severe burns and AIDS* [somatropin]

**Protuss** liquid ℞ *narcotic antitussive; expectorant* [hydrocodone bitartrate; potassium guaiacolsulfonate] 5•300 mg/5 mL

**Protuss-D** liquid ℞ *narcotic antitussive; decongestant; expectorant* [hydrocodone bitartrate; pseudoephedrine HCl; potassium guaiacolsulfonate] 5•30•300 mg/5 mL

**prourokinase** [see: saruplase]

**Provatene** soft gel perles (discontinued 1996) OTC *to reduce photosensitivity reaction* [beta-carotene] 15 mg

**Proventil** inhalation aerosol ℞ *bronchodilator* [albuterol] 90 μg/dose

**Proventil** tablets, Repetabs (extended-release tablets), syrup, solution for inhalation ℞ *bronchodilator* [albuterol sulfate] 2, 4 mg; 4 mg; 2 mg/5 mL; 0.083%

**Proventil HFA** CFC-free inhalation aerosol ℞ *bronchodilator* [albuterol] 90 μg/dose

**Provera** tablets ℞ *progestin for secondary amenorrhea or abnormal uterine bleeding* [medroxyprogesterone acetate] 2.5, 5, 10 mg

**Provigil** *investigational (orphan) analeptic for excessive daytime sleepiness of narcolepsy* [modafinil]

**Provir** ℞ *investigational antiviral for respiratory viruses*

**Provir** ℞ *investigational (Phase II) oral treatment for watery diarrhea*

**Proviron** *brand name for mesterolone, an androgen abused with anabolic steroid street drugs*

**Provisc** ℞ *investigational ophthalmic agent*

**provitamin A** [see: beta carotene]

**Provocholine** powder for reconstitution for inhalation ℞ *bronchoconstrictor for in vivo pulmonary function challenge test* [methacholine chloride] 100 mg/5 mL

**proxazole** USAN, INN *smooth muscle relaxant; analgesic; anti-inflammatory*

**proxazole citrate** USAN *smooth muscle relaxant; analgesic; anti-inflammatory*

**proxetil** INN *combining name for radicals or groups*

**proxibarbal** INN

**proxibutene** INN

**proxicromil** USAN, INN *antiallergic*

**proxifezone** INN

**Proxigel** OTC *topical oral anti-inflammatory/anti-infective for braces* [carbamide peroxide] 10%

**proxorphan** INN *analgesic; antitussive* [also: proxorphan tartrate]

**proxorphan tartrate** USAN *analgesic; antitussive* [also: proxorphan]

**Proxy 65** tablets ℞ *analgesic* [propoxyphene HCl; acetaminophen]

**proxymetacaine** INN, BAN *topical ophthalmic anesthetic* [also: proparacaine HCl]

**proxymetacaine HCl** [see: proparacaine HCl]

**proxyphylline** INN, BAN

**Prozac** Pulvules (capsules), liquid ℞ *selective serotonin reuptake inhibitor (SSRI) for depression, obsessive-compulsive disorder, and bulimia nervosa* [fluoxetine HCl] 10, 20 mg; 20 mg/5 mL

**prozapine** INN

**Prozine-50** IM injection ℞ *antipsychotic* [promazine HCl] 50 mg/mL

**Prulet** tablets OTC *laxative* [white phenolphthalein] 60 mg

**Pryme** ℞ *investigational vaccine for Lyme disease*

**PSC-833** *investigational adjunct to chemotherapy for multi–drug-resistant tumors*

**Pseudo** liquid OTC *nasal decongestant* [pseudoephedrine HCl] 30 mg/5 mL

**pseudocaine** *street drug slang for phenylpropanolamine, an adulterant for cutting crack*

**Pseudo-Car DM** syrup ℞ *antitussive; decongestant; antihistamine* [dextromethorphan hydrobromide; pseudoephedrine HCl; carbinoxamine maleate] 15•60•4 mg/5 mL

**Pseudo-Chlor** sustained-release capsules ℞ *decongestant; antihistamine* [pseudoephedrine HCl; chlorpheniramine maleate] 120•8 mg

**pseudoephedrine** INN, BAN *vasoconstrictor; nasal decongestant* [also: pseudoephedrine HCl]

**pseudoephedrine HCl** USAN, USP *vasoconstrictor; nasal decongestant* [also: pseudoephedrine] 30, 60 mg oral; 30 mg/5 mL oral

**pseudoephedrine HCl & carbinoxamine maleate** *decongestant; antihistamine* 60•4 mg/5 mL oral; 25•2 mg/mL oral

**pseudoephedrine polistirex** USAN *nasal decongestant*

**pseudoephedrine sulfate** USAN, USP *bronchodilator; nasal decongestant*

**Pseudo-Gest** tablets OTC *nasal decongestant* [pseudoephedrine HCl] 30, 60 mg

**Pseudo-Gest Plus** tablets OTC *decongestant; antihistamine* [pseudoephedrine HCl; chlorpheniramine maleate] 60•4 mg

*Pseudomonas* **immune globulin** [see: mucoid exopolysaccharide *Pseudomonas* hyperimmune globulin]

**pseudomonic acid A** [see: mupirocin]

**Pseudostat** ℞ *investigational (Phase II) theraccine for chronic bronchitis*

**psilocin** *a hallucinogenic street drug closely related to psilocybin*

**psilocybin** BAN *a hallucinogenic street drug derived from the Psilocybe mexicana mushroom* [also: psilocybine]

**psilocybine** INN, DCF *a hallucinogenic street drug derived from the Psilocybe mexicana mushroom* [also: psilocybin]

**psoralens** *a class of light-activated agents for the treatment of psoriasis*

**Psor-a-set** bar OTC *therapeutic skin cleanser; topical keratolytic* [salicylic acid] 2%

**Psorcon** cream, ointment ℞ *topical corticosteroidal anti-inflammatory* [diflorasone diacetate] 0.05%

**PsoriGel** OTC *topical antipsoriatic; antiseborrheic; antiseptic* [coal tar solution; alcohol 33%] 7.5%

**PsoriNail** liquid (discontinued 1994) OTC *topical antipsoriatic; antiseborrheic; antiseptic* [coal tar solution] 2.5%

**Psorion** cream (discontinued 1995) ℞ *topical corticosteroid* [betamethasone dipropionate] 0.05%

**psyllium husk** USP *bulk laxative*

**psyllium hydrocolloid** *bulk laxative*

**psyllium hydrophilic mucilloid** *bulk laxative*

**psyllium seed** [see: plantago seed]

**PTC (plasma thromboplastin component)** [see: factor IX]

**P.T.E.-4; P.T.E.-5** IV injection ℞ *intravenous nutritional therapy* [multiple trace elements (metals)]

**pterins** *a class of investigational antineoplastics*

**pteroyldiglutamic acid (PDGA)**

**pteroylglutamic acid (PGA)** [see: folic acid]

**PTFE (polytetrafluoroethylene)** [see: polytef]

**PTU (propylthiouracil)** [q.v.]

**puffy** *street drug slang* [see: PCP]

**pulborn** *street drug slang* [see: heroin]

**Pulmicort** Turbuhaler (dry powder in a metered dose inhaler) ℞ *intranasal steroidal anti-inflammatory* [budesonide] 200 μg/dose

**Pulmocare** ready-to-use liquid OTC *enteral nutritional therapy for pulmonary problems*

**pulmonary surfactant replacement, porcine** *investigational (orphan) for infant respiratory distress syndrome of prematurity*

**Pulmozyme** solution for nebulization ℞ *reduces respiratory viscoelasticity of sputum in cystic fibrosis (orphan)* [dornase alfa] 1 mg/mL

**pulse VAC (vincristine, actinomycin D, cyclophosphamide)** *chemotherapy protocol* [also: VAC]

**pulse VAC (vincristine, Adriamycin, cyclophosphamide)** *chemotherapy protocol* [also: VAC]

**Pulvule** (trademarked dosage form) *bullet-shaped capsule*

**pumice** USP *dental abrasive*

**pumitepa** INN

**Punctum Plug** ℞ *blocks the puncta and canaliculus to eliminate tear loss in keratitis sicca* [silicone plug]

**Puralube** ophthalmic ointment OTC *ocular moisturizer/lubricant* [white petrolatum; mineral oil]

**Puralube Tears** eye drops OTC *ocular moisturizer/lubricant* [polyvinyl alcohol; polyethylene glycol 400] 1%•1%

**pure** *street drug slang* [see: heroin]

**pure love** *street drug slang* [see: LSD]

**Purge** liquid OTC *stimulant laxative* [castor oil] 95%

**purified cotton** [see: cotton, purified]

**purified protein derivative (PPD) of tuberculin** [see: tuberculin]

**purified rayon** [see: rayon, purified]

**purified siliceous earth** [see: siliceous earth, purified]

**purified water** [see: water, purified]

*H*-**purin-6-amine** [see: adenine]

**purine nucleoside phosphorylase** *investigational (Phase III) treatment for psoriasis*

**Purinethol** tablets ℞ *antimetabolic antineoplastic for multiple leukemias* [mercaptopurine] 50 mg

**Purinol** ⒸⒶⓃ (U.S. product: Zyloprim) tablets ℞ *xanthine oxidase inhibitor for gout and hyperuricemia* [allopurinol] 100, 300 mg

**puromycin** USAN, INN *antineoplastic; antiprotozoal (Trypanosoma)*

**puromycin HCl** USAN *antineoplastic; antiprotozoal (Trypanosoma)*

**purple** *street drug slang* [see: ketamine HCl]

**purple barrels; purple flats; purple haze; purple ozoline** *street drug slang* [see: LSD]

**purple hearts** *street drug slang for Luminal Sodium (phenobarbital sodium), LSD, amphetamines, or various CNS depressants* [see: Luminal Sodium; phenobarbital sodium; LSD; amphetamines]

**purple rain** *street drug slang* [see: PCP]

**Purpose Alpha Hydroxy Moisture** lotion, cream OTC *moisturizer; emollient; exfoliant* [glycolic acid] 8%

**Purpose Dry Skin** cream OTC *moisturizer; emollient*

**Purpose Soap** bar OTC *therapeutic skin cleanser*

**PVA (polyvinyl alcohol)** [q.v.]

**PVB (Platinol, vinblastine, bleomycin)** *chemotherapy protocol*

**PVDA (prednisone, vincristine, daunorubicin, asparaginase)** *chemotherapy protocol*

**PVP; PVP-16 (Platinol, VP-16)** *chemotherapy protocol*

**P-V-Tussin** syrup ℞ *narcotic antitussive; decongestant; antihistamine* [hydrocodone bitartrate; pseudoephedrine HCl; chlorpheniramine maleate; alcohol 5%] 2.5•30•2 mg/5 mL

**P-V-Tussin** tablets ℞ *narcotic antitussive; antihistamine; expectorant* [hydrocodone bitartrate; phenindamine tartrate; guaifenesin] 5•25•200 mg

**Pyloriset** reagent kit for professional use *in vitro diagnostic aid for GI disorders*

**pyrabrom** USAN *antihistamine*

**pyradone** [see: aminopyrine]

**pyrantel** INN *anthelmintic for ascariasis (roundworm) and enterobiasis (pinworm)* [also: pyrantel pamoate]

**pyrantel pamoate** USAN, USP *anthelmintic for ascariasis (roundworm) and enterobiasis (pinworm)* [also: pyrantel]

**pyrantel tartrate** USAN *anthelmintic*

**pyrathiazine HCl** [see: parathiazine]

**pyrazinamide (PZA)** USP, INN, BAN *bactericidal; primary tuberculostatic* 500 mg oral

**pyrazinecarboxamide** [see: pyrazinamide]

**pyrazofurin** USAN *antineoplastic* [also: pirazofurin]

**pyrazoline** [see: antipyrine]

**pyrbenzindole** [see: benzindopyrine HCl]

**pyrbuterol HCl** [see: pirbuterol HCl]

**pyrethrins**

**pyribenzamine (PBZ)** [see: tripelennamine]

**pyricarbate** INN

**pyridarone** INN

**Pyridiate; Pyridiate No. 2** tablets ℞ *urinary analgesic* [phenazopyridine HCl] 100 mg; 200 mg

**4-pyridinamine** [see: fampridine]

**2-pyridine aldoxime methylchloride (2-PAM)** [see: pralidoxime chloride]

**3-pyridinecarboxamide** [see: niacinamide]

**3-pyridinecarboxylic acid** [see: niacin]

**4-pyridinecarboxylic acid hydrazide** [see: isoniazid]

**3-pyridinecarboxylic acid methyl ester** [see: methyl nicotinate]

**3-pyridinemethanol** [see: nicotinyl alcohol]

**2-pyridinemethanol** [see: piconol]

**3-pyridinemethanol tartrate** [see: nicotinyl tartrate]

**Pyridium** tablets ℞ *urinary analgesic* [phenazopyridine HCl] 100, 200 mg ⚠ Dyrenium; pyridoxine; pyrithione; pyritidium

**Pyridium Plus** tablets (discontinued 1993) ℞ *urinary analgesic; antispasmodic; sedative* [phenazopyridine HCl; hyoscyamine hydrobromide; butabarbital] 150•0.3•15 mg

**pyridofylline** INN

**pyridostigmine bromide** USP, INN *cholinergic; anticholinesterase muscle stimulant* ⚠ physostigmine

**pyridoxal** [see: pyridoxine HCl]

**pyridoxamine** [see: pyridoxine HCl]

**pyridoxine** INN *vitamin B$_6$; enzyme cofactor* [also: pyridoxine HCl] ⚠ pralidoxime; Pyridium

**pyridoxine HCl** USP *vitamin B$_6$; enzyme cofactor* [also: pyridoxine] 25, 50, 100 mg oral; 100 mg/mL injection ⚠ pralidoxime; Pyridium

**β-pyridylcarbinol** [see: nicotinyl alcohol]

**pyridylmethanol** *me+* [see: nicotinyl alcohol]

**9-[3-pyridylmethyl]-9-deazaguanine** *investigational (orphan) for cutaneous T-cell lymphoma*

**pyrilamine maleate** USP *anticholinergic; antihistamine; sleep aid* [also: mepyramine]

**pyrilamine tannate, phenylephrine tannate, and chlorpheniramine tannate** *antihistamine; decongestant* 25•25•8 mg oral

pyrimethamine USP, INN *malaria suppression and transmission control; folic acid antagonist*

pyrimethamine & sulfadiazine *Toxoplasma gondii encephalitis treatment (orphan)*

pyrimitate INN, BAN

**Pyrinex Pediculicide** shampoo OTC *pediculicide* [pyrethrins; piperonyl butoxide; deodorized kerosene] 0.2%•2%•0.8%

pyrinoline USAN, INN *antiarrhythmic*

**Pyrinyl** liquid OTC *pediculicide* [pyrethrins; piperonyl butoxide; deodorized kerosene] 0.2%•2%•0.8%

**Pyrinyl II** liquid OTC *pediculicide* [pyrethrins; piperonyl butoxide] 0.3%•3%

**Pyrinyl Plus** shampoo OTC *pediculicide* [pyrethrins; piperonyl butoxide] 0.3%•3%

pyrithen [see: chlorothen citrate]

pyrithione sodium USAN *topical antimicrobial* ⊇ Pyridium

pyrithione zinc USAN, INN, BAN *antibacterial; antifungal; antiseborrheic*

pyrithyldione INN

pyritidium bromide INN ⊇ Pyridium

pyritinol INN, BAN

pyrodifenium bromide [see: prifinium bromide]

pyrogallic acid [see: pyrogallol]

pyrogallol NF

pyrophendane INN

pyrophenindane [see: pyrophendane]

pyrovalerone INN *CNS stimulant* [also: pyrovalerone HCl]

pyrovalerone HCl USAN *CNS stimulant* [also: pyrovalerone]

pyroxamine INN *antihistamine* [also: pyroxamine maleate]

pyroxamine maleate USAN *antihistamine* [also: pyroxamine]

pyroxylin USP, INN *pharmaceutic necessity for collodion*

pyrrobutamine phosphate USP

pyrrocaine USAN, INN *local anesthetic*

pyrrocaine HCl NF

pyrrolifene INN *analgesic* [also: pyrroliphene HCl]

pyrrolifene HCl [see: pyrroliphene HCl]

pyrroliphene HCl USAN *analgesic* [also: pyrrolifene]

pyrrolnitrin USAN, INN *antifungal*

pyrroxane [now: proroxan HCl]

**Pyrroxate** capsules OTC *decongestant; antihistamine; analgesic* [phenylpropanolamine HCl; chlorpheniramine maleate; acetaminophen] 25•4•650 mg

pyrvinium chloride INN

pyrvinium embonate [see: pyrvinium pamoate]

pyrvinium pamoate USP *anthelmintic* [also: viprynium embonate]

pytamine INN

PZA (pyrazinamide) [q.v.]

PZI (protamine zinc insulin) [q.v.]

q'at; kat; khat *street drug slang for leaves of the Catha edulis plant* [see: *Catha edulis*, cathinone]

**Q.B.** liquid (discontinued 1993) ℞ *antiasthmatic; bronchodilator; expectorant* [theophylline; guaifenesin]

**Q-Pam** tablets (discontinued 1993) ℞ *skeletal muscle relaxant* [diazepam]

**QTest** test stick for home use OTC *in vitro diagnostic aid for urine pregnancy test*

**QTest Ovulation** test kit for professional use *in vitro diagnostic aid to predict ovulation time*

qua; quaa; quack; quad; quas *street drug slang for Quaalude (methaqualone; discontinued 1983)* [see: methaqualone]

quadazocine INN, BAN *opioid antagonist* [also: quadazocine mesylate]

quadazocine mesylate USAN *opioid antagonist* [also: quadazocine]

**Quadra-Hist** extended-release tablets (discontinued 1995) ℞ *decongestant; antihistamine* [phenylpropanolamine HCl; phenylephrine HCl; chlorpheniramine maleate; phenyltoloxamine citrate] 40•10•5•15 mg

**Quadra-Hist ER** syrup (discontinued 1993) ℞ *decongestant; antihistamine* [phenylpropanolamine HCl; phenylephrine HCl; phenyltoloxamine citrate; chlorpheniramine maleate]

**Quadra-Hist Pediatric** syrup (discontinued 1995) ℞ *pediatric decongestant and antihistamine* [phenylpropanolamine HCl; phenylephrine HCl; chlorpheniramine maleate; phenyltoloxamine citrate] 5•1.25•0.5•2 mg/5 mL

**Quadramet** IV injection ℞ *radiopharmaceutical for treatment of bone pain from osteoblastic metastatic tumors* [samarium Sm 153 lexidronam] 1850 MBq/mL (50 mCi/mL)

**Quadrinal** tablets ℞ *antiasthmatic; bronchodilator; decongestant; expectorant; sedative* [theophylline; ephedrine HCl; potassium iodide; phenobarbital] 65•24•320•24 mg

**quadrosilan** INN

**Quantaffirm** reagent kit for professional use *in vitro diagnostic aid for mononucleosis*

**quarter moon** *street drug slang* [see: hashish]

**quartz** *street drug slang for smokable speed* [see: amphetamines]

**Quarzan** capsules ℞ *anticholinergic; peptic ulcer treatment* [clidinium bromide] 2.5, 5 mg ℞ Questran

**quatacaine** INN

**quaternium-18 bentonite** [see: bentoquatam]

**quazepam** USAN, INN *sedative; hypnotic*

**quazinone** USAN, INN *cardiotonic*

**quazodine** USAN, INN *cardiotonic; bronchodilator*

**quazolast** USAN, INN *antiasthmatic; mediator release inhibitor*

**Queen Anne's lace** *street drug slang* [see: marijuana]

**Quelicin** IV or IM injection ℞ *neuromuscular blocker* [succinylcholine chloride] 20, 50, 100 mg/mL

**Quelidrine Cough** syrup OTC *antitussive; decongestant; antihistamine; expectorant* [dextromethorphan hydrobromide; ephedrine HCl; phenylephrine HCl; chlorpheniramine maleate; ammonium chloride; ipecac; alcohol 2%] 10 mg•5 mg•5 mg•2 mg•40 mg•0.005 mL per 5 mL

**Queltuss** tablets (discontinued 1993) OTC *antitussive; expectorant* [dextromethorphan hydrobromide; guaifenesin]

**Quercetin** tablets OTC *dietary supplement* [eucalyptus bioflavonoids] 50, 250 mg

**Questran** wax-coated tablets (discontinued 1994) ℞ *cholesterol-lowering antihyperlipidemic* [cholestyramine resin] 1 g ℞ Quarzan

**Questran; Questran Light** powder for oral suspension ℞ *cholesterol-lowering antihyperlipidemic; also used for biliary obstruction* [cholestyramine resin] 4 g/dose

**quetiapine fumarate** USAN *antipsychotic; dopamine $D_2$ and serotonin $5-HT_2$ receptor antagonists*

**Quibron; Quibron-300** capsules ℞ *antiasthmatic; bronchodilator; expectorant* [theophylline; guaifenesin] 150•90 mg; 300•180 mg

**Quibron Plus** elixir (discontinued 1993) ℞ *antiasthmatic; bronchodilator; decongestant; expectorant; sedative* [theophylline; ephedrine HCl; guaifenesin; butabarbital]

**Quibron-T** Dividose (multiple-scored tablets) ℞ *bronchodilator* [theophylline] 300 mg

**Quibron-T/SR** sustained-release Dividose (multiple-scored tablets) ℞ *bronchodilator* [theophylline] 300 mg

**Quick Care** solutions OTC *two-step chemical disinfecting system for soft contact lenses* [hydrogen peroxide-based]

**Quick Pep** tablets OTC *CNS stimulant; analeptic* [caffeine] 150 mg

**quicksilver** *street drug slang* [see: isobutyl nitrite]

**QuickVue** test cassettes for professional use *in vitro diagnostic aid for urine pregnancy test*

**Quiess** IM injection ℞ *anxiolytic* [hydroxyzine HCl] 50 mg/mL

**quifenadine** INN

**quiflapon sodium** USAN *leukotriene biosynthesis inhibitor for asthma and inflammatory bowel disease*

**quill** *street drug slang* [see: methamphetamine HCl; heroin; cocaine]

**quillifoline** INN

**quilostigmine** USAN *cholinesterase inhibitor for Alzheimer's disease*

**quinacainol** INN

**quinacillin** INN, BAN

**quinacrine HCl** USP *antimalarial; anthelmintic for giardiasis and cestodiasis (tapeworm)* [also: mepacrine] ⊘ quinidine

**Quinaglute** Dura-Tabs (sustained-release tablets) ℞ *antiarrhythmic* [quinidine gluconate] 324 mg

**Quinalan** sustained-release tablets ℞ *antiarrhythmic* [quinidine gluconate] 324 mg

**quinalbarbitone sodium** BAN *hypnotic; sedative* [also: secobarbital sodium]

**quinaldine blue** USAN *obstetric diagnostic aid*

**quinambicide** [see: clioquinol]

**Quinamm** tablets (discontinued 1996) ℞ *prevention and treatment of nocturnal leg cramps* [quinine sulfate] 260 mg

**quinapril** INN, BAN *antihypertensive; angiotensin-converting enzyme (ACE) inhibitor* [also: quinapril HCl]

**quinapril HCl** USAN *antihypertensive; angiotensin-converting enzyme (ACE) inhibitor* [also: quinapril]

**quinaprilat** USAN, INN *antihypertensive; angiotensin-converting enzyme (ACE) inhibitor*

**quinazosin** INN *antihypertensive* [also: quinazosin HCl]

**quinazosin HCl** USAN *antihypertensive* [also: quinazosin]

**quinbolone** USAN, INN *anabolic*

**quincarbate** INN

**quindecamine** INN *antibacterial* [also: quindecamine acetate]

**quindecamine acetate** USAN *antibacterial* [also: quindecamine]

**quindonium bromide** USAN, INN *antiarrhythmic*

**quindoxin** INN, BAN

**quinelorane** INN *antihypertensive; antiparkinsonian* [also: quinelorane HCl]

**quinelorane HCl** USAN *antihypertensive; antiparkinsonian* [also: quinelorane]

**quinestradol** INN, BAN

**quinestrol** USAN, USP, INN, BAN *estrogen*

**quinetalate** INN *smooth muscle relaxant* [also: quinetolate]

**quinethazone** USP, INN *diuretic; antihypertensive*

**quinetolate** USAN *smooth muscle relaxant* [also: quinetalate]

**quinezamide** INN

**quinfamide** USAN, INN *antiamebic*

**quingestanol** INN *progestin* [also: quingestanol acetate]

**quingestanol acetate** USAN *progestin* [also: quingestanol]

**quingestrone** USAN, INN *progestin*

**Quinidex** Extentabs (extended-release tablets) ℞ *antiarrhythmic* [quinidine sulfate] 300 mg

**quinidine** NF, BAN *antiarrhythmic* ⊘ clonidine; quinacrine; Quinatime; quinine

**quinidine gluconate** USP *antiarrhythmic* 324 mg oral; 80 mg/mL injection

**quinidine polygalacturonate** *antiarrhythmic*

**quinidine sulfate** USP *antiarrhythmic* 300 mg oral

**quinine** NF, BAN ⊘ quinidine

**quinine ascorbate** USAN *smoking deterrent*

**quinine biascorbate** [now: quinine ascorbate]

**quinine bisulfate** NF

**quinine dihydrochloride** NF *investigational anti-infective for pernicious malaria*

**quinine ethylcarbonate** NF

**quinine glycerophosphate** NF

**quinine HCl** NF

**quinine hydrobromide** NF

**quinine hypophosphite** NF

**quinine monohydrobromide** [see: quinine hydrobromide]

**quinine monohydrochloride** [see: quinine HCl]

**quinine monosalicylate** [see: quinine salicylate]

**quinine phosphate** NF

**quinine phosphinate** [see: quinine hypophosphite]

**quinine salicylate** NF

**quinine sulfate** USP *antimalarial schizonticide; treatment of nocturnal leg cramps* 200, 260, 325 mg oral

**quinine sulfate dihydrate** [see: quinine sulfate]

**quinine tannate** USP

**quinisocaine** INN [also: dimethisoquin HCl; dimethisoquin]

**quinocide** INN

**8-quinolinol** [see: oxyquinoline]

**8-quinolinol benzoate** [see: benzoxiquine]

**quinolizidines** *a class of antibiotics* [also called: norlupinanes]

**quinolones** *a class of antibiotics*

**Quinora** tablets ℞ *antiarrhythmic* [quinidine sulfate] 300 mg

**quinotolast** *investigational antiallergic/ antiasthmatic agent*

**quinoxyl** [see: chiniofon]

**quinpirole** INN *antihypertensive* [also: quinpirole HCl]

**quinpirole HCl** USAN *antihypertensive* [also: quinpirole]

**quinprenaline** INN *bronchodilator* [also: quinterenol sulfate]

**quinprenaline sulfate** [see: quinterenol sulfate]

**Quin-Release** sustained-release tablets ℞ *antiarrhythmic* [quinidine gluconate]

**Quinsana Plus** powder OTC *topical antifungal* [tolnaftate] 1%

**Quintabs** tablets OTC *vitamin supplement* [multiple vitamins; folic acid] ±•0.1 mg

**Quintabs-M** tablets OTC *vitamin/mineral/iron supplement* [multiple vitamins & minerals; iron; folic acid] ± •18•0.4 mg

**quinterenol sulfate** USAN *bronchodilator* [also: quinprenaline]

**quintiofos** INN, BAN

**3-quinuclidinol benzoate** [see: benzoclidine]

**quinuclium bromide** USAN, INN *antihypertensive*

**quinupramine** INN

**quinupristin** USAN, INN *streptogramin antibiotic bacteriostatic to gram-positive infections*

**quinupristin & dalfopristin** *two streptogramin antibiotics that are synergistically bactericidal to gram-positive infections; investigational (NDA filed) for pneumonia*

**quipazine** INN *antidepressant; oxytocic* [also: quipazine maleate]

**quipazine maleate** USAN *antidepressant; oxytocic* [also: quipazine]

**Quiphile** tablets (discontinued 1996) ℞ *prevention and treatment of nocturnal leg cramps* [quinine sulfate] 260 mg

**quisultazine** INN

**quisultidine** [see: quisultazine]

**Q-Vel** soft caplets (discontinued 1996) OTC *prevention and treatment of nocturnal leg cramps* [quinine sulfate] 64.8 mg

**r24 antibody** [see: monoclonal antibody r24]

**R 87,926** *investigational treatment for stroke*

**R 89,439** *investigational agent for HIV*

**R 93,777** *investigational treatment for irritable bowel syndrome*

**R 93,877** *investigational therapy for chronic constipation*

**R and R** *street drug slang for reds (Seconal Sodium; secobarbital sodium) and Ripple wine* [see: Seconal Sodium; secobarbital sodium; alcohol]

**R & C** shampoo OTC *pediculicide* [pyrethrins; piperonyl butoxide] 0.3%•3%

**R & D Calcium Carbonate/600 ℞** *investigational (orphan) for hyperphosphatemia of end-stage renal disease* [calcium carbonate]

**RA Lotion** OTC *topical acne treatment* [resorcinol; alcohol 43%] 3%

**rabeprazole** INN *antiulcerative; proton pump inhibitor* [also: rabeprazole sodium]

**rabeprazole sodium** USAN *investigational (Phase III) antiulcerative; proton pump inhibitor* [also: rabeprazole]

**rabies immune globulin (RIG)** USP *passive immunizing agent*

**rabies vaccine** USP *active immunizing agent* Challenge Virus Standard (CVS)

**rabies vaccine, adsorbed (RVA)** [see: rabies vaccine]

**rabies vaccine, HDCV (human diploid cell vaccine)** [see: rabies vaccine]

**racefemine** INN

**racefenicol** INN *antibacterial* [also: racephenicol]

**racehorse Charlie** *street drug slang* [see: cocaine; heroin]

**racemethadol** [see: dimepheptanol]

**racemethionine** USAN, USP *urinary acidifier* [also: methionine (the DL- form)]

**racemethorphan** INN, BAN

**racemetirosine** INN

**racemic amphetamine phosphate**

**racemic amphetamine sulfate** [see: amphetamine sulfate]

**racemic calcium pantothenate** [see: calcium pantothenate, racemic]

**racemoramide** INN, BAN

**racemorphan** INN

**racephedrine HCl** USAN

**racephenicol** USAN *antibacterial* [also: racefenicol]

**racepinefrine** INN *bronchodilator* [also: racepinephrine]

**racepinephrine** USP *bronchodilator* [also: racepinefrine]

**racepinephrine HCl** USP *bronchodilator*

**raclopride** INN, BAN

**ractopamine** INN *veterinary growth stimulant* [also: ractopamine HCl]

**ractopamine HCl** USAN *veterinary growth stimulant* [also: ractopamine]

**Radinyl** ℞ *investigational antineoplastic for breast cancer* [etanidazole]

**radio-chromated serum albumin** [see: albumin, chromated]

**radio-iodinated I 125 serum albumin** [see: albumin, iodinated]

**radio-iodinated I 131 serum albumin** [see: albumin, iodinated]

**radiomerisoprol $^{197}$Hg** [see: merisoprol Hg 197]

**radioselenomethionine $^{75}$Se** [see: selenomethionine Se 75]

**radiotolpovidone I 131** INN *hypoalbuminemia test; radioactive agent* [also: tolpovidone I 131]

**radium** *element (Ra)*

**radon** *element (Rn)*

**rafoxanide** USAN, INN *anthelmintic*

**ragweed** *street drug slang for inferior-quality marijuana or heroin* [see: marijuana; heroin]

**railroad weed** *street drug slang* [see: marijuana]

**rainbows** *street drug slang for Tuinal (amobarbital sodium + secobarbital sodium), which comes in multicolored striped capsules* [see: Tuinal; amobarbital sodium; secobarbital sodium]

**rainy day woman** *street drug slang for a marijuana cigarette* [see: marijuana]

**ralitoline** USAN, INN *anticonvulsant*

**raloxifene** INN *antiestrogen; investigational (NDA filed) treatment for postmenopausal osteoporosis* [also: raloxifene HCl]

**raloxifene HCl** USAN *antiestrogen; investigational (NDA filed) treatment for postmenopausal osteoporosis* [also: raloxifene]

**raltitrexed** USAN *investigational (Phase III) thymidylate synthase inhibitor for advanced colorectal cancer*

**raluridine** USAN *antiviral*

**Rambo** *street drug slang* [see: heroin]

**rambufaside** [see: meproscillarin]

**ramciclane** INN

**ramifenazone** INN

**ramipril** USAN, INN, BAN *antihypertensive; angiotensin-converting enzyme (ACE) inhibitor*

**ramiprilat** INN

**ramixotidine** INN

**ramnodigin** INN

**ramoplanin** USAN, INN *antibacterial antibiotic; investigational decontaminant for bowel surgery and wound infections*

**RAMP Urine hCG Assay** test kit for professional use (discontinued 1994) *in vitro diagnostic aid for urine pregnancy test* [monoclonal antibody-based enzyme immunoassay]

**Ramses** vaginal jelly OTC *spermicidal contraceptive* [nonoxynol 9] 5%

**Ramses Extra** premedicated condom OTC *spermicidal/barrier contraceptive* [nonoxynol 9] 15%

**Rane** street drug slang [see: cocaine; heroin]

**rangood** street drug slang for marijuana grown wild [see: marijuana]

**ranimustine** INN

**ranimycin** USAN, INN *antibacterial*

**ranitidine** USAN, INN, BAN *treatment of GI ulcers; histamine $H_2$ antagonist*

**ranitidine bismuth citrate** USAN *treatment of GI ulcers; histamine $H_2$ blocker* [also: ranitidine bismutrex]

**ranitidine bismutrex** BAN *treatment of GI ulcers; histamine $H_2$ blocker* [also: ranitidine bismuth citrate]

**ranitidine HCl** USP, JAN *treatment of GI ulcers; histamine $H_2$ antagonist* 15 mg/mL oral

**ranolazine** INN *antianginal* [also: ranolazine HCl]

**ranolazine HCl** USAN *antianginal; investigational treatment for peripheral artery disease* [also: ranolazine]

**Rapamune** ℞ *investigational adjunct for organ transplant and treatment for autoimmune diseases* [sirolimus]

**rapamycin** [now: sirolimus]

**RapidTest Strep** test kit for professional use (discontinued 1995) *in vitro diagnostic test for streptococcal antigens in throat swabs*

**RapidVue** test kit for home use OTC *in vitro diagnostic aid for urine pregnancy test*

**Rapimine** *investigational antihistamine for allergic conjunctivitis* [emedastine difumarate]

**rasagiline** INN

**rasagiline mesylate** USAN *antiparkinsonian; monoamine oxidase B (MAO-B) inhibitor*

**raspberry [syrup]** USP

**Rasta weed** street drug slang [see: marijuana]

**rathyronine** INN

**rattlesnake antivenin** [see: antivenin (Crotalidae) polyvalent]

**Raudixin** tablets (discontinued 1995) ℞ *antihypertensive; antipsychotic* [rauwolfia serpentina (whole root)] 50, 100 mg

**Rauverid** tablets (discontinued 1995) ℞ *antihypertensive; antipsychotic* [rauwolfia serpentina (whole root)] 50 mg

**rauwolfia derivatives** *all rauwolfia derivatives except reserpine were discontinued 1991–1995*

**rauwolfia serpentina** USP *antihypertensive; peripheral antiadrenergic*

**Rauzide** tablets ℞ *antihypertensive* [bendroflumethiazide; rauwolfia serpentina] 4•50 mg

**Ravocaine & Novocaine with Levophed** injection ℞ *injectable local anesthetic for dental procedures* [proproxycaine HCl; procaine; norepinephrine] 7.2•36•0.12 mg/1.8 mL

**Ravocaine & Novocaine with Neo-Cobefrin** injection (discontinued 1995) ℞ *injectable local anesthetic for dental procedures* [proproxycaine HCl; procaine; levonordefrin] 7.2•36•0.09 mg/1.8 mL

**raw** street drug slang [see: cocaine, crack]

**rayon, purified** USAN, USP *surgical aid*

**razinodil** INN

**razobazam** INN

**razoxane** INN, BAN

**⁸⁶Rb** [see: rubidium chloride Rb 86]

**RBC-CD4** *antiviral for HIV*

**rBPI-21 (bactericidal/permeability-increasing protein, recombinant)** *investigational (Phase III) agent for sepsis, hemorrhagic shock, and meningococcemia*

**rCD4 (recombinant soluble human CD4)** [see: CD4, recombinant soluble human]

**RCF** liquid OTC *hypoallergenic infant formula* [soy protein formula, carbohydrate free]

**Reabilan; Reabilan HN** ready-to-use liquid OTC *enteral nutritional therapy* [lactose-free formula]

**Reactine** ⒸⒶⓃ (U.S. product: Zyrtec) film-coated tablets, syrup ℞ *once-daily antihistamine* [cetirizine HCl] 5, 10 mg; 5 mg/5 mL

**reactrol** [see: clemizole HCl]

**ready rock** *street drug slang* [see: cocaine; cocaine, crack; heroin]

**rebamipide** INN

**Rebif** (commercially available in Italy) ℞ *investigational (orphan) for malignant melanoma, metastatic renal cell carcinoma, T-cell lymphoma, and Kaposi sarcoma* [interferon beta, recombinant]

**reboxetine** INN *investigational (Phase III) fast-acting antidepressant*

**recainam** INN, BAN *antiarrhythmic* [also: recainam HCl]

**recainam HCl** USAN *antiarrhythmic* [also: recainam]

**recainam tosylate** USAN *antiarrhythmic*

**recanescin** [see: deserpidine]

**Receptin** ℞ *investigational (Phase II) antiviral for AIDS; orphan status withdrawn 1997* [CD4, recombinant soluble human]

**reclazepam** USAN, INN *sedative*

**Reclomide** tablets ℞ *antidopaminergic; antiemetic for chemotherapy; peristaltic* [metoclopramide monohydrochloride monohydrate] 10 mg

**Recombigen HIV-1 LA Test** reagent kit for professional use *in vitro diagnostic aid for HIV-1 antibodies in blood, serum, or plasma* [latex agglutination test]

**recombinant alpha₁ antitrypsin** [see: alpha₁ antitrypsin, recombinant]

**recombinant antihemophilic factor** [see: antihemophilic factor, recombinant]

**recombinant factor VIIa** [see: factor VIIa, recombinant]

**recombinant factor VIII** [see: antihemophilic factor, recombinant]

**recombinant human CD4 immunoglobulin G** [CD4 immunoglobulin G, recombinant human]

**recombinant human deoxyribonuclease (rhDNase)** [see: dornase alfa]

**recombinant human erythropoietin** [see: erythropoietin, recombinant human]

**recombinant human growth hormone (rhGH)** [see: somatropin]

**recombinant human interferon beta** [see: interferon beta, recombinant human]

**recombinant human interleukin-1 receptor (rhIL-1R; rhu IL-1R)** [see: interleukin-1 receptor]

**recombinant human nerve growth factor (rhNGF)** [see: nerve growth factor]

**recombinant human serum albumin (rHSA)**

**recombinant human superoxide dismutase (SOD)** [see: superoxide dismutase, recombinant human]

**recombinant interferon alfa-2a** [see: interferon alfa-2a, recombinant]

**recombinant interferon alfa-2b** [see: interferon alfa-2b, recombinant]

**recombinant interferon beta** [see: interferon beta, recombinant]

**recombinant interleukin-2** [see: interleukin-2, recombinant]

**recombinant methionyl granulocyte CSF** [see: methionyl granulocyte CSF, recombinant]

**recombinant methionyl human granulocyte CSF** [see: methionyl human granulocyte CSF, recombinant]

**recombinant soluble human CD4 (rCD4)** [see: CD4, recombinant soluble human]

**recombinant tissue plasminogen activator (rtPA; rt-PA)** [see: alteplase]

**recombinant TNF receptor fusion protein** *investigational treatment for rheumatoid arthritis and septic shock*

**Recombinate** powder for IV injection ℞ *antihemophilic to correct coagulation deficiency* [antihemophilic factor, recombinant] 250, 500, 1000 IU

**Recombivax HB** adult IM injection, pediatric IM injection, adolescent/ high-risk infant IM injection, dialysis formulation ℞ *active immunizing agent for hepatitis B and hepatitis D* [hepatitis B virus vaccine, recombinant] 10 μg/mL; 2.5 μg/0.5 mL; 5 μg/0.5 mL; 40 μg/mL

**Recormon** ℞ *investigational blood cell growth factor* [erythropoietin]

**Rectacort** rectal suppositories ℞ *topical corticosteroidal anti-inflammatory* [hydrocortisone acetate] 10%

**Rectagene** rectal suppositories OTC *temporary relief of hemorrhoidal symptoms* [live yeast cell derivative; shark liver oil] 2000 SRF U/oz.

**Rectagene II** rectal suppositories OTC *temporary relief of hemorrhoidal symptoms* [bismuth subgallate; bismuth resorcin compound; benzyl benzoate; peruvian balsam; zinc oxide] 2.25%•1.75%•1.2%•1.8%•11%

**Rectagene Medicated Rectal Balm** ointment OTC *temporary relief of hemorrhoidal symptoms* [shark liver oil; phenyl mercuric nitrate; live yeast cell derivative] 3%•1:10 000•66.67 U/g

**Rectolax** suppositories OTC *laxative* [bisacodyl] 10 mg

**recycle** *street drug slang* [see: LSD]

**red and blues** *street drug slang* [see: Tuinal; amobarbital sodium; secobarbital sodium]

**red birds; red bullets** *street drug slang* [see: secobarbital sodium]

**red blood cells** [see: blood cells, red]

**red caps** *street drug slang* [see: cocaine, crack]

**red chicken** *street drug slang* [see: heroin]

**red chicken** *street drug slang for Chinese heroin* [see: heroin]

**red cross** *street drug slang* [see: marijuana]

**Red Cross Toothache** liquid OTC *topical oral analgesic* [eugenol] 85%

**red devil** *street drug slang for PCP or Seconal Sodium (secobarbital sodium) capsules* [see: PCP; Seconal Sodium; secobarbital sodium]

**red dirt** *street drug slang* [see: marijuana]

**red eagle** *street drug slang* [see: heroin]

**red ferric oxide** [see: ferric oxide, red]

**red phosphorus** *street drug slang for smokable speed* [see: amphetamines]

**red rum** *street drug slang (murder spelled backward) for a potent form of heroin* [see: heroin]

**red veterinarian petrolatum (RVP)** [see: petrolatum]

**Redi Vial** (trademarked packaging form) *dual-compartment vial*

**Redi Vial** (trademarked packaging form) *two-compartment vial*

**Rediject** (trademarked delivery system) *prefilled disposable syringe*

**Redipak** (trademarked packaging form) *unit dose or unit-of-issue package*

**redox-acyclovir** *orphan status withdrawn 1996*

**redox-penicillin G** *orphan status withdrawn 1996*

**redox-phenytoin** *orphan status withdrawn 1996*

**reds** *street drug slang* [see: Seconal Sodium; secobarbital sodium]

**reds and Ripple** *street drug slang for a combination of Seconal Sodium (secobarbital sodium) and Ripple wine* [see: Seconal Sodium; secobarbital sodium; alcohol]

**Reducin** ℞ *investigational (orphan) for nonoperative management of cutaneous fistulas of the GI tract and bleeding esophageal varices* [somatostatin]

**Redutemp** tablets OTC *analgesic; antipyretic* [acetaminophen] 500 mg

**Redux** capsules ℞ *anorexiant and appetite suppressant for long-term dieting* [dexfenfluramine HCl] 15 mg

**reefer** *street drug slang* [see: marijuana]

**Reese's Pinworm** soft gel capsules, liquid OTC *anthelmintic for ascariasis (roundworm) and enterobiasis (pinworm)* [pyrantel pamoate] 180 mg; 50 mg/mL

**ReFacto** *investigational (Phase III, orphan) for long-term hemophilia A treatment or for surgical procedures* [factor VIII, recombinant]

**Refludan** *investigational (orphan) for heparin-associated thrombocytopenia type II* [lepirudin]

**Refresh** eye drops OTC *ocular moisturizer/lubricant* [polyvinyl alcohol] 1.4%

**Refresh Plus** eye drops OTC *ocular moisturizer/lubricant* [carboxymethylcellulose] 0.5%

**Refresh P.M.** ophthalmic ointment OTC *ocular moisturizer/lubricant* [white petrolatum; mineral oil; lanolin]

**Regain** snack bar OTC *enteral nutritional therapy for impaired renal function* [essential amino acids] ☒ Rogaine

**Regitine** IV or IM injection ℞ *antihypertensive for pheochromocytoma* [phentolamine mesylate] 5 mg/mL

**Reglan** tablets, syrup, IV infusion ℞ *antidopaminergic; antiemetic for chemotherapy; peristaltic* [metoclopramide monohydrochloride monohydrate] 5, 10 mg; 5 mg/5 mL; 5 mg/mL ☒ Regonol

**Regonol** IM or IV injection ℞ *anticholinesterase muscle stimulant; muscle relaxant reversal* [pyridostigmine bromide] 5 mg/mL ☒ Reglan

**regramostim** USAN, INN *antineutropenic; hematopoietic stimulant; biologic response modifier; bone marrow stimulant*

**Regranex** *investigational recombinant platelet-derived growth factor B for chronic dermal ulcers* [becaplermin]

**Regroton** tablets ℞ *antihypertensive* [chlorthalidone; reserpine] 50•0.25 mg ☒ Hygroton

**Regulace** capsules OTC *laxative; stool softener* [casanthranol; docusate sodium] 30•100 mg

**Regular Iletin I** subcu injection OTC *antidiabetic* [insulin (beef-pork)] 100 U/mL

**Regular Iletin II (beef)** subcu injection (discontinued 1994) OTC *antidiabetic* [insulin]

**Regular Iletin II (pork)** subcu injection OTC *antidiabetic* [insulin] 100 U/mL

**Regular Iletin II U-500 (concentrated)** subcu or IM injection ℞ *antidiabetic* [insulin (pork)] 500 U/mL

**Regular Insulin** subcu injection (discontinued 1997) OTC *antidiabetic* [insulin (pork)] 100 U/mL

**regular P** *street drug slang* [see: cocaine, crack]

**Regular Purified Pork Insulin** subcu injection OTC *antidiabetic* [insulin] 100 U/mL

**Regulax SS** capsules OTC *stool softener* [docusate sodium] 100, 250 mg

**Reguloid** powder OTC *bulk laxative* [psyllium hydrophilic mucilloid] 3.4 g/tsp.

**Regutol** tablets (discontinued 1997) OTC *stool softener* [docusate sodium] 100 mg

**Rehydralyte** oral solution OTC *electrolyte replacement* [sodium, potassium, and chloride electrolytes]

**reindeer dust** *street drug slang* [see: heroin]

**Rela** sugar-coated tablets (discontinued 1993) ℞ *skeletal muscle relaxant* [carisoprodol]

**Relafen** film-coated tablets ℞ *antiarthritic; nonsteroidal anti-inflammatory drug (NSAID)* [nabumetone] 500, 750 mg

**Relaxadon** tablets (discontinued 1995) ℞ *GI anticholinergic; sedative* [atropine sulfate; scopolamine hydrobromide; hyoscyamine hydrobromide; phenobarbital] 0.0194•0.0065•0.1037•16.2 mg

**relaxin** *investigational agent to facilitate childbirth (clinical trials discontinued 1994); investigational (orphan) for progressive systemic sclerosis*

**Release-Tabs** (dosage form) *timed-release tablets*

**Relefact TRH** IV injection (name changed to Thyrel-TRH in 1995)

**Relief** eye drops OTC *topical ocular decongestant* [phenylephrine HCl] 0.12%

**relomycin** USAN, INN *antibacterial*

**remacemide** INN *neuroprotective anticonvulsant; investigational treatment for stroke and Huntington's disease* [also: remacemide HCl]

**remacemide HCl** USAN *neuroprotective anticonvulsant; investigational treatment for stroke and Huntington's disease* [also: remacemide]

**Remcol Cold** capsules (discontinued 1995) OTC *decongestant; antihistamine; analgesic* [phenylpropanolamine HCl; chlorpheniramine maleate; acetaminophen] 25•2•300 mg

**Remcol-C** capsules (discontinued 1995) OTC *antitussive; antihistamine; analgesic* [dextromethorphan hydrobromide; chlorpheniramine maleate; acetaminophen] 15•2•300 mg

**Remeron** coated tablets ℞ *tetracyclic antidepressant* [mirtazapine] 15, 30 mg

**remifentanil** INN, BAN *short-acting narcotic agonist analgesic* [also: remifentanil HCl]

**remifentanil HCl** USAN *short-acting narcotic agonist analgesic* [also: remifentanil]

**remikiren** INN

**remiprostol** USAN, INN *antiulcerative*

**Remisar** ℞ *investigational oncolytic and immunomodulator for bladder cancer and lymphoma* [bropirimine]

**remoxipride** USAN, INN, BAN *antipsychotic*

**remoxipride HCl** USAN *antipsychotic*

**Remular-S** tablets ℞ *skeletal muscle relaxant* [chlorzoxazone] 250 mg

**Remune** ℞ *investigational (Phase III) immunostimulant for HIV*

**Renacidin** powder for solution ℞ *bladder and catheter irrigant for apatite or struvite calculi (orphan)* [citric acid; d-gluconic acid lactone; magnesium hydroxycarbonate] 6.602•0.198•3.177 g/100 mL

**Renacidin Irrigation** solution ℞ *bladder and catheter irrigant for calcifications (orphan)* [citric acid; glucono-delta-lactone; magnesium carbonate]

**RenaGel** ℞ *investigational (Phase III) phosphate binding polymer to reduce serum phosphate levels in chronic kidney failure patients*

**RenAmin** IV infusion ℞ *nutritional therapy for renal failure* [multiple essential and nonessential amino acids; electrolytes]

**renanolone** INN

**Renese** tablets ℞ *diuretic; antihypertensive* [polythiazide] 1, 2, 4 mg

**Renese-R** tablets ℞ *antihypertensive* [polythiazide; reserpine] 2•0.25 mg

**Renografin-60; Renografin-76** injection ℞ *parenteral radiopaque agent* [diatrizoate meglumine; diatrizoate sodium] 52%•8%; 66%•10%

**Reno-M-30; Reno-M-60; Reno-M-Dip** intracavitary instillation ℞ *urologic radiopaque agent* [diatrizoate meglumine] 30%; 60%; 30%

**Renoquid** tablets ℞ *broad-spectrum bacteriostatic* [sulfacytine] 250 mg

**Renormax** tablets (discontinued 1995) ℞ *antihypertensive; ACE inhibitor* [spirapril] 3, 6, 12, 24 mg

**Renova** cream ℞ *retinoid for photodamage, fine wrinkles, mottled hyperpigmentation, and roughness of facial skin* [tretinoin] 0.05%

**Renovist; Renovist II** injection ℞ *parenteral radiopaque agent* [diatrizoate meglumine; diatrizoate sodium] 34.3%•35%; 28.5%•29.1%

**Renovue-Dip; Renovue-65** injection ℞ *parenteral renal radiopaque agent* [iodamide meglumine] 24%; 65%

**Rentamine Pediatric** oral suspension ℞ *pediatric antitussive, decongestant, and antihistamine* [carbetapentane tannate; phenylephrine tannate; ephedrine tannate; chlorpheniramine tannate] 30•5•5•4 mg/5 mL

**rentiapril** INN

**ReNu** solution OTC *rinsing/storage solution for soft contact lenses* [preserved saline solution]

**ReNu Effervescent Enzymatic Cleaner; ReNu Thermal Enzymatic Cleaner** tablets OTC *enzymatic cleaner for soft contact lenses* [subtilisin]

**ReNu Multi-Purpose** solution OTC *chemical disinfecting solution for soft contact lenses*

**renytoline** INN *anti-inflammatory* [also: paranyline HCl]

**renytoline HCl** [see: paranyline HCl]

**renzapride** INN, BAN

**ReoPro** IV injection ℞ *antiplatelet agent for acute arterial occlusive disorders (antianginal trials discontinued 1995)* [abciximab] 2 mg/mL

**Repan** tablets, capsules ℞ *analgesic; antipyretic; sedative* [acetaminophen; caffeine; butalbital] 325•40•50 mg
⃞ Riopan

**Repan CF** tablets ℞ *analgesic; antipyretic; sedative* [acetaminophen; butalbital] 650•50 mg

**Repetab** (trademarked dosage form) *extended-release tablet*

**repirinast** USAN, INN *antiallergic; antiasthmatic*

**Replens** vaginal gel OTC *lubricant* [glycerin; mineral oil]

**Replete** ready-to-use liquid OTC *enteral nutritional therapy* [lactose-free formula]

**Replistatin** ℞ *investigational antineoplastic and postsurgery coagulation restorer (heparin reversal)* [platelet factor 4, recombinant]

**rEPO (recombinant erythropoietin)** [see: epoetin alfa; epoetin beta]

**Reposans-10** capsules ℞ *anxiolytic* [chlordiazepoxide HCl] 10 mg

**repository corticotropin** [see: corticotropin, repository]

**Rep-Pred 40; Rep-Pred 80** injection (discontinued 1994) ℞ *glucocorticoid; anti-inflammatory; immunosuppressant* [methylprednisolone acetate] 40 mg/mL; 80 mg/mL

**repromicin** USAN, INN *antibacterial*

**Repronex** powder for IM injection ℞ *ovulation stimulant for women; spermatogenesis stimulant for men* [menotropins] 75, 150 IU/ampule

**reproterol** INN, BAN *bronchodilator* [also: reproterol HCl]

**reproterol HCl** USAN *bronchodilator* [also: reproterol]

**Resaid** sustained-release capsules ℞ *decongestant; antihistamine* [phenylpropanolamine HCl; chlorpheniramine maleate] 75•12 mg

**Rescaps-D S.R.** sustained-release capsules ℞ *antitussive; decongestant* [caramiphen edisylate; phenylpropanolamine HCl] 40•75 mg

**rescimetol** INN

**rescinnamine** NF, INN, BAN *antihypertensive; rauwolfia derivative*

**Rescon** liquid OTC *decongestant; antihistamine* [phenylpropanolamine HCl; chlorpheniramine maleate] 12.5•2 mg/5 mL

**Rescon** sustained-release capsules ℞ *decongestant; antihistamine* [pseudo-

ephedrine HCl; chlorpheniramine maleate] 120•12 mg

**Rescon JR** controlled-release capsules ℞ *pediatric decongestant and antihistamine* [pseudoephedrine HCl; chlorpheniramine maleate] 60•4 mg

**Rescon-DM** liquid OTC *antitussive; decongestant; antihistamine* [dextromethorphan hydrobromide; pseudoephedrine HCl; chlorpheniramine maleate] 10•30•2 mg/5 mL

**Rescon-ED** controlled-release capsules ℞ *decongestant; antihistamine* [pseudoephedrine HCl; chlorpheniramine maleate] 120•8 mg

**Rescon-GG** liquid OTC *decongestant; expectorant* [phenylephrine HCl; guaifenesin] 5•100 mg/5 mL

**Rescriptor** tablets ℞ *antiretroviral; non-nucleoside reverse transcriptase inhibitor (NNRTI) for HIV-1* [delavirdine mesylate] 100 mg

**Rescue Pak** (trademarked dosage form) *unit dose package*

**Rescula** ℞ *investigational (Phase III) antiglaucoma agent* [isopropyl unoprostone]

**Resectisol** solution ℞ *genitourinary irrigant* [mannitol] 5 g/100 mL

**reserpine** USP, INN *antihypertensive; peripheral antiadrenergic; rauwolfia derivative* 0.1, 0.25 mg oral

**resibufogenin** [see: bufogenin]

**Resinol** ointment OTC *topical poison ivy treatment* [calamine; zinc oxide; resorcinol] 6%•12%•2%

**resocortol butyrate** USAN *topical anti-inflammatory*

**Resol** oral solution OTC *electrolyte replacement* [sodium, potassium, chloride, calcium, magnesium, and phosphate electrolytes]

**Resolve/GP** solution OTC *cleaning solution for hard or rigid gas permeable contact lenses*

**resorantel** INN

**resorcin** [see: resorcinol]

**resorcin acetate** [see: resorcinol monoacetate]

**resorcin brown** NF

**resorcinol** USP *keratolytic; antifungal*

**resorcinol monoacetate** USP *antiseborrheic; keratolytic*

**Resource; Resource Plus** ready-to-use liquid OTC *enteral nutritional therapy* [lactose-free formula]

**Respa-1st** sustained-release tablets ℞ *decongestant; expectorant* [pseudoephedrine HCl; guaifenesin] 60•600 mg

**Respa-DM** sustained-release tablets ℞ *antitussive; expectorant* [dextromethorphan hydrobromide; guaifenesin] 30•600 mg

**Respa-GF** sustained-release tablets ℞ *expectorant* [guaifenesin] 600 mg

**Respahist** sustained-release capsules ℞ *decongestant; antihistamine* [pseudoephedrine HCl; brompheniramine maleate] 60•6 mg

**Respaire-60; Respaire-120** extended-release capsules ℞ *decongestant; expectorant* [pseudoephedrine HCl; guaifenesin] 60•200 mg; 120•250 mg

**Respalor** ready-to-use liquid OTC *enteral nutritional therapy for pulmonary problems*

**Respbid** sustained-release tablets ℞ *bronchodilator* [theophylline] 250, 500 mg

**RespiGam** IV infusion ℞ *preventative for respiratory syncytial virus (RSV) infections in high-risk infants (orphan)* [respiratory syncytial virus immune globulin (RSV-IG)] 2500 mg/dose (50 mg/mL)

**Respihaler** (trademarked delivery system) *oral inhalation aerosol*

**Respinol-G** film-coated tablets (discontinued 1994) ℞ *decongestant; expectorant* [phenylpropanolamine HCl; phenylephrine HCl; guaifenesin]

**Respiracult-Strep** culture paddles for professional use *in vitro diagnostic test for Group A streptococci from throat and nasopharyngeal sources*

**Respiralex** test kit for professional use *in vitro diagnostic test for Group A streptococcal antigens in throat and pharynx* [latex agglutination test]

**respiratory syncytial virus immune globulin (RSV-IG)** *preventative for respiratory syncytial virus (RSV) infections in high-risk infants (orphan)*

**Respirgard II** (trademarked delivery system) *nebulizer*

**Respivir** (name changed to RespiGam in 1994)

**Resporal** sustained-release tablets (discontinued 1993) OTC *decongestant; antihistamine* [pseudoephedrine sulfate; dexbrompheniramine maleate]

**Res-Q** powder (discontinued 1996) OTC *universal antidote* [activated charcoal; magnesium hydroxide; tannic acid] 50%•25%• ?

**Restore** powder OTC *bulk laxative* [psyllium hydrophilic mucilloid] 3.4 g/dose

**Restoril** capsules ℞ *sedative; hypnotic* [temazepam] 7.5, 15, 30 mg ⑨ Vistaril

**Retavase** powder for IV infusion ℞ *thrombolytic; tissue plasminogen activator (tPA) for acute myocardial infarction* [reteplase] 18.8 mg (10.8 IU)

**retelliptine** INN

**reteplase** INN *thrombolytic; tissue plasminogen activator (tPA) for acute myocardial infarction*

**Retin-A** cream, gel, liquid ℞ *topical keratolytic for acne* [tretinoin] 0.025%, 0.05%, 0.1% (0.01% available in Canada); 0.025%, 0.1%; 0.05%

**Retin-A Micro** gel ℞ *topical keratolytic for acne* [tretinoin] 0.1%

**retinamide, R-II** *investigational (orphan) for myelodysplastic syndrome*

**retinoic acid (all-*trans*-retinoic acid)** [see: tretinoin]

**9-*cis*-retinoic acid** *investigational (Phase I/III) for AIDS-related Kaposi sarcoma; investigational (Phase III, orphan) for acute promyelocytic leukemia and proliferative vitreoretinopathy*

**13-*cis*-retinoic acid** [see: isotretinoin]

**retinoids** *a class of antineoplastics chemically related to vitamin A*

**Retinol** cream OTC *moisturizer; emollient* [vitamin A] 100 000 IU

**retinol** INN, BAN *vitamin $A_1$*

**Retinol-A** cream OTC *moisturizer; emollient* [vitamin A palmitate] 10 000 IU/g

**Retrovector** ℞ *investigational (Phase II) gene therapy for asymptomatic HIV infection* [HIV immunotherapeutic (HIV-IT)]

**Retrovir** film-coated tablets, capsules, syrup, IV injection ℞ *nucleoside antiviral for HIV, AIDS, and AIDS-related complex (orphan)* [zidovudine] 300 mg; 100 mg; 50 mg/5 mL; 10 mg/mL

**revenast** INN

**reverse transcriptase (RT) inhibitors** *a class of antivirals that inhibit HIV replication* [reverse transcriptase is also known as DNA polymerase]

**reversible proton pump inhibitor** *investigational treatment for peptic ulcers*

**Reversol** IV or IM injection ℞ *myasthenia gravis treatment; antidote to curare-type overdose* [edrophonium chloride] 10 mg/mL

**Revex** IV, IM, or subcu injection ℞ *opioid antagonist for narcotic overdose* [nalmefene] 100 μg/mL, 1 mg/mL

**Rēv-Eyes** powder for eye drops ℞ *miotic to reverse iatrogenic mydriasis* [dapiprazole HCl] 0.5%

**ReVia** tablets ℞ *narcotic antagonist for opiate dependence or overdose (orphan) and alcoholism* [naltrexone HCl] 50 mg

**revospirone** INN, BAN

**Rexigen Forte** sustained-release capsules ℞ *anorexiant* [phendimetrazine tartrate] 105 mg

**Rexolate** IM injection ℞ *analgesic; antipyretic; anti-inflammatory; antirheumatic* [sodium thiosalicylate] 50 mg/mL

**Rezamid** lotion OTC *topical acne treatment* [sulfur; resorcinol; alcohol] 5%•2%•28%

**Rezine** tablets (discontinued 1995) ℞ *anxiolytic* [hydroxyzine HCl] 10, 25 ml

**Rezipas** ℞ *investigational (orphan) for ulcerative colitis* [aminosalicylic acid]

**Rezulin** film-coated tablets ℞ *thiazolidinedione antidiabetic; increases cell response to insulin without increasing insulin secretion* [troglitazone] 200, 400 mg

**R-Frone** ℞ *investigational (orphan) for metastatic renal cell carcinoma, malignant melanoma, and Kaposi sarcoma* [interferon beta, recombinant]

**RG 12525** *investigational leukotriene D4 antagonist for asthma*

**RG 12915** *investigational antiemetic for chemotherapy (clinical trials discontinued 1994)*

**RG 12986** *investigational antithrombotic* [recombinant human von Willebrand factor]

**RG 201** *investigational (Phase I) anti-infective for AIDS-related Pneumocystis carinii pneumonia (PCP)*

**RG 83894** *investigational antiviral for AIDS (clinical trials discontinued 1994)* [HIV immunotherapeutic]

**rGCR (recombinant glucocerebrosidase)** [see: glucocerebrosidase, recombinant retroviral vector]

**rG-CSF (recombinant granulocyte colony-stimulating factor)** [see: lenograstim]

**R-Gel** OTC *topical analgesic* [capsaicin] 0.025%

**R-Gen** elixir ℞ *expectorant* [iodinated glycerol] 60 mg/5 mL

**R-gene 10** IV injection ℞ *pituitary (growth hormone) function diagnostic aid* [arginine HCl] 10% (950 mOsm/L)

**RGG0853,E1A lipid complex** *investigational (orphan) for advanced ovarian cancer*

**rGM-CSF; rhGM-CSF; rhuGM-CSF (granulocyte-macrophage colony-stimulating factor)** [q.v.]

**rgp160; rgp160 IIIB; rgp160 MN (recombinant glycoprotein)** *investigational (Phase I/II) antiviral (treatment) and vaccine (preventative) for HIV* [also: AIDS vaccine]

**$Rh_0(D)$ immune globulin** USP *passive immunizing agent; treatment for immune thrombocytopenic purpura (orphan)*

**$Rh_0(D)$ immune human globulin** [now: $Rh_0(D)$ immune globulin]

**rhamnus purshiana** [see: cascara sagrada]

**rhDNase (recombinant human deoxyribonuclease)** [see: dornase alfa]

**Rheaban** caplets OTC *antidiarrheal; GI adsorbent* [activated attapulgite] 750 mg

**rhenium** *element (Re)*

**Rheomacrodex** IV infusion ℞ *plasma volume expander for shock due to hemorrhage, burns, or surgery* [dextran 40] 10%

**RheothRx Copolymer** ℞ *investigational therapy for heart attack and malaria; investigational (orphan) for sickle cell crisis and severe burns* [poloxamer 188]

**rheotran (45)** [see: dextran 45]

**Rhesonativ** IM injection (discontinued 1995) ℞ *obstetric Rh factor immunity suppressant* [Rh$_0$(D) immune globulin]

**rhetinic acid** [see: enoxolone]

**Rheumatex** slide tests for professional use *in vitro diagnostic aid for rheumatoid factor in the blood* ⃞ Rheumatrex

**Rheumaton** slide tests for professional use *in vitro diagnostic aid for rheumatoid factor in serum or synovial fluid*

**Rheumatrex** Dose Pack (tablets) ℞ *antirheumatic; antipsoriatic; antineoplastic for leukemia; investigational (orphan) for juvenile rheumatoid arthritis* [methotrexate sodium] 2.5 mg ⃞ Rheumatex

**Rheumox** ℞ *investigational nonsteroidal anti-inflammatory drug (NSAID)* [azapropazone]

**rhFSH (recombinant human follicle-stimulating hormone)** [see: menotropins]

**rhGH (recombinant human growth hormone)** [see: somatropin]

**rhIGF-1 (recombinant human insulin-like growth factor-1)** [now: mecasermin]

**rhIL-1R; rhu IL-1R (recombinant human interleukin-1 receptor)** [see: interleukin-1 receptor]

**rhIL-11 (recombinant human interleukin-11)** [see: interleukin-11, recombinant human]

**rhIL-12 (recombinant human interleukin-12)** [see: interleukin-12]

**Rhinall** nasal spray, nose drops OTC *nasal decongestant* [phenylephrine HCl] 0.25%

**Rhinatate** tablets ℞ *decongestant; antihistamine* [phenylephrine tannate; chlorpheniramine tannate; pyrilamine tannate] 25•8•25 mg

**Rhindecon** timed-release capsules (discontinued 1993) ℞ *nasal decongestant; diet aid* [phenylpropanolamine HCl] 75 mg

**Rhine** *street drug slang* [see: heroin]

**Rhinocaps** capsules OTC *decongestant; analgesic; antipyretic* [phenylpropanolamine HCl; acetaminophen; aspirin] 20•162•162 mg

**Rhinocort** nasal inhalation aerosol ℞ *intranasal steroidal anti-inflammatory* [budesonide] 32 μg/dose

**Rhinocort Aqua** ⒸⒶⓃ nasal spray ℞ *intranasal steroidal anti-inflammatory* [budesonide] 100 μg/spray

**Rhinocort Turbuhaler** ⒸⒶⓃ powder for nasal inhalation ℞ *intranasal steroidal anti-inflammatory* [budesonide] 100 μg/dose

**Rhinogesic** tablets (discontinued 1995) OTC *decongestant; antihistamine; analgesic* [phenylephrine HCl; chlorpheniramine maleate; acetaminophen; salicylamide] 5•2•150•250 mg

**Rhinolar** sustained-release capsules (discontinued 1995) ℞ *decongestant; antihistamine; anticholinergic* [phenylpropanolamine HCl; chlorpheniramine maleate; methscopolamine nitrate] 75•8•2.5 mg

**Rhinolar-EX; Rhinolar-EX 12** sustained-release capsules ℞ *decongestant; antihistamine* [phenylpropanolamine HCl; chlorpheniramine malelate] 75•8 mg; 75•12 mg

**Rhinosyn; Rhinosyn-PD** liquid OTC *decongestant; antihistamine* [pseudoephedrine HCl; chlorpheniramine maleate; alcohol] 60•4 mg/5 mL; 30•2 mg/5 mL

**Rhinosyn-DM** liquid OTC *antitussive; decongestant; antihistamine* [dextromethorphan hydrobromide; pseudoephedrine HCl; chlorpheniramine maleate; alcohol 1.4%] 15•30•2 mg/5 mL

**Rhinosyn-DMX** syrup OTC *antitussive; expectorant* [dextromethorphan hydrobromide; guaifenesin] 15•100 mg/5 mL

**Rhinosyn-X** liquid OTC *antitussive; decongestant; expectorant* [dextromethorphan hydrobromide; pseudoephedrine HCl; guaifenesin; alcohol 7.5%] 10•30•100 mg/5 mL

**rhNGF (recombinant human nerve growth factor)** [see: nerve growth factor]

**rhodine** [see: aspirin]

**rhodium** *element (Rh)*

**RhoGAM** IM injection ℞ *obstetric Rh factor immunity suppressant* [Rh₀(D) immune globulin] 300 μg

**rHSA (recombinant human serum albumin)**

**Rhuli** cream (discontinued 1994) OTC *topical poison ivy treatment* [benzocaine; calamine; camphor] 5%•3%•0.3%

**Rhuli** gel OTC *topical poison ivy treatment* [benzyl alcohol; menthol; camphor] 2%•0.3%•0.3%

**Rhuli** spray OTC *topical poison ivy treatment* [benzocaine; calamine; camphor] 5%•13.8%•0.7%

**rhythm** *street drug slang* [see: amphetamines]

**Rhythmin** sustained-release tablets ℞ *antiarrhythmic* [procainamide HCl]

**rib** *street drug slang* [see: Rohypnol; flunitrazepam]

**ribaminol** USAN, INN *memory adjuvant*

**ribavirin** USP, INN *antiviral for severe lower respiratory tract infections; investigational (Phase II/III) for HIV; investigational (orphan) for hemorrhagic fever with renal syndrome* [also: tribavirin]

**riboflavin** USP, INN *vitamin B₂; vitamin G; enzyme cofactor* 25, 50, 100 mg oral

**riboflavin 5′-phosphate sodium** USP *vitamin*

**riboflavine** [see: riboflavin]

**riboprine** USAN, INN *antineoplastic*

**ribostamycin** INN, BAN

**riboxamide** [see: tiazofurin]

**ricainide** [see: indecainide HCl]

**Ricelyte** oral solution (name changed to Infalyte in 1994)

**ricin (blocked) conjugated murine MAb (anti-MY9)** *investigational (orphan) for myeloid leukemia (including AML), ex vivo treatment of autol-*

ogous bone marrow in AML, and blast crisis in CML

**ricin (blocked) conjugated murine MAb (anti-B4)** *investigational (orphan) for B-cell lymphoma, leukemia, and treatment of bone marrow in non-T-cell ALL; clinical trials discontinued 1997*

**ricin (blocked) conjugated murine MAb (CD6)** *investigational (orphan) for T-cell leukemias, lymphomas, and other mature T-cell malignancies*

**ricin (blocked) conjugated murine MAb (N901)** *investigational (orphan) for small cell lung cancer*

**RID** liquid OTC *pediculicide* [pyrethrins; piperonyl butoxide; petroleum distillate] 0.3%•3•1.2%

**Rid-A-Pain** drops (discontinued 1994) OTC *topical oral anesthetic; antiseptic* [benzocaine; cetalkonium chloride; alcohol 20%] 2.5•0.02%

**Rid-A-Pain** gel OTC *topical oral anesthetic* [benzocaine] 10%

**Rid-A-Pain with Codeine** tablets (discontinued 1995) ℞ *narcotic analgesic* [codeine phosphate; acetaminophen; aspirin; caffeine; salicylamide] 1•97.2•226.8•32.4•32.4 mg

**Ridaura** capsules ℞ *antirheumatic; investigational antiasthmatic* [auranofin] 3 mg

**ridazolol** INN

**RIDD (recombinant interleukin-2, dacarbazine, DDP)** *chemotherapy protocol*

**Ridenol** elixir OTC *analgesic; antipyretic* [acetaminophen] 80 mg/5 mL

**ridogrel** USAN, INN, BAN *thromboxane synthetase inhibitor; investigational treatment for ulcerative colitis*

**rifabutin** USAN, INN *antiviral; antibacterial; for prevention of Mycobacterium avium complex (MAC) in advanced HIV patients (orphan)*

**Rifadin** capsules, powder for IV injection ℞ *tuberculostatic; (IV administration where oral use is not feasible is orphan)* [rifampin] 150, 300 mg; 600 mg ⬚ rifampin; Ritalin

**Rifamate** capsules ℞ *tuberculostatic* [rifampin; isoniazid] 300•150 mg

**rifametane** USAN, INN *antibacterial*

**rifamexil** USAN *antibacterial*

**rifamide** USAN, INN *antibacterial*

**rifampicin** INN, BAN, JAN *antibacterial* [also: rifampin]

**rifampin** USAN, USP *antibacterial; antituberculosis treatment (orphan)* [also: rifampicin] ⑨ Rifadin

**rifampin & isoniazid & pyrazinamide** *short-course treatment of tuberculosis (orphan)*

**rifamycin** INN, BAN

**rifamycin diethylamide** [see: rifamide]

**rifamycin M-14** [see: rifamide]

**rifapentine** USAN, INN, BAN *antibacterial; investigational (orphan) for tuberculosis and AIDS-related Mycobacterium avium complex (MAC)*

**Rifater** tablets ℞ *short-course treatment for tuberculosis (orphan)* [rifampin; isoniazid; pyrazinamide] 120•50•300 mg

**rifaxidin** [see: rifaximin]

**rifaximin** USAN, INN *antibacterial*

**rIFN-A (recombinant interferon alfa)** [see: interferon alfa-2a, recombinant]

**rIFN-α2 (recombinant interferon alfa-2)** see: interferon alfa-2b, recombinant

**rIFN-B (recombinant interferon beta)** [see: interferon beta-1b, recombinant]

**r-IFN-beta** ℞ *investigational (orphan) for malignant melanoma, metastatic renal cell carcinoma, T-cell lymphoma, and Kaposi sarcoma* [interferon beta, recombinant]

**rifomycin** [see: rifamycin]

**RIG (rabies immune globulin)** [q.v.]

**rilapine** INN

**rilmazafone** INN

**rilmenidine** INN

**rilopirox** INN

**rilozarone** INN

**Rilutek** film-coated tablets ℞ *amyotrophic lateral sclerosis (ALS) treatment (orphan); investigational (orphan) for Huntington's disease* [riluzole] 50 mg

**riluzole** USAN, INN *amyotrophic lateral sclerosis (ALS) treatment (orphan); investigational (orphan) for Huntington's disease*

**Rimactane** capsules ℞ *tuberculostatic* [rifampin] 300 mg

**Rimactane/INH** Dual Pack (two-product package) (discontinued 1996) ℞ *tuberculostatic* [rifampin (2 capsules); isoniazid (1 tablet)] 300 mg; 300 mg

**Rimadyl** ℞ *investigational nonsteroidal anti-inflammatory drug (NSAID); analgesic; antipyretic* [carprofen]

**rimantadine** INN *antiviral* [also: rimantadine HCl]

**rimantadine HCl** USAN *antiviral* [also: rimantadine]

**rimazolium metilsulfate** INN

**rimcazole** INN *antipsychotic* [also: rimcazole HCl]

**rimcazole HCl** USAN *antipsychotic* [also: rimcazole]

**rimexolone** USAN, INN, BAN *ophthalmic corticosteroidal anti-inflammatory*

**rimiterol** INN *bronchodilator* [also: rimiterol hydrobromide]

**rimiterol hydrobromide** USAN *bronchodilator* [also: rimiterol]

**rimoprogin** INN

**Rimso-50** solution for bladder instillation ℞ *anti-inflammatory for symptomatic relief of interstitial cystitis* [dimethyl sulfoxide (DMSO)] 50%

**Rinade B.I.D.** sustained-release capsules ℞ *decongestant; antihistamine* [pseudoephedrine HCl; chlorpheniramine maleate] 120•8 mg

**Ringer's injection** USP *fluid and electrolyte replenisher* [also: compound solution of sodium chloride]

**Ringer's injection, lactated** USP *fluid and electrolyte replenisher; systemic alkalizer* [also: compound solution of sodium lactate]

**Ringer's irrigation** USP *irrigation solution*

**Ringer's solution** [now: Ringer's irrigation]

**riodipine** INN

**Riopan** suspension OTC *antacid* [magaldrate] 540 mg/5 mL

**Riopan** tablets, chewable tablets (discontinued 1994) OTC *antacid* [magaldrate] 480 mg; 480 mg ⑨ Repan

**Riopan Plus** chewable tablets, oral suspension OTC *antacid; antiflatulent* [magaldrate; simethicone] 480•20, 1080•20 mg; 540•40, 1080•40 mg/5 mL

**Riopan Plus 2** chewable tablets, oral suspension (discontinued 1994) OTC *antacid; antiflatulent* [magaldrate; simethicone] 1080•30 mg; 216•6 mg/mL

**rioprostil** USAN, INN *gastric antisecretory*

**ripazepam** USAN, INN *minor tranquilizer*

**rippers** street drug slang [see: amphetamines]

**risedronate sodium** USAN *bisphosphonate calcium regulator*

**rismorelin porcine** USAN *growth stimulant for growth hormone deficiencies*

**risocaine** USAN, INN *local anesthetic*

**risotilide HCl** USAN *antiarrhythmic*

**Risperdal** tablets, oral solution ℞ *antipsychotic for schizophrenia; serotonin-dopamine antagonist* [risperidone] 1, 2, 3, 4 mg; 1 mg/mL

**risperidone** USAN, INN, BAN *neuroleptic; antipsychotic*

**ristianol** INN, BAN *immunoregulator* [also: ristianol phosphate]

**ristianol phosphate** USAN *immunoregulator* [also: ristianol]

**ristocetin** USP, INN, BAN

**Ritalin** tablets ℞ *CNS stimulant for attention deficit hyperactivity disorders (ADHD) and narcolepsy; also abused as a street drug* [methylphenidate HCl] 5, 10, 20 mg ☒ Ismelin; Rifadin

**Ritalin-SR** sustained-release tablets ℞ *CNS stimulant for attention deficit hyperactivity disorders (ADHD) and narcolepsy* [methylphenidate HCl] 20 mg

**ritanserin** USAN, INN, BAN *serotonin antagonist; investigational agent for various psychiatric illnesses and substance abuse* 10 mg oral

**ritiometan** INN

**ritodrine** USAN, INN *smooth muscle relaxant*

**ritodrine HCl** USAN, USP *smooth muscle relaxant; uterine relaxant* 0.3, 10, 15 mg/mL injection

**ritolukast** USAN, INN *antiasthmatic; leukotriene antagonist*

**ritonavir** USAN *antiviral; investigational (Phase III) HIV-1 and HIV-2 protease inhibitor*

**ritropirronium bromide** INN

**ritrosulfan** INN

**rituximab** *investigational (Phase III, orphan) treatment for non-Hodgkin's lymphoma*

**rizatriptan benzoate** USAN *investigational (Phase III) serotonin 5-HT receptor agonist for migraine*

**rizatriptan sulfate** USAN *serotonin 5-HT receptor agonist for migraine*

**rizolipase** INN

**RMP-7 (receptor-mediated permeabilizer)** *investigational (Phase III) for AIDS; investigational (Phase II) blood-brain barrier permeability-enhancing agent for carrying carboplatin to brain tumors*

**RMS** suppositories ℞ *narcotic analgesic; preoperative sedative and anxiolytic* [morphine sulfate] 10, 20, 30 mg

**rNPA (recombinant novel plasminogen activator)** [see: novel plasminogen activator]

**Ro 24-7429** *investigational antiviral for AIDS (clinical trials discontinued 1994)*

**Roaccutane** gel (French name for U.S. product Isotrex)

**roach** street drug slang for the butt of a marijuana cigarette [see: marijuana]

**roach 2; roaches** street drug slang [see: Rohypnol; flunitrazepam]

**road dope** street drug slang [see: amphetamines]

**Robafen AC Cough** syrup ℞ *narcotic antitussive; expectorant* [codeine phosphate; guaifenesin; alcohol 3.5%] 10•100 mg/5 mL

**Robafen CF** liquid OTC *antitussive; decongestant; expectorant* [dextromethorphan hydrobromide; phenylpropanolamine HCl; guaifenesin] 10•12.5•100 mg/5 mL

**Robafen DAC** syrup ℞ *narcotic antitussive; decongestant; expectorant* [codeine phosphate; pseudoephedrine HCl; guaifenesin; alcohol 1.4%] 10•30•100 mg/5 mL

**Robafen DM** syrup OTC *antitussive; expectorant* [dextromethorphan

hydrobromide; guaifenesin; alcohol
1.4%] 10•100 mg/5 mL

**RoBathol Bath Oil** OTC *bath emollient*

**Robaxacet** ℞ *investigational adjunct for
musculoskeletal pain* [methocarbamol;
acetaminophen] ⃞ Robaxisal

**Robaxin** tablets, IV or IM injection ℞
*skeletal muscle relaxant* [methocar-
bamol] 500, 750 mg; 100 mg/mL

**Robaxisal** tablets ℞ *skeletal muscle
relaxant; analgesic* [methocarbamol;
aspirin] 400•325 mg ⃞ Robaxacet

**robenidine** INN *coccidiostat for poultry*
[also: robenidine HCl]

**robenidine HCl** USAN *coccidiostat for
poultry* [also: robenidine]

**Robicap** (trademarked dosage form)
*capsule*

**Robicillin VK** tablets ℞ *bactericidal
antibiotic* [penicillin V potassium]
250, 500 mg

**Robimycin** Robitabs (enteric-coated
tablets) ℞ *macrolide antibiotic* [eryth-
romycin] 250 mg

**Robinul** tablets, IV or IM injection ℞
*anticholinergic; peptic ulcer treatment
adjunct; antisecretory* [glycopyrrolate]
1 mg; 0.2 mg/5 mL

**Robinul Forte** tablets ℞ *anticholinergic; peptic ulcer treatment adjunct;
antisecretory* [glycopyrrolate] 2 mg

**Robitab** (trademarked dosage form)
*tablet*

**Robitet** Robicaps (capsules) (discontinued 1997) ℞ *broad-spectrum antibiotic* [tetracycline HCl] 250, 500 mg

**Robitussin** syrup OTC *expectorant* [guai-
fenesin; alcohol 3.5%] 100 mg/5 mL

**Robitussin A-C** syrup ℞ *narcotic antitussive; expectorant* [codeine phosphate; guaifenesin; alcohol 3.5%]
10•100 mg/5 mL

**Robitussin Cold & Cough Liqui-
Gels** (capsules) OTC *antitussive; decongestant; expectorant* [dextromethor-
phan hydrobromide; pseudoephedrine
HCl; guaifenesin] 10•30•200 mg

**Robitussin Cough Calmers** lozenge
OTC *antitussive* [dextromethorphan
hydrobromide] 5 mg

**Robitussin Cough & Cold; Robitus-
sin Pediatric Cough & Cold** liq-

uid OTC *antitussive; decongestant*
[dextromethorphan hydrobromide;
pseudoephedrine HCl] 15•30 mg/5
mL; 7.5•15 mg/5 mL

**Robitussin Cough Drops** lozenge
OTC *mild topical anesthetic* [menthol]
7.4, 10 mg

**Robitussin Liquid Center Cough
Drops** lozenges OTC *topical antipruri-
tic/counterirritant; mild local anesthetic*
[menthol] 10 mg

**Robitussin Night Relief** liquid OTC
*antitussive; decongestant; antihista-
mine; analgesic* [dextromethorphan
hydrobromide; pseudoephedrine
HCl; pyrilamine maleate; acetamin-
ophen] 5•10•8.3•108.3 mg/5 mL

**Robitussin Pediatric** liquid OTC *antitussive* [dextromethorphan hydrobro-
mide] 7.5 mg/5 mL

**Robitussin Severe Congestion
Liqui-Gels** (capsules) OTC *expectorant; decongestant* [guaifenesin; pseudoephedrine HCl] 200•30 mg

**Robitussin-CF** liquid OTC *antitussive;
decongestant; expectorant* [dextrometh-
orphan hydrobromide; phenylpropanolamine HCl; guaifenesin; alcohol
4.75%] 10•12.5•100 mg/5 mL

**Robitussin-DAC** syrup ℞ *narcotic
antitussive; decongestant; expectorant*
[codeine phosphate; pseudoephedrine HCl; guaifenesin; alcohol 1.9%]
10•30•100 mg/5 mL

**Robitussin-DM** liquid OTC *antitussive;
expectorant* [dextromethorphan
hydrobromide; guaifenesin] 10•100
mg/5 mL

**Robitussin-PE** syrup OTC *decongestant; expectorant* [pseudoephedrine
HCl; guaifenesin; alcohol 1.4%] 30•
100 mg/5 mL

**Robomol-500; Robomol-750** tablets
(discontinued 1993) ℞ *skeletal muscle relaxant* [methocarbamol]

**roca** (Spanish for "rock") *street drug
slang* [see: cocaine, crack]

**Rocaltrol** capsules ℞ *treatment of
hypocalcemia in dialysis patients;
decreases severity of psoriatic lesions*
[calcitriol] 0.25, 0.5 μg

**rocastine** INN *antihistamine* [also: rocastine HCl]

**rocastine HCl** USAN *antihistamine* [also: rocastine]

**Rocephin** powder for IV or IM injection, ADD-vantage vials ℞ *cephalosporin-type antibiotic* [ceftriaxone sodium] 0.25, 0.5, 1, 2, 10 g

**Roche** *street drug slang* [see: Rohypnol; flunitrazepam]

**rochelle salt** [see: potassium sodium tartrate]

**rociverine** INN

**rock(s)** *street drug slang* [see: cocaine, crack]

**rocket** *street drug slang for a marijuana cigarette* [see: marijuana]

**rocket fuel** *street drug slang* [see: PCP]

**rocks; rox; rocks of hell** *street drug slang* [see: cocaine, crack]

**Rocky III** *street drug slang* [see: cocaine, crack]

**Rocky Mountain spotted fever vaccine** USP

**rocuronium bromide** INN, BAN *neuromuscular blocking agent*

**R.O.-Dexsone** ⓒᴬᴺ (U.S. product: Decadron Phosphate) eye drops ℞ *ophthalmic topical corticosteroidal anti-inflammatory* [dexamethasone sodium phosphate] 0.1%

**rodocaine** USAN, INN *local anesthetic*

**rodorubicin** INN

**rofelodine** INN

**Roferon-A** subcu or IM injection ℞ *antineoplastic for hairy cell leukemia, chronic myelogenous leukemia, and Kaposi sarcoma (orphan); hepatitis C treatment* [interferon alfa-2a (recombinant)] 3, 6, 9, 36 million IU/mL

**roflurane** USAN, INN *inhalation anesthetic*

**Rogaine for Men; Rogaine for Women** topical solution OTC *hair growth stimulant* [minoxidil] 2% ℗ Rēgain

**Rogenic** IM injection (discontinued 1994) ℞ *hematinic* [peptonized iron; vitamin B₁₂] 20•500 mg/mL

**Rogenic** slow-release tablets (discontinued 1994) OTC *hematinic* [ferrous fumarate, ferrous gluconate & ferrous sulfate; desiccated liver; multiple vitamins] 60•25• ≗ mg

**rogletimide** USAN, INN, BAN *antineoplastic; aromatase inhibitor*

**rokitamycin** INN

**Rolaids, Calcium Rich** chewable tablets OTC *antacid* [magnesium hydroxide; calcium carbonate] 80•412 mg

**Rolaids Antacid** chewable tablets (discontinued 1994) OTC *antacid* [dihydroxyaluminum sodium carbonate] 334 mg

**Rolaids Sodium Free** chewable tablets (discontinued 1994) OTC *antacid* [magnesium hydroxide; calcium carbonate]

**Rolatuss Expectorant** liquid ℞ *narcotic antitussive; decongestant; antihistamine; expectorant* [codeine phosphate; phenylephrine HCl; chlorpheniramine maleate; ammonium chloride; alcohol 5%] 9.85•5•2•33.3 mg/5 mL

**Rolatuss Plain** liquid OTC *decongestant; antihistamine* [phenylephrine HCl; chlorpheniramine maleate; alcohol 5%] 5•2 mg/5 mL

**Rolatuss with Hydrocodone** liquid ℞ *narcotic antitussive; decongestant; antihistamine* [hydrocodone bitartrate; phenylpropanolamine HCl; phenylephrine HCl; pyrilamine maleate; pheniramine maleate] 1.7•3.3•5•3.3•3.3 mg/5 mL

**roletamide** USAN, INN *hypnotic*

**rolgamidine** USAN, INN, BAN *antidiarrheal*

**rolicton** [see: amisometradine]

**rolicyclidine** INN

**rolicypram** BAN *antidepressant* [also: rolicyprine]

**rolicyprine** USAN, INN *antidepressant* [also: rolicypram]

**rolipram** USAN, INN *tranquilizer*

**rolitetracycline** USAN, USP, INN *antibacterial*

**rolitetracycline nitrate** USAN *antibacterial*

**rolling** *street drug slang* [see: MDMA]

**rolodine** USAN, INN *skeletal muscle relaxant*

**rolziracetam** INN, BAN

**romazarit** USAN, INN, BAN *anti-inflammatory; antirheumatic*

**Romazicon** IV injection ℞ *benzodiazepine antagonist to reverse anesthesia or treat overdose* [flumazenil] 0.1 mg/mL

**rometin** [see: clioquinol]

**romifenone** INN

**romifidine** INN

**romurtide** INN

**Romycin** topical solution (discontinued 1995) ℞ *topical antibiotic for acne* [erythromycin] 2%

**ronactolol** INN

**Rondamine-DM** pediatric drops ℞ *pediatric antitussive, decongestant, and antihistamine* [dextromethorphan hydrobromide; pseudoephedrine HCl; carbinoxamine maleate] 4•25•2 mg/5 mL

**Rondec** film-coated tablets, chewable tablets, syrup, pediatric drops ℞ *decongestant; antihistamine* [pseudoephedrine HCl; carbinoxamine maleate] 60•4 mg; 60•4 mg; 60•4 mg/5 mL; 25•2 mg/mL

**Rondec-DM** syrup, pediatric drops ℞ *antitussive; decongestant; antihistamine* [dextromethorphan hydrobromide; pseudoephedrine HCl; carbinoxamine maleate] 15•60•4 mg/5 mL; 4•25•2 mg/mL

**Rondec-TR** timed-release Filmtabs (film-coated tablets) ℞ *decongestant; antihistamine* [pseudoephedrine HCl; carbinoxamine maleate] 120•8 mg

**ronidazole** USAN, INN *antiprotozoal*

**ronifibrate** INN

**ronipamil** INN

**ronnel** USAN *systemic insecticide* [also: fenclofos; fenchlorphos]

**roofie; roofies** *street drug slang* [see: Rohypnol; flunitrazepam]

**rooms** *street drug slang for Psilocybe mushrooms* [see: psilocybin]

**roopies** *street drug slang* [see: Rohypnol; flunitrazepam]

**rooster** *street drug slang* [see: cocaine, crack]

**root** *street drug slang for a marijuana cigarette* [see: marijuana]

**rope** *street drug slang* [see: marijuana; Rohypnol; flunitrazepam]

**rophy; ropies; roples** *street drug slang* [see: Rohypnol; flunitrazepam]

**ropinirole** INN, BAN *antiparkinsonian* [also: ropinirole HCl]

**ropinirole HCl** USAN *antiparkinsonian* [also: ropinirole]

**ropitoin** INN *antiarrhythmic* [also: ropitoin HCl]

**ropitoin HCl** USAN *antiarrhythmic* [also: ropitoin]

**ropivacaine** INN *long-acting local anesthetic*

**ropivacaine HCl** *long-acting local anesthetic*

**ropizine** USAN, INN *anticonvulsant*

**roquinimex** USAN, INN *investigational (Phase II) immunomodulator for HIV; investigational (orphan) for bone marrow transplant for leukemia; clinical trials for MS discontinued 1997*

**Rosa** (Spanish for "rose" or "pink") *street drug slang* [see: amphetamines]

**rosamicin** [now: rosaramicin]

**rosamicin butyrate** [now: rosaramicin butyrate]

**rosamicin propionate** [now: rosaramicin propionate]

**rosamicin sodium phosphate** [now: rosaramicin sodium phosphate]

**rosamicin stearate** [now: rosaramicin stearate]

**rosaprostol** INN

**rosaramicin** USAN, INN *antibacterial*

**rosaramicin butyrate** USAN *antibacterial*

**rosaramicin propionate** USAN *antibacterial*

**rosaramicin sodium phosphate** USAN *antibacterial*

**rosaramicin stearate** USAN *antibacterial*

**rose bengal** *corneal injury and pathology diagnostic aid* 1.3 mg/strip

**rose bengal sodium ($^{131}$I)** INN *hepatic function test; radioactive agent* [also: rose bengal sodium I 131]

**rose bengal sodium I 125** USAN *radioactive agent*

**rose bengal sodium I 131** USAN, USP *hepatic function test; radioactive agent* [also: rose bengal sodium ($^{131}$I)]

**Rose Maria** *street drug slang* [see: marijuana]

**rose oil** NF *perfume*

**rose petal aqueous infusion** *ocular emollient*

**rose water, stronger** NF *perfume*

**rose water ointment** USP *emollient; ointment base*

**roses** *street drug slang for Benzedrine (amphetamine sulfate; discontinued 1982) tablets* [see: amphetamine sulfate]

**Rosets** ophthalmic strips OTC *corneal disclosing agent* [rose bengal] 1.3 mg

**rosin** USP

**rosoxacin** USAN, INN *antibacterial* [also: acrosoxacin]

**Ross SLD** powder for oral solution (discontinued 1994) OTC *oral nutritional supplement for patients on clear liquid diets*

**rosterolone** INN

**Rotacaps** (trademarked form) *encapsulated powder for inhalation*

**Rotalex** test kit for professional use (discontinued 1995) *in vitro diagnostic aid for fecal rotavirus* [latex agglutination test]

**rotamicillin** INN

**rotavirus vaccine** *investigational (NDA filed) immunization against diarrhea*

**rotoxamine** USAN, INN *antihistamine*

**rotoxamine tartrate** NF

**rotraxate** INN

**Rovamycine** ℞ *orphan status withdrawn 1994* [spiramycin]

**Rowasa** suppositories, rectal suspension enema ℞ *treatment of active ulcerative colitis, proctosigmoiditis and proctitis* [mesalamine] 500 mg; 4 g/60 mL

**rox; rocks; rocks of Hell** *street drug slang* [see: cocaine, crack]

**roxadimate** USAN, INN *sunscreen*

**Roxanne** *street drug slang* [see: cocaine; cocaine, crack]

**Roxanol** suppositories ℞ *narcotic analgesic* [morphine sulfate] 5, 10, 20, 30 mg

**Roxanol; Roxanol 100; Roxanol Rescudose; Roxanol UD** oral solution ℞ *narcotic analgesic* [morphine sulfate] 20 mg/mL; 100 mg/5 mL; 10 mg/2.5 mL; 20 mg/mL

**Roxanol SR** sustained-release tablets (name changed to Oramorph SR in 1994)

**roxarsone** USAN, INN *antibacterial*

**roxatidine** INN, BAN *antiulcerative* [also: roxatidine acetate HCl]

**roxatidine acetate HCl** USAN *antiulcerative for duodenal and gastric ulcers; histamine $H_2$ receptor antagonist* [also: roxatidine]

**Roxiam** (commercially available in the UK, Denmark, and Luxembourg) ℞ *investigational antipsychotic for schizophrenia (clinical trials discontinued 1994)* [remoxipride]

**roxibolone** INN

**Roxicet** tablets, oral solution ℞ *narcotic analgesic* [oxycodone HCl; acetaminophen] 5•325 mg; 5•325 mg/5 mL

**Roxicet 5/500** caplets ℞ *narcotic analgesic* [oxycodone HCl; acetaminophen] 5•500 mg

**Roxicodone** tablets, oral solution, Intensol (concentrated oral solution) ℞ *narcotic analgesic* [oxycodone HCl] 5 mg; 5 mg/5 mL; 20 mg/mL

**Roxilox** capsules ℞ *narcotic analgesic* [oxycodone HCl; acetaminophen] 5•500 mg

**Roxin** ℞ *investigational treatment for duodenal and gastric ulcers* [roxatidine acetate HCl]

**roxindole** INN

**Roxiprin** tablets ℞ *narcotic analgesic* [oxycodone HCl; oxycodone terephthalate; aspirin] 4.5•0.38•325 mg

**roxithromycin** USAN, INN *antibacterial*

**roxolonium metilsulfate** INN

**roxoperone** INN

**royal blues** *street drug slang* [see: LSD]

**Roz** *street drug slang* [see: cocaine, crack]

**RP 60180** *investigational kappa agonist for severe pain*

**RP 64477** *investigational intestinal ACAT inhibitor for hypercholesterolemia*

**rp24** *investigational antiviral for AIDS* [also: AIDS vaccine]

**rPF4 (recombinant platelet factor 4)** [see: platelet factor 4, recombinant]

**R/S** lotion OTC *topical acne treatment* [sulfur; resorcinol; alcohol] 5%•2%•28%

**RS 15385** *investigational alpha₂ adreno-receptor antagonist for male sexual dysfunction*

**RS 66271** *investigational osteoporosis treatment and preventative*

**RSV-IG (respiratory syncytial virus immune globulin)** [q.v.]

**RT (reverse transcriptase) inhibitors** [q.v.]

**R-Tannamine** tablets, pediatric oral suspension ℞ *decongestant; antihistamine* [phenylephrine tannate; chlorpheniramine tannate; pyrilamine tannate] 25•8•25 mg; 5•2•12.5 mg/5 mL

**R-Tannate** tablets, pediatric oral suspension ℞ *decongestant; antihistamine* [phenylephrine tannate; chlorpheniramine tannate; pyrilamine tannate] 25•8•25 mg; 5•2•12.5 mg/5 mL

**rtPA; rt-PA (recombinant tissue plasminogen activator)** [see: alteplase]

**Rubacell II** test for professional use (discontinued 1995) *in vitro diagnostic aid for rubella virus antibodies in serum or plasma* [passive hemagglutination (PHA) test]

**Rubazyme** reagent kit for professional use *in vitro diagnostic aid for rubella virus IgG antibodies in serum* [enzyme immunoassay (EIA)]

**rubbing alcohol** [see: alcohol, rubbing]

**rubbing isopropyl alcohol** [see: isopropyl alcohol, rubbing]

**rubella & mumps virus vaccine, live** *active immunizing agent for rubella and mumps*

**rubella virus vaccine, live** USP *active immunizing agent for rubella*

**rubeola vaccine** [see: measles virus vaccine, live]

**Rubesol-1000** IM or subcu injection (discontinued 1996) ℞ *antianemic; vitamin B₁₂ supplement* [cyanocobalamin] 1000 μg/mL

**Rubex** powder for IV injection ℞ *antineoplastic antibiotic* [doxorubicin HCl] 10, 50, 100 mg

**rubidium** *element (Rb)*

**rubidium chloride Rb 82** USAN *radioactive diagnostic aid for cardiac disease*

**rubidium chloride Rb 86** USAN *radioactive agent*

**Rubramin PC** IM or subcu injection ℞ *antianemic; vitamin B₁₂ supplement* [cyanocobalamin] 100, 1000 μg/mL

**ruderalis** *street drug slang, from a species of cannabis found in Russia* [see: cannabis]

**Rufen** film-coated tablets (discontinued 1995) ℞ *nonsteroidal anti-inflammatory drug (NSAID); antiarthritic; analgesic* [ibuprofen] 400, 600, 800 mg

**ruffies; ruffles** *street drug slang* [see: Rohypnol; flunitrazepam]

**rufloxacin** INN

**rufocromomycin** INN, BAN *antineoplastic* [also: streptonigrin]

**Ru-lets 500** film-coated tablets (discontinued 1995) OTC *vitamin/mineral supplement* [multiple vitamins and minerals] ≛

**Ru-lets M 500** film-coated tablets OTC *vitamin/mineral supplement* [multiple vitamins & minerals] ≛

**Rulid** ℞ *investigational macrolide antibiotic* [roxithromycin]

**RuLox** oral suspension OTC *antacid* [aluminum hydroxide; magnesium hydroxide] 225•200 mg/5 mL

**RuLox #1; RuLox #2** chewable tablets OTC *antacid* [aluminum hydroxide; magnesium hydroxide] 200•200 mg; 400•400 mg

**RuLox Plus** chewable tablets, oral suspension OTC *antacid; antiflatulent* [aluminum hydroxide; magnesium hydroxide; simethicone] 200•200•25 mg; 500•450•40 mg/5 mL

**Rum-K** liquid ℞ *potassium supplement* [potassium chloride] 30 mEq/15 mL

**running** *street drug slang* [see: MDMA]

**rush; rush snappers** *street drug slang* [see: isobutyl nitrite]

**Russian sickles** *street drug slang* [see: LSD]

**rutamycin** USAN, INN *antifungal*

**ruthenium** *element (Ru)*

**rutin** NF [also: rutoside]

**rutoside** INN [also: rutin]

**Ru-Tuss** liquid OTC *decongestant; antihistamine* [phenylephrine HCl;

chlorpheniramine maleate; alcohol 5%] 5•2 mg/5 mL

**Ru-Tuss** sustained-release tablets (discontinued 1995) ℞ *decongestant; antihistamine; anticholinergic* [phenylpropanolamine HCl; phenylephrine HCl; chlorpheniramine maleate; hyoscyamine sulfate; atropine sulfate; scopolamine hydrobromide] 50•25•8•0.19•0.04•0.01 mg

**Ru-Tuss II** slow-release capsules (discontinued 1995) ℞ *decongestant; antihistamine* [phenylpropanolamine HCl; chlorpheniramine maleate] 75•12 mg

**Ru-Tuss DE** prolonged-action film-coated tablets ℞ *decongestant; expectorant* [pseudoephedrine HCl; guaifenesin] 120•600 mg

**Ru-Tuss Expectorant** liquid OTC *antitussive; decongestant; expectorant* [dextromethorphan hydrobromide; pseudoephedrine HCl; guaifenesin; alcohol 10%] 10•30•100 mg/5 mL

**Ru-Tuss with Hydrocodone** liquid ℞ *narcotic antitussive; decongestant; antihistamine* [hydrocodone bitartrate; phenylpropanolamine HCl; phenylephrine HCl; pyrilamine maleate; pheniramine maleate; alcohol 5%] 1.7•3.3•5•3.3•3.3 mg/5 mL

**ruvazone** INN

**Ru-Vert-M** film-coated tablets ℞ *anticholinergic; antivertigo agent; motion sickness preventative* [meclizine HCl] 25 mg

**RVA (rabies vaccine, adsorbed)** [see: rabies vaccine]

**r-VIII SQ** ℞ *investigational antihemophilic* [recombinant factor VIII]

**RVP (red veterinarian petrolatum)** [see: petrolatum]

**RWJ 23989** *investigational retinoid for acne*

**RWJ 26091** *investigational retinoid for acne*

**RWJ 26127** *investigational treatment for osteoporosis*

**RxPak; ℞Pak** (trademarked form) *prescription package*

**Rymed** capsules ℞ *decongestant; expectorant* [pseudoephedrine HCl; guaifenesin] 30•250 mg

**Rymed** liquid OTC *decongestant; expectorant* [pseudoephedrine HCl; guaifenesin; alcohol 1.4%] 30•100 mg/5 mL

**Rymed-TR** long-acting caplets ℞ *decongestant; expectorant* [phenylpropanolamine HCl; guaifenesin] 75•400 mg

**Ryna** liquid OTC *decongestant; antihistamine* [pseudoephedrine HCl; chlorpheniramine maleate] 30•2 mg/5 mL

**Ryna-C** liquid ℞ *narcotic antitussive; decongestant; antihistamine* [codeine phosphate; pseudoephedrine HCl; chlorpheniramine maleate] 10•30•2 mg/5 mL

**Ryna-CX** liquid ℞ *narcotic antitussive; decongestant; expectorant* [codeine phosphate; pseudoephedrine HCl; guaifenesin] 10•30•100 mg/5 mL

**Rynatan** tablets, pediatric oral suspension ℞ *decongestant; antihistamine* [phenylephrine tannate; chlorpheniramine tannate; pyrilamine tannate] 25•8•25 mg; 5•2•12.5 mg/5 mL

**Rynatan-S** oral suspension ℞ *pediatric decongestant and antihistamine* [phenylephrine tannate; chlorpheniramine tannate; pyrilamine tannate] 5•2•12.5 mg/5 mL

**Rynatuss** tablets, pediatric suspension ℞ *antitussive; decongestant; antihistamine* [carbetapentane tannate; phenylephrine tannate; ephedrine tannate; chlorpheniramine tannate] 60•10•10•5 mg; 30•5•5•4 mg/5 mL

**Rythmol** film-coated tablets ℞ *antiarrhythmic* [propafenone HCl] 150, 225, 300 mg

# S

**S-2** solution for inhalation OTC *bronchodilator for bronchial asthma* [racepinephrine] 2.25%

**$^{35}$S** [see: sodium sulfate S 35]

**SA (salicylic acid)** [q.v.]

**SA (serum albumin)** [see: albumin, human]

**Saave +** capsules (discontinued 1993) OTC *dietary supplement* [multiple amino acids, vitamins, and minerals]

**sabeluzole** USAN, INN, BAN *anticonvulsant; antihypoxic; investigational treatment for Alzheimer's disease*

**Sabin vaccine** [see: poliovirus vaccine, live oral]

**Sabril** (commercially available in 40 foreign countries) ℞ *investigational anticonvulsant* [vigabatrin]

**S-A-C** tablets (discontinued 1995) OTC *analgesic; antipyretic; anti-inflammatory* [acetaminophen; salicylamide; caffeine] 150•230•30 mg

**Sacarasa** ℞ *orphan status withdrawn 1997* [sucrase]

**saccharin** NF *flavoring agent*

**saccharin calcium** USP *non-nutritive sweetener*

**saccharin sodium** USP *non-nutritive sweetener*

**sack** *street drug slang* [see: heroin]

**sacrament** *street drug slang* [see: LSD]

**sacred mushrooms** *street drug slang* [see: psilocybin]

**sacrosidase** *investigational (orphan) treatment for congenital sucrase-isomaltase deficiency*

**Saf-Clens** spray OTC *wound cleanser*

**Safe Tussin 30** liquid OTC *antitussive; expectorant* [dextromethorphan hydrobromide; guaifenesin] 15•100 mg/5 mL

**safflower oil** USP *oleaginous vehicle; essential fatty acid supplement*

**safingol** USAN *antipsoriatic; antineoplastic adjunct*

**safingol HCl** USAN *antipsoriatic; antineoplastic adjunct*

**safrole** USP

**St. Joseph Adult Chewable Aspirin** chewable tablets OTC *analgesic; antipyretic; anti-inflammatory* [aspirin] 81 mg

**St. Joseph Anti-Diarrheal for Children** liquid OTC *antidiarrheal; GI adsorbent* [attapulgite]

**St. Joseph Aspirin-Free Fever Reducer for Children** liquid (discontinued 1997) OTC *analgesic; antipyretic* [acetaminophen] 160 mg/5 mL

**St. Joseph Aspirin-Free for Children** chewable tablets (discontinued 1997) OTC *analgesic; antipyretic* [acetaminophen] 80 mg

**St. Joseph Aspirin-Free Infant Drops** (discontinued 1997) OTC *analgesic; antipyretic* [acetaminophen] 100 mg/mL

**St. Joseph Cold Tablets for Children** chewable tablets OTC *pediatric decongestant and analgesic* [phenylpropanolamine HCl; acetaminophen] 3.125•80 mg

**St. Joseph Complete Nighttime Cold Relief, Aspirin Free** liquid (discontinued 1993) OTC *pediatric decongestant, antihistamine, antitussive and analgesic* [pseudoephedrine HCl; chlorpheniramine maleate; dextromethorphan hydrobromide; acetaminophen]

**St. Joseph Cough Suppressant** syrup OTC *antitussive* [dextromethorphan hydrobromide] 7.5 mg/5 mL

**Saizen** powder for subcu or IM injection ℞ *growth hormone for congenital or renal-induced growth failure (orphan); investigational (orphan) for Turner syndrome and severe burns* [somatropin (recombinant)] 5 mg (15 IU) per vial

**SalAc** liquid OTC *topical keratolytic cleanser for acne* [salicylic acid] 2%

**salacetamide** INN

**salacetin** [see: aspirin]

**Sal-Acid** plaster OTC *topical keratolytic* [salicylic acid in a collodion-like vehicle] 40%

**Salacid 25%; Salacid 60%** ointment (discontinued 1994) ℞ *topical kera-*

*tolytic* [salicylic acid in a petroleum base] 25%; 60%

**Salactic Film** liquid OTC *topical keratolytic* [salicylic acid in a collodion-like vehicle] 17%

**salafibrate** INN

**Salagen** film-coated tablets ℞ *treatment for radiation-induced xerostomia (orphan); investigational (orphan) for keratoconjunctivitis sicca of Sjögren syndrome* [pilocarpine HCl] 5 mg

**salantel** USAN, INN *veterinary anthelmintic*

**Salazide; Salazide-Demi** tablets ℞ *antihypertensive* [hydroflumethiazide; reserpine]

**salazodine** INN

**Salazopyrin** (European name for U.S. product Azulfidine)

**salazosulfadimidine** INN [also: salazo-sulphadimidine]

**salazosulfamide** INN

**salazosulfapyridine** JAN *broad-spectrum bacteriostatic; anti-inflammatory for ulcerative colitis; antirheumatic* [also: sulfasalazine; sulphasalazine]

**salazosulfathiazole** INN

**salazosulphadimidine** BAN [also: salazosulfadimidine]

**salbutamol** INN, BAN *bronchodilator* [also: albuterol]

**salbutamol sulfate** JAN *bronchodilator* [also: albuterol sulfate]

**salcatonin** BAN *synthetic analog of calcitonin (salmon); calcium regulator; investigational osteoporosis treatment* [also: calcitonin salmon (synthesis)]

**salcetogen** [see: aspirin]

**Sal-Clens Acne Cleanser** gel OTC *topical keratolytic for acne* [salicylic acid] 2%

**salcolex** USAN, INN *analgesic; anti-inflammatory; antipyretic*

**saletamide** INN *analgesic* [also: salethamide maleate]

**saletamide maleate** [see: salethamide maleate]

**salethamide maleate** USAN *analgesic* [also: saletamide]

**saletin** [see: aspirin]

**Saleto** tablets OTC *analgesic; antipyretic; anti-inflammatory* [acetaminophen; aspirin; salicylamide; caffeine] 115• 210•65•16 mg

**Saleto CF** tablets OTC *antitussive; decongestant; analgesic* [dextromethorphan hydrobromide; phenylpropanolamine; acetaminophen] 10• 12.5•325 mg

**Saleto-200** tablets OTC *nonsteroidal anti-inflammatory drug (NSAID); antiarthritic; analgesic* [ibuprofen] 200 mg

**Saleto-400; Saleto-600; Saleto-800** tablets ℞ *nonsteroidal anti-inflammatory drug (NSAID); antiarthritic; analgesic* [ibuprofen] 400 mg; 600 mg; 800 mg

**Saleto-D** capsules OTC *decongestant; analgesic; antipyretic* [phenylpropanolamine HCl; acetaminophen; salicylamide; caffeine] 18•240•120•16 mg

**Salflex** film-coated tablets OTC *analgesic; antipyretic; anti-inflammatory; antirheumatic* [salsalate] 500, 750 mg

**salfluverine** INN

**salicain** [now: salicyl alcohol]

**salicin** USP

**salicyl alcohol** USAN *local anesthetic*

**salicylamide** USP *analgesic*

**salicylanilide** NF

**salicylate meglumine** USAN *antirheumatic; analgesic*

**salicylates** *a class of drugs that have analgesic, antipyretic, and anti-inflammatory effects*

**salicylazosulfapyridine** [now: sulfasalazine]

**salicylic acid (SA)** USP *keratolytic; antiseborrheic; antipsoriatic*

**salicylic acid, bimolecular ester** [see: salsalate]

**salicylic acid acetate** [see: aspirin]

**Salicylic Acid Acne Treatment** bar (discontinued 1995) OTC *medicated cleanser for acne* [salicylic acid] 2%

**Salicylic Acid and Sulfur Soap** bar OTC *medicated cleanser for acne* [salicylic acid; precipitated sulfur] 3%• 10%

**Salicylic Acid Cleansing** bar OTC *medicated cleanser for acne* [salicylic acid] 2%

**salicylic acid dihydrogen phosphate** [see: fosfosal]

**salicylsalicylic acid** [see: salsalate]

**Saligel** gel (discontinued 1994) OTC *topical keratolytic for acne* [salicylic acid; alcohol] 5%•14%

**saligenin** [now: salicyl alcohol]

**saligenol** [now: salicyl alcohol]

**salinazid** INN, BAN

**saline, lactated potassic** [see: potassic saline, lactated]

**saline solution (SS)** [also: normal saline]

**SalineX** nasal mist, nose drops OTC *nasal moisturizer* [sodium chloride (saline)] 0.4%

**saliniazid** [see: salinazid]

**salinomycin** INN, BAN

**Saliva Substitute** oral solution OTC *saliva substitute*

**Salivart** oral spray OTC *saliva substitute*

**Salix** lozenges OTC *saliva substitute*

**salmaterol** [see: salmeterol]

**salmefamol** INN, BAN

**salmeterol** USAN, INN, BAN *bronchodilator*

**salmeterol xinafoate** USAN *adrenergic; bronchodilator*

**salmisteine** INN

**salmon calcitonin** [see: salcatonin]

**Salmonine** subcu or IM injection ℞ *calcium regulator for hypercalcemia, Paget's disease, and postmenopausal osteoporosis* [calcitonin (salmon)] 200 IU/mL

**salmotin** [see: adicillin]

**salnacedin** USAN *topical anti-inflammatory*

**Salocol** tablets (discontinued 1995) OTC *analgesic; antipyretic; anti-inflammatory* [acetaminophen; aspirin; salicylamide; caffeine] 115•210•65•16 mg

**Sal-Oil-T** hair dressing ℞ *antipsoriatic; antiseborrheic; keratolytic* [coal tar; salicylic acid] 10%•6%

**salol** [see: phenyl salicylate]

**Salphenyl** capsules (discontinued 1995) OTC *decongestant; antihistamine; analgesic* [phenylephrine HCl; chlorpheniramine maleate; acetaminophen; salicylamide] 10•2•130•200 mg

**Sal-Plant** gel OTC *topical keratolytic* [salicylic acid in a collodion-like vehicle] 17%

**Salprofen** IV injection ℞ *investigational (orphan) for patent ductus arteriosus* [ibuprofen]

**salprotoside** INN

**salsalate** USAN, USP, INN, BAN *analgesic; antipyretic; anti-inflammatory; antirheumatic* 500, 750 mg oral

**Salsitab** film-coated tablets ℞ *analgesic; antipyretic; anti-inflammatory; antirheumatic* [salsalate] 500, 750 mg

**salt** *street drug slang* [see: heroin]

**salt and pepper** *street drug slang* [see: marijuana]

**Sal-Tropine** tablets ℞ GI *anticholinergic and antispasmodic* [atropine sulfate] 0.4 mg

**salty water** *street drug slang* [see: GHB]

**Saluron** tablets ℞ *diuretic; antihypertensive* [hydroflumethiazide] 50 mg

**Salutensin; Salutensin-Demi** tablets ℞ *antihypertensive* [hydroflumethiazide; reserpine] 50•0.125 mg; 25•0.125 mg ⑨ Diutensin

**saluzide** [see: opiniazide]

**salvarsan** [see: arsphenamine]

**salverine** INN

**Salzen** ℞ *investigational treatment for growth hormone deficiency and chronic renal insufficiency* [human growth hormone]

**samarium** *element (Sm)*

**samarium Sm 153 EDTMP (ethylenediaminetetramethylenephosphoric acid)** [see: samarium Sm 153 lexidronam]

**samarium Sm 153 lexidronam** USAN *radiopharmaceutical for treatment of bone pain from osteoblastic metastatic tumors*

**sancycline** USAN, INN *antibacterial*

**Sandimmune** gel capsules, oral solution, IV injection ℞ *immunosuppressant for allogenic kidney, liver, and heart transplants; investigational for many uses* [cyclosporine] 25, 50, 100 mg; 100 mg/mL; 50 mg/mL

**Sandimmune** ophthalmic ointment ℞ *investigational (orphan) for kerato-*

plasty graft rejection and corneal melting syndrome [cyclosporine] 2%

**Sandoglobulin** powder for IV infusion ℞ passive immunizing agent for HIV and idiopathic thrombocytopenic purpura (ITP) [immune globulin] 1, 3, 6, 12 g

**SandoPak** (trademarked packaging form) unit dose blister package

**Sandostatin** subcu or IV injection ℞ acromegaly; carcinoid tumors; vasoactive intestinal peptide tumors (VIPomas) [octreotide acetate] 0.05, 0.1, 0.2, 0.5, 1 mg/mL

**Sandostatin LAR** ℞ investigational antineoplastic for breast and colon cancer [octreotide acetate]

**Sandoz** street drug slang, a reference to the manufacturer [see: LSD]

**sandwich** street drug slang for two layers of cocaine with a layer of heroin [see: cocaine; heroin]

**sanfetrinem** INN, BAN antibacterial [also: sanfetrinem sodium]

**sanfetrinem cilexetil** USAN antibacterial

**sanfetrinem sodium** USAN antibacterial [also: sanfetrinem]

**sanguinarine chloride** [now: sanguinarium chloride]

**sanguinarium chloride** USAN, INN antifungal; antimicrobial; anti-inflammatory

**Sani-Pak** (trademarked packaging form) sanitary dispensing box

**Sani-Supp** suppositories OTC hyperosmolar laxative [glycerin]

**Sanitube** ointment (discontinued 1996) OTC venereal prophylactic [calomel; benzoxiquine; trolamine] 30% • ? • ?

**Sanorex** tablets ℞ anorexiant; investigational (orphan) treatment for Duchenne muscular dystrophy [mazindol] 1, 2 mg

**Sansert** tablets ℞ agent for migraine and vascular headaches [methysergide maleate] 2 mg

**Santa Marta** (Spanish for "Saint Marta") street drug slang [see: marijuana]

**santonin** NF

**Santyl** ointment ℞ topical enzyme for biochemical debridement [collagenase] 250 U/g

**saperconazole** USAN, INN, BAN antifungal

**saprisartan** INN, BAN antihypertensive; angiotensin II antagonist [also: saprisartan potassium]

**saprisartan potassium** USAN antihypertensive; angiotensin II antagonist [also: saprisartan]

**sapropterin** INN

**saquinavir** INN, BAN antiviral; HIV protease inhibitor [also: saquinavir mesylate]

**saquinavir mesylate** USAN antiviral; HIV protease inhibitor [also: saquinavir]

**sarafloxacin** INN, BAN anti-infective; DNA gyrase inhibitor [also: sarafloxacin HCl]

**sarafloxacin HCl** USAN anti-infective; DNA gyrase inhibitor [also: sarafloxacin]

**saralasin** INN antihypertensive [also: saralasin acetate]

**saralasin acetate** USAN antihypertensive [also: saralasin]

**Saratoga** ointment OTC astringent; antiseptic; wound protectant [zinc oxide; boric acid; eucalyptol]

**sarcolysin** INN

**L-sarcolysin** [see: melphalan]

**Sardo Bath & Shower** oil OTC bath emollient

**Sardoettes** towelettes OTC moisturizer; emollient

**sargramostim** USAN, INN, BAN antineutropenic for bone marrow transplant and graft delay (orphan); investigational (Phase III) for malignant melanoma; investigational AIDS cytokine

**Sarisol No. 2** tablets (discontinued 1993) ℞ sedative; hypnotic [butabarbital sodium]

**sarmazenil** INN

**sarmoxicillin** USAN, INN antibacterial

**Sarna Anti-Itch** foam, lotion OTC counterirritant [camphor; menthol] 0.5% • 0.5%

**saroten** [see: amitriptyline]

**sarpicillin** USAN, INN antibacterial

**saruplase** INN

**sassafras** street drug slang [see: marijuana]

**Sastid** cream OTC *keratolytic for acne* [precipitated sulfur; salicylic acid]

**Sastid (AL) Scrub** cream (discontinued 1994) OTC *abrasive cleanser for acne* [aluminum oxide; sulfur; salicylic acid] 20%•1.6%•1.6%

**Sastid Plain Therapeutic Shampoo & Acne Wash** (discontinued 1994) OTC *topical acne cleanser* [sulfur; salicylic acid] 1.6%•1.6%

**SAStid Soap** bar OTC *medicated cleanser for acne* [precipitated sulfur] 10%

**saterinone** INN

**sativa** *street drug slang, from a species of cannabis found in cool, damp climates* [see: cannabis]

**satranidazole** INN

**satumomab** INN, BAN *radiodiagnostic monoclonal antibody for ovarian and colorectal carcinoma* [also: indium In 111 satumomab pendetide]

**satumomab pendetide** [see: indium In 111 satumomab pendetide]

**savoxepin** INN

**SB-210396** *investigational (Phase III) anti-CD4 antibody for rheumatoid arthritis* [also: IDEC-CE9.1]

**SC (succinylcholine)** [see: succinylcholine chlorine]

**SC-49483** *investigational pro-drug that prevents the clumping of HIV cells which leads to drug resistance*

**SCA proteins (single-chain antigen-binding proteins)** *a class of investigational antineoplastics*

**Scabene** lotion, shampoo ℞ *scabicide; pediculicide* [lindane] 1%

**scabicides** *a class of agents effective against scabies*

**Scadan** scalp lotion OTC *antiseptic; antiseborrheic* [myristyltrimethylammonium bromide; stearyl dimethyl benzyl ammonium chloride] 1%•0.1%

**scaffle** *street drug slang* [see: PCP]

**scag** *street drug slang* [see: heroin]

**Scalpicin** liquid OTC *topical corticosteroid* [hydrocortisone] 1%

**scandium** *element (Sc)*

**scarlet fever streptococcus toxin**

**scarlet red** NF *promotes wound healing*

**Scarlet Red Ointment Dressings** *medication-impregnated gauze* ℞ *wound dressings* [scarlet red] 5%

**scat; scate** *street drug slang* [see: heroin]

**sCD4-PE40** [see: alvircept sudotox]

**SCF (stem cell factor)** [q.v.]

**Schamberg** lotion OTC *antiseptic; astringent; antifungal; counterirritant* [zinc oxide; menthol; phenol] 8.25%•0.25%•1.5%

**Schick test** [see: diphtheria toxin for Schick test]

**Schick test control** USP *dermal reactivity indicator*

**Schirmer Tear Test** ophthalmic strips OTC *diagnostic tear flow test aid*

**schmack; smack; schmeck; shmeck** *street drug slang* [see: heroin]

**schoolboy** *street drug slang* [see: cocaine; codeine]

**schoolboy scotch** *street drug slang for Scotch whiskey with codeine added* [see: codeine; alcohol]

**Schoolcraft** *street drug slang* [see: cocaine, crack]

**scissors** *street drug slang* [see: marijuana]

**Sclavo PPD Solution** intradermal injection (discontinued 1995) ℞ *tuberculosis skin test* [tuberculin purified protein derivative] 5 U/0.1 mL

**Sclavo Test-PPD** single-use intradermal puncture test device (discontinued 1995) ℞ *tuberculosis skin test* [tuberculin purified protein derivative] 5 U

**Scleromate** IV injection ℞ *sclerosing agent for varicose veins* [morrhuate sodium] 50 mg/mL

**Sclerosol** ℞ *investigational treatment for malignant pleural effusion via intrapleural thoracoscopy administration* [sterile aerosol talc]

**Sclerosol** ℞ *orphan status withdrawn 1994* [dimethyl sulfoxide (DMSO)]

**scoop** *street drug slang* [see: GHB]

**scopafungin** USAN *antibacterial; antifungal*

**Scope** mouthwash OTC *oral antiseptic* [cetylpyridinium chloride]

**scopolamine** *transdermal motion sickness preventative*

**scopolamine hydrobromide** USP *GI antispasmodic; anticholinergic; motion sickness preventative; cycloplegic; mydriatic* [also: hyoscine hydrobromide] 0.3, 0.4, 0.86, 1 mg/mL injection

**scopolamine methyl nitrate** [see: methscopolamine nitrate]

**scopolamine methylbromide** [see: methscopolamine bromide]

**scorpion** *street drug slang* [see: cocaine]

**Scott** *street drug slang* [see: heroin]

**Scottie; Scotty** *street drug slang* [see: cocaine; cocaine, crack]

**Scott's Emulsion** OTC *vitamin supplement* [vitamins A and D] 1250•100 IU/5 mL

**Scot-Tussin Allergy** liquid OTC *antihistamine* [diphenhydramine HCl] 12.5 mg/5 mL

**Scot-Tussin DM** liquid OTC *antitussive; antihistamine* [dextromethorphan hydrobromide; chlorpheniramine maleate] 15•2 mg/5 mL

**Scot-Tussin DM Cough Chasers** lozenges OTC *antitussive* [dextromethorphan hydrobromide] 2.5 mg

**Scot-Tussin Expectorant** sugar-free liquid OTC *expectorant* [guaifenesin; alcohol 3.5%] 100 mg/5 mL

**Scot-Tussin Original 5-Action Cold Formula** syrup, sugar-free liquid OTC *decongestant; antihistamine; analgesic* [phenylephrine HCl; pheniramine maleate; sodium citrate; sodium salicylate; caffeine citrate] 4.2•13.3•83.3•83.3•25 mg

**Scot-Tussin Senior Clear** liquid OTC *antitussive; expectorant* [dextromethorphan hydrobromide; guaifenesin] 15•200 mg/5 mL

**sCR1 (soluble complement receptor 1)** *investigational complement inhibitor for severe burns and adult respiratory distress syndrome*

**scramble** *street drug slang* [see: cocaine, crack]

**Scriptene** ℞ *investigational (Phase I) antiviral for AIDS* [zidovudine; didanosine]

**scrubwoman's kick** *street drug slang for inhaled cleaning fluid, especially*

*naphtha* [see: petroleum distillate inhalants]

**scruples** *street drug slang* [see: cocaine, crack]

**scuffle; skuffle** *street drug slang* [see: PCP]

**scuroforme** [see: butyl aminobenzoate]

**SD (streptodornase)** [q.v.]

**SD Polygam** (name changed to Polygam S/D in 1994)

**⁷⁵Se** [see: selenomethionine Se 75]

**Sea Mist** nasal spray OTC *nasal moisturizer* [sodium chloride (saline)] 0.65%

**Seale's Lotion Modified** OTC *topical acne treatment* [sulfur] 6.4%

**Sea-Omega 30; Sea-Omega 50** softgels OTC *dietary supplement* [omega-3 fatty acids] 1200 mg; 1000 mg

**SEB-324** *investigational anxiolytic and antidepressant*

**Sebacide Cleanser** liquid (discontinued 1994) OTC *topical acne cleanser* [parachlorometaxylenol] 0.35%

**Seba-Nil Cleansing Mask** scrub OTC *abrasive cleanser for acne*

**Seba-Nil Oily Skin Cleanser** liquid OTC *topical cleanser for acne* [alcohol; acetone]

**Sebaquin** shampoo (discontinued 1994) OTC *antiseborrheic; antimicrobial* [iodoquinol] 3%

**Sebasorb** liquid (discontinued 1994) OTC *topical acne treatment* [colloidal sulfur; salicylic acid; attapulgite] 2%•2%•10%

**Sebasorb** lotion OTC *topical keratolytic for acne* [salicylic acid; attapulgite] 2%•10%

**Sebex** shampoo OTC *antiseborrheic; keratolytic* [sulfur; salicylic acid] 2%•2%

**Sebex-T** shampoo OTC *antiseborrheic; antipsoriatic; keratolytic* [sulfur; salicylic acid; coal tar] 2%•2%•5%

**Sebizon** lotion ℞ *bacteriostatic; antiseborrheic* [sulfacetamide sodium] 10%

**Sebucare** hair lotion OTC *antiseborrheic; keratolytic* [salicylic acid; alcohol 61%] 1.8%

**Sebulex** shampoo (discontinued 1997) OTC *antiseborrheic; keratolytic* [sulfur; salicylic acid] 2%•2%

**Sebulex with Conditioners** shampoo OTC *antiseborrheic; keratolytic* [sulfur; salicylic acid] 2%•2%

**Sebulon** shampoo (discontinued 1997) OTC *antiseborrheic; antibacterial; antifungal* [pyrithione zinc] 2%

**Sebutone** cream shampoo, liquid shampoo (discontinued 1997) OTC *antiseborrheic; antipsoriatic; keratolytic* [coal tar; sulfur; salicylic acid] 0.5%•2%•2%

**SEC-579** *investigational anxiolytic and 5-HT₃ antagonist*

**secalciferol** USAN, INN, BAN *calcium regulator; investigational (orphan) for familial hypophosphatemic rickets*

**secbutabarbital sodium** INN *sedative; hypnotic* [also: butabarbital sodium]

**secbutobarbitone** BAN *sedative; hypnotic* [also: butabarbital]

**seccy; seggy** *street drug slang* [see: Seconal Sodium; secobarbital sodium]

**seclazone** USAN, INN *anti-inflammatory; uricosuric*

**secnidazole** INN, BAN

**secobarbital** USP, INN *hypnotic; sedative*

**secobarbital sodium** USP, JAN *hypnotic; sedative; also abused as a street drug* [also: quinalbarbitone sodium] 100 mg oral; 50 mg/mL injection

**Seconal Sodium** Pulvules (capsules) ℞ *sedative; hypnotic; also abused as a street drug* [secobarbital sodium] 100 mg

**secoverine** INN

**Secran** liquid OTC *vitamin supplement* [vitamins B₁, B₃, and B₁₂; alcohol 17%] 10 mg•10 mg•25 μg per 5 mL

**Secran Prenatal** tablets (discontinued 1995) ℞ *vitamin/calcium/iron supplement* [multiple vitamins; calcium; iron; folic acid] ≝•250•60•1 mg

**secretin** INN, BAN *pancreatic function diagnostic aid*

**Secretin Ferring** powder for IV injection ℞ *in vivo pancreatic function test* [secretin] 10 CU/mL

**Sectral** capsules ℞ *antihypertensive; antiarrhythmic; β-blocker* [acebutolol HCl] 200, 400 mg

**Secule** (trademarked packaging form) *single-dose vial*

**securinine** INN

**sedaform** [see: chlorobutanol]

**Sedapap-10** tablets ℞ *analgesic; antipyretic; sedative* [acetaminophen; butalbital] 650•50 mg

**sedatine** [see: antipyrine]

**sedecamycin** USAN, INN *veterinary antibacterial*

**sedeval** [see: barbital]

**sedoxantrone trihydrochloride** USAN *topoisomerase II inhibitor antineoplastic*

**seeds** *street drug slang* [see: marijuana]

**seganserin** INN, BAN

**seggy; seccy** *street drug slang* [see: Seconal Sodium; secobarbital sodium]

**seglitide** INN *antidiabetic* [also: seglitide acetate]

**seglitide acetate** USAN *antidiabetic* [also: seglitide]

**Seldane** tablets ℞ *nonsedating antihistamine* [terfenadine] 60 mg

**Seldane-D** sustained-release tablets ℞ *decongestant; antihistamine* [pseudoephedrine HCl; terfenadine] 120•60 mg

**Selecor** tablets ℞ *investigational antihypertensive; antianginal; β-blocker* [celiprolol HCl]

**Select-A-Jet** (trademarked delivery system) *syringe system*

**selective serotonin reuptake inhibitors (SSRIs)** *a class of oral antidepressants that inhibit neuronal uptake of 5-HT (serotonin), a CNS neurotransmitter*

**selegiline** INN, BAN *antiparkinsonian; investigational treatment for Alzheimer's disease* [also: selegiline HCl]

**selegiline HCl** USAN *antiparkinsonian (orphan); investigational treatment for Alzheimer's disease* [also: selegiline] 5 mg oral

**selenious acid** USP *dietary selenium supplement* 65.4 μg/mL injection

**selenium** *element (Se)*

**selenium dioxide, monohydrated** [see: selenious acid]

**selenium sulfide** USP *antifungal; antiseborrheic* 1%, 2.5% topical

**selenomethionine (⁷⁵Se)** INN *pancreas function test; radioactive agent* [also: selenomethionine Se 75]

selenomethionine Se 75 USAN, USP *pancreas function test; radioactive agent* [also: selenomethionine ($^{75}$Se)]

Sele-Pak IV injection ℞ *intravenous nutritional therapy* [selenious acid] 65.4 μg/mL

Selepen IV injection ℞ *intravenous nutritional therapy* [selenious acid] 65.4 μg/mL

Selestoject IV, IM injection (discontinued 1996) ℞ *glucocorticoid* [betamethasone sodium phosphate] 4 mg/mL

selfotel USAN N-methyl-D-aspartate (NMDA) antagonist for treatment of stroke-induced impairment

Seloken (foreign name for U.S. product Lopressor)

Seloken ZOC (foreign name for U.S. product Toprol XL)

selprazine INN

Selsun lotion/shampoo ℞ *antiseborrheic; antifungal* [selenium sulfide] 2.5%

Selsun Blue; Selsun Gold for Women lotion/shampoo OTC *antiseborrheic* [selenium sulfide] 1%

sematilide INN *antiarrhythmic* [also: sematilide HCl]

sematilide HCl USAN *antiarrhythmic* [also: sematilide]

semduramicin USAN, INN *coccidiostat*

semduramicin sodium USAN *coccidiostat*

Semicid vaginal suppositories OTC *spermicidal contraceptive* [nonoxynol 9] 100 mg

Semilente Iletin I subcu injection (discontinued 1994) OTC *antidiabetic* [insulin zinc (beef-pork)]

Semilente Insulin subcu injection (discontinued 1994) OTC *antidiabetic* [insulin zinc, prompt (beef)]

semisodium valproate BAN *anticonvulsant; antipsychotic for manic episodes; migraine prophylaxis* [also: divalproex sodium; valproate semisodium]

Semprex-D capsules ℞ *decongestant; antihistamine* [pseudoephedrine HCl; acrivastine] 60•8 mg

semustine USAN, INN *antineoplastic*

sen *street drug slang* [see: marijuana]

Senexon tablets OTC *laxative* [senna concentrate] 187 mg

seni *street drug slang for peyote* [see: mescaline]

Senilezol elixir ℞ *vitamin/iron supplement* [multiple B vitamins; ferric pyrophosphate] ≛•3.3 mg

senna USP *stimulant laxative*

Senna-Gen tablets OTC *stimulant laxative* [sennosides] 8.6 mg

sennosides USP *stimulant laxative*

Senokot tablets, granules, suppositories, syrup OTC *laxative* [senna concentrate] 187 mg; 326 mg/tsp.; 652 mg; 218 mg/5 mL

Senokot-S tablets OTC *laxative; stool softener* [docusate sodium; senna concentrate] 50•187 mg

Senokotxtra tablets OTC *laxative* [senna concentrate] 374 mg

Senolax tablets OTC *laxative* [senna concentrate] 187 mg

Sensitive Eyes; Sensitive Eyes Plus solution OTC *rinsing/storage solution for soft contact lenses* [preserved saline solution]

Sensitive Eyes Daily Cleaner; Sensitive Eyes Saline/Cleaning Solution OTC *surfactant cleaning solution for soft contact lenses*

Sensitive Eyes Drops OTC *rewetting solution for soft contact lenses*

Sensitivity Protection Crest toothpaste OTC *tooth desensitizer; dental caries preventative* [potassium nitrate; sodium fluoride]

Sensodyne, Original toothpaste (name changed to Sensodyne-SC in 1994)

Sensodyne Cool Gel toothpaste OTC *tooth desensitizer; dental caries preventative* [potassium nitrate; sodium fluoride]

Sensodyne Fresh Mint toothpaste OTC *tooth desensitizer; dental caries preventative* [potassium nitrate; sodium monofluorophosphate] ≛

Sensodyne-F toothpaste (name changed to Sensodyne Fresh Mint in 1994)

Sensodyne-SC toothpaste OTC *tooth desensitizer* [strontium chloride hexahydrate] 10%

SensoGARD gel OTC *topical oral anesthetic* [benzocaine] 20%

**Sensorcaine** injection ℞ *injectable local anesthetic* [bupivacaine HCl] 0.25%, 0.5%

**Sensorcaine** injection ℞ *injectable local anesthetic* [bupivacaine HCl; epinephrine] 0.25%•1:200 000; 0.5%•1:200 000

**Sensorcaine MPF** injection ℞ *injectable local anesthetic* [bupivacaine HCl] 0.25%, 0.5%, 0.75%

**Sensorcaine MPF** injection ℞ *injectable local anesthetic* [bupivacaine HCl; epinephrine] 0.25%•1:200 000, 0.5%•1:200 000, 0.75%•1:200 000

**Sensorcaine MPF Spinal** injection ℞ *injectable local anesthetic* [bupivacaine HCl] 0.75%

**Sentinel** test kit for professional use ℞ *urine test for HIV-1 antibodies*

**sepazonium chloride** USAN, INN *topical anti-infective*

**seperidol HCl** USAN *antipsychotic* [also: clofluperol]

**Seprafilm** hydrated gel film *to reduce the incidence, extent, and severity of postoperative adhesions* [sodium hyaluronate; carboxymethylcellulose]

**seprilose** USAN *antirheumatic*

**seproxetine HCl** USAN *antidepressant*

**Septa** ointment OTC *topical antibiotic* [polymyxin B sulfate; neomycin sulfate; bacitracin] 5000 U•3.5 mg•400 U per g ☑ Sepo; Septra

**SeptiGAM** ℞ *investigational antibacterial for Staphylococcus aureus-induced sepsis*

**Septi-Soft** solution ℞ *antiseptic; disinfectant* [triclosan] 0.25%

**Septisol** foam ℞ *bacteriostatic skin cleanser* [hexachlorophene; alcohol 56%] 0.23%

**Septisol** solution ℞ *antiseptic; disinfectant* [triclosan] 0.25%

**septomonab** [see: nebacumab]

**Septopal** polymethyl methacrylate (PMMA) beads on surgical wire ℞ *investigational (orphan) for chronic osteomyelitis* [gentamicin]

**Septra** tablets, oral suspension ℞ *anti-infective; antibacterial* [trimethoprim; sulfamethoxazole] 80•400 mg; 40•200 mg/5 mL ☑ Septa

**Septra DS** tablets ℞ *anti-infective; antibacterial* [trimethoprim; sulfamethoxazole] 160•800 mg

**Septra IV** infusion ℞ *anti-infective; antibacterial* [trimethoprim; sulfamethoxazole] 80•400 mg/5 mL

**Sequels** (trademarked dosage form) *sustained-release capsule or tablet*

**sequifenadine** INN

**seractide** INN *adrenocorticotropic hormone* [also: seractide acetate]

**seractide acetate** USAN *adrenocorticotropic hormone* [also: seractide]

**Ser-A-Gen** tablets (discontinued 1993) ℞ *antihypertensive* [hydrochlorothiazide; reserpine; hydralazine HCl]

**Ser-Ap-Es** tablets ℞ *antihypertensive* [hydrochlorothiazide; reserpine; hydralazine HCl] 15•0.1•25 mg ☑ Catapres

**seratrodast** USAN, INN *anti-inflammatory; antiasthmatic; thromboxane receptor antagonist*

**Serax** capsules, tablets ℞ *anxiolytic* [oxazepam] 10, 15, 30 mg; 15 mg ☑ Eurax; Urex; Xerac

**serazapine HCl** USAN *anxiolytic*

**Serc-16** tablets ℞ *treatment for vertigo due to Meniere syndrome* [betahistine]

**Sereine** solution OTC *cleaning solution for hard contact lenses* [note: one of three different products with the same name]

**Sereine** solution OTC *wetting solution for hard contact lenses* [note: one of three different products with the same name]

**Sereine** solution OTC *wetting/soaking solution for hard contact lenses* [note: one of three different products with the same name]

**serenity; serenity, tranquility, and peace** *street drug slang* [see: STP]

**Serentil** tablets, oral concentrate, IM injection ℞ *antipsychotic* [mesoridazine besylate] 10, 25, 50, 100 mg; 25 mg/mL; 25 mg/mL ☑ Surital

**Serevent** oral metered dose inhaler ℞ *twice-daily bronchodilator for asthma and bronchospasm* [salmeterol xinafoate] 25 μg/dose

**serfibrate** INN

**sergolexole** INN *antimigraine* [also: sergolexole maleate]

**sergolexole maleate** USAN *antimigraine* [also: sergolexole]

**serine (L-serine)** USAN, USP, INN *nonessential amino acid; symbols: Ser, S*

**L-serine diazoacetate** [see: azaserine]

**84-L-serineplasminogen activator** [see: monteplase]

**sermetacin** USAN, INN *anti-inflammatory*

**sermorelin** INN, BAN *growth hormone deficiency diagnosis and treatment* [also: sermorelin acetate]

**sermorelin acetate** USAN *pituitary diagnostic aid; investigational (orphan) for growth hormone deficiency, anovulation, and AIDS-related weight loss* [also: sermorelin]

**Sernyl** *street drug slang* [see: PCP]

**Seromycin** Pulvules (capsules) R̥ *tuberculostatic* [cycloserine] 250 mg

**Serophene** tablets R̥ *ovulation stimulant* [clomiphene citrate] 50 mg

**Seroquel** R̥ *investigational dopamine and serotonin antagonist for schizophrenia* [quetiapine fumarate]

**Serostim** powder for subcu injection R̥ *growth hormone for growth failure due to renal insufficiency and treatment of AIDS wasting syndrome or cachexia (orphan)* [somatropin] 5, 6 mg (15, 18 IU) per vial

**Seroxat** (European name for U.S. product Paxil)

**Serpalan** tablets (discontinued 1995) R̥ *antihypertensive; antipsychotic* [reserpine] 0.1, 0.25 mg

**Serpazide** tablets R̥ *antihypertensive* [hydrochlorothiazide; reserpine; hydralazine HCl]

**Serpico 21** *street drug slang* [see: cocaine]

**serrapeptase** INN

***Serratia marcescens* extract (polyribosomes)** *investigational (orphan) for primary brain malignancies*

**sertaconazole** INN

**sertindole** USAN, INN *antipsychotic; neuroleptic*

**sertraline** INN, BAN *selective serotonin reuptake inhibitor (SSRI) for depression and obsessive-compulsive disorder* [also: sertraline HCl]

**sertraline HCl** USAN *selective serotonin reuptake inhibitor (SSRI) for depression and obsessive-compulsive disorder* [also: sertraline]

**serum albumin (SA)** [see: albumin, human]

**serum albumin, iodinated ($^{125}$I) human** [see: albumin, iodinated I 125 serum]

**serum albumin, iodinated ($^{131}$I) human** [see: albumin, iodinated I 131 serum]

**serum fibrinogen (SF)** [see: fibrinogen, human]

**serum globulin (SG)** [see: globulin, immune]

**serum gonadotrophin** [see: gonadotrophin, serum]

**serum gonadotropin** [see: gonadotrophin, serum]

**serum prothrombin conversion accelerator (SPCA) factor** [see: factor VII]

**Serutan** powder, granules OTC *bulk laxative* [psyllium] 3.4 g/tsp.; 2.5 g/tsp.

**Serzone** tablets R̥ *antidepressant* [nefazodone HCl] 100, 150, 200, 250 mg

**sesame oil** NF *solvent; oleaginous vehicle*

**Sesame Street Complete** chewable tablets OTC *vitamin/mineral/calcium/iron supplement* [multiple vitamins and minerals; calcium; iron; folic acid; biotin] ≛•80•10•0.2•0.015 mg

**Sesame Street Plus Extra C** chewable tablets OTC *vitamin supplement* [multiple vitamins; folic acid] ≛•0.2 mg

**Sesame Street Plus Iron** chewable tablets OTC *vitamin/iron supplement* [multiple vitamins; iron; folic acid] ≛•10•0.2 mg

**Sesame Street Vitamins** chewable tablets (discontinued 1993) OTC *vitamin supplement* [multiple vitamins; folic acid] ≛•0.4 mg

**Sesame Street Vitamins and Minerals** (name changed to Sesame Street Complete in 1993)

**Sess** *street drug slang* [see: marijuana]

**setastine** INN

**setazindol** INN

**setiptiline** INN

**setoperone** USAN, INN *antipsychotic*

**sets** *street drug slang for a combination of Talwin (pentazocine HCl) and PBZ (pyribenzamine)* [see: Talwin; pentazocine HCl; tripelennamine]

**Seudotabs** tablets OTC *nasal decongestant* [pseudoephedrine HCl] 30 mg

**7 + 3 protocol (cytarabine, daunorubicin)** *chemotherapy protocol*

**7 + 3 protocol (cytarabine, idarubicin)** *chemotherapy protocol*

**7 + 3 protocol (cytarabine, mitoxantrone)** *chemotherapy protocol*

**seven fourteens** *street drug slang for Quaalude (methaqualone; discontinued 1983), from ID# 714 on the tablets* [see: methaqualone]

**7E3 MAb** [see: abciximab]

**7U85** *investigational antineoplastic*

**Seven-up** *street drug slang* [see: cocaine; cocaine, crack]

**sevirumab** USAN, INN *investigational (Phase I) antiviral for AIDS; orphan status withdrawn 1996*

**sevitropium mesilate** INN

**sevoflurane** USAN, INN *inhalation general anesthetic*

**sevopramide** INN

**sezolamide HCl** USAN *carbonic anhydrase inhibitor*

**sezz** *street drug slang* [see: marijuana]

**SF (serum fibrinogen)** [see: fibrinogen, human]

**SFC** lotion OTC *soap-free therapeutic skin cleanser*

**sfericase** INN

**SG (serum globulin)** [see: globulin, immune]

**SG (soluble gelatin)** [see: gelatin]

**SH 570** *investigational treatment for acne*

**shabu** *street drug slang* [see: cocaine; methamphetamine HCl; amphetamines; MDMA; PCP]

**shake** *street drug slang* [see: marijuana]

**shark liver oil** *emollient/protectant*

**She** *street drug slang* [see: cocaine]

**sheet rocking** *street drug slang for a combination of crack and LSD* [see: cocaine, crack; LSD]

**sheets** *street drug slang* [see: PCP]

**Sheik Elite** premedicated condom OTC *spermicidal/barrier contraceptive* [nonoxynol 9] 8%

**shellac** NF *tablet coating agent*

**Shepard's Cream Lotion; Shepard's Skin Cream** OTC *moisturizer; emollient*

**Sherm(s); Sherman(s)** *street drug slang for a tobacco cigarette laced with PCP* [see: PCP]

**shmeck; schmeck; schmack; smack** *street drug slang* [see: heroin]

**Shohl solution, modified (sodium citrate & citric acid)** *urinary alkalizer; compounding agent*

**shoot the breeze** *street drug slang* [see: nitrous oxide]

**short chain fatty acids** *investigational (orphan) for left-sided ulcerative colitis*

**'shrooms** *street drug slang for "mushrooms"* [see: psilocybin; psilocin]

**Shur-Clens** solution OTC *wound cleanser* [poloxamer 188] 20%

**Shur-Seal** vaginal gel OTC *spermicidal contraceptive (for use with a diaphragm)* [nonoxynol 9] 2%

**siagoside** INN

**Sibelium** ℞ *investigational (orphan) vasodilator for alternating hemiplegia* [flunarizine]

**Siblin** granules (discontinued 1997) OTC *bulk laxative* [blond psyllium seed coatings] 2.5 g/tsp.

**sibopirdine** USAN *cognition enhancer for Alzheimer's disease; nootropic*

**sibutramine** INN, BAN *anorectic; monoamine reuptake inhibitor antidepressant; investigational treatment for obesity* [also: sibutramine HCl]

**sibutramine HCl** USAN *anorectic; antidepressant; investigational treatment for obesity* [also: sibutramine]

**siccanin** INN

**Sickledex** test kit for professional use *in vitro diagnostic aid for hemoglobin S (sickle cell)*

**siddi** *street drug slang* [see: marijuana]

**sightball** *street drug slang* [see: cocaine, crack]

**Sigosix** ℞ *investigational treatment for radiation- or chemotherapy-induced thrombocytopenia* [recombinant human interleukin-6]

**SigPak** (trademarked packaging form) *unit-of-use package*

**Sigtab** tablets OTC *vitamin supplement* [multiple vitamins; folic acid] $\triangleq$•0.4 mg

**Sigtab-M** tablets OTC *vitamin/mineral/ calcium/iron supplement* [multiple vitamins & minerals; calcium; iron; folic acid; biotin] $\triangleq$•200•18•0.4• 0.045 mg

**siguazodan** INN, BAN

**Silace** syrup OTC *stool softener* [docusate sodium] 20 mg/5 mL

**Silace-C** syrup OTC *stimulant laxative; stool softener* [casanthranol; docusate sodium; alcohol 10%] 30•60 mg/15 mL

**SilaClean 20/20** solution (discontinued 1995) OTC *cleaning solution for hard contact lenses*

**Siladryl** elixir OTC *antihistamine* [diphenhydramine HCl] 12.5 mg/5 mL

**Silafed** syrup OTC *decongestant; antihistamine* [pseudoephedrine HCl; triprolidine HCl] 30•1.25 mg/5 mL

**silafilcon A** USAN *hydrophilic contact lens material*

**silafocon A** USAN *hydrophobic contact lens material*

**Silaminic Cold** syrup OTC *decongestant; antihistamine* [phenylpropanolamine HCl; chlorpheniramine maleate] 12.5•2 mg/5 mL

**Silaminic Expectorant** syrup OTC *decongestant; expectorant* [phenylpropanolamine HCl; guaifenesin; alcohol 5%] 12.5•100 mg/5 mL

**silandrone** USAN, INN *androgen*

**Silapap, Children's** liquid OTC *analgesic; antipyretic* [acetaminophen] 80 mg/2.5 mL

**Silapap, Infant's** drops OTC *analgesic; antipyretic* [acetaminophen] 100 mg/mL

**Sildec-DM** syrup, pediatric drops Ŗ *antitussive; decongestant; antihistamine* [dextromethorphan hydrobromide; pseudoephedrine HCl; carbinoxamine maleate] 15•60•4 mg/5 mL; 4•25•2 mg/mL

**Sildicon-E** pediatric drops OTC *pediatric decongestant and expectorant*

[phenylpropanolamine HCl; guaifenesin] 6.25•30 mg/mL

**Silfedrine, Children's** liquid OTC *nasal decongestant* [pseudoephedrine HCl] 30 mg/5 mL

**silibinin** INN

**silica, dental-type** NF *pharmaceutic aid*

**silica gel** [now: silicon dioxide]

**siliceous earth, purified** NF *filtering medium*

**silicic acid, magnesium salt** [see: magnesium trisilicate]

**silicon** element (Si)

**silicon dioxide** NF *dispersing and suspending agent*

**silicon dioxide, colloidal** NF *suspending agent; tablet and capsule diluent*

**silicone**

**Silicone No. 2** ointment OTC *skin protectant* [silicone; hydrophobic starch derivative] 10%• $\triangleq$

**silicone oil** [see: polydimethylsiloxane]

**silicristin** INN

**silidianin** INN

**Silly Putty** street drug slang [see: psilocybin; psilocin]

**silodrate** USAN *antacid* [also: simaldrate]

**Silphen Cough** syrup OTC *antihistamine; antitussive* [diphenhydramine HCl; alcohol 5%] 12.5 mg/5 mL

**Silphen DM** syrup OTC *antitussive* [dextromethorphan hydrobromide; alcohol 5%] 10 mg/5 mL

**Siltapp with Dextromethorphan HBr Cold & Cough** elixir Ŗ *antitussive; decongestant; antihistamine* [dextromethorphan hydrobromide; phenylpropanolamine HCl; brompheniramine maleate] 10•12.5• 2 mg/5 mL

**Sil-Tex** liquid Ŗ *decongestant; expectorant* [phenylpropanolamine HCl; phenylephrine HCl; guaifenesin; alcohol 5%] 20•5•100 mg/5 mL

**Siltussin** syrup OTC *expectorant* [guaifenesin; alcohol 3.5%] 100 mg/5 mL

**Siltussin DM** syrup OTC *antitussive; expectorant* [dextromethorphan hydrobromide; guaifenesin] 10•100 mg/5 mL

**Siltussin-CF** liquid OTC *antitussive; decongestant; expectorant* [dextromethorphan hydrobromide; phenylpropanolamine HCl; guaifenesin; alcohol 4.75%] 10•12.5•100 mg/5 mL

**Silvadene** cream ℞ *broad-spectrum bactericidal for adjunctive burn treatment* [silver sulfadiazine] 10 mg/g

**silver** *element (Ag)*

**silver nitrate** USP *ophthalmic neonatal anti-infective; strong caustic* 1% eye drops; 10%, 25%, 50%, 75% topical

**silver nitrate, toughened** USP *caustic*

**silver protein, mild** NF *ophthalmic antiseptic; ophthalmic surgical aid*

**silver sulfadiazine (SSD)** USAN, USP *broad-spectrum bactericidal; adjunct to burn therapy* [also: sulfadiazine silver]

**Simaal; Simaal II** gel (renamed Simaal Gel; Simaal Gel 2 in 1994)

**Simaal Gel; Simaal Gel 2** liquid OTC *antacid; antiflatulent* [aluminum hydroxide; magnesium hydroxide; simethicone] 200•200•20 mg/5 mL; 500•400•40 mg/5 mL

**simaldrate** INN *antacid* [also: silodrate]

**simethicone** USAN, USP *antiflatulent* 80 mg oral; 40 mg/0.6 mL oral

**simetride** INN

**simfibrate** INN

**Similac Low Iron** liquid, powder OTC *total or supplementary infant feeding*

**Similac PM 60/40 Low-Iron** liquid OTC *formula for infants predisposed to hypocalcemia* [whey formula with lowered mineral levels]

**Similac with Iron** liquid, powder OTC *total or supplementary infant feeding*

**Simple Simon** *street drug slang* [see: psilocybin; psilocin]

**simple syrup** [see: syrup]

**Simplet** tablets OTC *decongestant; antihistamine; analgesic* [pseudoephedrine HCl; chlorpheniramine maleate; acetaminophen] 60•4•650 mg ☒ Singlet

**Simron** soft gelatin capsules OTC *hematinic* [ferrous gluconate] 86 mg

**Simron Plus** capsules OTC *vitamin/iron supplement* [multiple vitamins; ferrous gluconate; folic acid] ±•10•0.1 mg

**simtrazene** USAN, INN *antineoplastic*

**simvastatin** USAN, INN, BAN *antihyperlipidemic; HMG-CoA reductase inhibitor*

**Sinapils** tablets OTC *decongestant; antihistamine; analgesic* [phenylpropanolamine HCl; chlorpheniramine maleate; acetaminophen; caffeine] 12.5•2•325•32.5 mg

**Sinarest; Sinarest Sinus** tablets OTC *decongestant; antihistamine; analgesic* [pseudoephedrine HCl; chlorpheniramine maleate; acetaminophen] 30•2•500 mg; 30•2•325 mg

**Sinarest, No Drowsiness** tablets OTC *decongestant; analgesic; antipyretic* [pseudoephedrine HCl; acetaminophen] 30•500 mg

**Sinarest 12 Hour** nasal spray OTC *nasal decongestant* [oxymetazoline HCl] 0.05%

**sincalide** USAN, INN *choleretic*

**Sine-Aid** tablets, caplets, gelcaps OTC *decongestant; analgesic; antipyretic* [pseudoephedrine HCl; acetaminophen] 30•500 mg

**Sine-Aid IB** caplets OTC *decongestant; analgesic* [pseudoephedrine HCl; ibuprofen] 30•200 mg

**sinefungin** USAN, INN *antifungal*

**Sinemet 10/100; Sinemet 25/100; Sinemet 25/250** tablets ℞ *antiparkinsonian* [carbidopa; levodopa] 10•100 mg; 25•100 mg; 25•250 mg

**Sinemet CR** sustained-release tablets ℞ *antiparkinsonian* [carbidopa; levodopa] 25•100, 50•200 mg

**Sine-Off Allergy/Sinus** caplets (name changed to Sine-Off Sinus Medicine in 1995)

**Sine-Off No Drowsiness Formula** caplets OTC *decongestant; analgesic; antipyretic* [pseudoephedrine HCl; acetaminophen] 30•500 mg

**Sine-Off Sinus Medicine** caplets OTC *decongestant; antihistamine; analgesic* [pseudoephedrine HCl; chlorpheniramine maleate; acetaminophen] 30•2•500 mg

**Sine-Off Sinus Medicine** tablets (discontinued 1995) OTC *decongestant; antihistamine; analgesic; antipyretic* [phenylpropanolamine HCl; chlorpheniramine maleate; aspirin] 12.5•2•325 mg

**Sinequan** capsules, oral concentrate ℞ *tricyclic antidepressant; anxiolytic* [doxepin HCl] 10, 25, 50, 75, 100, 150 mg; 10 mg/mL

**Sinex** nasal spray OTC *nasal decongestant* [phenylephrine HCl] 0.5%

**Sinex 12-Hour** nasal spray OTC *nasal decongestant* [oxymetazoline HCl] 0.05%

**Sinex Long-Acting** nasal spray (name changed to Sinex 12-Hour in 1994)

**single-chain antigen-binding proteins (SCA proteins)** *a class of investigational antineoplastics*

**Singlet for Adults** tablets OTC *decongestant; antihistamine; analgesic* [pseudoephedrine HCl; chlorpheniramine maleate; acetaminophen] 60•4•650 mg ⍰ Simplet

**Sinografin** intracavitary instillation ℞ *radiopaque agent* [diatrizoate meglumine; iodipamide meglumine] 52.7%•26.8%

**sinorphan** [now: ecadotril]

**sinse; sinsemilla** *street drug slang for a potent variety of marijuana* [see: marijuana]

**sintropium bromide** INN

**Sinubid** sustained-release tablets (discontinued 1993) ℞ *decongestant; antihistamine; analgesic* [phenylpropanolamine HCl; phenyltoloxamine citrate; acetaminophen]

**Sinufed** Timecelles (sustained-release capsules) ℞ *decongestant; expectorant* [pseudoephedrine HCl; guaifenesin] 60•300 mg

**Sinulin** tablets OTC *decongestant; antihistamine; analgesic* [phenylpropanolamine HCl; chlorpheniramine maleate; acetaminophen] 25•4•650 mg

**Sinumist-SR** sustained-release Capsulets (capsule-shaped tablet) ℞ *expectorant* [guaifenesin] 600 mg

**Sinupan** controlled-release capsules ℞ *decongestant; expectorant* [phenylephrine HCl; guaifenesin] 40•200 mg

**Sinus Headache & Congestion** tablets OTC *decongestant; antihistamine; analgesic* [pseudoephedrine HCl; chlorpheniramine maleate; acetaminophen] 30•2•500 mg

**Sinus Relief** tablets OTC *decongestant; analgesic* [pseudoephedrine HCl; acetaminophen] 30•325 mg

**Sinusol-B** subcu or IM injection ℞ *antihistamine; anaphylaxis* [brompheniramine maleate] 10 mg/mL

**SinuStat** capsules OTC *decongestant* [pseudoephedrine HCl]

**Sinustop Pro** capsules OTC *nasal decongestant* [pseudoephedrine HCl] 60 mg

**Sinutab Non-Drying** liquid capsules OTC *decongestant; expectorant* [pseudoephedrine HCl; guaifenesin] 30•200 mg

**Sinutab Sinus Allergy** caplets, tablets OTC *decongestant; antihistamine; analgesic* [pseudoephedrine HCl; chlorpheniramine maleate; acetaminophen] 30•2•500 mg

**Sinutab Without Drowsiness** caplets OTC *decongestant; analgesic; antipyretic* [pseudoephedrine HCl; acetaminophen] 30•500 mg

**Sinutab Without Drowsiness** tablets OTC *decongestant; analgesic; antipyretic* [pseudoephedrine HCl; acetaminophen] 30•325 mg; 30•500 mg

**Sinutrex** tablets (discontinued 1995) OTC *decongestant; antihistamine; analgesic* [pseudoephedrine HCl; chlorpheniramine maleate; acetaminophen] 30•2•500 mg

**SinuVent** long-acting tablets ℞ *decongestant; expectorant* [phenylpropanolamine HCl; guaifenesin] 75•600 mg

**Sirdalud** (foreign name for U.S. product Zanaflex)

**sirolimus** USAN *immunosuppressant*

**sisomicin** USAN, INN *antibacterial* [also: sissomicin]

**sisomicin sulfate** USAN, USP *antibacterial*

**sissomicin** BAN *antibacterial* [also: sisomicin]

**sitalidone** INN

**sitofibrate** INN

**sitogluside** USAN, INN *antiprostatic hypertrophy*

**sitosterols** NF

**Sitzmarks** capsules ℞ *GI contrast radiopaque agent* [radiopaque polyvinyl chloride] 20 rings

**619C** *investigational treatment for stroke*

**sixty-second trip** *street drug slang* [see: amyl nitrite]

**sizofiran** INN

**SK (streptokinase)** [q.v.]

**skee** *street drug slang* [see: opium]

**Skeeter Stik** liquid OTC *topical local anesthetic; counterirritant* [lidocaine; menthol] 4%•1%

**Skelaxin** tablets R *skeletal muscle relaxant* [metaxalone] 400 mg

**Skelid** tablets R *bisphosphonate bone resorption inhibitor for Paget's disease* [tiludronate disodium] 240 mg

**SK&F 97426** *investigational antihyperlipidemic*

**SK&F 106203** *investigational leukotriene antagonist for asthma*

**SK&F 110679** *orphan status withdrawn 1996*

**skid** *street drug slang* [see: heroin]

**skin respiratory factor (SRF)** *claimed to promote wound healing*

**Skin Shield** liquid OTC *skin protectant; topical local anesthetic* [dyclonine HCl; benzethonium chloride] 0.75%•0.2%

**Skinoren** (German name for U.S. product Azelex)

**skunk** *street drug slang* [see: marijuana]

**SL (sodium lactate)** [q.v.]

**slab** *street drug slang* [see: cocaine, crack]

**sleeper** *street drug slang* [see: heroin]

**Sleep-Eze 3** tablets OTC *antihistaminic sleep aid* [diphenhydramine HCl] 25 mg

**Sleepinal** capsules, soft gels OTC *antihistaminic sleep aid* [diphenhydramine HCl] 50 mg

**Sleepwell 2-nite** tablets OTC *antihistaminic sleep aid* [diphenhydramine HCl] 25 mg

**sleet** *street drug slang* [see: cocaine, crack]

**slick superspeed** *street drug slang* [see: methcathinone]

**slime** *street drug slang* [see: heroin]

**Slim-Mint** gum OTC *decrease taste perception of sweetness* [benzocaine] 6 mg

**Slo-bid** Gyrocaps (extended-release capsules) R *antiasthmatic; bronchodilator* [theophylline] 50, 75, 100, 125, 200, 300 mg

**Slocaps** (trademarked form) *sustained-release capsules*

**Slo-Niacin** controlled-release tablets OTC *nutritional supplement* [niacin] 250, 500, 750 mg

**Slo-phyllin** tablets, syrup, Gyrocaps (extended-release capsules) R *antiasthmatic; bronchodilator* [theophylline] 100, 200 mg; 80 mg/15 mL; 60, 125, 250 mg

**Slo-phyllin GG** capsules, syrup R *antiasthmatic; bronchodilator; expectorant* [theophylline; guaifenesin] 150•90 mg; 150•90 mg/15 mL

**Slo-Salt** slow-release tablets (discontinued 1993) OTC *sodium chloride replacement; dehydration preventative* [sodium chloride] 600 mg

**Slo-Salt-K** slow-release tablets OTC *sodium chloride/potassium replacement; dehydration preventative* [sodium chloride; potassium chloride] 410•150 mg

**slow channel blockers** *a class of coronary vasodilators that inhibit cardiac muscle contraction and slow electrocardial conduction velocity* [also called: calcium channel blockers; calcium antagonists]

**Slow Fe** slow-release tablets OTC *hematinic* [ferrous sulfate, dried] 160 mg

**Slow Fe with Folic Acid** slow-release tablets OTC *hematinic* [ferrous sulfate; folic acid] 50•0.4 mg

**Slow Fluoride** slow-release tablets R *investigational agent for postmenopausal osteoporosis* [sodium fluoride]

**Slow-K** controlled-release tablets R *potassium supplement* [potassium chloride] 600 mg (8 mEq)

**Slow-Mag** delayed-release enteric-coated tablets OTC *magnesium supplement* [magnesium chloride] 535 mg

**SLT** hair lotion OTC *antiseborrheic; antipsoriatic; keratolytic; antiseptic* [coal tar; salicylic acid; lactic acid; alcohol 65%] 2%•3%•5%

**Slyn-LL** sustained-release capsules (discontinued 1993) R *anorexiant* [phendimetrazine tartrate] 105 mg

**SMA Iron Fortified** liquid, powder (discontinued 1996) OTC *total or supplementary infant feeding*

**SMA Lo-Iron** liquid, powder (discontinued 1996) OTC *total or supplementary infant feeding*

**SMA with Whey** liquid (discontinued 1994) OTC *total or supplementary infant feeding* [whey protein formula]

**smack; schmack; shmeck; schmeck** *street drug slang* [see: heroin]

**smallpox vaccine** USP *active immunizing agent*

**SMART anti-tac; humanized anti-tac** [now: dacliximab]

**smears** *street drug slang* [see: LSD]

**SMF (streptozocin, mitomycin, flu-orouracil)** *chemotherapy protocol*

**smoke** *street drug slang for marijuana, crack, or a combination of heroin and crack* [see: marijuana; cocaine, crack; heroin]

**smoke Canada** *street drug slang* [see: marijuana]

**smoking** *street drug slang* [see: PCP]

**smoking gun** *street drug slang* [see: heroin; cocaine]

**SMX; SMZ (sulfamethoxazole)** [q.v.]

**SMZ-TMP (sulfamethoxazole & trimethoprim)** [q.v.]

**SN (streptonigrin)** [q.v.]

**snakebite antivenin** [see: antivenin, Crotalidae & Micrurus fulvius]

**snap** *street drug slang* [see: amphetamines]

**Snaplets-D** granules (discontinued 1995) OTC *pediatric decongestant and antihistamine* [phenylpropanolamine HCl; chlorpheniramine maleate] 6.25•1 mg/packet

**Snaplets-DM** granules OTC *pediatric antitussive and decongestant* [dextromethorphan hydrobromide; phenylpropanolamine HCl] 5•6.25 mg/packet

**Snaplets-EX** granules OTC *pediatric decongestant and expectorant* [phenylpropanolamine HCl; guaifenesin] 6.25•50 mg/packet

**Snaplets-FR** granules (discontinued 1997) OTC *analgesic; antipyretic* [acetaminophen] 80 mg/packet

**Snaplets-Multi** granules OTC *pediatric antitussive, decongestant, and antihistamine* [dextromethorphan hydrobro-

mide; phenylpropanolamine HCl; chlorpheniramine maleate] 5•6.25•1 mg/packet

**snappers** *street drug slang* [see: amyl nitrite; isobutyl nitrite]

**SnapTab** (trademarked dosage form) *scored tablet*

**SnET2** [see: tin ethyl etiopurpurin]

**sniff** *street drug slang for methcathinone, an inhalant, or to inhale cocaine* [see: methcathinone; petroleum distillate inhalants; cocaine]

**Snooze Fast** tablets OTC *antihistaminic sleep aid* [diphenhydramine HCl] 50 mg

**snop** *street drug slang* [see: marijuana]

**snort** *street drug slang for cocaine or inhalants* [see: cocaine; petroleum distillate inhalants]

**snorts** *street drug slang* [see: PCP]

**Sno-Strips** ophthalmic strips OTC *diagnostic tear flow test aid*

**snot** *street drug slang for the residue produced from smoking amphetamine* [see: amphetamines]

**snot balls** *street drug slang for rubber cement rolled into balls and burned* [see: petroleum distillate inhalants]

**snow** *street drug slang* [see: cocaine; heroin; amphetamines]

**snow bird** *street drug slang* [see: cocaine]

**snow pallets** *street drug slang* [see: amphetamines]

**snow seals** *street drug slang for a combination of cocaine and amphetamine* [see: cocaine; amphetamines]

**snow soke** *street drug slang* [see: cocaine, crack]

**snow white** *street drug slang* [see: cocaine]

**snowball** *street drug slang for a combination of cocaine and heroin* [see: cocaine; heroin]

**snowcones** *street drug slang* [see: cocaine]

**SNX-111** *investigational (Phase III) calcium-channel blocker for neurologic disorders due to severe head trauma*

**Soac-Lens** solution OTC *wetting/soaking solution for hard contact lenses*

**soap** *street drug slang* [see: GHB]

**soap, green** USP *detergent*

**soaper; Sopors** *street drug slang for Sopor (methaqualone; discontinued 1981)* [see: methaqualone]

**society high** *street drug slang* [see: cocaine]

**SOD (superoxide dismutase)** [see: orgotein]

**soda** *street drug slang for injectable cocaine* [see: cocaine]

**soda lime** NF *carbon dioxide absorbent*

**Soda Mint** tablets OTC *antacid* [sodium bicarbonate]

**sodium** *element (Na)*

**sodium acetate** USP *dialysis aid; electrolyte replenisher; pH buffer* 2, 4 mEq/mL (16.4%, 32.8%) injection

**sodium acetate trihydrate** [see: sodium acetate]

**sodium acetrizoate** INN, BAN [also: acetrizoate sodium]

**sodium acetylsalicylate** *analgesic*

**sodium acid phosphate** *urinary acidifier*

**sodium acid pyrophosphate** *urinary acidifier*

**sodium alginate** NF *suspending agent*

**sodium amidotrizoate** INN *radiopaque medium* [also: diatrizoate sodium; sodium diatrizoate]

**sodium aminobenzoate** [see: aminobenzoate sodium]

**sodium amylopectin sulfate** [see: sodium amylosulfate]

**sodium amylosulfate** USAN *enzyme inhibitor*

**sodium anoxynaphthonate** BAN *blood volume and cardiac output test* [also: anazolene sodium]

**sodium antimony gluconate** [see: sodium stibogluconate]

**sodium antimonylgluconate** BAN

**sodium apolate** INN, BAN *anticoagulant* [also: lyapolate sodium]

**sodium arsenate, exsiccated** NF

**sodium arsenate As 74** USAN *radioactive agent*

**sodium ascorbate** USP, INN *vitamin C; antiscorbutic* 500 mg oral; 1800 mg/½ tsp. oral; 222, 500 mg/mL injection

**sodium aurothiomalate** INN *antirheumatic* [also: gold sodium thiomalate]

**sodium aurotiosulfate** INN [also: gold sodium thiosulfate]

**sodium azodisalicylate** [now: olsalazine sodium]

**sodium benzoate** USAN, NF, JAN *antihyperammonemic; antifungal agent; preservative*

**sodium benzoate & sodium phenylacetate** *to prevent and treat hyperammonemia of urea cycle enzymopathy (orphan)*

**sodium benzyl penicillin** [see: penicillin G sodium]

**sodium bicarbonate** USP *electrolyte replenisher; systemic alkalizer; antacid* 325, 600, 650 mg oral; 0.5, 0.6, 0.9, 1 mEq/mL (4.2%, 5%, 7.5%, 8.4%) injection

**sodium biphosphate** *urinary acidifier; pH buffer*

**sodium bisulfite** NF *antioxidant*

**sodium bitionolate** INN *topical antiinfective* [also: bithionolate sodium]

**sodium borate** NF *alkalizing agent; antipruritic*

**sodium borocaptate ($^{10}$B)** INN *antineoplastic; radioactive agent* [also: borocaptate sodium B 10]

**sodium cacodylate** NF

**sodium calcium edetate** INN *heavy metal chelating agent* [also: edetate calcium disodium; sodium calciumedetate; calcium disodium edetate]

**sodium calciumedetate** BAN *heavy metal chelating agent* [also: edetate calcium disodium; sodium calcium edetate; calcium disodium edetate]

**sodium caprylate** *antifungal*

**sodium carbonate** NF *alkalizing agent*

**sodium chloride (NaCl)** USP *ophthalmic hypertonic; electrolyte replacement; abortifacient* [sterile isotonic solution] 650, 1000, 2250 mg oral; 0.45%, 0.9%, 3%, 5%, 14.6%, 23.4% injection

**0.45% sodium chloride (½ normal saline; ½ NS)** *electrolyte replacement*

**0.9% sodium chloride (normal saline; NS)** *electrolyte replacement* [also: saline solution]

**sodium chloride, compound solution of** INN *fluid and electrolyte replenisher* [also: Ringer's injection]

**sodium chloride Na 22** USAN *radio-active agent*

**sodium chondroitin sulfate** [see: chondroitin sulfate sodium]

**sodium chromate (⁵¹Cr)** INN *blood volume test; radioactive agent* [also: sodium chromate Cr 51]

**sodium chromate Cr 51** USAN *blood volume test; radioactive agent* [also: sodium chromate (⁵¹Cr)]

**sodium citrate** USP *systemic alkalizer; pH buffer; antacid; investigational (orphan) for leukapheresis procedures*

**sodium colistin methanesulfonate** [see: colistimethate sodium]

**sodium cyclamate** NF, INN

**sodium cyclohexanesulfamate** [see: sodium cyclamate]

**sodium dehydroacetate** NF *antimicrobial preservative*

**sodium dehydrocholate** INN [also: dehydrocholate sodium]

**sodium denyl** [see: phenytoin sodium]

**sodium diatrizoate** BAN *radiopaque medium* [also: diatrizoate sodium; sodium amidotrizoate]

**sodium dibunate** INN, BAN

**sodium dicloroacetate** *investigational (orphan) for lactic acidosis and homozygous familial hypercholesterolemia*

**sodium diethyldithiocarbamate** [see: ditiocarb sodium]

**sodium diiodomethanesulfonate** [see: dimethiodal sodium]

**sodium dioctyl sulfosuccinate** INN *stool softener; surfactant* [also: docusate sodium]

**sodium diphenylhydantoin** [see: phenytoin sodium]

**sodium diprotrizoate** INN, BAN [also: diprotrizoate sodium]

**Sodium Diuril** powder for IV injection ℞ *diuretic* [chlorothiazide] 500 mg

**sodium edetate** [see: edetate sodium]

**sodium etasulfate** INN *detergent* [also: sodium ethasulfate]

**sodium ethasulfate** USAN *detergent* [also: sodium etasulfate]

**sodium feredetate** INN [also: sodium ironedetate]

**sodium fluoride** USP *dental caries preventative; investigational agent for treat-*

ment of postmenopausal osteoporosis 1.1, 2.2 mg oral; 0.125 mg/drop oral

**sodium fluoride F 18** USP

**sodium fluoride & phosphoric acid** USP *dental caries prophylactic*

**sodium formaldehyde sulfoxylate** NF *preservative*

**sodium gammahydroxyburate** [see: sodium oxybate]

**sodium gentisate** INN

**sodium glucaspaldrate** INN, BAN

**sodium gluconate** USP *electrolyte replenisher*

**sodium glucosulfone** USP

**sodium glutamate**

**sodium glycerophosphate** NF

**sodium glycocholate** [see: bile salts]

**sodium gualenate** INN [also: azulene sulfonate sodium]

**sodium hyaluronate** [see: hyaluronate sodium]

**sodium hydroxide** NF *alkalizing agent*

**sodium hydroxybenzenesulfonate** [see: phenolsulphonate sodium]

**sodium 4-hydroxybutyrate** [see: sodium oxybate]

**sodium hypochlorite** USP, JAN *disinfectant; bleach; used for utensils and equipment*

**sodium hypochlorite, diluted** NF [also: antiformin, dental]

**sodium hypophosphite** NF

**sodium iodide** USP *dietary iodine supplement*

**sodium iodide (¹²³I)** JAN *thyroid function test; radioactive agent* [also: sodium iodide I 123]

**sodium iodide (¹²⁵I)** INN *thyroid function test; radioactive agent* [also: sodium iodide I 125]

**sodium iodide (¹³¹I)** JAN *antineoplastic for thyroid carcinoma; radioactive agent for hyperthyroidism* [also: sodium iodide I 131]

**sodium iodide I 123** USP *thyroid function test; radioactive agent* [also: sodium iodide (¹²³I)] 3.7, 7.4 MBq oral

**sodium iodide I 125** USAN, USP *thyroid function test; radioactive agent* [also: sodium iodide (¹²⁵I)]

**sodium iodide I 131** USAN, USP, INN *antineoplastic for thyroid carcinoma;*

*radioactive agent for hyperthyroidism*
[also: sodium iodide ($^{131}$I)] 0.75–100
mCi, 3.5–150 mCi oral

**sodium iodohippurate ($^{131}$I)** INN, JAN
*renal function test; radioactive agent*
[also: iodohippurate sodium I 131]

**sodium iodomethanesulfonate** [see:
methiodal sodium]

**sodium iopodate** JAN *cholecystographic
radiopaque medium* [also: ipodate
sodium; sodium iopodate]

**sodium iotalamate ($^{125}$I)** INN *radioactive agent* [also: iothalamate
sodium I 125]

**sodium iotalamate ($^{131}$I)** INN *radioactive agent* [also: iothalamate
sodium I 131]

**sodium iothalamate** BAN *radiopaque
medium* [also: iothalamate sodium]

**sodium ioxaglate** BAN *radiopaque
medium* [also: ioxaglate sodium]

**sodium ipodate** INN, BAN *cholecystographic radiopaque medium* [also: ipodate sodium; sodium iopodate]

**sodium ironedetate** BAN [also:
sodium feredetate]

**sodium lactate (SL)** USP *electrolyte
replenisher* 167 mEq/L (1/6 molar)
injection

**sodium lactate, compound solution
of** INN *electrolyte and fluid replenisher;
systemic alkalizer* [also: Ringer's injection, lactated]

**sodium lauryl sulfate** NF *surfactant/
wetting agent* [also: laurilsulfate]

**sodium lignosulfonate** [see: polignate sodium]

**sodium metabisulfite** NF *antioxidant*

**sodium metrizoate** INN *radiopaque
medium* [also: metrizoate sodium]

**sodium monododecyl sulfate** [see:
sodium lauryl sulfate]

**sodium monofluorophosphate** USP
*dental caries prophylactic*

**sodium monomercaptoundecahy-
dro-closo-dodecaborate** *investigational (orphan) for boron neutron capture therapy (BNCT) for glioblastoma
multiforme*

**sodium morrhuate** INN *sclerosing
agent* [also: morrhuate sodium]

**sodium nitrite** USP *antidote to cyanide
poisoning*

**sodium nitroferricyanide** [see:
sodium nitroprusside]

**sodium nitroferricyanide dihydrate**
[see: sodium nitroprusside]

**sodium nitroprusside** USP *emergency
antihypertensive* 50 mg/dose injection

**sodium noramidopyrine methane-
sulfonate** [see: dipyrone]

**sodium oxybate** USAN *adjunct to anesthesia; investigational (orphan) for narcolepsy, cataplexy, sleep paralysis, and
hypnagogic hallucinations*

**sodium oxychlorosene** [see: oxychlorosene sodium]

**sodium paratoluenesulfan chlora-
mide** [see: chloramine-T]

**Sodium P.A.S.** tablets (discontinued
1996) ℞ *tuberculostatic* [aminosali-
cylate sodium] 500 mg

**sodium penicillin G** [see: penicillin
G sodium]

**sodium pentosan polysulfate** [see:
pentosan polysulfate sodium]

**sodium perborate** *topical antiseptic/
germicidal*

**sodium perborate monohydrate**
USAN

**sodium pertechnetate Tc 99m**
USAN, USP *radioactive agent*

**sodium phenolate** [see: phenolate
sodium]

**sodium phenylacetate** USAN *antihyperammonemic*

**sodium phenylacetate & sodium
benzoate** *to prevent and treat hyperammonemia of urea cycle enzymopathy
(orphan)*

**sodium phenylbutyrate** USAN *antihyperammonemic for urea cycle disorders
(orphan); investigational (orphan) for
various sickling disorders*

**sodium phosphate ($^{32}$P)** INN *antineoplastic; antipolycythemic; neoplasm test*
[also: sodium phosphate P 32]

**sodium phosphate, dibasic** USP
*saline laxative; phosphorus replace-
ment; pH buffer*

**sodium phosphate, monobasic** USP
*phosphorus replacement; pH buffer*

**sodium phosphate P 32** USAN, USP *antipolycythemic; radiopharmaceutical antineoplastic for various leukemias and skeletal metastases* [also: sodium phosphate ($^{32}$P)] 0.67 mCi/mL

**sodium picofosfate** INN

**sodium picosulfate** INN

**sodium polyphosphate** USAN *pharmaceutic aid*

**sodium polystyrene sulfonate** USP *potassium-removing ion-exchange resin* 15 g/60 mL oral

**sodium propionate** NF *preservative; antifungal*

**sodium propionate hydrate** [see: sodium propionate]

**sodium 2-propylvalerate** [see: valproate sodium]

**sodium psylliate** NF

**sodium pyrophosphate** USAN *pharmaceutic aid*

**sodium radiochromate** [see: sodium chromate Cr 51]

**sodium rhodanate** [see: thiocyanate sodium]

**sodium salicylate (SS)** USP *analgesic; antipyretic; anti-inflammatory; antirheumatic* 325, 650 mg oral

**sodium starch glycolate** NF *tablet excipient*

**sodium stearate** NF *emulsifying and stiffening agent*

**sodium stearyl fumarate** NF *tablet and capsule lubricant*

**sodium stibocaptate** INN [also: stibocaptate]

**sodium stibogluconate** INN, BAN, DCF *investigational antiparasitic for leishmaniasis and trypanosomiasis*

**Sodium Sulamyd** eye drops, ophthalmic ointment Ŗ *ophthalmic bacteriostatic* [sulfacetamide sodium] 10%, 30%; 10%

**sodium sulfacetamide** [see: sulfacetamide sodium]

**sodium sulfate** USP *calcium regulator*

**sodium sulfate S 35** USAN *radioactive agent*

**sodium sulfocyanate** [see: thiocyanate sodium]

**sodium taurocholate** [see: bile salts]

**sodium tetradecyl (STD) sulfate** INN *sclerosing agent; investigational (orphan) for bleeding esophageal varices*

**sodium thiomalate, gold** [see: gold sodium thiomalate]

**sodium thiosalicylate** *analgesic; antipyretic; anti-inflammatory; antirheumatic* 50 mg/mL injection

**sodium thiosulfate** USP *antidote to cyanide poisoning; antiseptic; antifungal* 25% (250 mg/mL) IV injection

**sodium thiosulfate, gold** [see: gold sodium thiosulfate]

**sodium timerfonate** INN *topical anti-infective* [also: thimerfonate sodium]

**sodium trimetaphosphate** USAN *pharmaceutic aid*

**sodium tyropanoate** INN *cholecystographic radiopaque medium* [also: tyropanoate sodium]

**sodium valproate** [see: valproate sodium]

**Sodol** tablets Ŗ *skeletal muscle relaxant* [carisoprodol]

**Sodol Compound** tablets Ŗ *skeletal muscle relaxant; analgesic* [carisoprodol; aspirin] 200•325 mg

**sofalcone** INN

**Sofarin** tablets (discontinued 1995) Ŗ *anticoagulant* [warfarin sodium] 2, 2.5, 5 mg

**Sofenol 5** lotion OTC *moisturizer; emollient*

**Sof/Pro-Clean; Sof/Pro-Clean (s.a.)** solution (discontinued 1995) OTC *surfactant cleaning solution for soft contact lenses*

**Soft Mate Comfort Drops for Sensitive Eyes** OTC *rewetting solution for soft contact lenses*

**Soft Mate Consept** solution + aerosol spray OTC *two-step chemical disinfecting system for soft contact lenses* [hydrogen peroxide based] 3%

**Soft Mate Daily Cleaning for Sensitive Eyes** solution (discontinued 1995) OTC *surfactant cleaning solution for soft contact lenses*

**Soft Mate Disinfecting for Sensitive Eyes** solution OTC *chemical disinfecting solution for soft contact lenses*

**Soft Mate Enzyme Plus Cleaner** tablets (discontinued 1995) OTC *enzymatic cleaner for soft contact lenses*

**Soft Mate Hands Off Daily Cleaner** solution OTC *surfactant cleaning solution for soft contact lenses*

**Soft Mate Protein Remover** solution (discontinued 1993) OTC *surfactant cleaning solution for soft contact lenses*

**Soft Mate Saline for Sensitive Eyes** solution (discontinued 1995) OTC *rinsing/storage solution for soft contact lenses* [preserved saline solution]

**Soft Rinse 135** tablets (discontinued 1993) OTC *rinsing/storage solution for soft contact lenses* [sodium chloride for normal saline solution] 135 mg

**Soft Rinse 250** tablets (discontinued 1995) OTC *rinsing/storage solution for soft contact lenses* [sodium chloride for normal saline solution] 250 mg

**Soft Sense** lotion OTC *moisturizer; emollient*

**Softabs** (trademarked dosage form) *chewable tablets*

**softgels** (dosage form) *soft gelatin capsules*

**Soft-Stress** capsules (discontinued 1995) OTC *vitamin/mineral/calcium/ iron supplement* [multiple vitamins & minerals; calcium; iron; folic acid; biotin] ≐•50•4.5•0.05•≐ mg

**SoftWear** solution OTC *rinsing/storage solution for soft contact lenses* [preserved saline solution]

**sol particle immunoassay (SPIA)** *detects hCG in urine for pregnancy testing*

**solapsone** BAN [also: solasulfone]

**Solaquin** cream OTC *hyperpigmentation bleaching agent in a sunscreen base* [hydroquinone] 2%

**Solaquin Forte** cream, gel ℞ *hyperpigmentation bleaching agent; sunscreen* [hydroquinone; ethyl dihydroxypropyl PABA; dioxybenzone; oxybenzone] 4%•5%•3%•2%

**Solarase** ℞ *investigational (Phase III) topical treatment for actinic keratosis* [hyaluronate sodium; diclofenac potassium]

**Solarcaine** aerosol spray, lotion OTC *topical local anesthetic; antiseptic* [benzocaine; triclosan] 20%•0.13%

**Solarcaine** cream (name changed to Solarcaine Aloe Extra Burn Relief in 1995)

**Solarcaine Aloe Extra Burn Relief** spray, gel, cream OTC *topical local anesthetic* [lidocaine] 0.5%

**solasulfone** INN [also: solapsone]

**Solatene** capsules (discontinued 1996) ℞ *to reduce photosensitivity reaction* [beta-carotene] 30 mg

**soles** *street drug slang* [see: hashish]

**Solfoton** tablets, capsules ℞ *long-acting barbiturate sedative, hypnotic and anticonvulsant* [phenobarbital] 16 mg

**Solganal** IM injection ℞ *antirheumatic* [aurothioglucose] 50 mg/mL

**solpecainol** INN

**Soltice Quick-Rub** OTC *counterirritant* [methyl salicylate; camphor; menthol; eucalyptus oil]

**soluble complement receptor** [see: complement receptor type I, soluble recombinant human]

**soluble ferric pyrophosphate** [see: ferric pyrophosphate, soluble]

**soluble gelatin (SG)** [see: gelatin]

**Soluble T4** ℞ *orphan status withdrawn 1996* [CD4, human truncated 369 AA polypeptide]

**Solu-Cortef** powder for IV or IM injection ℞ *glucocorticoids* [hydrocortisone sodium succinate] 100, 250, 500, 1000 mg/vial

**Solu-Medrol** powder for IV or IM injection ℞ *glucocorticoid; anti-inflammatory; immunosuppressant* [methylprednisolone sodium succinate] 40, 125, 500, 1000, 2000 mg/vial

**Solumol** OTC *ointment base*

**Solurex** intra-articular, intralesional, soft tissue, or IM injection ℞ *glucocorticoids* [dexamethasone sodium phosphate] 4 mg/mL

**Solurex LA** intralesional, intra-articular, soft tissue, or IM injection ℞ *glucocorticoids* [dexamethasone acetate] 8 mg/mL

**Soluspan** (trademarked form) *injectable suspension*

**Soluvite C.T.** chewable tablets ℞ *pediatric vitamin supplement and dental caries preventative* [multiple vitamins; fluoride; folic acid] ± • 1 • 0.3 mg

**Soluvite-f** drops ℞ *pediatric vitamin supplement and dental caries preventative* [vitamins A, C, and D; fluoride] 1500 IU • 35 mg • 400 IU • 0.25 mg per 0.6 mL

**Solvent-G** OTC *liquid base*

**Solvet** (trademarked dosage form) *soluble tablet*

**solypertine** INN *antiadrenergic* [also: solypertine tartrate]

**solypertine tartrate** USAN *antiadrenergic* [also: solypertine]

**soma** (Italian for "burden" or "load") *street drug slang* [see: PCP]

**Soma** tablets ℞ *skeletal muscle relaxant* [carisoprodol] 350 mg

**Soma Compound** tablets ℞ *skeletal muscle relaxant; analgesic* [carisoprodol; aspirin] 200 • 325 mg

**Soma Compound with Codeine** tablets ℞ *skeletal muscle relaxant; analgesic* [carisoprodol; aspirin; codeine phosphate] 200 • 325 • 16 mg

**Somagard** ℞ *investigational (orphan) LHRH agonist for central precocious puberty* [deslorelin]

**somagrebove** USAN *veterinary galactopoietic agent*

**somalapor** USAN, INN, BAN *porcine growth hormone*

**somantadine** INN *antiviral* [also: somantadine HCl]

**somantadine HCl** USAN *antiviral* [also: somantadine]

**somatomax** *street drug slang* [see: GHB]

**somatomedin-C** [see: insulin-like growth factor-1]

**somatorelin** INN *growth hormone-releasing factor (GH-RF)*

**somatostatin (SS)** INN, BAN *growth hormone-release inhibiting factor; investigational (orphan) for cutaneous gastrointestinal fistulas and bleeding esophageal varices*

**somatotropin, human** [see: somatropin]

**Somatrel** ℞ *investigational (orphan) diagnostic aid for pituitary release of growth hormone* [NG-29 (code name—generic name not yet approved)]

**somatrem** USAN, INN, BAN *growth hormone for congenital growth failure (orphan) or due to chronic renal insufficiency; investigational (orphan) for Turner syndrome*

**somatropin** USAN, INN, BAN, JAN *growth hormone for congenital or renal-induced growth failure (orphan); investigational (orphan) for Turner syndrome, severe burns and AIDS* [also: human growth hormone]

**somatropin & glutamine** *investigational (orphan) for GI malabsorption due to short bowel syndrome*

**somavubove** USAN, INN *veterinary galactopoietic agent*

**somenopor** USAN *porcine growth hormone*

**sometribove** USAN, INN, BAN *veterinary growth stimulant*

**sometripor** USAN, INN, BAN *veterinary growth stimulant*

**somfasepor** USAN *veterinary growth stimulant*

**somidobove** USAN, INN *synthetic bovine growth hormone*

**Sominex** tablets, caplets OTC *antihistaminic sleep aid* [diphenhydramine HCl] 25 mg; 50 mg

**Sominex 2** tablets (name changed to Sominex in 1993)

**Sominex Pain Relief** tablets OTC *antihistaminic sleep aid; analgesic* [diphenhydramine HCl; acetaminophen] 25 • 500 mg

**SonoRx** ℞ *investigational ultrasound contrast agent* [cellulose]

**Soothaderm** lotion OTC *topical anesthetic; topical antihistamine; emollient* [pyrilamine maleate; benzocaine; zinc oxide] 2.07 • 2.08 • 41.35 mg/mL

**Soothe** eye drops (discontinued 1995) OTC *topical ocular decongestant/vasoconstrictor* [tetrahydrozoline HCl] 0.05%

**Soothers Throat Drops** lozenges (discontinued 1995) OTC *topical antipruritic/counterirritant; mild local anesthetic* [menthol] 2 mg

**sopecainol** [see: solpecainol]

**sopitazine** INN

**Sopors; soaper** *street drug slang for Sopor (methaqualone; discontinued 1981)* [see: methaqualone]

**Soprodol** tablets (discontinued 1993) ℞ *skeletal muscle relaxant* [carisoprodol]

**sopromidine** INN

**soquinolol** INN

**sorbic acid** NF *antimicrobial agent; preservative*

**sorbimacrogol laurate 300** [see: polysorbate 20]

**sorbimacrogol oleate 300** [see: polysorbate 80]

**sorbimacrogol palmitate 300** [see: polysorbate 40]

**sorbimacrogol stearate** [see: polysorbate 60]

**sorbimacrogol tristearate 300** [see: polysorbate 65]

**sorbinicate** INN

**sorbinil** USAN, INN, BAN *aldose reductase enzyme inhibitor*

**sorbitan laurate** INN *surfactant* [also: sorbitan monolaurate]

**sorbitan monolaurate** USAN, NF *surfactant* [also: sorbitan laurate]

**sorbitan monooleate** USAN, NF *surfactant* [also: sorbitan oleate]

**sorbitan monopalmitate** USAN, NF *surfactant* [also: sorbitan palmitate]

**sorbitan monostearate** USAN, NF *surfactant* [also: sorbitan stearate]

**sorbitan oleate** INN *surfactant* [also: sorbitan monooleate]

**sorbitan palmitate** INN *surfactant* [also: sorbitan monopalmitate]

**sorbitan sesquioleate** USAN, INN *surfactant*

**sorbitan stearate** INN *surfactant* [also: sorbitan monostearate]

**sorbitan trioleate** USAN, INN *surfactant*

**sorbitan tristearate** USAN, INN *surfactant*

**sorbitol** NF *flavoring agent; tablet excipient; urologic irrigant* 3%, 3.3%

**sorbitol (solution)** USP *flavoring agent; tablet excipient*

**Sorbitrate** tablets, sublingual tablets, chewable tablets ℞ *antianginal* [iso-sorbide dinitrate] 5, 10, 20, 30, 40 mg; 2.5, 5 mg; 5, 10 mg

**Sorbitrate SA** sustained-action tablets (discontinued 1995) ℞ *antianginal* [isosorbide dinitrate]

**Sorbsan** pads, wound packing ℞ *wound dressing* [calcium alginate fiber]

**Soretts** lozenges (discontinued 1993) OTC *topical oral anesthetic; antipruritic/counterirritant* [benzocaine; menthol] 32•0.5 mg

**Soriatane** ⒸⒶⓃ capsules ℞ *synthetic retinoid for psoriasis; investigational in the U.S.* [acitretin] 10, 25 mg

**sorivudine** USAN, INN, BAN *antiviral for varicella zoster and herpes zoster in immunocompromised patients; orphan status withdrawn 1997*

**sornidipine** INN

**SOSS-10** eye drops (discontinued 1993) ℞ *ophthalmic bacteriostatic* [sodium sulfacetamide]

**sotalol** INN, BAN *antiadrenergic (β-receptor)* [also: sotalol HCl]

**sotalol HCl** USAN *antiadrenergic (β-receptor) for ventricular arrhythmias (orphan)* [also: sotalol]

**soterenol** INN *adrenergic; bronchodilator* [also: soterenol HCl]

**soterenol HCl** USAN *adrenergic; bronchodilator* [also: soterenol]

**Sotradecol** IV injection, Dosette (unit-of-use injection) ℞ *sclerosing agent; investigational (orphan) for bleeding esophageal varices* [sodium tetradecyl sulfate] 1%, 3%

**Soviet gramicidin** [see: gramicidin S]

**Soyalac; I-Soyalac** liquid, powder OTC *hypoallergenic infant food* [soy protein formula]

**soybean oil** USP *pharmaceutic necessity*

**space base** *street drug slang for crack dipped in PCP or a hollowed-out cigar refilled with PCP and crack* [see: cocaine, crack; PCP]

**space cadet; space dust** *street drug slang for crack dipped in PCP* [see: cocaine, crack; PCP]

**spaglumic acid** INN

**Span C** tablets OTC *dietary supplement* [vitamin C; citrus & rose hips bioflavonoids] 200•300 mg

**Spancap No. 1** sustained-release capsules ℞ *CNS stimulant* [dextroamphetamine sulfate] 15 mg

**Spancaps** (dosage form) *timed-release capsules*

**Span-FF** controlled-release capsules OTC *hematinic* [ferrous fumarate] 325 mg

**Spanidin** *investigational (orphan) immunosuppressant for acute renal graft rejection* [gusperimus]

**Spansule** (trademarked dosage form) *sustained-release capsule*

**sparfloxacin** USAN, INN, BAN *fluoroquinolone antibacterial*

**sparfosate sodium** USAN *antineoplastic* [also: sparfosic acid]

**sparfosic acid** INN *antineoplastic* [also: sparfosate sodium]

**Sparine** tablets, Tubex (cartridge-needle unit for IM injection) ℞ *antipsychotic* [promazine HCl] 25, 50, 100 mg; 50 mg/mL

**sparkle plenty** *street drug slang* [see: amphetamines]

**sparklers** *street drug slang* [see: amphetamines]

**Sparkles** effervescent granules OTC *antacid; aid in endoscopic examination* [sodium bicarbonate; citric acid; simethicone] 2000•1500• $\stackrel{?}{=}$ mg/dose

**sparsomycin** USAN, INN *antineoplastic*

**sparteine** INN *oxytocic* [also: sparteine sulfate]

**sparteine sulfate** USAN *oxytocic* [also: sparteine]

**Spasmoject** IM injection (discontinued 1996) ℞ *gastrointestinal antispasmodic* [dicyclomine HCl] 10 mg/mL

**Spasmolin** capsules (discontinued 1995) ℞ *GI anticholinergic; sedative* [atropine sulfate; scopolamine hydrobromide; hyoscyamine hydrobromide; phenobarbital] 0.0194•0.0065•0.1037•16.2 mg

**Spasmolin** tablets ℞ *GI anticholinergic; sedative* [atropine sulfate; scopolamine hydrobromide; hyoscyamine hydrobromide; phenobarbital] 0.0194•0.0065•0.1037•16.2 mg

**Spasmophen** tablets, elixir (discontinued 1995) ℞ *GI anticholinergic; sedative* [atropine sulfate; scopolamine

hydrobromide; hyoscyamine hydrobromide; phenobarbital] 0.0194•0.0065•0.1037•15 mg; 0.0194•0.0065•0.1037•16.2 mg/5 mL

**Spasquid** elixir (discontinued 1995) ℞ *GI anticholinergic; sedative* [atropine sulfate; scopolamine hydrobromide; hyoscyamine hydrobromide; phenobarbital] 0.0194•0.0065•0.1037•16.2 mg/5 mL

**Spastosed** chewable tablets OTC *antacid* [calcium carbonate; magnesium carbonate]

**SPCA (serum prothrombin conversion accelerator) factor** [see: factor VII]

**spearmint** NF

**spearmint oil** NF

**Special K** *street drug slang* [see: ketamine HCl]

**special la coke** *street drug slang* [see: ketamine HCl]

**Specifid** ℞ *investigational antineoplastic for various B-cell lymphomas (clinical trials discontinued 1994)* [monoclonal antibodies]

**speckled birds; speckled eggs** *street drug slang* [see: amphetamines]

**specks** *street drug slang* [see: LSD]

**Spec-T** lozenges OTC *topical oral anesthetic* [benzocaine] 10 mg

**Spec-T Sore Throat/Cough Suppressant** lozenges OTC *topical oral anesthetic; antitussive* [benzocaine; dextromethorphan hydrobromide] 10•10 mg

**Spec-T Sore Throat/Decongestant** lozenges OTC *decongestant; topical oral anesthetic* [phenylpropanolamine HCl; phenylephrine HCl; benzocaine] 10.5•5•10 mg

**Spectazole** cream ℞ *topical antifungal* [econazole nitrate] 1%

**spectinomycin** INN *bactericidal antibiotic* [also: spectinomycin HCl]

**spectinomycin HCl** USAN, USP *bactericidal antibiotic* [also: spectinomycin]

**Spectrobid** film-coated tablets ℞ *penicillin-type antibiotic* [bacampicillin HCl] 400 mg

**Spectrobid** powder for oral suspension (discontinued 1997) ℞ *penicillin-type antibiotic* [bacampicillin HCl] 125 mg/5 mL

**Spectrocin Plus** ointment OTC *topical antibiotic; local anesthetic* [neomycin sulfate; polymyxin B sulfate; bacitracin; lidocaine] 5000 U•3.5 mg•400 U•5 mg per g

**Spectro-Jel** liquid OTC *soap-free therapeutic skin cleanser*

**speed** *street drug slang* [see: methamphetamine HCl; amphetamine; cocaine, crack; methcathinone]

**speed boat** *street drug slang for a combination of marijuana, PCP, and crack* [see: marijuana; PCP; cocaine, crack]

**speed for lovers** *street drug slang* [see: MDMA]

**speedball** *street drug slang for amphetamine or a combination of heroin and cocaine* [see: amphetamines; heroin; cocaine]

**spenbolic** [see: methandriol]

**spermaceti, synthetic** [see: cetyl esters wax]

**spermicides** *a class of topical contraceptive agents that kill the male sperm*

**Spersadex** ⒸⒶⓃ (U.S. product: Decadron Phosphate) eye drops ℞ *ophthalmic topical corticosteroidal anti-inflammatory* [dexamethasone sodium phosphate] 0.1%

**Spexil** ℞ *investigational broad-spectrum antibiotic for respiratory, gynecologic, and abdominal infections* [trospectomycin]

**Spherex** ℞ *investigational antineoplastic for liver metastases*

**Spherulin** intradermal injection ℞ *diagnostic aid for coccidioidomycosis* [coccidioidin] 1:100, 1:10

**SPIA (sol particle immunoassay)** [q.v.]

**spiclamine** INN

**spiclomazine** INN

**spider bite antivenin** [see: antivenin (Latrodectus mactans)]

**spider blue** *street drug slang* [see: heroin]

**Spider-Man Children's Chewable Vitamin Tablets** (discontinued 1993) OTC *vitamin supplement* [multiple vitamins; folic acid]

**spiperone** USAN, INN *antipsychotic*

**spiradoline** INN *analgesic* [also: spiradoline mesylate]

**spiradoline mesylate** USAN *analgesic* [also: spiradoline]

**spiramide** INN

**spiramycin** USAN, INN, BAN *antibacterial; orphan status withdrawn 1994* [also: acetylspiramycin]

**spirapril** INN, BAN *angiotensin-converting enzyme (ACE) inhibitor* [also: spirapril HCl]

**spirapril HCl** USAN *angiotensin-converting enzyme (ACE) inhibitor* [also: spirapril]

**spiraprilat** USAN, INN *angiotensin-converting enzyme (ACE) inhibitor*

**spirazine** INN

**spirazine HCl** [see: spirazine]

**spirendolol** INN

**spirgetine** INN

**spirilene** INN, BAN

**spirit of nitrous ether** [see: ethyl nitrite]

**Spiro-32** ℞ *investigational antineoplastic for colorectal cancer and rheumatoid arthritis* [spirogermanium]

**spirobarbital sodium**

**spirofylline** INN

**spirogermanium** INN, BAN *antineoplastic* [also: spirogermanium HCl]

**spirogermanium HCl** USAN *antineoplastic* [also: spirogermanium]

**spirohydantoin mustard** [now: spiromustine]

**spiromustine** USAN, INN *antineoplastic*

**Spironazide** tablets (discontinued 1993) ℞ *diuretic* [spironolactone; hydrochlorothiazide]

**spironolactone** USP, INN, BAN, JAN *potassium-sparing diuretic; aldosterone antagonist* 25 mg oral

**spiroplatin** USAN, INN, BAN *antineoplastic*

**spirorenone** INN

**spirotriazine HCl** [see: spirazine]

**spiroxamide** [see: spiroxatrine]

**spiroxasone** USAN, INN *diuretic*

**spiroxatrine** INN

**spiroxepin** INN

**Spirozide** tablets (discontinued 1994) ℞ *diuretic; antihypertensive* [spironolactone; hydrochlorothiazide] 25•25 mg

**spizofurone** INN

**SPL (staphage lysate)** [q.v.]

**splash** *street drug slang* [see: amphetamines]

**spliff** *street drug slang for a marijuana cigarette* [see: marijuana]

**splim** *street drug slang* [see: marijuana]

**splivins** *street drug slang* [see: amphetamines]

**SPL-Serologic types I and III** solution for subcu injection, nasal aerosol, nasal drop, oral, or topical irrigation ℞ *staphylococcal or polymicrobial vaccine* [staphage lysate (Staphylococcus aureus; Staphylococcus bacteriophage plaque-forming units)]

**Sporanox** capsules ℞ *systemic antifungal* [itraconazole] 100 mg

**Sporanox** oral solution ("swish and swallow") ℞ *antifungal for esophageal and oropharyngeal candidiasis* [itraconazole] 10 mg/mL

**spores** *street drug slang* [see: PCP]

**Sporidin-G** ℞ *investigational (orphan) for treatment of cryptosporidiosis infections in immunocompromised patients* [bovine immunoglobulin concentrate, Cryptosporidium parvum]

**Sports Spray** OTC *counterirritant; topical antiseptic* [methyl salicylate; menthol; camphor; alcohol 58%] 3.5%•10%•5%

**Sportscreme** OTC *topical analgesic* [trolamine salicylate] 10%

**Sportscreme Ice** gel OTC *topical analgesic; counterirritant* [trolamine; menthol] ≗•2%

**SPPG (sulfated polysaccharide peptidoglycan)** [see: tecogalan sodium]

**Spray-U-Thin** oral spray OTC *diet aid* [phenylpropanolamine HCl] 6.58 mg

**Sprinkle Caps** (trademarked form) *powder*

**sprodiamide** USAN *heart and CNS imaging aid for MRI*

**SPS** oral suspension ℞ *potassium-removing agent for hyperkalemia* [sodium polystyrene sulfonate] 15 g/60 mL

**S-P-T** "liquid" capsules ℞ *hypothyroidism; thyroid cancer* [pork thyroid, desiccated] 60, 120, 180, 300 mg

**squalane** NF *oleaginous vehicle*

**square mackerel** *street drug slang (from Florida)* [see: marijuana]

**square time Bob** *street drug slang* [see: cocaine, crack]

**squirrel** *street drug slang for LSD or a combination of cocaine, marijuana, and PCP for smoking* [see: LSD; cocaine; marijuana; PCP]

**$^{85}$Sr** [see: strontium chloride Sr 85]

**$^{85}$Sr** [see: strontium nitrate Sr 85]

**$^{85}$Sr** [see: strontium Sr 85]

**SRC Expectorant** liquid ℞ *narcotic antitussive; decongestant; expectorant* [hydrocodone bitartrate; pseudoephedrine HCl; guaifenesin; alcohol 12.5%] 5•60•200 mg/5 mL

**SRF (skin respiratory factor)** [q.v.]

**SS (saline solution)**

**SS (sodium salicylate)** [q.v.]

**SS (somatostatin)** [q.v.]

**SSD (silver sulfadiazine)** [q.v.]

**SSD; SSD AF** cream ℞ *broad-spectrum bactericidal for adjunctive burn treatment* [silver sulfadiazine] 10 mg/g

**SSKI** oral solution ℞ *expectorant* [potassium iodide] 1 g/mL

**SSRIs (selective serotonin reuptake inhibitors)** *a class of oral antidepressants that inhibit neuronal uptake of 5-HT (serotonin), a CNS neurotransmitter*

**S.T. 37** solution OTC *topical antiseptic* [hexylresorcinol] 0.1%

**S-T Cort** lotion ℞ *topical corticosteroid* [hydrocortisone] 0.5%

**S-T Forte 2** liquid ℞ *narcotic antitussive; antihistamine* [hydrocodone bitartrate; chlorpheniramine maleate] 2.5•2 mg/5 mL

**ST1-RTA immunotoxin (SR 44163)** *investigational (orphan) for graft vs. host disease and B-chronic lymphocytic leukemia*

**stable factor** [see: factor VII]

**stack** *street drug slang* [see: marijuana]

**Stadol** IV or IM injection ℞ *narcotic agonist-antagonist analgesic* [butorphanol tartrate] 1, 2 mg/mL

**Stadol NS** nasal spray ℞ *narcotic agonist-antagonist analgesic; antimigraine agent* [butorphanol tartrate] 10 mg/mL

**Stagesic** capsules ℞ *narcotic analgesic* [hydrocodone bitartrate; acetaminophen] 5•500 mg

**Stahist** sustained-release tablets ℞ *decongestant; antihistamine; anticholinergic* [phenylpropanolamine HCl; phenylephrine HCl; chlorpheniramine maleate; hyoscyamine sulfate; atropine sulfate; scopolamine hydrobromide] 50•25•8•0.19•0.04•0.01 mg

**stallimycin** INN *antibacterial* [also: stallimycin HCl]

**stallimycin HCl** USAN *antibacterial* [also: stallimycin]

**Stamoist E** sustained-release tablets ℞ *decongestant; expectorant* [pseudoephedrine HCl; guaifenesin] 120•500 mg

**Stamoist LA** sustained-release tablets ℞ *decongestant; expectorant* [phenylpropanolamine HCl; guaifenesin] 75•400 mg

**standard VAC** *chemotherapy protocol* [see: VAC standard (under VAC)]

**Stanford V (mechlorethamine, doxorubicin, vinblastine, vincristine, bleomycin, VePesid, prednisone)** *chemotherapy protocol*

**Stanley's stuff** *street drug slang* [see: LSD]

**stannous chloride** USAN *pharmaceutic aid*

**stannous fluoride** USP *dental caries prophylactic*

**stannous pyrophosphate** USAN *skeletal imaging aid*

**stannous sulfur colloid** USAN *bone, liver and spleen imaging aid*

**stanolone** BAN *investigational (orphan) for AIDS-wasting syndrome* [also: androstanolone]

**stanozolol** USAN, USP, INN, BAN *androgen; anabolic steroid*

**staphage lysate (SPL)** *active bacterin for staphylococcal infections*

**Staphcillin** powder for IV or IM injection ℞ *bactericidal antibiotic (penicillinase-resistant penicillin)* [methicillin sodium] 1, 4, 6, 10 g

***Staphylococcus aureus* vaccine** *investigational anti-infective for renal dialysis patients*

**star** *street drug slang for methcathinone or LSD blotter acid with star-shaped design* [see: methcathinone; LSD]

**starch** NF *dusting powder; pharmaceutic aid*

**starch, pregelatinized** NF *tablet excipient*

**starch, topical** USP *dusting powder*

**starch carboxymethyl ether, sodium salt** [see: sodium starch glycolate]

**starch glycerite** NF

**starch 2-hydroxyethyl ether** [see: hetastarch; pentastarch]

**stardust** *street drug slang* [see: cocaine; PCP]

**Star-Optic** eye wash (discontinued 1994) OTC *extraocular irrigating solution* [balanced saline solution]

**Star-Otic** ear drops OTC *antibacterial/ antifungal* [acetic acid; aluminum acetate; boric acid]

**star-spangled powder** *street drug slang* [see: cocaine]

**stat** *street drug slang* [see: methcathinone]

**Stat-Crit** electrode device for professional use *in vitro diagnostic aid for hemoglobin/hematocrit measurement*

**Staticin** topical solution ℞ *topical antibiotic for acne* [erythromycin] 1.5%

**statolon** USAN *antiviral* [also: vistatolon]

**Stat-One** gel OTC *topical antiseptic* [hydrogen peroxide] 3%

**Stat-One** gel OTC *topical antiseptic* [isopropyl alcohol] 70%

**Stat-Pak** (trademarked packaging form) *unit-dose package*

**Statrol** Drop-Tainers (eye drops), ophthalmic ointment (discontinued 1994) ℞ *ophthalmic antibiotic* [polymyxin B sulfate; neomycin sulfate] 16 250 U•3.5 mg per mL; 10 000 U•3.5 mg per g

**Statuss Expectorant** liquid ℞ *narcotic antitussive; decongestant; expectorant* [codeine phosphate; phenylpropanolamine HCl; guaifenesin; alcohol 5%] 10•12.5•100 mg/5 mL

**Statuss Green** liquid ℞ *narcotic antitussive; decongestant; antihistamine* [hydrocodone bitartrate; phenylpropanolamine HCl; phenylephrine HCl; pyrilamine maleate; pheni-

ramine maleate; alcohol 5%] 1.67•
3.3•5•3.3•3.3 mg/5 mL

**stavudine** USAN, INN *antiviral for HIV*

**Stay Trim** gum, mints (discontinued 1995) OTC *diet aid* [phenylpropanolamine HCl] 8.33 mg; 12.5 mg

**Stay-Brite** solution (discontinued 1993) OTC *cleaning solution for hard contact lenses*

**Stay-Wet** solution (discontinued 1995) OTC *wetting/rewetting solution for hard contact lenses*

**Stay-Wet 3; Stay-Wet 4** solution OTC *disinfecting/wetting/soaking solution for rigid gas permeable contact lenses*

**STD (sodium tetradecyl sulfate)** [q.v.]

**steaglate** INN *combining name for radicals or groups*

**STEAM (streptonigrin, thioguanine, cyclophosphamide, actinomycin, mitomycin)** *chemotherapy protocol*

**stearethate 40** [see: polyoxyl 40 stearate]

**stearic acid** NF *emulsion adjunct; tablet and capsule lubricant*

**stearyl alcohol** NF *emulsion adjunct*

**stearyl dimethyl benzyl ammonium chloride**

**stearylsulfamide** INN

**steffimycin** USAN, INN *antibacterial; antiviral*

**Stelazine** film-coated tablets, oral concentrate, IM injection ℞ *antianxiety; antipsychotic* [trifluoperazine HCl] 1, 2, 5, 10 mg; 10 mg/mL; 2 mg/mL

**stem cell factor (SCF)** *investigational (Phase III) agent for blood-related disorders and chemotherapy "rescue"*

**stems** *street drug slang* [see: marijuana]

**stenbolone** INN *anabolic steroid; also abused as a street drug* [also: stenbolone acetate]

**stenbolone acetate** USAN *anabolic steroid; also abused as a street drug* [also: stenbolone]

**Step 2** creme rinse OTC *for use following a pediculicide shampoo to remove lice eggs from hair*

**stepronin** INN

**Sterapred** tablets, Unipak (dispensing pack) ℞ *glucocorticoid* [prednisone] 5 mg

**Sterapred DS** tablets, Unipak (dispensing pack) ℞ *glucocorticoid* [prednisone] 10 mg

**stercuronium iodide** INN

**Sterecyt** ℞ *investigational antineoplastic for leukemia; investigational (orphan) for malignant non-Hodgkin's lymphomas* [prednimustine]

**Steri-Dose** (trademarked delivery system) *prefilled disposable syringe*

**Sterile Lens Lubricant** solution (discontinued 1993) OTC *rewetting solution for soft contact lenses*

**SteriNail** solution OTC *topical antifungal* [undecylenic acid; tolnaftate] ≟•≟

**Steri-Vial** (trademarked packaging form) *ampule*

**stevaladil** INN

**stibamine glucoside** INN, BAN

**stibocaptate** BAN [also: sodium stibocaptate]

**stibophen** NF

**stibosamine** INN

**stick** *street drug slang* [see: marijuana; PCP]

**sticks** *street drug slang for marijuana stems and waste* [see: marijuana]

**stilbamidine isethionate** [see: stilbamidine isetionate]

**stilbamidine isetionate** INN

**stilbazium iodide** USAN, INN *anthelmintic*

**stilbestroform** [see: diethylstilbestrol]

**stilbestrol** [see: diethylstilbestrol] ⑨ Stilphostrol

**stilbestronate** [see: diethylstilbestrol dipropionate]

**stilboestroform** [see: diethylstilbestrol]

**stilboestrol** BAN *estrogen* [also: diethylstilbestrol]

**stilboestrol DP** [see: diethylstilbestrol dipropionate]

**Stilnoct; Stilnox** (European name for U.S. product Ambien)

**stilonium iodide** USAN, INN *antispasmodic*

**Stilphostrol** tablets, IV injection ℞ *antineoplastic for prostatic carcinoma* [diethylstilbestrol diphosphate] 50 mg; 250 mg ℞ Disophrol; stilbestrol

**stilronate** [see: diethylstilbestrol dipropionate]

**Stimate** nasal spray ℞ *pituitary antidiuretic hormone for hemophilia A and von Willebrand's disease (orphan)* [desmopressin acetate] 150 μg (600 IU)/dose

**Stimulon QS-21** ℞ *investigational (Phase I/II) immune system stimulant for vaccines*

**Sting-Eze** concentrate OTC *topical antihistamine; antipruritic; anesthetic; bacteriostatic* [diphenhydramine HCl; camphor; phenol; benzocaine; eucalyptol]

**Stinging Insect Antigen No. 108** subcu or IM injection (discontinued 1993) ℞ *venom sensitivity testing (subcu); venom desensitization therapy (IM)* [bumblebee, honeybee, wasp, hornet, and yellow jacket antigen extracts]

**Sting-Kill** swabs OTC *topical local anesthetic* [benzocaine; menthol] 20%•1%

**stink weed** *street drug slang* [see: marijuana]

**stirimazole** INN, BAN

**stiripentol** USAN, INN *anticonvulsant*

**stirocainide** INN

**stirofos** USAN *veterinary insecticide*

**Stoko Gard** cream OTC *topical protection from the effects of poison ivy*

**stones** *street drug slang* [see: cocaine, crack]

**Stop** gel ℞ *topical dental caries preventative* [stannous fluoride] 0.4%

**storax** USP

**Storzfen** eye drops ℞ *ophthalmic decongestant/vasoconstrictor; mydriatic* [phenylephrine HCl] 2.5%

**Storzine 2** eye drops ℞ *antiglaucoma agent; direct-acting miotic* [pilocarpine HCl] 2%

**Storz-N-D** eye drops ℞ *topical ophthalmic corticosteroidal anti-inflammatory; antibiotic* [dexamethasone sodium phosphate; neomycin sulfate] 0.1%•0.35%

**Storz-N-P-D** eye drop suspension ℞ *topical ophthalmic corticosteroidal anti-inflammatory; antibiotic* [dexametha-

sone; neomycin sulfate; polymyxin B sulfate] 0.1%•0.35%•10 000 U/mL

**Storz-Sulf** eye drops ℞ *ophthalmic bacteriostatic* [sulfacetamide sodium] 10%

**STP** *street drug slang for the hallucinogen 2,5-dimethoxy-4-methylamphetamine (DOM), derived from amphetamine*

**stramonium** [see: jimsonweed]

**StrapKap** (dosage form) *piggyback vials*

**straw** *street drug slang for a marijuana cigarette* [see: marijuana]

**strawberry fields** *street drug slang* [see: LSD]

**Strep Detect** slide tests for professional use *in vitro diagnostic aid for streptococcal antigens in throat swabs*

**Streptase** powder for IV or intracoronary infusion ℞ *thrombolytic enzyme for lysis of thrombi and catheter clearance* [streptokinase] 250 000, 750 000, 1 500 000 IU ℞ Streptonase

**streptococcus immune globulin, group B** *investigational (orphan) for neonatal group B streptococcal infection*

**streptodornase (SD)** INN, BAN

**streptoduocin** USP

**streptogramins** *a class of antibiotics, isolated from Streptomyces pristinaspirales, used for gram-positive infections*

**streptokinase (SK)** INN *thrombolytic enzymes for myocardial infarction, thrombosis or embolism* ℞ Streptonase

**streptomycin** INN, BAN *aminoglycoside bactericidal antibiotic; primary tuberculostatic* [also: streptomycin sulfate]

**streptomycin sulfate** USP *aminoglycoside bactericidal antibiotic; primary tuberculostatic* [also: streptomycin]

**Streptonase-B** test kit for professional use *in vitro diagnostic test for DNAse-B streptococcal antigens in serum* ℞ Streptase; streptokinase

**streptoniazid** INN *antibacterial* [also: streptonicozid]

**streptonicozid** USAN *antibacterial* [also: streptoniazid]

**streptonigrin (SN)** USAN *antineoplastic* [also: rufocromomycin]

**Strepto-Sec** slide test for professional use (discontinued 1991) *in vitro diagnostic test for streptococcal antigens*

**streptovarycin** INN

**streptozocin** USAN, INN *nitrosourea-type alkylating antineoplastic for metastatic islet cell carcinoma of the pancreas*

**streptozotocin** [see: streptozocin]

**Streptozyme** slide tests for professional use *in vitro diagnostic test for streptococcal extracellular antigens in blood, plasma, and serum*

**Stress 600 with Zinc** tablets OTC *vitamin/mineral supplement* [multiple vitamins & minerals; folic acid; biotin] ± •400•45 μg

**Stress "1000"** tablets (discontinued 1993) OTC *vitamin supplement* [multiple vitamins]

**Stress B Complex** tablets OTC *vitamin/mineral supplement* [multiple vitamins & minerals; folic acid; biotin] ± •400•45 μg

**Stress B Complex with Vitamin C** timed-release tablets OTC *vitamin/mineral supplement* [multiple B vitamins; vitamin C; zinc] ± •300•15 mg

**Stress B with C** tablets (discontinued 1995) OTC *vitamin supplement* [multiple B vitamins; vitamin C; folic acid; biotin] ± •250 mg•50 μg•12.5 μg

**Stress Formula 500** tablets (discontinued 1993) OTC *vitamin supplement* [multiple vitamins; biotin; folic acid]

**Stress Formula 500 Plus Iron** tablets (discontinued 1993) OTC *vitamin/iron supplement* [ferrous fumarate; multiple B vitamins; vitamins C and E; folic acid; biotin] 27 mg• ± •500 mg•30 IU•0.4 mg•45 μg

**Stress Formula 500 Plus Zinc** tablets (discontinued 1993) OTC *vitamin/zinc supplement* [multiple vitamins; zinc; folic acid; biotin]

**Stress Formula 600** tablets OTC *vitamin supplement* [multiple vitamins; folic acid; biotin] ± •400•45 μg

**Stress Formula 600 plus Iron** tablets OTC *antianemic* [ferrous fumarate, dried; vitamins C and E; multiple B vitamins; folic acid]

**Stress Formula 600 plus Zinc** tablets (discontinued 1993) OTC *vitamin/mineral supplement* [multiple vitamins & minerals; folic acid; biotin]

**Stress Formula "605"** tablets (discontinued 1995) OTC *vitamin supplement* [multiple vitamins; folic acid; biotin] ± •400•45 μg

**Stress Formula "605" with Zinc** tablets (discontinued 1995) OTC *vitamin/mineral supplement* [multiple vitamins & minerals; folic acid; biotin] ± •400•45 μg

**Stress Formula Vitamins** capsules, tablets OTC *vitamin supplement* [multiple vitamins; folic acid; biotin] ± • 400•45 μg

**Stress Formula with Iron** film-coated tablets OTC *vitamin/iron supplement* [multiple B vitamins; vitamins C and E; ferrous fumarate; folic acid; biotin] ± •500 mg•30 IU•27 mg•0.4 mg•45 μg

**Stress Formula with Zinc** tablets OTC *vitamin/iron supplement* [multiple B vitamins; vitamins C and E; multiple minerals; folic acid; biotin] ± • 500 mg•30 IU• ± •0.4 mg•45 μg

**Stresscaps** capsules (discontinued 1995) OTC *vitamin supplement* [multiple B vitamins; vitamin C] ± •300 mg

**StressForm "605" with Iron** tablets OTC *vitamin/iron supplement* [multiple B vitamins; vitamins C and E; iron; folic acid; biotin] ± •605 mg•30 IU•27 mg•0.4 mg•45 μg

**Stresstabs** tablets OTC *vitamin supplement* [multiple vitamins; folic acid; biotin] ± •400•45 μg

**Stresstabs 600 with Iron** tablets OTC *antianemic* [ferrous fumarate, dried; vitamins E and C; multiple B vitamins; folic acid]

**Stresstabs Advanced Formula** tablets (name changed to Stresstabs in 1995)

**Stresstabs + Iron** film-coated tablets OTC *vitamin/iron supplement* [multiple B vitamins; vitamins C and E; ferrous fumarate; folic acid; biotin] ± •500 mg•30 IU•18 mg•0.4 mg•45 μg

**Stresstabs + Zinc** film-coated tablets OTC *vitamin/mineral supplement* [multiple vitamins & minerals; folic acid; biotin] ± •400•45 μg

**Stresstein** powder OTC *enteral nutritional therapy for moderate to severe*

*stress or trauma* [branched chain amino acids]

**Stri-Dex** pads OTC *topical keratolytic cleanser for acne* [salicylic acid; alcohol] 0.5%•28%, 2%•44%, 2%•54%

**Stri-Dex Cleansing** bar OTC *medicated cleanser for acne* [triclosan] 1%

**Stri-Dex Clear** gel OTC *topical acne treatment* [salicylic acid; alcohol] 2%•9.3%

**Stri-Dex Face Wash** solution OTC *antiseptic; disinfectant* [triclosan] 1%

**strinoline** INN

**Stromectol** tablets ℞ *anthelmintic for strongyloidiasis and onchocerciasis* [ivermectin] 6 mg

**strong ammonia solution** [see: ammonia solution, strong]

**Strong Iodine** solution, tincture ℞ *thyroid-blocking therapy; topical antimicrobial* [iodine; potassium iodide] 5%•10%; 7%•5%

**stronger rose water** [see: rose water, stronger]

**strontium** *element (Sr)*

**strontium chloride Sr 85** USAN *radioactive agent*

**strontium chloride Sr 89** USAN *radioactive agent; analgesic for metastatic bone pain*

**strontium nitrate Sr 85** USAN *radioactive agent*

**strontium salicylate** NF

**strontium Sr 85** USP

**Strovite** tablets ℞ *vitamin supplement* [multiple B vitamins; vitamin C; folic acid] ±•500•0.5 mg

**Strovite Plus** caplets ℞ *geriatric vitamin/mineral therapy* [multiple vitamins & minerals; folic acid; biotin] ±•800•150 μg

**strychnine** NF *an extremely poisonous CNS stimulant; occasionally abused as a street drug in combination with LSD*

**strychnine glycerophosphate** NF

**strychnine nitrate** NF

**strychnine phosphate** NF

**strychnine sulfate** NF

**strychnine valerate** NF

**Stuart Formula** tablets OTC *vitamin/mineral/iron supplement* [multiple vitamins & minerals; iron; folic acid] ±•18•0.1 mg

**Stuart Prenatal** tablets OTC *vitamin/calcium/iron supplement* [multiple vitamins; calcium; iron; folic acid] ±•200•60•0.8 mg

**Stuartinic** film-coated tablets (discontinued 1995) OTC *hematinic* [ferrous fumarate; multiple B vitamins; vitamin C] 100•±•500 mg

**Stuartnatal 1 + 1** tablets (name changed to Stuartnatal Plus in 1995)

**Stuartnatal Plus** tablets ℞ *vitamin/calcium/iron supplement* [multiple vitamins; calcium; iron; folic acid] ±•200•65•1 mg

**stuff** *street drug slang* [see: heroin]

**stugeron** [see: cinnarizine]

**stumblers** *street drug slang* [see: barbiturates]

**stutgin** [see: cinnarizine]

**Stye** ophthalmic ointment OTC *emollient* [white petrolatum; mineral oil; boric acid]

**Stye** ophthalmic ointment (discontinued 1995; replaced by Stye without yellow mercuric oxide) OTC *stye treatment (the FDA ruled yellow mercuric oxide "not safe and effective" in 1992)* [yellow mercuric oxide] 1%

**Stypto-Caine** solution OTC *to stop bleeding of minor cuts* [aluminum chloride; tetracaine HCl; oxyquinoline sulfate] 250•2.5•1 mg/g

**styramate** INN

**styronate resins**

**SU-101** *investigational (orphan) for malignant glioma and ovarian cancer*

**subathizone** INN

**subendazole** INN

**Sublimaze** IV or IM injection ℞ *narcotic analgesic; anesthetic* [fentanyl citrate] 0.05 mg/mL

**sublimed sulfur** [see: sulfur, sublimed]

**Sublingual B Total** drops OTC *vitamin supplement* [multiple B vitamins; vitamin C] ±•60 mg/mL

**substance F** [see: demecolcine]

**substance P antagonist** *investigational agent for pain, migraine, inflammatory diseases, asthma, and CNS diseases*

**substituted benzimidazoles** *a class of gastric antisecretory agents that inhibit the ATPase "proton pump" within the cell* [also called: proton pump inhibitors; ATPase inhibitors]

**Suby's G solution; Suby's solution G (citric acid, magnesium oxide, sodium carbonate)** *urologic irrigant to dissolve phosphatic calculi*

**succimer** USAN, INN, BAN *heavy metal chelating agent for lead poisoning (orphan); investigational (orphan) for mercury poisoning and cysteine kidney stones*

**succinchlorimide** NF

**succinimides** *a class of anticonvulsants*

**succinylcholine chloride** USP *neuromuscular blocker; muscle relaxant; anesthesia adjunct* [also: suxamethonium chloride] 20 mg/mL injection

**succinyldapsone** [see: succisulfone]

**succinylsulfathiazole** USP

**succisulfone** INN

**Succus Cineraria Maritima** *eye drops* ℞ *treatment for optic opacity caused by cataract* [aqueous/glycerin solution of senecio compositae, hamamelis water, and boric acid]

**suclofenide** INN, BAN

**Sucostrin** *IV or IM injection (discontinued 1996)* ℞ *muscle relaxant; anesthesia adjunct* [succinylcholine chloride] 20, 100 mg/mL

**Sucraid** ℞ *investigational (orphan) for congenital sucrase-isomaltase deficiency* [sacrosidase (sucrase)]

**sucralfate** USAN, INN, BAN *treatment of gastric ulcers; investigational (orphan) for oral mucositis and stomatitis following cancer radiation or chemotherapy* 1 g oral

**sucralose** BAN

**sucralox** INN, BAN

**sucrase** *orphan status withdrawn 1997* 🔊 sucrose

**Sucrets** *mouthwash/gargle (discontinued 1994)* OTC *topical antipruritic/counterirritant; mild local anesthetic* [dyclonine HCl] 0.1%

**Sucrets** *throat spray* OTC *topical antipruritic/counterirritant; mild local anesthetic* [dyclonine HCl] 0.1%

**Sucrets Children's Sore Throat; Vapor Lemon Sucrets; Sucrets Maximum Strength** *lozenges* OTC *topical antipruritic/counterirritant; mild local anesthetic* [dyclonine HCl] 1.2 mg; 2 mg; 3 mg

**Sucrets Cough Control; Sucrets 4-Hour Cough** *lozenges* OTC *antitussive* [dextromethorphan hydrobromide] 5 mg; 15 mg

**Sucrets Sore Throat** *lozenges* OTC *oral antiseptic* [hexylresorcinol] 2.4 mg

**sucrose** NF *flavoring agent; tablet excipient* 🔊 sucrose

**sucrose octaacetate** NF *alcohol denaturant*

**sucrosofate potassium** USAN *antiulcerative*

**Sudafed** *tablets* OTC *nasal decongestant* [pseudoephedrine HCl] 30, 60 mg

**Sudafed, Children's** *chewable tablets* OTC *nasal decongestant* [pseudoephedrine HCl] 15 mg

**Sudafed, Children's** *liquid (discontinued 1996)* OTC *nasal decongestant* [pseudoephedrine HCl] 30 mg/5 mL

**Sudafed 12 Hour Caplets** *extended-release tablets* OTC *nasal decongestant* [pseudoephedrine HCl] 120 mg

**Sudafed Cold & Cough** *liquid caps* OTC *antitussive; decongestant; expectorant; analgesic* [dextromethorphan hydrobromide; pseudoephedrine HCl; guaifenesin; acetaminophen] 10•30•100•250 mg

**Sudafed Cough** *syrup (discontinued 1996)* OTC *antitussive; decongestant; expectorant* [dextromethorphan hydrobromide; pseudoephedrine HCl; guaifenesin; alcohol 2.4%] 5•15•100 mg/5 mL

**Sudafed Plus** *liquid (discontinued 1996)* OTC *decongestant; antihistamine* [pseudoephedrine HCl; chlorpheniramine maleate] 30•2 mg/5 mL

**Sudafed Plus** *tablets* OTC *decongestant; antihistamine* [pseudoephedrine HCl; chlorpheniramine maleate] 60•4 mg

**Sudafed Severe Cold** *caplets, tablets* OTC *antitussive; decongestant; analgesic* [dextromethorphan hydrobro-

mide; pseudoephedrine HCl; aceta-
minophen] 15•30•500 mg

**Sudafed Sinus** tablets, caplets OTC
*decongestant; analgesic; antipyretic*
[pseudoephedrine HCl; acetamino-
phen] 30•500 mg

**Sudal 60/500; Sudal 120/600** film-
coated sustained-release tablets R
*decongestant; expectorant* [pseudo-
ephedrine HCl; guaifenesin] 60•500
mg; 120•600 mg

**Sudex** film-coated sustained-release
tablets (discontinued 1996) R *decongestant; expectorant* [pseudoephedrine
HCl; guaifenesin] 120•600 mg

**Sudex** tablets (discontinued 1997)
OTC *decongestant* [pseudoephedrine
HCl] 30 mg

**sudexanox** INN

**sudismase** INN

**sudoxicam** USAN, INN *anti-inflammatory*

**Sufenta** IV injection R *narcotic analgesic; anesthetic* [sufentanil citrate]
50 μg/mL

**sufentanil** USAN, INN, BAN *analgesic*

**sufentanil citrate** USAN *narcotic analgesic* 50 μg/mL

**sufosfamide** INN

**sufotidine** USAN, INN, BAN *antagonist
to histamine $H_2$ receptors*

**sugar** *street drug slang* [see: cocaine;
LSD; heroin]

**sugar, compressible** NF *flavoring
agent; tablet excipient*

**sugar, confectioner's** NF *flavoring
agent; tablet excipient*

**sugar, invert (50% dextrose & 50%
fructose)** USP *fluid and nutrient
replenisher; caloric replacement*

**sugar block** *street drug slang* [see:
cocaine, crack]

**sugar cubes; sugar lumps** *street drug
slang* [see: LSD]

**sugar spheres** NF *solid carrier vehicle*

**sugar weed** *street drug slang* [see: mari-
juana]

**Sulamyd** [see: Sodium Sulamyd]

**Sular** extended-release tablets R *calcium channel blocker for hypertension*
[nisoldipine] 10, 20, 30, 40 mg

**sulazepam** USAN, INN *minor tranquilizer*

**sulbactam** INN, BAN

**sulbactam benzathine** USAN *β-lactamase inhibitor; penicillin/cephalosporin
synergist*

**sulbactam pivoxil** USAN *β-lactamase
inhibitor; penicillin/cephalosporin synergist* [also: pivsulbactam]

**sulbactam sodium** USAN, USP *β-lactamase inhibitor; penicillin/cephalosporin
synergist*

**sulbenicillin** INN

**sulbenox** USAN, INN *veterinary growth
stimulant*

**sulbentine** INN

**sulbutiamine** INN [also: bisibutiamine]

**sulclamide** INN

**sulconazole** INN, BAN *antifungal* [also:
sulconazole nitrate]

**sulconazole nitrate** USAN, USP *antifungal* [also: sulconazole]

**Suldiazo** film-coated tablets (discontinued 1994) R *urinary anti-infective;
urinary analgesic* [sulfisoxazole;
phenazopyridine HCl] 500•50 mg

**sulergine** [see: disulergine]

**sulesomab** USAN *monoclonal antibody;
diagnostic aid for infectious lesions*
[also: technetium Tc 99m sulesomab]

**Sulf-10** eye drops R *ophthalmic bacteriostatic* [sulfacetamide sodium] 10%
2 Sulten-10

**Sulf-15** eye drops (discontinued 1995)
R *ophthalmic bacteriostatic* [sulfaceta-
mide sodium] 15%

**sulfabenz** USAN, INN *antibacterial; coccidiostat for poultry*

**sulfabenzamide** USAN, USP, INN *bacteriostatic antibiotic*

**sulfabromomethazine sodium** NF

**sulfacarbamide** INN [also: sulphaurea]

**sulfacecole** INN

**sulfacetamide** USP, INN *bacteriostatic
antibiotic*

**sulfacetamide sodium** USP *bacteriostatic antibiotic* 10%, 30% eye drops

**Sulfacet-R** lotion R *topical acne treatment* [sulfacetamide sodium; sulfur]
10%•5%

**sulfachlorpyridazine** INN

**sulfachrysoidine** INN

**sulfacitine** INN *antibacterial* [also: sul-
facytine]

**sulfaclomide** INN

**sulfaclorazole** INN

**sulfaclozine** INN

**sulfacombin** [see: sulfadiazine]

**sulfacytine** USAN *broad-spectrum bacteriostatic* [also: sulfacitine]

**sulfadiasulfone sodium** INN *antibacterial; leprostatic* [also: acetosulfone sodium]

**sulfadiazine** USP, INN, JAN *broad-spectrum sulfonamide bacteriostatic* [also: sulphadiazine] 500 mg oral

**sulfadiazine & pyrimethamine** *Toxoplasma gondii encephalitis treatment (orphan)*

**sulfadiazine silver** JAN *broad-spectrum bactericidal; adjunct to burn therapy* [also: silver sulfadiazine]

**sulfadiazine sodium** USP, INN *antibacterial* [also: sulphadiazine sodium]

**sulfadicramide** INN, DCF

**sulfadicrolamide** [see: sulfadicramide]

**sulfadimethoxine** NF [also: sulphadimethoxine]

**sulfadimidine** INN, BAN *antibacterial* [also: sulfamethazine]

**sulfadoxine** USAN, USP *bacteriostatic; antimalarial adjunct*

**sulfaethidole** NF, INN [also: sulphaethidole]

**sulfafurazole** INN *broad-spectrum sulfonamide bacteriostatic* [also: sulfisoxazole; sulphafurazole]

**sulfaguanidine** NF, INN

**sulfaguanole** INN

**sulfaisodimidine** [see: sulfisomidine]

**Sulfalax Calcium** capsules OTC *stool softener* [docusate calcium] 240 mg

**sulfalene** USAN, INN *antibacterial* [also: sulfametopyrazine]

**sulfaloxic acid** INN [also: sulphaloxic acid]

**sulfamates** *a class of anticonvulsants*

**sulfamazone** INN

**sulfamerazine** USP, INN *broad-spectrum bacteriostatic*

**sulfamerazine sodium** NF, INN

**sulfameter** USAN *antibacterial* [also: sulfametoxydiazine; sulfamethoxydiazine]

**sulfamethazine** USP *broad-spectrum bacteriostatic* [also: sulfadimidine]

**sulfamethizole** USP, INN, JAN *broad-spectrum sulfonamide bacteriostatic* [also: sulphamethizole] ⊕ sulfamethoxazole

**Sulfamethoprim** IV infusion ℞ *anti-infective; antibacterial* [trimethoprim; sulfamethoxazole] 16•80 mg/mL

**sulfamethoxazole (SMX; SMZ)** USAN, USP, INN, JAN *broad-spectrum sulfonamide bacteriostatic* [also: sulphamethoxazole; acetylsulfamethoxazole; sulfamethoxazole sodium] ⊕ sulfamethizole

**sulfamethoxazole sodium** JAN *broad-spectrum sulfonamide bacteriostatic* [also: sulfamethoxazole; sulphamethoxazole; acetylsulfamethoxazole]

**sulfamethoxydiazine** BAN *antibacterial* [also: sulfameter; sulfametoxydiazine]

**sulfamethoxypyridazine** USP, INN [also: sulphamethoxypyridazine]

**sulfamethoxypyridazine acetyl**

**sulfametin** [see: sulfameter]

**sulfametomidine** INN

**sulfametopyrazine** BAN *antibacterial* [also: sulfalene]

**sulfametoxydiazine** INN *antibacterial* [also: sulfameter; sulfamethoxydiazine]

**sulfametrole** INN, BAN

**Sulfamide** eye drop suspension (discontinued 1993) ℞ *topical ophthalmic corticosteroidal anti-inflammatory; bacteriostatic* [prednisolone acetate; sulfacetamide sodium]

**sulfamidothiodiazol** [see: glybuzole]

**sulfamonomethoxine** USAN, INN, BAN *antibacterial*

**sulfamoxole** USAN, INN *antibacterial* [also: sulphamoxole]

***p*-sulfamoylbenzoic acid** [see: carzenide]

**4′-sulfamoylsuccinanilic acid** [see: sulfasuccinamide]

**Sulfamylon** cream ℞ *broad-spectrum bacteriostatic* [mafenide acetate] 85 mg/g

**Sulfamylon** solution ℞ *broad-spectrum bacteriostatic; investigational (orphan) to prevent meshed autograft loss on burn wounds* [mafenide acetate]

**sulfanilamide** NF, INN *bacteriostatic antibiotic* 15% topical

**sulfanilanilide** [see: sulfabenz]
**sulfanilate zinc** USAN *antibacterial*
**N-sulfanilylacetamide** [see: sulfacetamide]
**N-sulfanilylacetamide monosodium salt monohydrate** [see: sulfacetamide sodium]
**N-*p*-sulfanilylphenylglycine sodium** [see: acediasulfone sodium]
**N-sulfanilylstearamide** [see: stearylsulfamide]
**4'-sulfanilylsuccinanilic acid** [see: succisulfone]
**sulfanilylurea** [see: sulfacarbamide]
**sulfanitran** USAN, INN, BAN *antibacterial; coccidiostat for poultry*
**sulfaperin** INN
**sulfaphenazole** INN [also: sulphaphenazole]
**sulfaphtalythiazol** [see: phthalysulfathiazole]
**sulfaproxyline** INN [also: sulphaproxyline]
**sulfapyrazole** INN, BAN *antibacterial* [also: sulfazamet]
**sulfapyridine** USP, INN *investigational (orphan) dermatitis herpetiformis suppressant* [also: sulphapyridine]
**sulfapyridine sodium** NF
**sulfaquinoxaline** INN, BAN
**sulfarsphenamine** NF, INN
**sulfasalazine** USAN, USP, INN *broad-spectrum bacteriostatic; anti-inflammatory for ulcerative colitis; antirheumatic* [also: sulphasalazine; salazosulfapyridine] 500 mg oral
**Sulfasim** ℞ *investigational (Phase I) immunomodulator for sulfamethoxazole allergy in AIDS patients*
**sulfasomizole** USAN, INN *antibacterial* [also: sulphasomizole]
**sulfastearyl** [see: stearylsulfamide]
**sulfasuccinamide** INN
**sulfasymazine** INN
**sulfated polysaccharide peptidoglycan (SPPG)** [see: tecogalan sodium]
**sulfathiazole** USP, INN *bacteriostatic antibiotic* [also: sulphathiazole] ② sulfisoxazole
**sulfathiazole sodium** NF
**sulfathiocarbamide** [see: sulfathiourea]
**sulfathiourea** INN

**sulfatolamide** INN
**Sulfatrim** oral suspension ℞ *anti-infective; antibacterial* [trimethoprim; sulfamethoxazole] 40•200 mg/5 mL ② Sulfa-Trip
**Sulfatrim DS** tablets ℞ *anti-infective; antibacterial* [sulfamethoxazole; trimethoprim] 160•800 mg
**Sulfa-Trip** vaginal cream (discontinued 1994) ℞ *broad-spectrum bacteriostatic* [sulfathiazole; sulfacetamide; sulfabenzamide; urea] ② Sulfatrim
**sulfatroxazole** INN
**sulfatrozole** INN
**sulfazamet** USAN *antibacterial* [also: sulfapyrazole]
**sulfinalol** INN *antihypertensive* [also: sulfinalol HCl]
**sulfinalol HCl** USAN *antihypertensive* [also: sulfinalol]
**sulfinpyrazone** USP, INN *uricosuric for gout* [also: sulphinpyrazone] 100, 200 mg oral
**sulfiram** INN [also: monosulfiram]
**sulfisomidine** [also: sulphasomidine]
**sulfisoxazole** USP, JAN *broad-spectrum sulfonamide bacteriostatic* [also: sulfafurazole; sulphafurazole] 500 mg oral ② sulfathiazole
**sulfisoxazole acetyl** USP *broad-spectrum bacteriostatic*
**sulfisoxazole diolamine** USAN, USP *broad-spectrum bacteriostatic*
**Sulfoam** shampoo OTC *antiseborrheic; keratolytic* [salicylic acid] 2%
**sulfobenzylpenicillin** [see: sulbenicillin]
**sulfobromophthalein sodium** USP *hepatic function test*
**sulfobromphthalein sodium** [see: sulfobromophthalein sodium]
**sulfogaiacol** INN *expectorant* [also: potassium guaiacolsulfonate]
**Sulfoil** liquid OTC *soap-free therapeutic skin cleanser* [sulfonated castor oil]
**sulfomyxin** USAN, INN *antibacterial* [also: sulphomyxin sodium]
**sulfonal** [see: sulfonmethane]
**sulfonamides** *a class of broad-spectrum bacteriostatic antibiotics effective against both gram-positive and gram-negative organisms*

**sulfonated hydrogenated castor oil** [see: hydroxystearin sulfate]

**sulfonethylmethane** NF

**sulfonmethane** NF

**sulfonterol** INN *bronchodilator* [also: sulfonterol HCl]

**sulfonterol HCl** USAN *bronchodilator* [also: sulfonterol]

**sulfonylureas** *a class of antidiabetic agents that stimulate insulin production in the pancreas*

**Sulforcin** lotion OTC *topical acne treatment* [sulfur; resorcinol; alcohol] 5%•2%•11.65%

**sulforidazine** INN

**sulfosalicylic acid**

**sulfoxone sodium** USP *antibacterial; leprostatic* [also: aldesulfone sodium]

**Sulfoxyl Regular; Sulfoxyl Strong** lotion ℞ *topical keratolytic for acne* [benzoyl peroxide; sulfur] 5%•2%; 10%•5%

**sulfur** *element (S)* [see: sulfur, precipitated; sulfur, sublimed]

**sulfur, precipitated** USP *scabicide; topical antibacterial; topical exfoliant*

**sulfur, sublimed** USP *scabicide; topical antibacterial; topical exfoliant*

**sulfur dioxide** NF *antioxidant*

**Sulfur Soap** bar OTC *medicated cleanser for acne* [precipitated sulfur] 10%

**sulfurated lime solution** [see: lime, sulfurated]

**sulfurated potash** [see: potash, sulfurated]

**sulfuric acid** NF *acidifying agent*

**sulfuric acid, aluminum ammonium salt, dodecahydrate** [see: alum, ammonium]

**sulfuric acid, aluminum potassium salt, dodecahydrate** [see: alum, potassium]

**sulfuric acid, aluminum salt, hydrate** [see: aluminum sulfate]

**sulfuric acid, barium salt** [see: barium sulfate]

**sulfuric acid, calcium salt** [see: calcium sulfate]

**sulfuric acid, copper salt pentahydrate** [see: cupric sulfate]

**sulfuric acid, disodium salt decahydrate** [see: sodium sulfate]

**sulfuric acid, magnesium salt** [see: magnesium sulfate]

**sulfuric acid, manganese salt** [see: manganese sulfate]

**sulfuric acid, zinc salt hydrate** [see: zinc sulfate]

**sulfurous acid, monosodium salt** [see: sodium bisulfite]

**sulglicotide** INN [also: sulglycotide]

**sulglycotide** BAN [also: sulglicotide]

**sulicrinat** INN

**sulindac** USAN, USP, INN, BAN *antiarthritic; nonsteroidal anti-inflammatory drug (NSAID); analgesic* 150, 200 mg oral

**sulisatin** INN

**sulisobenzone** USAN, INN *ultraviolet screen*

**sulmarin** USAN, INN *hemostatic*

**Sulmasque** mask OTC *antibacterial and exfoliant for acne* [sulfur] 6.4%

**sulmazole** INN

**sulmepride** INN

**sulnidazole** USAN, INN *antiprotozoal (Trichomonas)*

**sulocarbilate** INN

**suloctidil** USAN, INN, BAN *peripheral vasodilator*

**sulodexide** INN

**sulofenur** USAN, INN *antineoplastic*

**sulopenem** USAN, INN *antibacterial*

**sulosemide** INN

**sulotroban** USAN, INN, BAN *treatment for glomerulonephritis*

**suloxifen** INN *bronchodilator* [also: suloxifen oxalate]

**suloxifen oxalate** USAN *bronchodilator* [also: suloxifen]

**Sulperazon** ℞ *investigational antibiotic* [sulbactam; cefoperazone sodium]

**sulphabutin** [see: busulfan]

**sulphadiazine** BAN *broad-spectrum bacteriostatic* [also: sulfadiazine]

**sulphadiazine sodium** BAN *antibacterial* [also: sulfadiazine sodium]

**sulphadimethoxine** BAN [also: sulfadimethoxine]

**sulphaethidole** BAN [also: sulfaethidole]

**sulphafurazole** BAN *broad-spectrum sulfonamide bacteriostatic* [also: sulfisoxazole; sulfafurazole]

**sulphaloxic acid** BAN [also: sulfaloxic acid]

**sulphamethizole** BAN *broad-spectrum sulfonamide bacteriostatic* [also: sulfamethizole]

**sulphamethoxazole** BAN *broad-spectrum sulfonamide bacteriostatic* [also: sulfamethoxazole; acetylsulfamethoxazole; sulfamethoxazole sodium]

**sulphamethoxypyridazine** BAN [also: sulfamethoxypyridazine]

**sulphamoxole** BAN *antibacterial* [also: sulfamoxole]

**sulphan blue** BAN *lymphangiography aid* [also: isosulfan blue]

**sulphaphenazole** BAN [also: sulfaphenazole]

**sulphaproxyline** BAN [also: sulfaproxyline]

**sulphapyridine** BAN *dermatitis herpetiformis suppressant* [also: sulfapyridine]

**sulphasalazine** BAN *broad-spectrum bacteriostatic; anti-inflammatory for ulcerative colitis; antirheumatic* [also: sulfasalazine; salazosulfapyridine]

**sulphasomidine** BAN [also: sulfisomidine]

**sulphasomizole** BAN *antibacterial* [also: sulfasomizole]

**sulphathiazole** BAN *antibacterial* [also: sulfathiazole]

**sulphaurea** BAN [also: sulfacarbamide]

**sulphinpyrazone** BAN *uricosuric for gout* [also: sulfinpyrazone]

**sulphocarbolate sodium** [see: phenolsulphonate sodium]

**Sulpho-Lac** cream, soap OTC *antibacterial and exfoliant for acne* [sulfur] 5%

**Sulpho-Lac Acne Medication** cream OTC *antibacterial; exfoliant* [sulfur; zinc sulfate] 5%•27%

**sulphomyxin sodium** BAN *antibacterial* [also: sulfomyxin]

**sulphonal** [see: sulfonmethane]

**Sulphrin** eye drop suspension (discontinued 1993) ℞ *topical ophthalmic corticosteroidal anti-inflammatory; bacteriostatic* [prednisolone acetate; sulfacetamide sodium] 0.5%•10%

**Sulphrin** ophthalmic ointment (discontinued 1994) ℞ *topical ophthalmic corticosteroidal anti-inflammatory; bac-* *teriostatic* [prednisolone acetate; sulfacetamide sodium] 0.5%•10%

**sulpiride** USAN, INN *antidepressant*

**Sulpred** eye drop suspension ℞ *topical ophthalmic corticosteroidal anti-inflammatory; bacteriostatic* [prednisolone acetate; sodium sulfacetamide]

**sulprosal** INN

**sulprostone** USAN, INN *prostaglandin*

**Sulster** eye drops ℞ *ophthalmic topical corticosteroidal anti-inflammatory; bacteriostatic* [prednisolone sodium phosphate; sulfacetamide sodium] 0.25%•1%

**sultamicillin** USAN, INN, BAN *antibacterial*

**sulthiame** USAN *anticonvulsant* [also: sultiame]

**sultiame** INN *anticonvulsant* [also: sulthiame]

**sultopride** INN

**sultosilic acid** INN

**Sultrin Triple Sulfa** vaginal tablets, vaginal cream ℞ *broad-spectrum bacteriostatic* [sulfathiazole; sulfacetamide; sulfabenzamide] 172.5•143.75•184 mg; 3.42%•2.86%•3.7%

**sultroponium** INN

**sulukast** USAN, INN *antiasthmatic; leukotriene antagonist*

**sulverapride** INN

**Sumacal** powder OTC *carbohydrate caloric supplement* [glucose polymers]

**sumacetamol** INN, BAN

**sumarotene** USAN, INN *keratolytic*

**sumatriptan** INN, BAN *vascular serotonin receptor agonist for migraine and cluster headaches* [also: sumatriptan succinate]

**sumatriptan succinate** USAN *vascular serotonin receptor agonist for migraine and cluster headaches* [also: sumatriptan]

**sumetizide** INN

**Summer's Eve Disposable Douche** solution OTC *antifungal; vaginal cleanser and deodorizer; acidity modifier* [sodium benzoate; citric acid]

**Summer's Eve Disposable Douche; Summer's Eve Disposable Douche Extra Cleansing** solution

OTC *vaginal cleanser and deodorizer; acidity modifier* [vinegar (acetic acid)]

**Summer's Eve Feminine Bath** liquid OTC *for external perivaginal cleansing*

**Summer's Eve Feminine Powder** OTC *absorbs vaginal moisture* [cornstarch; benzethonium chloride]

**Summer's Eve Feminine Wash** liquid, wipes OTC *for external perivaginal cleansing*

**Summer's Eve Medicated Disposable Douche** solution OTC *antiseptic/germicidal; vaginal cleanser and deodorizer* [povidone-iodine] 0.3%

**Summer's Eve Post-Menstrual Disposable Douche** solution OTC *vaginal cleanser and deodorizer; acidity modifier* [monosodium phosphate; disodium phosphate]

**Sumycin** syrup ℞ *broad-spectrum antibiotic* [tetracycline HCl] 125 mg/5 mL

**Sumycin '250'; Sumycin '500'** capsules, tablets ℞ *broad-spectrum antibiotic* [tetracycline HCl] 250 mg; 500 mg

**sunagrel** INN

**suncillin** INN *antibacterial* [also: suncillin sodium]

**suncillin sodium** USAN *antibacterial* [also: suncillin]

**SunKist Multivitamins Complete, Children's** chewable tablets OTC *vitamin/mineral/iron supplement* [multiple vitamins & minerals; iron; folic acid; biotin] ± •18 mg•400 μg•40 μg

**SunKist Multi-Vitamins + Extra C** chewable tablets OTC *vitamin supplement* [multiple vitamins; folic acid] ± •0.3 mg

**SunKist Multivitamins + Iron, Children's** chewable tablets OTC *vitamin/iron supplement* [multiple vitamins; iron; folic acid] ± •15•0.3 mg

**SunKist Vitamin C** chewable tablets, caplets OTC *vitamin supplement* [ascorbic acid] 60, 250, 500 mg; 500 mg

**sunrise; sunshine** *street drug slang for yellow LSD* [see: LSD]

**Supac** tablets OTC *analgesic; antipyretic; anti-inflammatory* [acetaminophen; aspirin; caffeine] 160•230•32 mg

**super** *street drug slang* [see: PCP]

**super acid; super C** *street drug slang* [see: ketamine HCl]

**Super CalciCaps** tablets OTC *dietary supplement* [dibasic calcium phosphate; calcium gluconate; calcium carbonate; vitamin D] 400 mg (Ca)•42 mg (P)•133 IU

**Super CalciCaps M-Z** tablets OTC *dietary supplement* [vitamins A and D; multiple minerals] 1667 mg•133 IU• ±

**Super Calcium '1200'** softgels OTC *dietary supplement* [calcium; vitamin D] 600 mg•200 IU

**Super Citro Cee** sustained-release tablets OTC *dietary supplement* [ascorbic acid; lemon & rose hips bioflavonoids; rutin] 500•1000•50 mg

**Super Complex C-500 Caplets** OTC *dietary supplement* [ascorbic acid; various bioflavonoids; citrus hesperidin; rutin] 500•200•25•50 mg

**super cools; super kools** *street drug slang for PCP-laced cigarettes* [see: PCP]

**Super D** Perles (capsules) OTC *vitamin supplement* [vitamins A and D] 10 000•400 IU

**super grass; super weed** *street drug slang for PCP or marijuana laced with PCP* [see: marijuana; PCP]

**Super Hi Potency** tablets OTC *vitamin/mineral supplement* [multiple vitamins & minerals; folic acid; biotin] ± •0.4 mg•0.075 mg

**super ice** *street drug slang for smokable methamphetamine* [see: methamphetamine HCl]

**super joint** *street drug slang* [see: PCP]

**Super Quints-50** tablets OTC *vitamin supplement* [multiple B vitamins; folic acid; biotin] ± •400•50 μg

**super Sopors** *street drug slang for Parest (methaqualone; discontinued 1983)* [see: methaqualone]

**Superdophilus** powder OTC *dietary supplement; fever blister treatment; not generally regarded as safe and effective as an antidiarrheal* [Lactobacillus acidophilus] 2 billion U/g

**SuperEPA 1200; SuperEPA 2000** softgels OTC *dietary supplement* [omega-3 fatty acids] 1200 mg; 1000 mg

**superoxide dismutase (SOD)** [see: orgotein]

**Superplex-T** tablets OTC *vitamin supplement* [multiple B vitamins; vitamin C] ± • 500 mg

**supers** *street drug slang* [see: methaqualone]

**supidimide** INN

**Suplena** ready-to-use liquid OTC *enteral nutritional therapy for renal failure* [essential amino acids]

**Suppap-120; Suppap-650** suppositories (discontinued 1997) OTC *analgesic; antipyretic* [acetaminophen] 120 mg; 650 mg

**Suppap-325** suppositories (discontinued 1994) OTC *analgesic; antipyretic* [acetaminophen] 325 mg

**supper** *street drug slang for Sopor (methaqualone; discontinued 1981)* [see: methaqualone]

**Supprelin** subcu injection ℞ *gonadotropin-releasing hormone for central precocious puberty (orphan)* [histrelin acetate] 120, 300, 600 μg/0.6 mL

**Suppress** lozenges OTC *antitussive* [dextromethorphan hydrobromide] 7.5 mg

**Supprette** (trademarked dosage form) *suppository*

**Suprane** liquid for vaporization ℞ *inhalation general anesthetic* [desflurane]

**Suprax** film-coated tablets, powder for oral suspension ℞ *cephalosporin-type antibiotic* [cefixime] 200, 400 mg; 100 mg/5 mL

**Suprefact** ℞ *investigational antineoplastic for prostatic cancer* [buserelin acetate]

**suproclone** USAN, INN *sedative*

**suprofen** USAN, INN, BAN *ocular non-steroidal anti-inflammatory drug (NSAID); antimiotic*

**Supule** (trademarked dosage form) *suppository*

**suramin sodium** USP, BAN *investigational anti-infective for trypanosomiasis and onchocerciasis; investigational antineoplastic*

**Surbex** Filmtabs (film-coated tablets) OTC *vitamin supplement* [multiple B vitamins] ±

**Surbex 750 with Iron** Filmtabs (film-coated tablets) OTC *vitamin/iron supplement* [multiple B vitamins; vitamins C and E; ferrous sulfate, dried; folic acid] ± • 750 mg • 30 IU • 27 mg • 0.4 mg

**Surbex 750 with Zinc** Filmtabs (film-coated tablets) OTC *vitamin/zinc supplement* [multiple vitamins; zinc sulfate; folic acid] ± • 22.5 • 0.4 mg

**Surbex-T; Surbex with C** Filmtabs (film-coated tablets) OTC *vitamin supplement* [multiple B vitamins; vitamin C] ± • 500 mg; ± • 250 mg

**Surbu-Gen-T** film-coated tablets OTC *vitamin supplement* [multiple B vitamins; vitamin C] ± • 500 mg

**Sure Cell Chlamydia Test** reagent kit for professional use *in vitro diagnostic aid for Chlamydia trachomatis* [monoclonal antibody-based enzyme-linked immunosorbent assay (ELISA)]

**Sure Cell hCG-Urine Test** kit (name changed to Sure Cell Pregnancy in 1995)

**Sure Cell Herpes (HSV) Test** reagent kit for professional use *in vitro diagnostic aid for herpes simplex virus in genital, rectal, oral, or dermal swabs* [monoclonal antibody-based enzyme-linked immunosorbent assay (ELISA)]

**Sure Cell Pregnancy** test kit for professional use *in vitro diagnostic aid for urine pregnancy test* [monoclonal/polyclonal antibody ELISA test]

**Sure Cell Strep A Test** kit (name changed to Sure Cell Streptococci in 1995)

**Sure Cell Streptococci** test kit for professional use *in vitro diagnostic aid for Group A streptococcal antigens in blood and throat swabs* [enzyme-linked immunosorbent assay (ELISA)]

**SureLac** chewable tablets OTC *digestive aid for lactose intolerance* [lactase enzyme] 3000 U

**surface active extract of saline lavage of bovine lungs** [see: beractant]

**surfactant, human amniotic fluid derived** *orphan status withdrawn 1994* surfactant TA [see: beractant]

surfactant TA, modified bovine lung surfactant extract [see: beractant]

Surfak Liquigels (capsules) OTC *stool softener* [docusate calcium] 50, 240 mg

surfer *street drug slang* [see: PCP]

surfilcon A USAN *hydrophilic contact lens material*

Surfol Post-Immersion Bath Oil OTC *bath emollient*

surfomer USAN, INN *hypolipidemic*

Surgel vaginal gel OTC *lubricant* [propylene glycol; glycerin]

surgibone USAN *internal bone splint*

surgical catgut [see: suture, absorbable surgical]

surgical gut [see: suture, absorbable surgical]

Surgicel strips, Nu-knit pads ℞ *topical local hemostat for surgery* [oxidized cellulose]

suricainide INN *antiarrhythmic* [also: suricainide maleate]

suricainide maleate USAN, INN *antiarrhythmic* [also: suricainide]

suriclone INN, BAN

Surital IV injection (discontinued 1993) ℞ *barbiturate general anesthetic* [thiamylal sodium] 1, 5, 10 g ☒ Serentil

suritozole USAN, INN *antidepressant; investigational Alzheimer's treatment*

Surmontil capsules ℞ *tricyclic antidepressant* [trimipramine maleate] 25, 50, 100 mg

suronacrine INN *cholinesterase inhibitor* [also: suronacrine maleate]

suronacrine maleate USAN *cholinesterase inhibitor* [also: suronacrine]

Survanta suspension for intratracheal instillation ℞ *pulmonary surfactant for neonatal respiratory distress syndrome or respiratory failure (orphan)* [beractant] 25 mg/mL

Susano elixir ℞ *GI anticholinergic; sedative* [atropine sulfate; scopolamine hydrobromide; hyoscyamine hydrobromide; phenobarbital] 0.0194•0.0065•0.1037•16.2 mg/5 mL

Susano tablets (discontinued 1995) ℞ *GI anticholinergic; sedative* [phenobarbital; atropine sulfate; scopola-mine hydrobromide; hyoscyamine hydrobromide] 0.0194•0.0065•0.1037•16.2 mg

Sus-Phrine subcu injection ℞ *bronchodilator for bronchial asthma, bronchospasm and COPD; vasopressor for shock* [epinephrine] 1:200 (5 mg/mL)

Sustacal powder OTC *enteral nutritional therapy* [milk-based formula]

Sustacal pudding OTC *enteral nutritional therapy* [milk-based formula]

Sustacal ready-to-use liquid OTC *enteral nutritional therapy* [lactose-free formula]

Sustacal Basic; Sustacal Plus ready-to-use liquid OTC *enteral nutritional therapy* [lactose-free formula]

Sustacal HC ready-to-use liquid (discontinued 1994) OTC *high-calorie nutritional supplement* [lactose-free formula] 8 oz.

Sustagen powder OTC *enteral nutritional therapy* [milk-based formula]

Sustaire timed-release tablets ℞ *bronchodilator* [theophylline] 100, 300 mg

sutilains USAN, USP, INN, BAN *topical proteolytic enzymes for necrotic tissue debridement*

sutoprofen [see: suprofen]

suture, absorbable surgical USP *surgical aid*

suture, nonabsorbable surgical USP *surgical aid*

suxamethone [see: succinylcholine chloride]

suxamethonium chloride INN, BAN *neuromuscular blocking agent* [also: succinylcholine chloride]

suxemerid INN *antitussive* [also: suxemerid sulfate]

suxemerid sulfate USAN *antitussive* [also: suxemerid]

suxethonium chloride INN

suxibuzone INN

sweet birch oil [see: methyl salicylate]

sweet Jesus *street drug slang* [see: heroin]

sweet Lucy *street drug slang* [see: marijuana]

sweet orange peel tincture [see: orange peel tincture, sweet]

sweet spirit of nitre [see: ethyl nitrite]

**sweet stuff** *street drug slang* [see: heroin; cocaine]

**Sweet'n Fresh Clotrimazole-7** cream, vaginal suppositories OTC *antifungal* [clotrimazole] 1%; 100 mg

**sweets** *street drug slang* [see: amphetamines]

**swell up** *street drug slang* [see: cocaine, crack]

**Swim-Ear** ear drops OTC *antiseptic* [isopropyl alcohol] 95%

**Sygen** ℞ *investigational treatment for stroke, spinal cord injury, subarachnoid hemorrhage, and parkinsonism* [nerve growth factor GM$_1$ ganglioside]

**Syllact** powder OTC *bulk laxative* [psyllium seed husks] 3.3 g/tsp.

**Syllamalt** powder OTC *laxative* [malt soup extract; psyllium seed husks] 4•3 g/tsp.

**Symadine** capsules (discontinued 1996) ℞ *antiviral; antiparkinsonian agent* [amantadine HCl] 100 mg

**symclosene** USAN, INN *topical anti-infective*

**Symcor** ℞ *investigational treatment for hypertension and congestive heart failure* [tiamenidine]

**symetine** INN *antiamebic* [also: symetine HCl]

**symetine HCl** USAN *antiamebic* [also: symetine]

**Symmetrel** capsules, syrup ℞ *antiviral; antiparkinsonian agent* [amantadine HCl] 100 mg; 50 mg/5 mL

**sympatholytics** *a class of cardiovascular drugs that block the passage of impulses through the sympathetic nervous system* [also called: antiadrenergics]

**sympathomimetics** *a class of bronchodilators that relax the bronchial muscles, reducing bronchospasm* [also called: adrenergic agonists]

**Synacol CF** tablets OTC *antitussive; expectorant* [dextromethorphan hydrobromide; guaifenesin] 15•200 mg

**Synacort** cream ℞ *topical corticosteroid* [hydrocortisone] 1%, 2.5%

**Synalar** cream, ointment, topical solution ℞ *topical corticosteroid* [fluocinolone acetonide] 0.01, 0.25%; 0.025%; 0.01%

**Synalar-HP** cream ℞ *topical corticosteroid* [fluocinolone acetonide] 0.2%

**Synalgos-DC** capsules ℞ *narcotic analgesic* [dihydrocodeine bitartrate; aspirin; caffeine] 16•356.4•30 mg

**Synapton SR** ℞ *investigational (NDA filed) sustained-release cholinesterase inhibitor for Alzheimer's disease* [physostigmine]

**Synarel** nasal spray ℞ *gonadotropin-releasing hormone for central precocious puberty (orphan) and endometriosis* [nafarelin acetate] 2 mg/mL (200 μg/spray)

**Synemol** cream ℞ *topical corticosteroid* [fluocinolone acetonide] 0.025%

**Synercid** injection ℞ *investigational (NDA filed) semi-synthetic streptogramin antibiotic for iatrogenic infections* [quinupristin; dalfopristin]

**synestrin** [see: diethylstilbestrol]

**synnematin B** [see: adicillin]

**Synophylate-GG** syrup ℞ *antiasthmatic; bronchodilator; expectorant* [theophylline; guaifenesin; alcohol 10%] 150•100 mg/15 mL

**Synovir** ℞ *investigational (orphan) for graft vs. host disease, AIDS wasting, leprosy, and mycobacterial infections* [thalidomide]

**Syn-Rx** controlled-release tablets (14-day, 56-tablet treatment regimen) ℞ *decongestant; expectorant* [pseudoephedrine HCl; guaifenesin] 60•600 mg

**Synsorb-Pk** ℞ *investigational (Phase III, orphan) E. coli neutralizer for traveler's diarrhea and hemolytic uremic syndrome (HUS)* [8-methoxycarbonyloctyl oligosaccharides]

**synthestrin** [see: diethylstilbestrol]

**synthetic cocaine** *street drug slang* [see: PCP]

**synthetic lung surfactant** [see: colfosceril palmitate]

**synthetic paraffin** [see: paraffin, synthetic]

**synthetic spermaceti** [now: cetyl esters wax]

**synthetic THT** *street drug slang* [see: PCP]

**synthoestrin** [see: diethylstilbestrol]

**Synthroid** tablets, powder for injection ℞ *thyroid hormone* [levothyroxine sodium] 25, 50, 75, 88, 100, 112, 125, 150, 175, 200, 300 μg; 200, 500 μg ☑ Euthroid

**Syntocinon** IV, IM injection ℞ *induction of labor; postpartum bleeding; incomplete abortion* [oxytocin] 10 U/mL

**Syntocinon** nasal spray ℞ *initial milk let-down* [oxytocin] 40 U/mL

**synvinolin** [now: simvastatin]

**Synvisc** ℞ *investigational antiarthritic* [hylan fluid-gel mixture]

**Syprine** capsules ℞ *copper chelating agent for Wilson's disease (orphan)* [trientine HCl] 50 mg

**Syracol CF** tablets OTC *antitussive; expectorant* [dextromethorphan hydrobromide; guaifenesin] 15•200 mg

**syrosingopine** NF, INN, BAN

**syrup** NF *flavoring agent*

**syrup and beans** *street drug slang for a combination of Doriden (glutethimide; discontinued 1990) and codeine* [see: glutethimide; codeine]

**syrupus cerasi** [see: cherry juice]

**Syrvite** liquid OTC *vitamin supplement* [multiple vitamins] ±

**Sytobex** IM or subcu injection (discontinued 1994) ℞ *antianemic; vitamin B₁₂ supplement* [cyanocobalamin] 1000 μg/mL

**T-2 protocol (dactinomycin, doxorubicin, vincristine, cyclophosphamide, radiation)** *chemotherapy protocol*

**T₃ (liothyronine sodium)** [q.v.]

**T₄ (levothyroxine sodium)** [q.v.]

**T4, recombinant soluble human** *investigational (Phase I/II) antiviral for HIV*

**T4 endonuclease V (T4N5), liposome encapsulated** *investigational (orphan) for prevent cutaneous neoplasms in xeroderma pigmentosum*

**T-10 protocol (methotrexate, doxorubicin, cisplatin, bleomycin, cyclophosphamide, dactinomycin)** *chemotherapy protocol*

**T-88** *investigational treatment for gram-negative sepsis*

**T-3761** *investigational oral fluoroquinolone antibiotic*

**T-3762** *investigational injectable fluoroquinolone antibiotic*

**T30177** *investigational (Phase I) antiviral oligonucleotide for AIDS*

**T-61** ℞ *veterinary anesthesia; also for veterinary euthanasia* [embutramide]

**Tab-A-Vite** tablets OTC *vitamin supplement* [multiple vitamins; folic acid] ±•0.4 mg

**Tab-A-Vite + Iron** tablets OTC *vitamin/iron supplement* [multiple vitamins; iron; folic acid] ±•18•0.4 mg

**tabilautide** INN

**Tabloid** (trademarked dosage form) *tablet with raised lettering*

**Tabron** Filmseals (film-coated tablets) (discontinued 1996) ℞ *hematinic* [ferrous fumarate; multiple B vitamins; vitamins C and E; docusate sodium; folic acid] 100 mg•±•500 mg•30 IU•50 mg•1 mg

**tabs** *street drug slang* [see: LSD]

**Tabules** (dosage form) *tablets*

**tac** *street drug slang* [see: PCP]

**Tac-3** IM, intra-articular, intrabursal, intradermal injection ℞ *glucocorticoids* [triamcinolone acetonide] 3 mg/mL

**Tac-40** suspension ℞ *topical corticosteroid* [triamcinolone acetonide] 40 mg/mL

**Tacaryl** syrup (discontinued 1997) ℞ *antihistamine* [methdilazine HCl] 4 mg/5 mL

**Tacaryl** tablets, chewable tablets (discontinued 1994) ℞ *antihistamine* [methdilazine HCl] 8 mg; 4 mg

**Tace** capsules ℞ *hormone for estrogen replacement therapy or inoperable prostatic carcinoma* [chlorotrianisene] 12, 25 mg

**taclamine** INN *minor tranquilizer* [also: taclamine HCl]

**taclamine HCl** USAN *minor tranquilizer* [also: taclamine]

**tacrine** INN, BAN *reversible cholinesterase inhibitor; cognition adjuvant for Alzheimer's dementia* [also: tacrine HCl]

**tacrine HCl** USAN *reversible cholinesterase inhibitor; cognition adjuvant for Alzheimer's dementia* [also: tacrine]

**tacrolimus** USAN, INN *immunosuppressant*

**TAD (thioguanine, ara-C, daunorubicin)** *chemotherapy protocol* [also: DCT; DAT]

**Tagamet** film-coated tablets ℞ *gastric and duodenal ulcer treatment; for gastric hypersecretory conditions* [cimetidine] 200, 300, 400, 800 mg ⊇ Tegopen

**Tagamet** liquid, IV or IM injection, premixed injection ℞ *gastric and duodenal ulcer treatment; for gastric hypersecretory conditions* [cimetidine HCl] 300 mg/5 mL; 300 mg/2 mL; 300 mg/vial

**Tagamet 100** (British name for U.S. product Tagamet HB [in 100 mg strength])

**Tagamet CR** ℞ *investigational controlled-release gastric and duodenal ulcer treatment* [cimetidine]

**Tagamet HB** film-coated tablets OTC $H_2$ *antagonist for episodic heartburn and acid indigestion* [cimetidine] 100, 200 mg

**taglutimide** INN

**TA-HPV** ℞ *investigational (orphan) for cervical cancer* [vaccinia (human papillomavirus), recombinant]

**tail lights** *street drug slang* [see: LSD]

**taima** *street drug slang* [see: marijuana]

**taking a cruise** *street drug slang* [see: PCP]

**Takkouri** *street drug slang* [see: marijuana]

**Talacen** caplets ℞ *narcotic agonist-antagonist analgesic; antipyretic* [pentazocine HCl; acetaminophen] 25•650 mg

**talampicillin** INN *antibacterial* [also: talampicillin HCl]

**talampicillin HCl** USAN *antibacterial* [also: talampicillin]

**talastine** INN

**talbutal** USP, INN *sedative; hypnotic*

**talc** USP, JAN *dusting powder; tablet and capsule lubricant*

**talc, sterile aerosol** *investigational (orphan) treatment for malignant pleural effusions via intrapleural thoracoscopy administration*

**taleranol** USAN, INN *gonadotropin enzyme inhibitor*

**talinolol** INN

**talipexole** INN

**talisomycin** USAN, INN *antineoplastic*

**tall** *street drug slang* [see: Talwin; pentazocine HCl]

**tallimustine** INN *investigational antineoplastic for leukemia and solid tumors*

**tallysomycin A** [now: talisomycin]

**talmetacin** USAN, INN *analgesic; anti-inflammatory; antipyretic*

**talmetoprim** INN

**talniflumate** USAN, INN *anti-inflammatory; analgesic*

**talopram** INN *catecholamine potentiator* [also: talopram HCl]

**talopram HCl** USAN *catecholamine potentiator* [also: talopram]

**talosalate** USAN, INN *analgesic; anti-inflammatory*

**Taloxa** (foreign name for U.S. product Felbatol)

**taloximine** INN, BAN

**talsaclidine** INN

**talsaclidine fumarate** USAN *muscarinic $M_1$ agonist for Alzheimer's disease*

**talsupram** INN

**taltibride** [see: metibride]

**taltrimide** INN

**taludipine** [see: teludipine]

**taludipine HCl** (*previously used* USAN) [see: teludipine HCl]

**Talwin** IV, subcu or IM injection ℞ *narcotic agonist-antagonist analgesic; also abused as a street drug* [pentazocine lactate] 30 mg/mL

**Talwin Compound** caplets ℞ *narcotic agonist-antagonist analgesic; antipyretic; also abused as a street drug* [pentazocine HCl; aspirin] 12.5•325 mg

**Talwin NX** tablets ℞ *narcotic agonist-antagonist analgesic; also abused as a*

*street`drug* [pentazocine HCl; naloxone HCl] 50•0.5 mg

**Tambocor** tablets R *antiarrhythmic* [flecainide acetate] 50, 100, 150 mg

**tameridone** USAN, INN, BAN *veterinary sedative*

**tameticillin** INN

**tametraline** INN *antidepressant* [also: tametraline HCl]

**tametraline HCl** USAN *antidepressant* [also: tametraline]

**Tamine S.R.** sustained-release tablets R *decongestant; antihistamine* [phenylpropanolamine HCl; phenylephrine HCl; brompheniramine maleate] 15•15•12 mg

**tamitinol** INN

**tamoxifen** INN, BAN *antiestrogen; antineoplastic* [also: tamoxifen citrate]

**tamoxifen citrate** USAN, USP, JAN *antiestrogen antineoplastic for breast cancer; investigational for breast cancer prevention* [also: tamoxifen] 10 mg oral

**tampramine** INN *antidepressant* [also: tampramine fumarate]

**tampramine fumarate** USAN *antidepressant* [also: tampramine]

**Tamp-R-Tel** (trademarked packaging form) *tamper-evident cartridge-needle unit*

**tamsulosin** INN *alpha₁ antagonist for benign prostatic hypertrophy (BPH)* [also: tamsulosin HCl]

**tamsulosin HCl** USAN, JAN *alpha₁ antagonist for benign prostatic hypertrophy (BPH)* [also: tamsulosin]

**Tanac** gel OTC *topical oral anesthetic; vulnerary* [dyclonine HCl; allantoin] 1%•0.5%

**Tanac** liquid OTC *topical oral anesthetic; antiseptic* [benzocaine; benzalkonium chloride] 10%•0.12%

**Tanac Dual Core** stick OTC *topical oral anesthetic; antiseptic; astringent* [benzocaine; benzalkonium chloride; tannic acid] 7.5%•0.12%•6%

**Tanac Roll-On** liquid (discontinued 1994) OTC *topical oral anesthetic; antiseptic* [benzocaine; benzalkonium chloride] 5%•0.12%

**Tanafed** oral suspension R *decongestant; antihistamine* [pseudoephedrine

tannate; chlorpheniramine tannate] 75•4.5 mg/5 mL

**tandamine** INN *antidepressant* [also: tandamine HCl]

**tandamine HCl** USAN *antidepressant* [also: tandamine]

**tandospirone** INN, BAN *anxiolytic* [also: tandospirone citrate]

**tandospirone citrate** USAN *anxiolytic* [also: tandospirone]

**Tango & Cash** *street drug slang* [see: fentanyl]

**taniplon** INN

**tannic acid** USP, JAN *astringent; topical mucosal protectant*

**tannic acid acetate** [see: acetyltannic acid]

**tannin** [see: tannic acid]

**tannyl acetate** [see: acetyltannic acid]

**Tanoral** tablets R *decongestant; antihistamine* [phenylephrine tannate; chlorpheniramine tannate; pyrilamine tannate] 25•8•25 mg

**tantalum** *element (Ta)*

**Tao** capsules R *macrolide antibiotic* [troleandomycin] 250 mg

**taoryi edisylate** [see: caramiphen edisylate]

**Tapanol** tablets, caplets, gelcaps OTC *analgesic; antipyretic* [acetaminophen] 325, 500 mg; 500 mg; 500 mg

**Tapazole** tablets R *antithyroid agent* [methimazole] 5, 10 mg

**tape, adhesive** USP *surgical aid*

**taprostene** INN

**tar** [see: coal tar]

**tar** *street drug slang* [see: opium; heroin]

**Tarabine PFS** injection R *antineoplastic* [cytarabine]

**Taractan** IM injection (discontinued 1994) R *antipsychotic* [clorprothixene HCl] 12.5 mg/mL ⊡ Periactin; Tinactin

**Taractan** oral concentrate (discontinued 1994) R *antipsychotic* [clorprothixene lactate] 100 mg/5 mL

**Taractan** tablets (discontinued 1994) R *antipsychotic* [clorprothixene] 10, 25, 50, 100 mg

**Taraphilic Ointment** OTC *topical antipsoriatic; antiseborrheic* [coal tar] 1%

**tardust** *street drug slang* [see: cocaine]

**Targocid** (commercially available in 13 foreign countries) ℞ *investigational glycopeptide antibiotic* [teicoplanin]

**Targretin** oral, topical ℞ *investigational (Phase I/II) antineoplastic for AIDS-related Kaposi sarcoma* [LGD 1069 (code name—generic name not yet approved)] ② Tegopen; Tegrin

**Tarka** film-coated combination-release tablets ℞ *once-daily antihypertensive; ACE inhibitor; calcium channel blocker* [trandolapril (immediate release); verapamil HCl (extended release)] 2•180, 1•240, 2•240, 4•240 mg

**Tarlene** hair lotion OTC *antiseborrheic; antipsoriatic; keratolytic* [salicylic acid; coal tar] 2.5%•2%

**Tarsum** shampoo OTC *antipsoriatic; antiseborrheic; keratolytic* [coal tar; salicylic acid] 10%•5%

**tartar emetic** [see: antimony potassium tartrate]

**tartaric acid** NF *buffering agent*

**Tasmar** ℞ *investigational topical treatment for cutaneous actinic damage* [isotretinoin]

**tasosartan** USAN, INN *antihypertensive; angiotensin II antagonist*

**taste** *street drug slang for heroin or a small sample of drugs* [see: heroin]

**tasuldine** INN

**TAT antagonist** *investigational (Phase I/II) antiviral for HIV*

**Tauricyt** ℞ *investigational antineoplastic* [tauromustine]

**taurine** INN [also: aminoethylsulfonic acid]

**taurocholate sodium** [see: sodium taurocholate]

**taurolidine** INN, BAN *investigational antitoxin for the treatment of sepsis*

**tauromustine** INN *investigational treatment for renal cancer and multiple sclerosis*

**tauroselcholic acid** INN, BAN

**taurultam** INN, BAN

**Tavist** tablets, syrup ℞ *antihistamine* [clemastine fumarate] 2.68 mg; 0.67 mg/5 mL

**Tavist-1** tablets (discontinued 1997) OTC *antihistamine* [clemastine fumarate] 1.34 mg

**Tavist-D** film-coated sustained-release tablets OTC *decongestant; antihistamine* [phenylpropanolamine HCl; clemastine fumarate] 75•1.34 mg

**taxoids** *a class of antineoplastics*

**Taxol** IV infusion ℞ *antineoplastic for metastatic carcinoma of the ovary and breast and non-small cell lung cancer; investigational (orphan) for Kaposi sarcoma* [paclitaxel] 30 mg/5 mL

**Taxotere** IV infusion ℞ *antineoplastic for breast cancer; investigational for ovarian and lung cancers* [docetaxel] 20, 80 mg/vial

**tazadolene** INN *analgesic* [also: tazadolene succinate]

**tazadolene succinate** USAN *analgesic* [also: tazadolene]

**tazanolast** INN

**tazarotene** USAN, INN *retinoid pro-drug; topical keratolytic for acne and psoriasis*

**tazasubrate** INN, BAN

**tazeprofen** INN

**Tazicef** powder for IV or IM injection ℞ *cephalosporin-type antibiotic* [ceftazidime] 1, 2, 6 g

**Tazidime** powder for IV or IM injection ℞ *cephalosporin-type antibiotic* [ceftazidime] 0.5, 1, 2, 6 g

**tazifylline** INN *antihistamine* [also: tazifylline HCl]

**tazifylline HCl** USAN *antihistamine* [also: tazifylline]

**taziprinone** INN

**tazobactam** USAN, INN, BAN *β-lactamase inhibitor*

**tazobactam sodium** USAN *β-lactamase inhibitor*

**Tazocin** (European name for U.S. product Zosyn)

**tazofelone** USAN *investigational (Phase II) treatment for ulcerative colitis and Crohn's disease*

**tazolol** INN *cardiotonic* [also: tazolol HCl]

**tazolol HCl** USAN *cardiotonic* [also: tazolol]

**Tazorac** gel ℞ *retinoid pro-drug; topical keratolytic for acne and psoriasis* [tazarotene] 0.05%, 0.1%

**TBC-3B** *investigational (Phase I) vaccine for AIDS*

**TBC-CEA** ℞ *investigational cancer vaccine* [vaccinia virus vaccine for carcinoembryonic antigen (CEA)]

**T-birds** *street drug slang* [see: Tuinal; amobarbital sodium; secobarbital sodium]

**T-buzz** *street drug slang* [see: PCP]

**TBZ (thiabendazole)** [q.v.]

**TC (thioguanine, cytarabine)** *chemotherapy protocol*

**⁹⁹ᵐTc** [see: macrosalb (⁹⁹ᵐTc)]

**⁹⁹ᵐTc** [see: sodium pertechnetate Tc 99m]

**⁹⁹ᵐTc** [see: technetium Tc 99m albumin]

**⁹⁹ᵐTc** [see: technetium Tc 99m albumin aggregated]

**⁹⁹ᵐTc** [see: technetium Tc 99m albumin colloid]

**⁹⁹ᵐTc** [see: technetium Tc 99m albumin microaggregated]

**⁹⁹ᵐTc** [see: technetium Tc 99m antimony trisulfide colloid]

**⁹⁹ᵐTc** [see: technetium Tc 99m biciromab]

**⁹⁹ᵐTc** [see: technetium Tc 99m bicisate]

**⁹⁹ᵐTc** [see: technetium Tc 99m disofenin]

**⁹⁹ᵐTc** [see: technetium Tc 99m etidronate]

**⁹⁹ᵐTc** [see: technetium Tc 99m exametazine]

**⁹⁹ᵐTc** [see: technetium Tc 99m ferpentetate]

**⁹⁹ᵐTc** [see: technetium Tc 99m furifosmin]

**⁹⁹ᵐTc** [see: technetium Tc 99m gluceptate]

**⁹⁹ᵐTc** [see: technetium Tc 99m lidofenin]

**⁹⁹ᵐTc** [see: technetium Tc 99m mebrofenin]

**⁹⁹ᵐTc** [see: technetium Tc 99m medronate]

**⁹⁹ᵐTc** [see: technetium Tc 99m medronate disodium]

**⁹⁹ᵐTc** [see: technetium Tc 99m mertiatide]

**⁹⁹ᵐTc** [see: technetium Tc 99m oxidronate]

**⁹⁹ᵐTc** [see: technetium Tc 99m pentetate]

**⁹⁹ᵐTc** [see: technetium Tc 99m pentetate calcium trisodium]

**⁹⁹ᵐTc** [see: technetium Tc 99m (pyro- & trimeta-) phosphates]

**⁹⁹ᵐTc** [see: technetium Tc 99m pyrophosphate]

**⁹⁹ᵐTc** [see: technetium Tc 99m red blood cells]

**⁹⁹ᵐTc** [see: technetium Tc 99m sestamibi]

**⁹⁹ᵐTc** [see: technetium Tc 99m siboroxime]

**⁹⁹ᵐTc** [see: technetium Tc 99m succimer]

**⁹⁹ᵐTc** [see: technetium Tc 99m sulfur colloid]

**⁹⁹ᵐTc** [see: technetium Tc 99m teboroxime]

**⁹⁹ᵐTc** [see: technetium Tc 99m tetrofosmin]

**⁹⁹ᵐTc** [see: technetium Tc 99m tiatide]

**T-Caine** lozenges (discontinued 1993) OTC *topical oral anesthetic* [benzocaine] 5 mg

**TCC (trichlorocarbanilide)** [see: triclocarban]

**TC-CYT-380** *investigational imaging aid for breast cancer detection and staging*

**TC-CYT-380 fragment** *investigational imaging aid for non-small cell lung cancer detection and staging*

**TD; Td (tetanus & diphtheria [toxoids])** *the designation TD or DT denotes the pediatric vaccine; Td denotes the adult vaccine* [see: diphtheria & tetanus toxoids, adsorbed]

**T-Dry** sustained-release capsules (discontinued 1995) OTC *decongestant; antihistamine* [pseudoephedrine HCl; chlorpheniramine maleate] 120•12 mg

**tea** *street drug slang* [see: marijuana; PCP]

**TEAB (tetraethylammonium bromide)** [see: tetrylammonium bromide]

**teaberry oil** [see: methyl salicylate]

**TEAC (tetraethylammonium chloride)** [q.v.]

**Tear Drop** eye drops OTC *ocular moisturizer/lubricant* [polyvinyl alcohol]

**TearGard** eye drops OTC *ocular moisturizer/lubricant* [hydroxyethylcellulose]

**Teargen** eye drops OTC *ocular moisturizer/lubricant*

**Tearisol** eye drops OTC *ocular moisturizer/lubricant* [hydroxypropyl methylcellulose] 0.5%

**Tears Naturale; Tears Naturale II; Tears Naturale Free** eye drops OTC *ocular moisturizer/lubricant* [hydroxypropyl methylcellulose] 0.3%

**Tears Plus** eye drops OTC *ocular moisturizer/lubricant* [polyvinyl alcohol] 1.4%

**Tears Renewed** eye drops OTC *ocular moisturizer/lubricant* [hydroxypropyl methylcellulose] 0.3%

**Tears Renewed** ophthalmic ointment OTC *ocular moisturizer/lubricant* [white petrolatum; mineral oil]

**tease and bees; T's and B's; tees and bees** *street drug slang for a combination of Talwin (pentazocine HCl) and PBZ (pyribenzamine), used as a heroin substitute* [see: Talwin; pentazocine HCl; tripelennamine]

**tease and blues; T's and blues; tees and blues** *street drug slang for a combination of Talwin (pentazocine HCl) and PBZ (pyribenzamine), used as a heroin substitute* [see: Talwin; pentazocine HCl; tripelennamine]

**tease and peas; T's and P's; tees and pees** *street drug slang for a combination of Talwin (pentazocine HCl) and PBZ (pyribenzamine), used as a heroin substitute* [see: Talwin; pentazocine HCl; tripelennamine]

**Tebamide** suppositories, pediatric suppositories ℞ *anticholinergic; antiemetic* [trimethobenzamide HCl] 200 mg; 100 mg

**tebatizole** INN

**tebethion** [see: thioacetazone; thiacetazone]

**tebufelone** USAN, INN *analgesic; antiinflammatory*

**tebuquine** USAN, INN *antimalarial*

**tebutate** USAN, INN *combining name for radicals or groups*

**TEC (thiotepa, etoposide, carboplatin)** *chemotherapy protocol*

**tecata; Tecate** *street drug slang* [see: heroin]

**teceleukin** USAN, INN, BAN *immunostimulant; investigational (orphan) for metastatic renal cell cancer and metastatic malignant melanoma*

**TechneScan Q-12** ℞ *investigational radiodiagnostic aid for cardiac disease* [technetium Tc 99m furifosmin]

**technetium** *element (Tc)*

**technetium ($^{99m}$Tc) dimercaptosuccinic acid** JAN *diagnostic aid for renal function testing* [also: technetium Tc 99m succimer]

**technetium ($^{99m}$Tc) human serum albumin** JAN *radioactive agent*

**technetium ($^{99m}$Tc) labeled macroaggregated human albumin** JAN [also: macrosalb ($^{99m}$Tc)]

**technetium ($^{99m}$Tc) methylenediphosphonate** JAN *radioactive diagnostic aid for skeletal imaging* [also: technetium Tc 99m medronate]

**technetium ($^{99m}$Tc) phytate** JAN *radioactive agent*

**technetium Tc 99m albumin** USP *radioactive agent*

**technetium Tc 99m albumin aggregated** USAN, USP *radioactive diagnostic aid for lung imaging*

**technetium Tc 99m albumin colloid** USAN, USP *radioactive agent*

**technetium Tc 99m albumin microaggregated** USAN *radioactive agent*

**technetium Tc 99m antimelanoma murine MAb** *investigational (orphan) for diagnostic imaging agent for metastases of malignant melanoma*

**technetium Tc 99m antimony trisulfide colloid** USAN *radioactive agent*

**technetium Tc 99m apticide** *investigational (NDA filed) radiopharmaceutical diagnostic aid for acute venous thrombosis*

**technetium Tc 99m arcitumomab** USAN *radiopharmaceutical diagnostic aid for recurrent or metastatic thyroid and colorectal cancers*

**technetium Tc 99m bectumomab** *monoclonal antibody; investigational (Phase III, orphan) diagnostic aid for* non-Hodgkin's lymphoma and AIDS-related lymphoma [also: bectumomab]

**technetium Tc 99m biciromab** *radioactive diagnostic aid for deep vein thrombosis* [see: biciromab]

**technetium Tc 99m bicisate** USAN, INN, BAN *radioactive diagnostic aid for brain imaging*

**technetium Tc 99m disofenin** USP *radioactive diagnostic aid for hepatobiliary function testing*

**technetium Tc 99m DMSA (dimercaptosuccinic acid)** [see: technetium Tc 99m succimer]

**technetium Tc 99m DTPA (diethylenetriaminepentaacetic acid)** [see: technetium Tc 99m pentetate]

**technetium Tc 99m etidronate** USP *radioactive agent*

**technetium Tc 99m exametazine** USAN *radioactive agent*

**technetium Tc 99m ferpentetate** USP *radioactive agent*

**technetium Tc 99m furifosmin** USAN, INN *radioactive agent; diagnostic aid for cardiac disease*

**technetium Tc 99m gluceptate** USP *radioactive agent*

**technetium Tc 99m HSA (human serum albumin)** [see: technetium Tc 99m albumin]

**technetium Tc 99m iron ascorbate pentetic acid complex** [now: technetium Tc 99m ferpentetate]

**technetium Tc 99m lidofenin** USAN, USP *radioactive agent*

**technetium Tc 99m MAA (microaggregated albumin)** [see: technetium Tc 99m albumin aggregated]

**technetium Tc 99m MDP (methylenediphosphonate)** [see: technetium Tc 99m medronate]

**technetium Tc 99m mebrofenin** USAN, USP *radioactive agent*

**technetium Tc 99m medronate** USP *radioactive diagnostic aid for skeletal imaging* [also: technetium ($^{99m}$Tc) methylenediphosphonate]

**technetium Tc 99m medronate disodium** USAN *radioactive agent*

**technetium Tc 99m mertiatide** USAN *radioactive diagnostic aid for renal function testing*

**technetium Tc 99m murine MAb IgG$_2$a to B cell** [now: technetium Tc 99m bectumomab]

**technetium Tc 99m murine MAb to human alpha-fetoprotein (AFP)** *investigational (orphan) for diagnostic aid for AFP-producing tumors, hepatoblastoma, and hepatocellular carcinoma*

**technetium Tc 99m murine MAb to human chorionic gonadotropin (hCG)** *investigational (orphan) for diagnostic aid for hCG-producing tumors*

**technetium Tc 99m oxidronate** USP *radioactive diagnostic aid for skeletal imaging*

**technetium Tc 99m pentetate** USP *radioactive agent* [also: human serum albumin diethylenetriaminepentaacetic acid technetium ($^{99m}$Tc)]

**technetium Tc 99m pentetate calcium trisodium** USAN *radioactive agent*

**technetium Tc 99m pentetate sodium** [now: technetium Tc 99m pentetate]

**technetium Tc 99m (pyro- & trimeta-) phosphates** USP *radioactive agent*

**technetium Tc 99m pyrophosphate** USP, JAN *radioactive agent*

**technetium Tc 99m red blood cells** USAN *radioactive agent*

**technetium Tc 99m sestamibi** USAN, INN, BAN *radioactive/radiopaque diagnostic aid for cardiac perfusion imaging*

**technetium Tc 99m siboroxime** USAN, INN *radioactive diagnostic aid for brain imaging*

**technetium Tc 99m sodium gluceptate** [now: technetium Tc 99m gluceptate]

**technetium Tc 99m succimer** USP *diagnostic aid for renal function testing* [also: technetium ($^{99m}$Tc) dimercaptosuccinic acid]

**technetium Tc 99m sulesomab** *monoclonal antibody; diagnostic aid for infectious lesions* [also: sulesomab]

**technetium Tc 99m sulfur colloid (TSC)** USAN, USP *radioactive agent*

**technetium Tc 99m teboroxime** USAN, INN, BAN *radioactive/radio-opaque diagnostic aid for cardiac perfusion imaging*

**technetium Tc 99m tetrofosmin** *radioactive agent for cardiovascular imaging*

**technetium Tc 99m tiatide** BAN

**technetium Tc 99m TSC (technetium sulfur colloid)** [see: technetium Tc 99m sulfur colloid]

**technetium Tc 99m-labeled CEA scan** [see: arcitumomab]

**Techtide** [see: P829 Techtide]

**teclothiazide** INN, BAN

**teclozan** USAN, INN *antiamebic*

**Tecnu Poison Oak-N-Ivy** liquid OTC *topical poison ivy treatment* [deodorized mineral spirits] ℞

**tecogalan sodium** USAN *antiangiogenic antineoplastic*

**Teczem** film-coated extended-release tablets ℞ *antihypertensive* [diltiazem maleate; enalapril maleate] 180•5 mg

**Teddies and Bettys** *street drug slang for a combination of Talwin (pentazocine HCl) and PBZ (pyribenzamine), used as a heroin substitute* [see: Talwin; pentazocine HCl; tripelennamine]

**tedisamil** INN *investigational calcium channel blocker for ischemic heart disease and arrhythmias*

**Tedral** tablets, suspension (discontinued 1993) OTC *antiasthmatic; bronchodilator; decongestant; sedative* [theophylline; ephedrine HCl; phenobarbital] ℞ Teldrin

**Tedral SA** sustained-action tablets (discontinued 1993) ℞ *antiasthmatic; bronchodilator; decongestant; sedative* [theophylline; ephedrine HCl; phenobarbital]

**Tedrigen** tablets OTC *antiasthmatic; bronchodilator; decongestant; sedative* [theophylline; ephedrine HCl; phenobarbital] 120•22.5•7.5 mg

**tees and bees; T's and B's; tease and bees** *street drug slang for a combination of Talwin (pentazocine HCl) and PBZ (pyribenzamine), used as a heroin substitute* [see: Talwin; pentazocine HCl; tripelennamine]

**tees and blues; T's and blues; tease and blues** *street drug slang for a combination of Talwin (pentazocine HCl) and PBZ (pyribenzamine), used as a heroin substitute* [see: Talwin; pentazocine HCl; tripelennamine]

**tees and pees; T's and P's; tease and peas** *street drug slang for a combination of Talwin (pentazocine HCl) and PBZ (pyribenzamine), used as a heroin substitute* [see: Talwin; pentazocine HCl; tripelennamine]

**teeth** *street drug slang* [see: cocaine; cocaine, crack]

**tefazoline** INN

**tefenperate** INN

**tefludazine** INN

**teflurane** USAN, INN *inhalation anesthetic*

**teflutixol** INN

**tegafur** USAN, INN, BAN *antineoplastic*

**Tegison** capsules ℞ *systemic antipsoriatic* [etretinate] 10, 25 mg

**Tegopen** capsules, powder for oral solution ℞ *bactericidal antibiotic (penicillinase-resistant penicillin)* [cloxacillin sodium] 250, 500 mg; 125 mg/5 mL ℞ Tagamet; Tegrin; Targretin

**Tegretol** chewable tablets, tablets, oral suspension ℞ *anticonvulsant; analgesic for trigeminal neuralgia* [carbamazepine] 100 mg; 200 mg; 100 mg/5 mL ℞ Tegrin

**Tegretol-XR** extended-release tablets ℞ *anticonvulsant* [carbamazepine] 100, 200, 400 mg

**Tegrin for Psoriasis** cream, lotion, soap OTC *topical antipsoriatic; antiseborrheic; antiseptic* [coal tar solution] 5% ℞ Tegopen; Tegretol; Targretin

**Tegrin Medicated** gel shampoo, lotion shampoo OTC *antiseborrheic; antipsoriatic; antipruritic; antibacterial* [coal tar] 5%

**Tegrin Medicated Extra Conditioning; Advanced Formula Tegrin** shampoo OTC *antiseborrheic; antipsoriatic; antipruritic; antibacterial* [coal tar] 7%

**Tegrin-HC** ointment OTC *topical corticosteroid* [hydrocortisone] 1%

**Tegrin-LT** shampoo/conditioner OTC *pediculicide* [pyrethrins; piperonyl butoxide technical] 0.33%•3.15%

**T.E.H.** tablets (discontinued 1993) ℞ *antiasthmatic; bronchodilator; decongestant; anxiolytic* [theophylline; ephedrine sulfate; hydroxyzine HCl]

**teholamine** [see: aminophylline]

**TEIB (triethyleneiminobenzo-quinone)** [see: triaziquone]

**teicoplanin** USAN, INN, BAN *glycopeptide antibacterial antibiotic*

**teicoplanin A$_{2-1}$, A$_{2-2}$, A$_{2-3}$, A$_{2-4}$, A$_{2-5}$, and A$_{3-1}$** *components of teicoplanin*

**Tekron** ℞ *investigational antiglaucoma agent*

**Telachlor** timed-release capsules ℞ *antihistamine* [chlorpheniramine maleate] 8, 12 mg

**Teladar** cream ℞ *topical corticosteroid* [betamethasone dipropionate] 0.05%

**Teldrin** timed-release capsules OTC *antihistamine* [chlorpheniramine maleate] 12 mg ⊘ Tedral

**Teldrin 12-Hour Allergy Relief** sustained-release capsules OTC *decongestant; antihistamine* [phenylpropanolamine HCl; chlorpheniramine maleate] 75•8 mg

**Tel-E-Amp** (trademarked packaging form) *unit dose ampule*

**Tel-E-Dose** (trademarked packaging form) *unit dose package*

**Tel-E-Ject** (trademarked delivery system) *prefilled disposable syringe*

**telenzepine** INN

**Tel-E-Pack** (trademarked packaging form) *packaging system*

**Telepaque** tablets ℞ *oral cholecystographic radiopaque agent* [iopanoic acid] 500 mg

**Tel-E-Vial** (trademarked packaging form) *unit dose vial*

**telinavir** USAN *antiviral; HIV protease inhibitor*

**Teline; Teline-500** capsules (discontinued 1997) ℞ *broad-spectrum antibiotic* [tetracycline HCl] 250 mg; 500 mg

**tellurium** *element (Te)*

**teloxantrone** INN *antineoplastic* [also: teloxantrone HCl]

**teloxantrone HCl** USAN *antineoplastic* [also: teloxantrone]

**teludipine** INN, BAN *antihypertensive; calcium channel antagonist* [also: teludipine HCl]

**teludipine HCl** USAN *antihypertensive; calcium channel antagonist* [also: teludipine] [USAN previously used: taludipine HCl]

**temafloxacin** INN, BAN *antibacterial; microbial DNA topoisomerase inhibitor* [also: temafloxacin HCl]

**temafloxacin HCl** USAN *antibacterial; microbial DNA topoisomerase inhibitor* [also: temafloxacin]

**Temaril** tablets, syrup, Spansules (sustained-release capsules) (discontinued 1996) ℞ *antihistamine* [trimeprazine tartrate] 2.5 mg; 2.5 mg/5 mL; 5 mg ⊘ Demerol; Tepanil

**temarotene** INN

**tematropium methylsulfate** USAN *anticholinergic* [also: tematropium metilsulfate]

**tematropium metilsulfate** INN *anticholinergic* [also: tematropium methylsulfate]

**temazepam** USAN, INN *minor tranquilizer; hypnotic* 7.5, 15, 30 mg oral

**Temazin Cold** syrup OTC *decongestant; antihistamine* [phenylpropanolamine HCl; chlorpheniramine maleate] 12.5•2 mg/5 mL

**Tembid** (trademarked dosage form) *sustained-action capsule*

**temefos** USAN, INN *veterinary ectoparasiticide*

**temelastine** USAN, INN, BAN *antihistamine*

**Temelin** (Japanese name for U.S. product Zanaflex)

**Temicef** ℞ *investigational cephalosporin antibiotic* [cefodizime]

**temocapril HCl** USAN *antihypertensive*

**temocillin** USAN, INN, BAN *antibacterial*

**temodox** USAN, INN *veterinary growth stimulant*

**temoporfin** USAN, INN, BAN *photosensitizer for photodynamic cancer therapy*

**Temovate** ointment, gel, cream, scalp application ℞ *topical corticosteroidal anti-inflammatory* [clobetasol propionate] 0.05%

**Temovate Emollient** cream ℞ *topical corticosteroidal anti-inflammatory* [clobetasol propionate in an emollient base] 0.05%

**temozolomide** INN, BAN *investigational cytotoxic alkylating antineoplastic for malignant glioma*

**TEMP (tamoxifen, etoposide, mitoxantrone, Platinol)** *chemotherapy protocol*

**temple balls** *street drug slang* [see: hashish]

**Tempo** chewable tablets OTC *antacid; antiflatulent* [aluminum hydroxide; magnesium hydroxide; calcium carbonate; simethicone] 133•81•414• 20 mg

**Tempra, Children's** ⓒⒶⓃ syrup OTC *analgesic; antipyretic* [acetaminophen] 16 mg/mL

**Tempra 1** drops OTC *analgesic; antipyretic* [acetaminophen] 100 mg/mL

**Tempra 2** syrup OTC *analgesic; antipyretic* [acetaminophen] 160 mg/5 mL

**Tempra 3** chewable tablets OTC *analgesic; antipyretic* [acetaminophen] 80, 160 mg

**Tempule** (trademarked dosage form) *timed-release capsule or tablet*

**temurtide** USAN, INN, BAN *vaccine adjuvant*

**10 Benzagel; 5 Benzagel** gel ℞ *keratolytic for acne* [benzoyl peroxide] 10%; 5%

**10% LMD** IV injection ℞ *plasma volume expander for shock due to hemorrhage, burns, or surgery* [dextran 40] 10%

**tenamfetamine** INN

**ten-cent pistol** *street drug slang for a heroin dose laced with poison* [see: heroin]

**Tencet** capsules ℞ *analgesic; antipyretic; sedative* [acetaminophen; caffeine; butalbital] 325•40•50 mg

**Tencon** capsules ℞ *analgesic* [acetaminophen; butalbital] 650•50 mg

**tendamistat** INN

**Tenecrin** ℞ *investigational agent for cancer chemotherapy, infectious and autoimmune diseases* [tumor necrosis factor]

**Tenex** tablets ℞ *antihypertensive; anti-adrenergic* [guanfacine HCl] 1, 2 mg

**tenidap** USAN, INN *anti-inflammatory for osteoarthritis and rheumatoid arthritis; cytokine inhibitor*

**tenidap sodium** USAN, INN *anti-inflammatory for osteoarthritis and rheumatoid arthritis*

**tenilapine** INN

**teniloxazine** INN

**tenilsetam** INN

**teniposide** USAN, INN, BAN *antineoplastic for refractory childhood acute lymphocytic leukemia* (orphan)

**Ten-K** controlled-release tablets ℞ *potassium supplement* [potassium chloride] 750 mg (10 mEq)

**tenoate** INN *combining name for radicals or groups*

**tenocyclidine** INN

**Tenol-Plus** tablets (discontinued 1995) OTC *analgesic; antipyretic; anti-inflammatory* [acetaminophen; aspirin; caffeine] 250•250•65 mg

**tenonitrozole** INN

**Tenoretic 50; Tenoretic 100** tablets ℞ *antihypertensive* [chlorthalidone; atenolol] 25•50 mg; 25•100 mg

**Tenormin** tablets, IV injection ℞ *antianginal; antihypertensive; β-blocker* [atenolol] 25, 50, 100 mg; 5 mg/10 mL

**tenoxicam** USAN, INN, BAN *anti-inflammatory*

**tens** *street drug slang for 10 mg amphetamine tablets* [see: amphetamines]

**Tensilon** IV or IM injection ℞ *myasthenia gravis treatment; antidote to curare-type overdose* [edrophonium chloride] 10 mg/mL

**tension** *street drug slang* [see: cocaine, crack]

**Ten-Tab** (trademarked dosage form) *controlled-release tablet*

**Tenuate** tablets, Dospan (controlled-release tablets) ℞ *anorexiant* [diethylpropion HCl] 25 mg; 75 mg

**tenylidone** INN

**teoclate** INN *combining name for radicals or groups* [also: theoclate]

**teopranitol** INN

**teoprolol** INN

**T.E.P.** tablets OTC *antiasthmatic; bronchodilator; decongestant; sedative* [theophylline; ephedrine HCl; phenobarbital]

**Tepanil** tablets, Ten-tab (sustained-release tablets) (discontinued 1995) ℞ *anorexiant* [diethylpropion HCl] 25 mg; 75 mg ⌷ Temaril; Tofranil

**tepirindole** INN

**tepoxalin** USAN, INN *antipsoriatic; investigational anti-inflammatory for rheumatoid arthritis*

**teprenone** INN

**teprosilate** INN *combining name for radicals or groups*

**teprotide** USAN, INN *angiotensin-converting enzyme (ACE) inhibitor*

**Terak** ophthalmic ointment ℞ *ophthalmic antibiotic* [oxytetracycline HCl; polymyxin B sulfate] 5 mg•10 000 U per g

**Terazol 3** vaginal suppositories, vaginal cream ℞ *antifungal* [terconazole] 80 mg; 0.8%

**Terazol 7** vaginal cream ℞ *antifungal* [terconazole] 0.4%

**terazosin** INN, BAN *antihypertensive; $\alpha_1$-adrenergic blocker* [also: terazosin HCl]

**terazosin HCl** USAN *antihypertensive; $\alpha_1$-adrenergic blocker* [also: terazosin]

**terbinafine** USAN, INN, BAN *allylamine antifungal*

**terbinafine HCl** *allylamine antifungal*

**terbium** *element (Tb)*

**terbucromil** INN

**terbufibrol** INN

**terbuficin** INN

**terbuprol** INN

**terbutaline** INN, BAN *bronchodilator* [also: terbutaline sulfate]

**terbutaline sulfate** USAN, USP *bronchodilator* [also: terbutaline]

**terciprazine** INN

**terconazole** USAN, INN, BAN *antifungal*

**terephthalamidine** *investigational antineoplastic*

**terfenadine** USAN, USP, INN *antihistamine* 60 mg oral

**terfenadine carboxylate** *investigational antihistamine with fewer drug interactions than terfenadine (Seldane)*

**terflavoxate** INN

**terfluranol** INN

**terguride** INN *investigational dopamine agonist for central nervous system disorders*

**teriparatide** USAN, INN *diagnostic aid for hypocalcemia; anabolic osteoporosis treatment for women*

**teriparatide acetate** USAN, JAN *diagnostic aid for parathyroid-induced hypocalcemia (orphan)*

**terizidone** INN

**terlakiren** USAN *antihypertensive; renin inhibitor*

**terlipressin** INN, BAN *investigational (orphan) for bleeding esophageal varices*

**ternidazole** INN

**terodiline** INN, BAN, JAN *coronary vasodilator* [also: terodiline HCl]

**terodiline HCl** USAN *coronary vasodilator; investigational agent for urinary incontinence* [also: terodiline]

**terofenamate** INN

**teroxalene** INN *antischistosomal* [also: teroxalene HCl]

**teroxalene HCl** USAN *antischistosomal* [also: teroxalene]

**teroxirone** USAN, INN *antineoplastic*

**terpin hydrate** USP *(disapproved for use as an expectorant in 1991)* 85 mg/5 mL oral

**terpinol** [see: terpin hydrate]

**Terra-Cortril** eye drop suspension ℞ *topical ophthalmic corticosteroidal anti-inflammatory; antibiotic* [hydrocortisone acetate; oxytetracycline HCl] 1.5%•0.5%

**terrafungine** [see: oxytetracycline]

**Terramycin** capsules ℞ *tetracycline-type antibiotic* [oxytetracycline HCl] 250 mg ⌷ Garamycin

**Terramycin IM** injection ℞ *tetracycline-type antibiotic* [oxytetracycline; lidocaine] 50 mg•2%, 125 mg•2% per mL

**Terramycin with Polymyxin B** ophthalmic ointment ℞ *ophthalmic antibiotic* [oxytetracycline HCl; polymyxin B sulfate] 5 mg•10 000 U per g

**Tersaseptic** shampoo/cleanser OTC *soap-free therapeutic cleanser*

**tertatolol** INN, BAN

**tertiary amyl alcohol** [see: amylene hydrate]

*tert*-**pentyl alcohol** [see: amylene hydrate]

**Tesamone** IM injection R̶ *androgen replacement for delayed puberty or breast cancer* [testosterone] 100 mg/mL

**tesicam** USAN, INN *anti-inflammatory*

**tesimide** USAN, INN *anti-inflammatory*

**Teslac** tablets R̶ *adjunctive hormonal chemotherapy for advanced postmenopausal breast carcinoma* [testolactone] 50 mg

**TESPA (triethylenethiophosphoramide)** [see: thiotepa]

**Tessalon** Perles (capsules) R̶ *antitussive* [benzonatate] 100 mg

**Test Pack** kit for professional use *in vitro diagnostic aid for Group A streptococcal antigens in throat swabs* [enzyme immunoassay]

**Testandro** IM injection R̶ *androgen replacement for delayed puberty or breast cancer* [testosterone] 100 mg/mL

**Tes-Tape** reagent strips for home use (discontinued 1996) OTC *in vitro diagnostic aid for urine glucose*

**Test-Estro Cypionates** IM injection R̶ *estrogen/androgen for menopausal vasomotor symptoms* [estradiol cypionate; testosterone cypionate] 2•50 mg/mL

**Testex** IM injection (discontinued 1994) R̶ *androgen replacement for delayed puberty or breast cancer* [testosterone propionate] 100 mg/mL

**Testoderm; Testoderm with Adhesive** transdermal patch (for scrotal area) R̶ *hormone replacement therapy for hypogonadism* [testosterone] 4, 6 mg/day (10, 15 mg)

**testolactone** USAN, USP, INN *antineoplastic; androgen hormone* ⊡ testosterone

**Testone LA 100; Testone LA 200** IM injection (discontinued 1994) R̶ *androgen replacement for delayed puberty or breast cancer* [testosterone ethanate] 100 mg/mL; 200 mg/mL

**Testopel** pellets for subcu implantation R̶ *hormone replacement therapy for hypogonadism* [testosterone] 75 mg

**testosterone** USP, INN, BAN *androgen; investigational (orphan) for AIDS wasting and delay of growth and puberty in boys; investigational (Phase III) for testosterone deficiency in men* ⊡ testolactone

**Testosterone Aqueous** IM injection R̶ *androgen for hypogonadism, delayed puberty, and androgen-responsive metastatic cancers* [testosterone] 25, 50, 100 mg/mL

**testosterone cyclopentanepropionate** [see: testosterone cypionate]

**testosterone cyclopentylpropionate** [see: testosterone cypionate]

**testosterone cypionate** USP *parenteral androgen; sometimes abused as a street drug* 100, 200 mg/mL

**testosterone enanthate** USP *parenteral androgen; sometimes abused as a street drug* 100, 200 mg/mL injection

**testosterone heptanoate** [see: testosterone enanthate]

**testosterone ketolaurate** USAN, INN *androgen*

**testosterone 3-oxododecanoate** [see: testosterone ketolaurate]

**testosterone phenylacetate** USAN *androgen*

**testosterone propionate** USP *parenteral androgen; investigational (orphan) for vulvar dystrophies* 100 mg/mL injection

**TestPack** [see: Abbott TestPack]

**Testred** capsules R̶ *androgen for male hypogonadism, impotence and breast cancer* [methyltestosterone] 10 mg

**Testred Cypionate** IM injection (discontinued 1994) R̶ *androgen replacement for delayed puberty or breast cancer* [testosterone cypionate] 200 mg/mL

**Testrin PA** IM injection (discontinued 1994) R̶ *androgen replacement for delayed puberty or breast cancer* [testosterone enanthate] 200 mg/mL

**tetanus antitoxin** USP *passive immunizing agent*

**tetanus & gas gangrene antitoxins** NF

**tetanus & gas gangrene polyvalent antitoxin** [see: tetanus & gas gangrene antitoxins]

**tetanus immune globulin** USP *passive immunizing agent*

**tetanus immune human globulin** [now: tetanus immune globulin]

**tetanus toxoid** USP *active immunizing agent*

**tetanus toxoid, adsorbed** USP *active immunizing agent*

**tetiothalein sodium** [see: iodophthalein sodium]

**tetnicoran** [see: nicofurate]

**tetrabarbital** INN

**tetrabenazine** INN, BAN

**TetraBriks** (trademarked delivery form) *ready-to-use liquid containers*

**tetracaine** USP, INN *topical local anesthetic* [also: amethocaine]

**tetracaine HCl** USP, JAN *topical local anesthetic* [also: amethocaine HCl]

**Tetracap** capsules ℞ *broad-spectrum antibiotic* [tetracycline HCl] 250 mg

**tetrachloroethylene** USP

**tetrachloromethane** [see: carbon tetrachloride]

**tetracosactide** INN *adrenocorticotropic hormone* [also: cosyntropin; tetracosactrin]

**tetracosactrin** BAN *adrenocorticotropic hormone* [also: cosyntropin; tetracosactide]

**tetracycline** USP, INN, BAN *bacteriostatic antibiotic; antirickettsial*

**tetracycline HCl** USP *bacteriostatic antibiotic; antirickettsial* 100, 250, 500 mg oral; 125 mg/5 mL oral

**tetracycline phosphate complex** USP, BAN *antibacterial*

**tetracyclines** *a class of bacteriostatic, antimicrobial antibiotics*

**Tetracyn; Tetracyn 500** capsules ℞ *antibiotic* [tetracycline HCl]

**tetradecanoic acid, methylethyl ester** [see: isopropyl myristate]

**tetradonium bromide** INN

**tetraethylammonium bromide (TEAB)** [see: tetrylammonium bromide]

**tetraethylammonium chloride (TEAC)**

**tetraethylthiuram disulfide** [see: disulfiram]

**tetrafilcon A** USAN *hydrophilic contact lens material*

**tetraglycine hydroperiodide** *source of iodine for disinfecting water*

**tetrahydroaminoacridine (THA)** [see: tacrine HCl]

**tetrahydrocannabinol (THC)** [see: dronabinol]

**tetrahydrolipstatin** [see: orlistat]

**tetrahydrozoline** BAN *vasoconstrictor; nasal decongestant; topical ocular decongestant* [also: tetrhydrozoline HCl; tetryzoline] 0.05% eye drops

**tetrahydrozoline HCl** USP *vasoconstrictor; nasal decongestant; topical ocular decongestant* [also: tetryzoline; tetrahydrozoline]

**tetraiodophenolphthalein sodium** [see: iodophthalein sodium]

**Tetralan** syrup (discontinued 1997) ℞ *broad-spectrum antibiotic* [tetracycline HCl] 125 mg/5 mL

**Tetralan "250"; Tetralan-500** capsules (discontinued 1997) ℞ *broad-spectrum antibiotic* [tetracycline HCl] 250 mg; 500 mg

**tetrallobarbital** [see: butalbital]

**Tetram** capsules (discontinued 1996) ℞ *broad-spectrum antibiotic* [tetracycline HCl] 250 mg

**tetramal** [see: tetrabarbital]

**tetrameprozine** [see: aminopromazine]

**tetramethrin** INN

**tetramethylene dimethanesulfonate** [see: busulfan]

**tetramisole** INN *anthelmintic* [also: tetramisole HCl]

**tetramisole HCl** USAN *anthelmintic* [also: tetramisole]

**Tetramune** IM injection ℞ *pediatric vaccine for diphtheria, pertussis, tetanus and Haemophilus influenzae type b* [diphtheria & tetanus toxoids & whole-cell pertussis vaccine; Hemophilus b conjugate vaccine (DTwP-Hib)] 0.5 mL

**tetranitrol** [see: erythrityl tetranitrate]

**tetrantoin**

**TetraPaks** (trademarked delivery form) *ready-to-use open system containers*

**Tetrasine; Tetrasine Extra** eye drops OTC *topical ocular decongestant/vasoconstrictor* [tetrahydrozoline HCl] 0.05%

**tetrasodium ethylenediaminetetraacetate** [see: edetate sodium]

**tetrasodium pyrophosphate** [see: sodium pyrophosphate]

**tetrazepam** INN

**tetrazolast meglumine** USAN *antiallergic; antiasthmatic; investigational mediator-release inhibitor*

**tetridamine** INN *analgesic; anti-inflammatory* [also: tetrydamine]

**tetriprofen** INN

**tetrofosmin** USAN, INN, BAN *diagnostic aid*

**tetronasin** BAN [also: tetronasin 5930]

**tetronasin 5930** INN [also: tetronasin]

**tetroquinone** USAN, INN *systemic keratolytic*

**tetroxoprim** USAN, INN *antibacterial*

**tetrydamine** USAN *analgesic; anti-inflammatory* [also: tetridamine]

**tetrylammonium bromide** INN

**tetryzoline** INN *vasoconstrictor; nasal decongestant; topical ocular decongestant* [also: tetrahydrozoline HCl; tetrahydrozoline]

**tetryzoline HCl** [see: tetrahydrozoline HCl]

**Texacort** solution ℞ *topical corticosteroid* [hydrocortisone] 1%

**texacromil** INN

**Texas pot; Texas tea; Tex-mex** *street drug slang* [see: marijuana]

**6-TG (6-thioguanine)** [see: thioguanine]

**TG (thyroglobulin)** [q.v.]

**T-Gen** suppositories, pediatric suppositories ℞ *anticholinergic; antiemetic* [trimethobenzamide HCl] 200 mg; 100 mg

**T-Gesic** capsules ℞ *narcotic analgesic* [hydrocodone bitartrate; acetaminophen] 5•500 mg

**αTGI (α-triglycidyl isocyanurate)** [see: teroxirone]

**TH (theophylline)** [q.v.]

**TH (thyroid hormone)** [see: levothyroxine sodium]

**THA (tetrahydroaminoacridine)** [see: tacrine HCl]

**Thai sticks** *street drug slang for bundles of marijuana soaked in hashish oil or marijuana buds bound on short sections of bamboo* [see: marijuana; hashish]

**thalidomide** USAN, INN, BAN *sedative; hypnotic; investigational (Phase III, orphan) for GVHD, AIDS wasting, leprosy, and mycobacterial infections; investigational (Phase II) for various cancers*

**Thalitone** tablets ℞ *diuretic; antihypertensive* [chlorthalidone] 15, 25 mg

**thallium** *element (Tl)* 🔊 Valium

**thallous chloride Tl 201** USAN, USP *radiopaque medium; radioactive agent*

**Tham** IV infusion ℞ *corrects systemic acidosis associated with cardiac bypass surgery or cardiac arrest* [tromethamine] 18 g/500 mL (150 mEq/500 mL)

**thaumatin** BAN

**THC (tetrahydrocannabinol)** [see: dronabinol]

**THC (thiocarbanidin)**

**The Beast** *street drug slang* [see: heroin]

**The C** *street drug slang* [see: methcathinone]

**the devil** *street drug slang* [see: cocaine, crack]

**the witch** *street drug slang* [see: heroin]

**thebacon** INN, BAN

**Theelin Aqueous** IM injection (discontinued 1995) ℞ *estrogen replacement therapy; antineoplastic for prostatic and breast cancer* [estrone] 2 mg/mL

**theine** [see: caffeine]

**thenalidine** INN

**thenium closilate** INN *veterinary anthelmintic* [also: thenium closylate]

**thenium closylate** USAN *veterinary anthelmintic* [also: thenium closilate]

**thenyldiamine** INN

**thenylpyramine HCl** [see: methapyrilene HCl]

**Theo-24** timed-release capsules ℞ *bronchodilator* [theophylline] 100, 200, 300 mg

**Theobid** Duracaps (sustained-release capsules) ℞ *bronchodilator* [theophylline] 260 mg

**Theobid Jr.** Duracaps (sustained-release capsules) (discontinued 1996) ℞ *bronchodilator* [theophylline] 130 mg

**theobromine** NF
**theobromine calcium salicylate** NF
**theobromine sodium acetate** NF
**theobromine sodium salicylate** NF
**Theochron** extended-release tablets
℞ *bronchodilator* [theophylline] 100,
200, 300 mg
**theoclate** BAN *combining name for radicals or groups* [also: teoclate]
**Theoclear L.A.** extended-release capsules ℞ *bronchodilator* [theophylline]
130, 260 mg
**Theoclear-80** oral solution ℞ *bronchodilator* [theophylline] 80 mg/15
mL ☒ Theolair
**theodrenaline** INN, BAN
**Theodrine** tablets OTC *antiasthmatic;
bronchodilator; decongestant* [theophylline; ephedrine HCl] 120•22.5 mg
**Theo-Dur** extended-release tablets ℞
*bronchodilator* [theophylline] 100,
200, 300, 450 mg
**Theo-Dur Sprinkle** sustained-release
capsules (discontinued 1996) ℞
*bronchodilator* [theophylline] 50, 75,
125, 200 mg
**theofibrate** USAN *antihyperlipoproteinemic* [also: etofylline clofibrate]
**Theo-G** capsules (discontinued 1993)
℞ *antiasthmatic; bronchodilator; expectorant* [theophylline; guaifenesin]
**Theolair** tablets, liquid ℞ *antiasthmatic* [theophylline] 125, 250 mg; 80
mg/15 mL ☒ Theoclear; Thyrolar
**Theolair-SR** sustained-release tablets
℞ *antiasthmatic* [theophylline] 200,
250, 300, 500 mg
**Theolate** liquid ℞ *antiasthmatic; bronchodilator; expectorant* [theophylline;
guaifenesin] 150•90 mg/15 mL
**Theomax DF** pediatric syrup ℞ *antiasthmatic; bronchodilator; decongestant;
anxiolytic* [theophylline; ephedrine
sulfate; hydroxyzine HCl; alcohol
5%] 97.5•18.75•7.5 mg/15 mL
**Theo-Organidin** elixir (discontinued
1995) ℞ *antiasthmatic; bronchodilator; expectorant* [theophylline; iodinated glycerol] 8•2 mg/mL
**theophyldine** [see: aminophylline]
**theophyllamine** [see: aminophylline]

**Theophyllin KI** elixir ℞ *antiasthmatic; bronchodilator; expectorant*
[theophylline; potassium iodide] 80•
130 mg/15 mL
**theophylline (TH)** USP, BAN *bronchodilator* 100, 125, 200, 300 mg oral;
80 mg/15 mL oral
**theophylline aminoisobutanol** [see:
ambuphylline]
**theophylline calcium salicylate**
*bronchodilator*
**theophylline ethylenediamine** [now:
aminophylline]
**Theophylline Extended-Release**
tablets ℞ *bronchodilator* [theophylline] 450 mg
**theophylline monohydrate** [see: theophylline]
**theophylline olamine** USP
**theophylline sodium acetate** NF
**theophylline sodium glycinate** USP
*smooth muscle relaxant*
**Theo-R-Gen** elixir (discontinued
1993) ℞ *antiasthmatic; bronchodilator; expectorant* [theophylline; iodinated glycerol]
**Theo-Sav** controlled-release tablets ℞
*bronchodilator* [theophylline] 100,
200, 300 mg
**Theospan-SR** timed-release capsules
℞ *bronchodilator* [theophylline] 130,
260 mg
**Theostat 80** syrup ℞ *bronchodilator* [theophylline; alcohol 1%] 80 mg/15 mL
**Theotal** tablets (discontinued 1993)
OTC *antiasthmatic; bronchodilator;
decongestant; sedative* [theophylline;
ephedrine HCl; phenobarbital]
**Theovent** timed-release capsules ℞
*bronchodilator* [theophylline] 125,
250 mg
**Theo-X** controlled-release tablets ℞
*bronchodilator* [theophylline] 100,
200, 300 mg
**Thera Hematinic** tablets OTC *hematinic; vitamin supplement* [ferrous
fumarate; multiple vitamins; folic
acid] 66.7•≛•0.33 mg
**Thera Multi-Vitamin** liquid OTC *vitamin supplement* [multiple vitamins] ≛
**Therabid** tablets OTC *vitamin supplement* [multiple vitamins] ≛

**Therac** lotion OTC *topical acne treatment* [colloidal sulfur] 10%

**theraccines** *a class of vaccines with therapeutic action, usually used to help prevent the spread of cancer*

**TheraCys** freeze-dried suspension for intravesical injection ℞ *antineoplastic for urinary bladder cancer* [BCG vaccine, live] 27 mg

**TheraDerm-LRS** transdermal patch ℞ *investigational hormonal therapy for hypogonadism* [testosterone]

**Therafectin** ℞ *investigational (Phase III) anti-inflammatory for rheumatoid arthritis* [amiprilose]

**TheraFlu Flu, Cold & Cough; NightTime TheraFlu** powder for oral solution OTC *antitussive; decongestant; antihistamine; analgesic* [dextromethorphan hydrobromide; pseudoephedrine HCl; chlorpheniramine maleate; acetaminophen] 20•60•4•650 mg/packet; 30•60•4•1000 mg/packet ⑫ Thera-Flur

**TheraFlu Flu & Cold Medicine** powder for oral solution OTC *decongestant; antihistamine; analgesic* [pseudoephedrine HCl; chlorpheniramine maleate; acetaminophen] 60•4•650 mg/packet

**TheraFlu Non-Drowsy** powder for oral solution (name changed to TheraFlu Non-Drowsy Flu, Cold & Cough in 1995)

**TheraFlu Non-Drowsy Flu, Cold & Cough** powder for oral solution OTC *antitussive; decongestant; analgesic* [dextromethorphan hydrobromide; pseudoephedrine HCl; acetaminophen] 30•60•100 mg/packet

**TheraFlu Non-Drowsy Formula** caplets OTC *antitussive; decongestant; analgesic* [dextromethorphan hydrobromide; pseudoephedrine HCl; acetaminophen] 15•30•500 mg

**Thera-Flur; Thera-Flur-N** gel drops (for self-application) ℞ *dental caries preventative* [sodium fluoride] 1.1% ⑫ TheraFlu

**Theragenerix** tablets (name changed to Therapeutic in 1995)

**Theragenerix-H** tablets (name changed to Therapeutic-H in 1995)

**Theragenerix-M** tablets (name changed to Therapeutic-M in 1995)

**Thera-Gesic** cream OTC *counterirritant* [methyl salicylate; menthol] 15%•⸚

**Theragran** caplets OTC *vitamin supplement* [multiple vitamins; folic acid; biotin] ±•400•30 μg

**Theragran** liquid OTC *vitamin supplement* [multiple vitamins] ± ⑫ Phenergan

**Theragran AntiOxidant** softgels OTC *vitamin/mineral supplement* [vitamins A, C, and E; multiple minerals] 5000 IU•250 mg•200 IU•±

**Theragran Hematinic** tablets ℞ *hematinic; vitamin/mineral supplement* [ferrous fumarate; multiple vitamins and minerals; folic acid] 66.7•±•0.33 mg

**Theragran Stress Formula** tablets OTC *vitamin/iron supplement* [multiple B vitamins; vitamins C and E; ferrous fumarate; folic acid; biotin] ±•600 mg•30 IU•27 mg•0.4 mg•45 μg

**Theragran-M** caplets OTC *vitamin/mineral/calcium/iron supplement* [multiple vitamins & minerals; calcium; iron; folic acid; biotin] ±•40•27•0.4•0.03 mg

**Thera-Hist** powder (discontinued 1993) OTC *decongestant; antihistamine; analgesic* [pseudoephedrine HCl; chlorpheniramine maleate; acetaminophen]

**Thera-Hist** syrup OTC *decongestant; antihistamine* [phenylpropanolamine HCl; chlorpheniramine maleate] 12.5•2 mg/5 mL

**Thera-Ject** (trademarked delivery system) *prefilled disposable syringe*

**Thera-M** tablets OTC *vitamin/mineral/iron supplement* [multiple vitamins & minerals; iron; folic acid; biotin] ±•27 mg•0.4 mg•35 μg

**Theramine Expectorant** liquid OTC *decongestant; expectorant* [phenylpropanolamine HCl; guaifenesin] 12.5•100 mg/5 mL

**Theramycin Z** topical solution ℞ *topical antibiotic for acne* [erythromycin] 2%

**TheraPatch** transdermal patch OTC *external analgesic* [methyl salicylate; menthol; camphor]

**Therapeutic** tablets OTC *vitamin supplement* [multiple vitamins; folic acid; biotin] ± •400•30 µg

**Therapeutic B with C** capsules OTC *vitamin supplement* [multiple B vitamins; vitamin C] ± •300 mg

**Therapeutic Bath** lotion, oil OTC *moisturizer; emollient*

**Therapeutic Mineral Ice; Therapeutic Mineral Ice Exercise Formula** gel OTC *counterirritant* [menthol] 2%; 4%

**Therapeutic-H** tablets OTC *hematinic; vitamin supplement* [ferrous fumarate; multiple vitamins; folic acid] 66.7• ± •0.33 mg

**Therapeutic-M** tablets OTC *vitamin/ mineral/iron supplement* [multiple vitamins & minerals; iron; folic acid; biotin] ± •27 mg•0.4 mg•30 µg

**Theraplex T** shampoo OTC *antiseborrheic; antipsoriatic; antipruritic; antibacterial* [coal tar] 1%

**Theraplex Z** shampoo OTC *antiseborrheic; antibacterial; antifungal* [pyrithione zinc] 2%

**Theratope** ℞ *investigational (Phase III) therapeutic vaccine for recurrent or metastatic breast and colorectal cancer*

**Theravee** tablets OTC *vitamin supplement* [multiple vitamins; folic acid; biotin] ± •400•15 µg

**Theravee Hematinic** tablets OTC *hematinic; vitamin supplement* [ferrous fumarate; multiple vitamins; folic acid] 66.7• ± •0.33 mg

**Theravee-M** tablets OTC *vitamin/mineral/iron supplement* [multiple vitamins & minerals; iron; folic acid; biotin] ± •27 mg•0.4 mg•15 µg

**Theravim** tablets OTC *vitamin supplement* [multiple vitamins; folic acid; biotin] ± •400•35 µg

**Theravim-M** tablets OTC *vitamin/mineral/iron supplement* [multiple vitamins & minerals; iron; folic acid; biotin] ± •27 mg•0.4 mg•30 µg

**Theravir** ℞ *investigational anti-HIV drug* [monoclonal antibodies]

**Theravite** liquid OTC *vitamin supplement* [multiple vitamins] ± ⊡ Therevac

**Therems** tablets OTC *vitamin supplement* [multiple vitamins; folic acid; biotin] ± •400•15 µg

**Therems-M** tablets OTC *vitamin/mineral/iron supplement* [multiple vitamins & minerals; iron; folic acid; biotin] ± •27 mg•0.4 mg•30 µg

**Therevac-Plus** suppository enema OTC *laxative; stool softener* [docusate sodium; benzocaine] 283•20 mg ⊡ Theravite

**Therevac-SB** suppository enema OTC *laxative; stool softener* [docusate sodium] 283 mg

**Thermax** gel ℞ *investigational vulnerary for bed sores, chronic skin ulcers, and other wounds*

**Thermazene** cream ℞ *broad-spectrum bactericidal for adjunctive burn treatment* [silver sulfadiazine] 10 mg/g

**Theroxide** lotion (discontinued 1994) ℞ *topical keratolytic for acne* [benzoyl peroxide]

**Theroxide** wash (discontinued 1994) ℞ *topical keratolytic for acne* [benzoyl peroxide] 10%

**ThexForte** caplets OTC *vitamin supplement* [multiple B vitamins; vitamin C] ± •500 mg

**THF (thymic humoral factor)** [q.v.]

**thiabendazole (TBZ)** USAN, USP *anthelmintic for strongyloidiasis (threadworm), larva migrans, and trichinosis* [also: tiabendazole]

**thiabutazide** [see: buthiazide]

**thiacetarsamide sodium** INN

**thiacetazone** BAN [also: thioacetazone]

**Thiacide** film-coated tablets (discontinued 1994) ℞ *urinary anti-infective; acidifier* [methenamine mandelate; potassium acid phosphate] 500•250 mg ⊡ Dyazide; thiazides

**thialbarbital** INN [also: thialbarbitone]

**thialbarbitone** BAN [also: thialbarbital]

**thialisobumal sodium** [see: buthalital sodium]

**thiamazole** INN *thyroid inhibitor* [also: methimazole]

**thiambutosine** INN, BAN

**Thiamilate** enteric-coated tablets OTC *vitamin supplement* [thiamine HCl] 20 mg

**thiamine** INN *vitamin B₁; enzyme cofactor* [also: thiamine HCl]

**thiamine HCl** USP *vitamin B₁; enzyme cofactor* [also: thiamine] 50, 100, 250, 500 mg oral; 100 mg/mL injection

**thiamine mononitrate** USP *vitamin B₁; enzyme cofactor*

**thiamine propyl disulfide** [see: prosultiamine]

**thiamiprine** USAN *antineoplastic* [also: tiamiprine]

**thiamphenicol** USAN, INN, BAN *antibacterial*

**thiamylal** USP *barbiturate general anesthetic*

**thiamylal sodium** USP, JAN *barbiturate general anesthetic*

**thiazesim HCl** USAN *antidepressant* [also: tiazesim]

**thiazides** *a class of diuretic agents that increase urinary excretion of sodium and chloride in approximately equal amounts*

**thiazinamium chloride** USAN *antiallergic*

**thiazinamium metilsulfate** INN

**4-thiazolidinecarboxylic acid** [see: timonacic]

**thiazolsulfone** [see: thiazosulfone]

**thiazosulfone** INN

**thiazothielite** [see: antienite]

**thiazothienol** [see: antazonite]

**thiethylperazine** USAN, INN *antiemetic; antidopaminergic*

**thiethylperazine malate** USP *antiemetic; antipsychotic*

**thiethylperazine maleate** USAN, USP *antiemetic*

**thihexinol methylbromide** NF, INN

**thimerfonate sodium** USAN *topical anti-infective* [also: sodium timerfonate]

**thimerosal** USP *topical anti-infective; preservative (49% mercury)* [also: thiomersal] 1:1000 topical

**Thing** *street drug slang* [see: heroin; cocaine]

**thioacetazone** INN, DCF [also: thiacetazone]

**thiocarbanidin (THC)**

**thiocarlide** BAN [also: tiocarlide]

**thiocolchicine glycoside** [see: thiocolchicoside]

**thiocolchicoside** INN

**thiocyanate sodium** NF

**thiodiglycol** INN

**thiodiphenylamine** [see: phenothiazine]

**thiofuradene** INN

**thioguanine (6-TG)** USAN, USP *antimetabolic antineoplastic* [also: tioguanine] 40 mg oral

**thiohexallymal** [see: thialbarbital]

**thiohexamide** INN

**Thiola** sugar-coated tablets Ŗ *prevention of cystine nephrolithiasis in homozygous cystinuria (orphan)* [tiopronin] 100 mg

**thiomebumal sodium** [see: thiopental sodium]

**thiomersal** INN, BAN *topical anti-infective; preservative* [also: thimerosal]

**thiomesterone** BAN [also: tiomesterone]

**thiomicid** [see: thioacetazone; thiacetazone]

**thioparamizone** [see: thioacetazone; thiacetazone]

**thiopental sodium** USP, INN, JAN *barbiturate general anesthetic; anticonvulsant* [also: thiopentone sodium] 2%, 2.5% (20, 25 mg/mL) injection

**thiopentone sodium** BAN *general anesthetic; anticonvulsant* [also: thiopental sodium]

**thiophanate** BAN

**thiophosphoramide** [see: thiotepa]

**Thioplex** powder for IV, intracavitary, or intravesical injection Ŗ *alkylating antineoplastic for lymphomas and carcinoma of the breast, ovary, or bladder* [thiotepa] 15 mg

**thiopropazate** INN [also: thiopropazate HCl]

**thiopropazate HCl** NF [also: thiopropazate]

**thioproperazine** INN, BAN [also: thioproperazine mesylate]

**thioproperazine mesylate** [also: thioproperazine]

**thioproperazine methanesulfonate** [see: thioproperazine mesylate]

**thioridazine** USAN, USP, INN *antipsychotic; sedative*

**thioridazine HCl** USP *antipsychotic; sedative* 10, 15, 25, 50, 100, 150, 200 mg oral; 30, 100 mg/mL oral

**thiosalan** USAN *disinfectant* [also: tiosalan]

**Thiosulfil Forte** tablets ℞ *broad-spectrum sulfonamide bacteriostatic* [sulfamethizole] 500 mg

**thiosulfuric acid, disodium salt pentahydrate** [see: sodium thiosulfate]

**thiotepa** USP, INN, BAN, JAN *alkylating antineoplastic for lymphomas and carcinoma of the breast, ovary, or bladder*

**thiotetrabarbital** INN

**thiothixene** USAN, USP, BAN *antipsychotic* [also: tiotixene] 1, 2, 5, 10, 20 mg oral

**thiothixene HCl** USAN, USP *antipsychotic* 5 mg/mL oral

**thiouracil**

**thiourea** *antioxidant*

**thioxanthenes** *a class of antipsychotic agents*

**thioxolone** BAN [also: tioxolone]

**thiphenamil HCl** USAN *smooth muscle relaxant* [also: tifenamil]

**thiphencillin potassium** USAN *antibacterial* [also: tifencillin]

**thiram** USAN, INN *antifungal*

**thirteen** *street drug slang* [see: marijuana]

**Thiuretic** tablets (discontinued 1993) ℞ *diuretic; antihypertensive* [hydrochlorothiazide]

**thonzonium bromide** USAN, USP *detergent* [also: tonzonium bromide]

**thonzylamine HCl** USAN, INN

**Thorazine** tablets, Spansules (capsules), IV or IM injection, syrup, suppositories, concentrate ℞ *tranquilizer; antiemetic* [chlorpromazine] 10, 25, 50, 100, 200 mg; 30, 75, 150, 200, 300 mg; 25 mg/mL; 10 mg/5 mL; 25, 50 mg; 30, 100 mg/mL

**thorium** *element (Th)*

**thozalinone** USAN *antidepressant* [also: tozalinone]

**THQ (tetrahydroxybenzoquinone)** [see: tetroquinone]

**THR (trishydroxyethyl rutin)** [see: troxerutin]

**Threamine DM** syrup OTC *antitussive; decongestant; antihistamine* [dextro-

methorphan hydrobromide; phenylpropanolamine HCl; chlorpheniramine maleate] 10•12.5•2 mg/5 mL

**Threamine Expectorant** liquid OTC *decongestant; expectorant* [phenylpropanolamine HCl; guaifenesin; alcohol 5%] 12.5•100 mg/5 mL

**three hundreds** *street drug slang for Quaaludes (methaqualone; discontinued 1983), a reference to 300 mg tablets* [see: methaqualone]

**3 in 1 Toothache Relief** gum, liquid, lotion/gel OTC *topical oral anesthetic* [benzocaine]

**3118** *investigational antibacterial antibiotic*

**348U** *investigational antiviral*

**threes** *street drug slang* [see: Tylenol with Codeine No. 3; Empirin with Codeine No. 3]

**3TC** [now: lamivudine]

**threonine (L-threonine)** USAN, USP, INN *essential amino acid; investigational (orphan) for spasticity and amyotrophic lateral sclerosis; symbols: Thr, T* 500 mg oral

**Threostat** ℞ *investigational (orphan) for familial spastic paraparesis and amyotrophic lateral sclerosis* [L-threonine] ② Triostat

**Throat Discs** lozenges OTC *analgesic; counterirritant* [capsicum; peppermint oil]

**Thrombate III** ℞ *for thrombosis and pulmonary emboli of congenital AT-III deficiency (orphan)* [antithrombin III, human]

**thrombin** USP, INN *topical local hemostatic*

**Thrombinar** powder ℞ *topical local hemostatic for surgery* [thrombin] 1000, 5000, 50 000 U

**Thrombin-JMI** powder ℞ *topical local hemostatic for surgery* [thrombin] 10 000, 20 000, 50 000 U

**thrombinogen (prothrombin)**

**Thrombogen** powder ℞ *topical local hemostatic for surgery* [thrombin] 1000, 5000, 10 000, 20 000 U

**thrombolyse-inj 1500** *investigational tissue-cultured plasminogen activator for acute myocardial infarction*

**thrombolytics** *a class of enzymes that dissolve blood clots, used emergently to treat stroke, pulmonary embolus, and myocardial infarct*

**thromboplastin** USP

**Thrombostat** powder ℞ *topical local hemostatic for surgery* [thrombin] 5000, 10 000, 20 000 U

**thromboxane inhibitor** *investigational therapy for stroke and heart attack*

**thrust** *street drug slang* [see: isobutyl nitrite]

**thrusters** *street drug slang* [see: amphetamines]

**thulium** *element (Tm)*

**thumb** *street drug slang for a marijuana cigarette* [see: marijuana]

**Thylline-GG** tablets (discontinued 1995) ℞ *antiasthmatic; bronchodilator; expectorant* [dyphylline; guaifenesin] 200•200 mg

**thymalfasin** USAN *vaccine enhancer for hepatitis, cancer, and infectious diseases; investigational (Phase III, orphan) for chronic active hepatitis B*

**thymic hormone factor** *investigational agent for HIV, genital herpes, and hepatitis*

**thymic humoral factor, gamma 2** *investigational (Phase II) immunomodulator for HIV*

**thymidylate synthase (TS) inhibitors** *a class of folate-based antineoplastics*

**thymocartin** INN

**thymoctonan** INN *investigational antiviral for HIV infection, genital herpes, and chronic viral hepatitis*

**Thymoglobulin** ℞ *investigational (Phase III) immunosuppressant for kidney transplants* [anti-human thymocyte immunoglobulin, rabbit]

**thymol** NF *stabilizer; topical antiseptic*

**thymol iodide** NF

**Thymone** ℞ *investigational (orphan) for infant respiratory distress syndrome of prematurity* [protirelin]

**thymopentin** USAN, INN, BAN *immunoregulator; investigational (Phase III) for HIV*

**thymopoietin 32-36** [now: thymopentin]

**thymosin alpha-1** [now: thymalfasin]

**thymostimulin** INN *investigational (Phase III) immunomodulator for AIDS*

**thymotrinan** INN

**thymoxamine** BAN [also: moxisylyte]

**thymoxamine HCl** *orphan status withdrawn 1994*

**Thypinone** IV injection ℞ *in vivo thyroid function test* [protirelin] 500 μg/mL

**Thyrar** tablets ℞ *thyroid replacement therapy; hypothyroidism; thyroid cancer* [thyroid (bovine)] 30, 60, 120 mg ② Thyrolar

**Thyrel-TRH** IV injection ℞ *in vivo thyroid function test* [protirelin] 500 μg/mL

**Thyro-Block** tablets ℞ *thyroid-blocking therapy* [potassium iodide] 130 mg

**thyrocalcitonin** [see: calcitonin]

**Thyrogen** ℞ *thyroid-stimulating hormone; investigational (orphan) diagnostic aid for thyroid cancer* [thyrotropin]

**thyroglobulin (TG)** USAN, USP, INN *thyroid hormone*

**thyroid** USP *thyroid hormone* 15, 30, 60, 90, 120, 180, 240, 300 mg oral ② euthroid

**thyroid hormone (TH)** [see: levothyroxine sodium]

**thyroid-stimulating hormone (TSH)** [see: thyrotropin]

**Thyroid Strong** tablets ℞ *hypothyroidism; thyroid cancer* [thyroid, desiccated] 30, 60, 120, 180 mg

**Thyrolar-0.25; -0.5; -1; -2; -3** tablets ℞ *thyroid hormone therapy* [liotrix] 15 mg; 30 mg; 60 mg; 120 mg; 180 mg ② Theolair; Thyrar

**thyromedan HCl** USAN *thyromimetic* [also: tyromedan]

**thyropropic acid** INN

**thyrotrophic hormone** [see: thyrotrophin]

**thyrotrophin** INN *thyroid-stimulating hormone* [also: thyrotropin]

**thyrotropin** *thyroid-stimulating hormone; investigational (orphan) diagnostic aid for thyroid cancer* [also: thyrotrophin]

**thyrotropin-releasing hormone (TRH)** [see: protirelin]

**thyroxine** BAN *thyroid hormone* [also: levothyroxine sodium]

**D-thyroxine** [see: dextrothyroxine sodium]

**L-thyroxine** [see: levothyroxine sodium]

**thyroxine I 125** USAN *radioactive agent*

**thyroxine I 131** USAN *radioactive agent*

**Thytropar** powder for IM or subcu injection R *thyrotrophic hormone; in vivo thyroid function test* [thyrotropin] 10 IU

**TI-23** *investigational (Phase I) antiviral for cytomegalovirus retinitis*

**tiabendazole** INN *anthelmintic* [also: thiabendazole]

**Tiabex** *investigational anticonvulsant* [tiagabine HCl]

**tiacrilast** USAN, INN *antiallergic*

**tiacrilast sodium** USAN *antiallergic*

**tiadenol** INN

**tiafibrate** INN

**tiagabine** INN *investigational anticonvulsant*

**tiagabine HCl** USAN *anticonvulsant*

**Tiamate** extended-release film-coated tablets R *antihypertensive* [diltiazem maleate] 120, 180, 240 mg

**tiamenidine** USAN, INN *antihypertensive*

**tiamenidine HCl** USAN *antihypertensive*

**tiametonium iodide** INN

**tiamiprine** INN *antineoplastic* [also: thiamiprine]

**tiamizide** INN *diuretic; antihypertensive* [also: diapamide]

**tiamulin** USAN, INN *veterinary antibacterial*

**tiamulin fumarate** USAN *veterinary antibacterial*

**tianafac** INN

**tianeptine** INN

**tiapamil** INN, BAN *antagonist to calcium* [also: tiapamil HCl]

**tiapamil HCl** USAN *antagonist to calcium* [also: tiapamil]

**tiapirinol** INN

**tiapride** INN

**tiaprofenic acid** INN

**tiaprost** INN

**tiaramide** INN, BAN *antiasthmatic* [also: tiaramide HCl]

**tiaramide HCl** USAN *antiasthmatic* [also: tiaramide]

**Tiazac** extended-release capsules R *antihypertensive; antianginal; calcium channel blocker* [diltiazem HCl] 120, 180, 240, 300, 360 mg

**tiazesim** INN *antidepressant* [also: thiazesim HCl]

**tiazesim HCl** [see: thiazesim HCl]

**tiazofurin** USAN *antineoplastic* [also: tiazofurine]

**tiazofurine** INN *antineoplastic* [also: tiazofurin]

**Tiazole** R *investigational treatment for leukemia* [tiazofurin]

**tiazuril** USAN, INN *coccidiostat for poultry*

**tibalosin** INN

**tibenelast sodium** USAN *antiasthmatic; bronchodilator*

**tibenzate** INN

**tibezonium iodide** INN

**tibolone** USAN, INN, BAN *anabolic*

**tibric acid** USAN, INN *antihyperlipoproteinemic*

**tibrofan** USAN, INN *disinfectant*

**tic; tic tac** *street drug slang* [see: PCP]

**ticabesone** INN *glucocorticoid* [also: ticabesone propionate]

**ticabesone propionate** USAN *glucocorticoid* [also: ticabesone]

**Ticar** powder for IV or IM injection R *extended-spectrum penicillin-type antibiotic* [ticarcillin disodium] 1, 3, 6, 20, 30 g ⍰ Tigan

**ticarbodine** USAN, INN *anthelmintic*

**ticarcillin** INN *antibacterial* [also: ticarcillin disodium]

**ticarcillin cresyl sodium** USAN *antibacterial*

**ticarcillin disodium** USAN, USP *bactericidal antibiotic* [also: ticarcillin]

**Tice BCG** percutaneous injection for TB, intravesical injection for cancer R *tuberculosis immunizing agent; antineoplastic for bladder cancer* [BCG vaccine, Tice strain] 50 mg

**ticket; ticket to ride** *street drug slang* [see: LSD]

**ticlatone** USAN, INN *antibacterial; antifungal*

**Ticlid** film-coated tablets R *platelet aggregation inhibitor for stroke* [ticlopidine HCl] 250 mg

**ticlopidine** INN, BAN *platelet aggregation inhibitor* [also: ticlopidine HCl]

**ticlopidine HCl** USAN *platelet aggregation inhibitor* [also: ticlopidine]

**ticolubant** USAN *leukotriene B₄ receptor antagonist for psoriasis*

**Ticon** IM injection ℞ *anticholinergic; antiemetic* [trimethobenzamide HCl] 100 mg/mL

**ticrynafen** USAN *diuretic; uricosuric; antihypertensive* [also: tienilic acid]

**tidiacic** INN

**tiemonium iodide** INN, BAN

**tienilic acid** INN *diuretic; uricosuric; antihypertensive* [also: ticrynafen]

**tienocarbine** INN

**tienopramine** INN

**tienoxolol** INN

**tifemoxone** INN

**tifenamil** INN *smooth muscle relaxant* [also: thiphenamil HCl]

**tifenamil HCl** [see: thiphenamil HCl]

**tifencillin** INN *antibacterial* [also: thiphencillin potassium]

**tifencillin potassium** [see: thiphencillin potassium]

**tiflamizole** INN

**tiflorex** INN

**tifluadom** INN

**tiflucarbine** INN

**tiformin** INN [also: tyformin]

**tifurac** INN *analgesic* [also: tifurac sodium]

**tifurac sodium** USAN *analgesic* [also: tifurac]

**Tigan** capsules, suppositories, pediatric suppositories, IM injection ℞ *antiemetic* [trimethobenzamide HCl] 100, 250 mg; 200 mg; 100 mg; 100 mg/mL ▣ Ticar

**tigemonam** INN *antimicrobial* [also: tigemonam dicholine]

**tigemonam dicholine** USAN *antimicrobial* [also: tigemonam]

**tigestol** USAN, INN *progestin*

**tigloidine** INN, BAN

**tiglyl*pseudo*tropine** [see: tigloidine]

**tiglyltropeine** [see: tropigline]

**Tijuana** *street drug slang, a reference to a Mexican town on the U.S. border* [see: marijuana]

**tilactase** INN *digestive enzyme*

**Tilad** (Spanish name for U.S. product Tilade)

**Tilade** oral inhalation aerosol ℞ *respiratory anti-inflammatory; antiasthmatic; bronchoconstriction inhibitor* [nedocromil sodium] 1.75 mg/dose

**Tilarin** nasal spray (commercially available in Germany) ℞ *investigational antiasthmatic* [nedocromil sodium]

**Tilavist** eye drops ℞ *investigational treatment for allergic conjunctivitis* [nedocromil sodium]

**tilbroquinol** INN

**Tilcotil** ℞ *investigational analgesic for postoperative and menstrual pain and juvenile arthritis* [tenoxicam]

**tiletamine** INN *anesthetic; anticonvulsant* [also: tiletamine HCl]

**tiletamine HCl** USAN *anesthetic; anticonvulsant* [also: tiletamine]

**tilidate HCl** BAN *analgesic* [also: tilidine HCl; tilidine]

**tilidine** INN *analgesic* [also: tilidine HCl; tilidate HCl]

**tilidine HCl** USAN *analgesic* [also: tilidine; tilidate HCl]

**tiliquinol** INN

**tilisolol** INN

**tilmicosin** USAN, INN, BAN *veterinary antibacterial*

**tilmicosin phosphate** USAN *veterinary antibacterial*

**tilomisole** USAN, INN *immunoregulator*

**tilorone** INN *antiviral* [also: tilorone HCl]

**tilorone HCl** USAN *antiviral* [also: tilorone]

**tilozepine** INN

**tilsuprost** INN

**Tiltab** (trademarked dosage form) *film-coated tablets*

**tiludronate disodium** USAN *bisphosphonate bone resorption inhibitor for osteoporosis and Paget's disease*

**tiludronic acid** INN

**Timecap** (trademarked dosage form) *sustained-release capsule*

**Timecelle** (trademarked dosage form) *timed-release capsule*

**timefurone** USAN, INN *antiatherosclerotic*

**timegadine** INN

**Time-Hist** sustained-release capsules ℞ *decongestant; antihistamine* [pseudoephedrine HCl; chlorpheniramine maleate] 120•8 mg

**timelotem** INN

**Timentin** powder for IV injection ℞ *extended-spectrum penicillin-type antibiotic* [ticarcillin disodium; clavulanate potassium] 3•0.1 g

**timepidium bromide** INN

**Timespan** (trademarked dosage form) *timed-release tablets*

**Timesules** (dosage form) *sustained-release capsules*

**timiperone** INN

**timobesone** INN *topical adrenocortical steroid* [also: timobesone acetate]

**timobesone acetate** USAN *topical adrenocortical steroid* [also: timobesone]

**Timodal** ⓐ (U.S. product: Timoptic) eye drops ℞ *antiglaucoma agent (β-blocker)* [timolol maleate] 0.25%, 0.5%

**timofibrate** INN

**Timolide 10-25** tablets ℞ *antihypertensive* [timolol maleate; hydrochlorothiazide] 10•25 mg

**timolol** USAN, INN, BAN *antiadrenergic (β-receptor)* ⓢ atenolol

**timolol hemihydrate** *topical antiglaucoma agent (β-blocker)*

**timolol maleate** USAN, USP *antiadrenergic; topical antiglaucoma agent (β-blocker); migraine preventative* 5, 10, 20 mg oral; 0.25%, 0.5% eye drops

**timonacic** INN

**timoprazole** INN

**Timoptic** Ocumeter (eye drops), Ocudose (single-use eye drop dispenser) ℞ *topical antiglaucoma agent (β-blocker)* [timolol maleate] 0.25%, 0.5%

**Timoptic-XE** ophthalmic gel ℞ *topical once-daily antiglaucoma agent (β-blocker)* [timolol maleate] 0.25%, 0.5%

**Timpilo** ℞ *investigational treatment for glaucoma* [timolol; pilocarpine]

**Timunox** ℞ *investigational (Phase III) immunomodulator for asymptomatic HIV infection* [thymopoentin]

**tin** *element (Sn)*

**tin chloride dihydrate** [see: stannous chloride]

**tin ethyl etiopurpurin** *investigational (Phase III) treatment for various cancers by photodynamic therapy*

**tin fluoride** [see: stannous fluoride]

**tinabinol** USAN, INN *antihypertensive*

**Tinactin** cream, powder, spray powder, spray liquid, solution OTC *topical antifungal* [tolnaftate] 1% ⓢ Taractan

**Tinactin for Jock Itch** cream, spray powder OTC *topical antifungal* [tolnaftate] 1%

**tinazoline** INN

**TinBen** tincture OTC *skin protectant* [benzoin; alcohol 75% to 83%]

**TinCoBen** tincture OTC *skin protectant* [benzoin; aloe; alcohol 77%]

**Tincture of Green Soap** liquid OTC *antiseptic cleanser* [green soap; alcohol 28-32%]

**Tindal** sugar-coated tablets (discontinued 1995) ℞ *antipsychotic* [acetophenazine maleate] 20 mg

**Tine Test OT** [see: Tuberculin Tine Test, Old]

**Tine Test PPD** single-use intradermal puncture test device ℞ *tuberculosis skin test* [tuberculin purified protein derivative] 5 U

**Ting** cream, powder, spray powder, spray liquid OTC *topical antifungal* [tolnaftate] 1%

**tinidazole** USAN, INN *antiprotozoal*

**tinisulpride** INN

**tinofedrine** INN

**tinoridine** INN

**Tinver** lotion ℞ *topical antifungal; keratolytic; antipruritic; anesthetic* [sodium thiosulfate; salicylic acid; alcohol 10%] 25%•1%

**tinzaparin sodium** USAN, INN, BAN *anticoagulant; antithrombotic*

**T-inzole** ℞ *investigational antineoplastic for leukemia* [tizofurin]

**tiocarlide** INN [also: thiocarlide]

**tioclomarol** INN

**tioconazole** USAN, USP, INN, BAN, JAN *antifungal*

**tioctilate** INN

**tiodazosin** USAN, INN *antihypertensive*

**tiodonium chloride** USAN, INN *antibacterial*

**tiofacic** [see: stepronin]

**tioguanine** INN *antineoplastic* [also: thioguanine]

**tiomergine** INN

**tiomesterone** INN [also: thiomesterone]

**tioperidone** INN *antipsychotic* [also: tioperidone HCl]

**tioperidone HCl** USAN *antipsychotic* [also: tioperidone]

**tiopinac** USAN, INN *anti-inflammatory; analgesic; antipyretic*

**tiopronin** INN *prevention of cystine nephrolithiasis in homozygous cystinuria* (orphan)

**tiopropamine** INN

**tiosalan** INN *disinfectant* [also: thiosalan]

**tiosinamine** [see: allylthiourea]

**tiospirone** INN *antipsychotic* [also: tiospirone HCl]

**tiospirone HCl** USAN *antipsychotic* [also: tiospirone]

**tiotidine** USAN, INN *antagonist to histamine $H_2$ receptors*

**tiotixene** INN *antipsychotic* [also: thiothixene]

**tioxacin** INN

**tioxamast** INN

**tioxaprofen** INN

**tioxidazole** USAN, INN *anthelmintic*

**tioxolone** INN [also: thioxolone]

**tipentosin** INN, BAN *antihypertensive* [also: tipentosin HCl]

**tipentosin HCl** USAN *antihypertensive* [also: tipentosin]

**tipepidine** INN

**tipetropium bromide** INN

**tipindole** INN

**tipredane** USAN, INN, BAN *topical adrenocortical steroid*

**tiprenolol** INN *antiadrenergic (β-receptor)* [also: tiprenolol HCl]

**tiprenolol HCl** USAN *antiadrenergic (β-receptor)* [also: tiprenolol]

**tiprinast** INN *antiallergic* [also: tiprinast meglumine]

**tiprinast meglumine** USAN *antiallergic* [also: tiprinast]

**tipropidil** INN *vasodilator* [also: tipropidil HCl]

**tipropidil HCl** USAN *vasodilator* [also: tipropidil]

**tiprostanide** INN, BAN

**tiprotimod** INN

**tiqueside** USAN, INN *antihyperlipidemic*

**tiquinamide** INN *gastric anticholinergic* [also: tiquinamide HCl]

**tiquinamide HCl** USAN *gastric anticholinergic* [also: tiquinamide]

**tiquizium bromide** INN

**tirapazamine** USAN, INN *antineoplastic*

**tiratricol** INN

**tiratricol & levothyroxine sodium** *investigational (orphan) to suppress thyroid-stimulating hormone (TSH) in thyroid cancer*

**Tirend** tablets OTC *CNS stimulant; analeptic* [caffeine] 100 mg

**tirilazad** INN, BAN *lipid peroxidation inhibitor; 21-aminosteroid (lazaroid); antioxidant* [also: tirilazad mesylate]

**tirilazad mesylate** USAN *lipid peroxidation inhibitor; 21-aminosteroid (lazaroid); antioxidant* [also: tirilazad]

**tirofiban HCl** USAN *GPIIb/IIIa receptor inhibitor; antiplatelet/antithrombotic agent for unstable angina*

**tiropramide** INN

**tish** *street drug slang* [see: PCP]

**tisilfocon A** USAN *hydrophobic contact lens material*

**Tisit** liquid, shampoo OTC *pediculicide* [pyrethrins; piperonyl butoxide] 0.3%•2%; 0.3%•3%

**Tisit Blue** gel OTC *pediculicide* [pyrethrins; piperonyl butoxide; petroleum distillate] 0.3%•3%•1.2%

**tisocromide** INN

**TiSol** solution OTC *anesthetic and antimicrobial throat irrigation* [benzyl alcohol; menthol] 1%•0.04%

**tisopurine** INN

**tisoquone** INN

**tissue** *street drug slang* [see: cocaine, crack]

**tissue factor** [see: thromboplastin]

**tissue plasminogen activator (tPA; t-PA)** [see: alteplase]

**Tis-U-Sol** solution ℞ *sterile irrigant* [physiologic irrigating solution]

**Titan** solution OTC *cleaning solution for hard contact lenses*

**titanium** *element* (Ti)

**titanium dioxide** USP *topical protectant; astringent*

**titanium oxide** [see: titanium dioxide]

**titch** *street drug slang* [see: PCP]

**Titracid** chewable tablets (discontinued 1994) OTC *antacid* [calcium carbonate; glycine]

**Titradose** (trademarked dosage form) *scored tablet*

**Titralac** chewable tablets OTC *antacid* [calcium carbonate] 420, 750 mg

**Titralac Plus** chewable tablets, liquid OTC *antacid; antiflatulent* [calcium carbonate; simethicone] 420•21 mg; 500•20 mg/5 mL

**tivanidazole** INN

**tivazine** [see: piperazine citrate]

**tixadil** INN

**tixanox** USAN *antiallergic* [also: tixanoxum]

**tixanoxum** INN *antiallergic* [also: tixanox]

**tixocortol** INN *topical anti-inflammatory* [also: tixocortol pivalate]

**tixocortol pivalate** USAN *topical anti-inflammatory* [also: tixocortol]

**Tixogel VP** *investigational topical skin protectant for allergic contact dermatitis* [bentoquatam]

**tizabrin** INN

**tizanidine** INN, BAN *antispasmodic; central* $\alpha_2$ *agonist* [also: tizanidine HCl]

**tizanidine HCl** USAN, JAN *antispasmodic for multiple sclerosis and spinal cord injury (orphan); central* $\alpha_2$ *agonist* [also: tizanidine]

**tizofurin** *investigational antineoplastic for leukemia*

**tizolemide** INN

**tizoprolic acid** INN

**TJ-9** *investigational herbal compound (Sho-Saiko-To) adjunct for HIV*

**T-Koff** liquid R *narcotic antitussive; decongestant; antihistamine* [codeine phosphate; phenylpropanolamine HCl; phenylephrine HCl; chlorpheniramine maleate] 10•20•20•5 mg/5 mL

$^{201}$**Tl** [see: thallous chloride Tl 201]

**TLC A-60** *investigational vaccine adjuvant*

**TLC ABLC** R *investigational systemic antifungal for bone marrow transplants* [amphotericin B lipid complex (ABLC)]

**TLC C-53** *investigational cell adhesion antagonist for adult respiratory distress syndrome*

**TLC D-99** R *investigational antineoplastic for metastatic breast cancer* [liposome-encapsulated doxorubicin]

**TLC D-99** *investigational liposomal form of doxorubicin for Kaposi sarcoma*

**T-lymphotrophic virus antigens** [see: human T-lymphotropic virus type III (HTLV-III) gp-160 antigens]

**TMB (trimedoxime bromide)** [q.v.]

**TMP (trimethoprim)** [q.v.]

**TMP-SMZ (trimethoprim & sulfamethoxazole)** [q.v.]

**TNF (tumor necrosis factor)** [q.v.]

**TNK-tPA** R *investigational (Phase II) second-generation tissue plasminogen activator for the treatment of acute myocardial infarction*

**TNP-470** *investigational angiogenesis inhibitor for AIDS-related Kaposi sarcoma*

**TOAP (thioguanine, Oncovin, [cytosine] arabinoside, prednisone)** *chemotherapy protocol*

**tobacco** *dried leaves of the Nicotiana tabacum plant; sedative narcotic; emetic; diuretic; heart depressant; antispasmodic* [also see: nicotine]

**TobraDex** eye drop suspension R *topical ophthalmic corticosteroidal anti-inflammatory; antibiotic* [dexamethasone; tobramycin] 0.1%•0.3% ② Tobrex

**TobraDex** ophthalmic ointment R *topical ophthalmic corticosteroidal anti-inflammatory; antibiotic* [dexamethasone; tobramycin; chlorobutanol] 0.1%•0.3%•0.5%

**tobramycin** USAN, USP, INN, BAN *antibacterial antibiotic; investigational (Phase III, orphan) inhalation therapy for Pseudomonas aeruginosa in cystic fibrosis* 0.3% eye drops ② Trobicin

**tobramycin sulfate** USP *aminoglycoside bactericidal antibiotic* 10, 40 mg/mL injection

**Tobrex** Drop-Tainers (eye drops), ophthalmic ointment R *ophthalmic antibiotic* [tobramycin] 0.3%; 3 mg/g ② TobraDex

**tobuterol** INN

**tocainide** USAN, INN, BAN *antiarrhythmic*
**tocainide HCl** USP *antiarrhythmic*
**tocamphyl** USAN, INN *choleretic*
**tocofenoxate** INN
**tocofersolan** INN *vitamin E supplement* [also: tocophersolan]
**tocofibrate** INN
**tocolytics** *a class of drugs used to inhibit uterine contractions*
**tocopherol, *d*-alpha** [see: vitamin E]
**tocopherol, *dl*-alpha** [see: vitamin E]
**tocopherols, mixed** [see: vitamin E]
**tocopherols excipient** NF *antioxidant*
**tocophersolan** USAN *vitamin E supplement; orphan status withdrawn 1994* [also: tocofersolan]
**tocopheryl acetate, *d*-alpha** [see: vitamin E]
**tocopheryl acetate, *dl*-alpha** [see: vitamin E]
**tocopheryl acid succinate, *d*-alpha** [see: vitamin E]
**tocopheryl acid succinate, *dl*-alpha** [see: vitamin E]
**tocopheryl polyethylene glycol succinate (TPGS)** [see: tocophersolan]
**Today** vaginal sponge (discontinued 1995) OTC *spermicidal/barrier contraceptive* [nonoxynol 9] 1 g
**todralazine** INN, BAN
**tofenacin** INN *anticholinergic* [also: tofenacin HCl]
**tofenacin HCl** USAN *anticholinergic* [also: tofenacin]
**tofesilate** INN *combining name for radicals or groups*
**tofetridine** INN
**tofisoline**
**tofisopam** INN
**Tofranil** sugar-coated tablets, IM injection R̥ *tricyclic antidepressant; treatment for childhood enuresis* [imipramine HCl] 10, 25, 50 mg; 25 mg/2 mL ⑨ Tepanil
**Tofranil-PM** capsules R̥ *tricyclic antidepressant; treatment for childhood enuresis* [imipramine pamoate] 75, 100, 125, 150 mg
**tolamolol** USAN, INN *vasodilator; antiarrhythmic; antiadrenergic (β-receptor)*

**tolazamide** USAN, USP, INN, BAN *sulfonylurea-type antidiabetic* 100, 250, 500 mg oral
**tolazoline** INN *peripheral vasodilator* [also: tolazoline HCl]
**tolazoline HCl** USP *antihypertensive; peripheral vasodilator* [also: tolazoline]
**tolboxane** INN
**tolbutamide** USP, INN, BAN *sulfonylurea-type antidiabetic* 500 mg oral
**tolbutamide sodium** USP *diagnostic aid for diabetes*
**tolcapone** USAN, INN *antiparkinsonian*
**tolciclate** USAN, INN *antifungal*
**tolclotide** [see: disulfamide]
**toldimfos** INN, BAN
**Tolectin 200; Tolectin 600** tablets R̥ *nonsteroidal anti-inflammatory drug (NSAID); antiarthritic; analgesic* [tolmetin sodium] 200 mg; 600 mg
**Tolectin DS** capsules R̥ *nonsteroidal anti-inflammatory drug (NSAID); antiarthritic; analgesic* [tolmetin sodium] 400 mg
**Tolerex** powder OTC *enteral nutritional therapy* [lactose-free formula]
**tolfamide** USAN, INN *urease enzyme inhibitor*
**tolfenamic acid** INN, BAN
**Tolfrinic** film-coated tablets OTC *hematinic* [ferrous fumarate; cyanocobalamin; ascorbic acid] 200 mg•25 μg•100 mg
**tolgabide** USAN, INN, BAN *anticonvulsant*
**tolhexamide** [see: glycyclamide]
**tolimidone** USAN, INN *antiulcerative*
**Tolinase** tablets R̥ *sulfonylurea-type antidiabetic* [tolazamide] 100, 250, 500 mg ⑨ Orinase
**tolindate** USAN, INN *antifungal*
**toliodium chloride** USAN, INN *veterinary food additive*
**toliprolol** INN
**tolmesoxide** INN
**tolmetin** USAN, INN *nonsteroidal anti-inflammatory drug (NSAID); analgesic*
**tolmetin sodium** USAN, USP *antiarthritic; nonsteroidal anti-inflammatory drug (NSAID); analgesic* 200, 400, 600 mg oral
**tolnaftate** USAN, USP, INN, BAN *antifungal* 1% topical

**tolnapersine** INN

**tolnidamine** INN

**toloconium metilsulfate** INN

**tolofocon A** USAN *hydrophobic contact lens material*

**tolonidine** INN

**tolonium chloride** INN

**toloxatone** INN

**toloxichloral** [see: toloxychlorinol]

**toloxychlorinol** INN

**tolpadol** INN

**tolpentamide** INN, BAN

**tolperisone** INN, BAN

**tolpiprazole** INN, BAN

**tolpovidone I 131** USAN *hypoalbuminemia test; radioactive agent* [also: radiotolpovidone I 131]

**tolpronine** INN, BAN

**tolpropamine** INN, BAN

**tolpyrramide** USAN, INN *antidiabetic*

**tolquinzole** INN

**tolrestat** USAN, INN, BAN *aldose reductase inhibitor*

**toltrazuril** USAN, INN, BAN *veterinary coccidiostat*

**tolu balsam** USP *pharmaceutic aid*

***p*-toluenesulfone dichloramine** [see: dichloramine T]

**tolufazepam** INN

**toluidine blue O** [see: tolonium chloride]

**toluidine blue O chloride** [see: tolonium chloride]

**Tolu-Sed DM** syrup OTC *antitussive; expectorant* [dextromethorphan hydrobromide; guaifenesin; alcohol 10%] 10•100 mg/5 mL

**tolycaine** INN, BAN

**tomelukast** USAN, INN *antiasthmatic; leukotriene antagonist*

**Tomocat** concentrated suspension R̥ *GI contrast radiopaque agent* [barium sulfate] 5%

**tomoglumide** INN

**Tomosar** R̥ *investigational antineoplastic for breast, prostatic, and stomach cancers and lymphomas* [menogaril]

**tomoxetine** INN *antidepressant* [also: tomoxetine HCl]

**tomoxetine HCl** USAN *antidepressant* [also: tomoxetine]

**tomoxiprole** INN

**Tomudex** R̥ *investigational (Phase III) thymidylate synthase inhibitor for colorectal cancer* [raltitrexed]

**tonazocine** INN *analgesic* [also: tonazocine mesylate]

**tonazocine mesylate** USAN *analgesic* [also: tonazocine]

**toncho** *street drug slang for an octane booster, that is inhaled* [see: petroleum distillate inhalants]

**Tonocard** film-coated tablets R̥ *antiarrhythmic* [tocainide HCl] 400, 600 mg

**Tonopaque** powder for suspension R̥ *GI contrast radiopaque agent* [barium sulfate; sorbitol] 95%

**tonzonium bromide** INN *detergent* [also: thonzonium bromide]

**tooey; tuie; twoie** *street drug slang* [see: Tuinal; amobarbital sodium; secobarbital sodium]

**tooly** *street drug slang for toluene, which is inhaled* [see: petroleum distillate inhalants]

**toot** *street drug slang* [see: cocaine]

**Toothache** gel OTC *topical oral anesthetic* [benzocaine] ?

**Tootsie Roll** *street drug slang* [see: heroin]

**top gun** *street drug slang* [see: cocaine, crack]

**Topamax** coated tablets R̥ *broad-spectrum sulfamate anticonvulsant for partial-onset seizures; investigational (orphan) for Lennox-Gastaut syndrome* [topiramate] 25, 100, 200 mg

**topi** *street drug slang for peyote cactus* [see: mescaline]

**Topic** gel OTC *antipruritic; counterirritant* [benzyl alcohol; camphor; menthol; alcohol 30%] 5%•?•? ⊡ Topicort

**topical starch** [see: starch, topical]

**Topicort** ointment, cream, gel R̥ *topical corticosteroidal anti-inflammatory* [desoximetasone] 0.25%; 0.25%; 0.05% ⊡ Topic

**Topicort LP** cream R̥ *topical corticosteroidal anti-inflammatory* [desoximetasone] 0.05%

**Topicycline** solution R̥ *topical antibiotic for acne* [tetracycline HCl] 2.2 mg/mL

**topiramate** USAN, INN, BAN *broad-spectrum sulfamate anticonvulsant for partial-onset seizures; investigational (orphan) for Lennox-Gastaut syndrome*

**Toposar** IV injection ℞ *antineoplastic for testicular and small cell lung cancers* [etoposide; alcohol 30.5%] 20 mg/mL

**topotecan** INN, BAN *antineoplastic for ovarian cancer; DNA topoisomerase I inhibitor* [also: topotecan HCl]

**topotecan HCl** USAN *hormonal antineoplastic for ovarian cancer; DNA topoisomerase I inhibitor* [also: topotecan]

**toprilidine** INN

**Toprol XL** film-coated extended-release tablets ℞ *antihypertensive; long-term antianginal; β-blocker* [metoprolol succinate] 50, 100, 200 mg

**tops** *street drug slang for peyote* [see: mescaline]

**tops and bottoms** *street drug slang for a combination of Talwin (pentazocine HCl) and PBZ (pyribenzamine), used as a heroin substitute* [see: Talwin; pentazocine HCl; tripelennamine]

**topterone** USAN, INN *antiandrogen*

**TOPV (trivalent oral poliovirus vaccine)** [see: poliovirus vaccine, live oral]

**toquizine** USAN, INN *anticholinergic*

**Toradol** film-coated tablets, Tubex (cartridge-needle unit) for IM or IV injection ℞ *nonsteroidal anti-inflammatory drug (NSAID); analgesic for acute, moderately severe pain* [ketorolac tromethamine] 10 mg; 15, 30 mg/mL

**Toradol** gel, transdermal, IV injection ℞ *investigational nonsteroidal anti-inflammatory drug (NSAID)* [ketorolac tromethamine]

**torasemide** INN, BAN *loop diuretic* [also: torsemide]

**torbafylline** INN

**torch** *street drug slang* [see: marijuana]

**Torecan** tablets, IM injection, suppositories ℞ *antiemetic* [thiethylperazine maleate] 10 mg; 5 mg/mL; 10 mg

**toremifene** INN, BAN *antiestrogen; antineoplastic; investigational (orphan) for metastatic carcinoma of the breast and desmoid tumors* [also: toremifene citrate]

**toremifene citrate** USAN *antiestrogen; antineoplastic* [also: toremifene]

**toripristone** INN

**Tornalate** oral inhalation aerosol, inhalation solution ℞ *bronchodilator* [bitolterol mesylate] 0.8%; 0.2%

**torpedo** *street drug slang for chloral hydrate in an alcoholic beverage or a combination of crack and marijuana* [see: chloral hydrate; cocaine, crack; marijuana]

**torsemide** USAN *loop diuretic* [also: torasemide]

**tosactide** INN [also: octacosactrin]

**tosifen** USAN, INN *antianginal*

**tosilate** INN *combining name for radicals or groups* [also: tosylate]

**tosufloxacin** USAN, INN *antibacterial*

**tosulur** INN

**tosylate** USAN, BAN *combining name for radicals or groups* [also: tosilate]

**tosylchloramide sodium** INN [also: chloramine-T]

**Totacillin** capsules, powder for oral suspension ℞ *penicillin-type antibiotic* [ampicillin trihydrate] 250, 500 mg; 125, 250 mg/5 mL

**Totacillin-N** powder for IV or IM injection ℞ *penicillin-type antibiotic* [ampicillin sodium] 0.25, 0.5, 1, 2, 10 g

**Total** solution OTC *cleaning/soaking/wetting solution for hard contact lenses*

**Total Formula; Total Formula-2** tablets OTC *vitamin/mineral/iron supplement* [multiple vitamins & minerals; iron; folic acid; biotin] ±•20•0.4•0.3 mg

**Total Formula-3 without Iron** tablets OTC *vitamin/mineral supplement* [multiple vitamins & minerals; folic acid; biotin] ±•0.4•0.3 mg

**toughened silver nitrate** [see: silver nitrate, toughened]

**Touro A & H** timed-release capsules ℞ *decongestant; antihistamine* [pseudoephedrine HCl; brompheniramine maleate] 60•6 mg

**Touro Ex** sustained-release caplets ℞ *expectorant* [guaifenesin] 600 mg

**Touro LA** long-acting caplets ℞ *decongestant; expectorant* [pseudoephedrine HCl; guaifenesin] 120•500 mg

**toxoids** *a class of drugs used for active immunization that produce endogenous antibodies to toxins*

**toxy** *street drug slang* [see: opium]

**toys** *street drug slang* [see: opium]

**tozalinone** INN *antidepressant* [also: thozalinone]

**tPA; t-PA (tissue plasminogen activator)** [see: alteplase]

**TPCH (thioguanine, procarbazine, CCNU, hydroxyurea)** *chemotherapy protocol*

**TPDCV (thioguanine, procarbazine, DCD, CCNU, vincristine)** *chemotherapy protocol*

**TPGS (tocopheryl polyethylene glycol succinate)** [see: tocophersolan]

**T-Phyl** timed-release tablets R̲ *bronchodilator* [theophylline] 200 mg

**TPM Test** kit for professional use *in vitro diagnostic aid for Toxoplasma gondii antibodies in serum* [indirect hemagglutination test]

**TPN Electrolytes; TPN Electrolytes II; TPN Electrolytes III** IV admixture R̲ *intravenous electrolyte therapy* [combined electrolyte solution]

**traboxopine** INN

**Trac Tabs 2X** tablets R̲ *urinary anti-infective; analgesic; antispasmodic; acidifier* [methenamine; phenyl salicylate; atropine sulfate; hyoscyamine sulfate; benzoic acid; methylene blue] 120•30•0.06•0.03•7.5•6 mg

**tracazolate** USAN, INN, BAN *sedative*

**Trace Metals Additive in 0.9% NaCl** IV injection R̲ *intravenous nutritional therapy* [multiple trace elements (metals)]

**Tracelyte; Tracelyte II; Tracelyte with Double Electrolytes; Tracelyte II with Double Electrolytes** IV admixture R̲ *intravenous nutritional therapy* [multiple trace elements (metals); electrolytes]

**Tracer bG** reagent strips for home use (discontinued 1995) OTC *in vitro diagnostic aid for blood glucose*

**Tracrium** IV infusion R̲ *nondepolarizing neuromuscular blocker; adjunct to anesthesia* [atracurium besylate] 10 mg/mL

**tragacanth** NF *suspending agent*

**tragic magic** *street drug slang for crack dipped in PCP* [see: cocaine, crack; PCP]

**tralonide** USAN, INN *glucocorticoid*

**tramadol** INN *central analgesic* [also: tramadol HCl]

**tramadol HCl** USAN *central analgesic* [also: tramadol]

**tramazoline** INN *adrenergic* [also: tramazoline HCl]

**tramazoline HCl** USAN *adrenergic* [also: tramazoline]

**Trancopal** caplets R̲ *anxiolytic* [chlormezanone] 100, 200 mg

**Trandate** film-coated tablets, IV injection R̲ *antihypertensive; alpha- and beta-adrenergic blocking agent* [labetalol HCl] 100, 200, 300 mg; 5 mg/mL

**trandolapril** INN, BAN *antihypertensive; angiotensin converting enzyme (ACE) inhibitor*

**trandolaprilat** INN

**tranexamic acid** USAN, INN, BAN *systemic hemostatic; orphan status withdrawn 1996*

**tranilast** USAN, INN *antiasthmatic*

**trank** *street drug slang, from "tranquilizer"* [see: PCP]

**trans AMCHA (*trans*-aminomethyl cyclohexanecarboxylic acid)** [see: tranexamic acid]

**transcainide** USAN, INN *antiarrhythmic*

**transclomiphene** [now: zuclomiphene]

**Transderm Scōp** transdermal patch R̲ *motion sickness prevention* [scopolamine hydrobromide] 1.5 mg

**Transderm-Nitro** transdermal patch R̲ *antianginal* [nitroglycerin] 12.5, 25, 50, 75, 100 mg

**transforming growth factor beta 2** *investigational connective tissue growth stimulator; investigational (orphan) for full-thickness macular holes*

**Trans-Plantar** transdermal patch (name changed to Trans-Ver-Sal Plantar-Patch in 1995)

**trans-** JAN *topical antipruritic; mild local anesthetic; counterirritant* [also: camphor]

***trans*-retinoic acid** [see: tretinoin]

**Trans-Ver-Sal Adult-Patch; Trans-Ver-Sal Pedia-Patch; Trans-Ver-Sal Plantar-Patch** transdermal patch OTC *topical keratolytic* [salicylic acid] 15%

**trantelinium bromide** INN

**Tranxene** T-Tabs ("T"-imprinted tablets) ℞ *anxiolytic; minor tranquilizer; anticonvulsant adjunct* [clorazepate dipotassium] 3.75, 7.5, 15 mg

**Tranxene-SD** single-dose tablets ℞ *anxiolytic; minor tranquilizer; anticonvulsant adjunct* [clorazepate dipotassium] 11.25, 22.5 mg

**tranylcypromine** INN, BAN *antidepressant; MAO inhibitor* [also: tranylcypromine sulfate]

**tranylcypromine sulfate** USP *antidepressant; MAO inhibitor* [also: tranylcypromine]

**trapencaine** INN

**trapidil** INN

**trapymin** [see: trapidil]

**Trasylol** IV infusion ℞ *systemic hemostatic for coronary artery bypass graft (CABG) surgery (orphan)* [aprotinin] 10 000 KIU/mL (Kallikrein inhibitor units) ② Travasol

**TraumaCal** ready-to-use liquid OTC *enteral nutritional therapy for moderate to severe stress or trauma* [branched chain amino acids]

**Traum-Aid HBC** powder (discontinued 1994) OTC *oral nutritional supplement for trauma and sepsis* 125.8 g/packet

**Travase** ointment (discontinued 1996) ℞ *topical enzyme for biochemical debridement* [sutilains] 82 000 U/g

**Travasol 2.75% in 5% (10%, 25%) Dextrose; Travasol 4.25% in 5% (10%, 25%) Dextrose** IV infusion ℞ *total parenteral nutrition; peripheral parenteral nutrition* [multiple essential and nonessential amino acids; dextrose] ② Trasylol

**Travasol 3.5% (5.5%, 8.5%) with Electrolytes** IV infusion ℞ *total parenteral nutrition (all except 3.5%); peripheral parenteral nutrition (all)* [multiple essential and nonessential amino acids & electrolytes] ±

**Travasol 5.5% (8.5%, 10%)** IV infusion ℞ *total parenteral nutrition; peripheral parenteral nutrition* [multiple essential and nonessential amino acids] ±

**Travasorb Hepatic Diet** powder (discontinued 1996) OTC *enteral nutritional therapy for hepatic failure* [branched chain amino acids] ±

**Travasorb HN; Travasorb MCT; Travasorb STD** powder OTC *enteral nutritional therapy* [lactose-free formula]

**Travasorb Renal Diet** powder OTC *enteral nutritional therapy for acute renal failure* [essential amino acids] ±

**Travert** IV infusion ℞ *nonelectrolyte fluid and caloric replacement* [invert sugar (50% dextrose + 50% fructose) in water]

**5% Travert and Electrolyte No. 2; 10% Travert and Electrolyte No. 2** IV infusion ℞ *intravenous nutritional/electrolyte therapy* [combined electrolyte solution; invert sugar (50% dextrose + 50% fructose)]

**traxanox** INN

**Traypak** (trademarked packaging form) *multivial carton*

**trazitiline** INN

**trazium esilate** INN

**trazodone** INN *tetracyclic antidepressant* [also: trazodone HCl]

**trazodone HCl** USAN *tetracyclic antidepressant; used for panic disorders, aggressive behavior, and cocaine withdrawal* [also: trazodone] 50, 100, 150 mg oral

**trazolopride** INN

**trebenzomine** INN *antidepressant* [also: trebenzomine HCl]

**trebenzomine HCl** USAN *antidepressant* [also: trebenzomine]

**trecadrine** INN

**Trecator-SC** tablets ℞ *tuberculostatic* [ethionamide] 250 mg

**trefentanil HCl** USAN *analgesic*

**treloxinate** USAN, INN *antihyperlipoproteinemic*

**trenbolone** INN, BAN *veterinary anabolic steroid, also abused as a street drug* [also: trenbolone acetate]

**trenbolone acetate** USAN *veterinary anabolic steroid, also abused as a street drug* [also: trenbolone]
**trenbolone hexahydrobenzylcarbonate** *veterinary anabolic steroid, also abused as a street drug*
**Trendar** tablets (discontinued 1996) OTC *nonsteroidal anti-inflammatory drug (NSAID); antiarthritic; analgesic* [ibuprofen] 200 mg
**trengestone** INN
**trenizine** INN
**Trental** film-coated controlled-release tablets ℞ *hemorheologic agent to improve blood microcirculation in intermittent claudication* [pentoxifylline] 400 mg
**treosulfan** INN, BAN *investigational (orphan) for ovarian cancer*
**trepibutone** INN
**trepipam** INN *sedative* [also: trepipam maleate]
**trepipam maleate** USAN *sedative* [also: trepipam]
**trepirium iodide** INN
**treptilamine** INN
**trequinsin** INN
**trestolone** INN *antineoplastic; androgen* [also: trestolone acetate]
**trestolone acetate** USAN *antineoplastic; androgen* [also: trestolone]
**tretamine** INN, BAN [also: triethylenemelamine]
**trethinium tosilate** INN
**trethocanic acid** INN
**trethocanoic acid** [see: trethocanic acid]
**tretinoin** USAN, USP, INN, BAN *keratolytic; treat acute promyelocytic leukemia (orphan); investigational (orphan) for other leukemias and ophthalmic squamous metaplasia*
**Tretinoin APS** (Advanced Polymer System) controlled-release sponge ℞ *investigational keratolytic for acne* [tretinoin]
**Tretinoin LF** ℞ *investigational (Phase III) antineoplastic for promyelocytic leukemia and Kaposi sarcoma*
**tretoquinol** INN
**Trexan** tablets (name changed to ReVia in 1995)
**TRH (thyrotropin-releasing hormone)** [see: protirelin]
**Tri Vit with Fluoride** drops ℞ *pediatric vitamin supplement and dental caries preventative* [vitamins A, C, and D; fluoride] 1500 IU•35 mg•400 IU•0.25 mg, 1500 IU•35 mg•400 IU•0.5 mg per mL
**Triacana** ℞ *investigational (orphan) for suppression of thyroid-stimulating hormone (TSH) in thyroid cancer* [tiratricol; levothyroxine sodium]
**Triacet** cream ℞ *topical corticosteroid* [triamcinolone acetonide] 0.1%
**triacetin** USP, INN *antifungal*
**triacetyloleandomycin** BAN *macrolide bactericidal antibiotic* [also: troleandomycin]
**Triacin-C Cough** syrup ℞ *narcotic antitussive; decongestant; antihistamine* [codeine phosphate; pseudoephedrine HCl; triprolidine HCl; alcohol] 10•30•1.25 mg/5 mL
**triaconazole** [now: terconazole]
**Triad** capsules ℞ *sedative; analgesic* [acetaminophen; caffeine; butalbital] 325•40•50 mg
**Triafed** syrup (discontinued 1995) OTC *decongestant; antihistamine* [pseudoephedrine HCl; triprolidine HCl] 30•1.25 mg/5 mL ⑨ Trifed
**Triafed** tablets (discontinued 1994) OTC *decongestant; antihistamine* [pseudoephedrine HCl; triprolidine HCl] 60•2.5 mg
**Triafed with Codeine** syrup ℞ *narcotic antitussive; decongestant; antihistamine* [codeine phosphate; pseudoephedrine HCl; triprolidine HCl] 10•30•1.25 mg/5 mL
**triafungin** USAN, INN *antifungal*
**Triam Forte** IM injection ℞ *glucocorticoids* [triamcinolone diacetate] 40 mg/mL
**Triam-A** IM, intra-articular, intrabursal, intradermal injection ℞ *glucocorticoids* [triamcinolone acetonide] 40 mg/mL
**triamcinolone** USP, INN, BAN, JAN *corticosteroid* 4 mg oral ⑨ Triaminicin
**triamcinolone acetonide** USP, JAN *corticosteroid; inhalant for asthma*

0.025%, 0.1%, 0.5% topical; 40 mg/mL injection

**triamcinolone acetonide sodium phosphate** USAN *corticosteroid*

**triamcinolone benetonide** INN

**triamcinolone diacetate** USP, JAN *corticosteroid* 40 mg/mL injection

**triamcinolone furetonide** INN

**triamcinolone hexacetonide** USAN, USP, INN, BAN *corticosteroid*

**Triaminic** chewable tablets, syrup OTC *pediatric decongestant and antihistamine* [phenylpropanolamine HCl; chlorpheniramine maleate] 6.25•0.5 mg; 6.25•1 mg/5 mL ▣ Triaminicin; TriHemic

**Triaminic** oral infant drops ℞ *pediatric decongestant and antihistamine* [phenylpropanolamine HCl; pyrilamine maleate; pheniramine maleate] 20• 10•10 mg/mL

**Triaminic Allergy; Triaminic Cold** tablets OTC *decongestant; antihistamine* [phenylpropanolamine HCl; chlorpheniramine maleate] 25•4 mg; 12.5•2 mg

**Triaminic AM Cough & Decongestant Formula** liquid OTC *pediatric antitussive and decongestant* [dextromethorphan hydrobromide; pseudoephedrine HCl] 7.5•15 mg/5 mL

**Triaminic AM Decongestant Formula** syrup OTC *decongestant* [pseudoephedrine HCl] 15 mg/5 mL

**Triaminic Decongestant** oral infant drops OTC *pediatric decongestant* [pseudoephedrine HCl] 7.5 mg/0.8 mL

**Triaminic DM** syrup OTC *antitussive; decongestant* [dextromethorphan hydrobromide; phenylpropanolamine HCl] 5•6.25 mg/5 mL

**Triaminic DM Day time** ⊛ oral solution OTC *pediatric antitussive, decongestant, and expectorant* [dextromethorphan hydrobromide; phenylpropanolamine HCl; guaifenesin] 1.5•1.75•7.5 mg/mL

**Triaminic DM Night time for Children** ⊛ (U.S. product: Triaminic Night Light) liquid OTC *pediatric antitussive, decongestant, and antihistamine* [dextromethorphan hydrobromide;

pseudoephedrine HCl; chlorpheniramine maleate] 7.5•15•1 mg/5 mL

**Triaminic Expectorant** liquid OTC *decongestant; expectorant* [phenylpropanolamine HCl; guaifenesin] 6.25• 50 mg/5 mL

**Triaminic Expectorant DH** liquid ℞ *narcotic antitussive; decongestant; antihistamine; expectorant* [hydrocodone bitartrate; phenylpropanolamine HCl; pyrilamine maleate; pheniramine maleate; guaifenesin; alcohol 5%] 1.67•12.5•6.25•6.25•100 mg/5 mL

**Triaminic Expectorant with Codeine** liquid ℞ *narcotic antitussive; decongestant; expectorant* [codeine phosphate; phenylpropanolamine HCl; guaifenesin; alcohol 5%] 10•12.5•100 mg/5 mL

**Triaminic Nite Light** liquid OTC *pediatric antitussive, decongestant, and antihistamine* [dextromethorphan hydrobromide; pseudoephedrine HCl; chlorpheniramine maleate] 7.5•15•1 mg/5 mL

**Triaminic Sore Throat Formula** liquid OTC *pediatric antitussive, decongestant, and analgesic* [dextromethorphan hydrobromide; pseudoephedrine HCl; acetaminophen] 7.5•15• 160 mg/5 mL

**Triaminic TR** sustained-release tablets (discontinued 1993) ℞ *decongestant; antihistamine* [phenylpropanolamine HCl; pyrilamine maleate; pheniramine maleate]

**Triaminic-12** sustained-release tablets OTC *decongestant; antihistamine* [phenylpropanolamine HCl; chlorpheniramine maleate] 75•12 mg

**Triaminicin** tablets (name changed to Triaminicin Cold, Allergy, Sinus in 1993) ▣ triamcinolone; Triaminic

**Triaminicin Cold, Allergy, Sinus** tablets OTC *decongestant; antihistamine; analgesic* [phenylpropanolamine HCl; chlorpheniramine maleate; acetaminophen] 25•4•650 mg ▣ triamcinolone; Triaminic

**Triaminicol Multi-Symptom Cough and Cold** tablets OTC *antitussive; decongestant; antihistamine* [dextromethorphan hydrobromide; phenyl-propanolamine HCl; chlorpheniramine maleate] 10•12.5•2 mg

**Triaminicol Multi-Symptom Relief** liquid OTC *antitussive; decongestant; antihistamine* [dextromethorphan hydrobromide; phenylpropanolamine HCl; chlorpheniramine maleate] 10•12.5•2 mg/5 mL

**Triaminicol Multi-Symptom Relief Colds with Cough** liquid OTC *pediatric antitussive, decongestant, and antihistamine* [dextromethorphan hydrobromide; phenylpropanolamine HCl; chlorpheniramine maleate] 5•6.25•1 mg/5 mL

**Triamolone 40** IM injection ℞ *glucocorticoids* [triamcinolone diacetate] 40 mg/mL

**Triamonide 40** IM, intra-articular, intrabursal, intradermal injection ℞ *glucocorticoids* [triamcinolone acetonide] 40 mg/mL

**triampyzine** INN *anticholinergic* [also: triampyzine sulfate]

**triampyzine sulfate** USAN *anticholinergic* [also: triampyzine]

**triamterene** USAN, USP, INN, BAN, JAN *potassium-sparing diuretic* ⊡ trimipramine

**trianisestrol** [see: chlorotrianisene]

**Triaprin** capsules ℞ *analgesic; antipyretic; sedative* [acetaminophen; butalbital] 325•50 mg

**Tri-Aqua** tablets (discontinued 1993) OTC *diuretic* [caffeine; buchu, uva ursi, zea, and triticum extracts]

**Triasyn B** capsules, tablets (discontinued 1993) OTC *vitamin supplement* [vitamins B₁, B₂, and B₃]

**Triavil 2-10; Triavil 2-25; Triavil 4-10; Triavil 4-25; Triavil 4-50** tablets ℞ *antipsychotic; antidepressant* [perphenazine; amitriptyline HCl] 2•10 mg; 2•25 mg; 4•10 mg; 4•25 mg; 4•50 mg

**Tri-A-Vite F** drops ℞ *pediatric vitamin supplement and dental caries preventative* [vitamins A, C, and D; fluoride] 1500 IU•35 mg•400 IU•0.5 mg per mL

**Triaz** gel, skin cleanser ℞ *topical keratolytic for acne* [benzoyl peroxide] 6%, 10%; 10%

**triaziquone** INN, BAN

**triazolam** USAN, USP, INN *sedative; hypnotic* 0.125, 0.25 mg oral

**Triban; Pediatric Triban** suppositories ℞ *anticholinergic; antiemetic* [trimethobenzamide HCl; benzocaine] 200 mg•2%; 100 mg•2%

**Tri-Barbs** capsules (discontinued 1993) ℞ *sedative; hypnotic* [phenobarbital; butabarbital sodium; secobarbital sodium]

**tribasic calcium phosphate** [see: calcium phosphate, tribasic]

**tribavirin** BAN *antiviral for severe lower respiratory tract infections* [also: ribavirin]

**tribendilol** INN

**tribenoside** USAN, INN *sclerosing agent*

**Tribiotic Plus** ointment OTC *topical antibiotic; anesthetic* [polymyxin B sulfate; bacitracin; neomycin sulfate; lidocaine] 5000 U•500 U•3.5 mg•40 mg per g

**tribromoethanol** NF

**tribromomethane** [see: bromoform]

**tribromsalan** USAN, INN *disinfectant*

**tribuzone** INN

**tricalcium phosphate** [see: calcium phosphate, tribasic]

**Tricana** *investigational (orphan) to suppress thyroid-stimulating hormone (TSH) in thyroid cancer* [tiratricol; levothyroxine sodium]

**tricarbocyanine dye** [see: indocyanine green]

**tricetamide** USAN *sedative*

**Trichinella extract** USP

**Tri-Chlor** liquid ℞ *cauterant; keratolytic* [trichloroacetic acid] 80%

**trichlorethoxyphosphamide** [see: defosfamide]

**Trichlorex** tablets (discontinued 1993) ℞ *diuretic; antihypertensive* [trichlormethiazide]

**trichlorisobutylalcohol** [see: chlorobutanol]

**trichlormethiazide** USP, INN *diuretic; antihypertensive* 4 mg oral

**trichlormethine** INN [also: trimustine]

**trichloroacetic acid** USP *strong kerato-lytic/cauterant*

**trichlorocarbanilide (TCC)** [see: tri-clocarban]

**trichloroethylene** NF, INN

**trichlorofluoromethane** [see: trichlo-romonofluoromethane]

**trichlorofon** [see: metrifonate]

**trichloromonofluoromethane** NF *aerosol propellant*

**trichlorphon** [see: metrifonate]

**Trichophyton extract** *diagnosis and treatment of Trichophyton-induced skin infections*

**trichorad** [see: acinitrazole]

**trichosanthin** *investigational (Phase II) antiviral for AIDS and ARC*

**Trichotine Douche** powder OTC *anti-septic/germicidal; vaginal cleanser and deodorizer; acidity modifier* [sodium perborate]

**Trichotine Douche** solution OTC *antiseptic/germicidal; vaginal cleanser and deodorizer; acidity modifier* [sodium borate]

**triciribine** INN *antineoplastic* [also: tri-ciribine phosphate]

**triciribine phosphate** USAN *antineo-plastic* [also: triciribine]

**triclabendazole** INN

**triclacetamol** INN

**triclazate** INN

**triclobisonium chloride** NF, INN

**triclocarban** USAN, INN *disinfectant*

**triclodazol** INN

**triclofenate** INN *combining name for radicals or groups*

**triclofenol piperazine** USAN, INN *ant-helmintic*

**triclofos** INN *hypnotic; sedative* [also: triclofos sodium]

**triclofos sodium** USAN *hypnotic; seda-tive* [also: triclofos]

**triclofylline** INN

**triclonide** USAN, INN *anti-inflammatory*

**triclosan** USAN, INN, BAN *disinfectant/antiseptic*

**Tricodene Cough and Cold** liquid R̥ *narcotic antitussive; antihistamine* [codeine phosphate; pyrilamine mal-eate] 8.2●12.5 mg/5 mL

**Tricodene Forte; Tricodene NN** liq-uid OTC *antitussive; decongestant; antihistamine* [dextromethorphan hydrobromide; phenylpropanol-amine HCl; chlorpheniramine male-ate] 10●12.5●2 mg/5 mL

**Tricodene Pediatric Cough & Cold** liquid OTC *pediatric antitussive and decongestant* [dextromethorphan hydrobromide; phenylpropanol-amine HCl] 10●12.5 mg/5 mL

**Tricodene Sugar Free** liquid OTC *anti-tussive; antihistamine* [dextrometho-rphan hydrobromide; chlorphenir-amine maleate] 10●2 mg/5 mL

**Tricom** tablets (discontinued 1995) OTC *decongestant; antihistamine; anal-gesic* [pseudoephedrine HCl; chlor-pheniramine maleate; acetamino-phen] 60●4●650 mg

**Tricomin** R̥ *investigational hair growth enhancer* [peptide metal compound]

**tricosactide** INN

**Tricosal** film-coated tablets R̥ *analge-sic; antipyretic; antirheumatic* [choline magnesium trisalicylate] 500, 750, 1000 mg

**tricyclamol chloride** INN

**tricyclics** *a class of antidepressants*

**Triderm** cream R̥ *topical corticosteroid* [triamcinolone acetonide] 0.1%

**Tridesilon** cream, ointment R̥ *topical corticosteroidal anti-inflammatory* [des-onide] 0.05%

**Tridesilon Otic** [see: Otic Tridesilon]

**Tri-Desogen** R̥ *investigational triphasic oral contraceptive* [ethinyl estradiol; desogestrel]

**tridihexethyl chloride** USP *peptic ulcer adjunct*

**tridihexethyl iodide** INN

**Tridil** IV infusion R̥ *antianginal; periop-erative antihypertensive; for congestive heart failure with myocardial infarction* [nitroglycerin] 0.5, 5 mg/mL

**Tridione** capsules, Dulcets (chewable tablets) R̥ *anticonvulsant* [trimetha-dione] 300 mg; 150 mg

**Tridione** oral solution (discontinued 1995) R̥ *anticonvulsant* [trimetha-dione] 40 mg/mL

**Tridrate Bowel Evacuant Kit** oral solution + 3 tablets + 1 suppository OTC *pre-procedure bowel evacuant* [magnesium citrate (solution); bisacodyl (tablets and suppository)] 300 mL; 5 mg; 10 mg

**trientine** INN *chelating agent* [also: trientine HCl; trientine dihydrochloride]

**trientine dihydrochloride** BAN *chelating agent* [also: trientine HCl; trientine]

**trientine HCl** USAN, USP *copper chelating agent for Wilson's disease (orphan)* [also: trientine; trientine dihydrochloride]

**triethanolamine** [now: trolamine]

**triethyl citrate** NF *plasticizer*

**triethyleneiminobenzoquinone (TEIB)** [see: triaziquone]

**triethylenemelamine** NF [also: tretamine]

**triethylenethiophosphoramide (TSPA; TESPA)** [see: thiotepa]

**Trifed** tablets (discontinued 1995) ℞ *decongestant; antihistamine* [pseudoephedrine HCl; triprolidine HCl] 60•2.5 mg ⊡ Triafed

**Trifed-C Cough** syrup ℞ *narcotic antitussive; decongestant; antihistamine* [codeine phosphate; pseudoephedrine HCl; triprolidine HCl; alcohol 4.4%] 10•30•1.25 mg/5 mL

**trifenagrel** USAN, INN *antithrombotic*

**trifezolac** INN

**triflocin** USAN, INN *diuretic*

**Tri-Flor-Vite with Fluoride** drops ℞ *pediatric vitamin supplement and dental caries preventative* [vitamins A, C, and D; fluoride] 1500 IU•35 mg•400 IU•0.25 mg per mL'

**triflubazam** USAN, INN *minor tranquilizer*

**triflumidate** USAN, INN *anti-inflammatory*

**trifluomeprazine** INN, BAN

**trifluoperazine** INN *antipsychotic; sedative* [also: trifluoperazine HCl] 1, 2, 5, 10 mg oral; 10 mg/mL oral; 2 mg/mL injection

**trifluoperazine HCl** USP *antipsychotic; sedative* [also: trifluoperazine]

**N-trifluoroacetyl adriamycin-14-valerate** *investigational (orphan) for carcinoma in situ of the urinary bladder*

**trifluorothymidine** [see: trifluridine]

**trifluperidol** USAN, INN *antipsychotic*

**triflupromazine** USP, INN *antiemetic; antipsychotic; antidopaminergic*

**triflupromazine HCl** USP *antipsychotic; antiemetic*

**trifluridine** USAN, INN *ophthalmic antiviral*

**triflusal** INN

**triflutate** USAN, INN *combining name for radicals or groups*

**Trigesic** tablets (discontinued 1995) OTC *analgesic; antipyretic; anti-inflammatory* [acetaminophen; aspirin; caffeine] 125•230•30 mg

**trigevolol** INN

**α-triglycidyl isocyanurate (αTGI)** [see: teroxirone]

**TriHemic 600** film-coated tablets ℞ *hematinic* [ferrous fumarate; cyanocobalamin; ascorbic acid; vitamin E; intrinsic factor concentrate; docusate sodium; folic acid] 115 mg•25 μg•600 mg•30 IU•75 mg•50 mg•1 mg ⊡ Triaminic

**Trihexy-2; Trihexy-5** tablets ℞ *anticholinergic; antiparkinsonian agent* [trihexyphenidyl HCl] 2 mg; 5 mg

**trihexyphenidyl** INN *anticholinergic; antiparkinsonian* [also: trihexyphenidyl HCl; benzhexol]

**trihexyphenidyl HCl** USP *anticholinergic; antiparkinsonian* [also: trihexyphenidyl; benzhexol] 2, 5 mg oral

**TriHIBit** IM injection ℞ *immunization against diphtheria, tetanus, and pertussis* [diphtheria & tetanus toxoids & acellular pertussis vaccine (DTaP)]

**Tri-Hydroserpine** tablets ℞ *antihypertensive* [hydrochlorothiazide; reserpine; hydralazine HCl] 15•0.1•25 mg

**Tri-Immunol** IM injection ℞ *immunization against diphtheria, tetanus and pertussis* [diphtheria & tetanus toxoids & whole-cell pertussis vaccine, adsorbed (DTwP)] 0.5 mL

**triiodothyronine sodium, levo** [see: liothyronine sodium]

**Tri-K** liquid ℞ *potassium supplement* [potassium acetate; potassium bicarbonate; potassium citrate] 45 mEq/15 mL (K)

**trikates** USP *electrolyte replenisher*

**trikes and bikes; tricycles and bicycles** *street drug slang for a combination of Talwin (pentazocine HCl) and PBZ (pyribenzamine), used as a heroin substitute* [see: Talwin; pentazocine HCl; tripelennamine]

**Tri-Kort** IM, intra-articular, intrabursal, intradermal injection ℞ *glucocorticoids* [triamcinolone acetonide] 40 mg/mL

**Trilafon** tablets, oral concentrate, IV or IM injection ℞ *antipsychotic; antidopaminergic; antiemetic* [perphenazine] 2, 4, 8, 16 mg; 16 mg/5 mL; 5 mg/mL

**Trileptal** (commercially available in Argentina, Finland, and the Netherlands) ℞ *investigational antiepileptic* [oxcarbazepine]

**triletide** INN

**Tri-Levlen** tablets ℞ *triphasic oral contraceptive; emergency "morning after" contraceptive* [levonorgestrel; ethinyl estradiol] Phase 1: 0.05 mg•30 μg; Phase 2: 0.075 mg•40 μg; Phase 3: 0.125 mg•30 μg

**Trilisate** tablets, liquid ℞ *analgesic; antipyretic; anti-inflammatory; antirheumatic* [choline salicylate; magnesium salicylate] 500, 750, 1000 mg; 500 mg/5 mL

**trilithium citrate tetrahydrate** [see: lithium citrate]

**Trilog** IM, intra-articular, intrabursal, intradermal injection ℞ *glucocorticoids* [triamcinolone acetonide] 40 mg/mL

**Trilone** IM injection ℞ *glucocorticoids* [triamcinolone diacetate] 40 mg/mL

**trilostane** USAN, INN, BAN *adrenocortical suppressant; antisteroidal antineoplastic*

**Trimazide** capsules, suppositories, pediatric suppositories ℞ *anticholinergic; antiemetic* [trimethobenzamide HCl] 100 mg; 200 mg; 100 mg

**trimazosin** INN, BAN *antihypertensive* [also: trimazosin HCl]

**trimazosin HCl** USAN *antihypertensive* [also: trimazosin]

**trimebutine** INN

**trimecaine** INN

**Trimedine** liquid OTC *antitussive; decongestant; antihistamine* [dextromethorphan hydrobromide; phenylephrine HCl; chlorpheniramine maleate]

**trimedoxime bromide** INN

**trimegestone** USAN *progestin for postmenopausal hormone deficiency*

**trimeperidine** INN, BAN

**trimeprazine** BAN *antipruritic; antihistamine* [also: trimeprazine tartrate; alimemazine; alimemazine tratrate] ⊘ trimipramine

**trimeprazine tartrate** USP *antipruritic; antihistamine* [also: alimemazine; trimeprazine; alimemazine tratrate]

**trimeproprimine** [see: trimipramine]

**trimetamide** INN

**trimetaphan camsilate** INN *antihypertensive* [also: trimethaphan camsylate; trimetaphan camsylate]

**trimetaphan camsylate** BAN *antihypertensive* [also: trimethaphan camsylate; trimetaphan camsilate]

**trimetazidine** INN, BAN

**trimethadione** USP, INN *anticonvulsant* [also: troxidone]

**trimethamide** [see: trimetamide]

**trimethaphan camphorsulfonate** [see: trimethaphan camsylate] ⊘ trimethoprim

**trimethaphan camsylate** USP *emergency antihypertensive* [also: trimetaphan camsilate; trimetaphan camsylate]

**trimethidinium methosulfate** NF, INN

**trimethobenzamide** INN *antiemetic; anticholinergic* [also: trimethobenzamide HCl]

**trimethobenzamide HCl** USP *antiemetic; anticholinergic* [also: trimethobenzamide] 250 mg oral; 100, 200 mg suppositories; 100 mg/mL injection

**trimethoprim (TMP)** USAN, USP, INN, BAN *antibacterial antibiotic* 100, 200 mg oral ⊘ trimethaphan

**trimethoprim sulfate** USAN *antibacterial*

**trimethoquinol** [see: tretoquinol]

**trimethylammonium chloride carbamate** [see: bethanechol chloride]

**trimethylene** [see: cyclopropane]

**trimethyltetradecylammonium bromide** [see: tetradonium bromide]

**trimetozine** USAN, INN *sedative*

**trimetrexate** USAN, INN, BAN *antimetabolic antineoplastic; systemic antiprotozoal*

**trimetrexate glucuronate** USAN *antimetabolic antineoplastic for Pneumocystis carinii pneumonia of AIDS (orphan); investigational (orphan) for multiple other cancers*

**trimexiline** INN

**Triminol Cough** syrup OTC *antitussive; decongestant; antihistamine* [dextromethorphan hydrobromide; phenylpropanolamine HCl; chlorpheniramine maleate] 10•12.5•2 mg/5 mL

**Tri-Minulet** Ŗ *investigational triphasic oral contraceptive* [gestodene]

**trimipramine** USAN, INN *tricyclic antidepressant* ⊡ imipramine; triamterene; trimeprazine

**trimipramine maleate** USAN *tricyclic antidepressant*

**trimolide** [see: trimetozine]

**trimopam maleate** [now: trepipam maleate]

**trimoprostil** USAN, INN *gastric antisecretory*

**Trimo-San** vaginal jelly OTC *antibacterial; astringent; antipruritic* [oxyquinoline sulfate; boric acid; sodium borate] 0.025%•1%•0.7%

**Trimox '125'; Trimox '250'** powder for oral suspension Ŗ *penicillin-type antibiotic* [amoxicillin trihydrate] 125 mg/5 mL; 250 mg/5 mL

**Trimox '250'** capsules Ŗ *penicillin-type antibiotic* [amoxicillin trihydrate] 250 mg

**Trimox '500'** capsules (discontinued 1997) Ŗ *penicillin-type antibiotic* [amoxicillin trihydrate] 500 mg

**trimoxamine** INN *antihypertensive* [also: trimoxamine HCl]

**trimoxamine HCl** USAN *antihypertensive* [also: trimoxamine]

**Trimpex** tablets Ŗ *anti-infective; antibacterial* [trimethoprim] 100 mg

**Trimstat** tablets (discontinued 1996) Ŗ *anorexiant* [phendimetrazine tartrate] 35 mg

**trimustine** BAN [also: trichlormethine]

**Trinalin** Repetabs (repeat-action tablets) Ŗ *decongestant; antihistamine* [pseudoephedrine sulfate; azatadine maleate] 120•1 mg

**Trinasal** nasal spray Ŗ *investigational treatment for allergic rhinitis*

**Trind** liquid (discontinued 1995) OTC *decongestant; antihistamine* [phenylpropanolamine HCl; chlorpheniramine maleate; alcohol 5%] 12.5•2 mg/5 mL

**Trind-DM** liquid (discontinued 1994) OTC *antitussive; decongestant; antihistamine* [dextromethorphan hydrobromide; phenylpropanolamine HCl; chlorpheniramine maleate; alcohol]

**Tri-Nefrin** tablets OTC *decongestant; antihistamine* [phenylpropanolamine HCl; chlorpheniramine maleate] 25•4 mg

**trinitrin** [see: nitroglycerin]

**trinitrophenol** NF

**Tri-Norinyl** tablets Ŗ *triphasic oral contraceptive* [norethindrone; ethinyl estradiol] Phase 1: 0.5 mg•35 μg; Phase 2: 1 mg•35 μg; Phase 3: 0.5 mg•35 μg

**Trinsicon** capsules Ŗ *hematinic* [ferrous fumarate; cyanocobalamin; ascorbic acid; intrinsic factor concentrate; folic acid] 110 mg•15 μg• 75 mg•240 mg•0.5 mg

**Triofed** syrup OTC *decongestant; antihistamine* [pseudoephedrine HCl; triprolidine HCl] 30•1.25 mg/5 mL

**triolein I 125** USAN *radioactive agent*

**triolein I 131** USAN *radioactive agent*

**trional** [see: sulfonethylmethane]

**Triostat** IV injection Ŗ *thyroid hormone; treatment of myxedema coma or precoma (orphan)* [liothyronine sodium] 10 μg/mL ⊡ Threostat

**Triotann** pediatric oral suspension (discontinued 1995) Ŗ *decongestant; antihistamine* [phenylephrine tannate; chlorpheniramine tannate; pyrilamine tannate] 5•2•12.5 mg/5 mL

**Triotann** tablets Ŗ *decongestant; antihistamine* [phenylephrine tannate; chlorpheniramine tannate; pyrilamine tannate] 25•8•25 mg

**Tri-Otic** ear drops Ŗ *topical corticosteroid; topical local anesthetic; antiseptic*

[hydrocortisone; pramoxine HCl; chloroxylenol] 10•10•1 mg/mL

**trioxifene** INN *antiestrogen* [also: trioxifene mesylate]

**trioxifene mesylate** USAN *antiestrogen* [also: trioxifene]

**trioxsalen** USAN, USP *pigmentation agent for vitiligo; antipsoriatic* [also: trioxysalen]

**trioxyethylrutin** [see: troxerutin]

**trioxymethylene** [see: paraformaldehyde]

**trioxysalen** INN *pigmentation agent* [also: trioxsalen]

**trip** *street drug slang* [see: LSD; alpha-ethyltryptamine]

**Tri-Pain** tablets (discontinued 1995) OTC *analgesic; antipyretic; anti-inflammatory* [acetaminophen; aspirin; salicylamide; caffeine] 162•162•162•16.2 mg

**Tripalgen Cold** syrup (discontinued 1995) OTC *decongestant; antihistamine* [phenylpropanolamine HCl; chlorpheniramine maleate] 12.5•2 mg/5 mL

**tripamide** USAN, INN *antihypertensive; diuretic*

**triparanol** INN *(withdrawn from market)*

**Tripedia** IM injection R *immunization against diphtheria, tetanus and pertussis* [diphtheria & tetanus toxoids & acellular pertussis vaccine (DTaP)] 6.7 LfU•5 LfU• 46.8 μg per 0.5 mL

**tripelennamine** INN *antihistamine* [also: tripelennamine citrate]

**tripelennamine citrate** USP *antihistamine* [also: tripelennamine]

**tripelennamine HCl** USP *antihistamine* 50 mg oral

**Triphasil** tablets R *triphasic oral contraceptive; emergency "morning after" contraceptive* [levonorgestrel; ethinyl estradiol] Phase 1: 0.05 mg•30 μg; Phase 2: 0.075 mg•40 μg; Phase 3: 0.125 mg•30 μg

**Tri-Phen-Chlor** syrup, pediatric syrup, pediatric drops R *decongestant; antihistamine* [phenylpropanolamine HCl; phenylephrine HCl; chlorpheniramine maleate; phenyltoloxamine citrate] 20•5•2.5•7.5 mg/5 mL; 5•1.25•0.5•2 mg/5 mL; 5• 1.25•0.5•2 mg/mL

**Tri-Phen-Chlor T.R.** timed-release tablets R *decongestant; antihistamine* [phenylpropanolamine HCl; phenylephrine HCl; chlorpheniramine maleate; phenyltoloxamine citrate] 40•10•5•15 mg

**Tri-Phen-Mine** syrup, drops R *pediatric decongestant and antihistamine* [phenylpropanolamine HCl; phenylephrine HCl; chlorpheniramine maleate; phenyltoloxamine citrate] 5•1.25•0.5•2 mg/5 mL; 5•1.25• 0.5•2 mg/mL

**Tri-Phen-Mine S.R.** timed-release tablets R *decongestant; antihistamine* [phenylpropanolamine HCl; phenylephrine HCl; chlorpheniramine maleate; phenyltoloxamine citrate] 40•10•5•15 mg

**Triphenyl** syrup OTC *decongestant; antihistamine* [phenylpropanolamine HCl; chlorpheniramine maleate] 6.25•1 mg/5 mL

**Triphenyl Expectorant** liquid OTC *decongestant; expectorant* [phenylpropanolamine HCl; guaifenesin; alcohol 5%] 12.5•100 mg/5 mL

**Triple Antibiotic** ointment OTC *topical antibiotic* [polymyxin B sulfate; neomycin sulfate; bacitracin] 5000 U•3.5 mg•400 U per g

**Triple Antibiotic** ophthalmic ointment R *ophthalmic antibiotic* [polymyxin B sulfate; neomycin sulfate; bacitracin zinc] 5000 U•3.5 mg• 400 U per g

**Triple Antibiotic with HC** ophthalmic ointment (discontinued 1993) R *topical ophthalmic corticosteroidal anti-inflammatory; antibiotic* [hydrocortisone; neomycin sulfate; bacitracin zinc; polymyxin B sulfate]

**Triple Paste** ointment (discontinued 1993) OTC *topical diaper rash treatment* [zinc oxide; aluminum acetate]

**Triple Sulfa** vaginal cream R *broad-spectrum bacteriostatic* [sulfathiazole; sulfacetamide; sulfabenzamide] 3.42%•2.86%•3.7%

**triple sulfa (sulfathiazole, sulfaceta-mide, and sulfabenzamide)** [q.v.]

**Triple Sulfa No. 2** tablets (discontinued 1995) ℞ *broad-spectrum bacteriostatic* [trisulfapyrimidines] 500 mg

**Triple Vitamin ADC with Fluoride** drops ℞ *pediatric vitamin supplement and dental caries preventative* [vitamins A, C, and D; fluoride] 1500 IU•35 mg•400 IU•0.5 mg per mL

**Triple Vitamins with Fluoride** chewable tablets ℞ *vitamin supplement; dental caries preventative* [vitamins A, C, and D; fluoride]

**Triple X Kit** liquid + shampoo OTC *pediculicide* [pyrethrins; piperonyl butoxide; petroleum distillate] 0.3%•3%• ²⁄

**Triple-Gen** eye drop suspension (discontinued 1993) ℞ *topical ophthalmic corticosteroidal anti-inflammatory; antibiotic* [hydrocortisone; neomycin sulfate; polymyxin B sulfate]

**Triple-Vita-Flor** drops (discontinued 1993) ℞ *pediatric vitamin supplement and dental caries preventative* [multiple vitamins; fluoride]

**Triplevite with Fluoride** drops (discontinued 1993) ℞ *pediatric vitamin supplement and dental caries preventative* [multiple vitamins; fluoride]

**Triposed** tablets, syrup OTC *decongestant; antihistamine* [pseudoephedrine HCl; triprolidine HCl] 60•2.5 mg; 30•1.25 mg/5 mL

**tripotassium citrate monohydrate** [see: potassium citrate]

**trippers** *street drug slang* [see: LSD]

**triproamylin** [see: pramlintide]

**triprolidine** INN *antihistamine* [also: triprolidine HCl]

**triprolidine HCl** USP *antihistamine* [also: triprolidine] 1.25 mg/5 mL oral

**Triptone** long-acting caplets OTC *antinauseant; antiemetic; antivertigo; motion sickness preventative* [dimenhydrinate] 50 mg

**triptorelin** USAN, INN *antineoplastic*

**triptorelin pamoate** *antineoplastic; orphan status withdrawn 1996*

**trisaccharides A & B** *investigational (orphan) for newborn hemolytic disease and ABO blood incompatibility of organ or bone marrow transplants*

**Trisequens** ℞ *investigational osteoporosis treatment* [17-beta-estradiol; norethindrone acetate]

**trisodium citrate** [see: sodium citrate]

**trisodium citrate dihydrate** [see: sodium citrate]

**trisodium hydrogen ethylenediaminetetraacetate** [see: edetate trisodium]

**Trisoralen** tablets ℞ *taken before exposure to sunlight to enhance repigmentation* [trioxsalen] 5 mg

**Tri-Statin II** cream ℞ *topical corticosteroid; antifungal* [triamcinolone acetonide; nystatin] 0.1%•100 000 U per g

**Tristoject** IM injection ℞ *glucocorticoids* [triamcinolone diacetate] 40 mg/mL

**trisulfapyrimidines (a mixture of sulfadiazine, sulfamerazine, and sulfamethazine)** USP *broad-spectrum bacteriostatic*

**Tritan** tablets ℞ *decongestant; antihistamine* [phenylephrine tannate; chlorpheniramine tannate; pyrilamine tannate] 25•8•25 mg

**Tritann Pediatric** oral suspension (discontinued 1995) ℞ *pediatric antihistamine and decongestant* [phenylephrine tannate; chlorpheniramine tannate; pyrilamine tannate] 5•2•12.5 mg/5 mL

**Tri-Tannate** tablets, pediatric oral suspension ℞ *decongestant; antihistamine* [phenylephrine tannate; chlorpheniramine tannate; pyrilamine tannate] 25•8•25 mg; 5•2•12.5 mg/5 mL

**Tri-Tannate Plus Pediatric** oral suspension ℞ *pediatric antitussive, decongestant, and antihistamine* [carbetapentane tannate; phenylephrine tannate; ephedrine tannate; chlorpheniramine tannate] 30•5•5•4 mg/5 mL

**Tritec** film-coated tablets ℞ *histamine H₂ antagonist for duodenal ulcers with H. pylori infection* [ranitidine bismuth citrate] 400 mg

**tritheon** [see: acinitrazole]

**tritiated water** USAN *radioactive agent*

**Tri-Tinic** capsules ℞ *antianemic* [ferrous fumarate; intrinsic factor; vitamins $B_{12}$ and C; folic acid]

**tritiozine** INN

**tritoqualine** INN

**Triva Douche** powder OTC *antiseptic/germicidal; vaginal cleanser and deodorizer* [oxyquinoline sulfate] 2%

**trivalent oral poliovirus vaccine (TOPV)** [see: poliovirus vaccine, live oral]

**Tri-Vi-Flor** chewable tablets, drops ℞ *pediatric vitamin supplement and dental caries preventative* [vitamins A, C, and D; sodium fluoride] 2500 IU•60 mg•400 IU•1 mg; 1500 IU•35 mg•400 IU•0.25 mg, 1500 IU•35 mg•400 IU•0.5 mg per mL

**Tri-Vi-Flor with Iron** drops ℞ *pediatric vitamin/iron supplement and dental caries preventative* [vitamins A, C, and D; iron; sodium fluoride] 1500 IU•35 mg•400 IU•0.25 mg per mL

**Tri-Vi-Sol** drops OTC *pediatric vitamin supplement* [vitamins A, C, and D] 1500 IU•35 mg•400 IU per mL

**Tri-Vi-Sol with Iron** drops OTC *vitamin/iron supplement* [vitamins A, C, and D; ferrous sulfate] 1500 IU•35 mg•400 IU•10 mg per mL

**Trivitamin Fluoride** chewable tablets, drops ℞ *pediatric vitamin supplement and dental caries preventative* [vitamins A, C, and D; fluoride] 2500 IU•60 mg•400 IU•1 mg; 1500 IU•35 mg•400 IU•0.25 mg, 1500 IU•35 mg•400 IU•0.5 mg per mL

**Tri-Vitamin Infants' Drops** OTC *vitamin supplement* [vitamins A, C, and D] 1500 IU•35 mg•400 IU per mL

**Tri-Vitamin with Fluoride** drops ℞ *pediatric vitamin supplement and dental caries preventative* [vitamins A, C, and D; fluoride] 1500 IU•35 mg•400 IU•0.5 mg per mL

**trixolane** INN

**trizoxime** INN

**Trizyme** (ingredient) OTC *digestive enzymes* [amylolytic, proteolytic and cellulolytic enzymes (amylase; protease; cellulase)]

**Trobicin** powder for IM injection ℞ *antibiotic* [spectinomycin HCl] 400 mg/mL ⑨ tobramycin

**Trocaine** lozenges OTC *topical oral anesthetic* [benzocaine] 10 mg

**Trocal** lozenges OTC *antitussive* [dextromethorphan hydrobromide] 7.5 mg

**trocimine** INN

**troclosene potassium** USAN, INN *topical anti-infective*

**Trofan; Trofan-DS** tablets (discontinued 1993) OTC *dietary amino acid supplement* [L-tryptophan] 500 mg; 1000 mg

**trofosfamide** INN

**troglitazone** USAN, INN *thiazolidinedione antidiabetic; increases cell response to insulin without increasing insulin secretion*

**trolamine** USAN, NF *alkalizing agent; analgesic*

**troleandomycin** USAN, USP *macrolide bactericidal antibiotic; investigational (orphan) for severe asthma* [also: triacetyloleandomycin]

**trolnitrate** INN

**trolnitrate phosphate** [see: trolnitrate]

**tromantadine** INN

**trometamol** INN, BAN *alkalizer for cardiac bypass surgery* [also: tromethamine]

**tromethamine** USAN, USP *alkalizer for cardiac bypass surgery* [also: trometamol]

**Tronolane** anorectal cream OTC *topical local anesthetic* [pramoxine HCl] 1% ⑨ Tronothane

**Tronolane** rectal suppositories OTC *astringent; emollient* [zinc oxide] 11%

**Tronothane HCl** cream OTC *topical local anesthetic* [pramoxine HCl] 1% ⑨ Tronolane

**tropabazate** INN

**Tropamine +** capsules (discontinued 1993) OTC *dietary supplement* [multiple amino acids, vitamins, and minerals]

**tropanserin** INN, BAN *migraine-specific serotonin receptor antagonist* [also: tropanserin HCl]

**tropanserin HCl** USAN *migraine-specific serotonin receptor antagonist* [also: tropanserin]

**tropapride** INN

**tropatepine** INN

**tropenziline bromide** INN

**TrophAmine 6%; TrophAmine 10%** IV infusion ℞ *total parenteral nutrition; peripheral parenteral nutrition* [multiple essential and nonessential amino acids]

**Troph-Iron** liquid (name changed to Trophite + Iron in 1995)

**Trophite** liquid (discontinued 1995) OTC *vitamin supplement* [vitamins $B_1$ and $B_{12}$] 10 mg•25 μg per 5 mL

**Trophite + Iron** liquid OTC *hematinic* [ferric pyrophosphate; vitamins $B_1$ and $B_{12}$] 60 mg•30 mg•75 μg per 15 mL

**trophosphamide** [see: trofosfamide]

**Tropicacyl** eye drops ℞ *cycloplegic; mydriatic* [tropicamide] 0.5%, 1%

**tropicamide** USAN, USP, INN *ophthalmic anticholinergic; cycloplegic; short-acting mydriatic*

**tropigline** INN, BAN

**tropirine** INN

**tropisetron** INN, BAN *investigational treatment for nausea and vomiting related to chemotherapy*

**Tropi-Storz** eye drops ℞ *cycloplegic; mydriatic* [tropicamide] 0.5%, 1%

**tropodifene** INN

**tropp** *street drug slang* [see: cocaine, crack]

**troquidazole** INN

**trospectomycin** INN, BAN *broad-spectrum aminocyclitol antibiotic* [also: trospectomycin sulfate]

**trospectomycin sulfate** USAN *broad-spectrum aminocyclitol antibiotic* [also: trospectomycin]

**trospium chloride** INN

**trovafloxacin mesylate** USAN *investigational (Phase III) quinolone-type antibacterial*

**troxerutin** INN, BAN *vitamin $P_4$*

**troxidone** BAN *anticonvulsant* [also: trimethadione]

**troxipide** INN

**troxolamide** INN

**troxonium tosilate** INN [also: troxonium tosylate]

**troxonium tosylate** BAN [also: troxonium tosilate]

**troxundate** INN *combining name for radicals or groups*

**troxypyrrolium tosilate** INN [also: troxypyrrolium tosylate]

**troxypyrrolium tosylate** BAN [also: troxypyrrolium tosilate]

**truck drivers** *street drug slang, a reference to their use of amphetamines during long-distance runs* [see: amphetamines]

**T.R.U.E. Test** patch ℞ *diagnostic aid for contact dermatitis*

**Truphylline** suppositories ℞ *bronchodilator* [aminophylline] 250, 500 mg

**Truquant BR RIA** test for professional use *in vitro diagnostic aid for breast cancer recurrence* [radioimmunoassay (RIA) test for CA27.29 antigen]

**Trusopt** eye drops ℞ *topical carbonic anhydrase inhibitor for glaucoma* [dorzolamide HCl] 2%

**Trutol** oral liquid ℞ *glucose tolerance test beverage* [glucose]

**truxicurium iodide** INN

**truxipicurium iodide** INN

**trypaflavine** [see: acriflavine HCl]

**tryparsamide** USAN, INN

**trypsin, crystallized** USP *topical proteolytic enzyme; necrotic tissue debridement*

**Tryptacin** tablets (discontinued 1993) OTC *dietary amino acid supplement* [L-tryptophan] 500, 1000 mg

**tryptizol** [see: amitriptyline]

**tryptizol HCl** [see: amitriptyline HCl]

**tryptophan (L-tryptophan)** USAN, USP, INN *essential amino acid; serotonin precursor (The FDA has recalled all OTC tryptophan supplements.)*

**Trysul** vaginal cream ℞ *broad-spectrum bacteriostatic* [sulfathiazole; sulfacetamide; sulfabenzamide] 3.42%•2.86%•3.7%

**T's and blues; tees and blues; tease and blues** *street drug slang for a combination of Talwin (pentazocine HCl) and PBZ (pyribenzamine), used as a heroin substitute* [see: Talwin; pentazocine HCl; tripelennamine]

**T's and B's; tees and bees; tease and bees** *street drug slang for a combination of Talwin (pentazocine HCl) and PBZ (pyribenzamine), used as a* *heroin substitute* [see: Talwin; pentazocine HCl; tripelennamine]

**T's and P's; tees and pees; tease and peas** *street drug slang for a combination of Talwin (pentazocine HCl) and PBZ (pyribenzamine), used as a heroin substitute* [see: Talwin; pentazocine HCl; tripelennamine]

**TSC (technetium sulfur colloid)** [see: technetium Tc 99m sulfur colloid]

**T/Scalp** liquid OTC *topical corticosteroid* [hydrocortisone] 1%

**TSH (thyroid-stimulating hormone)** [see: thyrotropin]

**TSPA (triethylenethiophosphoramide)** [see: thiotepa]

**TST (tuberculin skin test)** [see: tuberculin]

**T-Stat** topical solution, medicated pads ℞ *topical antibiotic for acne* [erythromycin] 2%

**T-Tabs** (trademarked form) *"T"-imprinted tablets*

**tuaminoheptane** USP, INN *adrenergic; vasoconstrictor*

**tuaminoheptane sulfate** USP

**tuberculin** USP *dermal tuberculosis test*

**tuberculin, crude** [see: tuberculin]

**tuberculin, old (OT)** [see: tuberculin]

**tuberculin purified protein derivative (PPD)** [see: tuberculin]

**Tuberculin Tine Test, Old** single-use intradermal puncture test device ℞ *tuberculosis skin test* [old tuberculin] 5 U

**tuberculosis vaccine** [see: BCG vaccine]

**Tubersol** intradermal injection ℞ *tuberculosis skin test* [tuberculin purified protein derivative] 1, 5, 250 U/0.1 mL

**Tubex** (trademarked delivery system) *cartridge-needle unit*

**tubocurarine chloride** USP, INN, BAN *neuromuscular blocker; muscle relaxant* 3 mg (20 U)/mL injection

**tubocurarine chloride HCl pentahydrate** [see: tubocurarine chloride]

**tubulozole** INN *antineoplastic; microtubule inhibitor* [also: tubulozole HCl]

**tubulozole HCl** USAN, INN *antineoplastic; microtubule inhibitor* [also: tubulozole]

**tucaresol** INN, BAN *investigational (Phase I/II) immunopotentiator for HIV*

**Tucks; Tucks Take-Alongs** cleansing pads OTC *moisturizer and cleanser for the perineal area; astringent* [witch hazel; glycerin] 50%•10%

**Tucks Clear** gel OTC *astringent* [hamamelis water; glycerin] 50%•10%

**Tucks Hemorrhoidal** cream (discontinued 1995) OTC *astringent* [hamamelis water] 50%

**tuclazepam** INN

**tuie; tooey; twoie** *street drug slang* [see: Tuinal; amobarbital sodium; secobarbital sodium]

**Tuinal** Pulvules (capsules) ℞ *sedative; hypnotic; also abused as a street drug* [amobarbital sodium; secobarbital sodium] 50•50, 100•100 mg ⑤ Luminal; Tylenol

**tulobuterol** INN, BAN, JAN [also: tulobuterol HCl]

**tulobuterol HCl** JAN [also: tulobuterol]

**tulopafant** INN

**tumor necrosis factor (TNF)** *investigational (Phase I) antiviral for HIV; investigational treatment for septic shock* [also see: anti-TNF]

**tumor necrosis factor-binding protein I and II** *investigational (orphan) for symptomatic AIDS patients*

**Tums** liquid (discontinued 1994) OTC *antacid* [calcium carbonate] 200 mg/mL

**Tums; Tums E-X** chewable tablets OTC *antacid* [calcium carbonate] 500 mg; 750 mg

**Tums 500; Tums Ultra** chewable tablets OTC *antacid* [calcium carbonate] 1.25 g; 1 g

**Tums with Simethicone** liquid (discontinued 1994) OTC *antacid; antiflatulent* [calcium carbonate; simethicone] 200•6 mg/mL

**tungsten** *element (W)*

**Turbinaire** (trademarked delivery system) *nasal inhalation aerosol*

**turbo** *street drug slang for a combination of crack and marijuana* [see: cocaine, crack; marijuana]

**Turbuhaler** (trademarked delivery system) *dry powder in a metered-dose inhaler*

**turkey** *street drug slang* [see: cocaine; amphetamines]

**turnabout; turnarounds** *street drug slang, a reference to truckers' use of amphetamines for long-distance runs* [see: amphetamines]

**turosteride** INN

**turp** *street drug slang for an elixir of terpin hydrate and codeine (disapproved in 1991)* [see: terpin hydrate; codeine]

**Tusal** IM injection (discontinued 1994) ℞ *analgesic; antipyretic; antiinflammatory; antirheumatic* [sodium thiosalicylate] 50 mg/mL

**Tusibron** syrup OTC *expectorant* [guaifenesin; alcohol 3.5%] 100 mg/5 mL

**Tusibron-DM** syrup OTC *antitussive; expectorant* [dextromethorphan hydrobromide; guaifenesin] 15•100 mg/5 mL

**Tusquelin** syrup ℞ *antitussive; decongestant; antihistamine; analgesic* [dextromethorphan hydrobromide; phenylpropanolamine HCl; phenylephrine HCl; chlorpheniramine maleate; alcohol 5%] 15•5•5•2 mg/5 mL

**Tussafed** syrup, pediatric drops ℞ *antitussive; decongestant; antihistamine* [dextromethorphan hydrobromide; pseudoephedrine HCl; carbinoxamine maleate; menthol] 15•60•4 mg/5 mL; 4•25•2 mg/mL ℞ Tussafin

**Tussafin Expectorant** liquid ℞ *narcotic antitussive; decongestant; expectorant* [hydrocodone bitartrate; pseudoephedrine HCl; guaifenesin; alcohol 12.5%] 5•60•200 mg/5 mL ℞ Tussafed

**Tuss-Allergine Modified T.D.** capsules ℞ *antitussive; decongestant* [caramiphen edisylate; phenylpropanolamine HCl] 40•75 mg

**Tussanil DH** syrup ℞ *narcotic antitussive; decongestant; antihistamine* [hydrocodone bitartrate; phenyleph-

rine HCl; chlorpheniramine maleate; alcohol 5%] 2.5•10•4 mg/5 mL

**Tussanil DH** tablets ℞ *narcotic antitussive; decongestant; expectorant; analgesic* [hydrocodone bitartrate; phenylpropanolamine HCl; guaifenesin; salicylamide] 1.66•25•100•300 mg

**Tussanil Plain** syrup (discontinued 1995) ℞ *decongestant; antihistamine* [phenylephrine HCl; chlorpheniramine maleate; alcohol 5%] 10•4 mg/5 mL

**Tussar DM** syrup OTC *antitussive; decongestant; antihistamine* [dextromethorphan hydrobromide; pseudoephedrine HCl; chlorpheniramine maleate] 15•30•2 mg/5 mL

**Tussar SF; Tussar-2** liquid ℞ *narcotic antitussive; antihistamine; expectorant* [codeine phosphate; pseudoephedrine HCl; guaifenesin; alcohol 2.5%] 10•30•100 mg/5 mL

**Tuss-DM** tablets OTC *antitussive; expectorant* [dextromethorphan hydrobromide; guaifenesin] 10•200 mg

**Tussend** syrup ℞ *narcotic antitussive; decongestant; antihistamine* [hydrocodone bitartrate; pseudoephedrine HCl; chlorpheniramine maleate; alcohol 5%] 2.5•30•2 mg/5 mL

**Tussex Cough** syrup OTC *antitussive; decongestant; expectorant* [dextromethorphan hydrobromide; phenylephrine HCl; guaifenesin] 10•5•100 mg/5 mL ℞ Tussionex; Tussirex

**Tussgen** liquid (discontinued 1995) ℞ *narcotic antitussive; decongestant* [hydrocodone bitartrate; pseudoephedrine HCl; alcohol 5%] 5•60 mg/5 mL

**Tuss-Genade Modified** sustained-release capsules (discontinued 1995) ℞ *antitussive; decongestant* [caramiphen edisylate; phenylpropanolamine HCl] 40•75 mg

**Tussibron-DM** liquid (discontinued 1995) OTC *antitussive; expectorant* [dextromethorphan hydrobromide; guaifenesin] 15•100 mg/5 mL ℞ Tussigon

**Tussigon** tablets ℞ *narcotic antitussive; GI anticholinergic/antispasmodic* [hydrocodone bitartrate; homatropine methylbromide] 5•1.5 mg ℞ Tussibron

**Tussionex Pennkinetic** extended-release suspension ℞ *narcotic antitussive; antihistamine* [hydrocodone polistirex; chlorpheniramine polistirex] 10•8 mg/5 mL ℞ Tussex; Tussirex

**Tussi-Organidin** liquid (discontinued 1993; replaced by Tussi-Organidin NR ["Newly Reformulated"] in 1994) ℞ *narcotic antitussive; expectorant* [codeine phosphate; iodinated glycerol] 10•30 mg/5 mL ℞ Tussi-R-Gen

**Tussi-Organidin DM** liquid (discontinued 1993; replaced by Tussi-Organidin DM NR ["Newly Reformulated"] in 1994) ℞ *antitussive; expectorant* [dextromethorphan hydrobromide; iodinated glycerol] 10•30 mg/5 mL

**Tussi-Organidin DM NR; Tussi-Organidin DM-S NR** liquid (S includes a 10 mL oral syringe) ℞ *antitussive; expectorant* [dextromethorphan hydrobromide; guaifenesin] 10•100 mg/5 mL

**Tussi-Organidin NR; Tussi-Organidin-S NR** liquid (S includes a 10 mL oral syringe) ℞ *narcotic antitussive; expectorant* [codeine phosphate; guaifenesin] 10•100 mg/5 mL

**Tussirex** syrup, sugar-free liquid ℞ *narcotic antitussive; decongestant; antihistamine; expectorant; analgesic* [codeine phosphate; phenylephrine HCl; pheniramine maleate; sodium citrate; sodium salicylate; caffeine citrate] 10•4.17•13.33•83.3•83.33•25 mg/5 mL ℞ Tussex; Tussionex

**Tussi-R-Gen** liquid (discontinued 1994) ℞ *narcotic antitussive; expectorant* [codeine phosphate; iodinated glycerol] ℞ Tussi-Organidin

**Tussi-R-Gen DM** liquid (discontinued 1994) ℞ *antitussive; expectorant* [dextromethorphan hydrobromide; iodinated glycerol]

**Tuss-LA** sustained-release tablets ℞ *decongestant; expectorant* [pseudoephedrine HCl; guaifenesin] 120•500 mg

**Tusso-DM** liquid ℞ *antitussive; expectorant* [dextromethorphan hydrobromide; iodinated glycerol] 10•30 mg/5 mL

**Tussogest** extended-release capsules ℞ *antitussive; decongestant* [caramiphen edisylate; phenylpropanolamine HCl] 40•75 mg

**Tuss-Ornade** Spansules (sustained-release capsules), liquid (discontinued 1997) ℞ *antitussive; decongestant* [caramiphen edisylate; phenylpropanolamine HCl] 40•75 mg; 6.7•12.5 mg/5 mL

**Tusstat** syrup ℞ *antihistamine; antitussive* [diphenhydramine HCl; alcohol 5%] 12.5 mg/5 mL

**tutti-frutti** *street drug slang for a flavored cocaine developed in Brazil* [see: cocaine]

**tuvatidine** INN

**tuvirumab** USAN, INN *antiviral monoclonal antibody*

**TV-1203** *investigational antiparkinsonism agent*

**TVC-2 Dandruff Shampoo** OTC *antiseborrheic; antibacterial; antifungal* [pyrithione zinc] 2%

**T-Vites** tablets OTC *vitamin/mineral supplement* [multiple vitamins & minerals; biotin] ±•30 μg

**tweek** *street drug slang for methamphetamine-like substance* [see: methamphetamine HCl; amphetamines]

**tweeker** *street drug slang* [see: methcathinone]

**12 Hour** nasal spray OTC *nasal decongestant* [oxymetazoline HCl] 0.05%

**12 Hour Antihistamine Nasal Decongestant** sustained-release tablets (discontinued 1995) OTC *decongestant; antihistamine* [pseudoephedrine sulfate; dexbrompheniramine maleate] 120•6 mg

**12 Hour Cold** sustained-release capsules (discontinued 1995) OTC *decongestant; antihistamine* [phenylpropanolamine HCl; chlorpheniramine maleate] 75•4 mg

**12 Hour Cold** sustained-release tablets OTC *decongestant; antihistamine*

[pseudoephedrine sulfate; dexbrompheniramine maleate] 120•6 mg

**twenty-five** *street drug slang* [see: LSD]

**Twice-A-Day** nasal spray OTC *nasal decongestant* [oxymetazoline HCl] 0.05%

**Twilite** caplets OTC *antihistaminic sleep aid* [diphenhydramine HCl] 50 mg

**Twin-K** liquid ℞ *potassium supplement* [potassium gluconate; potassium citrate] 20 mEq/15 mL (K)

**twist; twistum** *street drug slang for a marijuana cigarette* [see: marijuana]

**TwoCal HN** ready-to-use liquid OTC *enteral nutritional therapy* [lactose-free formula]

**Two-Dyne** capsules ℞ *analgesic; antipyretic; sedative* [acetaminophen; caffeine; butalbital] 325•40•50 mg

**twoie; tuie; tooey** *street drug slang* [see: Tuinal; amobarbital sodium; secobarbital sodium]

**tybamate** USAN, NF, INN, BAN *minor tranquilizer*

**Ty-Cold** tablets (discontinued 1995) OTC *antitussive; decongestant; antihistamine; analgesic* [dextromethorphan hydrobromide; pseudoephedrine HCl; chlorpheniramine maleate; acetaminophen] 15•30•2•325 mg

**tyformin** BAN [also: tiformin]

**tylcalsin** [see: calcium acetylsalicylate]

**tylemalum** [see: carbubarb]

**Tylenol** tablets, caplets, gelcaps, liquid OTC *analgesic; antipyretic* [acetaminophen] 325, 500 mg; 325, 650 mg; 500 mg; 500 mg/15 mL ▣ Tuinal

**Tylenol, Children's** chewable tablets, liquid OTC *analgesic; antipyretic* [acetaminophen] 80 mg; 160 mg/5 mL

**Tylenol, Children's** ⒸⒶⓃ suspension OTC *analgesic; antipyretic* [acetaminophen] 32 mg/mL

**Tylenol Allergy Sinus** caplets, gelcaps OTC *decongestant; antihistamine; analgesic* [pseudoephedrine HCl; chlorpheniramine maleate; acetaminophen] 30•2•500 mg

**Tylenol Allergy Sinus NightTime** caplets OTC *decongestant; antihistamine; analgesic* [pseudoephedrine

HCl; diphenhydramine HCl; acetaminophen] 30•25•500 mg

**Tylenol Cold** effervescent tablets (discontinued 1995) OTC *decongestant; antihistamine; analgesic* [phenylpropanolamine HCl; chlorpheniramine maleate; acetaminophen] 12.5•2•325 mg

**Tylenol Cold, Children's** chewable tablets, liquid OTC *pediatric decongestant, antihistamine and analgesic* [pseudoephedrine HCl; chlorpheniramine maleate; acetaminophen] 7.5•0.5•80 mg; 15•1•160 mg/5 mL

**Tylenol Cold, Multi-Symptom** caplets, tablets OTC *antitussive; decongestant; antihistamine; analgesic* [dextromethorphan hydrobromide; pseudoephedrine HCl; chlorpheniramine maleate; acetaminophen] 10•30•2•325 mg

**Tylenol Cold & Flu** powder for oral solution (name changed to Tylenol Multi-Symptom Hot Medication in 1995)

**Tylenol Cold & Flu No Drowsiness** powder for oral solution (discontinued 1995) OTC *antitussive; decongestant; analgesic* [dextromethorphan hydrobromide; pseudoephedrine HCl; acetaminophen] 30•60•650 mg/packet

**Tylenol Cold Multi Symptom Plus Cough, Children's** liquid OTC *pediatric antitussive, decongestant, antihistamine, and analgesic* [dextromethorphan hydrobromide; pseudoephedrine HCl; chlorpheniramine maleate; acetaminophen] 5•15•1•160 mg/5 mL

**Tylenol Cold Night Time** liquid (discontinued 1995) OTC *decongestant; antihistamine; analgesic* [pseudoephedrine HCl; diphenhydramine HCl; acetaminophen; alcohol 10%] 2•1.66•21.66 mg

**Tylenol Cold No Drowsiness** caplets, gelcaps OTC *antitussive; decongestant; analgesic* [dextromethorphan hydrobromide; pseudoephedrine HCl; acetaminophen] 15•30•325 mg

**Tylenol Cold Plus Cough, Children's** chewable tablets OTC *antitussive; decongestant; antihistamine; analgesic* [dextromethorphan hydrobromide; pseudoephedrine HCl; chlorpheniramine maleate; acetaminophen] 2.5•7.5•0.5•80 mg

**Tylenol Cough** liquid (name changed to Multi-Symptom Tylenol Cough in 1995)

**Tylenol Cough, Multi-Symptom** liquid OTC *antitussive; analgesic* [dextromethorphan hydrobromide; acetaminophen; alcohol 5%] 10•216.7 mg/5 mL

**Tylenol Cough with Decongestant** liquid (name changed to Multi-Symptom Tylenol Cough with Decongestant in 1995)

**Tylenol Cough with Decongestant, Multi-Symptom** liquid OTC *antitussive; decongestant; analgesic* [dextromethorphan hydrobromide; pseudoephedrine HCl; acetaminophen; alcohol 5%] 10•20•200 mg/5 mL

**Tylenol Extended Relief** extended-release caplets OTC *analgesic; antipyretic* [acetaminophen] 650 mg

**Tylenol Flu** gelcaps OTC *antitussive; decongestant; analgesic* [dextromethorphan hydrobromide; pseudoephedrine HCl; acetaminophen] 15•30•500 mg

**Tylenol Flu NightTime** gelcaps, powder OTC *decongestant; antihistamine; analgesic* [pseudoephedrine HCl; diphenhydramine HCl; acetaminophen] 30•25•500 mg; 60•50•1000 mg/packet

**Tylenol Fruit** ⓒⓐⓝ; **Tylenol Junior Fruit** ⓒⓐⓝ chewable tablets OTC *analgesic; antipyretic* [acetaminophen] 80 mg; 160 mg

**Tylenol Headache Plus** caplets OTC *analgesic; antipyretic; antacid* [acetaminophen; calcium carbonate] 500•250 mg

**Tylenol Infants' Drops** solution OTC *analgesic; antipyretic* [acetaminophen] 100 mg/mL

**Tylenol Infants' Drops** ⓒⓐⓝ suspension OTC *analgesic; antipyretic* [acetaminophen] 80 mg/mL

**Tylenol Junior Strength** chewable tablets OTC *analgesic; antipyretic* [acetaminophen] 160 mg

**Tylenol Multi-Symptom Hot Medication** powder for oral solution OTC *antitussive; decongestant; antihistamine; analgesic* [dextromethorphan hydrobromide; pseudoephedrine HCl; chlorpheniramine maleate; acetaminophen] 30•60•4•650 mg/packet

**Tylenol No. 1, No. 2, No. 3, and No. 4** [see: Tylenol with Codeine]

**Tylenol PM** tablets, caplets, gelcaps OTC *antihistaminic sleep aid; analgesic* [diphenhydramine HCl; acetaminophen] 25•500 mg

**Tylenol Severe Allergy** caplets OTC *antihistamine; analgesic* [diphenhydramine HCl; acetaminophen] 12.5•500 mg

**Tylenol Sinus** tablets, caplets, geltabs, gelcaps OTC *decongestant; analgesic; antipyretic* [pseudoephedrine HCl; acetaminophen] 30•500 mg

**Tylenol with Codeine** elixir ℞ *narcotic analgesic* [codeine phosphate; acetaminophen] 12•120 mg/5 mL

**Tylenol with Codeine No. 1** tablets (discontinued 1994) ℞ *narcotic analgesic* [codeine phosphate; acetaminophen] 7.5•300 mg

**Tylenol with Codeine No. 2, No. 3, and No. 4** tablets ℞ *narcotic analgesic; sometimes abused as a street drug* [codeine phosphate; acetaminophen] 15•300 mg; 30•300 mg; 60•300 mg

**tylosin** INN, BAN

**Tylox** capsules ℞ *narcotic analgesic* [oxycodone HCl; acetaminophen] 5•500 mg

**tyloxapol** USAN, USP, INN, BAN *detergent; wetting agent; cleaner/lubricant for artificial eyes; investigational (orphan) for cystic fibrosis*

**Tympagesic** ear drops ℞ *topical local anesthetic; analgesic; decongestant* [benzocaine; antipyrine; phenylephrine HCl] 5%•5%•0.25%

**Typhim Vi** IM injection ℞ *typhoid vaccine for adults and children over 2* *years* [typhoid Vi capsular polysaccharide vaccine] 25µg/0.5 mL

**typhoid vaccine** USP *active bacterin for typhoid fever (Salmonella typhi Ty21a, attenuated)*

**Typhoid Vaccine (AKD)** subcu injection by jet injectors only ℞ *typhoid vaccine for military use only* [typhoid vaccine, acetone-killed and dried] 8 U/mL

**Typhoid Vaccine (H-P)** subcu injection (incompatible with jet injectors) ℞ *typhoid vaccine for adults and children* [typhoid vaccine, heat- and phenol-inactivated] 8 U/mL

**typhoid Vi capsular polysaccharide vaccine** *active bacterin for typhoid fever (Salmonella typhi Ty2, inactivated)*

**typhus vaccine** USP

**Tyrex-2** powder OTC *enteral nutritional therapy for tyrosinemia*

**Tyrodone** liquid ℞ *antitussive; decongestant* [hydrodocone bitartrate; pseudoephedrine HCl; alcohol 5%] 5•60 mg/5 mL

**tyromedan** INN *thyromimetic* [also: thyromedan HCl]

**tyromedan HCl** [see: thyromedan HCl]

**Tyromex-1** powder OTC *formula for infants with tyrosinemia type I*

**tyropanoate sodium** USAN, USP *cholecystographic radiopaque medium* [also: sodium tyropanoate]

**tyrosine (L-tyrosine)** USAN, USP, INN *nonessential amino acid; symbols: Tyr, Y*

**Tyrosum Cleanser** liquid, packets OTC *topical cleanser for acne* [isopropanol; acetone] 50%•10%

**tyrothricin** USP, INN *antibacterial*

**Tyzine** nasal spray, nose drops, pediatric drops ℞ *nasal decongestant* [tetrahydrozoline HCl] 0.1%; 0.1%; 0.05%

**U89** *investigational (Phase I/II) reverse transcriptase inhibitor for AIDS*

**U-10,483** *investigational treatment for diabetes*

**U-93,385** *investigational antidepressant and anxiolytic*

**U-96,988** *investigational protease inhibitor for HIV infections*

**U-98,222** *investigational treatment for Alzheimer's disease*

**U-98,950** *investigational treatment for Alzheimer's disease*

**UAA** sugar-coated tablets ℞ *urinary anti-infective; analgesic; antispasmodic; acidifier* [methenamine; phenyl salicylate; atropine sulfate; methylene blue; hyoscyamine sulfate; benzoic acid] 40.8•18.1•0.03•5.4•0.03•4.5 mg

**UAD** cream, lotion ℞ *topical anti-infective; corticosteroid* [clioquinol; hydrocortisone]

**UAD Otic** ear drop suspension ℞ *topical corticosteroidal anti-inflammatory; antibiotic* [hydrocortisone; neomycin sulfate; polymyxin B sulfate] 1%•5 mg•10 000 U per mL

**ubenimex** INN

**ubidecarenone** INN

**ubiquinone** [see: coenzyme Q10]

**ubisindine** INN

**UBT Breath Test for H. pylori** test for professional use *diagnostic aid for the detection of ulcers*

**Ucephan** oral solution ℞ *to prevent and treat hyperammonemia of urea cycle enzymopathy (orphan)* [sodium benzoate; sodium phenylacetate] 10•10 g/100 mL

**UCG Beta Slide Monoclonal II** slide tests for professional use *in vitro diagnostic aid for urine pregnancy test*

**UCG Slide** tests for professional use *in vitro diagnostic aid for urine pregnancy test* [latex agglutination test]

**U-Cort** cream (discontinued 1997) ℞ *topical corticosteroid* [hydrocortisone acetate] 1%

**UDIP** (trademarked packaging form) *unit-dose identification package*

**Uendex** ℞ *investigational (Phase II) antiviral for HIV and AIDS; investigational (orphan) for cystic fibrosis* [dextran sulfate]

**ufenamate** INN

**ufiprazole** INN

**U-Ject** (trademarked delivery system) *prefilled disposable syringe*

**UK-109,496** *investigational (Phase II) antifungal for HIV-related candidiasis and aspergillosis*

**Ulcerease** mouth rinse OTC *topical antipruritic/counterirritant; mild local anesthetic* [phenol] 0.6%

**uldazepam** USAN, INN *sedative*

**ulinastatin** INN

**ulobetasol** INN *topical corticosteroidal anti-inflammatory* [also: halobetasol propionate]

**ULR-LA** long-acting tablets ℞ *decongestant; expectorant* [phenylpropanolamine HCl; guaifenesin] 75•400 mg

**Ultane** liquid for vaporization ℞ *inhalation general anesthetic* [sevoflurane]

**ultimate** *street drug slang* [see: cocaine, crack]

**Ultiva** powder for IV infusion ℞ *narcotic analgesic; adjunct to anesthesia for surgery* [remifentanil HCl]

**Ultra Derm** lotion, bath oil OTC *moisturizer; emollient*

**Ultra KLB6** tablets OTC *dietary supplement* [vitamin $B_6$; multiple food supplements] 16.7•± mg

**Ultra Mide 25** lotion OTC *moisturizer; emollient; keratolytic* [urea] 25%

**Ultra Tears** eye drops OTC *ocular moisturizer/lubricant* [hydroxypropyl methylcellulose] 1%

**Ultra Vent** (trademarked delivery system) *jet nebulizer*

**Ultra Vita Time** tablets OTC *dietary supplement* [multiple vitamins, minerals, and food products; iron; folic acid; biotin] ±•6•0.4•1 mg

**UltraBrom** sustained-release capsules ℞ *decongestant; antihistamine* [pseudoephedrine HCl; brompheniramine maleate] 120•12 mg

**UltraBrom PD** timed-release capsules ℞ *pediatric decongestant and antihistamine* [pseudoephedrine HCl; brompheniramine maleate] 60•6 mg

**Ultracal** liquid OTC *enteral nutritional therapy* [lactose-free formula]

**Ultra-Care** solution + tablets OTC *two-step chemical disinfecting system for soft contact lenses* [hydrogen peroxide-based] 3%

**Ultracef** capsules, tablets (discontinued 1995) ℞ *cephalosporin-type antibiotic* [cefadroxil monohydrate] 500 mg; 1 g

**Ultracef** oral suspension (discontinued 1995) ℞ *cephalosporin-type antibiotic* [cefadroxil] 125, 250 mg/5 mL

**Ultra-Freeda; Ultra Freeda, Iron Free** tablets OTC *geriatric vitamin/mineral supplement* [multiple vitamins & minerals; folic acid; biotin] ±•270•100 μg

**UltraJect** prefilled syringe ℞ *narcotic analgesic* [morphine sulfate]

**Ultralan** liquid OTC *enteral nutritional therapy* [lactose-free formula]

**Ultralente Iletin I** subcu injection (discontinued 1994) OTC *antidiabetic* [insulin zinc (beef-pork)] 100 U/mL

**Ultralente Insulin** subcu injection (name changed to Ultralente U in 1994)

**Ultralente U** subcu injection (discontinued 1994) OTC *antidiabetic* [extended insulin zinc (beef)] 100 U/mL

**Ultram** film-coated tablets ℞ *central analgesic* [tramadol HCl] 50 mg

**Ultrase MT 12; Ultrase MT 20** capsules ℞ *digestive enzymes* [lipase, protease; amylase] 12 000•39 000•39 000 U; 20 000•65 000•65 000 U

**Ultrase MT 24** capsules (discontinued 1994) ℞ *digestive enzymes* [lipase, protease; amylase] 24 000•78 000•78 000 U

**Ultravate** ointment, cream ℞ *topical corticosteroidal anti-inflammatory* [halobetasol propionate] 0.05%

**Ultravist** IV injection ℞ *radiopaque imaging agent for the head, heart, peripheral vascular system, and genitourinary tract* [iopromide (source of iodine)] 311.7 (150), 498.72 (240), 623.4 (300), 768.86 (370) mg

**Ultrazyme Enzymatic Cleaner** effervescent tablets OTC *enzymatic cleaner for soft contact lenses* [subtilisin A]
**umespirone** INN
**Unasyn** powder for IV or IM injection ℞ *penicillin-type antibiotic* [ampicillin sodium; sulbactam sodium] 1•0.5, 2•1 g
**Uncle Miltie; Uncle Milty** *street drug slang* [see: Miltown; meprobamate]
**10-undecenoic acid** [see: undecylenic acid]
**10-undecenoic acid, calcium salt** [see: calcium undecylenate]
**undecoylium chloride-iodine**
**undecylenic acid** USP *antifungal*
**Unguentine** aerosol spray (discontinued 1995) OTC *topical local anesthetic* [benzocaine] 0.99 g/oz.
**Unguentine** ointment OTC *minor burn treatment* [phenol; zinc oxide; eucalyptus oil] 1%•≟•≟
**Unguentine Plus** cream OTC *topical local anesthetic* [lidocaine HCl; phenol] 2%•0.5%
**Unguentum Bossi** cream ℞ *topical antipsoriatic; anti-infective; bactericidal* [ammoniated mercury; methenamine sulfosalicylate; coal tar] 5%•2%•2%
**Uni-Ace** drops OTC *analgesic; antipyretic* [acetaminophen] 100 mg/mL
**Uni-Amp** (trademarked packaging form) *single-dose ampule*
**Unibase** OTC *ointment base*
**Uni-Bent Cough** syrup OTC *antihistamine; antitussive* [diphenhydramine HCl; alcohol 5%] 12.5 mg/5 mL
**Unicap** capsules, tablets OTC *vitamin supplement* [multiple vitamins; folic acid] ≛•0.4 mg
**Unicap Jr.** chewable tablets OTC *vitamin supplement* [multiple vitamins; folic acid] ≛•0.4 mg
**Unicap M; Unicap T** tablets OTC *vitamin/mineral/iron supplement* [multiple vitamins & minerals; iron; folic acid] ≛•18•0.4 mg
**Unicap Plus Iron** tablets OTC *vitamin/iron supplement* [multiple vitamins; iron; folic acid] ≛•22.5•0.4 mg
**Unicap Sr.** tablets OTC *vitamin/mineral/iron supplement* [multiple vitamins & minerals; iron; folic acid] ≛•10•0.4 mg
**Unicard** ℞ *investigational antihypertensive and vasodilator* [dilevalol]
**Unicomplex T & M** tablets OTC *vitamin/mineral/iron supplement* [multiple vitamins & minerals; iron; folic acid] ≛•18•0.4 mg
**Uni-Decon** sustained-release tablets ℞ *decongestant; antihistamine* [phenylpropanolamine HCl; phenylephrine HCl; chlorpheniramine maleate; phenyltoloxamine citrate] 40•10•5•15 mg
**Uni-Dur** extended-release tablets ℞ *once-daily antiasthmatic/bronchodilator* [theophylline] 400, 600 mg
**Unifiber** powder OTC *bulk laxative* [powdered cellulose]
**unifocon A** USAN *hydrophobic contact lens material*
**Unilax** capsules OTC *laxative; stool softener* [phenolphthalein; docusate sodium] 130•230 mg
**Unimatic** (trademarked delivery system) *prefilled disposable syringe*
**Uni-nest** (trademarked packaging form) *ampule*
**Unipak** (packaging form) *dispensing pack*
**Unipen** film-coated tablets, capsules, powder for IV or IM injection ℞ *bactericidal antibiotic (penicillinase-resistant penicillin)* [nafcillin sodium monohydrate] 500 mg; 250 mg; 0.5, 1, 2, 10 g ☒ Omnipen
**Uniphyl** timed-release tablets ℞ *bronchodilator* [theophylline] 400, 600 mg
**Unipres** tablets (discontinued 1996) ℞ *antihypertensive* [hydrochlorothiazide; reserpine; hydralazine HCl] 15•0.1•25 mg
**Uniquin** (foreign name for U.S. product Maxaquin)
**Uniretic** tablets ℞ *antihypertensive* [moexipril HCl; hydrochlorothiazide] 7.5•12.5, 15•25 mg
**Uni-Rx** (trademarked packaging form) *unit-dose containers and packages*
**Unisert** (trademarked dosage form) *suppository*

**Unisol; Unisol 4** solution OTC *rinsing/ storage solution for soft contact lenses* [preservative-free saline solution]

**Unisol Plus** aerosol solution OTC *rinsing/storage solution for soft contact lenses* [preservative-free saline solution]

**Unisom Nighttime Sleep-Aid** tablets OTC *antihistaminic sleep aid* [doxylamine succinate] 25 mg

**Unisom SleepGels** (capsules) OTC *antihistaminic sleep aid* [diphenhydramine HCl] 50 mg

**Unisom with Pain Relief** tablets OTC *antihistaminic sleep aid; analgesic* [diphenhydramine citrate; acetaminophen] 50•650 mg

**Unistep hCG** test kit for professional use *in vitro diagnostic aid for urine pregnancy test*

**Unitrol** timed-release capsules OTC *diet aid* [phenylpropanolamine HCl] 75 mg

**Unituss HC** syrup ℞ *narcotic antitussive; decongestant; antihistamine* [hydrocodone bitartrate; phenylephrine HCl; chlorpheniramine maleate] 2.5•5•2 mg/5 mL

**Uni-Tussin** syrup OTC *expectorant* [guaifenesin; alcohol 3.5%] 100 mg/5 mL

**Uni-Tussin DM** syrup OTC *antitussive; expectorant* [dextromethorphan hydrobromide; guaifenesin] 10•100 mg/5 mL

**Univasc** tablets ℞ *antihypertensive; angiotensin-converting enzyme (ACE) inhibitor* [moexipril HCl] 7.5, 15 mg

**Universal Antidote** (discontinued 1996) *general-purpose gastric adsorbent/ detoxicant* [activated charcoal; magnesium hydroxide; tannic acid] ²

**Univial** (trademarked form) *single-dose vials*

**Unizime** ℞ *investigational cephalosporin antibiotic* [cefodizime]

**unkie** street drug slang [see: morphine]

**Unna's boot** [see: Dome-Paste bandage]

**uppers; uppies** street drug slang [see: amphetamines]

**Uracid** capsules ℞ *urinary acidifier to control ammonia production* [racemethionine] 200 mg ☒ uracil; Urised; Urocit

**uracil mustard** USAN, USP *nitrogen mustard-type alkylating antineoplastic* [also: uramustine] ☒ Uracel; Uracid

**uradal** [see: carbromal]

**uralenic acid** [see: enoxolone]

**uramustine** INN, BAN *nitrogen mustard-type alkylating antineoplastic* [also: uracil mustard]

**Uranap; Uranap 500** capsules (discontinued 1993) OTC *urinary acidifier to control ammonia production; oral amino acid supplement* [racemethionine]

**uranin** [see: fluorescein sodium]

**uranium** *element (U)*

**urapidil** INN, BAN

**urea** USP *osmotic diuretic; keratolytic; emollient*

**urea peroxide** [see: carbamide peroxide]

**Ureacin-10** lotion OTC *moisturizer; emollient; keratolytic* [urea] 10%

**Ureacin-20** cream OTC *moisturizer; emollient; keratolytic* [urea] 20%

**Ureacin-40** cream (discontinued 1995) ℞ *for removal of dystrophic nails* [urea] 40%

**Ureaphil** IV infusion ℞ *osmotic diuretic* [urea] 40 g/150 mL

**Urecholine** tablets, subcu injection ℞ *cholinergic urinary stimulant for post-surgical and postpartum urinary retention* [bethanechol chloride] 5, 10, 25, 50 mg; 5 mg/mL

**uredepa** USAN, INN *antineoplastic*

**uredofos** USAN, INN *veterinary anthelmintic*

**urefibrate** INN

*p*-**ureidobenzenearsonic acid** [see: carbarsone]

**urethan** NF [also: urethane]

**urethane** INN, BAN [also: urethan]

**urethane polymers** [see: polyurethane foam]

**Urethrin** injection ℞ *investigational treatment of urinary incontinence*

**Urex** tablets ℞ *urinary bactericidal* [methenamine hippurate] 1 g ☒ Eurax; Serax

**Uricult** culture paddles for professional use *in vitro diagnostic aid for nitrate, uropathogens, or bacteria in the urine*

**uridine 5′-triphosphate** *investigational (orphan) for cystic fibrosis and primary ciliary dyskinesia*

**Uridon Modified** sugar-coated tablets ℞ *urinary anti-infective; analgesic; antispasmodic; acidifier* [methenamine; phenyl salicylate; atropine sulfate; methylene blue; hyoscyamine sulfate; benzoic acid] 40.8•18.1•0.03•5.4•0.03•4.5 mg

**Urimar-T** tablets ℞ *urinary anti-infective; antiseptic; analgesic; antispasmodic* [methenamine; sodium biphosphate; phenyl salicylate; methylene blue; hyoscyamine sulfate] 81.6•40.8•36.2•10.8•0.12 mg

**Urinary Antiseptic No. 2** tablets ℞ *urinary anti-infective; analgesic; antispasmodic; acidifier* [methenamine; phenyl salicylate; atropine sulfate; methylene blue; hyoscyamine sulfate; benzoic acid] 40.8•18.1•0.03•5.4•0.03•4.5 mg

**Urised** sugar-coated tablets ℞ *urinary anti-infective; analgesic; antispasmodic; acidifier* [methenamine; phenyl salicylate; atropine sulfate; methylene blue; hyoscyamine sulfate; benzoic acid] 40.8•18.1•0.03•5.4•0.03•4.5 mg ▣ Uracel; Uracid; Urispas

**Urisedamine** tablets ℞ *urinary anti-infective; antispasmodic* [methenamine mandelate; hyoscyamine] 500•0.15 mg

**Urispas** film-coated tablets ℞ *urinary antispasmodic* [flavoxate HCl] 100 mg (200 mg available in Canada) ▣ Urised

**Uristat** tablets ℞ *urinary analgesic* [phenazopyridine HCl] 95 mg

**Uristix; Uristix 4** reagent strips *in vitro diagnostic aid for multiple urine products*

**Uritab** tablets ℞ *urinary anti-infective; analgesic; antispasmodic; acidifier* [methenamine; phenyl salicylate; atropine sulfate; methylene blue; hyoscyamine; benzoic acid] 40.8•18.1•0.03•5.4•0.03•4.5 mg

**Uri-Tet** capsules (discontinued 1997) ℞ *antibacterial* [oxytetracycline HCl] 250 mg

**Uritin** tablets ℞ *urinary anti-infective; analgesic; antispasmodic; acidifier* [methenamine; phenyl salicylate;

atropine sulfate; methylene blue; hyoscyamine sulfate; benzoic acid] 40.8•18.1•0.03•5.4•0.03•4.5 mg

**Urobak** tablets ℞ *broad-spectrum bacteriostatic* [sulfamethoxazole] 500 mg

**Urobiotic-250** capsules (discontinued 1997) ℞ *urinary anti-infective* [oxytetracycline HCl; sulfamethizole; phenazopyridine HCl] 250•250•50 mg ▣ Otobiotic

**Urocit-K** tablets ℞ *urinary alkalizer; nephrolithiasis and hypocitruria prevention (orphan)* [potassium citrate] 5, 10 mEq ▣ Uracid

**urodilatin** *investigational atrial natriuretic peptide to prevent renal failure after heart transplant*

**Urodine** tablets (discontinued 1997) ℞ *urinary analgesic* [phenazopyridine HCl] 100, 200 mg

**urofollitrophin** BAN *follicle-stimulating hormone (FSH)* [also: urofollitropin]

**urofollitropin** USAN, INN *follicle-stimulating hormone (FSH); ovulation stimulant in polycystic ovarian disease (orphan)* [also: urofollitrophin]

**urogastrone** *investigational (orphan) for recovery from corneal transplant surgery*

**Urogesic** tablets ℞ *urinary analgesic* [phenazopyridine HCl] 100 mg

**Urogesic Blue** sugar-coated tablets ℞ *urinary anti-infective; antiseptic; analgesic; antispasmodic* [methenamine; sodium biphosphate; phenyl salicylate; methylene blue; hyoscyamine sulfate] 81.6•40.8•36.2•10.8•0.12 mg

**urokinase** USAN, INN, BAN, JAN *plasminogen activator; thrombolytic enzyme*

**Uro-KP-Neutral** film-coated tablets ℞ *phosphorus supplement* [disodium phosphate; dipotassium phosphate; monobasic sodium phosphate] 250 mg (P)

**Urolene Blue** tablets ℞ *urinary anti-infective/antiseptic; antidote to cyanide poisoning* [methylene blue] 65 mg

**Uro-Mag** capsules OTC *antacid; magnesium supplement* [magnesium oxide] 140 mg

**uronal** [see: barbital]

**Uro-Phosphate** film-coated tablets ℞ *urinary anti-infective; acidifier* [methenamine; sodium biphosphate] 300•434.78 mg

**Uroplus SS; Uroplus DS** tablets (discontinued 1994) ℞ *anti-infective; antibacterial* [trimethoprim; sulfamethoxazole] 80•400 mg; 160•800 mg

**Uroqid-Acid** sugar-coated tablets (discontinued 1994) ℞ *urinary anti-infective; acidifier* [methenamine mandelate; sodium acid phosphate] 350•200 mg

**Uroqid-Acid No. 2** film-coated tablets ℞ *urinary anti-infective; acidifier* [methenamine mandelate; sodium acid phosphate] 500•500 mg

**Uro-Ves** tablets (discontinued 1994) ℞ *urinary anti-infective; analgesic; antispasmodic; acidifier* [methenamine; phenyl salicylate; atropine sulfate; methylene blue; hyoscyamine; benzoic acid] 40.8•18.1•0.03•5.4•0.03•4.5 mg

**Urovist Cysto** intracavitary instillation ℞ *urologic radiopaque agent* [diatrizoate meglumine] 30%

**Urovist Meglumine DIU/CT** injection ℞ *parenteral renal radiopaque agent* [diatrizoate meglumine] 30%

**Urovist Sodium 300** injection ℞ *parenteral radiopaque agent* [diatrizoate sodium] 50%

**Ursinus** Inlay-Tabs (tablets) OTC *decongestant; analgesic; antipyretic* [pseudoephedrine HCl; aspirin] 30•325 mg

**Urso** ℞ *investigational (orphan) for primary biliary cirrhosis; investigational for hypercholesterolemia, type IIa and IIb* [ursodiol]

**ursodeoxycholic acid** INN, BAN *anticholelithogenic* [also: ursodiol]

**ursodiol** USAN *anticholelithogenic; investigational (orphan) for primary biliary cirrhosis; investigational for hypercholesterolemia, type IIa and IIb* [also: ursodeoxycholic acid]

**ursulcholic acid** INN

**Uticort** cream, lotion, gel (discontinued 1996) ℞ *topical corticosteroid* [betamethasone benzoate] 0.025%

**Utopiates** *street drug slang for various hallucinogens*

**Uvadex** ℞ *investigational (orphan) treatment of diffuse systemic sclerosis and to prevent rejection of cardiac allografts* [methoxsalen]

**Uzi** *street drug slang* [see: cocaine, crack]

**VA (vincristine, actinomycin D)** *chemotherapy protocol*

**VAAP (vincristine, asparaginase, Adriamycin, prednisone)** *chemotherapy protocol*

**VAB; VAB-I (vinblastine, actinomycin D, bleomycin)** *chemotherapy protocol*

**VAB-II (vinblastine, actinomycin D, bleomycin, cisplatin)** *chemotherapy protocol*

**VAB-III (vinblastine, actinomycin D, bleomycin, cisplatin, chlorambucil, cyclophosphamide)** *chemotherapy protocol*

**VAB-V (vinblastine, actinomycin D, bleomycin, cyclophosphamide, cisplatin)** *chemotherapy protocol*

**VAB-6 (vinblastine, actinomycin D, bleomycin, cyclophosphamide, cisplatin)** *chemotherapy protocol*

**VABCD (vinblastine, Adriamycin, bleomycin, CCNU, DTIC)** *chemotherapy protocol*

**VAC (vincristine, Adriamycin, cisplatin)** *chemotherapy protocol*

**VAC; VAC pulse; VAC standard (vincristine, actinomycin D, cyclophosphamide)** *chemotherapy protocol*

**VAC; VAC pulse; VAC standard (vincristine, Adriamycin, cyclophosphamide)** *chemotherapy protocol* [also: CAV]

**VACA (vincristine, actinomycin D, cyclophosphamide, Adriamycin)** *chemotherapy protocol*

**VACAD (vincristine, actinomycin D, cyclophosphamide, Adriamycin, dacarbazine)** *chemotherapy protocol*

**VACAdr-IfoVP (vincristine, actinomycin D, cyclophosphamide, Adriamycin, ifosfamide, VePesid)** *chemotherapy protocol*

**vaccines** *a class of drugs used for active immunization that consist of antigens which induce endogenous production of antibodies*

**vaccinia (human papillomavirus), recombinant** *investigational (orphan) for cervical cancer*

**vaccinia immune globulin (VIG)** USP *passive immunizing agent*

**vaccinia immune human globulin** [now: vaccinia immune globulin]

**VACP (VePesid, Adriamycin, cyclophosphamide, Platinol)** *chemotherapy protocol*

**VAD (vincristine, Adriamycin, dactinomycin)** *chemotherapy protocol*

**VAD (vincristine, Adriamycin, dexamethasone)** *chemotherapy protocol*

**Vademin-Z** capsules OTC *vitamin/mineral supplement* [multiple vitamins & minerals] ≜

**vadocaine** INN

**VAdrC (vincristine, Adriamycin, cyclophosphamide)** *chemotherapy protocol*

**VAD/V (vincristine, Adriamycin, dexamethasone, verapamil)** *chemotherapy protocol*

**VAFAC (vincristine, amethopterin, fluorouracil, Adriamycin, cyclophosphamide)** *chemotherapy protocol*

**Vaginex** vaginal cream OTC *topical antihistamine* [tripelennamine HCl]

**Vagisec Douche** solution R *vaginal cleanser and deodorizer*

**Vagisec Plus** vaginal suppositories R *antiseptic* [aminacrine HCl] 6 mg

**Vagisil** cream OTC *topical local anesthetic; antipruritic; antifungal* [benzocaine; resorcinol] 5%•2%

**Vagisil** powder OTC *absorbs vaginal moisture* [cornstarch; aloe]

**Vagistat-1** vaginal ointment in prefilled applicator OTC *antifungal* [tioconazole] 6.5%

**VAI (vincristine, actinomycin D, ifosfamide)** *chemotherapy protocol*

**valaciclovir** INN *antiviral for herpes zoster and herpes simplex* [also: valacyclovir HCl]

**valacyclovir HCl** USAN *antiviral for herpes zoster and herpes simplex* [also: valaciclovir]

**valconazole** INN

**valdetamide** INN

**valdipromide** INN

**valepotriate** [see: valtrate]

**Valergen 10** IM injection (discontinued 1995) R *estrogen replacement therapy for postmenopausal disorders; antineoplastic for prostatic cancer* [estradiol valerate in oil] 10 mg/mL

**Valergen 20; Valergen 40** IM injection R *estrogen replacement therapy for postmenopausal disorders; antineoplastic for prostatic cancer* [estradiol valerate in oil] 20 mg/mL; 40 mg/mL

**Valertest No. 1** IM injection R *estrogen/androgen for menopausal vasomotor symptoms* [estradiol valerate; testosterone enanthate] 4•90 mg/mL

**valethamate bromide** NF

**valine (L-valine)** USAN, USP, INN, JAN *essential amino acid; symbols: Val, V*

**valine & isoleucine & leucine** *investigational (orphan) for hyperphenylalaninemia*

**Valisone** ointment, cream, lotion R *topical corticosteroid* [betamethasone valerate] 0.1%

**Valisone Reduced Strength** cream R *topical corticosteroid* [betamethasone valerate] 0.01%

**Valium** tablets, IV or IM injection, Tel-E-Ject syringes R *sedative; anxiolytic; skeletal muscle relaxant; anticonvulsant adjunct; also abused as a street drug* [diazepam] 2, 5, 10 mg; 5 mg/mL; 10 mg ⧉ thallium; Valpin

**Valium Roche Oral** ⊛ tablets R *sedative; anxiolytic; skeletal muscle relaxant; anticonvulsant adjunct; also abused as a street drug* [diazepam] 5, 10 mg

**valnoctamide** USAN, INN *tranquilizer*

**valofane** INN

**valperinol** INN

**valproate pivoxil** INN

**valproate semisodium** INN *anticonvulsant; antipsychotic for manic episodes; migraine prophylaxis* [also: divalproex sodium; semisodium valproate]

**valproate sodium** USAN *anticonvulsant* 250 mg/5 mL oral

**valproic acid** USAN, USP, INN, BAN *anticonvulsant* 250 mg oral

**valpromide** INN

**Valrelease** sustained-release capsules (discontinued 1996) R *sedative; anxiolytic; skeletal muscle relaxant; anticonvulsant adjunct* [diazepam] 15 mg

**valsartan** USAN, INN *antihypertensive; angiotensin II receptor antagonist*

**Valsartan** R *investigational angiotensin II antagonist for cardiovascular disorders*

**valtrate** INN

**Valtrex** film-coated caplets R *antiviral for herpes zoster and herpes simplex* [valacyclovir HCl] 500 mg

**VAM (vinblastine, Adriamycin, mitomycin)** *chemotherapy protocol*

**VAM (VP-16-213, Adriamycin, methotrexate)** *chemotherapy protocol*

**VAMP (vincristine, actinomycin, methotrexate, prednisone)** *chemotherapy protocol*

**VAMP (vincristine, Adriamycin, methylprednisolone)** *chemotherapy protocol*

**VAMP (vincristine, amethopterin, mercaptopurine, prednisone)** *chemotherapy protocol*

**vanadium** *element (V)*

**Vancenase** Pockethaler (nasal inhalation aerosol) R *intranasal steroidal anti-inflammatory* [beclomethasone dipropionate] 42 μg/dose

**Vancenase AQ** nasal spray R *intranasal steroidal anti-inflammatory* [beclomethasone dipropionate] 0.084%

**Vanceril; Vanceril Double Strength** oral inhalation aerosol R *corticosteroid for bronchial asthma* [beclomethasone dipropionate] 42 μg/dose; 84 μg/dose

**Vancocin** Pulvules (capsules), powder for oral solution, powder for IV or IM injection R *glycopeptide-type antibiotic* [vancomycin HCl] 125, 250 mg; 1, 10 g; 0.5, 1, 10 g

**Vancoled** powder for IV or IM injection R *glycopeptide-type antibiotic* [vancomycin HCl] 0.5, 1, 5 g

**vancomycin** INN, BAN *tricyclic glycopeptide bactericidal antibiotic* [also: vancomycin HCl]

**vancomycin HCl** USP *tricyclic glycopeptide bactericidal antibiotic* [also: vancomycin] 500, 1000 mg/vial injection; 250 mg/5 mL oral

**vaneprim** INN

**Vanex Expectorant** liquid R *narcotic antitussive; decongestant; expectorant* [hydrocodone bitartrate; pseudoephedrine HCl; guaifenesin; alcohol 5%] 2.5•30•100 mg/5 mL

**Vanex Forte** sustained-release caplets R *decongestant; antihistamine* [phenylpropanolamine HCl; phenylephrine HCl; chlorpheniramine maleate; pyrilamine maleate] 50•10•4•25 mg

**Vanex-HD** liquid R *narcotic antitussive; decongestant; antihistamine* [hydrocodone bitartrate; phenylephrine HCl; chlorpheniramine maleate] 1.67•5•2 mg/5 mL

**Vanex-LA** long-acting tablets (discontinued 1996) R *decongestant; expectorant* [phenylpropanolamine HCl; guaifenesin] 75•400 mg

**Vanicream** OTC *cream base*

**vanilla** NF *flavoring agent*

**vanillin** NF *flavoring agent*

**N-vanillylnonamide** [see: nonivamide]

**N-vanillyloleamide** [see: olvanil]

**vanitiolide** INN

**Vanoxide** lotion OTC *topical keratolytic for acne* [benzoyl peroxide] 5%

**Vanoxide-HC** lotion R *keratolytic for acne; topical corticosteroid* [benzoyl peroxide; hydrocortisone] 5%•0.5%

**Vanquish** caplets OTC *analgesic; antipyretic; anti-inflammatory* [acetaminophen; aspirin; caffeine] 194•227•33 mg

**Vanseb** cream, lotion OTC *antiseborrheic; keratolytic* [sulfur; salicylic acid]

**Vanseb** shampoo (discontinued 1994) OTC *antiseborrheic; keratolytic* [sulfur; salicylic acid] 2%•1%

**Vanseb-T** cream shampoo, lotion shampoo (discontinued 1994) OTC *antiseborrheic; antipsoriatic; keratolytic* [coal tar; salicylic acid; sulfur] 5%•2%•1%

**Vansil** capsules ℞ *anthelmintic for schistosomiasis (flukes)* [oxamniquine] 250 mg

**Vanticon** (German name for U.S. product Accolate)

**Vantin** film-coated tablets, granules for suspension ℞ *cephalosporin-type antibiotic* [cefpodoxime proxetil] 100, 200 mg; 50, 100 mg/5 mL

**Vantol** ℞ *investigational beta blocker for hypertension* [bevantolol]

**vanyldisulfamide** INN

**VAP (vinblastine, actinomycin D, Platinol)** *chemotherapy protocol*

**VAP (vincristine, Adriamycin, prednisone)** *chemotherapy protocol*

**VAP (vincristine, Adriamycin, procarbazine)** *chemotherapy protocol*

**VAP (vincristine, asparaginase, prednisone)** *chemotherapy protocol*

**vapiprost** INN, BAN *antagonist to thromboxane $A_2$* [also: vapiprost HCl]

**vapiprost HCl** USAN *antagonist to thromboxane $A_2$* [also: vapiprost]

**Vaponefrin** solution for inhalation OTC *bronchodilator for bronchial asthma* [racepinephrine] 2%

**Vaporole** (trademarked dosage form) *crushable ampule for inhalation*

**vapreotide** USAN *antineoplastic*

**Vaqta** IM injection ℞ *immunization against hepatitis A virus (HAV)* [hepatitis A vaccine, inactivated] 25 U/0.5 mL (pediatric), 50 U/mL (adult)

**varicella virus vaccine** *live, attenuated vaccine for chickenpox*

**varicella-zoster immune globulin (VZIG)** USP *passive immunizing agent* 10%–18% (125 U/2.5 mL)

**Varivax** powder for subcu injection ℞ *vaccine for chickenpox* [varicella virus vaccine, live attenuated] 1350 PFU/0.5 mL

**Vascor** film-coated tablets ℞ *antianginal* [bepridil HCl] 200, 300, 400 mg

**Vascoray** injection ℞ *parenteral radiopaque agent* [iothalamate meglumine; iothalamate sodium] 52%•26%

**Vaseretic 5-12.5; Vaseretic 10-25** tablets ℞ *antihypertensive* [enalapril maleate; hydrochlorothiazide] 5•12.5 mg; 10•25 mg

**vasoactive intestinal polypeptide** *investigational treatment for male sexual dysfunction; investigational (orphan) for acute esophageal food impaction*

**Vasocidin** eye drops ℞ *ophthalmic topical corticosteroidal anti-inflammatory; bacteriostatic* [prednisolone sodium phosphate; sulfacetamide sodium] 0.25%•10% ② Vasodilan

**Vasocidin** ophthalmic ointment ℞ *ophthalmic topical corticosteroidal anti-inflammatory; bacteriostatic* [prednisolone acetate; sulfacetamide sodium] 0.5%•10%

**VasoClear** eye drops OTC *topical ocular decongestant/vasoconstrictor; ocular lubricant* [naphazoline HCl; polyvinyl alcohol; PEG 400] 0.02%•0.25%•1%

**VasoClear A** eye drops OTC *topical ocular decongestant; astringent* [naphazoline HCl; zinc sulfate] 0.02%•0.25%

**Vasocon Regular** eye drops ℞ *topical ocular decongestant/vasoconstrictor* [naphazoline HCl] 0.1%

**Vasocon-A** eye drops ℞ *topical ocular decongestant and antihistamine* [naphazoline HCl; antazoline phosphate] 0.05%•0.5%

**Vasoderm; Vasoderm-E** cream ℞ *topical corticosteroid* [fluocinonide]

**Vasodilan** tablets ℞ *peripheral vasodilator* [isoxsuprine HCl] 10, 20 mg ② Vasocidin

**vasodilators, peripheral** *a class of cardiovascular drugs that cause dilation of the blood vessels*

**Vasomax** ℞ *investigational (Phase III) oral treatment for erectile dysfunction* [phentolamine mesylate]

**vasopressin (VP)** USP, INN *posterior pituitary hormone; antidiuretic* 20 U/mL injection

**vasopressin tannate** USP *posterior pituitary hormone; antidiuretic*

**vasopressors** *a class of posterior pituitary hormones that raise blood pressure by causing contraction of capillaries and arterioles* [also called: vasopressins]

**Vasoprost** ℞ *investigational (orphan) prostaglandin for severe peripheral arterial occlusive disease* [alprostadil]

**Vasosulf** eye drops ℞ *ophthalmic bacteriostatic and decongestant* [sodium sulfacetamide; phenylephrine HCl] 15%•0.125% ℞ Velosef

**Vasotate HC** ear drops ℞ *topical corticosteroidal anti-inflammatory; antibacterial/antifungal* [hydrocortisone; acetic acid] 1%•2%

**Vasotec** tablets ℞ *antihypertensive; angiotensin-converting enzyme (ACE) inhibitor* [enalapril maleate] 2.5, 5, 10, 20 mg

**Vasotec I.V.** injection ℞ *antihypertensive; angiotensin-converting enzyme (ACE) inhibitor* [enalaprilat] 1.25 mg/mL

**Vasoxyl** IV or IM injection ℞ *vasopressor for hypotensive shock during surgery* [methoxamine HCl] 20 mg/mL

**VAT (vinblastine, Adriamycin, thiotepa)** *chemotherapy protocol*

**VATD; VAT-D (vincristine, ara-C, thioguanine, daunorubicin)** *chemotherapy protocol*

**VATH (vinblastine, Adriamycin, thiotepa, Halotestin)** *chemotherapy protocol*

**Vatronol** [see: Vicks Vatronol]

**VAV (VP-16-213, Adriamycin, vincristine)** *chemotherapy protocol*

**VaxSyn HIV-1** ℞ *investigational (orphan) antiviral (therapeutic, Phase II) and vaccine (preventative, Phase I) for HIV and AIDS* [gp160 antigens]

**VB (vinblastine, bleomycin)** *chemotherapy protocol*

**VBA (vincristine, BCNU, Adriamycin)** *chemotherapy protocol*

**VBAP (vincristine, BCNU, Adriamycin, prednisone)** *chemotherapy protocol*

**VBC (VePesid, BCNU, cyclophosphamide)** *chemotherapy protocol*

**VBC (vinblastine, bleomycin, cisplatin)** *chemotherapy protocol*

**VBD (vinblastine, bleomycin, DDP)** *chemotherapy protocol*

**VBM (vincristine, bleomycin, methotrexate)** *chemotherapy protocol*

**VBMCP (vincristine, BCNU, melphalan, cyclophosphamide, prednisone)** *chemotherapy protocol*

**VBMF (vincristine, bleomycin, methotrexate, fluorouracil)** *chemotherapy protocol*

**VBP (vinblastine, bleomycin, Platinol)** *chemotherapy protocol*

**VC (VePesid, carboplatin)** *chemotherapy protocol*

**VC (vincristine)** [q.v.]

**VC (vinorelbine, cisplatin)** *chemotherapy protocol*

**VCAP (vincristine, cyclophosphamide, Adriamycin, prednisone)** *chemotherapy protocol* [see also: V-CAP III]

**V-CAP III (VP-16-213, cyclophosphamide, Adriamycin, Platinol)** *chemotherapy protocol* [see also: VCAP]

**VCF** (vaginal contraceptive film) OTC *spermicidal contraceptive* [nonoxynol 9] 28%

**VCF (vincristine, cyclophosphamide, fluorouracil)** *chemotherapy protocol*

**V-Cillin K** powder for oral solution (discontinued 1997) ℞ *bactericidal antibiotic* [penicillin V potassium] 125, 250 mg/5 mL ℞ Bicillin; Wycillin

**V-Cillin K** tablets ℞ *bactericidal antibiotic* [penicillin V potassium] 125, 250, 500 mg ℞ Bicillin; Wycillin

**VCMP (vincristine, cyclophosphamide, melphalan, prednisone)** *chemotherapy protocol*

**VCP (vincristine, cyclophosphamide, prednisone)** *chemotherapy protocol*

**VCP 205** *investigational (Phase I) vaccine for HIV*

**VCR (vincristine)** [q.v.]

**VDA (vincristine, daunorubicin, asparaginase)** *chemotherapy protocol*

**V-Dec-M** sustained-release tablets ℞ *decongestant; expectorant* [pseudoephedrine HCl; guaifenesin] 120•500 mg

**VDP (vinblastine, dacarbazine, Platinol)** *chemotherapy protocol*

**VDP (vincristine, daunorubicin, prednisone)** *chemotherapy protocol*

**Vectrin** capsules ℞ *tetracycline-type antibiotic* [minocycline HCl] 50, 100 mg

**vecuronium bromide** USAN, INN, BAN *nondepolarizing neuromuscular blocker; muscle relaxant; adjunct to anesthesia*

**Veetids '125'; Veetids '250'** powder for oral solution ℞ *bactericidal antibiotic* [penicillin V potassium] 125 mg/5 mL; 250 mg/5 mL

**Veetids '250'; Veetids '500'** film-coated tablets ℞ *bactericidal antibiotic* [penicillin V potassium] 250 mg; 500 mg

**Vega** ℞ *investigational antiasthmatic* [ozagrel]

**vegetable oil, hydrogenated** NF *tablet and capsule lubricant*

**Vehicle/N; Vehicle/N Mild** OTC *lotion base*

**VeIP (Velban, ifosfamide, Platinol)** *chemotherapy protocol*

**Velban** powder for IV injection ℞ *antineoplastic for lung, breast and testicular cancers, lymphomas, sarcomas, and neuroblastoma* [vinblastine sulfate] 10 mg ⌦ Valpin

**Veldona** ℞ *investigational (Phase I) cytokine for AIDS*

**velnacrine** INN, BAN *cholinesterase inhibitor* [also: velnacrine maleate]

**velnacrine maleate** USAN *cholinesterase inhibitor* [also: velnacrine]

**Velosef** capsules, oral suspension, powder for IV or IM injection ℞ *cephalosporin-type antibiotic* [cephradine] 250, 500 mg; 125, 250 mg/5 mL; 250, 500, 1000, 2000 mg ⌦ Vasosulf

**Velosulin** subcu injection (discontinued 1994) OTC *antidiabetic* [insulin (pork)]

**Velosulin Human BR** subcu injection OTC *antidiabetic* [human insulin (semisynthetic)] 100 U/mL

**Veltane** tablets ℞ *antihistamine* [brompheniramine maleate] 4 mg

**Veltap** Lanatabs (sustained-release tablets), elixir (discontinued 1993) ℞ *decongestant; antihistamine* [phenylpropanolamine HCl; phenylephrine HCl; brompheniramine maleate]

**Velvachol** OTC *cream base*

**Vendona** ℞ *investigational cytokine for AIDS*

**venlafaxine** INN, BAN *antidepressant* [also: venlafaxine HCl]

**venlafaxine HCl** USAN *antidepressant* [also: venlafaxine]

**Venoglobulin-I** powder for IV infusion ℞ *passive immunizing agent for HIV and idiopathic thrombocytopenic purpura (ITP)* [immune globulin] 50 mg/mL

**Venoglobulin-S** IV infusion ℞ *passive immunizing agent for HIV and idiopathic thrombocytopenic purpura (ITP)* [immune globulin, solvent/detergent treated] 5%, 10%

**Venomil** subcu or IM injection ℞ *venom sensitivity testing (subcu); venom desensitization therapy (IM)* [extracts of honeybee, yellow jacket, yellow hornet, white-faced hornet, mixed vespid, and wasp venom]

**Ventolin** inhalation aerosol ℞ *bronchodilator* [albuterol] 90 μg/dose ⌦ phentolamine

**Ventolin** Rotacaps (capsules for inhalation), tablets, Nebules (solution for inhalation), syrup ℞ *bronchodilator* [albuterol sulfate] 200 μg; 2, 4 mg; 0.083%; 2 mg/5 mL

**Ventus** ℞ *investigational (Phase III) treatment for acute respiratory distress syndrome (ARDS)*

**VePesid** IV injection, capsules ℞ *antineoplastic for testicular and small cell lung cancers* [etoposide] 20 mg/mL; 50 mg

**Veracolate** tablets OTC *laxative* [phenolphthalein; cascara sagrada extract; capsicum oleoresin] 32.4•75•0.05 mg

**veradoline** INN *analgesic* [also: veradoline HCl]

**veradoline HCl** USAN *analgesic* [also: veradoline]

**veralipride** INN

**verapamil** USAN, INN, BAN *coronary vasodilator; calcium channel blocker*

**verapamil HCl** USAN, USP *antianginal; antiarrhythmic; antihypertensive; calcium channel blocker* 40, 80, 120, 180, 240 mg oral; 5 mg/2 mL injection

**veratrylidene-isoniazid** [see: verazide]

**verazide** INN, BAN

**Verazinc** capsules OTC *zinc supplement* [zinc sulfate] 220 mg

**Vercyte** tablets (discontinued 1994) ℞ *alkylating antineoplastic for polycythemia vera and chronic myelocytic leukemia* [pipobroman] 25 mg

**Verelan** sustained-release capsules ℞ *antihypertensive; calcium channel blocker* [verapamil HCl] 120, 180, 240, 360 mg

**Vergogel** gel (discontinued 1994) OTC *topical keratolytic* [salicylic acid in collodion] 17%

**Vergon** capsules OTC *anticholinergic; antihistamine; antivertigo agent; motion sickness preventative* [meclizine HCl] 30 mg

**verilopam** INN *analgesic* [also: verilopam HCl]

**verilopam HCl** USAN *analgesic* [also: verilopam]

**verlukast** USAN, INN *bronchodilator; antiasthmatic*

**Verluma** technetium Tc 99 prep kit ℞ *monoclonal antibody imaging agent for small cell lung cancer* [nofetumomab merpentan]

**Vermox** chewable tablets ℞ *anthelmintic for trichuriasis, enterobiasis, ascariasis, and uncinariasis* [mebendazole] 100 mg

**verofylline** USAN, INN *bronchodilator; antiasthmatic*

**veronal** [see: barbital]

**veronal sodium** [see: barbital sodium]

**Verr-Canth** liquid ℞ *topical keratolytic* [cantharidin] 0.7%

**Verrex** liquid ℞ *topical keratolytic* [salicylic acid; podophyllum] 30%•10%

**Verrusol** liquid (discontinued 1996) ℞ *topical keratolytic* [salicylic acid; podophyllum; cantharidin] 30%•5%•1%

**Versacaps** prolonged-action capsules ℞ *decongestant; expectorant* [pseudoephedrine HCl; guaifenesin] 60•300 mg

**Versed** IV or IM injection, Tel-E-Ject syringes ℞ *short-acting benzodiazepine general anesthetic adjunct for preoperative sedation* [midazolam HCl] 1, 5 mg/mL

**versetamide** USAN *stabilizer; carrier agent for gadoversetamide*

**Versiclear** lotion ℞ *topical antifungal; keratolytic; antipruritic; anesthetic* [sodium thiosulfate; salicylic acid; alcohol 10%] 25%•1%

**Vertab** capsules (discontinued 1995) OTC *antinauseant; antiemetic; antivertigo; motion sickness preventative* [dimenhydrinate] 50 mg

**verteporfin** USAN *antineoplastic (used with phototherapy); investigational (Phase I/II) treatment for age-related macular degeneration (AMD)*

**Verukan** solution (discontinued 1994) ℞ *topical keratolytic* [salicylic acid in flexible collodion; lactic acid] 17%•17%

**Verukan-HP** solution (discontinued 1994) ℞ *topical keratolytic* [salicylic acid in flexible collodion] 26%

**Vesanoid** capsules ℞ *antineoplastic retinoid to induce remission of acute promyelocytic leukemia (orphan); investigational (orphan) for other leukemias* [tretinoin] 10 mg

**Vesanoid** CAN (U.S. product: Retin-A) gelatin capsule ℞ *topical keratolytic for acne* [tretinoin] 10 mg

**vesnarinone** USAN, INN *cardiotonic; investigational inotropic for congestive heart failure*

**vesperal** [see: barbital]

**Vesprin** IV or IM injection ℞ *antipsychotic; antiemetic* [triflupromazine HCl] 10, 20 mg/mL

**vetrabutine** INN, BAN

**Vetuss HC** syrup ℞ *narcotic antitussive; decongestant; antihistamine* [hydrocodone bitartrate; phenylpropanolamine HCl; phenylephrine HCl; pyrilamine maleate; pheniramine maleate; alcohol 5%] 1.7•3.3•5•3.3•3.3 mg/5 mL

**Vexol** eye drop suspension Ŗ *ophthalmic topical corticosteroidal anti-inflammatory* [rimexolone] 1%

**V-Gan 25; V-Gan 50** injection (discontinued 1996) Ŗ *antihistamine; motion sickness; sleep aid; antiemetic; sedative* [promethazine HCl] 25 mg/mL; 50 mg/mL

**Viaflex** (trademarked form) *ready-to-use IV*

**Vianain** *investigational (orphan) proteolytic enzymes for debridement of severe burns* [ananain/comosain; bromelains]

**vibesate**

**Vibramycin** capsules, powder for IV injection Ŗ *tetracycline-type antibiotic* [doxycycline hyclate] 50, 100 mg; 100, 200 mg

**Vibramycin** powder for oral suspension Ŗ *tetracycline-type antibiotic* [doxycycline monohydrate] 25 mg/5 mL

**Vibramycin** syrup Ŗ *tetracycline-type antibiotic* [doxycycline calcium] 50 mg/5 mL

**Vibra-Tabs** tablets Ŗ *tetracycline-type antibiotic* [doxycycline hyclate] 100 mg

**VIC (VePesid, ifosfamide [with mesna rescue], carboplatin)** *chemotherapy protocol* [also: CVI]

**VIC (vinblastine, ifosfamide, CCNU)** *chemotherapy protocol*

**Vicam** injection Ŗ *parenteral vitamin therapy* [multiple B vitamins; vitamin C] ± •50 mg/mL

**Vicef** capsules OTC *vitamin/iron supplement* [multiple vitamins; iron; folic acid]

**Vicks 44 Non-Drowsy Cold & Cough** LiquiCaps (capsules) OTC *antitussive; decongestant* [dextromethorphan hydrobromide; pseudoephedrine HCl] 30•60 mg

**Vicks 44 Pediatric** syrup (name changed to Vicks Pediatric 44d Dry Hacking Cough and Head Congestion in 1994)

**Vicks 44D Cough & Head Congestion; Vicks Formula 44D Cough & Decongestant; Vicks Pediatric Formula 44d Cough & Decongestant** liquid OTC *antitussive; decongestant* [dextromethorphan

hydrobromide; pseudoephedrine HCl] 10•20 mg/5 mL; 10•20 mg/5 mL; 5•10 mg/5 mL

**Vicks 44E** liquid OTC *antitussive; expectorant* [dextromethorphan hydrobromide; guaifenesin] 6.7•66.7 mg/5 mL

**Vicks 44M Cold, Flu & Cough LiquiCaps** (capsules) OTC *antitussive; decongestant; antihistamine; analgesic* [dextromethorphan hydrobromide; pseudoephedrine HCl; chlorpheniramine maleate; acetaminophen] 10•30•2•250 mg

**Vicks Children's Cough** syrup (discontinued 1994) OTC *antitussive; expectorant* [dextromethorphan hydrobromide; guaifenesin]

**Vicks Cough Drops; Vicks Menthol Cough Drops** OTC *topical antipruritic/counterirritant; mild local anesthetic* [menthol] 10 mg; 8.4 mg

**Vicks Cough Silencers** lozenges OTC *antitussive; topical oral anesthetic* [dextromethorphan hydrobromide; benzocaine] 2.5•1 mg

**Vicks Dry Hacking Cough** syrup OTC *antitussive* [dextromethorphan hydrobromide; alcohol 10%] 15 mg/5 mL

**Vicks Ice Blue Throat Lozenges** (discontinued 1994) OTC *topical antipruritic/counterirritant; mild local anesthetic* [menthol]

**Vicks Inhaler** OTC *nasal decongestant* [l-desoxyephedrine] 50 mg

**Vicks NyQuil** products [see: NyQuil]

**Vicks Pediatric 44d Dry Hacking Cough and Head Congestion** syrup OTC *antitussive* [dextromethorphan hydrobromide] 15 mg/15 mL

**Vicks Pediatric Formula 44e** liquid OTC *antitussive; expectorant* [dextromethorphan hydrobromide; guaifenesin] 3.3•33.3 mg/5 mL

**Vicks Pediatric Formula 44m Multi-Symptom Cough & Cold** liquid OTC *pediatric antitussive, decongestant, and antihistamine* [dextromethorphan hydrobromide; pseudoephedrine HCl; chlorpheniramine maleate] 5•10•0.67 mg/5 mL

**Vicks Sinex** products [see: Sinex]

**Vicks Throat** lozenges (discontinued 1994) OTC *topical oral anesthetic; antiseptic* [benzocaine; cetylpyridinium chloride] 5•1.66 mg

**Vicks VapoRub** vaporizing ointment, cream OTC *counterirritant* [camphor; menthol; eucalyptus oil] 4.7%• 2.6%•1.2%

**Vicks Vatronol** nose drops (discontinued 1994) OTC *nasal decongestant* [ephedrine sulfate] 0.5%

**Vicks Vitamin C Drops** (lozenges) OTC *vitamin supplement* [sodium ascorbate & ascorbic acid] 60 mg

**Vicodin; Vicodin ES; Vicodin HP** tablets ℞ *narcotic analgesic* [hydrocodone bitartrate; acetaminophen] 5• 500 mg; 7.5•750 mg; 10•660 mg

**Vicodin Tuss** syrup ℞ *narcotic antitussive; expectorant* [hydrocodone bitartrate; guaifenesin] 5•100 mg/5 mL ② Hycodan; Hycomine

**Vicon Forte** capsules ℞ *vitamin/mineral supplement* [multiple vitamins & minerals; folic acid] ±•1 mg

**Vicon Plus** capsules OTC *vitamin/mineral supplement* [multiple vitamins & minerals] ±

**Vicon-C** capsules OTC *vitamin/mineral supplement* [multiple B vitamins & minerals; vitamin C] ±•300 mg

**vicotrope** [see: cosyntropin]

**Victors Dual Action Cough Drops; Victors Vapor Cough Lozenges** (discontinued 1994) OTC *antipruritic/ counterirritant; mild local anesthetic; antiseptic* [menthol; eucalyptus oil]

**vidarabine** USAN, USP, INN, BAN *antiviral* ② cytarabine

**vidarabine monohydrate** *antiviral*
**vidarabine phosphate** USAN *antiviral*
**vidarabine sodium phosphate** USAN *antiviral*

**Vi-Daylin** chewable tablets OTC *vitamin supplement* [multiple vitamins; folic acid] ±•0.3 mg

**Vi-Daylin ADC** drops OTC *vitamin supplement* [vitamins A, C, and D] 1500 IU•35 mg•400 IU per mL

**Vi-Daylin ADC Vitamins + Iron** drops OTC *vitamin/iron supplement* [vitamins A, C, and D; ferrous glu-

conate] 1500 IU•35 mg•400 IU•10 mg per mL

**Vi-Daylin Multivitamin** liquid, drops OTC *vitamin supplement* [multiple vitamins] ±

**Vi-Daylin Multivitamin + Iron** chewable tablets OTC *vitamin/iron supplement* [multiple vitamins; iron; folic acid] ±•12•0.3 mg

**Vi-Daylin Multivitamin + Iron** liquid, drops OTC *vitamin/iron supplement* [multiple vitamins; ferrous gluconate] ±•10 mg/5 mL; ±•10 mg/mL

**Vi-Daylin/F ADC** drops ℞ *pediatric vitamin supplement and dental caries preventative* [vitamins A, C, and D; sodium fluoride] 1500 IU•35 mg• 400 IU•0.25 mg per mL

**Vi-Daylin/F ADC + Iron** drops ℞ *pediatric vitamin/iron supplement and dental caries preventative* [vitamins A, C, and D; sodium fluoride; ferrous sulfate] 1500 IU•35 mg•400 IU• 0.25 mg•10 mg per mL

**Vi-Daylin/F Multivitamin** chewable tablets ℞ *pediatric vitamin supplement and dental caries preventative* [multiple vitamins; sodium fluoride; folic acid] ±•1•0.3 mg

**Vi-Daylin/F Multivitamin** drops ℞ *pediatric vitamin supplement and dental caries preventative* [multiple vitamins; sodium fluoride] ±•0.25 mg/mL

**Vi-Daylin/F Multivitamin + Iron** chewable tablets ℞ *pediatric vitamin/ iron supplement and dental caries preventative* [multiple vitamins; sodium fluoride; ferrous sulfate; folic acid] ± •1•12•0.3 mg

**Vi-Daylin/F Multivitamin + Iron** drops ℞ *pediatric vitamin/iron supplement and dental caries preventative* [multiple vitamins; sodium fluoride; ferrous sulfate] ±•0.25•10 mg/mL

**video head cleaner** *street drug slang* [see: butyl nitrite]

**Videx** chewable/dispersible tablets, powder for oral solution, powder for pediatric oral solution ℞ *antiviral for advanced HIV infection and AIDS* [didanosine] 25, 50, 100, 150 mg; 100, 167, 250, 375 mg/packet; 2, 4 g

**VIE (vincristine, ifosfamide, etoposide)** *chemotherapy protocol*

**vifilcon A** USAN *hydrophilic contact lens material*

**vifilcon B** USAN *hydrophilic contact lens material*

**Vi-Flor** [see: Poly-Vi-Flor; Tri-Vi-Flor]

**VIG (vaccinia immune globulin)** [q.v.]

**vigabatrin** USAN, INN, BAN *anticonvulsant for tardive dyskinesia*

**Vigomar Forte** tablets OTC *vitamin/mineral/iron supplement* [multiple vitamins & minerals; iron] ± • 12 mg

**Vigortol** liquid OTC *geriatric vitamin/mineral supplement* [multiple B vitamins & minerals; alcohol 18%] ±

**viloxazine** INN, BAN *bicyclic antidepressant* [also: viloxazine HCl]

**viloxazine HCl** USAN *bicyclic antidepressant; orphan status withdrawn 1994* [also: viloxazine]

**Viminate** liquid OTC *geriatric vitamin/mineral supplement* [multiple B vitamins & minerals] ±

**viminol** INN

**VIMRxyn** ℞ *investigational (Phase I) antiviral for HIV and AIDS* [hypericin (synthetic)]

**vinafocon A** USAN *hydrophobic contact lens material*

**vinbarbital** NF, INN [also: vinbarbitone]

**vinbarbital sodium** NF

**vinbarbitone** BAN [also: vinbarbital]

**vinblastine** INN *antineoplastic* [also: vinblastine sulfate]

**vinblastine sulfate** USAN, USP *antineoplastic* [also: vinblastine] 10 mg/vial, 1 mg/mL injection

**vinburnine** INN

**vinca alkaloids** *a class of natural antineoplastics*

**vincaleukoblastine sulfate** [see: vinblastine sulfate]

**vincamine** INN, BAN

**vincanol** INN

**vincantenate** [see: vinconate]

**vincantril** INN

**Vincasar PFS** IV injection ℞ *antineoplastic* [vincristine sulfate] 1 mg/mL

**vincofos** USAN, INN *anthelmintic*

**vinconate** INN

**vincristine (VC; VCR)** INN *antineoplastic* [also: vincristine sulfate]

**vincristine sulfate** USAN, USP *antineoplastic* [also: vincristine] 1 mg/mL injection

**vindeburnol** INN

**vindesine** USAN, INN, BAN *antineoplastic*

**vindesine sulfate** USAN, JAN *antineoplastic*

**vinegar** [see: acetic acid]

**vinepidine** INN *antineoplastic* [also: vinepidine sulfate]

**vinepidine sulfate** USAN *antineoplastic* [also: vinepidine]

**vinformide** INN

**vinglycinate** INN *antineoplastic* [also: vinglycinate sulfate]

**vinglycinate sulfate** USAN *antineoplastic* [also: vinglycinate]

**vinleurosine** INN *antineoplastic* [also: vinleurosine sulfate]

**vinleurosine sulfate** USAN *antineoplastic* [also: vinleurosine]

**vinmegallate** INN

**vinorelbine** INN *antineoplastic* [also: vinorelbine tartrate]

**vinorelbine tartrate** USAN *antineoplastic* [also: vinorelbine]

**vinpocetine** USAN, INN

**vinpoline** INN

**vinrosidine** INN *antineoplastic* [also: vinrosidine sulfate]

**vinrosidine sulfate** USAN *antineoplastic* [also: vinrosidine]

**vintiamol** INN

**vintoperol** INN

**vintriptol** INN

**vinyl alcohol polymer** [see: polyvinyl alcohol]

**vinyl ether** USP

**vinyl gamma-aminobutyric acid** [see: vigabatrin]

**vinylbital** INN [also: vinylbitone]

**vinylbitone** BAN [also: vinylbital]

**vinylestrenolone** [see: norgesterone]

**vinymal** [see: vinylbital]

**vinyzene** [see: bromchlorenone]

**vinzolidine** INN *antineoplastic* [also: vinzolidine sulfate]

**vinzolidine sulfate** USAN *antineoplastic* [also: vinzolidine]

**Vio-Bec Forte** film-coated tablets (discontinued 1993) ℞ *vitamin/mineral therapy* [multiple B vitamins; vitamins C and E; folic acid; multiple minerals]

**Vioform** cream, ointment OTC *topical antifungal; antibacterial* [clioquinol] 3%

**Vioform-Hydrocortisone; Vioform-Hydrocortisone Mild** cream, ointment (discontinued 1994) ℞ *topical corticosteroid; antifungal; antibacterial* [hydrocortisone; clioquinol] 1%• 3%; 0.5%•3%

**Viogen-C** capsules OTC *vitamin/mineral supplement* [multiple B vitamins & minerals; vitamin C] ≐•300 mg

**Viokase** tablets, powder ℞ *digestive enzymes* [lipase; protease; amylase] 8000•30 000•30 000 U; 16 800• 70 000•70 000 U/0.7 g

**viomycin** INN [also: viomycin sulfate]

**viomycin sulfate** USP [also: viomycin]

**Viopan-T** film-coated tablets (discontinued 1993) OTC *geriatric vitamin/mineral supplement* [multiple vitamins & minerals; folic acid; biotin]

**viosterol in oil** [see: ergocalciferol]

**VIP; VIP-1; VIP-2 (VePesid, ifosfamide [with mesna rescue], Platinol)** *chemotherapy protocol*

**VIP (vinblastine, ifosfamide [with mesna rescue], Platinol)** *chemotherapy protocol*

**VIP-B (VP-16, ifosfamide, Platinol, bleomycin)** *chemotherapy protocol*

**viprostol** USAN, INN, BAN *hypotensive; vasodilator*

**viprynium embonate** BAN *anthelmintic* [also: pyrvinium pamoate]

**viqualine** INN

**viquidil** INN

**Viquin Forte** cream ℞ *hyperpigmentation bleaching agent; sunscreen* [hydroquinone; padimate O; dioxybenzone; oxybenzone] 4%•8%•3%•2%

**Vira-A** IV infusion (discontinued 1995) ℞ *antiviral for herpes simplex and herpes zoster* [vidarabine monohydrate] 200 mg/mL

**Vira-A** ophthalmic ointment ℞ *ophthalmic antiviral* [vidarabine monohydrate] 3%

**Viracept** tablets, powder for oral solution ℞ *antiretroviral HIV-1 protease inhibitor* [nelfinavir mesylate] 250 mg; 50 mg/g

**Viractin** cream, gel OTC *topical anesthetic for cold sores and fever blisters* [tetracaine] 2%

**Viramune** tablets ℞ *antiviral; nonnucleoside reverse transcriptase inhibitor (NNRTI) for HIV-1* [nevirapine] 200 mg

**Viranol** gel (discontinued 1994) OTC *topical keratolytic* [salicylic acid; lactic acid] 12%• ≐

**Viranol Gel Ultra** (discontinued 1994) ℞ *topical keratolytic* [salicylic acid in a collodion-like vehicle] 26%

**Virazole** powder for inhalation aerosol ℞ *antiviral for severe lower respiratory tract infections; investigational (Phase II/III) for HIV; investigational (orphan) for hemorrhagic fever with renal syndrome* [ribavirin] 6 g/100 mL vial (20 mg/mL reconstituted)

**Virend** ℞ *investigational (Phase II) antiviral for AIDS-related genital herpes* [SP-303 (code name—generic name not yet assigned)]

**virginiamycin** USAN, INN *antibacterial; veterinary food additive*

**virginiamycin factor M$_1$** [see: virginiamycin]

**virginiamycin factor S** [see: virginiamycin]

**viridofulvin** USAN, INN *antifungal*

**Virilon** capsules ℞ *androgen for male hypogonadism, impotence and breast cancer* [methyltestosterone] 10 mg

**Virogen Herpes** slide test for professional use *in vitro diagnostic aid for herpes simplex virus antigen in lesions or cell cultures* [latex agglutination test]

**Virogen HSV Antibody** slide test for professional use (discontinued 1993) *in vitro diagnostic aid for herpes simplex virus antibodies in serum* [latex agglutination test]

**Virogen Rotatest** slide test for professional use *in vitro diagnostic aid for fecal rotavirus* [latex agglutination test]

**Virogen Rubella; Virogen Rubella Microlatex** slide test for professional use (discontinued 1995) *in vitro diagnostic aid for rubella virus antibodies in serum* [latex agglutination test]

**Viro-Med** tablets (discontinued 1995) OTC *antitussive; decongestant; antihistamine; analgesic* [dextromethorphan hydrobromide; pseudoephedrine HCl; chlorpheniramine maleate; acetaminophen] 15•30•2•500 mg

**Viroptic** Drop-Dose (eye drops) ℞ *ophthalmic antiviral* [trifluridine] 1%

**viroxime** USAN, INN *antiviral*

**viroxime component A** [see: zinviroxime]

**viroxime component B** [see: enviroxime]

**Virulizin** ℞ *investigational antineoplastic for melanoma*

**Viscoat** prefilled syringes ℞ *viscoelastic agent for ophthalmic surgery* [hyaluronate sodium; chondroitin sulfate sodium] 30•40 mg/mL

**Visine** eye drops (discontinued 1996) OTC *topical ocular decongestant/vasoconstrictor* [tetrahydrozoline HCl] 0.05%

**Visine A.C.** eye drops (name changed to Visine Allergy Relief in 1995)

**Visine Allergy Relief** eye drops OTC *topical ocular decongestant; astringent* [tetrahydrozoline HCl; zinc sulfate] 0.05%•0.25%

**Visine Extra** eye drops (name changed to Visine Moisturizing in 1995)

**Visine L.R.** eye drops OTC *topical ocular decongestant/vasoconstrictor* [oxymetazoline HCl] 0.025%

**Visine Moisturizing** eye drops OTC *topical ocular decongestant/vasoconstrictor; emollient* [tetrahydrozoline HCl; PEG 400] 0.05%•1%

**Vision Care Enzymatic Cleaner** tablets OTC *enzymatic cleaner for soft contact lenses* [pork pancreatin]

**Visipak** (trademarked packaging form) *reverse-numbered package*

**Visipaque** intra-arterial or IV injection ℞ *nonionic dimeric contrast agent for CECT, CT, x-ray and visceral digital subtraction angiography* [iodixanol] 270, 320 mg iodine/mL

**Visken** tablets ℞ *antihypertensive; β-blocker* [pindolol] 5, 10 mg

**visnadine** INN, BAN

**visnafylline** INN

**Vi-Sol** [see: Ce-Vi-Sol; Poly-Vi-Sol; Tri-Vi-Sol]

**Vistacon** IM injection ℞ *anxiolytic* [hydroxyzine HCl] 50 mg/mL

**Vistaject-25; Vistaject-50** IM injection (discontinued 1996) ℞ *anxiolytic* [hydroxyzine HCl] 25 mg/mL; 50 mg/mL

**Vistaquel 50** IM injection ℞ *anxiolytic* [hydroxyzine HCl] 50 mg/mL

**Vistaril** capsules, oral suspension ℞ *anxiolytic* [hydroxyzine pamoate] 25, 50, 100 mg; 25 mg/5 mL ☒ Restoril

**Vistaril** IM injection ℞ *anxiolytic* [hydroxyzine HCl] 25, 50 mg/mL

**vistatolon** INN *antiviral* [also: statolon]

**Vistazine 50** IM injection ℞ *anxiolytic* [hydroxyzine HCl] 50 mg/mL

**Vistide** IV infusion ℞ *nucleoside antiviral for AIDS-related cytomegalovirus retinitis* [cidofovir] 75 mg/mL

**Visual-Eyes** ophthalmic solution OTC *extraocular irrigating solution* [sterile isotonic solution]

**Vita Bee C-800** tablets (discontinued 1995) OTC *vitamin supplement* [multiple B vitamins; vitamins C and E] ≐ •800•45 mg

**Vita-bee with C** Captabs (capsule-shaped tablets) OTC *vitamin supplement* [multiple B vitamins; vitamin C] ≐ •300 mg

**Vita-Bob** softgel capsules OTC *vitamin supplement* [multiple vitamins; folic acid] ≐ •0.4 mg

**Vita-C** crystals OTC *vitamin supplement* [ascorbic acid] 4 g/tsp.

**VitaCarn** oral solution ℞ *carnitine replenisher for deficiency of genetic origin or end-stage renal disease (orphan)* [levocarnitine]

**Vit-A-Drops** eye drops (discontinued 1995) OTC *ocular moisturizer/lubricant* [vitamin A]

**Vita-Feron** tablets OTC *hematinic* [iron; folic acid; vitamin $B_{12}$] 150•0.8• 0.006 mg

**Vitafōl** film-coated caplets Ṟ *hematinic; vitamin supplement* [ferrous fumarate; multiple vitamins; folic acid] 65 mg• ± •1 mg

**Vitafōl** syrup Ṟ *hematinic* [ferric pyrophosphate; multiple B vitamins; folic acid] 90• ± •0.75 mg/15 mL

**Vita-Kaps** Filmtabs (film-coated tablets) (discontinued 1993) Ṟ *vitamin supplement* [multiple vitamins]

**VitaKaps-M** Filmtabs (film-coated tablets) (discontinued 1993) OTC *vitamin/mineral/iron supplement* [multiple vitamins & minerals; iron]

**Vita-Kid** chewable wafers OTC *vitamin supplement* [multiple vitamins; folic acid] ± •0.3 mg

**Vital B-50** timed-release tablets OTC *vitamin supplement* [multiple B vitamins; folic acid; biotin] ± •100•50 µg

**Vital High Nitrogen** powder OTC *enteral nutritional therapy* [lactose-free formula] 79 g

**Vitalets** chewable tablets OTC *vitamin/mineral/iron supplement* [multiple vitamins & minerals; iron; biotin] ± • 10 mg•25 µg

**VitalEyes** capsules (discontinued 1995) OTC *vitamin/mineral supplement* [vitamins A, C, and E; multiple minerals] 10 000 IU•200 mg• 100 IU• ±

**Vitalize SF** liquid OTC *hematinic* [ferric pyrophosphate; multiple B vitamins; lysine] 66• ± •300 mg/15 mL

**vitamin A** USP *vitamin; antixerophthalmic; topical emollient* 10 000, 25 000, 50 000 IU oral

**vitamin A acid** [see: tretinoin]

**vitamin A palmitate**

**vitamin A$_1$** [see: retinol]

**Vitamin B Complex 100** injection Ṟ *parenteral vitamin therapy* [multiple B vitamins] ±

**vitamin B$_1$** [see: thiamine HCl]

**vitamin B$_1$ mononitrate** [see: thiamine mononitrate]

**vitamin B$_2$** [see: riboflavin]

**vitamin B$_3$** [see: niacin; niacinamide]

**vitamin B$_5$** [see: calcium pantothenate]

**vitamin B$_6$** [see: pyridoxine HCl]

**vitamin B$_8$** [see: adenosine phosphate]

**vitamin B$_{12}$** [now: cyanocobalamin; hydroxocobalamin]

**vitamin B$_c$** [see: folic acid]

**vitamin B$_t$** [see: carnitine]

**vitamin C** [see: ascorbic acid]

**vitamin D (vitamins D$_2$ and/or D$_3$)** [see: ergocalciferol (D$_2$); cholecalciferol (D$_3$)]

**vitamin D$_1$** [see: dihydrotachysterol]

**vitamin D$_2$** [see: ergocalciferol]

**vitamin D$_3$** [see: cholecalciferol]

**vitamin E** USP *vitamin E supplement; topical emollient* 100, 200, 400, 500, 600, 1000 IU oral

**vitamin E-TPGS (tocopheryl polyethylene glycol succinate)** [see: tocophersolan]

**vitamin G** [see: riboflavin]

**vitamin H** [see: biotin]

**vitamin K$_1$** [see: phytonadione]

**vitamin K$_2$** [see: menaquinone]

**vitamin K$_3$** [see: menadione]

**vitamin K$_4$** [see: menadiol sodium diphosphate]

**vitamin M** [see: folic acid]

**vitamin P** [see: bioflavonoids]

**vitamin P$_4$** [see: troxerutin]

**vitamin Q** *street drug slang for Quaalude (methaqualone; discontinued 1983)* [see: methaqualone]

**Vitamin-Mineral Supplement** liquid OTC *vitamin/mineral supplement* [multiple B vitamins & minerals; alcohol 18%] ±

**vitamins A & D (topical)** *emollient*

**Vitaneed** liquid OTC *enteral nutritional therapy* [lactose-free formula]

**Vita-Plus E** softgels OTC *vitamin supplement* [vitamin E] 400 IU

**Vita-Plus G** softgel capsules OTC *geriatric vitamin/mineral supplement* [multiple vitamins & minerals]

**Vita-Plus H** softgel capsules OTC *vitamin/mineral/iron supplement* [multiple vitamins & minerals; iron] ± •13.4 mg

**Vita-PMS; Vita-PMS Plus** tablets OTC *vitamin/mineral supplement; digestive enzymes* [multiple vitamins & minerals; folic acid; biotin; amylase; protease; lipase; betaine acid HCl]

± •0.33 mg• 10.4 μg• 2500 U• 2500
U• 200 U• 16.7 mg

**Vitarex** tablets OTC *vitamin/mineral/
iron supplement* [multiple vitamins &
minerals; iron] ± •15 mg

**Vite E** cream OTC *emollient* [vitamin
E] 50 mg/g

**Vitec** cream OTC *emollient* [vitamin E]

**Vitinoin** ⓒ (U.S. product: Retin-A)
cream, gel Ɍ *topical keratolytic for
acne* [tretinoin] 0.025%, 0.05%,
0.1%; 0.025%

**Vitrasert** intraocular implant (5–8
months' duration) Ɍ *investigational
(orphan) antiviral for AIDS-associated cytomegalovirus retinitis* [ganci-
clovir] 4.5 mg

**Vitron-C** chewable tablets OTC *hematinic* [ferrous fumarate; ascorbic acid]
66• 125 mg ▣ Vytone

**Vitron-C-Plus** tablets OTC *hematinic*
[ferrous fumarate; ascorbic acid]
132• 250 mg

**Vivactil** film-coated tablets Ɍ *tricyclic
antidepressant* [protriptyline HCl] 5,
10 mg

**Viva-Drops** eye drops OTC *ocular mois-
turizer/lubricant*

**Vivalan** Ɍ *orphan status withdrawn
1994* [viloxazine HCl]

**Vivarin** tablets OTC *CNS stimulant;
analeptic* [caffeine] 200 mg

**Vivelle** transdermal patch Ɍ *estrogen
replacement therapy for postmenopausal disorders* [estradiol] 37.5, 50, 75,
100 μg/day

**Vivonex T.E.N.** powder OTC *enteral
nutritional therapy* [lactose-free formula]

**Vivotif Berna** enteric-coated capsules
Ɍ *typhoid fever vaccine* [typhoid vac-
cine] 2–6 × 10⁹ viable CFU + 5–50
× 10⁹ nonviable cells

**Vi-Zac** capsules OTC *vitamin/zinc supplement* [vitamins A, C, and E; zinc]
5000 IU• 500 mg• 50 mg• 18 mg

**VLA-4** *investigational anti-inflammatory*

**V-Lax** powder OTC *bulk laxative* [psyl-
lium hydrophilic mucilloid] 50%

**VLP (vincristine, L-asparaginase,
prednisone)** *chemotherapy protocol*

**VM (vinblastine, mitomycin)** *chemotherapy protocol*

**VM-26** [see: teniposide]

**VM-26PP (teniposide, procarba-
zine, prednisone)** *chemotherapy
protocol*

**VMAD (vincristine, methotrexate,
Adriamycin, actinomycin D)** *chemotherapy protocol*

**VMCP (vincristine, melphalan,
cyclophosphamide, prednisone)**
*chemotherapy protocol*

**VMP (VePesid, mitoxantrone, pred-
nimustine)** *chemotherapy protocol*

**VOCAP (VP-16-213, Oncovin,
cyclophosphamide, Adriamycin,
Platinol)** *chemotherapy protocol*

**vodka acid** *street drug slang* [see: LSD]

**volatile nitrites** *amyl nitrite, butyl
nitrite, and isobutyl nitrite vapors that
produce coronary stimulant effects,
abused as street drugs* [see also: nitrous
oxide; petroleum distillate inhalants]

**volazocine** USAN, INN *analgesic*

**Volmax** extended-release tablets Ɍ *bronchodilator* [albuterol sulfate] 4, 8 mg

**Voltaren** delayed-release enteric-
coated tablets Ɍ *nonsteroidal anti-
inflammatory drug (NSAID); antiarthritic; analgesic* [diclofenac sodium]
25, 50, 75 mg

**Voltaren** eye drops Ɍ *ocular nonsteroidal anti-inflammatory drug
(NSAID) for postoperative treatment
following cataract extraction* [diclo-
fenac sodium] 0.1%

**Voltaren** ⓒ tablets, suppositories Ɍ
*nonsteroidal anti-inflammatory drug
(NSAID); antiarthritic; analgesic* [diclo-
fenac sodium] 25, 50 mg; 50, 100 mg

**Voltaren OTC** OTC *investigational
OTC strength* [diclofenac sodium]

**Voltaren Rapide** ⓒ (U.S. product:
Cataflam) tablets Ɍ *nonsteroidal anti-
inflammatory drug (NSAID); antiarthritic; analgesic for primary dysmenorrhea* [diclofenac potassium] 50 mg

**Voltaren SR** ⓒ (U.S. product:
Voltaren XR) slow-release tablets Ɍ
*once-daily antiarthritic for osteoarthritis
and rheumatoid arthritis* [diclofenac
sodium] 75, 100 mg

**Voltaren XR** extended-release tablets R *once-daily antiarthritic for osteoarthritis and rheumatoid arthritis* [diclofenac sodium] 100 mg

**von Willebrand's factor** [see: antihemophilic factor]

**Vontrol** tablets R *antiemetic; antivertigo agent* [diphenidol HCl] 25 mg ⊡ Bontril

**vorozole** USAN, INN, BAN *antineoplastic; aromatase inhibitor*

**vortel** [see: clorprenaline HCl]

**VōSol HC Otic** ear drops R *topical corticosteroidal anti-inflammatory; antibacterial/antifungal* [hydrocortisone; acetic acid] 1%•2%

**VōSol Otic** ear drops R *antibacterial/antifungal* [acetic acid] 2%

**votumumab** USAN *monoclonal antibody for cancer imaging and therapy*

**voxergolide** INN

**Voxsuprine** tablets R *peripheral vasodilator* [isoxsuprine HCl] 10, 20 mg

**VP (vasopressin)** [q.v.]

**VP (vincristine, prednisone)** *chemotherapy protocol*

**VP + A (vincristine, prednisone, asparaginase)** *chemotherapy protocol*

**VPB (vinblastine, Platinol, bleomycin)** *chemotherapy protocol*

**VPBCPr (vincristine, prednisone, vinblastine, chlorambucil, procarbazine)** *chemotherapy protocol*

**VPCA (vincristine, prednisone, cyclophosphamide, ara-C)** *chemotherapy protocol*

**VPCMF (vincristine, prednisone, cyclophosphamide, methotrexate, fluorouracil)** *chemotherapy protocol*

**VP-L-asparaginase (vincristine, prednisone, L-asparaginase)** *chemotherapy protocol*

**VPP (VePesid, Platinol)** *chemotherapy protocol*

**V-TAD (VePesid, thioguanine, ara-C, daunorubicin)** *chemotherapy protocol*

**Vumon** IV infusion R *antineoplastic for acute lymphoblastic leukemia (orphan) and bladder cancer* [teniposide] 50 mg (10 mg/mL)

**V.V.S.** vaginal cream R *broad-spectrum bacteriostatic* [sulfathiazole; sulfacetamide; sulfabenzamide] 3.42%• 2.86%•3.7%

**VX-478** *investigational (Phase III) antiviral protease inhibitor for HIV and AIDS* [also: 141W94]

**Vytone** cream R *topical corticosteroid; antifungal; antibacterial* [hydrocortisone; iodoquinol] 1%•1% ⊡ Hytone; Vitron

**VZIG (varicella-zoster immune globulin)** [q.v.]

**wac; wack** *street drug slang for PCP or marijuana laced with PCP* [see: marijuana; PCP]

**wacky dust** *street drug slang* [see: cocaine]

**wacky terbacky; wacky weed** *street drug slang* [see: marijuana]

**wafer** *street drug slang* [see: LSD]

**wake-ups** *street drug slang* [see: amphetamines]

**wallbangers** *street drug slang for Quaalude (methaqualone; discontinued 1983)* [see: methaqualone]

**Wampole One-Step hCG** test kit for professional use (discontinued 1995) *in vitro diagnostic aid for urine/serum pregnancy test*

**warfarin** INN, BAN *coumarin-derivative anticoagulant* [also: warfarin potassium]

**warfarin potassium** USP *coumarin-derivative anticoagulant* [also: warfarin]

**warfarin sodium** USP *coumarin-derivative anticoagulant*

**Wart Remover** liquid OTC *topical keratolytic* [salicylic acid in flexible collodion] 17%

**Wart-Off** liquid OTC *topical keratolytic* [salicylic acid in flexible collodion] 17%

**water** *street drug slang* [see: methamphetamine HCl; PCP]

**water, purified** USP *solvent*

**water, tritiated** [see: tritiated water]

**water moccasin snake antivenin** [see: antivenin (Crotalidae) polyvalent]

**water O 15** USAN *radioactive diagnostic aid for vascular disorders*

**[¹⁵O]water** [see: water O 15]

**water-d₂** [see: deuterium oxide]

**wave** *street drug slang* [see: cocaine, crack]

**wax, carnauba** NF *tablet-coating agent*

**wax, emulsifying** NF *emulsifying and stiffening agent*

**wax, microcrystalline** NF *stiffening and tablet-coating agent*

**wax, white** NF *stiffening agent* [also: beeswax, white]

**wax, yellow** NF *stiffening agent* [also: beeswax, yellow]

**weasel dust** *street drug slang* [see: cocaine]

**wedding bells** *street drug slang* [see: LSD]

**wedge** *street drug slang* [see: LSD]

**weed** *street drug slang* [see: marijuana; PCP]

**weed tea** *street drug slang for a tea made from marijuana waste* [see: marijuana]

**Wehdryl** injection (discontinued 1996) ℞ *antihistamine; motion sickness preventative; sleep aid; antiparkinsonian* [diphenhydramine HCl] 50 mg/mL

**Wehgen** IM injection (discontinued 1996) ℞ *estrogen replacement therapy; antineoplastic for prostatic and breast cancer* [estrone] 2 mg/mL

**Wehless** capsules, Timecelles (sustained-release capsules) (discontinued 1996) ℞ *anorexiant* [phendimetrazine tartrate] 35 mg; 105 mg

**Weightrol** tablets (discontinued 1996) ℞ *anorexiant* [phendimetrazine tartrate] 35 mg

**Wellbutrin** tablets ℞ *antidepressant* [bupropion HCl] 75, 100 mg

**Wellbutrin SR** sustained-release film-coated tablets ℞ *antidepressant; also used for smoking cessation and ADD in adults and children* [bupropion HCl] 50, 100, 150 mg

**Wellcovorin** powder for IV infusion ℞ *leucovorin "rescue" after methotrexate therapy (orphan)* [leucovorin calcium] 100 mg/vial

**Wellcovorin** tablets ℞ *leucovorin "rescue" after methotrexate therapy (orphan); antidote to folic acid antagonist overdose* [leucovorin calcium] 5, 25 mg

**Wellferon** ℞ *investigational (Phase III) cytokine for HIV; investigational (orphan) for human papillomavirus in severe respiratory papillomatosis* [interferon alfa-n1]

**Wesprin** tablets (discontinued 1994) OTC *analgesic; antipyretic; anti-inflammatory; antirheumatic* [aspirin (buffered with aluminum hydroxide and magnesium hydroxide)] 325 mg

**West Coast turnaround** *street drug slang, a reference to truckers' use of amphetamines for long-distance runs* [see: amphetamines]

**Westcort** ointment, cream ℞ *topical corticosteroid* [hydrocortisone valerate] 0.2%

**Wet-N-Soak** solution OTC *rewetting solution for rigid gas permeable contact lenses*

**Wet-N-Soak Plus** solution OTC *disinfecting/wetting/soaking solution for rigid gas permeable contact lenses* [note: RGP contact indication different from hard contact indication for same product]

**Wet-N-Soak Plus** solution OTC *wetting/soaking solution for hard contact lenses* [note: hard contact indication different from RGP contact indication for same product]

**Wetting** solution OTC *wetting solution for hard contact lenses*

**Wetting & Soaking** solution OTC *disinfecting/wetting/soaking solution for rigid gas permeable contact lenses* [note: one of two different products with the same name]

**Wetting & Soaking** solution OTC *wetting/soaking solution for hard contact*

*lenses* [note: one of two different products with the same name]

**whack** *street drug slang for a combination of PCP and heroin* [see: PCP; heroin]

**wheat** *street drug slang* [see: marijuana]

**wheat germ oil** [see: vitamin E]

**when-shee** *street drug slang* [see: opium]

**whiffenpoppers** *street drug slang* [see: amyl nitrite]

**whippets** *street drug slang* [see: nitrous oxide]

**white** *street drug slang* [see: amphetamines]

**white ball** *street drug slang* [see: cocaine, crack]

**white beeswax** [see: beeswax, white]

**white boy** *street drug slang* [see: heroin]

**White Cloverine Salve** ointment OTC *skin protectant* [white petrolatum] 97%

**White Cod Liver Oil Concentrate** capsules, chewable tablets OTC *vitamin supplement* [vitamins A, D, and E] 10 000•400• $\stackrel{\perp}{=}$ IU; 4000•200• $\stackrel{\perp}{=}$ IU

**White Cod Liver Oil Concentrate with Vitamin C** chewable tablets OTC *vitamin supplement* [vitamins A, C, and D] 4000 IU•50 mg•200 IU

**white cross** *street drug slang* [see: methamphetamine HCl; amphetamines]

**white dust** *street drug slang* [see: LSD]

**white ghost** *street drug slang* [see: cocaine, crack]

**white girl** *street drug slang* [see: cocaine; heroin]

**white horizon** *street drug slang* [see: PCP]

**white horse** *street drug slang* [see: cocaine]

**white junk** *street drug slang* [see: heroin]

**white lady** *street drug slang* [see: cocaine; heroin]

**white lightning** *street drug slang* [see: LSD]

**white lotion** USP *astringent; topical protectant*

**white mineral oil** [see: petrolatum, white]

**white mosquito** *street drug slang* [see: cocaine]

**white nurse** *street drug slang* [see: heroin]

**white ointment** [see: ointment, white]

**white Owsley; Owsley's acid; Owsley** *street drug slang* [see: LSD]

**white petrolatum** [see: petrolatum, white]

**white phenolphthalein** [see: phenolphthalein]

**white powder** *street drug slang* [see: cocaine; PCP]

**white stuff** *street drug slang* [see: heroin]

**white sugar** *street drug slang* [see: cocaine, crack]

**white tornado** *street drug slang* [see: cocaine, crack]

**white wax** [see: wax, white]

**white-haired lady** *street drug slang* [see: marijuana]

**whiteout** *street drug slang* [see: isobutyl nitrite]

**whites** *street drug slang for Benzedrine (amphetamine sulfate; discontinued 1982) or other amphetamines* [see: amphetamine sulfate; amphetamines]

**Whitfield's** ointment OTC *topical antifungal; keratolytic* [benzoic acid; salicylic acid] 6%•3%

**Whitfield's ointment** [see: benzoic & salicylic acids]

**whiz bang** *street drug slang for a combination of cocaine and heroin* [see: cocaine; heroin]

**whole blood** [see: blood, whole]

**whole root rauwolfia** [see: rauwolfia serpentina]

**whore pills** *street drug slang for Quaalude (methaqualone; discontinued 1983)* [see: methaqualone]

**Wibi** lotion OTC *moisturizer; emollient*

**widow spider species antivenin** [now: antivenin (Latrodectus mactans)]

**Wigraine** suppositories ℞ *migraine-specific vasoconstrictor* [ergotamine tartrate; caffeine; tartaric acid] 2•100•21.5 mg

**Wigraine** tablets ℞ *migraine-specific vasoconstrictor* [ergotamine tartrate; caffeine] 1•100 mg

**wild cat** *street drug slang for a combination of methcathinone and cocaine* [see: methcathinone; cocaine]

**wild cherry syrup** USP

**WIN 59010** *investigational liver imaging aid for MRI*

**window glass; window pane** *street drug slang* [see: LSD]

**WinGel** chewable tablets, liquid (discontinued 1994) OTC *antacid* [aluminum hydroxide; magnesium hydroxide] 180•180 mg; 36•32 mg/mL

**wings** *street drug slang* [see: heroin; cocaine]

**WinRho SD** IV or IM injection ℞ *obstetric Rh factor immunity suppressant; treatment for immune thrombocytopenic purpura (orphan)* [Rh₀(D) immune globulin] 600, 1500 IU (120, 300 μg)

**Winstrol** tablets ℞ *anabolic steroid for hereditary angioedema* [stanozolol] 2 mg

**wintergreen oil** [see: methyl salicylate]

**Wintersteiner's compound F** [see: hydrocortisone]

**witch** *street drug slang* [see: heroin; cocaine]

**witch hazel** [see: hamamelis water]

**witch hazel** *street drug slang* [see: heroin]

**wobble weed** *street drug slang* [see: PCP]

**wolf** *street drug slang* [see: PCP]

**wollie** *street drug slang for rocks of crack rolled into a marijuana cigarette* [see: cocaine; crack; marijuana]

**Women's Daily Formula** capsules OTC *vitamin/calcium/iron supplement* [multiple vitamins; calcium; iron; folic acid] ±•450•25•0.4 mg

**Wonder Ice** gel OTC *counterirritant* [menthol] 5.25%

**wonder star** *street drug slang* [see: methcathinone]

**Wondra** lotion OTC *moisturizer; emollient* [lanolin]

**wood creosote** [see: creosote carbonate]

**woolah** *street drug slang for a hollowed-out cigar refilled with marijuana and crack* [see: marijuana; cocaine; crack]

**woolas** *street drug slang for a cigarette laced with cocaine or a marijuana ciga-rette sprinkled with crack* [see: cocaine; cocaine, crack; marijuana]

**woolies; wooly blunts** *street drug slang for PCP or a combination of marijuana and crack* [see: PCP; marijuana; cocaine, crack]

**Woolley's antiserotonin** [see: benanserin HCl]

**worm** *street drug slang* [see: PCP]

**wrecking crew** *street drug slang* [see: cocaine, crack]

**Wyamine Sulfate** IV or IM injection ℞ *vasopressor for hypotensive shock* [mephentermine sulfate] 15, 30 mg/mL

**Wyamycin S** film-coated tablets (discontinued 1994) ℞ *macrolide antibiotic* [erythromycin stearate] 250, 500 mg

**Wyanoids Relief Factor** rectal suppositories OTC *emollient* [cocoa butter; shark liver oil] 79%•3%

**Wycillin** IM injection, Tubex (cartridge-needle units) ℞ *bactericidal antibiotic* [penicillin G procaine] 600 000, 1 200 000, 2 400 000 U ⊡ Bicillin; V-Cillin

**Wydase** IV or subcu injection, powder for injection ℞ *adjuvant to increase absorption and dispersion of injected drugs* [hyaluronidase] 150 U/mL; 150, 1500 U ⊡ Lidex

**Wygesic** tablets ℞ *narcotic analgesic* [propoxyphene HCl; acetaminophen] 65•650 mg

**Wymox** capsules, powder for oral suspension ℞ *penicillin-type antibiotic* [amoxicillin trihydrate] 250, 500 mg; 125, 250 mg/5 mL

**Wyseal** (trademarked dosage form) *film-coated tablet*

**Wytensin** tablets ℞ *antihypertensive* [guanabenz acetate] 4, 8 mg

**Xact** ℞ *investigational treatment for the symptoms of menopause, including osteoporosis* [norethindrone acetate; ethinyl estradiol]

**Xalatan** eye drops ℞ *prostaglandin agonist for glaucoma and ocular hypertension* [latanoprost] 0.005% (50 μg/mL)

**xamoterol** USAN, INN, BAN *cardiac stimulant*

**xamoterol fumarate** USAN *cardiac stimulant*

**Xanax** tablets ℞ *anxiolytic* [alprazolam] 0.25, 0.5, 1, 2 mg ☒ Zantac

**Xanax SR; Xanax XR** ℞ *investigational sustained-release anxiolytic* [alprazolam]

**xanomeline** USAN *cholinergic agonist for Alzheimer's disease*

**xanomeline tartrate** USAN *cholinergic agonist for Alzheimer's disease*

**xanoxate sodium** USAN *bronchodilator*

**xanoxic acid** INN

**xanthan gum** NF *suspending agent*

**xanthines, xanthine derivatives** *a class of bronchodilators*

**xanthinol niacinate** USAN *peripheral vasodilator* [also: xantinol nicotinate]

**xanthiol** INN

**xanthiol HCl** [see: xanthiol]

**xanthocillin** BAN [also: xantocillin]

**xanthotoxin** [see: methoxsalen]

**xantifibrate** INN

**xantinol nicotinate** INN *peripheral vasodilator* [also: xanthinol niacinate]

**xantocillin** INN [also: xanthocillin]

**xantofyl palmitate** INN

**¹²⁷Xe** [see: xenon Xe 127]

**¹³³Xe** [see: xenon Xe 133]

**Xeloda** ℞ *investigational (Phase II) antineoplastic for colorectal cancer* [capecitabine]

**xemilofiban HCl** USAN *antianginal; prevents reocclusion of coronary arteries after PTCA*

**xenalamine** [see: xenazoic acid]

**xenaldial** [see: xenygloxal]

**xenalipin** USAN, INN *hypolipidemic*

**xenazoic acid** INN

**xenbucin** USAN, INN *antihypercholesterolemic*

**xenbuficin** [see: xenbucin]

**Xenical** ℞ *investigational adjunct to weight loss* [orlistat]

**xenipentone** INN

**xenon** *element (Xe)*

**xenon (¹³³Xe)** INN *radioactive agent* [also: xenon Xe 133]

**xenon Xe 127** USP *diagnostic aid; medicinal gas; radioactive agent*

**xenon Xe 133** USAN, USP *radioactive agent* [also: xenon (¹³³Xe)]

**xenthiorate** INN

**xenygloxal** INN

**xenyhexenic acid** INN

**xenysalate** INN, BAN *topical anesthetic; antibacterial; antifungal* [also: biphenamine HCl]

**xenysalate HCl** [see: biphenamine HCl]

**xenytropium bromide** INN

**Xerac** gel (discontinued 1994) OTC *antibacterial and exfoliant for acne* [microcrystalline sulfur] 4% ☒ Serax

**Xerac AC** liquid ℞ *topical cleanser for acne* [aluminum chloride hexahydrate; anhydrous ethyl alcohol] 6.25%•96%

**Xerac BP5; Xerac BP10** gel (discontinued 1994) OTC *topical keratolytic for acne* [benzoyl peroxide] 5%; 10%

**Xeroderm** lotion OTC *moisturizer; emollient*

**Xero-Lube** oral spray (discontinued 1994) OTC *saliva substitute*

**xibenolol** INN

**xibornol** INN, BAN

**xilobam** USAN, INN *muscle relaxant*

**ximoprofen** INN

**xinafoate** USAN, INN, BAN *combining name for radicals or groups*

**X-ing** *street drug slang, from the slang "ecstasy"* [see: MDMA]

**xinidamine** INN

**xinomiline** INN

**xipamide** USAN, INN *antihypertensive; diuretic*

**xipranolol** INN

**XomaZyme-791** ℞ *orphan status withdrawn 1996* [anti-TAP-72 immunotoxin]

**XomaZyme-CD5 Plus** ℞ *investigational treatment for graft vs. host disease, rheumatoid arthritis, and type 1 diabetes* [anti-CD5 monoclonal antibodies]

**XomaZyme-CD7 Plus** ℞ *investigational antineoplastic for T-cell malignancies* [4MRTA (code name— generic name not yet approved)]

**XomaZyme-H65** ℞ *orphan status withdrawn 1997* [CD5-T lymphocyte immunotoxin]

**XomaZyme-Mel** ℞ *investigational antineoplastic for melanoma*

**Xomen** ℞ *investigational treatment for sepsis* [monoclonal antibody E5]

**xorphanol** INN *analgesic* [also: xorphanol mesylate]

**xorphanol mesylate** USAN *analgesic* [also: xorphanol]

**Xotic** ear drops (name changed to Zoto-HC in 1994)

**X-Prep** liquid OTC *pre-procedure bowel evacuant* [senna extract; alcohol 7%] 74 mL

**X-Prep Bowel Evacuant Kit-1** liquid, tablet & suppository in a kit OTC *pre-procedure bowel evacuant* [X-Prep liquid (q.v.); Senokot-S tablets (q.v.); Rectolax suppository (q.v.)]

**X-Prep Bowel Evacuant Kit-2** liquid, granules & suppository in a kit OTC *pre-procedure bowel evacuant* [X-Prep liquid (q.v.); Citralax granules (q.v.); Rectolax suppository (q.v.)]

**XRT (x-ray therapy)** *adjunct to chemotherapy* [not a pharmaceutical agent]

**X-Seb** shampoo OTC *antiseborrheic; keratolytic* [salicylic acid] 4%

**X-Seb Plus** shampoo OTC *antiseborrheic; keratolytic; antibacterial; antifungal* [salicylic acid; pyrithione zinc] 2%•1%

**X-seb T** shampoo OTC *antiseborrheic; antipsoriatic; keratolytic* [coal tar; salicylic acid] 10%•4%

**X-seb T Plus** shampoo OTC *antiseborrheic; antipsoriatic; keratolytic* [coal tar; salicylic acid; menthol] 10%•3%•1%

**xylamidine tosilate** INN *serotonin inhibitor* [also: xylamidine tosylate]

**xylamidine tosylate** USAN *serotonin inhibitor* [also: xylamidine tosilate]

**xylazine** INN *analgesic; veterinary muscle relaxant* [also: xylazine HCl]

**xylazine HCl** USAN *analgesic; veterinary muscle relaxant* [also: xylazine]

**xylitol** NF *sweetened vehicle*

**Xylocaine** injection ℞ *local anesthetic* [lidocaine HCl] 0.5%, 1%, 2%

**Xylocaine** liquid, solution, ointment, jelly ℞ *mucous membrane anesthetic* [lidocaine HCl] 5%; 4%; 5%; 2%

**Xylocaine** ointment OTC *topical local anesthetic* [lidocaine] 2.5%

**Xylocaine 10% Oral** spray ℞ *mucous membrane anesthetic* [lidocaine HCl] 10%

**Xylocaine HCl** injection ℞ *injectable local anesthetic* [lidocaine HCl; dextrose] 1.5%•7.5%

**Xylocaine HCl** injection ℞ *injectable local anesthetic* [lidocaine HCl; epinephrine] 0.5%•1:200 000, 1%•1:100 000, 1%•1:200 000, 2%•1:50 000, 2%•1:100 000, 2%•1:200 000

**Xylocaine HCl IV for Cardiac Arrhythmias** IV injection, IV admixture ℞ *antiarrhythmic* [lidocaine HCl] 1%, 2%, 4%, 20%

**Xylocaine MPF** injection ℞ *injectable local anesthetic* [lidocaine HCl] 0.5%, 1%, 1.5%, 2%, 4%

**Xylocaine MPF** injection ℞ *injectable local anesthetic* [lidocaine HCl; epinephrine] 1%•1:200 000, 1.5%•1:200 000, 2%•1:200 000

**Xylocaine MPF** injection ℞ *injectable local anesthetic* [lidocaine HCl; glucose] 5%•7.5%

**Xylocaine Viscous** solution ℞ *mucous membrane anesthetic* [lidocaine HCl] 2%

**xylocoumarol** INN

**xylofilcon A** USAN *hydrophilic contact lens material*

**xylometazoline** INN, BAN *vasoconstrictor; nasal decongestant* [also: xylometazoline HCl]

**xylometazoline HCl** USP *vasoconstrictor; nasal decongestant* [also: xylometazoline]

**Xylo-Pfan** tablets OTC *intestinal function test* [xylose] 25 g

**xylose (D-xylose)** USP *intestinal function test*

**xyloxemine** INN

**yahoo; yeaho** *street drug slang* [see: cocaine, crack]

**Yale** *street drug slang* [see: cocaine, crack]

**yatren** [see: chiniofon]

**169Yb** [see: pentetate calcium trisodium Yb 169]

**169Yb** [see: ytterbium Yb 169 pentetate]

**yeast, dried** NF

**yeast cell derivative** *claimed to promote wound healing*

**Yeast-Gard** vaginal suppositories OTC *for vaginal irritations, itching, and burning* [pulsatilla 28x]

**Yeast-Gard; Yeast-Gard Sensitive Formula** vaginal cream OTC *topical local anesthetic; keratolytic; antifungal* [benzocaine; resorcinol] 20%•3%; 5%•2%

**Yeast-Gard Medicated Disposable Douche Premix** solution OTC *antifungal; vaginal cleanser and deodorizer; acidity modifier* [sodium benzoate; lactic acid]

**Yeast-Gard Medicated Douche; Yeast-Gard Medicated Disposable Douche** solution OTC *antiseptic/germicidal; vaginal cleanser and deodorizer* [povidone-iodine] 10%; 0.3%

**Yeast-X** powder OTC *absorbs vaginal moisture; astringent* [cornstarch; zinc oxide]

**Yeast-X** vaginal suppositories OTC *for vaginal irritations, itching, and burning* [pulsatilla 28x]

**yeh** *street drug slang* [see: marijuana]

**Yelets** tablets OTC *vitamin/mineral/iron supplement* [multiple vitamins & minerals; ferrous fumarate; folic acid] ±•20•0.1 mg

**yellow** *street drug slang* [see: LSD]

**yellow bam** *street drug slang* [see: methamphetamine HCl]

**yellow beeswax** [see: beeswax, yellow]

**yellow dimples** *street drug slang* [see: LSD]

**yellow ferric oxide** [see: ferric oxide, yellow]

**yellow fever** *street drug slang* [see: PCP]

**yellow fever vaccine** USP *active immunizing agent for yellow fever*

**yellow jackets** *street drug slang, a reference to the capsule color* [see: Nembutal Sodium; pentobarbital sodium]

**yellow mercuric oxide** [see: mercuric oxide, yellow]

**yellow ointment** [see: ointment, yellow]

**yellow petrolatum** JAN *ointment base; emollient/protectant* [also: petrolatum]

**yellow phenolphthalein** [see: phenolphthalein, yellow]

**yellow precipitate** [see: mercuric oxide, yellow]

**yellow submarine** *street drug slang, a reference to the Beatles' song* [see: marijuana; Nembutal Sodium; pentobarbital sodium]

**yellow sunshine** *street drug slang* [see: LSD]

**yellow wax** [see: wax, yellow]

**yen pok** *street drug slang for an opium pellet (for smoking)* [see: opium]

**yen shen suey** *street drug slang for opium wine* [see: opium]

**yerba** (Spanish for "herb" or "grass") *street drug slang* [see: marijuana]

**yerba mala** (Spanish for "bad herb" or "bad grass") *street drug slang for a combination of PCP and marijuana* [see: PCP; marijuana]

**yerba santa** [see: eriodictyon]

**yesca; yesco** (Spanish for "tinder") *street drug slang* [see: marijuana]

**yeso** (Spanish for "chalk") *street drug slang* [see: cocaine]

**YF-Vax** subcu injection R *yellow fever vaccine* [yellow fever vaccine] 0.5 mL

**yimyom** *street drug slang* [see: cocaine, crack]

**Yocon** tablets ℞ *no approved uses; sympatholytic; mydriatic; aphrodisiac* [yohimbine HCl] 5.4 mg

**Yodoxin** tablets, powder ℞ *amebicide* [iodoquinol] 210, 650 mg; 25 g

**yohimbic acid** INN

**yohimbine HCl** *alpha$_2$-adrenergic blocker; claimed to be an aphrodisiac; no FDA-sanctioned uses* 5.4 mg oral

**Yohimex** tablets ℞ *no approved uses; sympatholytic; mydriatic; aphrodisiac* [yohimbine HCl] 5.4 mg

**Your Choice Non-Preserved Saline** solution OTC *rinsing/storage solution for soft contact lenses* [preservative-free saline solution]

**Your Choice Sterile Preserved Saline** solution OTC *rinsing/storage solution for soft contact lenses* [preserved saline solution]

**ytterbium** *element (Yb)*

**ytterbium Yb 169 pentetate** USP *radioactive agent*

**yttrium** *element (Y)*

**yuppie psychedelic** *street drug slang* [see: MDMA]

**Yurelax** (Spanish name for U.S. product Flexeril)

**Yutopar** IV infusion ℞ *uterine relaxant to arrest preterm labor* [ritodrine HCl] 10, 15 mg/mL

**Yutopar** tablets (discontinued 1995) ℞ *uterine relaxant to arrest preterm labor* [ritodrine HCl] 10 mg

# Z

**zabicipril** INN

**Zacatecas purple** ("zacate" is Spanish for "hay") *street drug slang for marijuana from Mexico* [see: marijuana]

**zacopride** INN *antiemetic; peristaltic stimulant* [also: zacopride HCl]

**zacopride HCl** USAN, INN *antiemetic; peristaltic stimulant* [also: zacopride]

**Zacutex** IV injection ℞ *investigational (Phase III) platelet activating factor (PAF) antagonist for acute pancreatitis* [lexipafant]

**Zadaxin** ℞ *investigational (Phase III) vaccine enhancer for lung cancer and chronic hepatitis B* [thymalfasin]

**Zaditen** ℞ *investigational antiasthmatic* [ketotifen]

**zafirlukast** USAN, INN, BAN *antiasthmatic; leukotriene receptor antagonist (LTRA)*

**zafuleptine** INN

**Zagam** film-coated tablets ℞ *once-daily broad-spectrum fluoroquinolone antibiotic* [sparfloxacin] 200 mg

**zalcitabine** USAN *antiviral for AIDS (orphan)*

**zaleplon** USAN *sedative; hypnotic*

**zalospirone** INN *anxiolytic* [also: zalospirone HCl]

**zalospirone HCl** USAN *anxiolytic* [also: zalospirone]

**zaltidine** INN, BAN *antagonist to histamine H$_2$ receptors* [also: zaltidine HCl]

**zaltidine HCl** USAN *antagonist to histamine H$_2$ receptors* [also: zaltidine]

**zambi** *street drug slang* [see: marijuana]

**zamifenacin** INN, BAN *investigational treatment for irritable bowel syndrome*

**Zanaflex** tablets ℞ *antispasmodic for multiple sclerosis and spinal cord injury (orphan)* [tizanidine HCl] 4 mg

**zanamivir** *investigational (Phase III) treatment for influenza*

**zankiren HCl** USAN *antihypertensive*

**Zanosar** powder for IV injection ℞ *nitrosourea-type alkylating antineoplastic for metastatic islet cell carcinoma of pancreas* [streptozocin] 1 g (100 mg/mL)

**zanoterone** USAN *antiandrogen*

**Zantac** film-coated tablets, syrup, IV or IM injection ℞ *gastric and duodenal ulcer treatment; histamine H$_2$ antagonist* [ranitidine HCl] 150, 300 mg; 15 mg/mL; 0.5, 25 mg/mL ☒ Xanax

**Zantac 75** tablets OTC *treatment of episodic heartburn; histamine H$_2$ antagonist* [ranitidine HCl] 75 mg

**Zantac EFFERdose** effervescent tablets, effervescent granules ℞ *gastric and duodenal ulcer treatment; histamine H$_2$ antagonist* [ranitidine HCl] 150 mg; 150 mg/packet

**Zantac GELdose** capsules ℞ *gastric and duodenal ulcer treatment; histamine H$_2$ antagonist* [ranitidine HCl] 150, 300 mg

**Zantryl** capsules ℞ *anorexiant* [phentermine HCl] 30 mg

**zapizolam** INN

**zaprinast** INN, BAN

**zardaverine** INN

**Zarontin** capsules, syrup ℞ *anticonvulsant* [ethosuximide] 250 mg; 250 mg/5 mL ⊡ Zaroxolyn

**Zaroxolyn** tablets ℞ *diuretic; antihypertensive* [metolazone] 2.5, 5, 10 mg ⊡ Zarontin; Zeroxin

**Zartan** capsules (discontinued 1995) ℞ *cephalosporin-type antibiotic* [cephalexin monohydrate] 500 mg

**zatosetron** INN *antimigraine; investigational selective serotonin antagonist for anxiety and schizophrenia* [also: zatosetron maleate]

**zatosetron maleate** USAN *antimigraine; investigational selective serotonin antagonist for anxiety and schizophrenia* [also: zatosetron]

**Zavedos** (European name for U.S. product Idamycin)

**Z-Bec** tablets OTC *vitamin/zinc supplement* [multiple vitamins; zinc sulfate] ≛•22.5 mg

**ZBT Baby** powder OTC *topical diaper rash treatment* [talc]

**ZD 0490** *investigational immunotoxin for colorectal cancer*

**ZD 0870** *investigational broad-spectrum systemic antifungal*

**ZD 2079** *investigational treatment for diabetes and obesity*

**ZD 2138** *investigational 5-lipoxygenase inhibitor for rheumatoid arthritis and asthma*

**ZD 3523** *investigational leukotriene receptor antagonist for asthma*

**ZD 7288** *investigational sinoatrial node modulator for angina*

**ZE Caps** soft capsules OTC *dietary supplement* [vitamin E; zinc gluconate] 200•9.6 mg

**Zeasorb-AF** powder OTC *topical antifungal* [miconazole nitrate] 2%

**Zebeta** film-coated tablets ℞ *antihypertensive; β-blocker* [bisoprolol fumarate] 5, 10 mg

**Zecnil** ℞ *investigational (orphan) for secreting cutaneous gastrointestinal fistulas and bleeding esophageal varices* [somatostatin]

**Zefazone** powder for IV injection ℞ *cephalosporin-type antibiotic* [cefmetazole sodium] 1, 2 g

**zein** NF *coating agent*

**Zeisin** Autohaler (metered-dose inhaler) ℞ *investigational antiasthmatic*

**Zemuron** IV injection ℞ *neuromuscular blocking agent for anesthesia* [rocuronium bromide] 10 mg/mL

**zen** *street drug slang* [see: LSD]

**Zenapax** *investigational (Phase III, orphan) preventative for acute renal allograft rejection and acute graft vs host disease following bone marrow transplant* [dacliximab]

**Zenate, Advanced Formula** film-coated tablets ℞ *vitamin/iron supplement* [multiple vitamins; iron; folic acid] ≛•65•1 mg

**Zenate Prenatal** film-coated tablets (name changed to Advanced Formula Zenate in 1994)

**zenazocine mesylate** USAN *analgesic*

**Zeneca 182,780** *investigational steroidal antiestrogen for breast cancer*

**Zeneca 200,880** *investigational treatment for adult respiratory distress syndrome*

**zepastine** INN

**Zephiran Chloride** tincture, tincture spray, aqueous solution, towelettes, disinfectant concentrate OTC *topical antiseptic* [benzalkonium chloride] 1:750; 1:750; 1:750; 1:750; 17%

**zephirol** [see: benzalkonium chloride]

**Zephrex** film-coated tablets ℞ *decongestant; expectorant* [pseudoephedrine HCl; guaifenesin] 60•400 mg

**Zephrex LA** timed-release tablets ℞ *decongestant; expectorant* [pseudoephedrine HCl; guaifenesin] 120•600 mg

**zeranol** USAN, INN *anabolic*

**Zerit** capsules, oral solution, powder for oral solution ℞ *antiviral for HIV infection* [stavudine] 15, 20, 30, 40 mg; 1 mg/mL; 1 mg/mL

**zero** *street drug slang* [see: opium]

**Zeroxin-5; Zeroxin-10** gel (discontinued 1994) ℞ *topical keratolytic for acne* [benzoyl peroxide] 5%; 10% ⊡ Zaroxolyn

**Zestoretic** tablets ℞ *antihypertensive* [hydrochlorothiazide; lisinopril] 12.5•10, 25•20 mg

**Zestril** tablets ℞ *antihypertensive; angiotensin-converting enzyme (ACE) inhibitor for CHF and acute MI* [lisinopril] 2.5, 5, 10, 20, 40 mg

**Zetar** shampoo OTC *antiseborrheic; antipsoriatic; antipruritic; antibacterial* [coal tar] 1%

**Zetar Emulsion** bath oil ℞ *antipsoriatic; antiseborrheic; antipruritic; emollient* [coal tar] 30%

**zetidoline** INN, BAN

**Zetran** IV or IM injection (discontinued 1996) ℞ *sedative; anxiolytic; skeletal muscle relaxant; anticonvulsant adjunct* [diazepam] 5 mg/mL

**Z-gen** tablets OTC *vitamin/zinc supplement* [multiple vitamins; zinc] ±•22.5 mg

**Ziac** tablets ℞ *antihypertensive* [hydrochlorothiazide; bisoprolol fumarate] 6.25•2.5, 6.25•5, 6.25•10 mg

**zidapamide** INN

**zidometacin** USAN, INN *anti-inflammatory*

**zidovudine** USAN, INN, BAN *nucleoside antiviral for AIDS and AIDS-related complex (orphan)*

**zifrosilone** USAN *acetylcholinesterase inhibitor for Alzheimer's disease*

**zigzag man** *street drug slang* [see: LSD; marijuana]

**Zilactin Medicated** gel OTC *astringent for oral canker and herpes lesions* [tannic acid; alcohol 80%] 7%

**Zilactin-B Medicated** gel OTC *topical oral anesthetic* [benzocaine; alcohol 76%] 10%

**Zilactin-L** liquid OTC *topical local anesthetic* [lidocaine] 2.5%

**Zilactol Medicated** liquid (discontinued 1993) OTC *astringent for pre-emergent oral herpes lesions* [tannic acid]

**ZilaDent** gel (discontinued 1995) OTC *topical oral anesthetic* [benzocaine; alcohol 74.9%] 6%

**zilantel** USAN, INN *anthelmintic*

**zileuton** USAN, INN, BAN *5-lipoxygenase inhibitor; leukotriene receptor inhibitor; for prophylaxis and chronic treatment of asthma*

**zilpaterol** INN

**zimeldine** INN, BAN *antidepressant* [also: zimeldine HCl]

**zimeldine HCl** USAN *antidepressant* [also: zimeldine]

**zimelidine HCl** [now: zimeldine HCl]

**zimidoben** INN

**Zinacef** powder for IV or IM injection ℞ *cephalosporin-type antibiotic* [cefuroxime sodium] 0.75, 1.5, 7.5 g

**zinc** *element* (Zn)

**Zinc 15** tablets OTC *zinc supplement* [zinc sulfate] 66 mg

**zinc acetate** USP *investigational (orphan) copper blocking/complexing agent for Wilson's disease*

**zinc acetate, basic** INN

**zinc acetate dihydrate** [see: zinc acetate]

**zinc bacitracin** [see: bacitracin zinc]

**zinc caprylate** *antifungal*

**zinc carbonate** USAN *zinc supplement*

**zinc chloride** USP *astringent; dentin desensitizer; dietary zinc supplement*

**zinc chloride Zn 65** USAN *radioactive agent*

**zinc complex bacitracins** [see: bacitracin zinc]

**zinc gelatin** USP

**zinc gluconate** USP *dietary zinc supplement* 10, 15, 50, 78 mg oral

**Zinc Lozenges** OTC *topical anti-infective to relieve sore throat* [zinc citrate and zinc gluconate] 23 mg

**zinc mesoporphyrin** [see: hemin and zinc mesoporphyrin]

**zinc oleate** NF

**zinc oxide** USP, JAN *astringent; topical protectant; emollient; antiseptic* 20% *topical*

**zinc peroxide, medicinal** USP

**zinc phenolsulfonate** NF *not generally regarded as safe and effective as an antidiarrheal*

**zinc propionate** *antifungal*

**zinc pyrithione** [see: pyrithione zinc]

**zinc stearate** USP *dusting powder; tablet and capsule lubricant; antifungal*

**zinc sulfate** USP, JAN *ophthalmic astringent; dietary zinc supplement* 200, 250 mg *oral*; 1, 5 mg/mL *injection*

**zinc sulfate heptahydrate** [see: zinc sulfate]

**zinc sulfate monohydrate** [see: zinc sulfate]

**zinc sulfocarbolate** [see: zinc phenolsulfonate]

**zinc undecylenate** USP *antifungal*

**zinc valerate** USP

**Zinc-220** capsules OTC *zinc supplement* [zinc sulfate] 220 mg

**Zinca-Pak** IV injection ℞ *intravenous nutritional therapy* [zinc sulfate] 1, 5 mg/mL

**Zincate** capsules ℞ *zinc supplement* [zinc sulfate] 220 mg

**zinc-eugenol** USP

**Zincfrin** Drop-Tainers (eye drops) OTC *topical ocular decongestant; astringent* [phenylephrine HCl; zinc sulfate] 0.12%•0.25%

**Zincon** shampoo OTC *antiseborrheic; antibacterial; antifungal* [pyrithione zinc] 1%

**Zincvit** capsules ℞ *vitamin/mineral supplement* [multiple vitamins and minerals; folic acid] ±•1 mg

**zindotrine** USAN, INN *bronchodilator*

**zindoxifene** INN

**Zinecard** powder for IV drip or push ℞ *cardioprotectant for doxorubicin-induced cardiomyopathy (orphan)* [dexrazoxane] 250, 500 mg/vial

**zinoconazole** INN *antifungal* [also: zinoconazole HCl]

**zinoconazole HCl** USAN *antifungal* [also: zinoconazole]

**zinostatin** USAN, INN *antineoplastic*

**zinterol** INN *bronchodilator* [also: zinterol HCl]

**zinterol HCl** USAN *bronchodilator* [also: zinterol]

**zinviroxime** USAN, INN *antiviral*

**zip** *street drug slang* [see: cocaine]

**zipeprol** INN

**ziprasidone** *investigational antipsychotic for schizophrenia*

**ziprasidone HCl** *antipsychotic*

**Ziradryl** lotion OTC *topical antihistamine; astringent; antiseptic* [diphenhydramine HCl; zinc oxide; alcohol 2%] 1%•2%

**zirconium** *element* (Zr)

**zirconium oxide** *astringent*

**Zithromax** tablets, powder for oral suspension, powder for IV or IM injection ℞ *macrolide antibiotic* [azithromycin] 250, 600 mg; 100, 200 mg/5 mL, 1 g/packet; 500 mg

**Zithromax** ⒸⒶⓃ capsules, tablets, powder for oral suspension ℞ *macrolide antibiotic* [azithromycin] 250 mg; 250 mg; 300, 600 mg/15 mL, 900 mg/22.5 mL

**Zixoryn** ℞ *investigational (orphan) for neonatal hyperbilirubinemia* [flumecinol]

**$^{65}$Zn** [see: zinc chloride Zn 65]

**ZNP** cleansing bar OTC *antiseborrheic; antibacterial; antifungal* [pyrithione zinc] 2%

**zocainone** INN

**Zocor** tablets ℞ *cholesterol-lowering antihyperlipidemic; HMG-CoA reductase inhibitor; reduces mortality in coronary heart disease* [simvastatin] 5, 10, 20, 40 mg

**Zodeac-100** tablets ℞ *hematinic; vitamin/mineral supplement* [ferrous fumarate; multiple vitamins & minerals; folic acid; biotin] 60 mg• ±•1 mg•300 μg

**zofenopril** INN, BAN *angiotensin-converting enzyme (ACE) inhibitor* [also: zofenopril calcium]

**zofenopril calcium** USAN *angiotensin-converting enzyme (ACE) inhibitor* [also: zofenopril]

**zofenoprilat** INN *antihypertensive* [also: zofenoprilat arginine]

**zofenoprilat arginine** USAN *antihypertensive* [also: zofenoprilat]

**zoficonazole** INN

**Zofran** film-coated tablets, IV infusion ℞ *5-HT₃ antagonist; antiemetic for chemotherapy and radiotherapy; investigational anxiolytic and Alzheimer treatment* [ondansetron HCl] 4, 8 mg; 2 mg/mL, 32 mg/50 mL

**zol** *street drug slang for a marijuana cigarette* [see: marijuana]

**Zoladex** subcu implant in preloaded syringe ℞ *palliative hormonal chemotherapy for prostatic carcinoma, breast cancer, and endometriosis* [goserelin acetate] 3.6 mg (1-month implant), 10.8 mg (3-month implant)

**zolamine** INN *antihistamine; topical anesthetic* [also: zolamine HCl]

**zolamine HCl** USAN *antihistamine; topical anesthetic* [also: zolamine]

**zolazepam** INN, BAN *sedative* [also: zolazepam HCl]

**zolazepam HCl** USAN *sedative* [also: zolazepam]

**zoledronate disodium** USAN *bone resorption inhibitor for osteoporosis*

**zoledronate trisodium** USAN *bone resorption inhibitor for osteoporosis*

**zoledronic acid** USAN *bone resorption inhibitor for osteoporosis*

**zolenzepine** INN

**zolertine** INN *antiadrenergic; vasodilator* [also: zolertine HCl]

**zolertine HCl** USAN *antiadrenergic; vasodilator* [also: zolertine]

**Zolicef** powder for IV or IM injection ℞ *cephalosporin-type antibiotic* [cefazolin sodium] 0.5, 1 g

**zolimidine** INN

**zolimomab aritox** USAN *anti-T lymphocyte monoclonal antibody*

**zoliprofen** INN

**zoliridine** [see: zolimidine]

**zolmitriptan** USAN *serotonin 5-HT₁D agonist for migraine*

**Zoloft** film-coated tablets ℞ *selective serotonin reuptake inhibitor (SSRI) for depression and obsessive-compulsive disorder* [sertraline HCl] 25, 50, 100 mg

**Zoloft** ⓒ capsules ℞ *selective serotonin reuptake inhibitor (SSRI) for depression and obsessive-compulsive disorder* [sertraline HCl] 25, 50, 100 mg

**zoloperone** INN

**zolpidem** INN, BAN *imidazopyridine-type sedative/hypnotic* [also: zolpidem tartrate]

**zolpidem tartrate** USAN *imidazopyridine-type sedative/hypnotic* [also: zolpidem]

**Zolyse** ophthalmic solution (discontinued 1993) ℞ *enzymatic zonulolytic for intracapsular lens extraction* [chymotrypsin] 750 U

**zombie** *street drug slang* [see: PCP]

**zombie weed** *street drug slang for PCP or marijuana laced with PCP* [see: PCP; marijuana]

**zomebazam** INN

**zomepirac** INN, BAN *analgesic; anti-inflammatory* [also: zomepirac sodium]

**zomepirac sodium** USAN, USP *analgesic; anti-inflammatory* [also: zomepirac]

**zometapine** USAN *antidepressant*

**Zonalon** cream ℞ *topical antihistamine/antipruritic* [doxepin HCl] 5%

**Zonavir** ℞ *investigational treatment for varicella zoster virus* [5-propynylarabinofuranosyluracil]

**Zone-A** lotion, cream (discontinued 1993) ℞ *topical corticosteroid; anesthetic* [hydrocortisone acetate; pramoxine]

**Zone-A Forte** lotion, cream ℞ *topical corticosteroid; local anesthetic* [hydrocortisone acetate; pramoxine] 2.5%•1%

**zoniclezole** INN *anticonvulsant* [also: zoniclezole HCl]

**zoniclezole HCl** USAN *anticonvulsant* [also: zoniclezole]

**zonisamide** USAN, INN, BAN *anticonvulsant*

**Zonite Douche** solution concentrate OTC *antiseptic; antipruritic/counterirritant; vaginal cleanser and deodorizer* [benzalkonium chloride; menthol; thymol]

**zoom** *street drug slang for PCP or marijuana laced with PCP* [see: PCP; marijuana]

**zopiclone** INN, BAN *sedative; hypnotic*

**zopolrestat** USAN *antidiabetic; aldose reductase inhibitor*

**zorbamycin** USAN *antibacterial*

**ZORprin** Zero Order Release tablets ℞ *analgesic; antipyretic; anti-inflammatory; antirheumatic* [aspirin] 800 mg

**zorubicin** INN *antineoplastic* [also: zorubicin HCl]

**zorubicin HCl** USAN *antineoplastic* [also: zorubicin]

**Zostrix; Zostrix-HP** cream OTC *topical analgesic* [capsaicin] 0.025%; 0.075%

**Zosyn** powder for IV injection ℞ *extended-spectrum penicillin-type antibiotic* [piperacillin sodium; tazobactam sodium] 2•0.25, 3•0.375, 4•0.5 g

**zotepine** INN *investigational antipsychotic*

**Zoto-HC** ear drops ℞ *topical corticosteroidal anti-inflammatory; antibacterial; local anesthetic* [hydrocortisone; chloroxylenol; pramoxine HCl] 10%•1%•10%

**Zovia** tablets ℞ *monophasic oral contraceptive* [ethynodiol diacetate; ethinyl estradiol] 1 mg•35 μg; 1 mg•50 μg

**Zovirax** powder for IV infusion ℞ *antiviral for herpes infections* [acyclovir sodium] 500, 1000 mg

**Zovirax** tablets, capsules, oral suspension, ointment ℞ *antiviral for herpes simplex, herpes zoster, and adult-onset chickenpox; investigational for AIDS* [acyclovir] 400, 800 mg; 200 mg; 200 mg/5 mL; 5%

**Zovirax OTC** *investigational (awaiting approval) OTC formulation for recurrent genital herpes* [acyclovir]

**zoxazolamine** NF, INN

**zucapsaicin** USAN *topical analgesic*

**zuclomifene** INN

**zuclomiphene** USAN

**zuclopenthixol** INN, BAN

**Zumenon; Zumeston** ℞ *investigational treatment of postmenopausal symptoms* [estrogen; progestogen]

**Zurinol** tablets ℞ *uricosuric for gout* [allopurinol]

**Zyban** film-coated sustained-release tablets ℞ *non-nicotine aid to smoking cessation* [bupropion HCl] 100, 150 mg

**Zydone** capsules ℞ *narcotic analgesic* [hydrocodone bitartrate; acetaminophen] 5•500 mg

**Zyflo** film-coated tablets ℞ *5-lipoxygenase inhibitor; leukotriene receptor inhibitor; prophylaxis and treatment for chronic asthma* [zileuton] 600 mg

**zylofuramine** INN

**Zyloprim** injection ℞ *antineoplastic for leukemia, lymphoma, and solid tumor malignancies (orphan)* [allopurinol sodium]

**Zyloprim** tablets ℞ *xanthine oxidase inhibitor for gout and hyperuricemia* [allopurinol] 100, 300 mg

**Zymacap** capsules OTC *vitamin supplement* [multiple vitamins; folic acid] ±•0.4 mg

**Zymase** capsules containing enteric-coated spheres ℞ *digestive enzymes* [lipase; protease; amylase] 12 000•24 000•24 000 U

**Zyprexa** film-coated tablets ℞ *thienobenzodiazepine antipsychotic for schizophrenia and other psychotic disorders* [olanzapine] 5, 7.5, 10 mg

**Zyrkamine** *investigational (orphan) for non-Hodgkin's lymphoma* [mitoguazone]

**Zyrtec** film-coated tablets, syrup ℞ *once-daily antihistamine* [cetirizine HCl] 5, 10 mg; 5 mg/5 mL

# Sound-Alikes

Listed below are 967 pairs of drugs that sound alike or sufficiently alike that they may be confused in transcription. The list is not all-inclusive, and we would appreciate hearing of any additions the reader might suggest. These sound-alikes have also been included in the main section of the book where appropriate. Look for the "ear" icon (🔊).

| | |
|---|---|
| A-Caine | Anocaine |
| Accurbron | Accutane |
| Accutane | Accurbron |
| Achromycin | actinomycin |
| Achromycin | Aureomycin |
| Actidil | Actifed |
| Actifed | Actidil |
| actinomycin | Achromycin |
| actinomycin | Aureomycin |
| Adapin | Atabrine |
| Adapin | Ativan |
| Adapin | Betapen |
| adrenaline | adrenalone |
| adrenalone | adrenaline |
| Advil | Avail |
| Aerolone | Aralen |
| Aerolone | Arlidin |
| Afrin | Afrinol |
| Afrin | aspirin |
| Afrinol | Afrin |
| Agoral | Argyrol |
| Ak-Mycin | Akne-Mycin |
| Akne-Mycin | Ak-Mycin |
| Alamag | Alma-Mag |
| Aldactazide | Aldactone |
| Aldactone | Aldactazide |
| Aldomet | Aldoril |
| Aldoril | Aldomet |
| Aldoril | Elavil |
| Allergan | allergen |
| Allergan | Auralgan |
| allergen | Allergan |
| allergen | Auralgan |
| Alma-Mag | Alamag |
| ALOMAD | Alomide |
| Alomide | ALOMAD |
| Ambenyl | Aventyl |
| Amicar | Amikin |

| | |
|---|---|
| Amikin | Amicar |
| amitriptyline | nortriptyline |
| amoxapine | amoxicillin |
| amoxapine | Amoxil |
| amoxicillin | amoxapine |
| Amoxil | amoxapine |
| Anafranil | enalapril |
| Analbalm | Analpram |
| Analpram | Analbalm |
| Ancobon | Oncovin |
| Anocaine | A-Caine |
| Anturane | Artane |
| Anusol | Aplisol |
| APAC | APAP |
| APAP | APAC |
| Aplisol | Anusol |
| Aplisol | Apresoline |
| Appedrine | aprindine |
| Appedrine | ephedrine |
| Apresoline | Aplisol |
| Apresoline | Priscoline |
| aprindine | Appedrine |
| aprindine | ephedrine |
| ara-C | ERYC |
| Aralen | Aerolone |
| Aralen | Arlidin |
| Argyrol | Agoral |
| Aricept | Erycette |
| Arlidin | Aerolone |
| Arlidin | Aralen |
| Artane | Anturane |
| aspirin | Afrin |
| Atabrine | Adapin |
| Atarax | Marax |
| atenolol | timolol |
| Ativan | Adapin |
| Ativan | Avitene |
| Auralgan | Allergan |
| Auralgan | allergen |
| Aureomycin | Achromycin |
| Aureomycin | actinomycin |
| Avail | Advil |
| Aventyl | Ambenyl |
| Aventyl | Bentyl |
| Avitene | Ativan |
| Azlin | Mezlin |
| azolimine | Azulfidine |
| Azulfidine | azolimine |
| Bacid | Banacid |
| bacitracin | Bacitrin |
| bacitracin | Bactrim |
| Bacitrin | bacitracin |

| | |
|---|---|
| Bactocill | Pathocil |
| Bactrim | bacitracin |
| Banacid | Bacid |
| Banophen | Barophen |
| Banthine | Brethine |
| Barophen | Banophen |
| Belladenal | belladonna |
| Belladenal | Benadryl |
| belladonna | Belladenal |
| Beminal | Benemid |
| Benadryl | Belladenal |
| Benadryl | Bentyl |
| Benadryl | Benylin |
| Benadryl | Caladryl |
| Benemid | Beminal |
| Benoxyl | PanOxyl |
| Bentyl | Aventyl |
| Bentyl | Benadryl |
| Bentyl | Bontril |
| Benylin | Benadryl |
| Benylin | Betalin |
| Betagan | Betagen |
| Betagen | Betagan |
| Betalin | Benylin |
| Betapen | Adapin |
| Betapen | Phenaphen |
| Bichloracetic acid | dichloroacetic acid |
| Bicillin | V-Cillin |
| Bicillin | Wycillin |
| bleomycin | Cleocin |
| boil | Boyol |
| Bonain | Bonine |
| Bonine | Bonain |
| Bontril | Bentyl |
| Bontril | Vontrol |
| Boyol | boil |
| Brethine | Banthine |
| Bretylol | Brevital |
| Brevital | Bretylol |
| Bromfed | Bromphen |
| Bromophen | Bromphen |
| Bromphen | Bromfed |
| Bromphen | Bromophen |
| Broncholate | Brondelate |
| Brondecon | Bronitin |
| Brondelate | Broncholate |
| Bronitin | Brondecon |
| butabarbital | butalbital |
| butalbital | butabarbital |
| butalbital | Butibel |
| Butazolidin | Butisol |
| Butibel | butalbital |

| | |
|---|---|
| Butisol | Butazolidin |
| Byclomine | Hycomine |
| Bydramine | Hydramine |
| Caladryl | Benadryl |
| Calamox | Camalox |
| calcitonin | calcitriol |
| calcitriol | calcitonin |
| Camalox | Calamox |
| Capastat | Cepastat |
| Capitrol | captopril |
| captopril | Capitrol |
| Catapres | Catarase |
| Catapres | Combipres |
| Catapres | Ser-Ap-Es |
| Catarase | Catapres |
| cefazolin | cephalexin |
| cefazolin | cephalothin |
| cefotaxime | cefoxitin |
| cefoxitin | cefotaxime |
| ceftizoxime | cefuroxime |
| cefuroxime | ceftizoxime |
| Cefzil | Kefzol |
| Cepastat | Capastat |
| cephalexin | cefazolin |
| cephalexin | cephalothin |
| cephalothin | cefazolin |
| cephalothin | cephalexin |
| cephapirin | cephradine |
| cephradine | cephapirin |
| chlorpheniramine | chlorphentermine |
| chlorphentermine | chlorpheniramine |
| cimetidine | dimethicone |
| claretin | Claritin |
| claretin | Clarityne |
| Claritin | claretin |
| Claritin | Clarityne |
| Clarityne | claretin |
| Clarityne | Claritin |
| Cleocin | bleomycin |
| Cleocin | Lincocin |
| Clinoxide | clioxanide |
| Clinoxide | Clipoxide |
| clioxanide | Clinoxide |
| Clipoxide | Clinoxide |
| clomiphene | clonidine |
| clonidine | clomiphene |
| clonidine | Klonopin |
| clonidine | quinidine |
| clotrimazole | co-trimoxazole |
| co-trimoxazole | clotrimazole |
| Codafed | Codaphen |
| Codaphen | Codafed |

| | |
|---|---|
| Codegest | Codehist |
| Codehist | Codegest |
| codeine | Kaodene |
| Colestid | colistin |
| colestipol | colistin |
| colistin | Colestid |
| colistin | colestipol |
| Combipres | Catapres |
| Cort-Dome | Cortone |
| Cortenema | quart enema |
| Cortin | Cotrim |
| cortisone | Cortizone |
| Cortizone | cortisone |
| Cortone | Cort-Dome |
| Cotrim | Cortin |
| Coumadin | Kemadrin |
| cytarabine | vidarabine |
| dacarbazine | Dicarbosil |
| dacarbazine | procarbazine |
| dactinomycin | daunorubicin |
| Dalmane | Dialume |
| danthron | Dantrium |
| Dantrium | danthron |
| Daranide | Daraprim |
| Daraprim | Daranide |
| Daricon | Darvon |
| Darvocet-N | Darvon-N |
| Darvon | Daricon |
| Darvon-N | Darvocet-N |
| daunorubicin | dactinomycin |
| daunorubicin | doxorubicin |
| Decaderm | Decadron |
| Decadron | Decaderm |
| Decadron | Percodan |
| Deconal | Deconsal |
| Deconsal | Deconal |
| Delacort | Delcort |
| Delcort | Delacort |
| Demerol | Demulen |
| Demerol | dicumarol |
| Demerol | Dymelor |
| Demerol | Temaril |
| Demolin | Demulen |
| Demulen | Demerol |
| Demulen | Demolin |
| Dermacort | DermiCort |
| DermiCort | Dermacort |
| deserpidine | desipramine |
| Desferal | Disophrol |
| desipramine | deserpidine |
| desoximethasone | dexamethasone |
| Desoxyn | digitoxin |

| | |
|---|---|
| Desoxyn | digoxin |
| dexamethasone | desoximethasone |
| Dexedrine | dextran |
| dextran | Dexedrine |
| dextran | dextrin |
| dextrin | dextran |
| Dialume | Dalmane |
| Dicarbosil | dacarbazine |
| dichloroacetic acid | Bichloracetic acid |
| dicumarol | Demerol |
| digitoxin | Desoxyn |
| digitoxin | digoxin |
| digoxin | Desoxyn |
| digoxin | digitoxin |
| Dilantin | Dilaudid |
| Dilaudid | Dilantin |
| Dimacol | dimercaprol |
| dimenhydrinate | diphenhydramine |
| dimercaprol | Dimacol |
| Dimetabs | Dimetane |
| Dimetabs | Dimetapp |
| Dimetane | Dimetabs |
| Dimetapp | Dimetabs |
| dimethicone | cimetidine |
| diphenhydramine | dimenhydrinate |
| Diphenylin | Dyphenylan |
| Disophrol | Desferal |
| Disophrol | disoprofol |
| Disophrol | Stilphostrol |
| disoprofol | Disophrol |
| Ditropan | Intropin |
| Diutensen | Salutensin |
| dobutamine | dopamine |
| Dommanate | Dramanate |
| Donnagel | Donnatal |
| Donnatal | Donnagel |
| Donnazyme | Entozyme |
| dopamine | dobutamine |
| dopamine | Dopram |
| Dopar | Dopram |
| Dopram | dopamine |
| Dopram | Dopar |
| doxepin | Doxidan |
| Doxidan | doxepin |
| doxorubicin | daunorubicin |
| Dramanate | Dommanate |
| Dyazide | Thiacide |
| Dyazide | thiazides |
| Dymelor | Demerol |
| Dymelor | Pamelor |
| Dyphenylan | Diphenylin |
| Dyrenium | Pyridium |

| | |
|---|---|
| Ecotrin | Edecrin |
| Edecrin | Ecotrin |
| Edecrin | Ethaquin |
| Elavil | Aldoril |
| Elavil | Enovil |
| Elavil | Equanil |
| Elavil | Mellaril |
| emetine | Emetrol |
| Emetrol | emetine |
| Endal | Intal |
| Enduron | Imuran |
| Enduron | Inderal |
| Enduronyl | Inderal |
| Enovil | Elavil |
| Entozyme | Donnazyme |
| ephedrine | Appedrine |
| ephedrine | aprindine |
| Epifrin | epinephrine |
| Epifrin | EpiPen |
| Epinal | Epitol |
| epinephrine | Epifrin |
| EpiPen | Epifrin |
| Epitol | Epinal |
| Equanil | Elavil |
| erythromycin | clarithromycin |
| ERYC | ara-C |
| Erycette | Aricept |
| Esidrix | Lasix |
| Esimil | Estinyl |
| Esimil | Isomil |
| Estinyl | Esimil |
| Estraderm | Estradurin |
| Estradurin | Estraderm |
| Estratab | Ethatab |
| ethacridine | ethacrynic |
| ethacrynic | ethacridine |
| Ethaquin | Edecrin |
| Ethatab | Estratab |
| ethinamate | ethionamide |
| ethionamide | ethinamate |
| Eurax | Serax |
| Eurax | Urex |
| Euthroid | Synthroid |
| Euthroid | thyroid |
| Eutonyl | Eutron |
| Eutron | Eutonyl |
| Evac-Q-Kit | Evac-Q-Kwik |
| Evac-Q-Kwik | Evac-Q-Kit |
| Feosol | Feostat |
| Feosol | Fer-in-Sol |
| Feosol | Festal |
| Feostat | Feosol |

| | |
|---|---|
| Fer-in-Sol | Feosol |
| Festal | Feosol |
| Festal | Festalan |
| Festalan | Festal |
| Feverall | Fiberall |
| Fiberall | Feverall |
| Fioricet | Lorcet |
| Fiorinal | Florinef |
| Flaxedil | Flexeril |
| Flexeril | Flaxedil |
| Florinef | Fiorinal |
| fluocinolone | fluocinonide |
| fluocinonide | fluocinolone |
| folacin | Fulvicin |
| Fostex | pHisoHex |
| Fulvicin | folacin |
| Fulvicin | Furacin |
| Furacin | Fulvicin |
| Gamastan | Garamycin |
| Gantanol | Gantrisin |
| Gantrisin | Gantanol |
| Garamycin | Gamastan |
| Garamycin | kanamycin |
| Garamycin | Terramycin |
| Gelfoam | Ger-O-Foam |
| Genapap | Genatap |
| Genatap | Genapap |
| gentamicin | Jenamicin |
| gentamicin | kanamycin |
| Ger-O-Foam | Gelfoam |
| glucose | Glutose |
| Glutose | glucose |
| Glycotuss | Glytuss |
| Glytuss | Glycotuss |
| Gonak | Gonic |
| Gonic | Gonak |
| guaifenesin | guanfacine |
| guanethidine | guanidine |
| guanfacine | guaifenesin |
| guanidine | guanethidine |
| Guiatuss | Guiatussin |
| Guiatussin | Guiatuss |
| Haldol | Halenol |
| Haldol | Halog |
| Halenol | Haldol |
| Halog | Haldol |
| Halotestin | Halotex |
| Halotestin | Halotussin |
| Halotex | Halotestin |
| Halotussin | Halotestin |
| Hespan | Histastan |
| Hexadrol | Hexalol |

| | |
|---|---|
| Hexalen | Hexalol |
| Hexalol | Hexadrol |
| Hexalol | Hexalen |
| Hiprex | Hispril |
| Hispril | Hiprex |
| Histastan | Hespan |
| Histastan | Histatime |
| Histatime | Histastan |
| Hycodan | Hycomine |
| Hycodan | Vicodin |
| Hycomine | Byclomine |
| Hycomine | Hycodan |
| Hycomine | Vicodin |
| Hydergine | Hydramine |
| Hydramine | Bydramine |
| Hydramine | Hydergine |
| Hydramine | Hydramyn |
| Hydramine | Hytramyn |
| Hydramyn | Hydramine |
| Hydropane | Hydropine |
| Hydrophen | Hydropine |
| Hydropine | Hydropane |
| Hydropine | Hydrophen |
| Hygroton | Regroton |
| Hyper-Tet | HyperHep |
| Hyper-Tet | Hyperstat |
| HyperHep | Hyper-Tet |
| HyperHep | Hyperstat |
| Hyperstat | Hyper-Tet |
| Hyperstat | HyperHep |
| Hyperstat | Nitrostat |
| Hytone | Vytone |
| Hytramyn | Hydramine |
| Ilosone | inosine |
| Imferon | imipramine |
| Imferon | Imuran |
| imipramine | Imferon |
| imipramine | Norpramin |
| imipramine | trimipramine |
| Imuran | Enduron |
| Imuran | Imferon |
| Inderal | Enduron |
| Inderal | Enduronyl |
| Inderal | Inderide |
| Inderide | Inderal |
| Indocin | Lincocin |
| Indocin | Minocin |
| inosine | Ilosone |
| insulin | inulin |
| Intal | Endal |
| Intropin | Ditropan |
| Intropin | Isoptin |

| | |
|---|---|
| inulin | insulin |
| Ismelin | Ritalin |
| Isomil | Esimil |
| Isoptin | Intropin |
| Isopto Carpine | Isopto Eserine |
| Isopto Eserine | Isopto Carpine |
| Isordil | Isuprel |
| Isuprel | Isordil |
| K-LOR | Kaochlor |
| K-LOR | Klor |
| kanamycin | Garamycin |
| kanamycin | gentamicin |
| Kaochlor | K-LOR |
| Kaodene | codeine |
| kaolin | Kaon |
| Kaon | kaolin |
| Kaopectate | Kapectalin |
| Kapectalin | Kaopectate |
| Kay Ciel | KCl |
| KCl | Kay Ciel |
| Keflet | Keflex |
| Keflet | Keflin |
| Keflex | Keflet |
| Keflex | Keflin |
| Keflin | Keflet |
| Keflin | Keflex |
| Kefzol | Cefzil |
| Kemadrin | Coumadin |
| Kenalog | Ketalar |
| Ketalar | Kenalog |
| Klonopin | clonidine |
| Klor | K-LOR |
| Klotrix | Liotrix |
| Komex | Koromex |
| Koromex | Komex |
| lanolin | Lanoline |
| Lanoline | lanolin |
| Lanoxin | Levoxine |
| Lasix | Esidrix |
| Lasix | Lidex |
| levallorphan | levorphanol |
| levodopa | methyldopa |
| levorphanol | levallorphan |
| levothyroxine | liothyronine |
| Levoxine | Lanoxin |
| Lidex | Lasix |
| Lidex | Lidox |
| Lidex | Wydase |
| Lidox | Lidex |
| Lincocin | Cleocin |
| Lincocin | Indocin |
| liothyronine | levothyroxine |

| | |
|---|---|
| Liotrix | Klotrix |
| Loniten | clonidine |
| Lorcet | Fioricet |
| Lotrimin | Otrivin |
| Luminal | Tuinal |
| LuVax | Luvox |
| Luvox | LuVax |
| Maalox | Marax |
| Mandol | nadolol |
| Marax | Atarax |
| Marax | Maalox |
| Marcaine | Narcan |
| mazindol | mebendazole |
| Mebaral | Medrol |
| Mebaral | Mellaril |
| mebendazole | mazindol |
| Meclan | Meclomen |
| Meclan | Mezlin |
| Meclomen | Meclan |
| Medrol | Mebaral |
| Mellaril | Elavil |
| Mellaril | Mebaral |
| Mellaril | Moderil |
| meperidine | meprobamate |
| mephenytoin | Mephyton |
| mephenytoin | Mesantoin |
| Mephyton | mephenytoin |
| Mephyton | methadone |
| meprobamate | meperidine |
| Meprospan | Naprosyn |
| Mesantoin | mephenytoin |
| Mesantoin | Mestinon |
| Mesantoin | Metatensin |
| Mestinon | Mesantoin |
| Mestinon | Metatensin |
| Metahydrin | Metandren |
| Metandren | Metahydrin |
| metaproterenol | metoprolol |
| Metatensin | Mesantoin |
| Metatensin | Mestinon |
| metaxalone | metolazone |
| methadone | Mephyton |
| methenamine | methionine |
| methionine | methenamine |
| methixene | methoxsalen |
| methoxsalen | methixene |
| methyldopa | levodopa |
| metolazone | metaxalone |
| Metopirone | metyrapone |
| metoprolol | metaproterenol |
| metyrapone | Metopirone |
| metyrapone | metyrosine |

| | |
|---|---|
| metyrosine | metyrapone |
| Mezlin | Azlin |
| Mezlin | Meclan |
| MICRhoGAM | microgram |
| microgram | MICRhoGAM |
| Midrin | Mydfrin |
| Milontin | Miltown |
| Milontin | Mylanta |
| Miltown | Milontin |
| Minocin | Indocin |
| Minocin | Mithracin |
| Minocin | niacin |
| Mithracin | Minocin |
| mithramycin | mitomycin |
| mitomycin | mithramycin |
| mitomycin | Mity-Mycin |
| mitomycin | Mutamycin |
| Mity-Mycin | mitomycin |
| Moban | Mobidin |
| Moban | Modane |
| Mobidin | Moban |
| Modane | Moban |
| Modane | Mudrane |
| Moderil | Mellaril |
| Modicon | Mylicon |
| Moi-Stir | moisture |
| moisture | Moi-Stir |
| Monocete | Monoket |
| Mono-Chlor | Monocor |
| Monocor | Mono-Chlor |
| Monoket | Monocete |
| Mudrane | Modane |
| Mutamycin | mitomycin |
| Myambutol | Nembutal |
| Mydfrin | Midrin |
| Mydfrin | Myfedrine |
| Myfedrine | Mydfrin |
| Mylanta | Milontin |
| Myleran | Mylicon |
| Mylicon | Modicon |
| Mylicon | Myleran |
| nadolol | Mandol |
| Naldecon | Nalfon |
| Nalfon | Naldecon |
| Naprosyn | Meprospan |
| Naprosyn | naproxen |
| Naprosyn | Natacyn |
| naproxen | Naprosyn |
| Narcan | Marcaine |
| Nardil | Norinyl |
| Natacyn | Naprosyn |
| Nembutal | Myambutol |

| | |
|---|---|
| Neomixin | neomycin |
| neomycin | Neomixin |
| niacin | Minocin |
| Nicobid | Nitro-Bid |
| Nilstat | Nitrostat |
| Nilstat | nystatin |
| Nitro-Bid | Nicobid |
| nitroglycerin | Nitroglyn |
| Nitroglyn | nitroglycerin |
| Nitrostat | Hyperstat |
| Nitrostat | Nilstat |
| Nitrostat | nystatin |
| Norinyl | Nardil |
| Norlutate | Norlutin |
| Norlutin | Norlutate |
| Norpramin | imipramine |
| nortriptyline | amitriptyline |
| nystatin | Nilstat |
| nystatin | Nitrostat |
| Omnipen | Unipen |
| Oncovin | Ancobon |
| Ophthochlor | Ophthocort |
| Ophthocort | Ophthochlor |
| Orabase | Orinase |
| Oracin | orarsan |
| Oracin | Orasone |
| orarsan | Oracin |
| orarsan | Orasone |
| Orasone | Oracin |
| Orasone | orarsan |
| Oretic | Oreton |
| Oreton | Oretic |
| Orex | Ornex |
| Orinase | Orabase |
| Orinase | Ornade |
| Orinase | Ornex |
| Orinase | Tolinase |
| Ornade | Orinase |
| Ornade | Ornex |
| Ornex | Orex |
| Ornex | Orinase |
| Ornex | Ornade |
| Ortho-Creme | Orthoclone |
| Orthoclone | Ortho-Creme |
| Otobiotic | Urobiotic |
| Otrivin | Lotrimin |
| oxymetazoline | oxymetholone |
| oxymetholone | oxymetazoline |
| oxymetholone | oxymorphone |
| oxymorphone | oxymetholone |
| Pamelor | Dymelor |
| Panarex | Panorex |

| | |
|---|---|
| Panasol | Panscol |
| Panorex | Panarex |
| PanOxyl | Benoxyl |
| Panscol | Panasol |
| Pantopon | Parafon |
| Parafon | Pantopon |
| paramethadione | paramethasone |
| paramethasone | paramethadione |
| Pathilon | Pathocil |
| Pathocil | Bactocill |
| Pathocil | Pathilon |
| Pathocil | Placidyl |
| Pavabid | Pavased |
| Pavased | Pavabid |
| Pavatine | Pavatym |
| Pavatym | Pavatine |
| Paverolan | Pavulon |
| Pavulon | Paverolan |
| penicillamine | penicillin |
| penicillin | penicillamine |
| penicillin | Polycillin |
| Pentazine | Phenazine |
| pentobarbital | phenobarbital |
| Pentothal | pentrinitrol |
| pentrinitrol | Pentothal |
| Percodan | Decadron |
| Perdiem | Pyridium |
| Periactin | Taractan |
| Persantine | Pertofrane |
| Pertofrane | Persantine |
| Phazyme | Pherazine |
| phenacetin | phenazocine |
| Phenaphen | Betapen |
| Phenaphen | Phenergan |
| Phenazine | Pentazine |
| Phenazine | phenelzine |
| Phenazine | Phenoxine |
| Phenazine | Pherazine |
| phenazocine | phenacetin |
| phenelzine | Phenazine |
| phenelzine | Phenylzin |
| Phenergan | Phenaphen |
| Phenergan | Theragran |
| phenobarbital | pentobarbital |
| Phenoxine | Phenazine |
| phentermine | phentolamine |
| phentolamine | phentermine |
| phentolamine | Ventolin |
| Phenylzin | phenelzine |
| Pherazine | Phazyme |
| Pherazine | Phenazine |
| pHisoHex | Fostex |

| | |
|---|---|
| physostigmine | pyridostigmine |
| physostigmine | Prostigmin |
| piperacetazine | piperazine |
| piperazine | piperacetazine |
| piracetam | piroxicam |
| piroxicam | piracetam |
| Pitocin | Pitressin |
| Pitressin | Pitocin |
| Placidyl | Pathocil |
| Pod-Ben | Podoben |
| Podoben | Pod-Ben |
| Podoben | Podofin |
| Podofin | Podoben |
| Podofin | podophyllin |
| podophyllin | Podofin |
| Polycillin | penicillin |
| Ponstel | Pronestyl |
| pralidoxime | pramoxine |
| pralidoxime | pyridoxine |
| Pramosone | pramoxine |
| pramoxine | pralidoxime |
| pramoxine | Pramosone |
| Pravachol | Primacor |
| prazepam | prazepine |
| prazepam | Prazosin |
| prazepine | prazepam |
| Prazosin | prazepam |
| prednisolone | prednisone |
| prednisone | prednisolone |
| Primacor | Pravachol |
| Priscoline | Apresoline |
| procaine | Procan |
| Procan | procaine |
| procarbazine | dacarbazine |
| Prolene | proline |
| proline | Prolene |
| promazine | Promethazine |
| Promethazine | promazine |
| Pronestyl | Ponstel |
| Prostigmin | physostigmine |
| Protamine | Protopam |
| Protopam | Protamine |
| Psorex | Serax |
| Pyridium | Dyrenium |
| Pyridium | pyridoxine |
| Pyridium | pyrithione |
| Pyridium | pyritidium |
| pyridostigmine | physostigmine |
| pyridoxine | pralidoxime |
| pyridoxine | Pyridium |
| pyrithione | Pyridium |
| pyritidium | Pyridium |

| | |
|---|---|
| quart enema | Cortenema |
| Quarzan | Questran |
| Questran | Quarzan |
| quinacrine | quinidine |
| Quinatime | quinidine |
| quinidine | clonidine |
| quinidine | quinacrine |
| quinidine | Quinatime |
| quinidine | quinine |
| quinine | quinidine |
| Regain | Rogaine |
| Reglan | Regonol |
| Regonol | Reglan |
| Regroton | Hygroton |
| Repan | Riopan |
| Resperol | Risperdal |
| Resperol | Restoril |
| Restoril | Resperol |
| Restoril | Vistaril |
| Rheumatex | Rheumatrex |
| Rheumatrex | Rheumatex |
| Rifadin | rifampin |
| Rifadin | Ritalin |
| rifampin | Rifadin |
| Riopan | Repan |
| Risperdal | Resperol |
| Ritalin | Ismelin |
| Ritalin | Rifadin |
| Robaxacet | Robaxisal |
| Robaxisal | Robaxacet |
| Rogaine | Regain |
| Salutensin | Diutensen |
| Sepo | Septa |
| Septa | Sepo |
| Septa | Septra |
| Septra | Septa |
| Ser-Ap-Es | Catapres |
| Serax | Eurax |
| Serax | Psorex |
| Serax | Urex |
| Serax | Xerac |
| Serentil | Surital |
| Simplet | Singlet |
| Singlet | Simplet |
| Soprodol | Sopronol |
| Sopronol | Soprodol |
| stilbestrol | Stilphostrol |
| Stilphostrol | Disophrol |
| Stilphostrol | stilbestrol |
| Streptase | Streptonase |
| streptokinase | Streptonase |
| Streptonase | Streptase |

| | |
|---|---|
| Streptonase | streptokinase |
| sucrase | sucrose |
| sucrose | sucrase |
| Sulf-10 | Sulten-10 |
| Sulfa-Trip | Sulfatrim |
| sulfamethizole | sulfamethoxazole |
| sulfamethoxazole | sulfamethizole |
| sulfathiazole | sulfisoxazole |
| Sulfatrim | Sulfa-Trip |
| sulfisoxazole | sulfathiazole |
| Sulten-10 | Sulf-10 |
| Surital | Serentil |
| Synthroid | Euthroid |
| Tagamet | Tegopen |
| Taractan | Periactin |
| Taractan | Tinactin |
| Tedral | Teldrin |
| Tegopen | Tagamet |
| Tegopen | Tegrin |
| Tegretol | Tegrin |
| Tegrin | Tegopen |
| Tegrin | Tegretol |
| Teldrin | Tedral |
| Temaril | Demerol |
| Temaril | Tepanil |
| Tepanil | Temaril |
| Tepanil | Tofranil |
| Terramycin | Garamycin |
| testolactone | testosterone |
| testosterone | testolactone |
| thallium | Valium |
| Theoclear | Theolair |
| Theocolate | Theolate |
| Theolair | Theoclear |
| Theolair | Thyrolar |
| Theolate | Theocolate |
| Thera-Flur | TheraFlu |
| TheraFlu | Thera-Flur |
| Theragran | Phenergan |
| Theravite | Therevac |
| Therevac | Theravite |
| Thiacide | Dyazide |
| Thiacide | thiazides |
| thiazides | Dyazide |
| thiazides | Thiacide |
| Threostat | Triostat |
| Thyrar | Thyrolar |
| thyroid | Euthroid |
| Thyrolar | Theolair |
| Thyrolar | Thyrar |
| Ticar | Tigan |
| Tigan | Ticar |

| | |
|---|---|
| timolol | atenolol |
| Tinactin | Taractan |
| TobraDex | Tobrex |
| tobramycin | Trobicin |
| Tobrex | TobraDex |
| Tofranil | Tepanil |
| Tolinase | Orinase |
| Topic | Topicort |
| Topicort | Topic |
| Trasylol | Travasol |
| Travasol | Trasylol |
| Triafed | Trifed |
| triamcinolone | Triaminicin |
| Triaminic | Triaminicin |
| Triaminic | TriHemic |
| Triaminicin | triamcinolone |
| Triaminicin | Triaminic |
| triamterene | trimipramine |
| Trifed | Triafed |
| TriHemic | Triaminic |
| trimeprazine | trimipramine |
| trimethaphan | trimethoprim |
| trimethoprim | trimethaphan |
| trimipramine | imipramine |
| trimipramine | triamterene |
| trimipramine | trimeprazine |
| Triostat | Threostat |
| Trobicin | tobramycin |
| Tronolane | Tronothane |
| Tronothane | Tronolane |
| Tuinal | Luminal |
| Tuinal | Tylenol |
| Tussafed | Tussafin |
| Tussafin | Tussafed |
| Tussex | Tussionex |
| Tussex | Tussirex |
| Tussi-Organidin | Tussi-R-Gen |
| Tussi-R-Gen | Tussi-Organidin |
| Tussionex | Tussex |
| Tussionex | Tussirex |
| Tussirex | Tussex |
| Tussirex | Tussionex |
| Tylenol | Tuinal |
| Unipen | Omnipen |
| Uracel | uracil |
| Uracel | Urised |
| Uracid | uracil |
| Uracid | Urised |
| Uracid | Urocit |
| uracil | Uracel |
| uracil | Uracid |
| Urex | Eurax |

| | |
|---|---|
| Urex | Serax |
| Urised | Uracel |
| Urised | Uracid |
| Urised | Urispas |
| Urispas | Urised |
| Urobiotic | Otobiotic |
| Urocit | Uracid |
| V-Cillin | Bicillin |
| V-Cillin | Wycillin |
| Valium | thallium |
| Valium | Valpin |
| Valmid | Valpin |
| Valpin | Valium |
| Valpin | Valmid |
| Valpin | Valprin |
| Valpin | Velban |
| Valprin | Valpin |
| Vasocidin | Vasodilan |
| Vasodilan | Vasocidin |
| Vasosulf | Velosef |
| Velban | Valpin |
| Velosef | Vasosulf |
| Ventolin | phentolamine |
| Vicodin | Hycodan |
| Vicodin | Hycomine |
| vidarabine | cytarabine |
| Vigran | Wigraine |
| Vistaril | Restoril |
| Vitron | Vytone |
| Vontrol | Bontril |
| Vytone | Hytone |
| Vytone | Vitron |
| Wigraine | Vigran |
| Wycillin | Bicillin |
| Wycillin | V-Cillin |
| Wydase | Lidex |
| Xanax | Zantac |
| Xerac | Serax |
| Zantac | Xanax |
| Zarontin | Zaroxolyn |
| Zarontin | Zentron |
| Zaroxolyn | Zarontin |
| Zaroxolyn | Zeroxin |
| Zentron | Zarontin |
| Zeroxin | Zaroxolyn |

# Investigational Code Names

A code name is a temporary identification assigned to a product by the manufacturer. The number or letter-number combination is used while the substance is undergoing testing, before a generic name is given. Code names appearing in this appendix (1) have had a generic name assigned within the past five years, or (2) are currently undergoing testing with a generic name not yet assigned, or (3) have had testing discontinued within the past five years. Code names appearing here without generic names are also listed alphabetically in the main section of this book. Information about ongoing testing or the date testing was discontinued may be obtained there.

| | |
|---|---|
| 1069C | generic not yet assigned—see main list |
| 10 80 07 | omoconazole nitrate |
| 10-EDAM | edatrexate |
| 129Y83 | colfosceril palmitate |
| 12C | velaresol |
| 1370U | generic not yet assigned—see main list |
| 141W94 | generic not yet assigned—see main list |
| 142780 | generic not yet assigned—see main list |
| 1592U89 | abacavir succinate |
| 256U87 HCl | valacyclovir HCl |
| 3118 | generic not yet assigned—see main list |
| 311C90 | zolmitriptan |
| 348U | generic not yet assigned—see main list |
| 3TC | lamivudine |
| 403U | generic not yet assigned—see main list |
| 4197X-RA | generic not yet assigned—see main list |
| 447C | generic not yet assigned—see main list |
| 4MRTA | generic not yet assigned—see main list |
| 51W89 | cisatracurium besylate |
| 520C9x22 | generic not yet assigned—see main list |
| 566C | atovaquone |
| 566C80 | atovaquone |
| 589C | tucaresol |
| 5A8 | generic not yet assigned—see main list |
| 619C | generic not yet assigned—see main list |
| 7-OMEN | menogaril |
| 7U85 | generic not yet assigned—see main list |
| 882 | generic not yet assigned—see main list |
| 882C | generic not yet assigned—see main list |
| 88BV59 | votumumab |
| 935U83 | raluridine |
| A-16686 | ramoplanin |
| A-33547.HCl.$H_2O$ | remoxipride HCl |
| A-3508.HCl | mirfentanil HCl |

| | |
|---|---|
| A-3665.HCl | trefentanil HCl |
| A-73001 | seratrodast |
| A-75200 mesylate | napitane mesylate |
| A-77000 | pazinaclone |
| AA-2414 | seratrodast |
| AA-673 | amlexanox |
| Abbott-56620 | sarafloxacin HCl |
| Abbott-57135 (sarafloxacin) | sarafloxacin HCl |
| Abbott-64077 | zileuton |
| Abbott 70569.1 | tiagabine HCl |
| Abbott 70569 HCl | tiagabine HCl |
| Abbott-72517 | zankiren HCl |
| Abbott-73001 | seratrodast |
| Abbott-76745 | fenleuton |
| Abbott-84538 | ritonavir |
| ABC 12/3 | doxofylline |
| ABT-001 | seratrodast |
| ABT-538 | ritonavir |
| ABT-569 | tiagabine HCl |
| ABT-719 | generic not yet assigned—see main list |
| AC001 | amlintide |
| AC0137 | pramlintide |
| AC 137 | generic not yet assigned—see main list |
| AC625 | generic not yet assigned—see main list |
| ACA-147 | generic not yet assigned—see main list |
| ACC-9653-010 | fosphenytoin sodium |
| AD-439 | generic not yet assigned—see main list |
| AD-519 | generic not yet assigned—see main list |
| ADR-529 | dexrazoxane |
| AE-0047 | generic not yet assigned—see main list |
| AF102B | generic not yet assigned—see main list |
| AF 1934 (lysine) | bendazac |
| AF 2838 | bindarit |
| AG-1343 | nelfinavir mesylate |
| AG331 | metesind glucuronate |
| AG-337 | generic not yet assigned—see main list |
| AGN 190168 | tazarotene |
| AGN 190342-LF | brimonidine tartrate |
| AHR-11748 | dezinamide |
| AI204 | generic not yet assigned—see main list |
| AJ-2615 | monatepil maleate |
| AL-3432A | emedastine difumarate |
| AL-4862 | brinzolamide |
| AL-721 | generic not yet assigned—see main list |
| ALO 2184 | resocortol butyrate |
| ALO4943A | olopatadine HCl |
| ALRT 1057 | 9-cis-retinoic acid |
| ALVAC-120TMG | generic not yet assigned—see main list |
| ALVAC-HIV 1 | generic not yet assigned—see main list |
| AMI-121 | ferumoxsil |
| AMI-227 | generic not yet assigned—see main list |
| AMI-25 | ferumoxides |

| | |
|---|---|
| AN021 | tizanidine HCl |
| AN-051 | dezinamide |
| ANA-756 | generic not yet assigned—see main list |
| antibiotic 273a$_1$ | paldimycin |
| APL 400-020 | generic not yet assigned—see main list |
| AR-121 | nystatin liposomal |
| AR-177 | generic not yet assigned—see main list |
| AR-623 | generic not yet assigned—see main list |
| ARI-509 | generic not yet assigned—see main list |
| AS-013 | generic not yet assigned—see main list |
| AT-4140 | sparfloxacin |
| AY-22989 | sirolimus |
| AZT-P-ddI | zidovudine + didanosine |
| B1 61.012 | sargramostim |
| B19036/7 | gagobenate dimeglumine |
| BASF 52404 | linarotene |
| BAY i 3930 | isomalt |
| BAY w 6228 | cerivastatin sodium |
| BAY w 6240 | factor VIII (rDNA) |
| BAY X 1352 | nerelimomab |
| BAY y 7432 | ecadotril |
| BB-2516 | marimastat |
| BB-882 | lexipafant |
| BB-94 | batimastat |
| BBM-2478A | elsamitrucin |
| BCX-34 | peldesine |
| BEC-2 | generic not yet assigned—see main list |
| BG8967 | bivalirudin |
| BIIP 20 XX | apaxifylline |
| BI-L-239 | enofelast |
| BILA 2011 BS | palinavir |
| BIM-23014C | lanreotide acetate |
| BIRG 0587 | nevirapine |
| BIRM-270 | ontazolast |
| BI-RR-0001 | enlimomab |
| BM01.004 | metipranolol |
| BM 06.019 | epoetin beta |
| BM 14802 | generic not yet assigned—see main list |
| BM 41.440 | ilmofosine |
| BMS 180048 | avitriptan fumarate |
| BMS 180048-02 | avitriptan fumarate |
| BMS-180194 | lobucavir |
| BMS-180291 | ifetroban |
| BMS-180291-02 | ifetroban sodium |
| BMS 181101 | generic not yet assigned—see main list |
| BMS-181173 | gusperimus trihydrochloride |
| BMS-181339-01 | paclitaxel |
| BMS-186091 | ammonium lactate |
| BMS-186295 | irbesartan |
| BMY-05763-1-D | dexsotalol HCl |
| BMY 13754 | nefazodone HCl |
| BMY 14802 | generic not yet assigned—see main list |

| | |
|---|---|
| BMY-25801-01 | batanopride HCl |
| BMY-27857 | stavudine |
| BMY-28090 | elsamitrucin |
| BMY-28100-03-800 | cefprozil |
| BMY-28142 2HCl.H$_2$O | cefepime HCl |
| BMY-30056 | halobetasol propionate |
| BMY-40327 | modecainide |
| BMY 40481 | etoposide phosphate |
| BMY-40900 | didanosine |
| BMY-42215-1 | gusperimus trihydrochloride |
| BMY-45622 | generic not yet assigned—see main list |
| BP 1.02; S.049 | ecadotril |
| BRL-38227 | levcromakalim |
| BRL-39123 | penciclovir |
| BRL-42810 | famciclovir |
| BRL 43694 | granisetron |
| BRL 43694A | granisetron HCl |
| BRL 46470 | generic not yet assigned—see main list |
| BRL 4910F | mupirocin calcium |
| BRL55834 | generic not yet assigned—see main list |
| BRL 61063 | cipamfylline |
| BTS 54524 | sibutramine HCl |
| BTS67,583 | generic not yet assigned—see main list |
| BTS 7706 | debropol |
| BW 12C | generic not yet assigned—see main list |
| BW256U | valacyclovir |
| BY 1023 | pantoprazole |
| C-1 | edrecolomab |
| C-4 | imciromab pentetate |
| c7E3 | abciximab |
| CARN 750 | acemannan |
| CAS 936 | pirsidomine |
| CB 7432 | idoxifene |
| CCD 1042 | ganaxolone |
| CD 271 | adapalene |
| CDDD 3602 | tematropium methylsulfate |
| CDDD 5604 | loteprednol etabonate |
| CEN 000029 | priliximab |
| CEP 1538 | modafinil |
| GCA 18809 | azamethiphos |
| CGP 14,458 | halobetasol propionate |
| CGP 25827A | formoterol |
| CGP 30694 | edatrexate |
| CGP 32349 | formestane |
| CGP 39393 | desirudin |
| CGP 42446 | zoledronic acid |
| CGP 42446A | zoledronate disodium |
| CGP 42446B | zoledronate trisodium |
| CGP 45840B | diclofenac potassium |
| CGP 48933 | valsartan |
| CGP 57701 | generic not yet assigned—see main list |
| CGS 13429A | batelapine maleate |

| | |
|---|---|
| CGS 16949A | fadrozole HCl |
| CGS 18416A | zoniclezole HCl |
| CGS 19755 | selfotel |
| CGS 20267 | letrozole |
| CHX-3673 | amlexanox |
| CI-1020 | generic not yet assigned—see main list |
| CI-9148 | cysteamine HCl |
| CI 925 | moexipril HCl |
| CI-946 | ralitoline |
| CI-958 | sedoxantrone trihydrochloride |
| CI-960 HCl | clinafloxacin HCl |
| CI-977 | enadoline HCl |
| CI-978 | sparfloxacin |
| CI-979 | milameline HCl |
| CI-980 | generic not yet assigned—see main list |
| CI-981 | atorvastatin calcium |
| CI-982 | fosphenytoin sodium |
| CI-983 | cefdinir |
| CI-988 | generic not yet assigned—see main list |
| CI-991 | troglitazone |
| CL09 | icomethasone enbutate |
| CL 108,756 | brocresine |
| CL 184,116 | porfimer sodium |
| CL 184,824 | alovudine |
| CL 186,815 | biapenem |
| CL 273,547 | ocinaplon |
| CL 284,846 | zaleplon |
| CL 286,558 | zeniplatin |
| CL 287,110 | enloplatin |
| CL 291,894 | somagrebove |
| CL 297,939 | bisoprolol fumarate |
| CL 307,782 | levoleucovorin calcium |
| CL 318,952 | verteporfin |
| CL 81,587 | avoparcin |
| CNS 1102 | aptiganel HCl |
| CP-0127 | deltibant |
| CP-116,517-27 | alatrofloxacin mesylate |
| CP-118,954-11 | icopezil maleate |
| CP-148,623 | pamaqueside |
| CP-66,248 | tenidap |
| CP-70,429 | sulopenem |
| CP-70,490-09 | enazadrem phosphate |
| CP-72,133 | ilonidap |
| CP-72,467-2 | englitazone sodium |
| CP-73,850 | zopolrestat |
| CP-80,794 | terlakiren |
| CP-86,325-2 | darglitazone sodium |
| CP-88,059 | ziprasidone |
| CP-88,059-1 | ziprasidone HCl |
| CP-88,818 | tiqueside |
| CP-99,219-27 | trovafloxacin mesylate |
| CPC-111 | generic not yet assigned—see main list |

| | |
|---|---|
| CPC-211 | generic not yet assigned—see main list |
| CPT-11 | irinotecan |
| CRL 40476 | modafinil |
| CS-045 | troglitazone |
| CS-622 | temocapril HCl |
| CT 1501R | lisofylline |
| CTX | lornoxicam |
| CY-1503 | generic not yet assigned—see main list |
| CY-1787 | generic not yet assigned—see main list |
| CY-1899 | generic not yet assigned—see main list |
| CY 216 | nadroparin calcium |
| CYT-103 $^{111}$In | indium In 111 satumomab pendetide |
| CYT-103-Y-90 | generic not yet assigned—see main list |
| CYT-356 | capromab pendetide |
| CYT-356-In-111 | generic not yet assigned—see main list |
| CYT-356-Y-90 | generic not yet assigned—see main list |
| CYT-372-In-111 | generic not yet assigned—see main list |
| CYT-424 | samarium Sm 153 lexidronam penta-sodium |
| d4T | stavudine |
| DAU6215CL | itasetron |
| DCL Hb | hemoglobin crosfumaril |
| DMP 266 | generic not yet assigned—see main list |
| DMP-504 | generic not yet assigned—see main list |
| DMP 728 | generic not yet assigned—see main list |
| DMP 777 | generic not yet assigned—see main list |
| DMP 840 | bisnafide dimesylate |
| DN-2327 | pazinaclone |
| DO6 | lexipafant |
| DR-3355 | levofloxacin |
| DS 103-282 | tizanidine HCl |
| DS-4152 | tecogalan sodium |
| DTC 101 | generic not yet assigned—see main list |
| DTPA-SMS | pentetreotide |
| DuP 128 | lecimibide |
| DuP 753 | losartan potassium |
| DuP 921 | sibopirdine |
| DUP 937 | teloxantrone HCl |
| DUP 941 | losoxantrone |
| DuP 996 | linopirdine |
| DyDTPA-BMA | sprodiamide |
| E-2020 | generic not yet assigned—see main list |
| E-3810 | rabeprazole sodium |
| EF9 | temoporfin |
| EL10 | dehydroepiandrosterone |
| EL-970 | fampridine |
| EV2-7 | sevirumab |
| FC 41-12 | perflenapent + perflisopent |
| FCE 21336 | cabergoline |
| FCF 89 | roquinimex |
| FG-10571 | panadiplon |
| FGN-1 | generic not yet assigned—see main list |

| | |
|---|---|
| FK-037 | generic not yet assigned—see main list |
| FK-1052 | generic not yet assigned—see main list |
| FK-143 | generic not yet assigned—see main list |
| FK-176 | generic not yet assigned—see main list |
| FK-201 | quinotolast |
| FK-224 | generic not yet assigned—see main list |
| FK-3311 | generic not yet assigned—see main list |
| FK-366 | generic not yet assigned—see main list |
| FK-409 | generic not yet assigned—see main list |
| FK-453 | generic not yet assigned—see main list |
| FK-480 | generic not yet assigned—see main list |
| FK 482 | cefdinir |
| FK-506 | tacrolimus |
| FK-508 | generic not yet assigned—see main list |
| FK-565 | generic not yet assigned—see main list |
| FK-613 | generic not yet assigned—see main list |
| FK-739 | generic not yet assigned—see main list |
| FK-780 | generic not yet assigned—see main list |
| FK-906 | generic not yet assigned—see main list |
| FLA 731(–) | remoxipride HCl |
| FPL64170 | generic not yet assigned—see main list |
| FPL67085 | generic not yet assigned—see main list |
| FUT-175 | nafamostat mesylate |
| G-101 | erythromycin salnacedin |
| G-201 | salnacedin |
| G-203 | fluocinonide |
| GEM 91 | generic not yet assigned—see main list |
| GER-11 | pimagedine HCl |
| GG-167 | zanamivir |
| GI147211C | lurtotecan dihydrochloride |
| GI 87084B | remifentanil HCl |
| GL-701 | dehydroepiandrosterone |
| GLQ 223 | trichosanthin |
| GM 6001 | generic not yet assigned—see main list |
| GMC 89-107 | regramostim |
| GP-1-110 | acadesine |
| gp120 | generic not yet assigned—see main list |
| gp 160 | generic not yet assigned—see main list |
| GP-2-121-3 | arbutamine HCl |
| GR109714X | lamivudine |
| GR 114297A | picumeterol fumarate |
| GR 114297X (picumeterol) | picumeterol fumarate |
| GR 116526X | isotretinoin anisatil |
| GR 122311X | ranitidine bismuth citrate |
| GR 138950C | saprisartan potassium |
| GR 32191B | vapiprost HCl |
| GR 33343 G | salmeterol xinafoate |
| GR 68755C | alosetron HCl |
| GR 81225C | galdansetron HCl |
| GR 85478 | generic not yet assigned—see main list |
| GR 85548A | naratriptan HCl |
| GR 87442 N | luroseron mesylate |

| | |
|---|---|
| GR92132 | troglitazone |
| GR 69153X | cefetecol |
| GRF1-44 | generic not yet assigned—see main list |
| GS-0504 | cidofovir |
| GS-0840 | adefovir dipivoxil |
| GS 393 | generic not yet assigned—see main list |
| GS 504 | generic not yet assigned—see main list |
| GS 840 | adefovir dipivoxil |
| GV 104326B | sanfetrinem sodium |
| GV 118819X | sanfetrinem cilexetil |
| GW-80126 | seprilose |
| H 168/68 sodium | omeprazole sodium |
| H65-RTA | zolimomab aritox |
| H 93/26 succinate | metoprolol succinate |
| HA-1A | nebacumab |
| HBY097 | generic not yet assigned—see main list |
| HGP-1 | loteprednol etabonate |
| HGP-30 | generic not yet assigned—see main list |
| HGP-6 | tematropium methylsulfate |
| HNK-20 | generic not yet assigned—see main list |
| HOE 077 | lufironil |
| HOE 140 | icatibant acetate |
| HOE 18 680 | embutramide |
| HOE 296b | ciclopirox |
| HOE 490 | glimepiride |
| HP 290 | quilostigmine |
| HP 749 | besipirdine HCl |
| HP 873 | iloperidone |
| HPA-23 | generic not yet assigned—see main list |
| HR111V-sulfate | cefquinome sulfate |
| HR 221 (as sodium) | cefodizime |
| HU-211 | generic not yet assigned—see main list |
| HWA 285 | propentofylline |
| Hyal-ct 1101 | generic not yet assigned—see main list |
| ICI 139603 | tetronasin |
| ICI 176,334 | bicalutamide |
| ICI 204,219 | zafirlukast |
| ICI 204,636 | quetiapine fumarate |
| ICI D1033 | anastrozole |
| ICRF-187 | dexrazoxane |
| IDEC-C2B8 | rituximab |
| IDEC-CE9.1 | generic not yet assigned—see main list |
| IMMU-4 | arcitumomab |
| IMMU-LL2 | bectumomab |
| IMMU-MN3 | sulesomab |
| IP 302 sodium | citicoline sodium |
| IP 456 | pagoclone |
| ISIS 2105 | generic not yet assigned—see main list |
| ISIS 2922 | generic not yet assigned—see main list |
| K 12148 | lifibrol |
| Kabi 2234 | generic not yet assigned—see main list |
| KNI-272 | generic not yet assigned—see main list |

| | |
|---|---|
| KP-363 | butenafine HCl |
| KW4679 | olopatadine HCl |
| L1 | deferiprone |
| L-627 | biapenem |
| L-668,019 | verlukast |
| L-696,229 | generic not yet assigned—see main list |
| L-697,661 | generic not yet assigned—see main list |
| L-735,524 | indinavir sulfate |
| LAS 30451 | pancopride |
| LDI-200 | generic not yet assigned—see main list |
| Leo 1031 | prednimustine |
| LFA3TIP | generic not yet assigned—see main list |
| LGD 1069 | generic not yet assigned—see main list |
| LJ C10,627 | biapenem |
| LM-427 | rifabutin |
| LS 2616 | roquinimex |
| Lu 23-174 | sertindole |
| LY031537 | ractopamine HCl |
| LY170053 | olanzapine |
| LY170680 | sulukast |
| LY177370 phosphate | tilmicosin phosphate |
| LY186641 | sulofenur |
| LY 201116 | ameltolide |
| LY206243 lactobionate | levdobutamine lactobionate |
| LY207506 | dobutamine lactobionate |
| LY210448 HCl | dapoxetine HCl |
| LY 213829 | tazofelone |
| LY215229 HCl | seproxetine HCl |
| LY237733 | amesergide |
| LY246708 | xanomeline |
| LY246708 tartrate | xanomeline tartrate |
| LY248686 HCl | duloxetine HCl |
| LY253351 | tamsulosin HCl |
| LY264618 | lometrexol sodium |
| LY275585 | insulin lyspro |
| LY277359 | zatosetron maleate |
| LY 293111 | generic not yet assigned—see main list |
| LY293404 | rismorelin porcine |
| LY294468 sulfate | efegatran sulfate |
| LY295337 | basifungin |
| LY307640 sodium | rabeprazole sodium |
| LY 333334 | teriparatide |
| MAB35 | indium In 111 altumomab pentetate |
| MAK 195 F | generic not yet assigned—see main list |
| MC 903 | calcipotriene |
| MDL 100,240 | generic not yet assigned—see main list |
| MDL 11,939 | glemanserin |
| MDL 16,455A | fexofenadine HCl |
| MDL 18,962 | plomestane |
| MDL-201129 | beraprost sodium |
| MDL-201229 | beraprost |
| MDL 201,404 | generic not yet assigned—see main list |

| | |
|---|---|
| MDL 26,024G0 | tetrazolast meglumine |
| MDL 26,479 | suritozole |
| MDL 27,192 | generic not yet assigned—see main list |
| MDL 28,314 | generic not yet assigned—see main list |
| MDL 28,574 | generic not yet assigned—see main list |
| MDL 62,198 | ramoplanin |
| MDL 62,769 | rifamexil |
| MDL 72,222 | bemesetron |
| MDL 72,974A | mofegiline HCl |
| MDL 73,005EF | binospirone mesylate |
| MDL 73,147EF | dolasetron mesylate |
| MDL 73,745 | zifrosilone |
| MDL 73,945 | camiglibose |
| MEDI 493 | generic not yet assigned—see main list |
| MEDR-640 | generic not yet assigned—see main list |
| MF 934 | rufloxacin |
| MK-0462 | rizatriptan benzoate |
| MK-233 | dexibuprofen lysine |
| MK-383 | generic not yet assigned—see main list |
| MK-397 | eprinomectin |
| MK-462 | generic not yet assigned—see main list |
| MK-476 | montelukast sodium |
| MK-499 | generic not yet assigned—see main list |
| MK-507 | dorzolamide HCl |
| MK-591 | quiflapon sodium |
| MK-639 | indinavir sulfate |
| MK790 | levomethadyl acetate HCl |
| MK-793 | diltiazem maleate |
| MK-966 | generic not yet assigned—see main list |
| MK-A462 | rizatriptan sulfate |
| ML-1129 | beraprost sodium |
| ML-1229 | beraprost |
| MP-1177 | gadoversetamide |
| MP-1196 | versetamide |
| MP-1554 | technetium Tc 99m furifosmin |
| MP-1727 | indium In 111 pentetreotide |
| MR6S4 | sevoflurane |
| MSI-78 | generic not yet assigned—see main list |
| MSL-109 | sevirumab |
| MY-5116 | repirinast |
| NE-10064 | azimilide dihydrochloride |
| NE 11740 | tebufelone |
| NE-58095 | risedronate sodium |
| NG-29 | generic not yet assigned—see main list |
| NGD 91-1 | generic not yet assigned—see main list |
| NK 204 | basifungin |
| NKT-01 | gusperimus trihydrochloride |
| NNC-05-0328 | tiagabine HCl |
| NO-05-0328 | tiagabine HCl |
| NXX-066 | quilostigmine |
| OK-B7 | generic not yet assigned—see main list |
| OLX-102 | generic not yet assigned—see main list |

| | |
|---|---|
| OM 401 | generic not yet assigned—see main list |
| OMS No 1825 | azamethiphos |
| ONO-1078 | generic not yet assigned—see main list |
| OP 21-23 | parnaparin sodium |
| OPC-14117 | generic not yet assigned—see main list |
| OPC-14597 | aripiprazole |
| OPC-17116 | grepafloxacin HCl |
| OPC-31 | aripiprazole |
| ORG 10172 | danaparoid sodium |
| ORG 2969 | desogestrel |
| ORG 3236 | etonogestrel |
| Org 32489 | generic not yet assigned—see main list |
| Org 6216 | rimexolone |
| ORG7417 | resocortol butyrate |
| ORG 9426 | rocuronium bromide |
| P-280 | generic not yet assigned—see main list |
| P-3232 | somfasepor |
| P-3895 | somfasepor |
| P53 | tetrofosmin |
| P-5604 | loteprednol etabonate |
| P829 | generic not yet assigned—see main list |
| P83 6029A | velnacrine maleate |
| PC1020 acetate | prezatide copper acetate |
| PD 81565 | pentostatin |
| PDA-641 | generic not yet assigned—see main list |
| PE1-1 | tuvirumab |
| PEM-420 | generic not yet assigned—see main list |
| PHXA41 | latanoprost |
| PIXY321 | milodistim |
| PMD-387 | crilvastatin |
| PPI-002 | generic not yet assigned—see main list |
| PR-122 | redox phenytoin |
| PR-225 | redox acyclovir |
| PR-239 | redox penicillin G |
| PR-320 | molecusol & carbamazepine |
| PSC-833 | generic not yet assigned—see main list |
| Q-12 | technetium Tc 99m furifosmin |
| R106-1 | basifungin |
| R 55104 | erbulozole |
| R 60844 | irtemazole |
| R 64947 | noberastine |
| R 66905 | saperconazole |
| R 68070 | ridogrel |
| R 72063 | loreclezole |
| R 75231 | draflazine |
| R 75251 | liarozole HCl |
| R 77975 | pirodavir |
| R 79598 | ocaperidone |
| R-837 | imiquimod |
| R 83842 | vorozole |
| R 85246 | liarozole fumarate |
| R 87 926 | generic not yet assigned—see main list |

| | |
|---|---|
| R 89 439 | generic not yet assigned—see main list |
| R 91,274 | alniditan dihydrochloride |
| R 93,777 | generic not yet assigned—see main list |
| R 93,877 | generic not yet assigned—see main list |
| RBC-CD4 | generic not yet assigned—see main list |
| RG 12525 | generic not yet assigned—see main list |
| RG 12561 | dalvastatin |
| RG-12915 | generic not yet assigned—see main list |
| RG 12986 | generic not yet assigned—see main list |
| RG 201 | generic not yet assigned—see main list |
| RG 83606 | diltiazem HCl |
| RG 83894 | generic not yet assigned—see main list |
| RGG0853,E1A | generic not yet assigned—see main list |
| rgp160 | generic not yet assigned—see main list |
| rgp160 MN | generic not yet assigned—see main list |
| RGW-2938 | prinoxodan |
| RJW 49004 | cedelizumab |
| RJW 60235 | becaplermin |
| r-metHuG-CSF | filgrastim |
| RMP-7 | generic not yet assigned—see main list |
| Ro 01-6794/706 | dextrorphan HCl |
| Ro 03-7355/000 | avizafone |
| Ro 09-1978/000 | capecitabine |
| Ro 14-9706/000 | sumarotene |
| Ro 15-1570/000 | etarotene |
| Ro 16-6028/000 | bretazenil |
| Ro 18-0647/002 | orlistat |
| Ro 19-6327/000 | lazabemide |
| Ro 24-2027/000 | zalcitabine |
| Ro 24-5913 | cinalukast |
| Ro 24-7375 | dacliximab |
| Ro 24-7429 | generic not yet assigned—see main list |
| Ro 31-8959 | saquinavir |
| Ro 31-8959/003 | saquinavir mesylate |
| Ro 40-5967/001 | mibefradil dihydrochloride |
| Ro 40-7592 | tolcapone |
| Ro 42-1611 | arteflene |
| Ro 44-9883/000 | lamifiban |
| Ro 46-6240/000 | napsagatran |
| Ro 47-0203/029 | bosentan |
| rp24 | generic not yet assigned—see main list |
| RP 27267 | zopiclone |
| RP 31264 | suriclone |
| RP 5337 | spiramycin |
| RP 54274 | rulizole |
| RP 54476 | dalfopristin |
| RP 54563 | enoxaparin sodium |
| RP 56976 | docetaxel |
| RP 57669 | quinupristin |
| RP 60180 | generic not yet assigned—see main list |
| RP 60475 | intoplicine |
| RP 62203 | fanserin |

| | |
|---|---|
| RP 62955 | pagoclone |
| RP 64305 | ebastine |
| RP 64477 | generic not yet assigned—see main list |
| RP 73401 | piclamilast |
| RS-10085-197 | moexipril HCl |
| RS 15385 | generic not yet assigned—see main list |
| RS-15385-197 | delequamine HCl |
| RS-21607-197 | azalanstat dihydrochloride |
| RS 25259 | palonosetron HCl |
| RS-26306 | ganirelix acetate |
| RS-61443 | mycophenolate mofetil |
| RS 66271 | generic not yet assigned—see main list |
| RS-87476-000 | lifarizine |
| RU 23908 | nilutamide |
| RU 27987 | trimegestone |
| RU35926 | milameline HCl |
| RU 38486 | mifepristone |
| RU 44570 | trandolapril |
| RU 486 | mifepristone |
| RU 882 | inocoterone acetate |
| RWJ-17021 | topiramate |
| RWJ 21757 | loroxibine |
| RWJ 23989 | generic not yet assigned—see main list |
| RWJ 24517 | carsatrin succinate |
| RWJ 24834 | linarotene |
| RWJ-25213 | levofloxacin |
| RWJ 29091 | generic not yet assigned—see main list |
| RWJ 26127 | generic not yet assigned—see main list |
| RWJ 26251 | cladribine |
| RWJ 28299 | immune globulin intravenous pente-tate |
| RWJ 37796 | mazapertine succinate |
| R-(–)-YM-12617 | tamsulosin HCl |
| S-041 | gadodiamide |
| S-043 | sprodiamide |
| S26308 | imiquimod |
| SB-209247 | ticolubant |
| SB-210396 | generic not yet assigned—see main list |
| SB-223030 | idoxifene |
| SC-40230 | bidisomide |
| SC-48834 | remiprostol |
| SC-49483 | generic not yet assigned—see main list |
| SC-52151 | telinavir |
| SC-52458 | forasartan |
| SC-54684A | xemilofiban HCl |
| SC-55389A | droxinavir HCl |
| SC-57099B | orbofiban acetate |
| SC-58635 | celecoxib |
| SC-66110 | eplerenone |
| Sch 39300 | molgramostim |
| SCH 40054 HCl | nemazoline HCl |
| SCY-Er | erythromycin salnacedin |

| | |
|---|---|
| SDZ 215-811 | pentetreotide |
| SDZ 215-811s | pentetreotide |
| SDZ ILE 964 | muplestim |
| SDZ MSL 109 | sevirumab |
| SDZ OST 577 | tuvirumab |
| SEB-324 | generic not yet assigned—see main list |
| SEC-579 | generic not yet assigned—see main list |
| SF-R11 | bovactant |
| SGP 3 | unifocon A |
| SH 570 | generic not yet assigned—see main list |
| SK&F 101468-A | ropinirole HCl |
| SK&F 104353-Q | pobilukast edamine |
| SKF 105657 | epristeride |
| SK&F 10623 | generic not yet assigned—see main list |
| SK&F 106615-A2 | altiprimod dihydrochloride |
| SK&F 108566 | eprosartan |
| SK&F 108566-J | eprosartan mesylate |
| SK&F 110679 | generic not yet assigned—see main list |
| SK&F 96022 | pantoprazole |
| SK&F 97426 | generic not yet assigned—see main list |
| SK&F S-104846-A | topotecan HCl |
| SM-7338 | meropenem |
| Sms2PA | strontium chloride Sr 89 |
| SNX-111 | generic not yet assigned—see main list |
| SP-303 | generic not yet assigned—see main list |
| SPC-100270 | safingol |
| SPC-100271 | safingol HCl |
| SPC-101210 | cedefingol |
| SPM 925 | moexipril HCl |
| SQ 26,703 | zofenoprilat arginine |
| SQ 27,519 | fosinoprilat |
| SQ 29,852 | ceronapril |
| SQ 32,097 | technetium Tc 99m siboroxime |
| SQ 32,692 | gadoteridol |
| SQ 32,756 | sorivudine |
| SQ 33,248 | calteridol calcium |
| SQ 34,514 | lobucavir |
| SR 25990 C | clopidogrel |
| SR 33557 | fantofarone |
| SR 41319B | tiludronate disodium |
| SR 47436 | irbesartan |
| SR 96225 | adenosine |
| ST1512/SO4 | hexoprenaline sulfate |
| SU-101 | generic not yet assigned—see main list |
| SUD919CL2Y | pramipexole |
| T2G1s | biciromab |
| T30177 | generic not yet assigned—see main list |
| T-3761 | generic not yet assigned—see main list |
| T-3762 | generic not yet assigned—see main list |
| T-88 | generic not yet assigned—see main list |
| TBC-3B | generic not yet assigned—see main list |
| TC-CYT-380 | generic not yet assigned—see main list |

| | |
|---|---|
| TC-CYT-380 fragment | generic not yet assigned—see main list |
| THR 221 (as sodium) | cefodizime |
| TI-23 | generic not yet assigned—see main list |
| TJ-9 | generic not yet assigned—see main list |
| TLC A-60 | generic not yet assigned—see main list |
| TLC ABLC | generic not yet assigned—see main list |
| TLC C-53 | generic not yet assigned—see main list |
| TLC D-99 | generic not yet assigned—see main list |
| TNF MAb | nerelinomab |
| TNP-470 | generic not yet assigned—see main list |
| TP-1 | thymostimulin |
| TV-1203 | generic not yet assigned—see main list |
| TVP-1012 | rasagiline mesylate |
| U-101.440E | irinotecan HCl |
| U-10,483 | generic not yet assigned—see main list |
| U-70226E | ibutilide fumarate |
| U-73,975 | adozelesin |
| U-77779 | bizelesin |
| U-78875 | panadiplon |
| U-78,938 | dexormaplatin |
| U-80244 | carzelesin |
| U-82127 | alexomycin |
| U-85,855 | alvircept sudotox |
| U-87201E | atevirdine mesylate |
| U-88943E | artilide fumarate |
| U89 | generic not yet assigned—see main list |
| U-90152S | delavirdine mesylate |
| U-93,385 | generic not yet assigned—see main list |
| U-95376 | premafloxacin |
| U-96988 | generic not yet assigned—see main list |
| U-98079A | itasetron |
| U-98222 | generic not yet assigned—see main list |
| U-98528E | pramipexole |
| U-98950 | generic not yet assigned—see main list |
| UDCG-115 | pimobendan |
| UF-021 | isopropyl unoprostone |
| UK-109,496 | generic not yet assigned—see main list |
| UK-14304-18 | brimonidine tartrate |
| UK-61260-27 | nanterinone |
| UK-67,994 | doramectin |
| UK-68,798 | dofetilide |
| UK-76654-2 (as fumarate) | zamifenacin |
| UK-79,300 | candoxatril |
| UK-80067 | modipafant |
| UK-88060 | espatropate |
| VCP 205 | generic not yet assigned—see main list |
| VLA-4 | generic not yet assigned—see main list |
| VUAB6453 (SPOFA) | metipranolol |
| VX-105 | arginine butyrate |
| VX-478 | generic not yet assigned—see main list |
| W-554 | felbamate |
| WAL 2014 FU | talsaclidine fumarate |

| | |
|---|---|
| WAY-ACA-147 | eldacimibe |
| WAY-ANA-756 | tasosartan |
| WAY-ARI-509 | minalrestat |
| WAY-PDA-641 | filaminast |
| WAY-PEM-420 | dexpemedolac |
| WAY-SEC-579 | mirisetron maleate |
| WIN 22118 | pegorgotein |
| Win 49,596 | zanoterone |
| WIN 59010 | generic not yet assigned—see main list |
| Win 59075 | tirapazamine |
| WY-44,635 sodium | cefpiramide sodium |
| WY-47791 HCl | carvotroline HCl |
| WY-47846 HCl | zalospirone HCl |
| WY-48252 | ritolukast |
| WY-48314 | lexithromycin |
| WY-50324 HCl | adatanserin HCl |
| WY-90493 RD | ardeparin sodium |
| XA41 | latanoprost |
| YM-12617-1 | tamsulosin HCl |
| YM617 | tamsulosin HCl |
| YN-72 | sorivudine |
| Z 1282 | fosfomycin tromethamine |
| ZCE025 | indium In 111 altumomab |
| ZD 0490 | generic not yet assigned—see main list |
| ZD 0870 | generic not yet assigned—see main list |
| ZD1033 | anastrozole |
| ZD 1694 | raltitrexed |
| ZD2079 | generic not yet assigned—see main list |
| ZD 2138 | generic not yet assigned—see main list |
| ZD 3523 | generic not yet assigned—see main list |
| ZD5077 | quetiapine fumarate |
| ZD 7288 | generic not yet assigned—see main list |
| Zeneca 182,780 | generic not yet assigned—see main list |
| Zeneca 200,880 | generic not yet assigned—see main list |
| ZK 35760 | iopromide |
| ZK 62498 | azelaic acid |
| ZM 204,636 | quetirapine fumarate |

APPENDIX **C**
# Abbreviations Used with Medications and Dosages

| Abbreviation | Literally | Meaning |
|---|---|---|
| a.c. | ante cibum | before meals or food |
| ad | ad | to, up to |
| A.D., AD | auris dextra | right ear |
| ad lib. | ad libitum | at pleasure |
| A.L. | auris laeva | left ear |
| a.m., A.M. | ante meridiem | morning |
| Aq. | aqua | water |
| A.S., AS | auris sinistra | left ear |
| A.U., AU* | auris uterque | each ear |
| b.i.d. | bis in die | twice daily |
| b.m. | bowel movement | |
| cc, cm³ | cubic centimeter | |
| d. | die | day |
| et | et | and |
| g | gram(s) | |
| gt. (plural gtt.) | gutta (plural guttae) | a drop (drops) |
| h. | hora | hour |
| h.s. | hora somni | at bedtime |
| IM† | intramuscular | |
| IV† | intravenous | |
| mcg, μg | microgram(s) | |
| mg | milligram(s) | |
| mEq | milliequivalent(s) | |
| mL, ml | milliliter(s) | |
| O.D. | oculus dexter | right eye |
| O.L. | oculus laevus | left eye |
| O.S. | oculus sinister | left eye |
| O.U.§ | oculus uterque | each eye |
| p.c. | post cibum | after meals |
| p.m., P.M. | post meridiem | afternoon or evening |
| p.o. | per os | by mouth |
| p.r.n. | pro re nata | as needed |
| q.a.d. | quaque alterni die | every other day |
| q.d. | quaque die | every day |
| q.h. | quaque hora | every hour |
| q.i.d. | quater in die | four times a day |
| q.o.d. | | every other day |
| q.s. | quantum satis | sufficient quantity |
| q.s. ad | quantum satis ad | a sufficient quantity to make |
| Rx, Rx | recipe | take; a recipe |

| Abbreviation | Literally | Meaning |
| --- | --- | --- |
| Sig. | signetur | label |
| s.o.s. | si opus sit | if there is need |
| stat | statim | at once, immediately |
| t.i.d. | ter in die | three times a day |
| tsp. | teaspoonful | |
| μg, mcg | microgram(s) | |

---

[*] Although some references have aures unitas (Latin, both ears), this cannot be justified by classical Latin.

[†] Some references suggest that IM and IV be typed with periods to distinguish from Roman numerals, but we believe context is sufficient to make this distinction.

[§] Although some references have oculi unitas (Latin, both eyes), this cannot be justified by classical Latin.

# Therapeutic Drug Levels

| Drug | Class | Serum Levels<br>metric units (SI units) |
|------|-------|----------------------|
| amantadine | antiviral | 300 ng/mL |
| amikacin | aminoglycoside | 16-32 μg/mL |
| amiodarone | antiarrhythmic | 0.5-2.5 μg/mL |
| amitriptyline | antidepressant | 110-250 ng/mL |
| amoxapine | antidepressant | 200-500 ng/mL |
| amrinone | cardiotonic | 3.7 μg/mL |
| bretylium | antiarrhythmic | 0.5-1.5 μg/mL |
| bupropion | antidepressant | 25-100 ng/mL |
| carbamazepine | anticonvulsant | 4-12 μg/mL (17-51 μmol/L) |
| chloramphenicol | antibiotic | 10-20 μg/mL (31-62 μmol/L) |
| chlorpromazine | antipsychotic | 30-500 ng/mL |
| clomipramine | antidepressant | 80-100 ng/mL |
| cyclosporine | immunosuppressive | 250-800 ng/mL (whole blood, RIA*) |
| trough values: | | 50-300 ng/mL (plasma, RIA*) |
| desipramine | antidepressant | 125-300 ng/mL |
| digitoxin | antiarrhythmic | 9-25 μg/L (11.8-32.8 nmol/L) |
| digoxin | antiarrhythmic | 0.5-2.2 ng/mL (0.6-2.8 nmol/L) |
| disopyramide | antiarrhythmic | 2-8 μg/mL (6-18 μmol/L) |
| doxepin | antidepressant | 100-200 ng/mL |
| flecainide | antiarrhythmic | 0.2-1 μg/mL |
| fluphenazine | antipsychotic | 0.13-2.8 ng/mL |
| gentamicin | aminoglycoside | 4-8 μg/mL |
| haloperidol | antipsychotic | 5-20 ng/mL |
| hydralazine | antihypertensive | 100 ng/mL |
| imipramine | antidepressant | 200-350 ng/mL |
| kanamycin | aminoglycoside | 15-40 μg/mL |
| lidocaine | antiarrhythmic | 1.5-6 μg/mL (4.5-21.5 μmol/L) |
| lithium | antipsychotic | 0.5-1.5 mEq/L (0.5-1.5 mmol/L) |
| maprotiline | antidepressant | 200-300 ng/mL |
| mexiletine | antiarrhythmic | 0.5-2 μg/mL |
| netilmicin | aminoglycoside | 6-10 μg/mL |
| nortriptyline | antidepressant | 50-150 ng/mL |
| perphenazine | antipsychotic | 0.8-1.2 ng/mL |

| Drug | Class | Serum Levels<br>*metric units (SI units)* |
|---|---|---|
| phenobarbital | anticonvulsant | 15-40 µg/mL (65-172 µmol/L) |
| phenytoin | anticonvulsant | 10-20 µg/mL (40-80 µmol/L) |
| primidone | anticonvulsant | 5-12 µg/mL (25-46 µmol/L) |
| procainamide | antiarrhythmic | 4-8 µg/mL (17-34 µmol/L) |
| propranolol | antiarrhythmic | 50-200 ng/mL (190-770 nmol/L) |
| protriptyline | antidepressant | 100-200 ng/mL |
| quinidine | antiarrhythmic | 2-6 µg/mL (4.6-9.2 µmol/L) |
| salicylate | analgesic | 100-200 mg/L (725 1448 µmol/L) |
| streptomycin | aminoglycoside | 20-30 µg/mL |
| sulfonamide | antibiotic | 5-15 mg/dL |
| terbutaline | bronchodilator | 0.5-4.1 ng/mL |
| theophylline | bronchodilator | 10-20 µg/mL (55-110 µmol/L) |
| thiothixene | antipsychotic | 2-57 ng/mL |
| tobramycin | aminoglycoside | 4-8 µg/mL |
| tocainide | antiarrhythmic | 4-10 µg/mL |
| trazodone | antidepressant | 800-1600 ng/mL |
| valproic acid | anticonvulsant | 50-100 µg/mL (350-700 µmol/L) |
| vancomycin | antibiotic | 30-40 ng/mL (peak) |
| verapamil | antiarrhythmic | 0.08-0.3 µg/mL |

* radioimmunoassay

# The Most Prescribed Drugs

| Drug | Class/Indications |
|------|-------------------|
| Accupril (quinapril HCl) | antihypertensive, ACE inhibitor |
| acetaminophen with codeine | analgesic, anti-inflammatory |
| Adalat CC (nifedipine) | antianginal, antihypertensive |
| albuterol sulfate | bronchodilator |
| alprazolam | anxiolytic, sedative |
| Altace (ramipril) | antihypertensive, ACE inhibitor |
| Ambien (zolpidem tartrate) | sedative, hypnotic |
| amoxicillin trihydrate | antibiotic |
| Amoxil (amoxicillin trihydrate) | antibiotic |
| atenolol | antiadrenergic |
| Atrovent (ipratropium bromide) | bronchodilator |
| Augmentin (amoxicillin trihydrate, clavulanate potassium) | antibiotic |
| Axid (nizatidine) | antiulcer, $H_2$ antagonist |
| Azmacort (triamcinolone acetonide) | corticosteroid for asthma |
| Bactroban (mupirocin) | topical antibiotic |
| Beconase AQ (beclomethasone dipropionate) | steroidal anti-inflammatory |
| Biaxin (clarithromycin) | antibiotic |
| BuSpar (buspirone HCl) | anxiolytic |
| Calan SR (verapamil HCl) | antianginal, antiarrhythmic, antihypertensive |
| Capoten (captopril) | antihypertensive, ACE inhibitor |
| Cardizem CD (diltiazem HCl) | antihypertensive, antianginal |
| Cardura (doxazosin mesylate) | antihypertensive, antiadrenergic |
| carisoprodol | skeletal muscle relaxant |
| cefaclor | antibiotic |
| Ceftin (cefuroxime axetil) | antibiotic |
| Cefzil (cefprozil) | antibiotic |
| cephalexin | antibiotic |
| cimetidine | antiulcer |
| Cipro (ciprofloxacin) | antibiotic |
| Claritin (loratadine) | antihistamine |
| Claritin-D (loratadine, pseudoephedrine sulfate) | antihistamine, decongestant |
| clonidine | antihypertensive |
| Coumadin (warfarin sodium) | anticoagulant |
| Cozaar (losartan potassium) | antihypertensive |
| cyclobenzaprine HCl | skeletal muscle relaxant |
| Cycrin (medroxyprogesterone acetate) | progestin |
| Darvocet-N 100 (propoxyphene napsylate, acetaminophen) | narcotic analgesic |
| Daypro (oxaprozin) | NSAID |

| | |
|---|---|
| Deltasone (prednisone) | glucocorticoid |
| Demulen 1/35 (ethynodiol diacetate, ethinyl estradiol) | monophasic oral contraceptive |
| Depakote (divalproex sodium) | anticonvulsant |
| Desogen (ethinyl estradiol, desogestrel) | monophasic oral contraceptive |
| diazepam | anxiolytic, skeletal muscle relaxant |
| diclofenac potassium/diclofenac sodium | NSAID |
| dicyclomine HCl | antispasmodic, anticholinergic |
| Diflucan (fluconazole) | systemic antifungal |
| Dilacor XR (diltiazem HCl) | antihypertensive |
| Dilantin (phenytoin sodium) | anticonvulsant |
| doxycycline hyclate | antibacterial |
| Duricef (cefadroxil monohydrate) | antibiotic |
| Dyazide (hydrochlorothiazide, triamterene) | diuretic, antihypertensive |
| Effexor (venlafaxine) | antidepressant |
| Elocon (mometasone furoate) | topical corticosteroid |
| Ery-Tab (erythromycin) | antibiotic |
| Erythrocin Stearate (erythromycin stearate) | antibiotic |
| Estrace (estradiol) | topical estrogen |
| Estraderm (estradiol) | estrogen replacement |
| Flonase (fluticasone propionate) | steroidal anti-inflammatory |
| Floxin (ofloxacin) | antibiotic |
| Fosamax (alendronate sodium) | postmenopausal osteoporosis treatment |
| furosemide | diuretic, antihypertensive |
| gemfibrozil | antihyperlipidemic |
| Genora 1/35 (norethindrone, ethinyl estradiol) | monophasic oral contraceptive |
| glipizide | antidiabetic |
| Glucophage (metformin HCl) | antidiabetic |
| Glucotrol XL (glipizide) | antidiabetic |
| glyburide | antidiabetic |
| Glynase (glyburide) | antidiabetic |
| guaifenesin with phenylpropanolamine | expectorant, decongestant |
| Humulin 70/30, N, R (human insulin) | antidiabetic |
| hydrochlorothiazide | diuretic, antihypertensive |
| hydrocodone with acetaminophen | antitussive, analgesic |
| Hytrin (terazosin HCl) | antihypertensive |
| ibuprofen | NSAID |
| Imdur (isosorbide mononitrate) | antianginal |
| Imitrex (sumatriptan succinate) | antimigraine |
| K-Dur (potassium chloride) | potassium supplement |
| Klonopin (clonazepam) | anticonvulsant |
| Klor-Con (potassium chloride) | potassium supplement |
| Lanoxin (digoxin) | antiarrhythmic |
| Lasix (furosemide) | diuretic |
| Lescol (fluvastatin sodium) | antihyperlipidemic |
| Levoxyl (levothyroxine sodium) | thyroid hormone |
| Lodine (etodolac) | NSAID, analgesic, antiarthritic |
| Loestrin Fe (norethindrone acetate, ethinyl estradiol, ferrous fumarate) | monophasic oral contraceptive with iron |

| | |
|---|---|
| Lo/Ovral (ethinyl estradiol, norgestrel) | monophasic oral contraceptive |
| Lopressor (metoprolol tartrate) | antianginal, antihypertensive, beta blocker |
| Lorabid (loracarbef) | antibiotic |
| lorazepam | anxiolytic, tranquilizer |
| Lotrisone (betamethasone dipropionate, clotrimazole) | topical corticosteroid, antifungal |
| Macrobid (nitrofurantoin macrocrystals, nitrofurantoin monohydrate) | urinary antibacterial |
| medroxyprogesterone | progestin |
| methylphenidate HCl | CNS stimulant for ADHD |
| methylprednisolone | corticosteroidal anti-inflammatory |
| metoprolol tartrate | antiadrenergic |
| Mevacor (lovastatin) | antihyperlipidemic |
| Monopril (fosinopril sodium) | antihypertensive, ACE inhibitor |
| naproxen sodium | NSAID, antiarthritic, analgesic |
| neomycin/polymyxin/hydrocortisone | antibiotic, steroidal anti-inflammatory |
| Nitro-Dur (nitroglycerin) | antianginal |
| Nitrostat (nitroglycerin) | antianginal |
| Norvasc (amlodipine) | antianginal, antihypertensive |
| Ortho-Cept (ethinyl estradiol, desogestrel) | monophasic oral contraceptive |
| Ortho-Cyclen (norgestimate, ethinyl estradiol) | monophasic oral contraceptive |
| Ortho-Novum 1/35 (norethindrone, ethinyl estradiol) | monophasic oral contraceptive |
| Ortho-Novum 7/7/7 (norethindrone, ethinyl estradiol) | triphasic oral contraceptive |
| Ortho Tri-Cyclen (norgestimate, ethinyl estradiol) | triphasic oral contraceptive |
| Oruvail (ketoprofen) | NSAID, antiarthritic, analgesic |
| Paxil (paroxetine HCl) | antidepressant |
| Pepcid (famotidine) | antiulcer |
| Phenergan (promethazine HCl) | antihistamine, antiemetic, sedative |
| phentermine | anorexiant, CNS stimulant |
| Pondimin (fenfluramine HCl) | anorexiant, CNS depressant |
| potassium chloride | potassium supplement |
| Pravachol (pravastatin sodium) | antihyperlipidemic |
| prednisone | corticosteroidal anti-inflammatory |
| Premarin (conjugated estrogen) | estrogen replacement |
| Prempro (conjugated estrogens, medroxyprogesterone acetate) | hormone replacement therapy |
| Prevacid (lansoprazole) | antisecretory, antiulcer |
| Prilosec (omeprazole) | antiulcer |
| Principen (ampicillin trihydrate) | antibiotic |
| Prinivil (lisinopril) | antihypertensive, ACE inhibitor |
| Procardia XL (nifedipine) | antianginal, antihypertensive |
| promethazine with codeine | narcotic antitussive, antihistamine |
| Propacet 100 (propoxyphene napsylate, acetaminophen) | narcotic analgesic |
| propoxyphene napsylate with acetaminophen | narcotic analgesic |

| | |
|---|---|
| Propulsid (cisapride) | gastroesophageal reflux |
| Proventil aerosol (albuterol) | bronchodilator |
| Prozac (fluoxetine HCl) | antidepressant |
| Relafen (namubetone) | NSAID, antiarthritic |
| Retin-A (tretinoin) | topical keratolytic |
| Risperdal (risperidone) | antipsychotic |
| Ritalin (methylphenidate HCl) | CNS stimulant for ADHD |
| Roxicet (oxycodone HCl, acetaminophen) | narcotic analgesic |
| Seldane (terfenadine) | antihistamine |
| Seldane-D (terfenadine, pseudoephedrine HCl) | antihistamine, decongestant |
| Serevent (salmeterol xinafoate) | antiasthmatic, bronchodilator |
| Sumycin (tetracycline HCl) | antibiotic |
| Suprax (cefixime) | antibiotic |
| Synthroid (levothyroxine sodium) | thyroid replacement |
| Tegretol (carbamazepine) | anticonvulsant |
| temazepam | tranquilizer, hypnotic |
| Tenormin (atenolol) | antianginal, antihypertensive, beta blocker |
| Terazol (terconazole) | antifungal |
| Timoptic (timolol maleate) | antiglaucoma |
| Toprol XL (metoprolol succinate) | antihypertensive, antianginal |
| Trental (pentoxifylline) | hemorrheologic to improve circulation |
| triamterene with hydrochlorothiazide | diuretic, antihypertensive |
| Tri-Levlen (levonorgestrel, ethinyl estradiol) | triphasic oral contraceptive |
| trimethoprim with sulfamethoxazole | anti-infective, antibacterial |
| Trimox (amoxicillin trihydrate) | antibiotic |
| Triphasil (levonorgestrel, ethinyl estradiol) | triphasic oral contraceptive |
| Trusopt (dorzolamide HCl) | glaucoma treatment |
| Ultram (tramadol HCl) | analgesic |
| Vancenase AQ (beclomethasone dipropionate) | steroidal anti-inflammatory |
| Vanceril (beclomethasone dipropionate) | corticosteroid for bronchial asthma |
| Vasotec (enalaprilat maleate) | antihypertensive, ACE inhibitor |
| Veetids (penicillin V potassium) | antibiotic |
| verapamil HCl | antianginal, antiarrhythmic, calcium channel blocker |
| Verelan (verapamil HCl) | antianginal, antiarrhythmic, calcium channel blocker |
| Xanax (alprazolam) | anxiolytic |
| Zantac (ranitidine HCl) | antiulcer |
| Zestril (lisinopril) | antihypertensive |
| Ziac (hydrochlorothiazide, bisoprolol fumarate) | antihypertensive |
| Zithromax (azithromycin dihydrate) | antibiotic |
| Zocor (simvastatin) | antihyperlipidemic |
| Zoloft (sertraline) | antidepressant |
| Zovirax (acyclovir) | antiviral |
| Zyrtec (cetirizine HCl) | antihistamine |

**Dropped from the previous list:**

| | |
|---|---|
| Advil, Children's (ibuprofen) | NSAID, antiarthritic, analgesic |
| amitriptyline HCl | antidepressant |
| Carafate (sucralfate) | antiulcer |
| Cardizem (diltiazem HCl) | antihypertensive, antianginal |
| Ceclor (cefaclor) | antibiotic |
| Compazine (prochlorperazine maleate) | antiemetic, tranquilizer |
| Cotrim DS (sulfamethoxazole, trimethoprim) | anti-infective, antibacterial |
| DiaBeta (glyburide) | antidiabetic |
| E.E.S. (erythromycin ethylsuccinate) | antibiotic |
| erythromycin base | antibiotic |
| Fiorinal with Codeine (codeine phosphate, acetaminophen, caffeine, butalbital) | narcotic analgesic, sedative |
| Glucotrol (glipizide) | antidiabetic |
| Hismanal (astemizole) | antihistamine |
| Lorcet (hydrocodone bitartrate, acetaminophen) | narcotic analgesic |
| Lorcet Plus (hydrocodone bitartrate, acetaminophen) | narcotic analgesic |
| Lotensin (benazepril HCl) | antihypertensive, ACE inhibitor |
| Lozol (indapamide) | antihypertensive, diuretic |
| Micronase (glyburide) | antidiabetic |
| Motrin (ibuprofen) | NSAID, antiarthritic, analgesic |
| Motrin, Childen's (ibuprofen) | NSAID, antiarthritic, analgesic |
| Nasacort (triamcinolone acetonide) | corticosteroidal anti-inflammatory |
| Nizoral (ketoconazole) | systemic antifungal |
| nortriptyline HCl | tricyclic antidepressant |
| PCE [polymer-coated erythromycin] | antibiotic |
| Penicillin-VK (penicillin V potassium) | antibiotic |
| Provera (medroxyprogesterone acetate) | progestin |
| sulfamethoxazole with trimethoprim | anti-infective, antibacterial |
| Theo-Dur (theophylline) | bronchodilator |
| Toradol (ketorolac tromethamine) | NSAID |
| Tylenol with Codeine (acetaminophen, codeine phosphate) | analgesic |
| Valium (diazepam) | sedative, skeletal muscle relaxant, anticonvulsant adjunct |
| Ventolin (albuterol sulfate) | bronchodilator |
| Vicodin (hydrocodone bitartrate, acetaminophen) | narcotic analgesic |
| Voltaren (diclofenac sodium) | NSAID, antiarthritic, analgesic |